HANDBOOK OF
CLINICAL AUDIOLOGY

FOURTH EDITION

HANDBOOK OF
CLINICAL
AUDIOLOGY

FOURTH EDITION

EDITOR

JACK KATZ, Ph.D.

Professor
Department of Communicative Disorders and Sciences
University at Buffalo
State University of New York
Buffalo, New York

ASSOCIATE EDITORS

WILMA LAUFER GABBAY, M.S.
SARALYN GOLD, Ph.D.
LARRY MEDWETSKY, M.S.
ROGER A. RUTH, Ph.D.

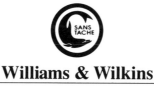

Williams & Wilkins

BALTIMORE • PHILADELPHIA • HONG KONG
LONDON • MUNICH • SYDNEY • TOKYO
A WAVERLY COMPANY

Editor: John P. Butler
Managing Editor: Linda S. Napora
Copy Editor: Gillian C. Sowell
Illustration Planner: Wayne Hubbel
Production Coordinator: Anne Stewart Seitz

Accurate indications, adverse reactions, and dosage schedules for drugs are provided in this book, but it is possible that they may change. The reader is urged to
review the package information data of the manufacturers of the medications
mentioned.

Printed in the United States of America

First Edition 1972

Library of Congress Cataloging in Publication Data

Handbook of clinical audiology / Jack Katz, editor : associate
    editors, Wilma Laufer Gabbay . . . [et al.]. — 4th ed.
        p.   cm.
    Includes bibliographical references and indexes.
    ISBN 0-683-04548-2
    1. Hearing disorders. 2. Audiology. I. Katz, Jack. II. Gabbay,
Wilma Laufer.
    [DNLM: 1. Hearing Disorders.   WV 270 H2363 1994]
RF290.H36 1994
617.8′9—dc20
DNLM/DLC
for Library of Congress   93-3629
                                                                   CIP

94 95 96 97 98
1 2 3 4 5 6 7 8 9 10

To Irma

PREFACE

Over 20 years ago the first edition of the *Handbook of Clinical Audiology* appeared on bookshelves. The field has changed so much during this time and, certainly, from the early days of audiology that our pioneers would hardly recognize the contents of the audiology suite and the measurements we now use. Much of this metamorphosis is reflected in the three previous editions of the *Handbook* and is culminated with our present level of development in this fourth edition. The complex and dynamic field of audiology is continually changing. Thus, these four volumes of "*HOCA*," like the other books in our field, provide important snapshots of where we are.

It is our purpose to keep HOCA a thorough, broad reflection of the science-art of clinical audiology (while housing it between a single set of covers). To do so, it was necessary to find contributors who view the field from varying prospectives, with proper respect for other points of view. To make the task more difficult, this book is used as both a text and a reference by those in high-tech clinical laboratories, as well as those in communities with much more limited instrumentation, and by people in audiology as well as those in otology and other related fields.

To provide a broad, current view of the field, regrettably we had to combine or elminate chapters from the previous edition so newly developing areas could be added. The final effort to include as much information as possible into this book required that the publisher increase the page size.

We are fortunate to have a remarkable group of contributors. They offer their understanding of the field and have added their research data and clinical observations. They come from all segments of our field. They are diagnosticians and rehabilitationists, clinicians and researchers, younger and older, male and female, and of primary interest to the reader, they are all teachers. I am grateful to them for their efforts and believe that the reader will be impressed with the wealth and variety of information contained in this volume.

I owe a great many thanks to the four associate editors who have advised, encouraged, disagreed, and agreed with me on many of the technical, practical, and philosophical decisions that had to be made. Each also helped to review and edit approximately one-quarter of the chapters. The associate editors are Wilma Gabbay, Saralyn Gold, Larry Medwetsky, and Roger Ruth. In addition, I would like to mention the considerable amount of input and planning that Roger Ruth had in the physiology section and that Larry Medwetsky contributed to the two aural rehabilitation sections. I am also grateful to my wife, Irma, for helping with *all* aspects of the book.

It is our collective hope that this fourth edition of the *Handbook of Clinical Audiology* will provide the reader with a firm basis for understanding and/or practicing audiology. We hope to have stimulated thought, provoked discussion, and provided useful references for further study. Finally, I should mention to the new student that audiology is a fascinating and rewarding field. We presume that our enthusiasm for our work has come through loudly and clearly.

CONTRIBUTORS

KATHRYN A. BARRETT, Ph.D.
Assistant Professor
Division of Communication Disorders
University of North Carolina-Greensboro
Greensboro, North Carolina

MICHAEL G. BLOCK, Ph.D.
Associate Professor and Chairperson
Department of Audiology
National Technical Institute for the Deaf at Rochester
  Institute of Technology
Rochester, New York

FLINT A. BOETTCHER, Ph.D.
Assistant Professor
Department of Otolaryngology
Medical University of South Carolina
Charleston, South Carolina

STEVEN P. BORNSTEIN, Ph.D.
Associate Professor
Department of Communication Disorders
School of Health and Human Services
Univeristy of New Hampshire
Durham, New Hampshire

KATHRYN E. BRIGHT, Ph.D.
Associate Professor
Department of Communication Disorders
University of Northern Colorado
Greeley, Colorado

MICHAEL A. BRUNT, Ph.D.
Associate Professor
Department of Speech Pathology and Audiology
Illinois State University
Normal, Illinois

JOAN M. BURLEIGH, M.A.
Director, Center for Central Auditory Research
Engineering Research Center
Colorado State University
Fort Collins, Colorado

Lt. Col. DAVID CHANDLER, Ph.D.
Chief of Audiology
Madigan Army Medical Center
Tacoma, WA

ANN E. CLOCK, Ph.D.
Post Doctoral Associate
Department of Neuroscience
University of Florida
College of Medicine
Health Sciences Center
Gainesville, Florida

JAMES J. DEMPSEY, Ph.D.
Associate Professor
Director of Audiology
Department of Communication Disorders
Southern Connecticut State University
New Haven, Connecticut

DONALD D. DIRKS, Ph.D.
Professor
Department of Head and Neck Surgery (Audiology)
UCLA School of Medicine
Los Angeles, California

JOHN D. DURRANT, Ph.D.
Professor of Otolaryngology and Communication
Director of Audiology
Montefiore University Hospital
University of Pittsburgh
Pittsburgh, Pennsylvania

JOHN A. FERRARO, Ph.D.
Professor and Chairman, Hearing and Speech Department
Associate Dean, School of Allied Health
University of Kansas Medical Center
Kansas City, Kansas

SANDRA ABBOTT GABBARD, M.A. CCC-A
Clinical Audiologist and Instructor
Department of Otolaryngology
University of Colorado Health Sciences Center
Denver, Colorado

IRVIN A. GINSBERG, M.D.
Chief of Otology
Buffalo Otological Group
Buffalo, New York

THOMAS G. GIOLAS, Ph.D.
Dean of Graduate School
Director of Research
Department of Communication Science
University of Connecticut
Storrs, Connecticut

BEVERLY A. GOLDSTEIN, Ph.D.
Vice President, Professional Services
Harmony Hearing Aids Co.
Northfield Center, Ohio

DAVID S. GREEN, Ph.D.
Professor Emeritus-Communication Disorders
Southern Connecticut State University
New Haven, Connecticut

JAMES W. HALL III, Ph.D.
Director of Vanderbilt Balance and Hearing Center
Division of Hearing and Speech Sciences
Department of Otolaryngology
School of Medicine
Vanderbilt University
Nashville, Tennessee

DONALD HENDERSON, Ph.D.
Professor
Department of Communication Disorders and Sciences
Hearing Research Laboratory
University of Buffalo
State University of New York
Buffalo, New York

TERRY HNATH-CHISOLM, Ph.D.
Assistant Professor of Audiology
Department of Communication Sciences and Disorders
University of South Florida
Tampa, Florida

WILLIAM R. HODGSON, Ph.D.
Professor
Department of Speech and Hearing Sciences
University of Arizona
Tucson, Arizona

LYNN E. HUERTA, Ph.D.
Program Administrator
Hearing Program
Division of Communication Sciences and Disorders
National Institute on Deafness and Other Communication
    Disorders
Rockville, Maryland

RAYMOND H. HULL, Ph.D.
Professor of Communicative Disorders and Sciences
The Wichita State University
Wichita, Kansas

LARRY E. HUMES, Ph.D.
Professor and Director of Audiology
Department of Speech and Hearing Sciences
Indiana University
Bloomington, Indiana

ROBERT G. IVEY, Ph.D.
Clinical Audiology Centre
London, Ontario, Canada

JANET R. JAMIESON, Ph.D.
Assistant Professor
Department of Educational Psychology and Special
    Education
University of British Columbia
Vancouver, British Columbia, Canada

JACK KATZ, Ph.D.
Professor
Department of Communicative Disorders and Sciences
University at Buffalo
State University of New York
Buffalo, New York

PAUL KILENY, Ph.D.
Professor and Director
Division of Audiology and Electrophysiology
Department of Otolaryngology
University of Michigan Hospital
Ann Arbor, Michigan

MICHELE KLIMOVITCH, M.S.
Assistant to the Principal and Speech Language
    Pathologists
Lake Drive School of Hearing Impaired Children
Mt. Lakes, New Jersey

NINA KRAUS, Ph.D.
Director, Evoked Potentials Laboratory
Associate Professor
Communication Sciences, Neurobiology, and
    Otolaryngology
Northwestern University
Evanston, Illinois

LLOYD LAMB, Ph.D.
Starkey Laboratories
Austin, Texas

SAMUEL F. LYBARGER, B.S.
Acoustical Consultant
McMurray, Pennsylvania

JANE R. MADELL, Ph.D.
Director, Communicative Disorders
Long Island College Hospital
Professor, Clinical Otolaryngology
State University of New York Health Sciences Center
Brooklyn, New York

FREDERICK N. MARTIN, Ph.D.
Jamail Centennial Professor
Communication Sciences and Disorders
The University of Texas at Austin
Austin, Texas

THERESE McGEE, Ph.D.
Associate Director
Evoked Potentials Laboratory
Research Associate Professor
Northwestern University
Evanston, Illinois

LAURA S. McKIRDY, Ph.D.
Project Director
Lake Drive School for Hearing Impaired Children
Mt. Lakes, New Jersey

LARRY MEDWETSKY, M.S.
Director of Audiology
Al Sigl Center
Rochester, New York

WILLIAM MELNICK, Ph.D.
Professor of Emeritus
Department of Otolaryngology
The Ohio State University
Columbus, Ohio

JOSEPH J. MONTANO, Ed.D.
Director, Department of Communication Disorders
Manhattan Eye, Ear & Throat Hospital
New York, New York

H. GUSTAV MUELLER, Ph.D.
Research Associate, University of Northern Colorado
Clinical Faculty
University of Colorado Health Sciences Center
Denver, Colorado
Adjunct Associate Professor
Vanderbilt University
Nashville, Tennessee
Senior Audiology Consultant
Siemens Hearing-Instruments, U.S.A.

FRANK E. MUSIEK, Ph.D.
Professor of Otolaryngology and Neurology
Dartmouth-Hitchcock Medical Center
Lebanon, New Hampshire

ANNA K. NÁBĚLEK, Ph.D.
Research Professor
Audiology and Speech Pathology Department
University of Tennessee
Knoxville, Tennessee

IGOR V. NÁBĚLEK, Ph.D.
Professor
Audiology and Speech Pathology Department
University of Tennessee
Knoxville, Tennessee

CRAIG W. NEWMAN, Ph.D.
Coordinator, Clinical Audiology Services
Division of Audiology
Henry Ford Hospital
Detroit, Michigan

JERRY L. NORTHERN, Ph.D.
Director of Audiology
University Hospital
Professor of Otolaryngology/Pediatrics
University of Colorado Health Sciences Center
Denver, Colorado

SUSAN J. NORTON, Ph.D., CCC-A
Director, Research and Clinical Audiology
Children's Hospital and Medical Center
Associate Professor
Department of Otolaryngology-Head and Neck Surgery
University of Washington School of Medicine
Seattle, Washington

JOHN P. PENROD, Ph.D.
Audiologist in Private Practice
Audiology Associates of North Florida
Tallahassee, Florida

MARTIN S. ROBINETTE, Ph.D.
Professor of Audiology
Mayo Medical School
Audiology Section Head
Mayo Clinic
Rochester, Minnesota

MARK ROSS, Ph.D.
Professor Emeritus
University of Connecticut
Storrs, Connecticut

ROGER A RUTH, Ph.D.
Professor and Director
Communication Disorders
University of Virginia Health Sciences Center
Charlottesville, Virginia

RICHARD J. SALVI, Ph.D.
Professor
Department of Communicative Disorders and Sciences
Hearing Research Laboratory
University at Buffalo
State University of New York
Buffalo, New York

ZAHRL G. SCHOENY, Ph.D.
Director of Audiology
Speech Language Hearing Center
University of Virginia
Charlottesville, Virginia

MITCHELL K. SCHWABER, M.D.
Associate Professor
Division of Hearing and Speech Science
Department of Otolaryngology
School of Medicine
Nashville, Tennessee

NEIL T. SHEPARD, Ph.D.
Associate Professor and Director
Vestibular Testing Center
Department of Otolaryngology
University of Michigan Medical Center
Ann Arbor, Michigan

WAYNE J. STAAB, Ph.D.
Acoustical Consultant
Phoenix, Arixona

LISA J. STOVER, Ph.D.
Post Doctorate Research Fellow
Boys Town National Research Hospital
Omaha, Nebraska

RICHARD E. TALBOTT, Ph.D.
Associate Dean
College of Health and Public Affairs
University of Central Florida
Orlando, Florida

STEVEN A. TELIAN, M.D.
Associate Professor and Director
Division of Neurotology
Department of Otolaryngology
University of Michigan Medical Center
Ann Arbor, Michigan

BRUCE A. WEBER, Ph.D.
Associate Professor
Audiology Program
Duke University Medical Center
Durham, North Carolina

BARBARA E. WEINSTEIN, Ph.D.
Associate Professor
Director, Audiology Program
Lehman College, CUNY
Bronx, New York
Faculty, Hunter/Mt. Sinai Geriatric Education Center
New York, New York

THOMAS P. WHITE, M.A.
Assistant Professor
Department of Communicative Disorders and Sciences
University at Buffalo
State University of New York
Buffalo, New York

LAURA ANN WILBER, Ph.D.
Professor of Audiology and Hearing Sciences
Northwestern University
Evanston, Illinois

LORIN WILDE, M.S.
Doctoral Candidate
Department of Electrical and Computer Science (Speech
    Communication Group)
Massachusetts Institute of Technology
Cambridge, Massachusetts

TERRY L. WILEY, Ph.D.
Professor
Department of Communicative Disorders
University of Wisconsin—Madison
Madison, Wisconsin

JACK A. WILLEFORD, Ph.D.
Professor Emeritus of Audiology
Colorado State University
Fort Collins, Colorado

PHILLIP A. YANTIS, Ph.D.
Professor Emeritus
Department of Speech and Hearing Sciences
University of Washington
Seattle, Washington

CAROLYN V. YOUNG, M.A.
Audiology Services Coordinator
Institute for the Study of Developmental Disabilities
The University of Illinois at Chicago
Chicago, Illinois

ROBERT L. ZIMMERMAN, Ph.D.
Chief, Audiology-Speech Pathology Service
Veterans Administration Medical Center
Buffalo, New York

CONTENTS

NATURE OF AUDITORY DISORDERS

CHAPTER 1

Clinical Audiology

Jack Katz

Twenty years ago (1972) the first edition of the *Handbook of Clinical Audiology (HOCA)* appeared on the scene. At that time there was neither much variety in textbooks for graduate students in clinical audiology nor a good selection of general reference books for the professional. At the present time the situation is quite different. There are many excellent texts from which to choose and a variety of reference works dealing with clinical audiology. Nevertheless, *HOCA* continues to enjoy a unique status among audiologists. It is considered one of the field's classic graduate textbooks and a standard reference for clinical procedures and approaches.

The purpose of *HOCA* remains, as in the past, (*a*) to provide information across the broad scope of the profession in a single volume, and (*b*) to offer clear and accurate information from authoritative contributors. The book provides the reader not only with the details of clinical procedures and their theoretical bases, but also with a wealth of clinical and research knowledge gathered by the writers.

Because each edition of *HOCA* has attempted to provide a reasonably complete and detailed review of clinical audiology, a study of the contents of the four editions provides a view of the dynamics in this field. One reflection of the growth that has taken place in audiology over the past 20 years is that each edition has attempted to include more and more information between its covers. The nature and focus of the discipline has also continued to change. The gradual evolution—and occasional revolution—have permitted the field of audiology to grow in size and strength. Audiology continues to develop new and improved procedures while perfecting those already in use. Clients and patients benefit when professionals and students keep abreast of current knowledge of how the auditory system works, what happens when it breaks down, and what approaches are effective in ameliorating the problems.

Each edition of the *Handbook of Clinical Audiology* has reflected the expanding scope of the field and, perhaps in some ways, *HOCA* has influenced those developments. For example, the first edition had an emphasis on physiological diagnostic procedures that was unusual for that time. The contribution on immittance was one of the earliest book chapters on this topic. Another physiological chapter dealt with galvanic skin response (GSR) au-

diometry, a procedure that has been abandoned for ethical purposes rather than any lack of effectiveness (Knox,. 1978). Early principles of electroencephalographic audiometry were discussed in a separate chapter. This contribution to *HOCA* predated the introduction of the computer into audiological measurement. Nevertheless, even 20 years ago there were signs that electrophysiology would offer the audiologist certain insights and capabilities that behavioral methods could not. A chapter on vestibular measurement was one of the early ones on this topic.

The first edition had four chapters devoted to central testing for purposes of site-of-lesion testing. This was unusually heavy emphasis on that topic 20 years ago. A related chapter involved the area of auditory processing in learning-disabled children. The latter was one of the very early chapters that encouraged audiologists to become involved in the evaluation and management of central auditory processing problems.

In contrast, this edition of *Handbook of Clinical Audiology* has 11 chapters devoted to physiological functions. Three are basic chapters while eight provide the clinical applications. The single immittance chapter of the first edition has been expanded to three and the evoked electrophysiological response chapter has now grown to six. Only the vestibular testing portion has remained a single chapter, however, the present chapter is far more detailed in basic aspects and discusses many newer techniques and insights.

In *HOCA*, while we present new and potentially important approaches at the forefront of the field, we also provide historically relevant material. Historical information gives us an understanding of where we are by allowing us to appreciate our origins. More importantly, an older technique in experienced hands generally can be more effective than a newer technique in inexperienced hands. We hold that the philosophy and practice of broadening one's ability is more advantageous than narrowing it merely for the sake of the modern. I believe that many of the old and less-popular procedures now being discarded by audiologists are still useful when applied effectively; in specific cases. For example, even some of our best tests (e.g., auditory brainstem response (ABR), acoustic reflex) have limitations for diagnostic purposes in the presence of various hearing losses. Often these same losses are less problematic when using the older procedures and, in fact, the greater losses typically render the older tests more effective.

PROFESSIONAL GROWTH OF AUDIOLOGY

It is interesting to view the growth and development of audiology as a profession. When I first became aware of this field over 35 years ago, audiology was a junior and somewhat silent partner in the field of communicative disorders. The number of audiologists was very small relative to those in speech pathology. In fact, relatively few audiologists came directly into the field; many moved over from speech pathology by simply changing their focus.

Audiology and speech pathology also differed in their makeup. Speech pathology had relatively equal numbers of male and female practitioners, but audiology was overwhelmingly male. In the three succeeding decades speech-language pathology has become predominantly, though not exclusively, a female profession, and audiology is now two-thirds female (ASHA, 1991). This is a marked shift even from the time of the second edition of *HOCA* in 1978 when audiologists were equally likely to be male or female.

It will be interesting to see if the trend toward greater and greater representation of women in audiology will continue. It is my hope that audiology will remain a desirable profession for both men and women (and not gender-typed as nursing and engineering often were, as female and male professions, respectively).

Unlike the silent partner of old, audiologists have become more vocal and have started to establish their own agenda. This is evident in the American Speech-Language-Hearing Association action declaring audiology to be a distinct profession from speech-language pathology (ASHA, 1990). In the meantime audiologists have begun to make headway in associating audiology with other professions (e.g., American Auditory Society). A more recent development has been the formation of an organization exclusively for audiologists. The organization, the American Academy of Audiology has grown remarkably in size and importance in the past few years (Northern, 1991). While it is unclear how quickly and how far audiology will distance itself from speech-language pathology, the trend is obvious and strong.

One of the ways in which audiology has started on its independent course is in the area of education and training. Other professions, such as medicine, psychology, and optometry provide useful models for shaping the education of audiologists. A need is perceived for more education in the basic sciences in the training of audiologists and for a requirement of more and varied clinical experience before a student graduates.

For many years the master's degree has been the entry level into the profession. At present the master's is the highest academic degree held by about 80% of audiologists who responded to a recent survey (ASHA, 1991). An outgrowth of the concerns about graduate and undergraduate education has been the call for a professional doctorate degree. This degree would serve as the entry point into the profession—at the doctorate level (American Academy Audiology, 1991). The proposed degree is the Doctor of Audiology or Au.D. The Au.D. would replace the master's as the entry level degree for audiology professionals and would serve alongside the Ph.D., which would remain the research degree in audiology.

At this writing, the Au.D. is not imminent. Nevertheless, the thrust of this movement is forcing educators to reexamine their educational programs. The most immediate effect of the efforts for establishing an Au.D. degree is to encourage programs to upgrade the master's degree and perhaps to add basic sciences to the undergraduate curricula. If the Au.D. becomes a viable degree, the impact on the profession and the other degrees now offered will be profound.

ABOUT THIS EDITION

We would like to think that each edition of *HOCA* has been superior to its predecessor. Although space limitations forced the elimination of some excellent material that was used in the third edition (i.e., general medical considerations, legal aspects of the profession, and the glossary), new chapters have been added in this edition to keep abreast of the developments in the field. The entirely new chapters include (*a*) the physiological basis of hearing and hearing loss, (*b*) electrocochleography, (*c*) otoacoustic emissions, and (*d*) cochlear implants and vibrotactile aids.

In addition, some chapters have been combined (e.g., various tests of cochlear function) and others expanded (e.g., counseling and guidance for the hearing impaired). All chapters have been updated as needed.

The 49 chapters of *Handbook of Clinical Audiology, Fourth Edition* are divided into seven sections. The first section is Nature of Auditory Disorders, which sets the stage for the clinical chapters to follow. This section includes two chapters on medical fields (otology and neurology) that relate closely to audiology and a chapter that deals with recent information from animal research that helps us to understand normal hearing and hearing loss. Another chapter is on psychoacoustics as it relates to our understanding of clinical tests and disorders. The final chapter in the first section is on calibration of equipment.

The second section is devoted to behavioral procedures that are used to study hearing function of the peripheral auditory system. This section covers standard air- and bone-conduction threshold testing, speech audiometry, tests of cochlear and retrocochlear function, and the use of clinical masking. This section is followed by one with similar information that is directed toward the study of central auditory function. These chapters include an overview of the area followed by specific procedures using non-speech tests, monosyllabic and spondaic words, and finally sentence tests.

Section four is devoted to physiological procedures. One subsection involves immittance (dealing with both admittance and impedance measurements). These chapters are introduced by an overview and a discussion of the basic principles of immittance. The two diagnostic chapters emphasize tympanometry and acoustic reflex testing but cover newer applications as well. The second subsection on evoked physiological procedures is introduced by a presentation of fundamentals and a review of procedures. Separate chapters discuss electrocochleography, ABR for neural monitoring, ABR for threshold estimation, middle and late evoked responses, and otoacoustic emissions. The final chapter in that section deals with measurement of vestibular function.

Section five involves special populations and applications. This section includes chapters on testing infants and young children, screening procedures in schools, auditory perceptual disorders, and study of the developmentally disabled. It also provides information about educational audiology, industrial audiology, pseudohypacusis, and presbycusis.

The sixth section concerns itself with management, beginning with a chapter that reviews all aspects of aural rehabilitation. The other chapters in this section deal with the impact of hearing impairment, counseling the hearing impaired and their families, the use of assistive listening devices, and, finally, considerations of room acoustics as it relates to speech perception.

The last section deals with sensory aids and training of the hearing-impaired person. The first of these chapters is on the characteristics and use of amplification. Two additional hearing aid chapters deal with evaluation procedures and dispensing of hearing aids. There is a chapter on cochlear implants and vibrotactile aids to complete the subsection on amplification. The last three chapters involve aural rehabilitation of children, of adults, and of the elderly. These include both traditional and new approaches in therapy and education.

Among the major changes in the present edition of *HOCA* is a heavier emphasis on electrophysiological measurements and (re)habilitation and management of the hearing impaired. These cohesive sections reflect the current status, with an eye toward the future, in two burgeoning areas of audiology. The addition of chapters on electrocochleography and otoacoustic emissions helps to round out the completely updated section on electrophysiological measurement. Over the past several years the management of hearing impairment has undergone important changes as well. The importance of hearing aid dispensing and the impact of new hearing aid designs and approaches are depicted in the management and sensory aids sections. Among the sensory aids discussed are cochlear implants, which have become an accepted method for improving hearing functions. In some cases, vibrotactile aids may be recommended instead. These current issues are thoughtfully discussed in a new chapter in the sensory aids section.

The 60 different authors with the aid of five editors have tried to make this book clear, accurate and up-to-date. It is our hope that this comprehensive text will provide the breadth of understanding needed by students and professionals in the field of audiology leading up to the twenty-first century.

REFERENCES

American Academy of Audiology. Position paper: the American Academy of Audiology and the Professional Doctorate (Au.D.). Audiology Today 1991;3:10–12.

ASHA. Legislative Council Report—LC 7-89. ASHA 1990;32:18.

ASHA. Results of 1989 ASHA Audiology Opinion Survey. Audiology Update 1991;10(1):9–11.

Knox AW. Electrodermal audiometry. In Katz J, Ed. Handbook of Clinical Audiology. Baltimore: Williams & Wilkins, 1978:304–310.

Northern J. President's message. Audiology Today 1991;3:2–3.

CHAPTER 2

Otologic Disorders and Examination

Irwin A. Ginsberg and Thomas P. White

RELATIONSHIP BETWEEN OTOLOGY AND AUDIOLOGY

Both audiology and otolaryngology have become sophisticated and highly specialized disciplines. The advances in one profession are often linked to advances in the other. As audiology has increased in its ability to study and rehabilitate the hearing impaired it has assumed a greater and greater importance to the practice of otolaryngology. Philosophic differences and misunderstandings between these allied professions that restrict their reciprocal contributions to one another must reduce the quality of care to the patient. In the past, some physicians failed to appreciate the contributions of the audiologist. With the technologic advances and development of expertise over the past two decades, this no longer seems to be likely. Rather, the otolaryngologist must rely increasingly on the judgment and contributions of the audiologist.

Likewise, the audiologist should value the input of the otologist in the evaluation of the patient with hearing impairment. Diagnostic audiology is not without error. It cannot detect all auditory pathology. Audiometric studies have their greatest strength when supported by the otologic examination. The practice of each discipline should be in conjunction with each other, not to the exclusion of the other. It is the otologic-audiologic team that will provide the patient with the highest quality care.

Otology and audiology are young professions, and the level of sophistication that we take so casually for granted was not even suspected a few years ago. The audiometer is about 60 years old (Bunch, 1943). Recruitment was first reported by Fowler in 1936; Bekesy described automatic audiometry in 1947; the short increment sensitivity index (SISI) was devised by Jerger et al in 1959; American National Standards Institute (ANSI) specifications for audiometers were adopted in 1969; marked advancements were made in the clinical application of the electroacoustic immittance concept in the 1960s, auditory brainstem response (ABR) measurements in the 1970s, and otoacoustic emissions in the 1990s. As recently as the 1940s, many otologists dismissed bone-conduction measurements as unreliable and of no value. The Lempert fenestration operation was reported in 1938. Rosen reported the stapes mobilization renaissance in 1953. Tympanoplasty was first described by Wullstein in 1953. Ultrasound labyrinthectomy in Ménière's disease dates back to 1953 (Arslan, 1953). Shea (1958) performed the first stapedectomy in the late 1950s. Translabyrinthine surgery in acoustic neurinomas was reported by House in 1961. The first reported cochlear implants for sensory-neural hearing loss were in 1971 by Michelson. Various implant procedures including those involving the middle ear, the mastoid, and refined cochlear implants evolved in the 1980s and 1990s. The refinements in otologic treatment have been inextricably associated with the refinements in diagnostic audiology. Audiologic procedures have been based on otologic knowledge, and their importance is dependent upon the medical and surgical skill of the otolaryngologist.

ANATOMY AND PHYSIOLOGY OF THE EAR

When one pictures the ear, it is the pinna that comes to mind (Fig. 2.1). In fact, beyond the auricle the ear is all but surrounded by bone and not outwardly visible. The auricle is essentially vestigial and serves little real function. Its major contribution is to serve as a sound collector and add slightly to the efficiency of hearing. In animals such as the fennel fox, the auricle continues to serve an important function.

In humans, the advancing sound front enters the external auditory canal directly striking the tympanic membrane. Movement of the drum displaces the malleus, which, in turn, moves the incus and stapes. They transfer the sound energy into the inner ear through the oval window, which holds the footplate of the stapes by means of the annular ligament. For this transfer of energy to be efficient, the middle ear space, which houses the ossicles, must function at atmospheric pressure. This pressure equalization is maintained by a functioning eustachian tube.

To this point, all of the sound energy is contained in the air-filled spaces of the external and middle ear. From the stapes inward, the pathway for sound is in fluid-filled spaces. In order to simplify the mechanism of hearing, one may picture sound as a compression wave through two and one-half turns of the scala vestibuli of the cochlea to its apex (Fig. 2.2). At this point, the direc-

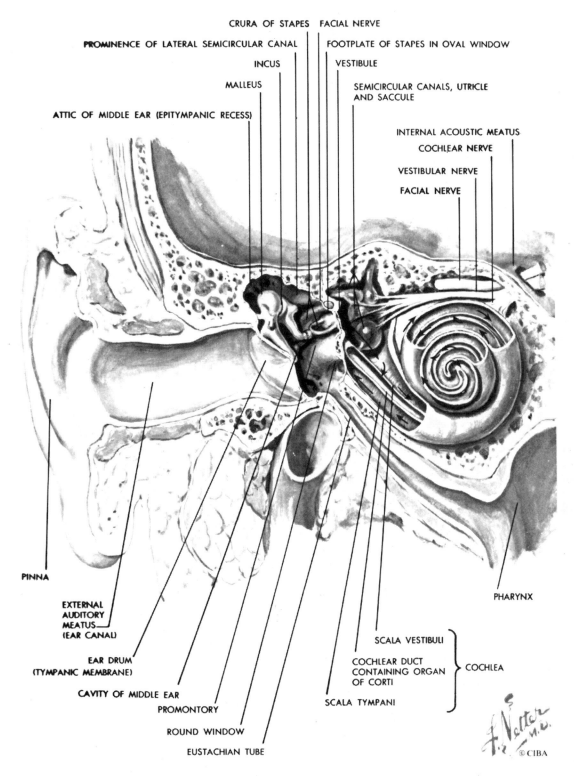

Figure 2.1. Pathway of sound reception.

tion of the compression wave is reversed, sending the energy back through the two and one-half turns of the scala tympani. The compression is relieved by the flexible round window membrane. As the stapes footplate moves inward, the round window moves outward 180° out of phase. The traveling compression wave sends a corresponding wave motion along the basilar membrane. This membrane holds the organ of Corti, often referred to as the end organ of hearing. Corti's organ is actually contained in the scala media, a fluid-filled chamber located between the scala tympani and the scala vestibuli. The traveling wave with associated distortion of the basilar membrane puts forces on the hair cells producing the potential of the nerve impulse. This potential innervates first fibers of the cochlear nerve that then join into a nerve trunk in the modiolus or "core" of the cochlea. These small electrical potentials then travel to the spiral ganglion, to the nuclei of the brainstem, and ultimately to the auditory cortex of the brain (Fig. 2.3).

Each part of the ear, the external, the middle, and the inner ear, has its own separate functions. The external ear essentially conducts the sound energy to the middle ear. The middle ear amplifies the speech frequencies and increases the efficiency of energy transmission so that the sound energy can get from the air-filled external world to the fluid-filled inner ear. Normally, when sound energy is directed to an air-water interface, most of the energy is reflected and does not penetrate. This accounts for the difficulty in speaking to someone who is swimming under water. The middle ear accomplishes transmission of sound energy through the air-water interface between the external ear and the inner ear by several mechanisms. The most important is the areal relationship. The area of the tympanic membrane is much greater than that of the stapes footplate. All of the sound energy striking the drum is therefore selectively funneled through the ossicular chain to the smaller footplate; the force per unit area is, therefore, much greater on the footplate, averaging about 25 dB in added hearing efficiency. The so-called lever action of the ossicular chain is of little effect, perhaps adding 2.5 dB to hearing efficiency. For this reason, reconstructive surgery of the ossicular chain may be accomplished with a single nonarticulated structure, forming a unified column. This type of middle ear structure is found as a columella in birds. The presence of an intact tympanic membrane is important since its very presence prevents the advancing sound front from passing through the middle ear and striking the round window membrane simultaneously with the inward movement of the stapes. This would, of course, destroy the 180° out-of-phase relationship. The development of the middle ear in some air-breathing animals is a fascinating occurrence. Fish,

living in a fluid-filled environment, do not need a middle ear. This is because the impedance between the fluid environment to the fluid-filled inner ear is already matched. It is interesting to note that, in the course of evolution, humans traded the gill-developing structures of the fish for a middle ear, since they no longer had to breathe underwater but had to live and hear on land. One glance at the developing head of a human fetus is illustrative of this evolutionary trade.

It is remarkable that the complex pathway of energy transmission should afford such tremendous sensitivity in the normal ear. A snapping twig may be heard and identified from a mile away, despite the fact that the tiny amount of energy is dissipated over a surface of 2 miles in diameter. From this wide area, the acoustic energy at the tympanic membrane alone is responsible for actuating the complex mechanism. It is said that at threshold the tympanic membrane moves only one-tenth the diameter of a hydrogen molecule, a movement too slight to imagine. Add to this sensitivity the nuances of pitch and quality to which the ear is at the same time attuned. Humans have a truly remarkable receptor that one never tires of studying.

THE AUDIOLOGIC EXAMINATION

Before the audiologist proceeds with the evaluation, two common problems must be ruled out. These are the presence of a collapsing external auditory canal and the presence of obstructing cerumen. Each of these problems can produce spurious conductive hearing loss. In order to eliminate these potential problems, the audiologist must be familiar with the use of the otoscope and should check the external auditory canal before testing is begun. This examination should be carried out routinely. Initially, concern should be directed to the appearance of the entrance of the external auditory canal. The pressure of a test earphone can produce a valve-like closing of the meatus, so complete as to produce a significant conductive hearing loss as shown in Figure 2.4. In order to determine if a collapse may occur while under test, pressure should be exerted by the fingers onto the auricle, pressing it to the head. An MC-41 ear cushion may also be used as suggested by Lynn (1967). If the opening closes, remedial action should be taken. A device should be inserted into the opening to prevent it from collapsing while the test earphone is in place. This may be either a piece of small diameter tubing or an impedance probe tip (Bryde and Feldman, 1980).

Once the opening is examined, the ear canal itself should be inspected. The purpose for this is to see if the tympanic membrane can be visualized. The speculum should be introduced gently into the canal and directed around the complete circumference of the canal for ori-

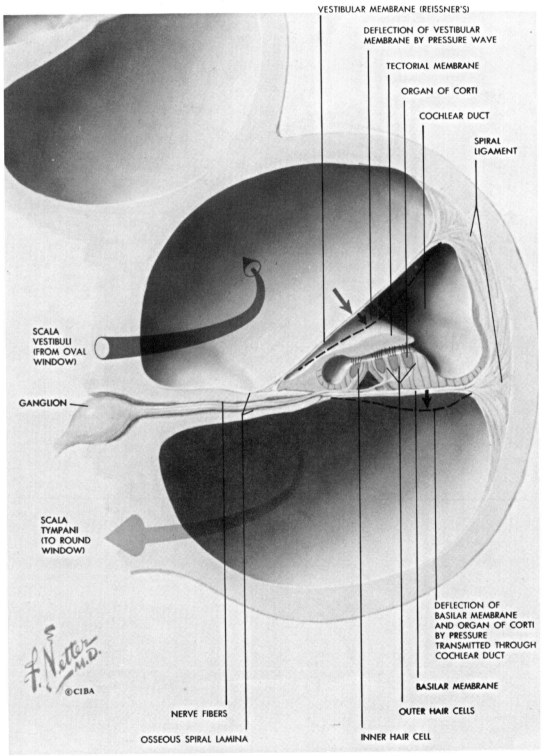

Figure 2.2. Transmission of sound across cochlear duct stimulating hair cells.

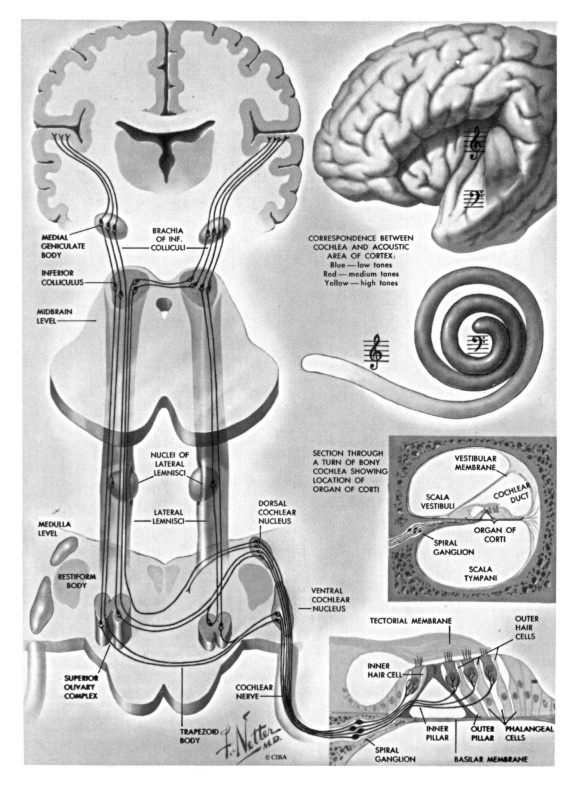

Figure 2.3. Central pathways of hearing.

entation. What the audiologist should be asking is, "Can I see the tympanic membrane?" It should not be the audiologist's responsibility to describe the drum appearance or make diagnostic statements. If any portion of the tympanic membrane is visible, the audiometric examination should be carried out. Except in rare instances, the cerumen must totally block the canal for its effect to be realized. Occasionally, cerumen on the tympanic membrane will affect puretone and tympanometric results. The audiometric examination would have to be repeated if removal of the cerumen proves necessary. If otoscopic examination reveals the presence of impacted cerumen, it must be removed. The old idea that appreciable conductive losses cannot be caused by cerumen plugs is not true, and losses of as much as 40 dB are possible (Fig. 2.5). If the audiologist is unsure if the canal is impacted, the presence of a normally shaped, normal middle-ear-pressure tympanogram will rule out a blocked ear canal.

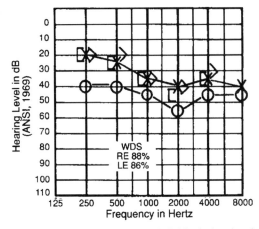

Figure 2.4. Audiometric findings of individual showing influence of collapsed canal while under test (right ear).

THE OTOLOGIC EXAMINATION

The otologic examination is preceded by a carefully taken case history. In the case of hearing impairment, the time of onset, whether the loss was gradual or sudden, and the presence or absence of associated symptoms—especially vertigo, tinnitus, discharge, or pain—should be noted. It should also include the family history, exposure to noise, previous ear or head trauma, and use of ototoxic drugs. A skillfully obtained case history is invaluable.

The physical examination is limited to the external ear and the tympanic membrane. Only when the tympanic membrane is not intact can the middle ear be visualized. Examination of the middle and inner is, under normal circumstances, dependent upon functional tests or sophisticated x-ray techniques.

Examination begins with a careful inspection of the auricle to determine whether congenital deformities are present. The external auditory canal should be checked for patency, foreign bodies, infections, or bony or soft tissue growths. The tympanic membrane should be studied for the presence or absence of normal landmarks. This should include the integrity of the tympanic membrane as well as its color and position. The otologic examination is enhanced by the use of the various tuning fork tests to give an overall impression of the function of the ear. In those ears in which visualization is difficult, the use of the otologic microscope is invaluable.

DISORDERS OF THE EXTERNAL EAR

Congenital

Congenital problems of the external ear can be rather serious and are normally discovered early because of the high visibility of the deformities. One may have a pure canal atresia (absence of the external auditory canal), with a normal auricle and with a normal middle and inner ear, or a canal atresia that is only part of the

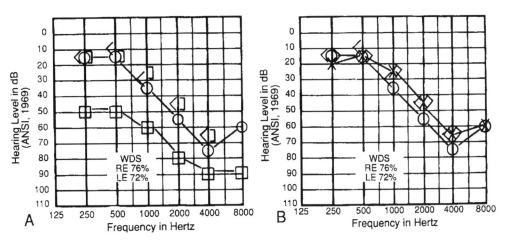

Figure 2.5. Hearing test results of patient showing effects of impacted cerumen, left ear (**A**) and results after removal of impacted cerumen (**B**).

problem and where some or all of the other portions of the ear are involved. Many times the atresia is associated with malformation of the auricle, such as microtia and multiple rudimentary auricular anlagen presenting as auricular tags or accessory auricles. Whenever one sees these obvious external deformities, one must immediately suspect associated deformities in the middle or inner ears. Because the embryology of the ear is complex, involving all three germ layers, and because all germ layers develop in a synchronized manner, when one of these "gets out of step" the development of the others may also be affected. It is this interrelationship that results in the myriad possible combinations of malformations.

The interrelationships of deformities due to embryologic mishap at first seem strange but quickly make sense when the embryology is understood. Abnormalities of the mandible associated with hearing loss, as in Treacher Collins syndrome, result because of the common first branchial arch origin of the mandible, malleus, and incus (Schuknecht, 1974).

X-ray studies using polytomographic techniques show the presence of an air-filled middle ear space, the status of the ossicular chain and the presence of a bony atresia plate that provide the otosurgeon with valuable preoperative information. The reconstruction of an ear with congenital atresia has some serious risks to the facial nerve and the inner ear and may frequently entail the need for multiple surgical procedures. As a general rule, complete unilateral atresia with a normal opposite ear provides insufficient hearing handicap to warrant a surgical approach.

Audiometric studies are of prime importance in planning the management of these patients. What is the status of the inner ear? Is there an intact cochlea and an intact neural mechanism? If so, it is merely a question of establishing a conducting mechanism. In cases of partial atresia where a drum is present, immittance studies may be of great help. The audiologist can help determine whether any surgical attempts should be made (Fig. 2.6).

Acquired

Otitis Externa

Otitis externa, usually a bacterial infection of the external ear canal skin and erroneously referred to as a fungus infection, can cause a conductive hearing loss. If the swelling of the canal is so marked that it obstructs the canal or if the discharge is so copious, a conductive element will result. Usually, however, the canal skin is red with some edema and only a small amount of discharge. In such a case there is no resulting hearing loss. Some varieties of otitis externa are associated only with dry,

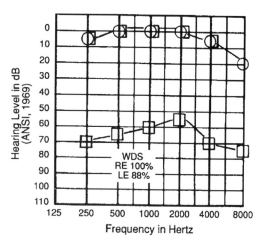

Figure 2.6. Audiometric results of 14-year-old boy with congenital atresia, left ear.

scaling canal skin with little discharge and little swelling. These obviously have no audiologic effect. The treatment of otitis externa should be topical antibiotics or soaks. Systemic antibiotics are not effective.

Foreign Body Obstruction

Obstruction of the external canal by foreign bodies can produce a conductive impairment, especially in children. Small foreign bodies have no audiologic consequences; thus a hearing loss discovered on routine school audiometry rarely is caused by this problem. The foreign object would have to be totally obstructing, such as a bead or pencil eraser. Foreign bodies should always be considered in cases of unilateral conductive loss, but their presence is soon discovered on otoscopy. Removal of foreign bodies should be left to the otologist to minimize the chances of injury to the sound-conducting mechanism.

Osteoma, Hyperostosis, Exostosis

Growths of the bony external canal are common and rarely produce a hearing loss. They can occur as either osteomas, which are discrete rounded excrescences of bone, or as a diffuse bony narrowing of the canal called hyperostosis. Osteomas usually occur close to the tympanic membrane. They usually are small, whitish, rounded masses and on cursory examination may be confused with the whitish, pearly cholesteatoma that occurs in the attic of the ear. A closer look reveals that they are in fact lateral to Shrapnell's membrane. Ordinarily they are too small to cause any degree of canal obstruction and are best left untreated. Uncommonly they may become large and completely obstructing, in which case they must be removed. An exostosis is a bony growth of the external ear canal, usually producing a smooth round mass or multiple mass. Exostoses are covered with canal skin and are hard on palpation. They must not be confused with middle ear polyps that are seen in the external canal as soft, shiny, rounded masses covered with moist mucous membrane and that have a totally different significance and effect on hearing. Hyperostosis also must be completely obstructing to produce a change in the puretone thresholds. Bony growths of the canal should be removed only if they are large enough to be obstructing.

DISORDERS OF THE MIDDLE EAR

Congenital

Congenital anomalies of the middle ear frequently occur with congenital atresia. Whenever an abnormality of the auricle or meatus is present, suspicion of the middle ear anomaly should be high. One of the most common anomalies is that of a fused malleus and incus. Sometimes, the incus is solidly fixed to the posterior bony annulus by a bony bridge. There may be a congenital stapes fixation frequently associated with a grossly deformed stapes. Other varieties of more minor congenital defects exist. These include absence of the stapedius tendon, completely uncovered facial nerves, aberrant courses of the facial nerve, and partial bony plate formation in the region of the bony annulus. Hearing loss, of course, will depend on the degree of abnormality of ossicular transmission as well as on the degree of abnormality of the associated inner ear structures.

The audiologist can help establish the indication for surgical reconstruction and, with the help of immittance measurements, can predict the pathology. Quite often, there is a normal but shallow tympanogram and absent acoustic reflexes (Fig. 2.7). Air-bone gaps of 60 dB are not infrequent in patients with a congenitally malformed middle ear.

Acquired

Acute Otitis Media

Acute otitis media is frequently associated with respiratory infection that ascends the eustachian tube. The usual offending bacteria are *Streptococcus*, *Pneumococcus*, or *Haemophilus influenzae*. It almost always results in a conductive hearing loss during its exudative stage and during the recovery stage until the middle ear is again well ventilated. A certain number of these cases do not go to complete resolution, and a conductive loss may persist because of unresolved or unevacuated products of infection. Treatment with appropriate antibiotics must continue for at least 12 days. Sterile fluid may persist with an effect on hearing.

The audiometric findings are important in determining further course of treatment. Certainly, it is extremely important for the otologist to know whether or not a conductive loss persists. If one does, treatment must be extended. Tympanometric studies play an extremely important role as negative middle ear pressure or fluid may exist without a significant hearing loss, as shown in Figure 2.8.

The importance of the use of tympanometry in assessing these cases cannot be overemphasized. Individuals presenting results as shown in Figure 2.8 will pass routine audiometric screening.

Since middle ear pressure determinations have been made, the question arises as to how abnormal should the pressure be to warrant treatment? No absolute value can be given. No matter what degree of abnormality, it must be correlated with the history, physical examination, and the audiologic data. A pressure of −100 mm in the absence of a history of recurrent ear infection or hearing loss can be treated with "scientific neglect" and merely be observed over a period of time. If, however, there is a middle ear pressure of only −50 mm and there are recur-

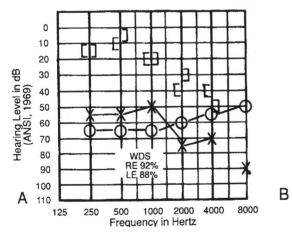
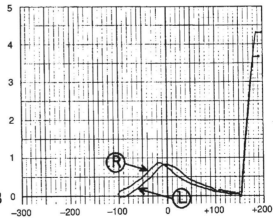

Figure 2.7. Audiogram (**A**) and tympanogram (**B**) of 11-year-old boy with surgically confirmed, bilateral, congenital stapes fixation.

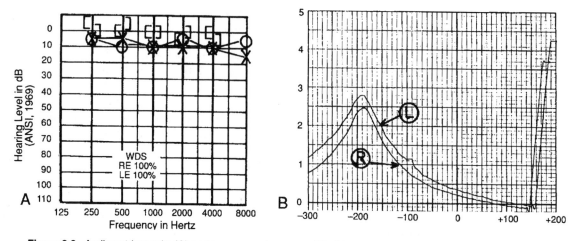

Figure 2.8. Audiometric results (**A**) and tympanometry curves (**B**) of 5-year-old girl with bilateral acute otitis media.

rent episodes of infection and hearing loss, more vigorous methods of intervention may be warranted. Like any findings, abnormal immittance measurements are only a part of the picture.

Chronic Otitis Media

Tympanic Membrane Perforation. It is from cases of acute otitis media that cases of chronic otitis media arise. Some infections are caused by particularly virulent organisms that, early in the course of the infection, can produce destruction of drum substance with a resulting perforation. Sometimes a perforation results because of a long-standing, low-grade infection or as the sequela of an incompletely treated acute otitis media.

The effect on audiometric findings can be very protean indeed. Not only is the size of the perforation important in determining the degree of hearing loss, but its location as well. The larger the perforation, the more the loss of sound pressure that can be transmitted to the inner ear. If the perforation is small but located directly over the round window, the loss may be even greater than that due to a larger perforation located elsewhere. In some cases, surprisingly large perforations may be associated with relatively small losses (Fig. 2.9). For example, the round window could be getting a valuable amount of sound protection either from a strategically placed band of mucosa or a collection of thick mucus or discharge. The perforation may, of course, be associated with an interrupted ossicular chain, in which case the advancing sound front strikes the mobile stapes directly, producing a loss of 30 to 40 dB. A large equivalent volume measurement using impedance can indicate the presence of a perforation that may even escape visualization on otoscopy.

Perforations of the tympanic membrane may be closed through a surgical technique known as tympano-

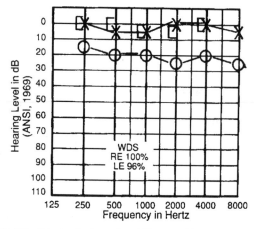

Figure 2.9. Hearing test results of 50-year-old man with a large central tympanic membrane perforation, left ear.

plasty. The drum may be partially or completely replaced, usually using grafts of tissue taken from the fascia covering the temporalis muscle. Other substances, including vein, have also been used. If the ossicular chain is involved, the tympanoplasty must include reconstruction of the sound-conducting mechanism.

Incus Necrosis. In some cases, subacute rather than acute infection can result in ossicular damage with incus necrosis. The lenticular process and lower half of the long process of the incus most frequently are involved when the ossicular chain is damaged. Long-standing infection leaves the ear with defects in the tympanic membrane, damage to the ossicular chain or both. Surprisingly, an intact drum in the presence of a discontinuous ossicular chain can be responsible for a 60 dB loss since its very presence prevents the sound wave from striking the stapes directly.

Myringostapediopexy. A perforation may be present with an incus necrosis but the drum remnant may have attached itself to the stapes head, producing a spontaneous "tympanoplasty" known as a myringostape-diopexy. In this case, if the perforation is not large and is not located directly over the round window, the hearing loss may be very slight or nonexistent. This may occur despite the appearance of a seriously damaged tympanic membrane.

Malleus Head Fixation. A very small amount of disease in the middle ear may cause a considerable conductive hearing loss. Such is the case of malleus head fixation resulting from either otitis media or new bone growth. The malleus head becomes fixed to the attic wall, markedly increasing impedance and producing a loss that might easily be mistaken for otosclerosis. Diagnostically, it is not possible to distinguish these cases from otosclerosis. When malleus head fixation is present, tympanoplasty with removal of the malleus head is performed with simultaneous reconstruction of the ossicular chain.

Tympanosclerosis. Tympanosclerosis is a form of scarring, often associated with long-standing infection. A tympanic membrane perforation may be small or even healed, and yet the conductive hearing loss might be great because of masses of tympanosclerosis that have formed about the ossicular chain causing fixation. Large cartilage-like masses or plaques can grow anywhere in the middle ear, involving the mucosa and ossicles. Such masses may produce fixation of the malleus and incus, fixation of the stapes, or even fixation of the tympanic membrane. Thus, with tympanosclerosis, the tympanic membrane may be intact and yet demonstrate a large conductive loss.

Audiometric studies would reveal an air-bone gap, low compliance, and absent stapedial reflexes on immittance measurements. Tympanometry may even reveal curves typical of otitis media with a flat configuration and no pressure peak.

Cholesteatoma. In some ears, associated with long periods of negative middle ear pressure and with recurring infection, one will find a cyst called a cholesteatoma. Such cysts are squamous-lined and usually begin in the attic of the ear, extending into the mastoid antrum, sometimes all the way to the mastoid tip. Cholesteatomas are filled with cast-off epithelial debris and slowly increase in size. They erode the bone they contact and can produce serious intracranial complications if they erode through the dura of the middle or posterior fossa of the skull, through the lateral sinus, or into the lateral semicircular canal. They may also produce a facial paralysis if the facial nerve is eroded in the middle ear or mastoid. Discharge has usually been present for many years and usually has a foul smell. Dizziness and true vertigo may result if the lateral semicircular canal is involved. Cholesteatomas often destroy ossicular structures, and it is common to see the long process of the incus and all

of the stapes superstructures destroyed, leaving only a stapes footplate. The footplate itself may be destroyed. The squamous tissue may extend to the most remote recesses of the ear, even into the innermost portion of the temporal bone.

Depending on how extensive the cholesteatomatous process is and depending on its exact location and the structures it involves, the hearing loss may vary from slight to total. A small cholesteatoma may be present in the attic of the ear, completely surrounding the elements of the ossicular chain without affecting hearing thresholds. Sometimes a member of the ossicular chain may be destroyed, and yet the hearing remains fairly good with the cholesteatoma itself bridging the gap and helping in sound transmission (Fig. 2.10). Since the cholesteatoma must be removed as a potentially fatal disease, it may in situations like these be necessary to lose hearing in order to eradicate the cyst.

There are essentially two types of chronic middle ear disease. One type is not dangerous, and the other is quite dangerous. A central tympanic membrane perforation, a break in the ossicular chain or a malleus fixation, for example, will not cause serious complications if untreated. Treatment consists of controlling any infection by local and systemic approaches followed by a reconstructive tympanoplasty if desired. Cholesteatomatous disease, however, is potentially serious, and its very presence demands surgical removal.

It is usually necessary to enter both the mastoid and the middle ear at the time of surgery in order to properly expose and remove all of the cyst. This can result in decreased hearing as a result of the surgery, and a secondary procedure may be planned at the time of the original removal. A secondary tympanoplasty would be appropriate 1 year later as a reconstructive procedure with the goal of hearing improvement. On rare occa-

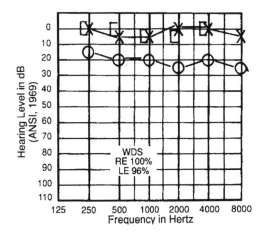

Figure 2.10. Audiometric results of 34-year-old woman with large cholesteatoma, right ear.

sions, when the cyst is small and easily removed, it might be possible to remove the cyst and during the same procedure reconstruct the drum and ossicular chain in a one-step mastoid-tympanoplasty. These cases must be followed carefully for many years to be certain there is no recurrence of the cyst. A few years ago, the ear surgeon was pleased if infection could be controlled, the discharge stopped and the ear made safe. As ear surgery has progressed, the goals are now higher, and hearing improvement is more to be expected.

Careful audiometric and immittance measurements are of great value in assessing the efficiency of the treatment. The audiologic evaluation is important for determining the baseline hearing. Accurate air- and bone-conduction thresholds will support surgical intervention and assist in estimating the maximum amount of hearing improvement that can be expected. Recent refinements in the application of immittance measurements also help the surgeon anticipate the pathology to expect at surgery. The authors wish to stress that normal audiometric and tympanometric studies do not rule out the presence of a cholesteatoma. The diagnosis is a clinical one and not based on x-ray or audiometric findings.

Polyp. In some cases of chronic otitis media with perforation, the middle ear mucosa may become so thick and hypertrophied that polypoid changes can occur and actual polyps may form. These may extend through the perforation and be seen as a mass in the external canal. Polyps, as opposed to bone exostoses, are soft, shiny and covered with mucosa. In cases of polypoid, chronic otitis media there may be a severely damaged middle ear with damage to the ossicular chain resulting in a conductive loss affected further by the very presence of the polyp. Merely removing the polyp and not correcting the underlying disease is rarely recommended. The surgery should be directed to the middle ear and sometimes the mastoid.

Serous Otitis Media

Serous or secretory otitis media is the most common cause of conductive loss in children and has increased in occurrence in recent years. Although one might be tempted to believe that the increased incidence represents cases previously missed and that the figures indicate better diagnosis, this would probably be an incorrect conclusion. Politzer described the entity over 100 years ago and even developed and used vulcanite collar-button tubes for ventilation (Noyes, 1869). The condition was known to exist then, and although some cases may have been missed due to the absence of modern diagnostic audiologic techniques, it seems apparent that fewer cases actually existed.

The causes of serous otitis media are variable, including infection and allergy. All that is known with any degree of certainty is that the middle ear is not ventilating, presumably because of eustachian tube dysfunction.

If the tube is not functioning or is blocked by swollen membranes or adenoid mass, the air is trapped in the middle ear and partly absorbed. This causes the middle ear pressure to be less than atmospheric pressure. The pressure on the external surface of the tympanic membrane is therefore greater and pushes inward on the membrane, stiffening the conducting system and causing a conductive hearing loss that is slightly greater in the low frequencies. If the pressure remains negative for a long period of time, fluid forms in the middle ear, producing a conductive hearing loss, usually greater in the high frequencies. Combination effects of both factors are often the result.

Once the stage has been set and the middle ear is under negative pressure, a vicious cycle is established. The histology of the mucosa in the middle ear undergoes structural changes, and a pavement type of epithelium becomes secretory and glandular in nature. The longer the ear is not ventilating, the greater these changes. The greater these changes, the more adverse the effect on ventilation since the eustachian tube is obstructed by even thicker secretions. The physician's diagnosis may be fairly simple with obvious fluid seen on otoscopic examination. In other cases, it might be difficult to recognize any abnormality of the tympanic membrane and yet a significant conductive hearing loss may be present (Fig. 2.11). It is in these cases that the audiometric workup is most valuable to the otolaryngologist.

In treating short-term cases, a conservative approach might be tried with eustachian tube inflation (politzerization) and decongestant medication. In cases of recurrent long-standing serous otitis media, this mode of treatment usually fails. The best approach is to perform a myringotomy and insertion of a ventilation tube, which in a sense replaces the function of the inoperative eustachian tube. The tube is usually placed in the anteroinferior quadrant of the tympanic membrane where the movement is least, reducing the risk of extrusion. After tubes have remained in place for a sufficient length of time, the mucosa may return to normal, with resumption of normal hearing. Audiometric and tympanometric follow-up, after the tubes have been extruded or have been removed, will determine the success of the treatment. Continued temporizing therapy for more than several months may lead to other middle ear pathology, and a conductive deficit may still be present even after complete control of the middle ear fluid. This may be due to the presence of an incus necrosis, tympanosclerosis, or cholesteatoma.

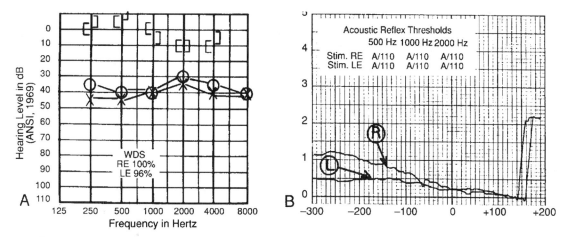

Figure 2.11. Audiometric findings (**A**) and tympanograms (**B**) of 7-year-old girl with bilateral serous otitis media.

Audiologically, in serous otitis media, the air-conduction curve initially will show a greater loss in the high frequencies and spread to the low frequencies as the duration of the problem increases. Eventually it assumes a flat configuration. Bone-conduction responses may be depressed slightly in the high frequencies. Tympanometry is exceedingly helpful, showing in advanced cases a relatively flat curve and in less severe cases merely negative pressure with diminished compliance. Tympanograms are especially helpful because they may reveal the presence of middle ear fluid when physical observation through otoscopy may not. A normal-appearing tympanic membrane may not reveal the presence of middle ear fluid and conversely, an abnormal-appearing membrane may incorrectly suggest middle ear fluid. Acoustic reflexes will be absent as the problem increases in severity. Audiometric and tympanometric follow-up after ventilation tube insertion helps in assessing the efficiency of treatment.

Otosclerosis

One of the most interesting of all ear diseases is otosclerosis. It is this disease and the exciting surgical developments concerning it that sparked the entire renaissance in the surgery of the ear.

Valsalva, in 1741, was the first to report that ankylosis or fixation of the stapes could cause hearing impairment. In 1857, Toynbee and others observed, in a large number of postmortem examinations done on patients who were known to have been hard-of-hearing, that ankylosis of the stapes was a common cause of hearing loss (Schuknecht, 1974). Politzer, in 1893, determined that this ankylosis was due to a particular disease of the bone forming the otic capsule and not to chronic middle ear catarrh as previously thought (Schuknecht, 1974). The cause of this bony growth still remains unknown, but certain characteristics are consistent with its

presence. A comprehensive computer analysis of 2405 surgically confirmed cases of otosclerosis (Ginsberg et al., 1979) verified the previously known fact that it occurs twice as often in women as in men. Results also showed that tinnitus is present approximately 50% of the time, and the average age when the hearing impairment was noticed was 36 years. The condition is aggravated in a good number of cases by pregnancy. Hearing loss is insidious in onset. It is slowly progressive and in most cases largely conductive, audiometrically. Many cases show a significant sensory-neural component due to the disease itself and increased in degree by the mechanical effect on bone conduction. This latter effect, known as the Carhart notch (Carhart, 1950) adds an apparent but not real bone-conduction loss of 5 dB at 500 Hz, 10 dB at 1000 Hz, 15 dB at 2000 Hz, and 5 dB at 4000 Hz. Ginsberg et al. (1979) indicate that the mechanical effect on bone conduction is greater than previously realized. They found the effect to be approximately 15 dB at 500 Hz, 15 dB at 1000 Hz, 20 dB at 2000 Hz, and 15 dB at 4000 Hz. Because of this effect, the prognosticated degree of hearing improvement following stapedectomy can be adjusted upward.

The actual bone changes in otosclerosis consist of a simultaneous laying down of new bone with a concomitant resorption of the older bone producing a spongy type of bone. This abnormal bone may occur anywhere in the otic capsule and depending on where it occurs will determine whether the hearing loss is conductive, sensory-neural, mixed or not present at all. If none of the elements of hearing is involved, one may have otosclerosis of the temporal bone and not be aware of it. This might account for negative family histories in some patients with otosclerosis. The main site of predilection for otosclerosis is that portion of the oval window just anterior to the footplate causing it to become fixed in position and wedged posteriorly.

The tympanic membranes are almost always normal except in those few cases, especially in younger adults, where the increased vascularity of the actively growing bone is reflected through the drum as a pink discoloration. This sign is known as the Schwartze sign and is very inconsistent. It has also been referred to as the "flamingo flush." Since the drum is almost always normal, one must depend on the history and the audiometric findings, the latter of which have characteristic features.

Audiometric results augmented by immittance measurements are of great help in establishing the diagnosis of otosclerosis. The presence of a significant air-bone gap and the absence of acoustic reflexes with a normally shaped (sometimes shallow) tympanogram with normal middle ear pressure support a diagnosis of otosclerosis and are indispensable as indications for surgery (Fig. 2.12). The classical example is a conductive impairment with a greater loss in the low frequencies than in the high frequencies, which follows the impedance formula for stiffness (Berlin and Cullen, 1980). The less typical case is a patient with a mixed loss and a greater or lesser degree of sensory-neural involvement.

It might be well to stress that all surgery for hearing improvement depends upon the ability of the audiologist to identify consistently the existence and the size of the air-bone gap. The preoperative bone-conduction curve is the target for the otosurgeon, and everything possible must be done in the testing to determine it accurately. In these cases, every aspect of bone-conduction measurement must be carefully controlled in order to avoid false estimates of the remaining cochlear potential.

Trauma

Various degrees of damage to the conductive mechanism may result from mechanical trauma, although most damage to the drum or ossicular chain results from infection. A blow to the ear with the open palm (frequently in play) may easily produce a traumatic perforation, a hemotympanum (a collection of blood in the middle ear) or damage to the ossicular chain (Fig. 2.13). Other common causes of the problem include entry of foreign objects into the external auditory canal including cotton tip swabs and twigs. Most recently, the popularity of racquetball has contributed to the occurrence of ear trauma. More patients are being seen who report being hit on the auricle with the ball. Examination often shows the presence of a tympanic membrane perforation due to the force of the ball striking the opening of the external auditory canal.

In severe cases of head trauma, sensory-neural elements also may be damaged. This can result in an irreversible hearing loss that can be total in some cases. Patients have been seen with such a hearing loss directly related to contact sports such as football. In this type of case, proper counseling of the patient is warranted in order to assure protection to the hearing in the unaffected ear.

Glomus tumors arise from glomus bodies along the course of the tympanic branches of the ninth and tenth cranial nerves. They are extremely vascular and depending on their location are called glomus tympanicum or glomus jugulare tumors.

Glomus tympanicum tumors usually arise in the middle ear, frequently on the floor of the promontory and are easily and successfully removed surgically through a transmeatal approach. Glomus jugulare tumors are usually more extensive. Arising in the region of the jugular bulb, they may erode through the floor of the middle ear and present as middle ear tumors. They may also invade anywhere in the temporal bone as well as in the vessels of the neck. Evaluation of the extent of glomus

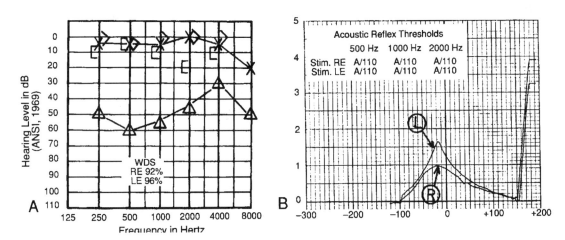

Figure 2.12. Results of audiometric (**A**) and tympanometric (**B**) studies performed on 46-year-old woman with surgically confirmed otosclerosis, right ear.

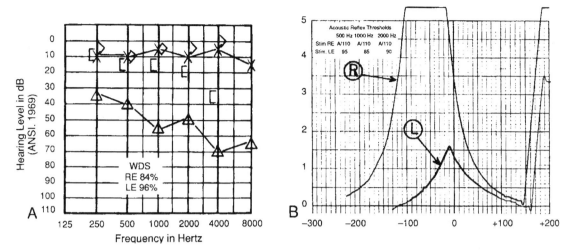

Figure 2.13. Hearing test results (**A**) and tympanograms (**B**) of 14-year-old girl with reported history of head trauma and subsequent surgically confirmed ossicular discontinuity, right ear.

jugulare tumors has become very precise with the advent of sophisticated imaging techniques including magnetic resonance imaging (MRI). Surgical removal alone is often unsuccessful and radiation treatment is generally necessary to control the tumor often without the hope of complete eradication but hopefully long-range control and survival.

Often the presenting symptom is pulsating tinnitus, synchronous with the heart beat, which is explained by the great vascularity of the tumor. Pain is rarely a complaint. Otoscopic examination may show a red mass filling the entire middle ear or the lower portion of the middle ear. Multiple cranial nerve deficits may also be present in more invasive tumors and intracranial extension is not rare. The tumors are rarely malignant and rarely metastasize. Conductive hearing loss may be present depending on the degree of involvement of the tumor and its affect on the ossicular chain. Neural elements may also be involved producing mixed deafness at times with a great sensory-neural component.

DISORDERS OF THE INNER EAR

Congenital Hearing Loss

Hereditary hearing loss may be defined as those cases in which the causative factors are present in the genetic make-up of the fertilized ovum. Congenital loss, on the other hand, means merely that the impairment was present at birth and includes both hereditary as well as acquired cases. These acquired cases have causative factors acting while the fetus was in utero but not contained in germ cells.

Hereditary hearing loss may be transmitted as a dominant or recessive characteristic. It may be associated with other stigmata such as renal involvement, degenerative disease of the nervous system, albinism, mental retardation, and metabolic abnormalities. There are many names of syndromes to describe various combinations of abnormalities such as Alport's, Waardenburg's, and Hurler's syndromes (Northern and Downs, 1984). The diagnosis of any particular entity can rarely be made from audiometric findings alone but is the result of the total clinical picture.

Some examples of congenital hearing loss that are acquired in utero and their etiologies are maternal rubella in the first and second trimesters of pregnancy, and the breakdown of red blood cells with resulting neonatal jaundice, most often the result of erythroblastosis fetalis (Rh incompatibility). In addition, sensory-neural hearing loss may be due to birth injury often associated with anoxia, drug ingestion by the mother (e.g., thalidomide or quinine) and significant degrees of prematurity (possibly because many premature infants have periods of hypoxia).

The diagnosis of a hearing loss in the young infant is quite difficult and challenging. The otologist can do little more than observe gross reflexes. It falls to the audiologist to determine and quantify the hearing loss. Behavioral testing has been supplemented recently with the use of immittance measurements and auditory brainstem response testing. Immittance measurements have helped greatly in assessing middle ear function and objectively predicting the presence and degree of hearing loss (Jerger et al., 1974). Auditory brainstem response and otoacoustic emissions procedures have contributed additional capabilities in assessing the auditory system of infants (see Chapter 25, Auditory Brainstem Response: Threshold Estimation and Auditory Screening; and Chapter 29, Otoacoustic Emissions).

Acquired Hearing Loss

Ménière's Disease

Many patients who consult an otologist do not complain of a hearing loss but rather of imbalance, dizziness, or vertigo. What must be determined first is whether true vertigo (hallucination of movement) is present. Unless it is, the likelihood of a peripheral or labyrinthine cause is remote. Complaints of "dizziness" by which the patient means weakness, "blacking out," or loss of consciousness are not otitic in origin.

The typical clinical picture of Ménière's disease includes (*a*) episodic true rotatory vertigo, (*b*) low-frequency roaring tinnitus, (*c*) a "fullness" or a sense of pressure in the offending ear, and (*d*) nausea and vomiting. During the period of vertigo, there is usually a definite hearing loss that may fluctuate to near normal levels. There may be marked intolerance to loud sounds. The attacks come suddenly and in clusters, usually followed by periods of complete freedom from them. The symptoms of hearing loss need not be noticed by the patient. Conversely, there may be periods of hearing impairment without associated vertigo.

After a complete history has been taken to establish a pattern that is sufficiently characteristic to suggest Ménière's disease, the patient should be referred to the audiologist in hopes that a characteristic audiometric pattern will also appear. When a hearing loss is present, it usually begins as a low frequency, sensory-neural impairment that tends to flatten over a long period of time (Fig. 2.14). A small number of cases can present first as a high frequency loss and later show flattening as the low frequencies are affected. In more than 80% of the cases the disease is unilateral, and recruitment can be determined by the alternate binaural loudness balance test (ABLB) (Fowler, 1936). Complete or even over-recruitment is the rule in this disease. Discrimination scores are usually depressed and in keeping with the degree of sensory-neural loss. There is absence of tone decay and usually a high SISI score. Hearing thresholds will fluctuate from day to day and this fact may be noted by both the audiologist and the patient. Immittance studies may help to confirm these findings. The presence of recruitment is indicated by a positive stapedial reflex produced by stimulus levels in the affected ear at or nearly equal to those levels required to elicit the reflex in the unaffected ear (Metz, 1946). This occurs despite the reduced hearing levels. The auditory brainstem response will show a normal central conduction time consistent with cochlear pathology (Glasscock et al., 1981).

Unless the audiometric findings and the otologic picture match a reasonably typical clinical picture, the diagnosis is in doubt. Using the phrase "Ménière's syn-

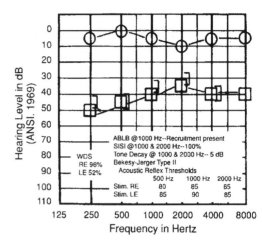

Figure 2.14. Audiogram indicating findings obtained in a 47-year-old man with diagnosed Ménière's disease, left ear.

drome" rather than "Ménière's disease" to indicate an atypical case may be a dangerous practice. It tends to serve as a "wastebasket" term for incompletely understood cases. The diagnosis of Ménière's disease must be a definite one—indicating endolymphatic hydrops only because similar symptoms may be caused by other disorders. Histologically, Ménière's disease almost always shows dilation of the endolymphatic spaces—the result of an increased volume of endolymph. It is not a syndrome; it is a diseased state.

The cause of Ménière's disease is unknown. Whenever a disease has an unknown cause, there are many different approaches to its treatment, and each approach has its own proponents. There is no universally accepted medical or dietary treatment for Ménière's disease at this time. Because the disease is cyclical and has many spontaneous remissions, whatever medication or diet used last might be thought to be effective. Various medications can and should be tried, however, if for no other reason than to buy time and hope for remission. If the vertigo becomes intolerable and is compatible with a normal life, then a surgical approach will be needed. The most reliable surgical procedure for elimination of the vertigo is a labyrinthectomy, but the residual hearing is lost. Therefore, unless the hearing is totally useless (remembering the possibility that it could fluctuate upward), a more conservative approach should be used in order to preserve the hearing.

Noise-Induced Hearing Loss

More and more attention has been given to the adverse effects of noise on the human organism. As civilization has "progressed" the noise in human environment has increased. The adverse effects of noise are widespread with respect to human physiology and produce changes

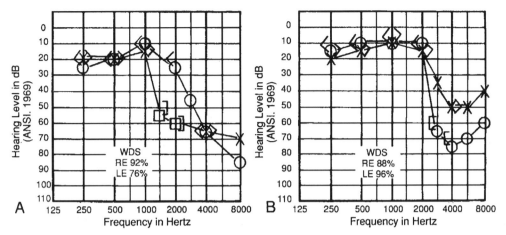

Figure 2.15. Audiometric findings of 44-year-old, right-handed man (**A**) and 46-year-old, left-handed woman (**B**) with significant history of noise exposure from rifle fire.

in many biosystems other than the ear. It is, however, the ear that concerns us here.

Traumatic noise levels almost invariably affect the threshold at 4000 Hz. As the exposure continues, the damage extends to either side of this area, and the loss for 4000 Hz increases. The pathologic process involves outer hair cell damage first as it progressively involves the other cells of the cochlea and later the inner hair cells. Finally, as reported by Siebenmann and Yoshii in 1908, the cochlear neurons may atrophy.

Industrial hearing loss resulting from noise exposure is usually equal bilaterally. Hearing impairment induced by the noise of gunfire may show different degrees of loss in each ear. A right-handed rifleman shooting a shotgun exposes his left ear to more sound than his right because of the proximity of the breech to the left ear and vice versa (Fig. 2.15). This may be a good lead in attempting to determine the cause of a particular loss and may, for example, reveal that a case of industrial hearing loss was in fact due to many years of skeet and trap shooting. There is no therapy for this type of loss, and prevention is the only possible approach. This requires cooperation on the part of the employee as well as the employer. Hearing conservation programs in industry must be supported vigorously by both groups.

Drug-Induced Hearing Loss

Certain ototoxic drugs have a propensity for causing cochlear or vestibular damage. The more common drugs that are particularly toxic to the ear are certain antibiotics, salicylates, and quinine. Streptomycin, dihydrostreptomycin, kanamycin, neomycin, gentamicin, viomycin and more recently, cis-platinum have been shown to be ototoxic and should therefore be utilized in treatment only when there is not a less toxic or nontoxic drug available. Streptomycin is essentially vestibulotoxic

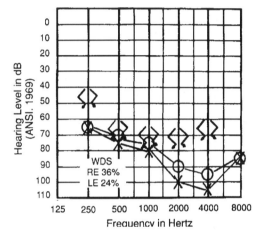

Figure 2.16. Puretone and speech discrimination results of 52-year-old man who had received large doses of neomycin, producing subsequent sensory-neural hearing loss.

while dihydrostreptomycin usually is more toxic to the cochlea (Schuknecht, 1974). Neither is exclusively so. Neomycin and kanamycin are essentially cochleotoxic, whereas gentamicin and viomycin seem to be more vestibulotoxic. Ordinarily, losses due to streptomycin are not as severe as those due to kanamycin and neomycin, which usually produce profound hearing loss as shown in Figure 2.16. In addition to the antibiotics mentioned above, other compounds can have a deleterious effect on hearing. Most recently cis-platinum, which is used in the treatment of carcinoma of the head and neck, has been shown to be ototoxic. When any ototoxic drug is administered, audiometric monitoring is indicated.

Virus-Induced Hearing Loss

The inner ear may be affected both by specific and nonspecific viruses. The viruses of measles and mumps are well-known offenders. The measles virus usually produces moderate to severe bilateral losses involving both the cochlear and vestibular systems. Mumps usually causes a total unilateral loss with no involvement of the vestibular system. Uncommonly, it may cause a high frequency loss only. Mumps infections may not be suspected in the absence of the typical parotid swelling and yet be the cause of sudden deafness. To determine that the mumps virus is the etiologic agent requires antibody studies. The group of viruses that, for example, can be the cause of respiratory infections may also be carried by the blood to the cochlea, producing a viral cochleitis. This can cause a sudden loss, but fortunately in some cases there has been partial to complete recovery.

Presbycusis

Presbycusis is a sensory-neural hearing loss due to degenerative changes of aging. It is the most common cause of sensory-neural loss in the adult population. Chapter 37, Presbycusis, and Chapter 49, Assisting the Older Client, deal specifically with this problem. Recent statistics show that hearing impairment can occur in as many as 25% of those in the 65–70 age category. This can increase to 40% of those over 75 (Powers and Powers, 1978). The degenerative effects of aging on hearing involve a variety of locations and cell types in the inner ear with nonspecific effects on puretone thresholds. It is for this reason that presbycusis in some may cause profound difficulties, while in others the deficit is small.

Sudden Hearing Loss

Although usually characterized by gradual onset with slow progression, sensory-neural hearing loss may also have a sudden onset. Sudden hearing loss of known cause may be due to drugs, trauma, infection, or disease. Those cases of sudden loss without apparent etiology have been explained by two hypotheses. The first is viral labyrinthitis, producing changes in the inner ear similar to those caused by known viral invaders such as the virus of mumps. Evidence of viral labyrinthitis as a likely cause of sudden hearing loss is that respiratory infection often seems to precede the hearing loss. The second hypothesis is that of vascular occlusion causing abrupt interruption of blood supply. The fact that sudden loss occurs at any age tends to mitigate against this as a frequent factor. Sudden hearing loss can also be attributed to rupture of the round window membrane but is usually associated with a definite history of trauma.

Sudden hearing loss is usually associated with tinnitus and sometimes with vertigo. If the latter symptom is present it usually disappears in a relatively short time, but the hearing loss tends to be irreversible. The loss may be moderate or severe and is almost always unilateral. Re-

covery occurs in less than half of the cases, and the value of any specific therapy is open to question.

When a patient presents with the history of sudden hearing loss following respiratory infection, the cause could be the sensory-neural loss described or otitis media producing a conductive loss. The audiologist can easily differentiate these disorders. Before the otologist proceeds with the inference that it is a eustachian tube or middle ear problem an audiometric assessment should be obtained, sparing the patient from much treatment foredoomed to failure.

Although one cannot be certain of the etiology, hospitalization with a regimen of intravenous medication is felt to increase the chances of recovery. Although some patients may recover spontaneously, a protocol of treatment is recommended over a do-nothing approach. It is generally accepted that sudden hearing loss is a medical emergency.

PROFOUND COCHLEAR HEARING LOSS AND COCHLEAR IMPLANT

Until the mid-1970s (Luxford and Brackmann, 1985), there was little in the armamentarium of the otologist or audiologist that offered any significant help for the individual with profound-to-total sensory-neural deafness. Cochlear implantation provides a form of a solution for those individuals. Electrical stimulation of the cochlea and residual nerve elements offers limited but significant help ranging from identification of environmental sounds to varying degrees of closed- and open-set speech identification.

Many patients who have been implanted are functioning with much improved communication skills. After several years of cochlear implant experience, it appears that the best candidate is one who is postlingually deafened for a short period of time and is well motivated and psychologically suited for such an approach. A good support system involving family members as well as professional involvement is of utmost importance (Owens, 1989). For a more detailed discussion of this area, see Chapter 46, Cochlear Implants and Tactile Aids.

DISORDERS OF THE RETROCOCHLEAR SYSTEM

Not many years ago the otologist had to be content with the audiologist telling only whether the loss was conductive, sensory-neural or mixed. As audiology evolved it has become possible to determine where the site of lesion occurs in the sensory-neural pathway. Immittance and ABR measurements have recently added a new dimension to locating dysfunction. Cochlear, retrocochlear, and central lesions can be identified in an ever-increasing percentage of cases. When dealing with conductive losses the otologist looks to the audiologist not only for the site of lesion but for the size of the air-bone gap. When dealing with sensory-neural hearing loss the otologist looks to the audiologist to determine the site of pathology. The audiologist and otologist working as a team can discover early cerebellopontine angle tumors such as acoustic neurinomas and through their cooperative efforts actually perform a lifesaving function.

Acoustic Neurinoma

The patient who presents with a suspected acoustic neurinoma will, due to the site of pathology, reveal a negative otologic examination. It is the accurate completion of the case history, reported symptomatology, and the accumulation of accurate test results that form the clinical picture of this retrocochlear problem. The reported duration of the problem may be short, or it may have been present for a long period of time. The patient will usually complain of unilateral hearing loss, tinnitus, and forms of imbalance. This is usually described not as vertigo, but as unsteadiness.

When the audiometric findings suggest a retrocochlear site, the case must be thoroughly investigated in an attempt to discover or rule out the presence of an acoustic neurinoma. The skilled audiologist is crucial in investigating the presence of one of these tumors. In this respect, a unilateral sensory-neural hearing loss should be considered a potential acoustic neurinoma until proven otherwise. The audiologist should in this case have a high index of suspicion and perform a complete battery of audiometric studies that help to determine the site of lesion. This may include the traditional tests that have been used to distinguish cochlear from retrocochlear losses (Fig. 2.17). Absence of recruitment, positive tone decay, a low SISI score, and inordinately poor word discrimination ability are all indicative of a possible retrocochlear pathology. These tests should be supplemented by immittance measurements and ABR testing. The absence of the acoustic reflex, or its presence with acoustic reflex decay, is a highly positive indication of a retrocochlear problem. Lengthened central conduction time on the ABR or absence of waves after the eighth nerve response (wave I) completes the comprehensive studies suggesting retrocochlear dysfunction.

Electronystagmography (ENG) is of great help in establishing retrocochlear disease. Characteristically, but not invariably, the caloric response on the affected side is severely depressed or absent in the ear with retrocochlear hearing loss. The study of retrocochlear pathology again points out the need for close cooperation between the otologist and the audiologist and a mutual understanding of the two disciplines. Corroboration should be further provided by x-rays of the internal audi-

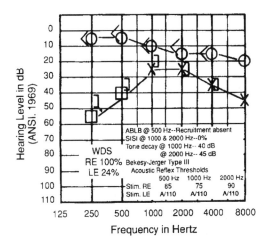

Figure 2.17. Results of audiologic studies carried out on 44-year-old woman with surgically confirmed cerebellopontine angle tumor, left side.

tory meatus and enhanced computed tomography (CT). A relatively new technique that provides remarkable visualization is MRI.

Other

Whenever the test battery indicates a retrocochlear site of lesion, one must remember that processes other than acoustic neurinomas may be responsible for the test results. These may include viral neuronitis, trauma, hemorrhage, meningioma, or neurologic disorders such as multiple sclerosis. While audiometric studies cannot distinguish these lesions, tests of central auditory dysfunction can confirm specific areas of involvement. Results of these tests should be supplemented with a neurologic evaluation including computerized x-ray techniques.

CONCLUSION

A realization of the complexity of the ear and its neural pathways and an awareness of the many disorders that involve the auditory system make us very much aware of the diagnostic effort that must be made to define the pathology in any given case. The otologist can view only the outer ear up to the tympanic membrane or the middle ear. Deeper portions are hidden from view and may be examined functionally by the audiologist. State-of-the-art otologic diagnosis is practiced by the audiologist-otologist team. It is the responsibility of otologists to treat conditions of the ear medically or surgically to the best of their ability. When hearing impairment remains, audiologists are called upon to ease the burden of the hearing handicap by using their expertise to select an appropriate amplification system, supplemented with counseling and principles of aural rehabilitation.

REFERENCES

American National Standards Institute. American National Standard Specifications for Audiometers. New York: ANSI, S3.6-1969, 1970.

Arslan M. Treatment of Ménière's syndrome by direct application of ultrasound waves in the vestibular system. In Proceedings of the Fifth International Congress in Otolaryngology. 1953:629–635.

Bekesy GV. A new audiometer. Acta Otolaryngol 1947;35:411–422.

Berlin C and Cullen J. 1980. The physical basis of impedance measurement. In Jerger J and Northern J, Eds. Clinical Impedance Audiometry. Acton, MA: American Electromedics, 1980.

Bryde RL and Feldman AS. An approach to the management of the collapsing ear canal. Paper presented at the American Speech-Language-Hearing Association Convention, Detroit, 1980

Bunch CC. Clinical Audiometry. St. Louis, MO: CV Mosby, 1943.

Carhart R. Clinical application of bone conduction audiometry. Arch Otolaryngol 1950;51:798–807.

Fowler EP. A method for the early detection of otosclerosis. Arch Otolaryngol 1936;24:731–741.

Ginsberg IA, Hoffman SR, Stinizano GD, and White TP. Stapedectomy—in-depth analysis of 2405 cases. Laryngoscope 1979; 88:1999–2016.

Glasscock M, Jackson G, and Josey A. 1981. Brainstem Electric Response Audiometry. New York: Brian C Decker, 1981.

House W. Surgical exposure of the internal auditory canal and its contents through the middle cranial fossa. Laryngoscope 1961; 71:1363–1385.

Jerger J, Burney P, Mauldin L, and Crump B. Predicting hearing loss from the acoustic reflex. J Speech Hear Disord 1974;39:11–22.

Jerger JF, Shedd J, and Harford ER. On the detection of extremely small changes in sound intensity. Arch Otolaryngol 1959;69:200–211.

Lempert J. Improvement of hearing in cases of otosclerosia: a new one-stage surgical technic. Arch Otolaryngol 1938;28:42–97.

Luxford WM and Brackman DE. The history of cochlear implants. In Gray RF, Ed. Cochlear Implants. San Diego: College Hill Press, 1985.

Lynn GE. A test to detect collapse of the external ear canal. J Speech Hear Disord 1967;32:273–274.

Metz D. The acoustic impedance measures on normal and pathological ears. Acta Otolaryngol 1946;63(Suppl):1–254.

Michelson RP. Electrical stimulation of the human cochlea. Arch Otolaryngol 1971;93:317–323.

Northern JL and Downs M. Hearing in Children, 3rd ed. Baltimore: Williams & Wilkins, 1984.

Noyes HD. Otitis media following the use of a bougie in the eustachian tube—introduction of an eyelet into the membrano tympani. Trans Am Otol Soc 1869:55–61.

Owens E. Present status of adults with cochlear implants. In Owens E and Kessler D, Eds. Cochlear Implants in Young Deaf Children. Boston: College Hill Press, 1989.

Powers JK and Powers EA. Hearing problems of elderly persons: social consequences and prevalence. ASHA 1978;20:79–83.

Rosen S. Mobilization of the stapes to restore hearing in otosclerosis. N Y State J Med 1953;53:2650–2653.

Schuknecht HF. Pathology of the Ear. Cambridge, MA: Harvard University Press, 1974.

Shea JJ. A fenestration of the oval window. Ann Otol Rhinol Laryngol 1958;67:932–951.

Siebenmann F and Yoshii U. Demonstration von experimentellen Akustischen Schaedigungen des Gehoroganes. Verb Dtsch Ges Otolog 1908;17:114–118.

Valsalva AM. Opera, hoc est, tractus de humana. Venice, Pitteri, 1741.

Wullstein J. Die tympanoplaskid als gehroverbessernde operation bei otitis media chronica und irh resultate. In Proceedings of the Fifth International Congress on Oto-Rhino-Laryngology. 1953; 108:104–118.

CHAPTER 3

Neurologic Disorders and Examination

Robert L. Zimmerman

In many settings audiologists work closely with neurologists to evaluate the hearing of patients with neurologic symptoms and contribute to the differential diagnoses of the site of lesion. The audiologist obtains behavioral (psychophysical) responses and corroborates this information with electrophysiologic information. Thus, the audiologic evaluation incorporates the interpretation of patient-stated perceptions as well as electrical responses that can be measured from the patient.

The basic battery of audiologic procedures is described in detail elsewhere in *Handbook of Clinical Audiology*. This chapter provides the audiologist with preliminary but necessary knowledge about all patients seen for purposes of differential diagnosis. Numerous test procedures are also available that help to focus on the area(s) of the auditory system that are of the greatest concern in a particular patient. Many of these central procedures are described in this volume and will be discussed in relation to case studies at the end of the chapter.

For the audiologist who works with neurology patients, one of the biggest benefits has come from the advances in electronics (e.g., microchips and microcomputers). By using such equipment the audiologist is able to measure minute electrical responses (often less than 1 nanovolt or 0.000001 volt) or analyze larger potentials from the auditory system. Temporal and amplitude characteristics are available for the audiologist's evaluation. Included in the test battery for neurologic patients are physiologic procedures such as electronystagmography, acoustic reflex measurement, and auditory brainstem response.

ANATOMY

Understanding of the anatomy of the auditory system is important for appreciating its basic structure and its underlying electrical network.

We shall begin our discussion at the level of axons and dendrites and conclude with disorders of the central auditory system and case studies.

Axons and Dendrites

In the body, transmission of electrical impulses is carried out through nerve tissue. Cell bodies in the central ner-

vous system (CNS) have a characteristic color that prompts the name gray matter. Among other sites, gray matter is found in the cerebral cortex, the outer layers of the brain. Cell bodies have two basic types of protrusions—axons and dendrites. These structures provide for the direction of travel of the electrical impulse. Each neuron has one axon which is made of white matter and allows impulses to travel away from the main cell body. Transmission of a signal toward the cell body is achieved through a dendrite. There are three basic types of neurons classified on the basis of structure.

The simplest type of neuron, the bipolar neuron, has one dendrite and one axon. The unipolar neuron has one axon which carries the signal away from the cell body. This axon splits after leaving the cell body with one branch functioning as an axon and the other as a dendrite. The multipolar neuron has a multiple dendritic input and the output of a single axon.

There is a one-way flow of electrical activity in the neuronal system. This is because each neuron has just one axon. However, the information in the nervous system must not only travel to the brain, but must return. Adjustment signals must be continually sent to organs and muscles to maintain body function. Because of this one-way-transmission characteristic and the need for a two-way system, two separate sets of neurons are required. These systems are referred to as afferent and efferent. Sensory, or afferent neurons, transmit information to the brain and CNS. Motor, or efferent neurons, transmit signals from the CNS to an organ or muscle.

Auditory afferent pathways which transmit from the cochlea to the cortex have a return efferent representation from the cortex to the cochlea. In addition to the afferent and efferent neurons a third group of neurons called the connector neurons act as relays between efferent and afferent pathways within the CNS.

Afferent Pathways

Afferent neurologic auditory pathways effectively begin with the first synapse at the cochlear nucleus (*1* on Fig. 3.1). The tonotopic organization of the basilar membrane is continual throughout the cells and synapses of the afferent pathways. As many as 30,000 nerve fibers connect the inner and outer hair cells to the brain-

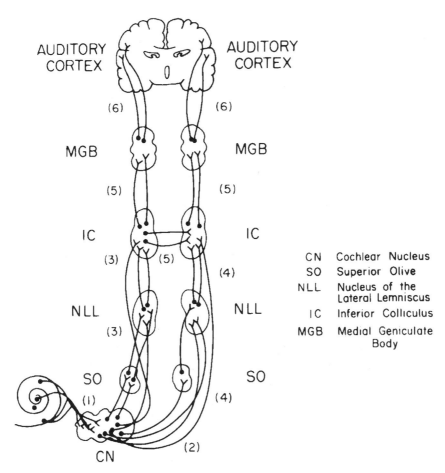

Figure 3.1. Afferent auditory system from cochlear to auditory cortex of the brain. Synapses within the major nuclei are shown.

stem. These nerve fibers enter the brainstem at the level of the pons and terminate with secondary neurons in one of the divisions of the cochlear nucleus (Mountcastle, 1980). The cochlear nucleus is divided into three separate sections (Brugge, 1980; Warr, 1982). These divisions include the dorsal cochlear nucleus, the anteroventral cochlear nucleus, and the posteroventral cochlear nucleus.

Figure 3.1 shows a rough schematic of the synaptic connections of the afferent auditory system. Some of the second-order fibers cross the midline (*2*) and synapse in the superior olivary complex on the opposite side. Others bypass the superior olivary complex and synapse across the midline at the inferior colliculus. While some ipsilateral neurons synapses occur at the lateral lemniscus and the inferior colliculus (IC) (*3*), a large number of neurons from the cochlear nucleus extend contralaterally to the lateral lemniscus (*4*) (Mountcastle, 1980). Thus, there is parallel bilateral representation to the IC (*3* and *4*).

At the IC, the auditory pathway goes both ipsilaterally and contralaterally (*5*). The contralateral pathway crosses the commissure of the IC to the IC and medial geniculate body (MGB) on the opposite side. The brachium of the inferior colliculus is the ipsilateral pathway to the MGB. There are three major divisions of the MGB of the thalamus. The areas are the ventral, medial, and dorsal divisions. The primary projections to the auditory areas of the cortex are from the ventral division (*6*).

The medial geniculate nucleus is the thalamic transfer region for the auditory system. The large afferent bundle to the medial geniculate nucleus is the brachium of the IC, which contains auditory fibers from different origins (IC, lateral lemniscus, and superior olivary complex). Under certain conditions, sensory evoked potentials can be used to map the central representation of the sensory system (Poggio and Mountcastle, 1980)

In experiments utilizing a cat, the auditory reception area of the cortex has been shown to occupy the transverse portion of the temporal gyrus of Heschl. This primary auditory cortical area (AI), sometimes referred to as the primary projection area, is unequivocally auditory cortex (Whitfield, 1982). The second important auditory area (AII) is located anterior to AI and continues the tonotopic organization initially seen in the cochlea. Tonturi (1968) completed studies in the dog that indicated at least four auditory areas of the cortex. One area, the posterior ectosylvian area, was found not to be directly stimulated from the cochlea. This implies that there are auditory pathways other than those measurable and described by conventional axon-dendrite synapse activity.

In humans, Brodmann's areas 41 and 42 have been shown to be associated with auditory response. In waking humans, when this area was stimulated, the illusion of auditory reception was expressed. This sensation was typically referred to the contralateral ear (Penfield and Rasmussen, 1950). Luria (1973) indicated that, in addition to the primary auditory reception areas, the secondary areas are quite important in the differentiation of acoustic stimuli presented together. These areas are also necessary to distinguish between consecutive sounds of different pitch. He further suggested that lesions in these areas of the left temporal cortex result in language reception problems. Lesions of the right temporal areas usually result in difficulties with musical recognition.

Efferent Pathways

The afferent auditory pathways have been, for the most part, well described. Efferent pathways, however, have not been described as thoroughly, but are mentioned throughout the literature. The primary evaluation and study of the efferent system have been done with animals. The inferior portion of the efferent system was first described by Rasmussen in the early 1940's (1942, 1946). The olivocochlear bundle (efferent system) of Rasmussen originates at or adjacent to the superior olivary complex and terminates at or near the hair cells within the contralateral cochlea. Mountcastle (1980) described the auditory neurologic pathway structure as one of an ascending and descending parallel system. That is, the efferent system descends in the reverse manner in order to provide a control of the afferent transmission originating at the cochlea. Absolute definition of this system has not been possible because of the multiple nerve fibers that require delineation. Continued research in this area will certainly change part of our interpretation of the function of this portion of the auditory pathway.

NEUROLOGIC EXAMINATION

The neurologic examination is a comprehensive evaluation of the patient. A complete history is taken. This includes an elaboration of the primary neurologic complaints and the history of these complaints. In addition, personal and family health histories are taken, especially neurologic and psychiatric histories. This inquiry should include questions of altered affect, cognition, memory, motor and sensory disturbances, as well as autonomic disturbances.

Basic Medical Examination

If a general medical examination has not been completed, the neurologist will proceed to carry out such an examination and appraisal of many different regions, including the head (ears, nose, throat), heart, endocrine changes, vasomotor responses, and cerebrovascular system. During this segment of the physical examination, size, pulsations, and tenderness of the superficial temporal, facial, and suborbital arteries are observed. Listening to the blood flow through the common carotid and carotid bifurcation with a stethoscope completes the physical examination.

The patient's mental status is assessed by observing the level of consciousness and attention span. The patient's affect, intellectual performance, and memory capabilities are important factors in overall health and well-being. Evaluation of these factors is carried out by assessing orientation to time, place, and person, abstract thinking rate, insight, judgment, and problem-solving abilities. These factors are also important in the patient's ability to understand the diagnosis and its ramifications and to follow the prescribed therapeutic program. Evaluations of the patient's motor programming abilities, perceptual patterns (visual, auditory, tactile), and central language functions provide further information about the patient's status.

Cranial Nerves

The neurologic examination continues with evaluation of cranial nerve I. The sense of smell is generally assessed with distinguishing items such as coffee and tobacco, or aromatic substances such as oil of cloves or peppermint. The visual apparatus reflecting the function of cranial nerves II, III, IV, and VI can be evaluated by checking visual acuity, visual sclera, cornea, lens, and fundus. The size and shape of the pupils, accommodation reflex, and direct and consensual reflexes are observed as are the extraocular muscles, optatokinetic nystagmus, and oculocephalic reflexes. Evaluation of facial sensation, jaw muscles, corneal reflexes, and jaw jerk helps to determine whether cranial nerve V is intact. Taste, facial symmetry, and voluntary movement of the facial muscles test seventh nerve function.

The eighth (acoustic) nerve is routinely assessed by the neurologist through use of tuning forks. The combination of the Weber and Rinne tests generally enable the examiner to differentiate a "nerve loss" from a conductive impairment and to determine the ear with the greater conductive or the least sensory-neural loss. The vestibular portion of the eighth nerve is assessed by caloric stimulation. Observation of palatal movement and symmetry, swallowing and precipitating a gag reflex will show the integrity of cranial nerves IX and X. The spinal accessory nerve (XI) is checked through the movements of the head left and right against resistance (examiner's hand). Having the patient shrug shoulders against resistance further demonstrates the integrity of cranial nerve XI. The hypoglossal nerve (XII) is evaluated by observing the tongue at rest on the floor of the mouth, then slightly protruded, and finally fully protruded. A deviation indicates paresis on the side toward which the tongue turns. The use of the tongue blade to provide resistance will provide further information about the strength of the tongue.

Motor Coordination

Motor speech is evaluated essentially by a sample of contextual speech. Assessment is made of respiration, phonation, resonation, articulatory precision, phrase length and prosody. Diadochokinetic rate and capacity for prolonged phonation can be quickly evaluated by having the patient rapidly repeat "pah," "tah," "kah," and sustain phonation.

The general motor survey of the appendicular and truncal motor systems includes observation and evaluation of posture, habituation of sitting and standing, righting reflexes, and the Romberg test, which differentiates between peripheral and cerebellar ataxia. An increase in the clumsiness of movement or gait when the patient's eyes are closed indicates a peripheral problem. The examiner can glean more information from an assessment of general mobility and observation for tremor, tics, mannerisms, and impairment of fast or slow voluntary movement.

Patient arm and leg coordination is evaluated by observing rapid alternating muscle movements in both pronation and supination. Further investigation of synergy and accuracy is made with the patient's eyes both open and closed; abnormalities seen in these tasks are consistent with cerebellar disease. A general muscle survey with emphasis on size, strength, structural symmetry, bulk, and tone provides essential information about the patient's overall health status.

Reflex, Motor, and Sensory Evaluation

Examination of the patient's involuntary reflexes is also made. This segment of the examination looks at both superficial and myotatic (stretching and extending) reflex activity. Superficial reflex activity of cranial nerves V, VII, IX, and X can be easily elicited by the corneal and the palatopharyngeal reflexes.

An extensive neurologic examination is necessary because of the difficult problems generally referred to the neurologist. The fundamental questions of location and etiology are the first that need to be answered. Further, the discovery of any inconsistency or weakness may give an indication as to the cause of the patient's primary complaint. Many times, however, several disease processes contribute to the central problem and act in concert to generate the malady. The effectiveness of the examination is dependent on the examiner's knowledge of anatomy and physiology and ability to devise tasks to assess the function of various systems. Only after a thorough examination can appropriate laboratory studies be ordered to augment and substantiate the findings.

ELECTROPHYSIOLOGIC MEASUREMENTS

Electroencephalography

Recording the electrical activity of the central and peripheral nervous systems became clinically applicable with the availability of electronic amplifiers and recording equipment. Perhaps the most widely used diagnostic test of the central nervous system is the electroencephalogram (EEG). The EEG examination records electrical activity from 8, 12, or even 16 channels through electrodes that are affixed to the scalp in a standard arrangement.

Normal EEG variants can be seen at all stages. EEG interpretation is based on the consistency of various waveforms seen in the different age groups. The repetition of the various waveform activities over time is referred to as rhythm. The waveform activity and rhythm are also classified by amplitude. The alpha rhythm is the starting point for analyzing the awake EEG. This rhythm has a lower limit of 8 Hz, which generally appears by the age of 3, and reaches a frequency of 9 to 12 Hz by the age of 16, then decreases with advancing age. It is felt that there is a relationship between EEG and cerebral blood flow. In addition to alpha rhythm, mu rhythm activity can be associated with the sensorimotor cortex as can beta activity.

The diagnosis of petit mal epilepsy is defined by thrice per second spike-wave activity (Most and Low, 1973). This tracing may be recorded even in the absence of clinically observable seizures. Usually, petit mal is diagnosed by clinical examination in addition to the EEG tracings. The distinctive spike-wave EEG configuration, however, is generally present in patients with this problem.

Intracranial tumor identification can be shown in many cases because of a characteristic slow wave activity (1–3 waves/sec) near the site of the neoplasm (Most and Low, 1973). This slow wave activity caused by a tumor can be characterized by a higher than normal voltage. The characteristic slow wave activity and higher than normal electrical output are also present with vascular disease. The EEG may not show focal slow wave activity in every tumor case nor in every case of vascular disease, but it can be of valuable assistance in identifying these pathologies.

Evoked Response

Stimulation of the sensory receptors or nerves produces action potentials that conform to an expected pattern when using certain stimulus parameters. The evoked responses have generally been shown to be highly consistent and reproducible between individuals. This noninvasive tool has proven to be a useful diagnostic technique for assessment of the auditory, visual, and somatosensory systems.

Somatosensory Evoked Potentials

Somatosensory evoked potentials (SEPs) can be detected over the entire body. Clinical evaluation has been limited to peripheral nerve action potentials. The SEP allows information to be obtained from peripheral nerves, spinal cord, brainstem, and cerebral cortex. The SEP response latencies are classified into three main time frames. The long latency, greater than a 75-msec response, is easily recognized in waveforms appearing in EEG tracings. The middle latency, 30 to 75 msec, and the early latency period, less than 30 msec, are more difficult to record and require sophisticated electronics. This equipment averages the evoked response over time and allows the low intensity responses of the early and middle latency period to be graphically displayed and latency periods to be quantified.

Visual Evoked Response

One of the more recent additions to the diagnostic neurology test battery is the visual evoked response (VER). VERs are obtained by recording responses elicited in patients viewing shifting patterns on a television screen or other suitable visual device. These pattern-shifting visual evoked responses (PSVERs) are even less variable than those obtained through auditory stimulation. The VER tracing is referred to as P100. This response was so named because the waveform is positive at occipital scalp locations and appears about 100 msec after the pattern shift. These potentials can be affected by very minor disturbances of the visual pathways. PSVER has been found to be more effective than clinical evaluations in defining optic neuritis and is a major tool in diagnosing multiple sclerosis. In addition, visual evoked potentials have been shown to demonstrate abnormal tracings with pathologies other than demyelinating diseases including glaucoma and various amblyopias. Maturational changes and assessment of functional problems can be determined using PSVER techniques.

Auditory Brainstem Responses

The "bumps" reported by Jewett (1970) when click stimuli were delivered to the ear of a cat have been shown to be the cochlear nerve response and brainstem response that follow the afferent auditory nerve pathways (see Chapter 22). Auditory brainstem response (ABR) testing has become a commonly accepted neurologic diagnostic procedure (see Chapters 24). The audiologist must be able to recognize the normal ABR response parameters and the variations in these responses. Chiappa et al (1979) described six possible category variations in normal ABR waveform morphology (structure). Absolute waveform and interpeak latency norms should be established for each laboratory and patient population. The reader is referred to Fria (1980) for a review of the history and literature concerning ABR.

Acoustic Reflex

The acoustic reflex is the result of an evoked response precipitated by an acoustic stimulus. While not directly measured using the methodology employed in ABR, PSVER, and SEP, the acoustic reflex measurements reflect the same degree of reproducibility and consistency. Because of this, the evaluation of the acoustic reflex of patients with suspected neurologic disease can add another bit of information to the overall diagnostic picture (see Chapter 21). In addition to the measurement of the acoustic reflex and the stability of this response, the reflex latency period relative to the onset of acoustic stimulus has been investigated. The acoustic reflex latency measurement, like SEP, seems to show considerable variability across subjects, and thus determination of an abnormal response may be considerably more difficult than with other evoked response tests.

NUCLEAR MEDICINE

Transmission of electrical signals through nerves requires an intact structure and one that is not interfered with by other structures (e.g., tumors). The imaging techniques used in nuclear medicine employ a radioactive compound linked to a pharmaceutical chosen to: (*a*) concentrate in a particular organ once injected into the body, (*b*) not concentrate in a particular organ, or (*c*) allow the monitoring of the arrival and subsequent elimination of the pertechnetate. Specialized radiation detectors are used to obtain structural images of data describing time functions. The detectors transform emitted radiation into visible light. This light is then amplified and processed so that an accurate structural analysis is permitted. In addition, this process is enhanced through the use of computers that allow image sequencing, radiation counting, averaging and analysis of intensity and rate, giving a three-dimensional effect to the study.

Radionuclide brain scanning has been used since the 1950s in the study of neurologic disease. A primary use of this diagnostic tool has been in the detection of space-occupying lesions in the cerebral hemispheres and the cerebellum. A space-occupying lesion in the brain leads to breakdown in the blood-brain barrier. This results in a "hot spot" on the brain scan image where the radioactive material concentrates. Cerebrovascular accidents are shown by a positive image. There is, however, a time relationship that must be observed. That is, for the first few days after a stroke the scan will be negative. Then for a period of 1 to 2 weeks there will be a positive uptake of the pertechnetate followed by a tendency to return to normal.

Brain scan procedures are approximately 90% accurate in the detection of space-occupying pathologies and the procedure has little associated morbidity. The conventional brain-scanning apparatus is being replaced by the γ camera. This instrument can be in the form of a mobile unit that offers bedside utility and monitoring activity in intensive care units or operating rooms.

RADIOLOGIC STUDIES

Neuroradiology

Conventional radiographic studies have historically utilized a controlled source of ionizing radiation to produce tomographs. Tomographs are "x-rays" that show structures under study and eliminate interference of the surrounding tissues. Utilizing a computer with this technique—computerized tomography (CT)—has enhanced the resolution of these pictures, enabling not only the visualization of the ossicles but also the identification of the eighth nerve. Because the normal anatomy is shown with definition, abnormalities can be better identified.

Regular tomography needs a "thin slice" in order to identify structures. The use of 1.5 to 2 mm collimation has been shown to work best for small structure identification. If the computerized radiographic study is less than this optimum, resolution of the images is lost to electronic "noise." That is, there is reduction in the amount of signal being transmitted and this information is amplified to fill the display, causing the "noise."

In addition to focusing the study on a particular area, contrast material can be used to enhance the images and, thus this abnormal tissue is more easily recognized.

Almost all acoustic nerve tumors can be enhanced (Taylor, 1982). This is important because these tumors are sometimes difficult to differentiate from the surrounding tissue. Enhancement can also be done using air or oil injected into the posterior fossa. Air has proven to be an excellent contrast agent and permits the use of various collimations.

Most tumors of the acoustic nerve are found in the cerebellopontine angle (Taylor, 1982). Current audiometric procedures, particularly ABR, help in early identification of these disorders. Of course, radiographic evidence of these neoplasms is needed for verification and to define the surgical approach to be followed. CT scan is the primary diagnostic tool used in the workup of these tumors. The use of plain films with CT has a diagnostic accuracy of about 90%.

Positron Emission Tomography

Positron emission tomography (PET) is an imaging technology that utilizes data from positron-emitting radionuclides usually bound with biochemical substances and injected into the patient. PET does not expose the patient to as much radioactivity as other diagnostic methods.

This reduction in radioactivity exposure is achieved by utilizing radionuclides with relatively short half life periods (see Table 3.1). PET scan reading are very accurate because the radioactive material is emitted from the area in question.

Among the disorders that can be evaluated utilizing PET scan techniques are stroke, parkinsonism, Huntington's chorea, mania, depression, schizophrenia, and epilepsy. Further definitive information about a number of diseases, including multiple sclerosis and its therapeutic management, has been obtained.

PET is valuable in early diagnosis. It can identify chemical changes and measure the size of an object prior to apparent structural changes detectable by CT and magnetic resonance imaging (MRI) scans. The limiting validation of the PET system is approximately 1 to 6 mm.

Table 3.1.
Some of the More Common Material used for PET Scans.

Element	Half Life in Minutes
Bromine 75	101
Carbon 11	20.4
Fluorine 18	109.7
Gallium 68	88.1
2-deoxy-D-glucose	20
Nitrogen 13	9.96
Oxygen 15	2.07

PET is a good technique for studying in vivo physiology and biochemistry in humans and animals. These images are functional representations of brain activity and behavioral or pharmacological responses that can be measured in both normal individuals and patients with cerebral pathology (see Fig. 3.2).

Magnetic Resonance Imaging

The most recent development in imaging techniques involves the use of a magnetic field. Magnetic resonance imaging does not use x-rays, isotopes, ultrasound, sources of ionization, contrast materials, invasive techniques, or any of the factors associated with typical diagnostic imaging that account for potentially detrimental effects. The procedure has better image quality than even the newest CT scanners. In addition, MRI can detect bone marrow while disregarding the bone structure, determine chemical changes associated with neoplasms, and identify and trace blood flow.

The MRI scanner is basically the same as a CT scanner with a magnetic gantry substituted for the x-ray source. The image is generated by varying the magnetic field surrounding an object (i.e., a human subject). The magnetic pulse of a certain frequency will excite only one cross-sectional plane through the body. The thickness of this cross-sectional plane is related to the frequency of the magnetic pulse. A radio frequency magnetic pulse is used to excite the nuclei in the subject, and a radio frequency receiver coil picks up the signal emitted by the nuclei. This signal is then amplified and mixed with a frequency synthesizer output to produce an audio frequency signal containing the same information as the original sound received by the radio frequency coil. This information is then digitized and stored in a computer for retrieval and image production. Unlike conventional CT images and nuclear medicine displays, MRI computer image displays can utilize color to show minute differences in signal intensity and thus depict small changes more efficiently. The MRI unit relies heavily on the computer programming capacity. This dependence on "software" rather than "hardware" to improve the capacity of the MRI unit should improve the cost effectiveness and the useful lifetime of the scanner. Figures 3.3 and 3.4 present a MRI of a patient with a large acoustic neuroma. This neoplasm is shown to be approximately ½ by 2 ½ cm. This irregularly shaped tumor is located in and essentially conforms to the space of the posterior fossa, medial to the medulla, lateral to the petrous ridge, and inferior to the cerebellum.

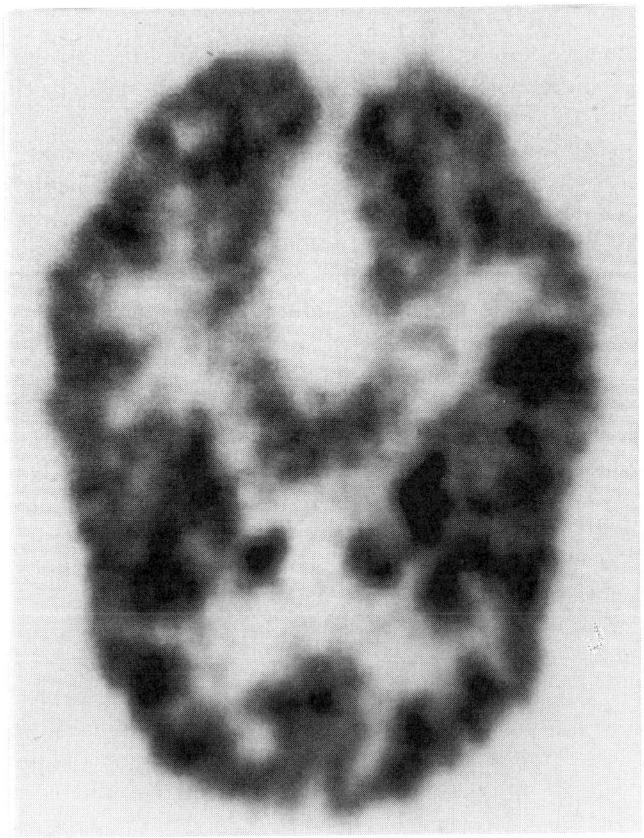

Figure 3.2. PET scan of a normal patient using 2 deoxy-D-glucose.

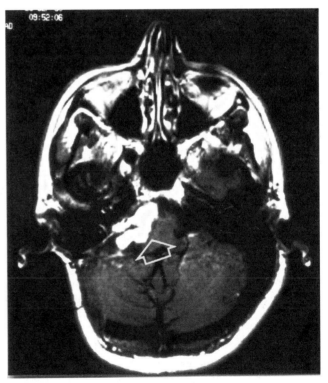

Figure 3.3. MRI tracing of (patient described in Case 2) an irregularly shaped acoustic neuroma approximately 1/2 – 2 1/2 cm.

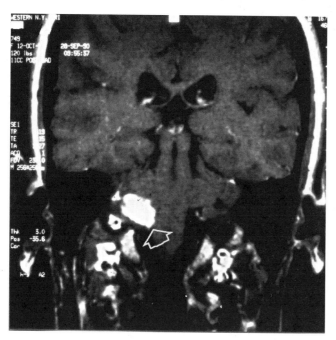

Figure 3.4. MRI (patient described in Case 2) from different angle (frontal).

NEUROLOGIC DISORDERS

Multiple Sclerosis

Multiple sclerosis (MS) can affect any sensory or motor system in the body including hearing. No certain cause for MS is known at this time. There is, however, more and more evidence that the cause is either a virus or a defense mechanism altered by a viral infection. MS can begin from early childhood to middle age. The age of onset is not easily determined because the neurologist usually does not see the patient until after the disease is established. This is due to the intermittent nature of the symptoms.

Clinical features of MS include certain combinations which are indicative of this disease. Typically, nystagmus, intention or action tremor is present. However, these symptoms are not evidenced in the early stages.

Almost all patients with MS at some time or another demonstrate problems with the optic nerve. Ocular difficulties include complaints of blurring of vision and/or diplopia (double vision) without obvious, clinically observable difficulties in ocular movements.

Laboratory findings with MS patients vary from one individual to another and from time to time. There may be increased protein values in the cerebrospinal fluid (CS), normal CS pressure, increased white cell count, and increased gamma globulins. EEG tracings are usually abnormal during the acute stage (typically characterized by abnormal slow waves) and normal during remissions. However, EEG findings are not particularly

of diagnostic value because of the variability from patient to patient.

Evoked response testing in patients with suggested MS is currently *a valuable* diagnostic tool. Results of these tests generally show abnormal peak waveform latencies in PSVER regardless of the results of the ophthalmologic evaluation. ABR results are variable and range from normal responses to increased peak waveform latencies and/or morphologic abnormalities. SEPs typically show delays or are not recordable using certain montages.

The diagnosis of MS is made when symptoms appear, disappear, and then reappear and can be referred simultaneously to several areas. No truly effective treatment for MS has been developed. Adrenocorticotrophic hormone (ACTH) and cortical steroids have been used in some cases during the acute stage with some temporary success. Recent studies on beta interferon suggest that is slows the progression of multiple sclerosis. Although it is not a cure it is the first new treatment since ACTH therapy was initiated 20 years ago.

Tumors

Neoplasms may be found in any body tissue structure. Audiology, however, has been primarily concerned with intracranial tumors. These intracranial structures can be intra-axial or extra-axial. That is, their points of origin are either inside or outside the brainstem. Audiologists probably encounter the acoustic neuroma—an intracranial tumor that affects the reception and interpretation of the acoustic signal—most frequently. This is a benign neoplasm that generally arises from the Schwann cells in the myelin sheath of the vestibular portion of the eighth nerve. This tumor grows into the internal acoustic canal and, with time, affects the auditory portion of the eighth nerve. Once the growth of this tumor has reached the posterior fossa, other cranial nerves and the cerebellum can be involved. Prior to an evagination into the brainstem area, however, detection and diagnosis of this tumor are quite often difficult. The audiometric test battery complement for diagnosis of this problem includes tests for recruitment/decruitment, speech discrimination, acoustic reflexes, and acoustic reflex decay abnormalities. In recent years ABR has been the primary audiological approach to diagnosis of eight nerve tumors.

Neurologic examination of the patient with suspected acoustic neuroma will typically include evaluation of the corneal reflex, diadochokinetic movement, and the peripheral motor system (i.e., heel to shin and finger to nose movements). This problem is also sometimes reflected by dysarthric or slurred speech. Because of the origin of the problem, a caloric test can be used to evaluate vestibular function. More recently, a minimal caloric stimulation technique, electronystagmography (ENG), has been utilized instead of maximum stimulation. With the ENG procedure, a quantifiable record of the patient's responses is obtained during and after caloric stimulation. As a general rule, acoustic neuromas occur unilaterally. With certain conditions, namely von Recklinghausen's disease (neurofibromatosis), acoustic neuromas may be manifested bilaterally. This inherited condition is characterized by multiple tumors of the spinal and cranial nerves, tumors of the skin, and subcutaneous pigmentation.

In addition, many other extra-axial tumors can affect the auditory system. Among these neoplasms are cholesteatomas, meningiomas, astrocytomas, and hemangiomas. Cholesteatoma is one of the more common extra-axial tumors. This neoplasm is generally associated with chronic otitis media or conditions that precipitate systemic infection. Upper respiratory problems and infections may contribute to the growth of this tumor. It is associated with a chronic drainage condition present in the external auditory meatus. The tumor occurs when the natural healing process of the tympanic membrane is abnormal and a sac-like growth develops into the middle ear cavity. If left unchecked, this growth can erode the ossicular chain and the mastoid process, and eventually the structure could extend into the meninges.

Meningiomas arise from the endothelium of the dura mater and are small- to large-sized structures that press on the surrounding areas. These tumors can invade the dura mater and sometimes the bones of the skull. They are said to constitute 10 to 15% of the intracranial tumors that are referred to large neurosurgical clinics (Merritt, 1979). This neoplasm is generally more common in adult females than in males and can be, but is not typically, associated with the internal auditory canal. This tumor is most commonly associated with the olfactory system and the optic nerve.

Astrocytomas of the brainstem or cerebellum occur primarily in patients under 30. This is a glioma that grows very slowly and can invade multiple sections of the cranial nervous system. Typically, it is a unilateral problem that can affect the patient's hearing and the facial nerve and may precipitate a unilateral palatal weakness. The course of this disease is progressive but may at times show improvement and remission. The progressive nature can be associated with multiple cranial nerve involvement and noted patient limb spasticity.

Hemangiomas are vascular abnormalities that assume two basic forms, capillary and cavernous. These lesions typically appear in early childhood and are not generally intracranial, but often involve the bones of the skull or spinal column. The lesions tend to grow progressively larger, causing headaches, jacksonian seizures, and focal neurologic signs after the inner area of the skull is penetrated. Hemangiomas are also found in the skin of the auricle. The hemangioma lesions generally do not reduce in size spontaneously and usually necessitate active treatment. To retard their course, surgical excision or radiation has been shown to be effective.

Vascular Disease

Each cerebral hemisphere has blood supplied by the anterior (internal carotid artery) and the posterior (vertebral-basilar) arteries. A vascular accident is the interruption of this blood supply due to hemorrhage, thrombosis, or embolus involving the cerebral blood vessels. Cerebrovascular disease then involves any of the arteries or veins that supply blood to the brain. With blood vessel obstruction or hemorrhage the cessation of blood circulation and oxygen supply to the brain is affected. If this condition lasts for a period of 25 to 30 seconds, ischemia (response to deficiency of oxygen) develops. If this condition continues for a period of 4 to 5 minutes, irreversible damage occurs and brain metabolism is permanently altered.

The most common vascular accident involves the middle cerebral artery. Vascular accidents involving this blood supply generally cause a hemiparesis on the side of the body opposite the accident. There are three major types of cerebrovascular accidents (CVA): hemorrhage, thrombosis, and embolus. Hemorrhage usually occurs during periods of activity (not necessarily strenuous) or as a result of cranial trauma. Laboratory results usually show blood in the CSF. Thrombosis is the most common form of CVA. This CVA can be preceded by transient ischemic attacks (TIAs) with the actual final CVA seemingly not directly related to the original TIA. The occurrence of the CVA due to thrombosis can be associated with the resting state.

Common causes of infarction (area of necrosis due to lack of oxygen) are atherosclerosis and embolism. It is believed that a buildup of atherosclerotic plaque gives way, causing a "clot" to be propagated within the arterial system. This material finally occludes a distant artery causing an ischemia and subsequent infarction.

This sequence of events could be the cause of some cases of sudden hearing loss, and also of the unilateral loss of vestibular function. Thrombosis of the internal auditory artery may also be aggravated by vascular malformations. Frequently, along with the hearing loss and/or dizziness/unsteadiness, there is an associated dysarthria and/or dysphasia. Specific vascular disorders include Wallenberg's syndrome or posterior inferior cerebellar artery thrombosis. Presenting symptoms include vertigo, ipsilateral facial paresthesia (burning or tingling sensation), numbness, dysphagia, and ipsilateral incoordination. Nystagmus and vertigo are probably due to vestibular nuclei involvement. No hearing loss has been reported for this syndrome.

The anterior internal carotid artery lies rostral to the eighth nerve and supplies the cerebellum and dorsolateral pons. Presenting symptoms of thrombosis of this artery include ipsilateral facial paresthesia, ipsilateral incoordination, ipsilateral loss of facial pain, ipsilateral deafness, and ipsilateral facial paresis. This thrombosis is sometimes noticed postoperatively after acoustic neuroma removal.

CASE STUDIES

Case 1

A 26-year-old male patient gave a history of a hearing loss in the left ear lasting for a period of 1 week in the spring of 1979. At this time, he also noticed he could not run as far as he was accustomed to (3 miles/day). In May of 1980, he reported that he had a numbness in his left hand and the loss of hearing in his right ear. He further indicated that long walks caused fatigue, and any significant physical activity lasting 1 or 2 hours caused fatigue that required 4 to 5 hours' rest. In July of 1981, he had side-by-side diplopia when exerting himself in temperatures over 80°F. In April of 1992, he felt a change in the rhythm and articulation of his speech. Two weeks prior to admission to the hospital, he noted increased imbalance and more problems with his speech.

The general medical examination was completed on admission showing a well-developed, well-nourished male in no acute distress. The neurologic evaluation showed equal right and left end-point gaze nystagmus, no intranuclear ophthalmoplegia, full visual fields, normal vessels, and no hemorrhages or exudates. There was a mild optic nerve atrophy. Gait was wide based; he could not tandem walk; one-leg stands were defective bilaterally. Coordination showed a left-sided dysmetria. Sensation was essentially normal except for a decreased vibratory sense. Muscle grip seemed to be normal. Reflexes for the upper right extremities were more active than the left. There was a positive left Babinski reflex and absent abdominal reflexes on the left side. There was a right Hoffmann reflex and no other pathologic reflex.

The Weber test lateralized to the left with air conduction greater than bone conduction bilaterally. Otoscopic evaluation showed normal tympanic membranes. Audiometric assessment showed normal right ear puretone thresholds at 250 Hz and 500 Hz (≤20 dB) with a precipitous drop to 85–90 dB through the remaining octaves. Left ear puretone thresholds were ≤10 dB except for a 50-dB loss at 4 kHz. Speech discrimination scores were 0% right ear and 96% left ear. Tympanometry showed type A tracings bilaterally. Acoustic reflexes were present bilater-

ally. These reflexes were recorded stimulating the better ear (left) for both measurements; that is, using an ipsilateral and also contralateral stimulus to elicit responses.

ABR tracing was normal in the left ear with normal central auditory pathway tracing times. An abnormal right ABR with waveforms I and III was present with fair definition. Because of poor waveform morphology, waveforms II, IV, V, VI, and VII were not distinguishable. Thus, ABR tracings could not be interpreted from the waveform cephalid to the superior olivary complex and above, indicating brainstem auditory pathway dysfunction (see Fig. 3.5).

Short latency somatosensory evoked potential testing was completed on this patient. It showed normal responses to right median nerve stimulation. For the left median nerve stimulation, there was no consistent waveform, implying dysfunction of the central portions of the left median nerve's sensory projection from the spinal cord to the brainstem, thalamus, and cortex.

The diagnosis of multiple sclerosis was made on the basis of the clinical neurologic examination and laboratory data. Multiple sclerosis usually involves multiple CNS lesions. The patient's hospital course was benign. He was given a course of ACTH medication intramuscularly. While on ACTH, he improved slightly and stated that he felt himself to be more stable in walking. The patient was discharged with a cane for walking and no medication.

Case 2

A 67-year-old male patient had been seen in the ear-nose-throat clinic for treatment of chronic nasal polyps and sinusitis since 1976. Audiometric assessment during the treatment period showed a mild to moderate bilat-

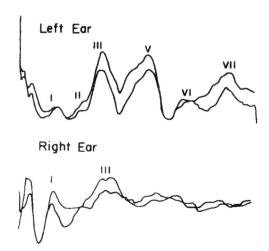

Figure 3.5. ABRs for patient with multiple sclerosis. Identifiable wavers are labeled. Trace for left ear (unaffected side) is normal both in latencies and morphology. Right ear (affected side) shows normal wave I, delayed wave III, and no other clearly identifiable waveforms.

eral high frequency sensory-neural hearing loss. Speech reception thresholds were within the expected normal (≤15 dB HL) range bilaterally. Speech discrimination scores (at 40 dB SL) were normal.

Tympanometry showed type A bilaterally with maximum compliance at 0 mm H_2O with absent acoustic reflexes. This patient then presented to the ear-nose-throat clinic in December 1979 complaining of decreased hearing in his right ear. Audiometric assessment showed a moderate to severe sensory-neural loss in the right ear with essentially no change in threshold data for the left ear. Speech reception thresholds and discrimination ability were unchanged for this patient's left ear. Right ear puretone thresholds showed a rather marked dip at 2 kHz (60 dB) and recovery at 4 kHz (20 dB). Speech reception thresholds and discrimination scores were not obtainable when testing the right ear. Positive tone decay was shown in the right ear at 2 kHz (30 dB in 30 seconds) and 4 kHz (25 dB in 30 seconds). Ten-percent short-increment sensitivity index scores were obtained at 2 kHz and 4 kHz. Bekesy tracings for the right ear were type III.

Electronystagmography showed a reduced right vestibular response. Optokinetic stimulation yielded asymmetrical tracings. The patient reported diplopia during right gaze testing.

The general medical examination at the time of admission was unremarkable. At the time of the examination, the patient was alert and well oriented.

Neurologic examination showed a right sixth nerve weakness present with diplopia on looking to the right. The right corneal reflex was diminished with hypalgesia of the right side of the face. No facial weakness was noted, and the other cranial nerve responses were normal. The motor reflexes were symmetrical. A truncal ataxia was present with the patient deviating to the right on walking. There was no dysmetria (abnormal voluntary muscle control). This patient demonstrated gait ataxia, especially on turning.

CT sections with and without contrast enhancement showed a well-defined and rounded tumor of right cerebellopontine angle, measuring 33 mm in diameter. Its anterior aspect was adjacent to the basilar artery. The internal auditory canals were symmetrical and normal in size and shape. The CT scan showed the fourth ventricle to be of normal size and slightly displaced toward the left. The lateral and third ventricle showed moderately diffuse dilation, apparently obstructive hydrocephalus secondary to the presence of the tumor (see Fig. 3.6).

After surgical removal of the neoplasm, audiometric follow-up testing showed a severe sensory-neural hearing loss in the right ear with no functional speech reception or discrimination and unchanged left ear audiometric results.

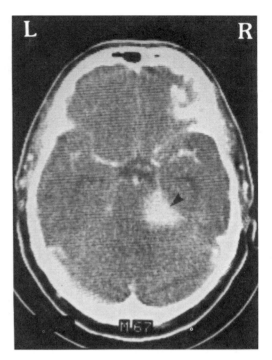

Figure 3.6. CT scan of brain of patient with right cerebellopontine angle tumor. Right lateral ventricle is not visible.

Case 3

A 65-year-old male reported a several month history of progressive hearing loss and difficulty with balance while walking. This patient further complained of a loud ringing tinnitus in his right ear.

Audiometric assessment showed a severe relatively flat sensoryneural hearing loss in his right ear with poor speech discrimination. He said that speech stimulis were loud enough but hard to understand. Ipsilateral acoustic reflexes were absent. A positive SupraThreshold Adaptation Test (STAT) result suggested a retrocochlear problem.

The ABR procedure showed increased latencies for waves I and II in the right ear and absent waves III, IV, and V. Left ear ABR testing yielded essentially normal results (see Table 3.2).

Table 3.2
Brainstem Auditory Response Latencies for Case 3

Left ear	Latencies (in msec)	Right ear	Latencies (in msec)
I	1.76	I	2.12
II	3.26	II	3.68
III	4.12	III	Absent
IV	4.96	IV	Absent
V	5.60	V	Absent
I-III	2.36	I-III	NA
III-V	1.48	III-V	NA
I-V	3.84	I-V	NA

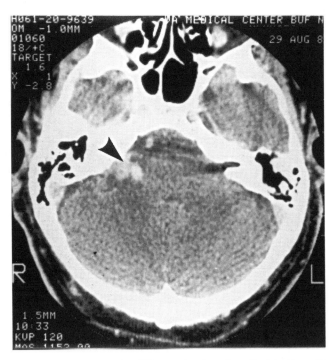

Figure 3.7. Preoperative CT scan (patient described in Case 3) showing a 3 cm space-occupying lesion.

CT findings showed a fairly large acoustic neuroma measuring approximately 3 cm and extending into the intercranial cavity. Figure 3.7 shows this patient's preoperative radiograph.

Acknowledgments

Selected photographic material was provided by: L. Jacobs, M.D., Head, Department of Neurology, Buffalo General Hospital, Buffalo, New York; and J.M. Gona, M.D., Chief, Nuclear Medicine, V.A. Medical Center, Buffalo, New York

REFERENCES

Brugge JF. Neurophysiology of the central auditory and vestibular systems. In Paparella MM and Shumrick DA, Eds. Otolaryngology, Vol. l. Philadelphia: WB Saunders, 1980:253–296.

Chiappa RH, Gladstone KJ, and Young ER. Brainstem auditory evoked responses in 50 normal human subjects. Arch Neurol 1979;36:81–87.

Coleman E. Positron tomography, a case for reimbursements. Applied Radiology 1989;Sept:39–48.

D'Agincourt L. Diagnostic imaging, PETS diagnostic process widens its clinical appeal, Diagnostic Imaging 1989;Oct:90–99.

Fria TJ. The audiotory brainstem response: background and clinical applications. In Monographs in Contemporary Audiology, Vol. 2. Minneapolis: Educational Publications Division, Maico Hearing Instruments, 1980.

Hoffman EJ., Phelps ME. Positron Emission Tomography: Principles and Quantitation in Phelps ME. Mazziotta JC. and Schelbert HR. Positron Emission Tomography and Autoradiography. New York: Raven Press, 1986:237–286.

Jewett DL. Volume conducted potentials in response to auditory stimuli as detected by averaging in the cat. Electroencephalogr Clin Neurophysiol 1970;28:609–619.

Luria AR. The Working Brain. London: Allen Lane, Penguin Press, 1973.

Mazziotta JC. and Phelps ME. Positron Emission Tomography Studies of the Brain in Phelps ME., Mazziotta JC. and Schelbert HR. Positron Emission Tomography and Autoradiography. New York: Raven Press, 1986:493–580.

Merritt HH. A Textbook of Neurology, 6th ed. Philadelphia: Lea & Febiger, 1979.

Most M and Low MP. The EEG Handbook. Anaheim, CA: Beckman Instruments, 1973.

Mountcastle VB. Central nervous mechanisms in hearing. In Mountcastle VB, Ed. Medical Physiology, 14th ed. Vol. l. St. Louis: CV Mosby, 1980:457–480.

Niedermeyer E. and Lopes da Silva F. Electroencephalography Basic Principles, Clinical Applications and Related Fields Baltimore-Munich: Urban and Schwarzenberg 1982.

Penfield W and Rasmussen G. The Cerebral Cortex of Man. New York: Macmillan, 1950.

Poggio GF and Mountcastle VB. Functional organization of the thalamus and cortex. In Mountcastle VB, Ed. Medical Physiology, 14th ed. Vol. l. St. Louis: CV Mosby, 1980:271–298.

Raichle ME. Positron emission tomography. Annals Rev Neuroscience 1983:249–267.

American National Standards Institute. American National Standard Specifications for Audiometers. New York: ANSI, S3.6-1969.

Rasmussen GL. An efferent cochlear bundle. Anat Rec 1942;82:441.

Rasmussen GL. The olivary peduncle and other fiber projections of the superior olivary complex. J Comp Neurol 1946;84:141.

Reivich M and Ataul A, Eds. Positron Emission Tomography. New York: Alan R Liss, 1985.

Report of the Committee on Methods of Clinical Examination in Electroencephalography. The ten twenty electrode system. Electroencephalogr Clin Neurophysiol 1957;10:371–375.

Taylor S. The petrous temporal bone (including the cerebellopontine angle). Radiol Clin North Am 1982;20:67–86.

Tonturi AR. Anatomy and physiology of the auditory cortex. In Rasmussen GL, Ed. Neural Mechanisms of the Auditory Vestibular System. Springfield, IL: Charles C Thomas, 1968:181–200.

Warr WB. Parallel ascending pathways from the cochlear nucleus.

Whitfield IC. 1982. Coding in the auditory cortex. In Neff WD, Ed. Contributions to Sensory Physology, Vol. 6. New York: Academic Press, 1982:159˜2D178.

Wolf AP and Fowler JS. Positron Emitter—Labeled Radiotranees—Chemical Conditions in Positron Emission Tomography. New York: Alan R Liss, 1985:63, 80.

CHAPTER 4

Neurophysiologic Correlates of Sensory-Neural Hearing Loss

Donald Henderson, Richard J. Salvi, Flint A. Boettcher, and Ann E. Clock

Sensory-neural hearing loss (SNHL) is characterized by elevated puretone thresholds and reduced speech recognition, particularly in noisy environments. In addition, many patients with SNHL also suffer from other symptoms such as tinnitus, abnormal loudness recruitment, and impaired temporal processing of sound. Although the clinical symptoms of sensory-neural hearing loss have been well documented, there is as yet no cure for the problem. Patients with SNHL are typically fitted with a hearing aid that compensates for the loss in sensitivity. However, a hearing aid does not compensate for other distortions in hearing, and, therefore, patients continue to have difficulty understanding acoustic information, especially speech sounds in noisy or reverberant environments. The less-than-optimal performance achieved with hearing aids is, in part, a reflection of distortions in auditory processing (e.g., recruitment or rapid growth of loudness, poor temporal resolution, poor frequency resolution). These may arise from cochlear damage that alters the neural code to the auditory nerve which is then relayed to the central nervous system. In order to understand the basic hearing impairment and the limitations of conventional amplification, it is critical to understand some of the neurophysiological correlates of SNHL.

It is well known that the cochlea can be damaged by intense noise, ototoxic drugs, aging, viral infections, and other agents. The resulting injury to or loss of inner hair cells (IHCs), outer hair cells (OHCs), supporting cells, and the vascular supply to the cochlea can significantly alter the neural code flowing out of the cochlea into the central nervous system. In addition, the pattern of neural activity within the central auditory pathway itself may be altered as a result of peripheral damage. The goal of this chapter is to describe some of the fundamental changes that occur in the pattern of neural activity within the auditory pathway as a result of SNHL. However, to provide a perspective on the physiology changes the normal pattern of neural activity within the auditory nerve is reviewed.

RESPONSES OF NORMAL AUDITORY NERVE FIBERS

Sound enters the cochlea at the oval window as a result of movement of the stapes footplate. The cochlea is tonotopically organized: high-frequency signals produce maximum movement of the basilar membrane near the basal end whereas low-frequency sounds produce maximum movement near the apex. Movement of the basilar membrane results in bending of the hair cell stereocilia which in turn leads to the depolarization (alteration of the electrical potential) of the hair cells (Davis, 1958). Depolarization of the hair cells leads to the release of neurotransmitters from the hair cell. This results in all-or-none spike discharges that can be recorded from auditory nerve fibers. Hudspeth (1985) provides an excellent summary of physiology and the process of transducing sound into a meaningful neural code. This chapter is focused on the next step in the process of hearing, namely the response of auditory nerve fibers and central auditory neurons in normal and impaired ears.

The afferent portion of the auditory nerve consists of 30,000 to 50,000 auditory nerve fibers that lead from the cochlea to the central auditory system. There are roughly three times as many OHCs as IHCs, but only a small proportion of auditory nerve fibers (5–10%) synapse on OHCs. Each of these VIII nerve fibers contacts approximately 20 OHCs, as illustrated in Figure 4.1 (Spoendlin, 1972). Unfortunately, almost nothing is known about the functional characteristics of the fibers that contact OHCs. The situation is much different at the IHC. Most auditory nerve fibers (90–95%) contact only a single IHC; thus, the response of each fiber reflects the output from a relatively discrete region of the organ of Corti. Furthermore, all auditory nerve fibers that respond to acoustic stimulation have been found to contact IHCs (Robertson, 1984) Therefore, virtually all of the sensory information flowing out of the auditory nerve into the central auditory system comes from IHCs.

If all of the afferent information comes from the IHCs, then what is the role of the OHC? Although there are many more OHCs than IHCs, it appears that the OHCs transmit relatively little sensory information to the central nervous system through afferent fibers (Robertson, 1984). Recent studies have shown that OHCs are motile and can elongate or shorten in a slow, sustained manner or oscillate rapidly at frequencies as high as 8

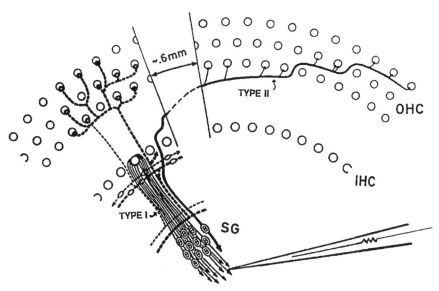

Figure 4.1. Schematic diagram of the cat's auditory nerve and organ of Corti. Recording electrode contacts a single auditory nerve fiber as the nerve exits the internal auditory meatus before it enters the cochlear nucleus. Adapted from Spoendlin H. Stuctural basis of peripheral frequency analysis. In Plomp R, and Smoorenburg GF, Eds. Frequency Analysis and Periodicity Detection in Hearing. Leiden: A.W. Sijthoff, 1970.

kHz (Brownell, 1990; Ashmore, 1987). Thus, the OHCs are now believed to act primarily like a motor system rather than to provide sensory input to the central auditory pathway. OHC motility is believed to contribute significantly to the exquisite sensitivity of the ear and the sharp mechanical tuning of the basilar membrane.

Neurophysiologists have correlated auditory sensation and perception with the output of the cochlea and auditory nerve. Two approaches have been used to understand the neurophysiological basis of sensation: gross evoked potentials and single neuron recordings. Neurologists and audiologists have measured the gross evoked potentials from the cochlea (electrocochleography) and brainstem (auditory brainstem response [ABR]). Both of these measures are clinically useful but are difficult to interpret because they are based on the summed activity of many auditory neurons. To better understand the effects of cochlear loss on neural processing, it is important to examine the activity of single auditory neurons.

Spontaneous Activity

When a microelectrode is inserted into the auditory nerve, one can record the all-or-none spike discharges (action potentials) from a single auditory nerve fiber. Most auditory nerve fibers produce spontaneous action potentials (Fig. 4.2 inset) at irregular time intervals in the absence of controlled acoustic stimulation. As shown in Fig. 4.2, the spontaneous discharge rates (SR) of the majority of units (physiological recordings from single neurons are typically referred to as "single units") vary

from 0 to 120 spikes per second. The SR distribution is typically bimodal with one peak near 70 sp/s and a second, larger peak below 10 sp/s. Relatively few fibers have SRs between 20 and 30 sp/s (Liberman, 1978; Salvi et al., 1983a). Tinnitus, or the perception of sound without acoustic stimulation, is a symptom frequently associated with SNHL. Since spontaneous activity occurs in the absence of acoustic stimulation, it has been suggested that hearing-impaired listeners may have regions of the cochlea that produce aberrant patterns of spontaneous activity that could give rise to the perception of tinnitus. To pursue this possibility, the distribution of spontaneous activity in the VIII nerve of chinchillas exposed to high levels of noise will be examined in a later section.

Sensitivity and Frequency Selectivity

When tone bursts of the appropriate frequency and intensity are presented to the ear, the discharge rate of an auditory nerve fiber increases above its spontaneous rate (Fig. 4.3 top). The sound level at which the firing rate in response to the tone burst exceeds the spontaneous rate (SR) is referred to as the threshold of the unit. If threshold for a fiber is measured over a wide range of frequencies, a tuning curve or frequency-threshold curve can be obtained. The tuning curves shown in Fig. 4.3 were obtained from six different neurons from a chinchilla. (The general shape of the tuning curve is very similar across all mammalian species, therefore it is reasonable to expect neurons of the VIII nerve of humans to respond essentially the same way.) Each tuning curve may

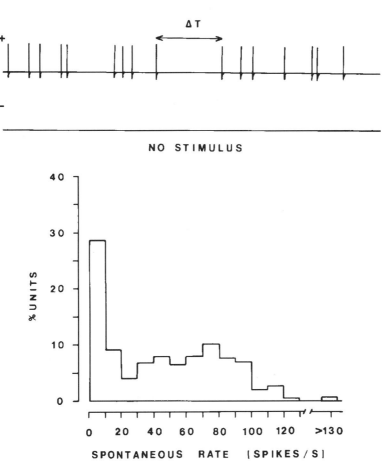

Figure 4.2. Top: Spike train for one auditory nerve fiber in the absence of controlled acoustic stimulation. Spontaneous rate (SR) is defined as the number of spikes per second when the ear is not stimulated. Bottom: Distribution of spontaneous rates from a sample (N = 144) of chinchilla single auditory nerve fibers. Reprinted with permission from Salvi RJ, Henderson D, and Hamernik RP. Physiological bases of sensorineural hearing loss. In Tobias JB, and Schubert ED, Eds. Hearing Research and Theory, Vol. 2. New York: Academic Press, 1983.

be thought of as an "audiogram" for a single unit. Note that each fiber is extremely sensitive to a narrow range of frequencies at the tip of each curve. The characteristic frequency (CF) refers to the frequency at which the threshold is lowest. The tuning curves shown in Fig. 4.3 have CFs that range from approximately 400 Hz to 15,000 Hz. If tuning curves are measured from a representative sample of units in the auditory nerve, their CFs would cover the entire frequency range of hearing. The thresholds of the most sensitive units would correspond to the subject's behavioral audiogram. In subjects with SNHL it is interesting to see if the distribution of single unit CFs approximate the audiogram, for example are there elevated or absent thresholds in the region of the hearing loss.

When tuning curves are plotted on a logarithmic frequency scale, a fiber with a high CF has a tuning curve with a low-threshold, a sharply-tuned tip near CF, a steep high frequency tail, and a high-threshold, broadly-tuned, low-frequency tail. By contrast, the tuning curves of fibers with low CFs are more symmetrical and broadly tuned than those from high CF units (Kiang, 1965). Thus, a normal unit acts like a narrowly-tuned bandpass filter that passes only those signals near CF and rejects extraneous noise outside the skirts of the filter. It has been suggested that a listener's ability to discriminate a signal from a noisy background is a reflection of the tuned response of the basilar membrane and the auditory nerve fibers. An increase in the bandwidth of these tuned filters could compromise a listener's ability to detect a signal embedded in noise because the filter would pass more noise and decrease the signal-to-noise ratio.

In a single animal, at a given frequency, there is generally a wide range of thresholds across a sample of units. Typically, units with the lowest SR have the highest

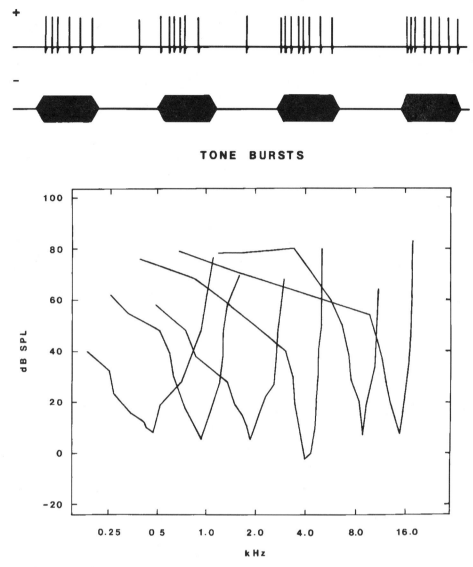

Figure 4.3. Top panel: Spike train for one auditory nerve fiber recorded during the presentation of a series of tone bursts. Threshold at a given frequency is defined as the level at which neural firing increases just above spontaneous rate. Bottom: Individual neuron frequency tuning curves (FTC), for six chinchilla auditory nerve fibers with different characteristic frequencies. Reprinted with permission from Salvi RJ, Henderson D, Hamernik RP, and Ahroon WA 1983. Neural correlates of sensorineural hearing loss. Ear and Hearing 1983;4:115–129.

(poorest) thresholds whereas those with the highest SR have the lowest (best) threshold (Liberman, 1978; Salvi et al., 1982). Because the thresholds of the most sensitive units closely match the behavioral audiogram (Salvi et al., 1982), it would be important to know if the thresholds at CF also correspond to the behavioral audiogram in animals with SNHL.

Temporal Response Patterns

The precise time at which the spike discharges occur during a particular presentation may vary from one stimulus presentation to the next (Fig. 4.3, top); however, if the same tone burst is presented many times, a post-stimulus time (PST) histogram can be calculated. The PST shows the total number of spikes that occurred at various times during the tone burst presentations. Fig. 4.4 (left) shows a series of PST histograms obtained with 50 tone bursts at the CF of a nerve fiber using sound levels between 18 dB sound pressure level (SPL) (near threshold) and 58 dB SPL. The histograms shown in Fig. 4.4 consist of a series of 1 ms time bins; each bin shows the total number of spikes that occurred during a particular 1 ms interval of the 200 ms tone burst. Virtually all of the units in the auditory nerve have PST histograms with the same general shape as shown in Fig. 4.4. The PST histograms show a

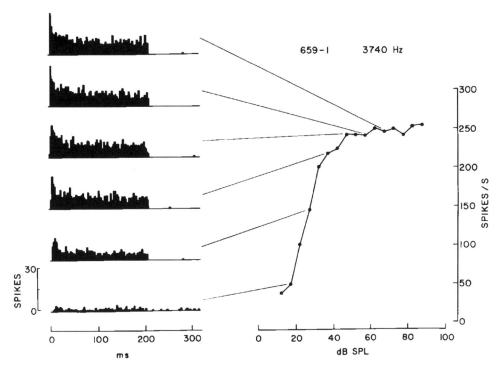

Figure 4.4. Series of post stimulus time histograms (PST) for a chinchilla auditory nerve fiber. Each histogram was collected at a different SPL using a 200 ms tone burst. Right panel: The change in firing rate with increased stimulus level, or rate-level function, was derived from the PST histograms in the left panel and presented as the number of spikes per second. Reprinted with permission from Salvi RJ, Henderson D, and and Hamernik RP. Physiological bases of sensorineural hearing loss. In Tobias JB, and Schubert ED, Eds. Hearing Research and Theory, Vol. 2. New York: Academic Press, 1983.

sharp peak near stimulus onset (high probability of a spike discharge occurring) followed by a gradual decay to a plateau approximately 15–50 ms after stimulus onset.

The discharge patterns observed in response to long duration stimuli may be relevant to the important psychophysical process of temporal integration. The behavioral threshold of a tone partially depends on the duration of the stimulus. The auditory system appears to be able to integrate the acoustic energy in a stimulus so that a short-duration stimulus results in a poorer threshold than a long-duration stimulus. Typically, a 10–15 dB improvement in quiet threshold occurs as stimulus duration increases from 10 ms to 500 ms (Plomp and Bouman, 1959; Zwislocki, 1960). A number of studies have reported that listeners with SNHL have a reduced capacity to temporally integrate acoustic information. Therefore, one might expect to see a change in the neural correlates of temporal integration in cochlear hearing loss (Jerger, 1955; Wright, 1968; Henderson, 1969; Solecki and Gerken, 1990).

Intensity Coding

When the stimulus level exceeds the neuron's threshold, the discharge rate of the typical unit rapidly increases over a 30–50 dB range and then plateaus or saturates (Sachs and Abbas, 1974). For the particular unit shown in Fig. 4.4 (right), the discharge rate increased from approximately 30 sp/s at 15 dB SPL to approximately 250 sp/s at 50 dB SPL; further increases in sound level failed to produce an increase in firing rate. The neural data pose a dilemma since the dynamic range of a single fiber is much smaller than the ear's dynamic range for coding loudness which is over 100 dB (Hellman and Zwislocki, 1961). Clearly, a single auditory nerve fiber is unable to encode the entire range of loudness that the organism can distinguish. Recall that nerve fibers with high spontaneous rates of activity have low thresholds and vice-versa. Presumably, loudness is encoded by a complicated set of neural responses. For a given frequency, as a stimulus is increased above the "behavioral" threshold, a population of nerve fibers with low thresholds (high SR) increase their firing rate. As the stimulus intensity is further increased, neurons with a CF equal to the stimulus but with moderate-to-high thresholds (low SR) begin to fire as well as neurons with adjacent CFs (Viemeister, 1983). Because cochlear losses generally result in abnormally rapid loudness growth, one might expect to find both (*a*) systematic changes in the way single auditory nerve fibers encode changes in stimulus level, and (*b*) the rate at which adjacent neurons are recruited into activity.

Latency of Neural Response

In clinical audiology, the most common electrophysiological measure of peripheral activity is Wave I of the auditory brainstem response (ABR) and the whole-nerve action potential (AP) in electrocochleography (ECochG). The latency of the AP or Wave I is closely related to neural firing of auditory nerve fibers. As illustrated in Fig. 4.5 (top), the latency of the AP is measured from the time of stimulus onset to the first peak of the waveform. The bottom of Fig. 4.5 shows that the AP latency decreases as stimulus intensity increases. To appreciate how these evoked potentials are generated, it is useful to examine the discharge patterns of auditory nerve fibers to the same type of click stimuli that are used to elicit the AP or Wave I. Fig. 4.6 (inset) shows the PST histogram obtained from an auditory nerve fiber (CF of 1 kHz) using click stimuli. The latency (L) of the first peak in the PST histogram is related to the unit's CF. As shown in Fig. 4.6, units with low CFs have longer latencies than units with high CF. This orderly increase in latency presumably reflects the longer time it takes for the mechanical disturbance to propagate to the lower frequency regions along the cochlear partition (von Bekesy, 1960; Robles et al., 1976). The high frequency components of the click are analyzed in the basal region of the cochlea which has a short response time, whereas the low frequencies are analyzed in the apex of the cochlea which has a long response time.

Neural Adaptation

After an auditory nerve fiber is stimulated by an acoustic stimulus, its response to subsequent stimuli will initially be depressed and then gradually recover toward its unadapted state. The time course of recovery from adaptation can be evaluated with a forward masking stimulus paradigm (Fig. 4.7 inset). A masking tone is used to adapt the unit and then a probe tone is used to assess the degree to which the unit's firing rate is depressed at various time intervals (ΔT) between masker offset and probe onset. Figure 4.7 (bottom right) shows a series of PST histograms from a normal auditory nerve fiber collected with a forward masking paradigm. When the masker-probe interval was very short, the response to the probe was low, but as the masker-probe interval increased the probe response increased. The degree of neural adaptation can be expressed as the ratio of the probe response in the masked condition compared to the unmasked condition (Fig. 4.7 left). Thus, a probe response magnitude of 100% would reflect no masking and 0% would reflect complete masking. As the masker-probe interval increases the probe response increases and reaches a maximum of approximately 100% at a ΔT of 150 ms.

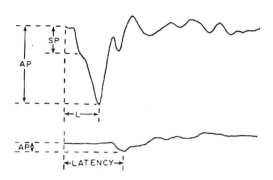

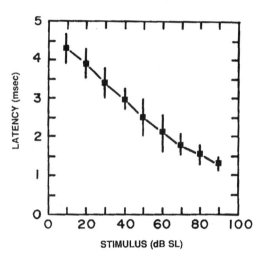

Figure 4.5. Top panel: Recordings of human AP responses with high level (top) and low level (bottom) stimulation. The measurement of peak latency spans from onset of the stimulus to the point of maximum voltage (L). Bottom panel: AP latency measured as a function of stimulus level. Reprinted with permission from Glattke TJ. Short-latency auditory evoked potentials: fundamental bases & clinical applications. Austin: Pro-ed, Inc., 1983.

The recovery of a neuron's firing rate following the presentation of a masker (adaptor tone) may be closely linked to the process of forward masking in psychophysics. In forward masking, the listener is required to detect a short duration probe tone that follows a high-level masking stimulus. At short masker-probe intervals, the threshold is greatly elevated relative to the probe's threshold in quiet. As the temporal separation of the masker and probe increases, the threshold of the probe approaches the threshold in quiet at approximately 100–200 ms (Elliott, 1962; Plomp, 1964). Interestingly, the time course of forward masking is known to be prolonged in listeners with SNHL (Cudahy, 1982; Nelson and Freyman, 1987) and this could contribute to abnormal processing of complex signals such as speech (e.g., the recognition of consonants following a high intensity vowel). Given that forward masking is prolonged in hearing impaired listeners, one might expect to see

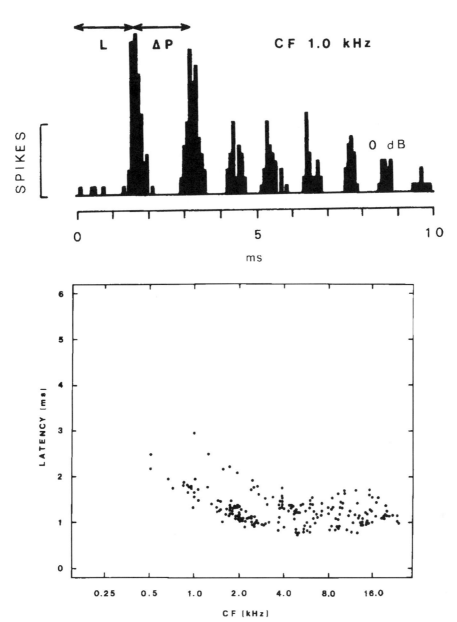

Figure 4.6. Comparison of individual auditory nerve latencies as a function of characteristic frequency (CF). Top: PST histogram for one auditory nerve fiber with a CF of 1 kHz collected using a series of click stimuli. Latency (L) equals the time from stimulus onset to first peak in PST histogram. ΔP equals the time interval between peaks (ΔP = 1/CF). Reprinted with permission from Salvi RJ, Henderson D, and Hamernik RP. Physiological bases of sensorineural hearing loss. In Tobias JB, and Schubert ED, Eds. Hearing Research and Theory, Vol. 2. New York: Academic Press, 1983.

changes in the rate at which auditory nerve fibers recover from adaptation.

EFFECTS OF SENSORY-NEURAL HEARING LOSS ON NEURAL CODING

The preceding section focused on the discharge patterns of auditory nerve fibers in normal animals and alluded to how these discharge patterns might be related to various aspects of hearing such as threshold, frequency selectivity, loudness, and temporal processing.

The following section will describe how the discharge patterns of auditory nerve fibers change in animals suffering from SNHL induced by acoustic overstimulation or ototoxic drugs. One of the main goals is to correlate the changes in neural activity with many of the common symptoms associated with SNHL, e.g., tinnitus, poor speech discrimination in noise, the breakdown in temporal integration, and loudness recruitment. In addition, the physiological results will be related to the underlying cochlear histopathologies.

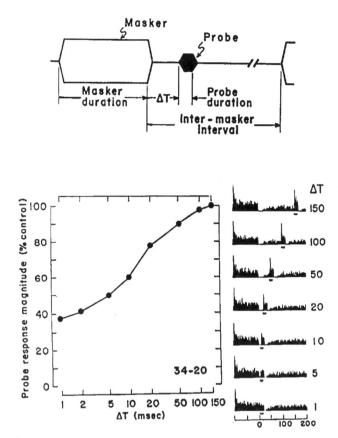

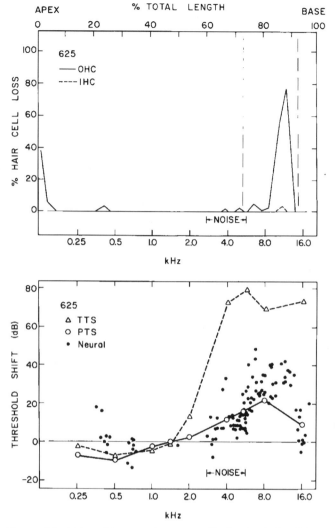

Figure 4.7. Top: Forward masking stimulus paradigm. ΔT equals the time between masker offset and probe onset. Bottom: PST histogram series and recovery function for an auditory nerve fiber collected with a forward masking paradigm. Reprinted with permission from Harris D, and Dallos P. Properties of auditory nerve responses in the absence of outer hair cells. J. Neurophysiol. 1978;41:365–383.

Threshold Shift

In normal animals, the thresholds of the most sensitive units parallel the behavioral audiogram. Thus, in animals with SNHL, one would expect the amount of hearing loss measured behaviorally to correlate with the neural threshold shifts. However, this relationship can be quite variable. Figs. 4.8 and 4.9 illustrate this point using data from two chinchillas exposed for 5 days to an octave band noise centered at 4 kHz at 86 dB SPL. The data in Fig. 4.8 (bottom) shows a close correlation between the permanent threshold shift (PTS) and the average neural threshold shifts. The neural and behavioral thresholds shifts are both elevated by as much as 20 dB between 6 and 15 kHz, but return to normal values at higher and lower frequencies. The upper panel is a cytocochleogram which shows hair cell loss plotted as a function of position and place of frequency analysis within the cochlea. Histological analysis of the cochlea from this animal revealed a relatively discrete loss of OHCs at approximately 80–90% of the distance from the apex of

Figure 4.8. Cytocochleogram (upper panel), showing hair cell loss as a function of distance along the cochlea, and behavioral (temporary threshold shift or permanent threshold shift) and neural thresholds (lower panel) for one chinchilla exposed for 5 days to an octave band of noise centered at 4.0 kHz (86 dB SPL). The cochleogram shows a discrete loss of OHCs in the 9-12 kHz region of the cochlea. The behavioral audiogram (PTS) shows a 20 dB shift in sensitivity which is paralleled by the neural sensitivity shift of 20 dB or greater. Reprinted with permission from Salvi RJ, Henderson D, Hamernik RP, and Ahroon WA. Neural correlates of sensorineural hearing loss. Ear and Hearing 1983;4:115–129.

the cochlea. This position in the chinchilla cochlea corresponds to a frequency of 8–14 kHz (Eldredge et al., 1981). In this case, the behavioral and neural threshold shifts are in good agreement. The data are also interesting from a clinical perspective in that the maximum hearing loss and hair cell damage occur more than a half-octave above the exposure frequency in agreement with previous reports (Davis et al., 1950); this suggests that the half-octave shift phenomenon has its origins in the cochlea.

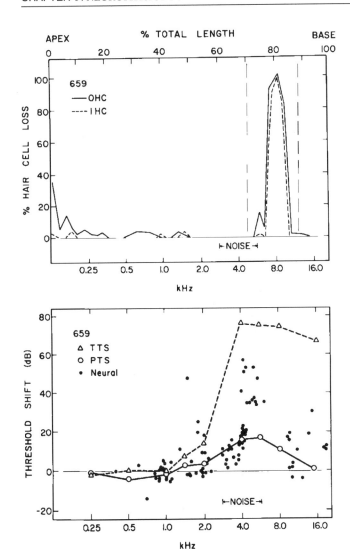

Figure 4.9. Cytocochleogram (upper panel) and behavioral and neural thresholds (lower panel) for one chinchilla exposed for 5 days to an octave band of noise centered at 4.0 kHz (86 dB SPL). The cochleogram shows a discrete loss of both IHC and OHC. The behavioral audiogram (PTS) is the same as Fig. 8, but there is a complete absence of neurons in the 7 to 12 kHz region. Reprinted with permission from Salvi RJ, Henderson D, and Hamernik RP. Physiological bases of sensorineural hearing loss. In Tobias JB, and Schubert ED, Eds. Hearing Research and Theory, Vol. 2. New York: Academic Press, 1983.

The physiological and histological data obtained from another chinchilla (Fig. 4.9) exposed to the same noise are distinctly different even though the behavioral thresholds for both animals are nearly identical (compare Fig. 4.8 and 4.9). The behavioral PTS for the animals shown in Fig. 4.9 (bottom) was roughly 15 to 20 dB between 4 and 8 kHz. However, in this subject, no units were found with CFs between 5.7 and 11.2 kHz. Histological analysis of the cochlea of this animal revealed an almost complete absence of IHCs and OHCs in the fre-

quency range where no recordings were obtained. An obvious question is "How did the animal detect 8 kHz tones without hair cells or nerve fibers tuned to this frequency?" The answer is not as obscure as it may seem at first if one recalls that a unit can respond to low-frequency tones presented in the "tail" of the tuning curve.

Tuning and Frequency Selectivity

Most listeners with SNHL have great difficulty in discriminating speech sounds particularly in a background of noise. This deterioration in speech perception has been linked to a more fundamental measure of hearing, namely the breakdown in frequency selectivity, i.e., the ability to extract one signal in the presence of other extraneous sounds (Tyler et al., 1982; Wightman, 1981). One of the most direct psychophysical measures of frequency selectivity is the psychophysical tuning curve (PTC). The PTC is obtained by having the listener detect a low-level probe tone of fixed frequency. A masking tone is introduced and increased in level until it just abolishes the detection of the probe (masked threshold). Masked thresholds are then obtained over a range of frequencies in order to map out the PTC. The shapes of the PTC are remarkably similar to the neural tuning curves shown in Fig. 4.3. The masked thresholds of the PTC are lowest near the probe frequency and increase rapidly as the frequency separation between masker and probe increases.

PTCs and neural tuning curves have been measured in animals with noise-induced PTS (Salvi et al., 1982). Figure 4.10 shows data from a chinchilla which developed approximately 20 to 30 dB of PTS between 1 and 4 kHz after being exposed for 5 days to a 95 dB SPL, octave band of noise centered at 0.5 kHz. The neural threshold shifts in this animal paralleled the behavioral threshold shifts. Each panel of Fig. 4.10 shows a PTC (dashed lines) plus a representative neural tuning curve (solid lines) from four different frequency regions. The PTCs and neural tuning curves in regions of normal hearing, 8 and 16 kHz, have low-threshold, narrowly-tuned tips and high-threshold, broadly-tuned tails. By contrast, the PTCs and neural tuning curves located within the region of greatest hearing loss, have high thresholds and are very broadly tuned. PTCs and neural tuning curves on the high-frequency edge of the hearing loss, 4 kHz, show an intermediate loss of sensitivity and tuning.

The changes in tuning curve shape have been correlated with different cochlear pathologies (Liberman et al., 1986). The trends that have emerged from numerous studies are illustrated in Fig. 4.11 using the surface diagrams of the organ of Corti (Fig. 4.11 left) and the auditory nerve fiber tuning curves (Fig. 4.11 right) from

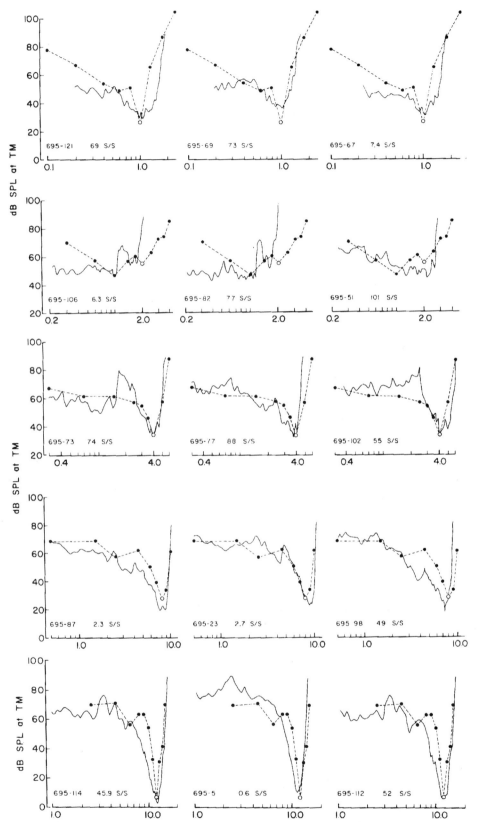

Figure 4.10. Psychophysical tuning curves (dashed lines) measured in a chinchilla for four different frequency regions. The solid lines represent neural tuning curves corresponding to the same frequency regions. Reprinted with permission from Hamernik RP, Henderson D, and Salvi RJ, Eds. New perspectives on noise-induced hearing loss, New York: Raven Press, 1982.

normal (solid lines) and noise-exposed (dotted lines) animals. The data in the upper half of Fig. 4.11 illustrates what happens to the neural tuning curves when damage is confined primarily to the IHCs. In this case, the OHCs are intact and have normal looking stereocilia. By contrast, the IHCs, although present, have missing or damaged stereocilia. Auditory nerve fibers that innervate regions of the cochlea with this type of pathology have elevated thresholds in both the tip and tail regions of the tuning curve but have relatively sharply tuned tips.

The bottom half of Fig. 4.11 illustrates what happens to the neural tuning curves when damage is confined

primarily to the OHCs. In this particular case, all of the OHCs have been destroyed and replaced by "X-shaped" scars formed by the phalangeal processes of Deiters' cells. All of the IHCs are present and their stereocilia appear normal. Auditory nerve fibers which innervate regions of the cochlea with this type of pathology have tuning curves (dotted lines) which show considerable loss of sensitivity near the tip region and a slight improvement in sensitivity in the tail of the tuning curves. The net result of these changes is a unit with a broadly-tuned "U-shaped" tuning curve with no obvious tip. Results such as these suggest that the OHCs primarily improve the sensitivity near the tip of the tuning curve.

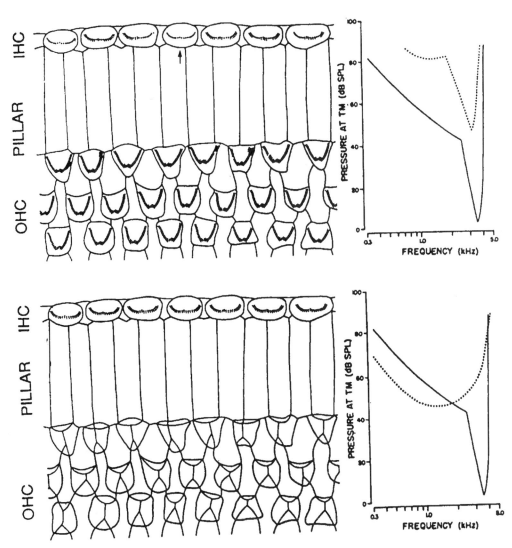

Figure 4.11. Upper panel: Camera lucida view of the organ of Corti of a cat with normal outer hair cells and damaged inner hair cells. Upper right panel shows a tuning curve from a normal animal (solid) and one from the damaged region of the organ of Corti (dashed) shown on the left. Lower panel: Camera lucida view of the organ of Corti of a cat with normal inner hair cells and complete loss of outer hair cells. Lower right panel shows a normal tuning curve (solid) and an abnormal tuning curve (dashed) recorded from the organ of Corti shown on the left. Reprinted with permission from Liberman MC, Dodds LW, and Learson DA, Structure-function correlates in noise-damaged ears: a light and electron-microscopic study. In Salvi RJ, Henderson D, Hamernik RP, and Colletti V, Eds. Basic and Applied aspects of Noise-Induced Hearing Loss. New York: Plenum Press, 1986.

In addition to the examples shown above, there are other cases where varying amounts of damage occur to both IHCs and OHCs. When this occurs, there will not only be a loss of sensitivity and tuning in the tip, but also an additional loss of sensitivity in the tail of the tuning curve (Liberman et al., 1986). The loss of tuning poses a significant problem for hearing-impaired listeners because background noise entering the tail of the tuning curve is just as effective in exciting the unit as noise with frequencies near the tip of the tuning curve, i.e., the neuron in damaged ears no longer responds selectively to tones near the CF. Although a hearing aid can compensate for losses in sensitivity (e.g., Fig. 4.11, top); it can not correct for the loss of frequency selectivity that typically occurs when the OHCs are damaged by high level noise or ototoxic drugs (Fig. 4.11 bottom).

Intensity Coding and Loudness Recruitment

Loudness recruitment, which is a common clinical symptom of cochlear hearing loss, refers to the abnormally rapid growth of loudness with increasing stimulus level (Hallpike and Hood, 1960). The reduced "dynamic" range of sound levels between threshold and uncomfortable sound levels poses a problem in hearing aid fitting.

The abnormally rapid growth of loudness was originally thought to be due to an abnormally rapid increase in firing rate once the neural threshold was exceeded in ears with cochlear damage. The left panel of Fig. 4.12 shows the predictions for this model. The dashed line and filled circles show the rate-level function for a typical auditory nerve fiber from a normal hearing chinchilla. The firing rate of the unit increases over roughly a 25 dB range and then saturates at approximately 300 sp/s. The solid line shows the predicted rate-level function for an auditory nerve fiber from an ear with cochlear hearing loss; the threshold is increased relative to the normal function. However, once threshold is exceeded, the discharge rate increases rapidly so that the firing rate soon reaches the saturation discharge rate of the normal unit. Thus, the slope of the rate-level function is extremely steep and the dynamic range quite narrow relative to normal units. In order to evaluate this model, discharge rate-level functions were measured from a large sample of auditory nerve fibers obtained from animals that had been exposed for 5 days to a 95 dB SPL octave band of noise centered at 0.5 kHz and were compared to discharge rate-level functions for normal animals. Units obtained from the noise-exposed chinchillas had thresholds that were approximately 30–60 dB higher than those from normal hearing animals (abscissa, Fig. 4.12 right). Even though there was a significant threshold shift, the slopes of the discharge rate-level functions (Fig. 4.12 upper right) and the saturation discharge rates (Fig. 4.12 lower right) were virtually identical to those from normal animals (Salvi et al., 1983a,b). Similar findings have been observed by others (Kiang et al., 1970; Harris and Dallos, 1978) and it may be concluded that animals with impaired ears have essentially the same input-output functions for auditory nerve fibers as normal animals. Thus, one cannot account for loudness recruitment in terms of abnormal rate-level functions of single fibers in the auditory nerve.

An alternative explanation for loudness recruitment is based on how the total amount of neural activity in a population of auditory nerve fibers increases with the level of the stimulus, i.e., the rate at which new neurons are "recruited" into the population of responding neurons as intensity increases. This model relies on the fact that auditory nerve fiber tuning curves become much broader near the tip (Fig. 4.13 top right) and threshold sometimes improves in the tail of the tuning curve in subjects with cochlear hearing loss (Kiang et al., 1970; Evans, 1976). Fig. 4.13 (upper panel) illustrates the model. The dashed line represents the signal frequency. As the height of the line increases (i.e., stimulus level increases), it cuts across additional tuning curves and activates more units. The upper left graph shows schematics of tuning curves from normal animals; the upper right from animals with SNHL. As the dashed line reaches the level to excite a neuron tuned to that frequency, it can be seen that the broad tuning curves allow for more neurons to be activated over smaller sound-level increments. This model was evaluated using the data from a group of chinchillas with 40–60 dB of noise-induced hearing loss (Fig. 4.13 bottom) (Salvi et al., 1983b). A standard frequency of 2 kHz was systematically increased in level. In the normal ears (solid line), the percentage of activated units gradually increases as the stimulus level is raised (Fig. 4.13 bottom). In the noise exposed ears (dashed line), there is a loss of sensitivity; however, once threshold is exceeded the percentage of fibers in the active population increases rapidly as stimulus level is increased.

More recent evoked potential studies suggest that the central auditory pathway may also be involved in loudness recruitment. Fig. 4.14 shows the evoked response input/output functions recorded with chronic electrodes implanted at different levels of the auditory pathway. The input/output functions shown in Fig. 4.14 were obtained with 1 kHz tone bursts and measurements were made before and after the animal was exposed to an intense 2 kHz puretone (Salvi et al., 1991). The exposure resulted in a significant hearing loss at the high frequencies (60–70 dB) with moderate to no loss below 2 kHz. Twenty-four hours after the exposure, the compound action potential recorded from the round window showed a loss of sensitivity and a signifi-

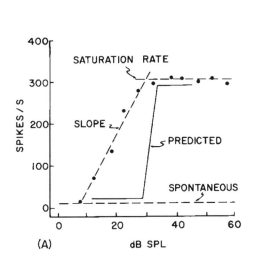

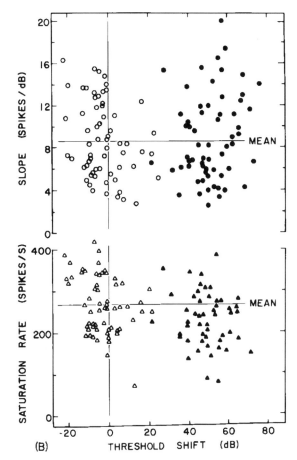

Figure 4.12. Left panel: Model of recruitment based on changes in nerve fiber rate-level function slopes. In the normal ears, neural firing rate increases with intensity over a 20 to 40 dB range (dashed line). In the ear with sensorineural loss, it is assumed that the range between the threshold and saturation rate is compressed (solid line) in an analogous fashion to the compressed range of hearing that is present in recruitment. If recruitment is encoded in the firing pattern of the VIII nerve, then it is reasonable to expect the rate-level slopes to be steeper in the impaired ears compared to the normal ears. The empirical data in the right panel do not support this model. Right panel: Rate-level function slopes (upper) and maximal firing rate of auditory nerve fibers recorded from normal and hearing-impaired chinchillas. The data from normal ears are plotted as open symbols (scattered around an average normal threshold shift of 0 dB) and the data from impaired ears are plotted as closed symbols. The mean slope and saturation rates are plotted as horizontal lines; it is clear that the average slope and saturation rates did not vary as a function of hearing loss. Reprinted with permission from Salvi RJ, Henderson D, Hamernik RP, and Ahroon WA. 1983. Neural correlates of sensorineural hearing loss. Ear and Hearing 1983;4:115–129.

cant reduction in the maximum amplitude of the AP (Fig. 4.14 left). Recordings made from the cochlear nucleus (CN) showed a loss in sensitivity and a reduction in maximum amplitude similar to that observed with the AP (Fig. 4.14 middle). The evoked response from the inferior colliculus (IC) also showed a loss in sensitivity after the exposure; however, in this case the maximum amplitude of the evoked response from the IC was much larger than normal, i.e., the maximum amplitude of the evoked response was "enhanced" (right). It is also important to note that the slope of the input/output function from the IC was much steeper than normal, whereas the slope of the AP and CN input/output functions were shallower than normal after the exposure. The "enhanced" evoked response amplitudes typi-

cally occur only at frequencies on the low-frequency side of the hearing loss.

What physiological mechanisms could be responsible for the enhanced evoked response amplitudes in the central auditory pathway? One mechanism that could potentially lead to enhanced evoked response amplitudes in the central auditory system is an alteration of the balance of excitation and inhibition in the central auditory neurons. Many units in the CN and IC have single-tone inhibitory sidebands (frequency-intensity combinations that decrease SR) located above and below the excitatory response area of the tuning curve; auditory nerve fibers do not have such inhibitory response areas. Sounds that activate the inhibitory sidebands of a CNS neuron may limit the maximum discharge rates of that neuron at high

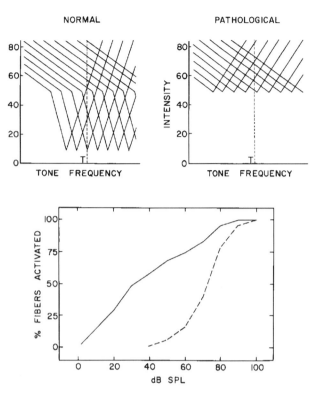

Figure 4.13. Upper panel: Model of recruitment based on abnormal tuning curves. Lower panel: Percentage of nerve fibers excited by a tone in a population of normal auditory nerve fibers (solid line) and a population of auditory nerve fibers from hearing impaired chinchillas (dashed line). Reprinted with permission from Evans EF, Wilson JP, and Borerwe TA. Animal models of tinnitus. In Evred E, and Lawrenson G, Eds. Tinnitus Bath: The Pitman Press, 1981.

intensities. Recent data from our lab suggest that if the inhibitory inputs to a unit in the central auditory pathway are selectively eliminated by acoustic trauma, an increase in the maximum firing rate of the unit at CF may occur. Fig. 4.15 shows the discharge rate-level functions measured with stimulation at a unit's CF (8892 Hz) and with stimulation at a frequency located in an inhibitory sideband above CF (12717 Hz). The pre-exposure rate-level function obtained at CF (Fig. 4.15, top) shows an increase in firing rate as stimulus level is increased, whereas the pre-exposure rate level function obtained in the inhibitory sideband above CF (Fig. 4.15, bottom) shows a decrease in firing rate as stimulus level increases. After the traumatizing tone was presented in the inhibitory response area, the discharge rate-level function measured above CF showed no decrease in firing rate with increased levels of stimulation, which reflects a complete loss of inhibition (Fig. 4.15, bottom). By contrast, the discharge rate-level function measured at CF (Fig. 4.15, top) showed little or no change at low stimulus levels; however, the firing rate at suprathreshold levels increased significantly ("enhancement") after the exposure. This increase in the maximum firing rate could be related to the enhanced evoked response amplitudes seen after acoustic trauma. Furthermore, it is conceivable that the enhanced neural activity observed in the central auditory pathway may be related to loudness recruitment.

Neural Adaptation and Temporal Resolution

The time course of forward masking is known to be prolonged in listeners with SNHL (Cudahy, 1982; Nelson and Freyman, 1987) and it is conceivable that this is related to

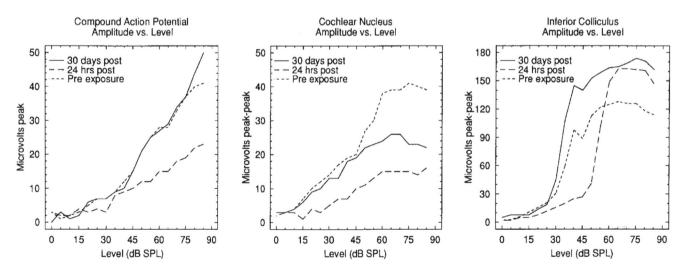

Figure 4.14. Input-output function for evoked potentials measured at the round window (compound action potential), cochlear nucleus (CN) and inferior colliculus (IC) before and after exposure to traumatic noise. Reprinted with permission from Salvi RJ, Powers NL,

Saunders SS, Boettcher FA, and Clock AE. Enhancement of evoked response amplitude and single unit activity after noise exposure. In Dancer A, Henderson D, Salvi RJ, and Hamernik RP, Eds. Noise-Induced Hearing Loss. Toronto: B.C. Decker, 1991.

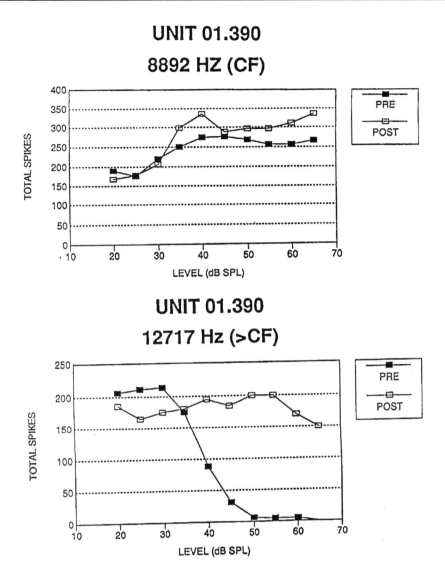

Figure 4.15. Rate-level functions of a CN unit measured at the CF (top) and one-half octave above the CF (bottom) of the unit. At each of the two frequencies, the rate-level functions were determined before (filled squares) and immediately after (open squares) exposure to a continuous tone (12717 Hz, 105 dB SPL) for 5 minutes. Note that the 12717 Hz tone inhibited the firing rate of the unit at high intensities before exposure, but the firing rate to 12717 Hz did not vary with intensity following trauma. The firing rate to the 8892 Hz tones increased significantly at high levels following the high-frequency trauma. Reprinted with permission from Salvi RJ, Powers NL, Saunders SS, Boettcher FA, and Clock AE. Enhancement of evoked response amplitude and single unit activity after noise exposure. In Dancer A, Henderson D, Salvi RJ, and Hamernik RP, Eds. Noise-Induced Hearing Loss. Toronto: B.C. Decker, 1991.

an abnormally slow rate of recovery from short-term adaptation in auditory nerve fibers. In order to evaluate this hypothesis, the forward masking stimulus paradigm was used to study the time course of recovery from short-term adaptation in auditory nerve fibers obtained from chinchillas with 30–60 dB of noise-induced temporary threshold shift (Salvi et al., 1986a, b). The data shown in Fig. 4.16 were obtained with a masker tone presented 40 dB above each unit's threshold and a probe tone presented 10 dB above threshold. Note that the normalized probe rate (ratio of the masked firing rate to the unmasked firing rate; a normalized probe rate of 1.0 suggests no masking and 0.0 suggests complete masking) increases as the time interval between masker and probe increases; however, the normalized probe rate is depressed to a greater extent and recovers more slowly in noise-exposed animals than in normal animals. This prolonged recovery from short-term adaptation could potentially account for poor temporal resolution as demonstrated by prolonged forward masking functions in listeners with SNHL.

Temporal Integration

Normal-hearing listeners typically show a 10–15 dB improvement in threshold as stimulus duration increases from 10 to 500 ms (Fig. 4.17 upper left); however this im-

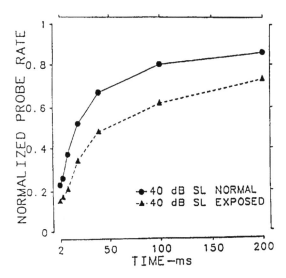

Figure 4.16. Forward-masking data from a single auditory nerve fiber in the chinchilla using a masking tone 40 dB above unit threshold and a probe tone 10 dB above threshold. Normalized probe rate (see text) increases as the time interval between masker and probe increases but shows slower recovery from adaptation in noise-exposed animals. Reprinted with permission from Salvi RJ, Saunders SS, Ahroon WA, Shivapuja BG, and Arehole S. Psychophysical and physiological aspects of auditory temporal processing in listeners with noise-induced sensorineural hearing loss. In Salvi RJ, Henderson D, Hamernik RP, and Colletti V, Eds. Basic and Applied aspects of Noise-Induced Hearing Loss. New York: Plenum Press, 1986

provement in threshold with increasing stimulus duration is greatly reduced in listeners with cochlear hearing loss (Wright, 1968; Henderson, 1969; Watson and Gengel, 1969; Solecki and Gerken, 1990). In order to account for this reduction in temporal integration, Wright (1968) suggested that cochlear hearing loss causes an abnormally rapid decay in the neural output of the cochlea (Fig. 4.17 lower left). According to this model, the centrally-located neural integrator will now have fewer spike discharges to summate over time; thus, there will be less improvement in threshold with increasing stimulus duration. In order to evaluate this hypothesis, the PST histograms from animals with 40–60 dB of hearing loss were evaluated for signs of abnormal adaptation (Salvi et al., 1983a, b). Gross inspection of the histograms shown in Fig. 4.17 (right) indicates that the decay in firing rate over time is within normal limits (see Fig. 4.4). Thus, the reduction in temporal summation cannot be explained on the basis of an abnormally rapid decay in the neural output of the cochlea (Wright, 1968).

An alternative explanation for the reduction in temporal integration with cochlear hearing loss involves a change in the "central integrator" (Zwislocki, 1960) and is supported by psychophysical studies involving electrical stimulation of the CN and IC (Gerken et al., 1991). In normal hearing animals, the behavioral thresholds for detecting electrical stimuli delivered to the CN or IC

show a temporal integration-like effect in which thresholds improve with increasing stimulus duration. Since the behavioral responses were elicited with electrical stimulation of the auditory brainstem (thus the stimulation bypassed the cochlea), one would assume that the threshold of detection would be unaffected by cochlear damage. However, after damaging the cochlea, the electrical stimulation thresholds showed little improvement with progressively longer stimuli, thus temporal integration of electrical stimuli was virtually abolished. One interpretation of these results is that peripheral damage must affect the centrally located integration process.

Latency Shift

The absolute and relative latency shifts of the waveforms obtained with ECochG and ABR are routinely utilized in the diagnosis of hearing disorders. However, interpretation of latency measures is complicated by the fact that the gross potentials depend on the temporal and spatial overlap of many different neural generators. Thus, an understanding of how cochlear hearing loss affects the response latencies of the individual auditory nerve fibers would help in interpreting the latency shifts of wave I of the ABR or the AP of the electrocochleogram. The effects of cochlear hearing loss on the response latencies of individual auditory nerve fibers is illustrated in Fig. 4.18 (upper panels) using the PST histograms obtained with click stimuli. Results are shown for two units with CFs of approximately 1 kHz; the data in upper right of Fig. 4.18 is from a normal animal whereas that in the upper left is from a noise-exposed animal with a flat hearing loss of approximately 30–50 dB. Stimulus level is expressed in dB of attenuation of the click where 0 dB corresponds to approximately 100 dB peak SPL. In the normal animal (Fig. 4.18, *top right*), the latency to the first peak systematically decreases from approximately 4 ms near threshold (arrow) to approximately 1.5 ms at the highest stimulus level. This progressive decrease in latency is absent in the histograms obtained from the noise-exposed animals (Fig. 4.18, *top left*). The latency to the first peak of the histogram near threshold (arrow) is approximately 1.5 ms. In other words, the neural latencies in ears with cochlear hearing loss are virtually the same as those from normal ears at the same SPL; however, the neural latencies at threshold would be shorter in the noise-exposed ears than in normals. Even though the neural latencies are the same for a given sound level (e.g., 10 dB attenuation), the shapes of the PST histograms are drastically different.

Similar trends were seen in the latency of the N_1 response of the AP recorded from the round window (Fig. 4.18, *bottom*). In normal animals, the latency of the AP systematically decreases from approximately 2 ms near threshold (80 dB of attenuation) to approximately 1 ms

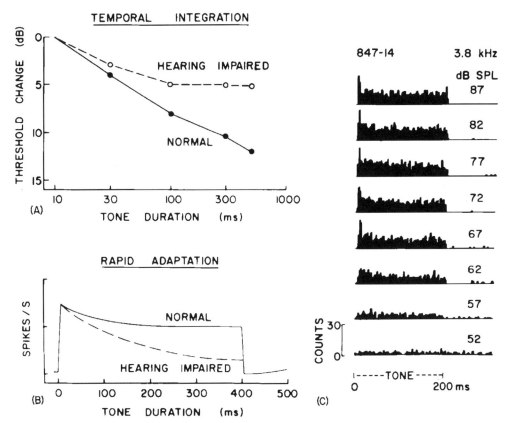

Figure 4.17. Upper left panel shows the approximate change in threshold with increasing stimulus duration for normal and hearing-impaired listeners. The lower panel represents a hypothetical model to account for the reduction in temporal integration. The model predicts an abnormally rapid decay (dashed line) in neural output for hearing-impaired listeners. The series of PST histograms (right panel) from one animal with 40–60 dB of hearing loss does not indicate an abnormal rapid decay in neural output over time. Reprinted with permission from Salvi RJ, Henderson D, and Hamernik RP. Physiological bases of sensorineural hearing loss. In Tobias JB, and Schubert ED, Eds. Hearing Research and Theory, Vol. 2. New York: Academic Press, 1983.

at high stimulus levels. However, in the noise-exposed ear (open circles), the latency is quite short (1 ms) near threshold (35 dB attenuation) and shows little change in latency with increasing stimulus level. Thus, both the latency of the AP as well as the latency of individual auditory nerve fibers seems to be closely linked to stimulus level rather than to how high the stimulus level is above threshold.

In some individuals with sensory-neural hearing loss, the AP or wave I latency may appear prolonged near threshold, but then the latency suddenly catches up (recruitment-like behavior) with the normal latency intensity function. How should this recruitment-like behavior of the AP or wave I be interpreted in light of the preceding AP and single unit data? When the wave I or AP latency is prolonged, then the response presumably is originating from a region of the cochlea that is apical (lower frequency) of the region that typically generates the response in a normal ear. When the click level is increased, energy "spills over" into more basal (high frequency) regions of the cochlea with elevated thresholds. The re-

sponse latencies of high-CF units are shorter than those of low-CF units (Fig. 4.5), consequently there is a sudden reduction in the latency of the AP at levels of stimulation high enough to excite the basal part of the cochlea.

SUMMARY AND CONCLUSIONS

In the past 10–15 years, auditory physiologists have begun to examine the changes in neural coding that accompany SNHL. It is now apparent from both psychophysical and physiological studies that SNHL involves more than a simple loss of sensitivity. Rather, a complex series of changes occurs in the neural coding of sound which in turn gives rise to a myriad of auditory perceptual distortions in the hearing-impaired listener. While a conventional hearing aid may be able to compensate for the loss in sensitivity, it can not correct for the loss in frequency selectivity, the reduction in temporal summation, the change in the latency of the neural responses, and the abnormally rapid growth of neural activity observed within the central auditory pathway.

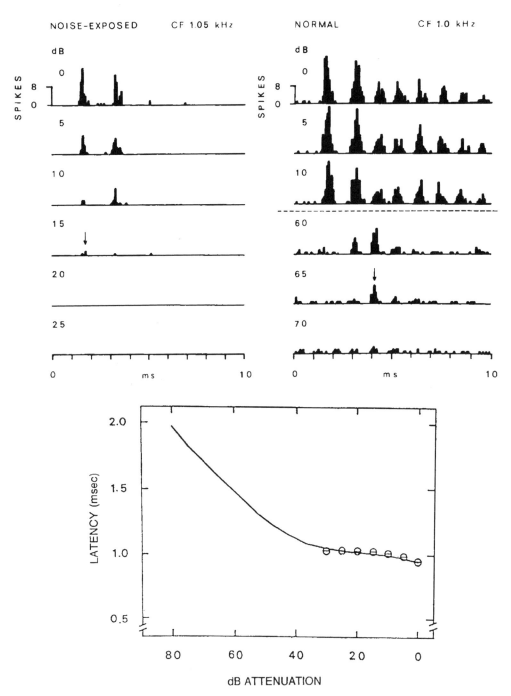

Figure 4.18. Upper panels: PST histograms collected from a noise-exposed (left) and normal chinchilla (right) using click stimuli. Note that the signal level is presented in dB of attenuation; thus, a lower number represents an intense sound and vice-versa. The right panel shows multiple peaks in the histograms which are a reflection of the "ringing" of the basilar membrane. The left panel, showing histograms from an impaired ear, has few peaks, reflecting an increase in damping of the basilar membrane and concomitant decrease in frequency selectivity in the impaired ear. Lower panel: Latency-intensity function for the whole-nerve action potential in a normal (solid line) and noise-exposed (circles) animal. Reprinted with permission from Salvi RJ, Henderson D, and Hamernik RP. Single auditory nerve fiber and action potential latencies in normal and noise-treated chinchillas. Hearing Research 1979;1:237–251.

Acknowledgments

The authors of this chapter have been supported by grants from the National Institutes of Health, National Institute of Occupational Safety and Health, National Science Foundation, and Deafness Research Foundation.

REFERENCES

Ashmore JF. A fast motile response in guinea-pig outer hair cells: the cellular basis of the cochlear amplifier. Nature 1987;322:368–371.

von Bekesy GV. Experiments in Hearing. New York: Wiley, 1960.

Brownell WE. Outer hair cell electromotility and otoacoustic emissions. Ear Hearing 1990;11:82–92.

Corwin JT, and Cotanche DA. Regeneration of sensory hair cells after acoustic trauma. Science 1988;240:1772–1774.

Cudahy E. (1982) Changes in the temporal processing of acoustic signals in hearing-impaired listeners. In Hamernik RP, Henderson D, and Salvi RJ, Eds. New Perspectives on Noise-Induced Hearing Loss. New York: Raven Press, 1982.

Davis H. A model for transducer action in the cochlea. Cold Spring Harbor Symp Quant Biol 1958;30:181–190.

Davis H, Morgan CT, Hawkins JE, Galambos R, and Smith FW. Temporary deafness following exposure to loud tones and noise. Acta Oto-Laryngol 1950;(Suppl)88:

Eldredge DH, Mills JH, and Bohne BA. A frequency-position map for the chinchilla cochlea. J Acoust Soc Am 1981;69:1091–1095

Elliott LL. Backward and forward masking of probe tones of different frequencies. J Acoust Soc Am 1962;34:1116–1117.

Evans EF. Temporary sensorineural hearing losses and 8th nerve changes. In Henderson D, Hamernik RP, Dosanjh DS, and Mills JH, Eds. Effects of Noise on Hearing. New York: Raven Press, 1976:199–224.

Evans EF, Wilson JP, and Borerwe TA (1981) Animal models of tinnitus. In: Evred E, and Lawrenson G, Eds. Tinnitus. Bath: The Pitman Press, 1981

Gerken GM, Solecki JM, and Boettcher FA. Temporal integration of electrical stimulation of auditory nuclei in normal-hearing and hearing-impaired cat. Hear Res 1991;53:101–112.

Glattke TJ. (1983) Short-latency auditory evoked potentials: fundamental bases & clinical applications. Austin: Pro-ed, Inc., 1983.

Hallpike CS, and Hood JD. (1960) Observations on the neurological mechanism of the loudness recruitment phenomenon. Acta Oto-Laryngol 1960;50:472–486.

Harris JD, Haines HL, and Meyers CK. Loudness perception for pure tones and speech. Arch Otolaryngol 1952;55:107–133.

Harris D and Dallos P. Properties of auditory nerve responses in the absence of outer hair cells. J Neurophysiol 1978;41:365–383.

Hellman RP, and Zwislocki JJ. (1961) Some factors affecting the estimation of loudness of loudness. J Acoust Soc Am 1961;33:687–694.

Henderson D. (1969) Temporal summation of acoustic signals by the chinchilla. J Acoust Soc Am 1969;46:474–475.

Hudspeth AJ. The cellular basis of hearing: the biophysics of hair cells. Science 1985;230:745–752.

Jerger JF. Influence of stimulus duration on the pure-tone threshold during recovery from auditory fatigue. J Acoust Soc Am 1955;27:121–124.

Kiang NYS. Discharge Patterns of Single Fibers in the Cat's Auditory Nerve. Cambridge, MA: M.I.T. Press, 1965: Research Monograph No. 35.

Kiang NYS, Moxon EC, and Levine RA. Auditory-nerve activity in cats with normal and abnormal cochleas. In Wolstenholme GEW, and Knight J, Eds. Sensorineural Hearing Loss. London: Churchill, 1970.

Liberman MC. Auditory-nerve response from cats raised in a low-noise chamber. J Acoust Soc Am 1978;63:442–455.

Liberman MC, Dodds LW, and Learson DA. Structure-function correlation in noise-damaged ears: a light and electron-microscopic study. In Salvi RJ, Henderson D, Hamernik RP, and Colletti V, Eds.

Basic and Applied Aspects of Noise-Induced Hearing Loss. Plenum Press, New York: Plenum Press, 1986.

Nelson DA, and Freyman RL. Temporal resolution in sensorineural hearing impaired listeners. J Acoust Soc Am 1987;81:709–720.

Plomp R. Rate of decay of auditory sensation. J Acoust Soc Am 1964;36:277–282.

Plomp R, and Bowman MA. Relation between hearing threshold and duration for tone pulses. J Acoust Soc Am 1959;31:749–758.

Robertson D (1984) Horseradish peroxidase injection of physiologically characterized afferent and efferent neurones in the guinea pig spiral ganglion. Hearing Res 1984;15:113–121.

Robles L, Rhode WS, and Geisler CD. Transient response of the basilar membrane measured in squirrel monkeys using the Mossbauer effect. J Acoust Soc Am 1976;59:926–939.

Sachs MB, and Abbas P. Rate versus level functions for auditory-nerve fibers in cats: tone-burst stimuli. J Acoust Soc Am 1974;56: 1835–1847.

Salvi RJ, Henderson D, and Hamernik RP. Single auditory nerve fiber and action potential latencies in normal and noise-treated chinchillas. Hearing Res 1979;1:237–251.

Salvi RJ, Perry J, Hamernik RP, and Henderson D. Relationship between cochlear pathologies and auditory nerve and behavioral responses following acoustic trauma. In Hamernik RP, Henderson D, and Salvi RJ, Eds. New Perspectives on Noise-Induced Hearing Loss. New York: Raven Press, 1982.

Salvi RJ, Henderson D, Hamernik R, and Ahroon WA. Neural correlates of sensorineural hearing loss. Ear and Hearing 1983a;4:115–129.

Salvi R, Henderson D, and Hamernik RP. Physiological bases of sensorineural hearing loss. In Tobias JV, and Schubert ED, Eds. Hearing Research and Theory, Vol. 2. New York: Academic Press, 1983b.

Salvi RJ, Saunders SS, Ahroon WA, Shivapuja BG, and Arehole S. 1986 Psychophysical and physiological aspects of auditory temporal processing in listeners with noise-induced sensorineural hearing loss. In Salvi RJ, Henderson D, Hamernik RP, and Colletti V, Eds. Basic and Applied Aspects of Noise-Induced Hearing Loss. New York: Plenum Press, 1986.

Salvi RJ, Powers NL, Saunders SS, Boettcher FA, and Clock AE. Enhancement of evoked response amplitude and single unit activity after noise exposure. In Dancer A, Henderson D, Salvi RJ, and Hamernik RP, Eds. Effects of Noise on the Auditory System. Toronto: BC Decker, 1991.

Solecki J, and Gerken G. Auditory temporal integration in the normal-hearing and hearing-impaired cat. J Acoust Soc Am 1990;88: 779–785.

Spoendlin H. 1970 Structural basis of peripheral frequency analysis. In Plomp R, Smoorenburg GF, Eds. Frequency Analysis and Periodicity Detection in Hearing. Leiden: A.W. Sijthoff, 1970.

Spoendlin H. 1972 Innervation densities of the cochlea. Acta Otolaryngol 1972;73:235–248.

Tyler R, Summerfield Q, Wood EJ, and Fernandes MA. Psychoacoustic and phonetic temporal processing in normal and hearing-impaired listeners. J Acoust Soc Am 1982;72:740–752.

Viemeister NF. 1983 Auditory intensity discrimination at high frequencies in the presence of noise. Science 1983;221:1206–1208.

Watson CS, and Gengel RW. Signal duration and signal frequency in relation to auditory sensitivity. J Acoust Soc Am 1969;46:989–997.

Wightman FL. Psychoacoustic correlates of hearing loss. In Hamernik RP, Henderson D, and Salvi RJ, Eds. New Perspectives on Noise-Induced Hearing Loss. New York: Raven Press, 1981.

Wright HN. The effect of sensorineural hearing loss on threshold-duration functions. J Speech Hear Res 1968;11:842–852.

Zwislocki J. Theory of temporal auditory summation. J Acoust Soc Am 1960;32:1046–1060.

CHAPTER 5

Psychoacoustic Considerations in Clinical Audiology

Larry E. Humes

It is the purpose of this chapter to provide the reader with a general understanding and appreciation of the psychoacoustic foundations of clinical audiology. Many contemporary tests evolved out of careful consideration of these foundations.

This is true for basic tests, such as puretone air-conduction procedures (Chapter 7), as well as more advanced special tests such as the Short Increment Sensitivity Index (Chapter 11) and the Masking Level Difference (Chapter 15). A full appreciation of many test procedures can be gained only by having a general understanding of the scientific bases underlying them. Such an understanding is even more essential if the audiologist trained today is to deal effectively with the test procedures of tomorrow.

The present chapter has been divided into three primary sections. Following a brief review of psychophysical methods, the chapter will discuss the perception of sound by normal-hearing listeners. The excitation pattern concept will be described as a unifying framework. The final section provides a few illustrations of the application of the excitation pattern concept to the interpretation of data from hearing-impaired listeners.

PSYCHOPHYSICAL METHODS

Classical Psychophysical Methods

Psychoacoustics is itself a field within a broader discipline known as psychophysics. Psychophysics is the study of the relation between a physical stimulus and the sensation it produces in the subject. In the case of psychoacoustics, the stimulus is an acoustic signal and the sensation is an auditory one. Fechner is generally given credit for the founding of the field of psychophysics with the publication of his German text, *Element der Psychophysik* in 1860.

If one is to study the relation between the physical stimulus and the sensation it elicits, then some means must be developed to quantify both the stimulus and the sensation. For the sensory modalities with which Fechner was concerned, quantification of the physical stimulus was straightforward. For example, in his investigation of the perceived heaviness of various objects, the weight of the object was determined easily. The quantification of the magnitude of sensation, however, was more difficult. Fechner chose an indirect method to measure or scale sensation. To estimate the magnitude of sensation indirectly, two basic sets of measurements were required; the absolute threshold and the difference threshold. Both thresholds were statistical concepts that were thought to represent points of transition along the scale of sensation. Absolute threshold represented the transition from no sensation to the onset of sensation, while the difference threshold represented a transition from one magnitude of sensation to a just noticeable change in sensation (either an increase or decrease).

Fechner developed three procedures to measure these two thresholds. These procedures have come to be known as: (*a*) the method of limits, (*b*) the method of adjustment, and (*c*) the method of constant stimuli. Each of these methods is described briefly here with emphasis on their use to measure the so-called absolute threshold of hearing. The reader should bear in mind, however, that these same procedures can be readily applied to difference thresholds.

In the method of limits, the listener is presented with an acoustic signal at an intensity predetermined by the investigator. The listener then either responds "Yes," indicating perception of the signal, or simply fails to respond, indicating that the signal was not perceived. Ascending and descending series are presented in an alternating fashion. In an ascending series, the intensity begins below the anticipated threshold and the intensity of successive stimuli is increased on each trial. For descending series, the intensity of the initial stimulus is above the estimated threshold and the intensity is decreased for successive trials. Ascending and descending series are typically alternated for a total of at least 10 series of trials (five ascending, five descending) with the initial and final intensity for each series varied. Figure 5.1 illustrates four series of stimulus presentation for the method of limits. Responses from the listener are recorded for each trial in a series. A transition point in the responses from either "Yes" to no response (descending series) or no response to "Yes" (ascending series) is observed, and the stimulus intensity corresponding to this transition is recorded. The mean of the

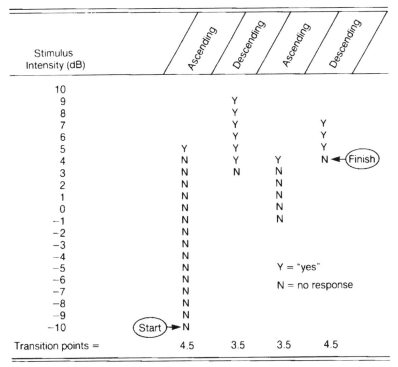

Stimulus Intensity (dB)	Ascending	Descending	Ascending	Descending
10				
9		Y		
8		Y		
7		Y		Y
6		Y		Y
5	Y	Y		Y
4	N	Y	Y	N ← (Finish)
3	N	N	N	
2	N		N	
1	N		N	
0	N		N	
−1	N		N	
−2	N			
−3	N			
−4	N			
−5	N		Y = "yes"	
−6	N		N = no response	
−7	N			
−8	N			
−9	N			
−10	(Start) → N			
Transition points =	4.5	3.5	3.5	4.5

* Mean threshold value = 4.0

Figure 5.1. Illustration of four series of trials, alternating ascending and descending, for the method of limits. For each series a transition point is recorded which marks the boundary between the two response categories ("Yes" and no response). The mean of these transition points corresponds to threshold. (Adapted from Gescheider, 1976.)

10 or more intensities, one at each transition point, defines the absolute threshold for a particular acoustic stimulus. The absolute threshold measured in this manner defines the stimulus intensity that yields a "Yes" response approximately 50% of the time.

In the method of limits, the experimenter controls the intensity of the stimulus and its presentation. In the method of adjustment, on the other hand, the listener plays an active role in the control of stimulus intensity. The experimenter typically determines the initial intensity of the stimulus for the trial and the listener adjusts the intensity accordingly. When the initial intensity is below anticipated threshold, the trial is an ascending one and the listener increases the intensity until the previously inaudible stimulus is made audible. Conversely, when the initial intensity of the stimulus is above the estimated threshold, the trial is a descending one and the subject's task is to decrease the intensity until the initially audible sound is rendered just inaudible. As shown in Figure 5.2, ascending and descending trials are typically alternated. The final intensity setting selected by the listener on each trial is then recorded by the experimenter. The mean of several intensity settings is then calculated and serves as the absolute threshold for the particular stimulus being utilized. If the distribution of intensity settings or adjustments made by the lis-

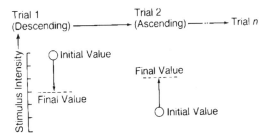

Figure 5.2. Schematic illustration of the method of adjustment. *Trial 1* is a descending one in which stimulus intensity begins above threshold and the subject adjusts the level until the signal can just no longer be heard. *Trial 2,* on the other hand, is an ascending one. Mean of the final values corresponds to threshold.

tener is a normal distribution, then the mean of this distribution represents the intensity corresponding to 50% "Yes" responses.

In the third classical psychophysical procedure developed by Fechner, the method of constant stimuli, the listener again assumes a passive role in the manipulation of stimulus intensity, as was the case for the method of limits. Unlike the previous two methods, the method of constant stimuli does not incorporate ascending and descending approaches to threshold. Rather, stimulus intensity is selected randomly for each trial, usually from a set of at least 10 intensities. Each intensity occurs several times (at least 10) and the percentage of trials to which the listener responds "Yes," indicating perception of the sound, is recorded for each intensity. The result is typically an ogive or S-shaped function relating percentage of "Yes" responses to stimulus intensity as shown in Figure 5.3. Threshold is defined with this procedure as the intensity corresponding to 50% "Yes" responses. Ideally, the intensities are positioned such that half yield percentage "Yes" values below 50% and half yield percentages above 50%. In addition, it is not desirable to have more than one or two intensities that yield 100% or 0% "Yes" responses.

If one considers reliablity of the data and the time required for determination of threshold as two continua along which these three classical psychophysical procedures can be evaluated, then the following general statements can be made. The method of adjustment requires the least amount of time to provide an estimate of threshold, but tends to yield less reliable data. The reliability of the data obtained with this procedure can be increased considerably by increasing the number of stimulus trials. This is done, however, at the expense of increased time of administration. The method of constant stimuli, on the other hand, perhaps provides the most reliable measure of threshold, but is the most time consuming of three classical procedures. The method of limits is intermediate along these two continua (Gescheider, 1976).

Many of the test procedures used in the clinical setting employ some version of one of these three classical psychophysical methods. They have usually been modified, however, to make them more efficient. The particular modifications of these procedures are described in many of the other chapters of this book.

The clinician should be aware that the absolute threshold or difference threshold measured with one of

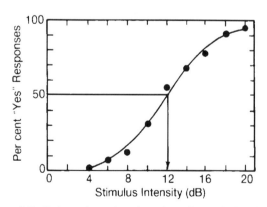

Figure 5.3. S-shaped or ogive-shaped psychometric function relating percentage of "Yes" responses to stimulus intensity as determined by the method of constant stimuli. The stimulus intensity corresponding to 50% "Yes" responses is considered to represent threshold. The threshold in this case is slightly greater than 12 dB.

the classical techniques generally is *not* considered to be an uncontaminated measure of sensory function. Rather, thresholds measured with these procedures could be altered considerably by biasing the subject through various means, such as the use of different sets of instructions or different schedules of reinforcement for correct and incorrect responses. The magnitude of sensation evoked within the sensory system during the signal presentations should remain unchanged under these manipulation, yet the threshold is noticeably affected. Hence, the threshold value measured is affected by factors other than the sensitivity of the auditory system. For the psychophysicist, other response measures are available that allow one to estimate sensitivity independent of contaminating subject biases (e.g., Green and Swets, 1974). At present, the time required to administer these procedures is too great for clinical application. For the audiologist, adaptations of the classical psychophysical procedures have proven to be valid, reliable, efficient tools to measure various aspects of hearing in clinical settings, as long as care is used in instructing listeners and administering the procedures in a standard fashion.

Adaptive Methods

The efficiency of threshold measurement procedures has been increased considerably in recent years by the use of adaptive test strategies (Zwislocki et al., 1958; Levitt, 1971). In adaptive methodologies, the signal intensity used in a particular trial is determined by the subject's previous responses. Notice in the example of the classical method of limits shown in Figure 5.1, for instance, that the ascending and descending series frequently started at intensities well beyond the intensity at which the listener changed response. In this sense then, much of the test time was wasted on stimulus presentations that were either well above or well below threshold. An adaptive modification of the method of limits, however, would reverse the direction of stimulus change as soon as the response changed. This is illustrated in Figure 5.4. Note that the stimulus level on a given trial is determined by the immediately preceding response. The threshold estimated in this way is identical to that obtained with the classical method of limits (Fig. 5.1), but fewer trials are required. Adaptive methodologies currently enjoy wide popularity among researchers and clinicians alike.

Scaling Procedures

Threshold procedures grew out of Fechner's attempts to quantify the magnitude of sensation indirectly. Another set of procedures, known generally as direct scaling techniques, attempts to measure sensation directly.

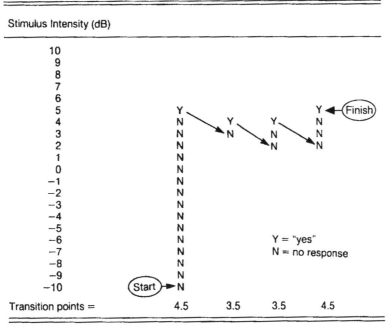

Stimulus Intensity (dB)

Y = "yes"
N = no response

Transition points = 4.5 3.5 3.5 4.5

* Mean threshold value = 4.0

Figure 5.4. An illustration of an adaptive version of the method of limits (illustrated previously in Fig. 5.1). Note the fewer number of trials required to estimate threshold here as compared to Figure 5.1.

These were developed primarily by another notable psychophysicist, S.S. Stevens, and are reviewed in detail by Stevens (1975). Scaling techniques are used most frequently in the study of hearing to measure the sensation of loudness, though they have also been used to quantify other sensations, such as pitch. The results from one of these procedures, magnitude estimation, are shown in Figure 5.5. In the magnitude estimation technique illustrated here, subjects simply assign numbers to the perceived loudness of a series of stimuli. In this case, the signals differed only in intensity. The average results fall along a straight line when plotted on log-log coordinates. Comparable results have been obtained for other sensations, such as brightness, vibration on the finger tip, and electric shock. In all cases, a straight line fits the average data very well, when plotted on log-log coordinates. From these extensive data, a law was developed that relates the perceived magnitude of sensation (S) to the physical intensity of the stimulus (I) in the following manner: $S = kI^x$, where k is an arbitrary constant and x is an exponent or power that varies with the sensation under investigation. This law is known as Stevens' power law. A convenient feature of a power function plotted on log-log coordinates is that the slope of the line fit to the data is the exponent, x. To obtain appropriate exponent values, average data from at least 10 subjects should be used. Scaling techniques have been used only sparingly by audiologists (Thalmann, 1965), although there appears to be renewed interest in

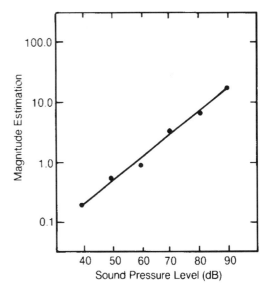

Figure 5.5. An illustration of the magnitude estimation procedure applied to the scaling of loudness. Subjects were presented with each intensity (40, 50, 60, 70, 80 and 90 dB SPL) in random order and simply asked to estimate its loudness by assigning a number to it. The data points represent the average data from a group of normal-hearing young adults. The x-axis is a dB scale which makes it logarithmic in nature. The y-axis is also a log scale. Note that when plotted on log-log coordinates a straight line can be fit to the data.

their clinical application (Harris and Goldstein, 1980; Barry and Kidd, 1981; Lawson and Chail, 1982; Knight and Margolis, 1984).

Matching Methods

Finally, a procedure that has been used extensively in psychoacoustics to measure auditory sensation via the subject's response is the matching procedure. The matching procedure maintains some features of classical threshold procedures and scaling procedures in that the technique is similar to that of the method of adjustment (one of the classical psychophysical methods), but its goal is to quantify a subjective attribute of sound, such as loudness or pitch. The matching procedures enable the experimenter to determine a set of stimulus parameters that all yield the same subjective sensation. A puretone fixed at 1000 Hz and 70 dB SPL (sound pressure level), for example, may be presented to one ear of a listener and a second puretone of 8000 Hz presented to the other ear in an alternating fashion. The subject controls the intensity of the 8000-Hz tone until it is judged to be equal in loudness to the 1000-Hz, 70-dB SPL reference tone. The starting intensity of the 8000-Hz tone is varied from trial to trial by the experimenter with an equal number of ascending and descending trials employed. Data in the literature indicate that the 8000-Hz tone would have to be set to 80 or 85 dB SPL to achieve a loudness match in the case presented above. The Alternate Binaural Loudness Balance (ABLB) test represents the most common clinical application of the matching procedure (see Chapter 11). Recent interest in the loudness and pitch of tinnitus has resulted in increased utilization of the matching technique.

Let us now examine how these procedures have been applied to the study of the perception of sound. The next section provides a cursory discussion and review of the literature. First, a conceptual framework will be developed from which a variety of psychoacoustic phenomena can be understood.

THE PERCEPTION OF SOUND BY NORMAL-HEARING LISTENERS

The Excitation-Pattern Concept

Excitation patterns have proven to be a useful conceptual framework with which to describe many psychoacoustic phenomena (Zwicker, 1970, Moore, 1982). It is not necessary to tie this concept to a particular physiologic response, such as the amplitude of displacement of the basilar membrane, the amount of shearing force along the hair cells, the amplitude of receptor potentials within the hair cells, or the response of the auditory nerve fibers (in either discharge rate or degree of synchronization). For the moment, any of these physiologic responses of the inner ear or auditory nerve can be envisioned as the event underlying the excitation process. Figure 5.6 shows several excitation patterns at six different places along the length of the cochlea. For any given pattern, the height of the pattern reflects the amount of excitation evoked by the stimulus at that particular place. Thus, those patterns having a peak at the apex represent excitation patterns for low frequencies while those with peaks at the base reflect stimulation by high-frequency puretones. Again, where this excitation occurs in the auditory periphery is not an issue. The series of excitation patterns located between the base and apex in Figure 5.6 illustrates the change in excitation associated with change in frequency, whereas the three patterns located in the middle reflect the effect of different sound pressure levels of the stimulus. Note that as sound level increases the excitation pattern becomes increasingly asymmetrical with excitation spreading more on the high frequency side than on the low frequency side of the pattern.

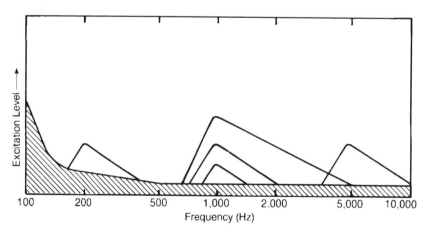

Figure 5.6. Schematic illustration of excitation patterns produced within the auditory system by puretones of various frequencies and intensities. The shaded area represents internal noise within the auditory system. The *triangular excitation patterns* are centered at 200, 1000, and 5000 Hz. Three patterns are shown at 1000 Hz representing three different intensities of the 1000-Hz tone. Thus, frequency is indicated by the horizontal position of the peak while intensity is represented by the vertical position of the peak of the excitation pattern.

Hearing Threshold

The excitation pattern provides a helpful conceptualization of several psychoacoustic phenomena. Figure 5.7, for example, illustrates the application of this concept to the measurement of the absolute threshold for hearing. The *shaded* low-level excitation represents the presence of random sensory noise that is presumed to be present at all times in the auditory system. For example, random spontaneous activity of nerve fibers might be the source of this internal noise background. The two excitation patterns at the extreme left in Figure 5.7A illustrate the excitation evoked by a low-frequency (200 Hz) puretone presented at two different levels; the lower one (*solid*) is just below threshold while the upper one (*open*) is at threshold. The *open patterns* in the center (1000 Hz) and at the right (5000 Hz) illustrate excitation patterns at threshold for middle- and high-frequency sounds. It is apparent that, for the patterns at threshold at each frequency, at the place associated with the point of maximum excitation (the peak of the excitation pattern), the excitation associated with the tone exceeds that of the internal noise, resulting in the detection of that tone.

The actual results obtained from measurement of hearing threshold at various frequencies are depicted in Figure 5.7 (Sivian and White, 1933). Note that the sound pressure level required for detection varies with frequency, especially below 500 Hz and above 8,000 Hz. It is apparent that the contour of the hearing threshold has a minimum in the 2,000 to 4,000 Hz range. This is attributable, in large part, to the amplification of signals in this frequency range by the outer ear. The range of audibility of the normal-hearing human ear is described frequently as 20 to 20,000 Hz. That is, frequencies above or below this range cannot be heard by the normal human ear.

Masking

The excitation-pattern concept is also helpful in understanding the phenomenon of masking. The masking of

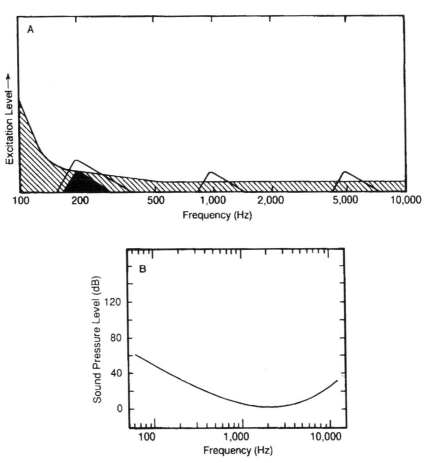

Figure 5.7. A, Schematic representation of excitation patterns corresponding to hearing thresholds at 200, 1000, and 5000 Hz. Two intensities are illustrated at 200 Hz. The *solid triangle* represents an intensity below threshold. Note that the tone's excitation never exceeds the excitation resulting from the internal noise. The *open triangles* at each frequency represent an intensity corresponding to threshold in which the excitation associated with the tone just exceeds the excitation resulting from the internal noise. **B,** Actual hearing thresholds obtained by Sivian and White (1933).

puretone signals by noise, for example, has been studied extensively. To consider the results that have been obtained, however, we must first examine some important acoustic parameters of the masking noise. Briefly, there are two measures of intensity that can be used to describe the amplitude of a noise. These two measures are the total power (TP) and the noise power per unit bandwidth or spectral density (N_o). The total power is the quantity measured by most measuring devices, such as sound level meters. The spectral density of the noise, on the other hand, is not measured directly. Rather, it is calculated from the following formula: N_o in dB = TP in dB–10 log BW, where N_o in dB = spectrum level, TP in dB = total power and BW = bandwidth of the noise. The spectrum level represents the average noise power in a 1-Hz band.

For broad-band noise, the spectrum level determines the masking produced by that noise at various frequencies. This is illustrated with the help of the excitation-pattern concept in Figure 5.8A. The masking at two different noise-masker intensities is illustrated here. The two levels of excitation of the broad-band masker are illustrated by the *horizontal solid lines* labeled *x* and *y*. The

open excitation patterns represent tones at masked threshold, while the *solid patterns* reflect the tone at threshold without the masker present. Note that the peak of the tone's excitation pattern at masked threshold just exceeds the excitation produced by the noise in all cases, indicating that the tone is just detectable. The left pattern illustrates a case in which the lower noise level (*x*) is too low to exceed the internal noise associated with quiet threshold. Thus, even though the noise is presented to the listener's ear, it fails to produce any masking. That is, the threshold for the tone with the noise is the same as that without the noise. This noise, therefore, is not an effective masker for the puretone signal. Masking is produced, however, at 1000 and 5000 Hz for the low level noise masker (*x*). The more intense noise masker (*y*) resulted in a masked threshold greater than quiet threshold at all three frequencies. Hence, the more intense noise is an effective masker at all three frequencies. Once the masking noise becomes an effective masker by producing a measurable amount of masking, an increase in noise level is followed by an equivalent increase in puretone threshold. That is 20-dB increase in noise level is followed by a 20-dB increase in masking.

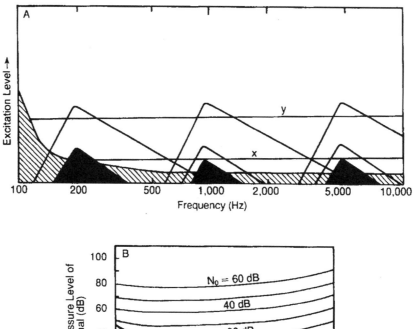

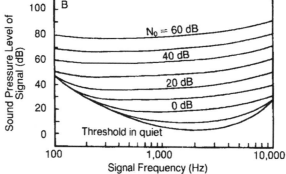

Figure 5.8. A, Excitation patterns at 200, 1000 and 5000 Hz in quiet (*solid triangles*) and in the presence of a broad-band masker at two different levels. The excitation produced by the two broad-band masker levels is represented by the *horizontal solid lines* labeled *x* and *y* (*x* < *y*). See the text for further details. **B**, Quiet threshold and masked threshold for a variety of noise levels as measured by Hawkins and Stevens (1950).

Figure 5.8B illustrates data obtained from one of the early studies of masking produced by broad-band noise (Hawkins and Stevens, 1950). These data have been replicated several times since then. The *lowest curve* in this figure depicts the threshold in quiet while all other *curves* represent masked thresholds obtained for various intensities of the noise masker. These intensities are expressed as the spectrum level of the masker. Note that the lowest noise levels are not effective maskers at low frequencies. At all frequencies, however, once the noise becomes an effective masker, a 10-dB increase in noise intensity produces a 10-dB increase in masked threshold for the puretone. Once the noise level that just begins to produce effective masking (0 dB effective masking) is determined, the desired amount of masking can be produced by simply increasing the noise level by a corresponding amount.

How might the masking produced by a noise be affected by decreasing the bandwidth of the noise? The excitation pattern concept can be used once again to provide some insight into the answer. Consider the three cases depicted in Figure 5.9. Panel **A** depicts the puretone signal at masked threshold in a broad-band noise of specified spectrum level. Panel **B** depicts the excitation pattern underlying the masked threshold for a noise masker that has the same spectrum level (reflected by the height of the noise's excitation pattern) but a narrower bandwidth. The *dashed horizontal lines labeled BW* reflect the bandwidth of the masker. Note that only the peak of the puretone signal's excitation pattern is detectable as was the case for the broad-band noise in **A.** Masked threshold remains unchanged as reflected in the height of the excitation patterns for the puretone in **A** and **B.** In Panel **C,** the bandwidth of the noise has been narrowed still further while the spectrum level remains the same. Note now that the tone's excitation pattern extends beyond that of the narrower masking noise in several places. Thus, this narrow-band masker is not effectively masking the puretone signal. The level of the puretone must be decreased to return it to masked threshold. Masked threshold, therefore, decreases for the narrow bandwidth depicted in **C.**

Figure 5.9**D** illustrates data obtained several decades ago from a masking experiment like the one just described (Fletcher, 1940). The results of this experiment, referred to frequently as the "band-narrowing" experiment, have also been replicated several times. Masked threshold in dB SPL is plotted as a function of the bandwidth of the masker in Hz. Results for two different puretone frequencies are shown. The *open circles* represent data for a 1000-Hz puretone, and the *solid circles* depict results for a 4000-Hz puretone. When the band of masking noise was narrowed, the tone always remained in the center of the noise and the spectrum level of the

noise was held constant. For a 4000-Hz puretone, for example, the signal intensity had to be about 24 dB greater than the spectrum level of a broad-band noise to be detected by the listener. This is illustrated by the *solid circle* in **D** at the far right (BW = 8000 Hz). For the same broad-band masking noise, a puretone at a frequency of 1000 Hz must be 18 dB greater than the spectrum level of the noise to be detected. For both frequencies, masked threshold remains the same as bandwidth decreases down to some bandwidth called the critical bandwidth (*CBW* in **D**). Continued decreases in bandwidth beyond the critical bandwidth reduce the masking produced by the noise as reflected by the decrease in masked threshold.

The critical bandwidth, first derived from the band-narrowing masking experiment, has proven to be a concept that applies to a wide variety of psychoacoustic phenomena. For the audiologist, one of the most important implications drawn from the band-narrowing experiment just described is that a band of noise having a bandwidth just exceeding the critical bandwidth is as effective a masker for a puretone centered in the noise as a broad-band noise of the same spectrum level. As described in Chapter 8, the audiologist frequently needs to introduce masking into a patient's ear. A broad-band masking noise can be uncomfortably loud to a patient. The loudness of the noise, however, can be reduced by decreasing the bandwidth of the noise while maintaining the same spectrum level. Hence, a masking noise having a bandwidth only slightly greater than the critical bandwidth will be just as effective as a broad-band noise in terms of its masking capability, but much less loud. The narrower band of noise, therefore, would be more appropriate for use with patients.

Loudness

Loudness is another psychoacoustic phenomenon that can be at least partially understood by means of the excitation-pattern concept. The effects of signal bandwidth on loudness alluded to above in the masking example, for instance, have been described in detail utilizing the excitation-pattern concept (Zwicker and Scharf, 1965). Basically, as the bandwidth of the stimulus increases beyond the critical bandwidth, an increasing number of adjacent critical bands are stimulated, resulting in an increase in loudness. Thus, broad-band signals are louder than narrow-band signals of the same spectrum level.

Loudness for puretones also varies with frequency. This has been established using the matching procedure described previously. Figure 5.10**A** depicts so-called equal loudness contours that have been derived with this technique (Robinson and Dadson, 1956). A given contour displays the sound pressure levels required at vari-

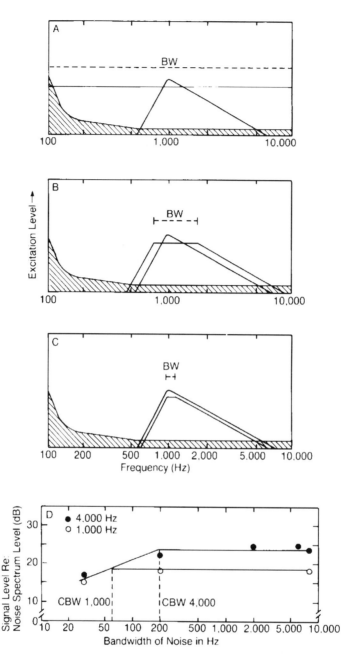

Figure 5.9. Schematic illustration of the critical bandwidth as measured in the band-narrowing experiment. **A,** Masked threshold for tone at 1000 Hz in broad-band noise. *Horizontal dashed line* labeled *BW* corresponds to bandwidth of noise masker. **B,** Spectrum level of noise (vertical displacement of noise masker) is same as in **A,** but bandwidth is narrowed as indicated by *dashed line* labeled *BW*. The tone's triangular excitation pattern is the same as in **A.** There is no change in masked threshold. **C,** Bandwidth of the masking noise is narrowed further. If the tone at 1000 Hz remains at the same intensity as in **A** and **B,** as is shown in **C,** the tone would be more easily detected. Tone intensity would need to be decreased below that shown in **C** to keep the tone at threshold (just detectable). **D,** Data from band-narrowing or band-limiting experiment obtained by Fletcher (1940) for puretones at 1000 and 4000 Hz. The *solid lines* were fit to the data by Fletcher. Note that at both signal frequencies masked threshold is unchanged for a wide range of bandwidths until a particular bandwidth, the critical bandwidth (*CBW*), is reached. As bandwidth decreases below the CBW, the tone becomes easier to hear and masked threshold decreases.

ous frequencies so as to match the loudness of a 1000-Hz puretone at the level indicated by the contour. For example, note that on the *curve* labeled *20* the function coincides with a sound pressure level of 20 dB SPL at 1000 Hz while the *curve* labeled *60* corresponds to 60 dB SPL at 1000 Hz. The contour labeled *60* indicates those combinations of frequencies and intensities that were matched in loudness to a 60-dB SPL 1000-Hz puretone.

All combinations of stimulus intensity and frequency lying along that contour are said to have a loudness level of 60 phons. Thus, a 100-Hz puretone at 70 dB SPL (*point A*) in Figure 5.10**A** and a 5000-Hz tone at 55 dB SPL (*point B*) are equivalent in loudness to 60-dB SPL 1000-Hz puretone. All three of those stimuli have a loudness level of 60 phons.

Notice in Figure 5.10**A** that stimulus intensity would have to be increased 115 dB to go from a loudness level of 5 phons (threshold) to 120 phons at 1000 Hz, but only roughly a 100-dB increase is required at 100 Hz to span that same change in loudness. From this we can conclude that loudness grows more rapidly at low frequencies. That is, it took only a 100-dB increase in sound level to go from a sound that was just audible (5 phons) to one that was uncomfortably loud (120 phons) at 100 Hz, whereas an increase of 115 dB was needed to cover this same range of loudness at 1000 Hz. Moore (1982) has indicated that the excitation pattern concept can assist in understanding this phenomenon. Figure 5.10**B** illustrates a low-frequency and high-frequency excitation pattern in Moore's scheme. Low-frequency excitation patterns are broader than those for high frequency signals, especially at high intensities. This is represented

schematically in the excitation patterns of Figure 5.10**B**. The *dashed excitation patterns* depict the excitation associated with a higher stimulus level. Notice that the amount of change at a given location is the same for both high and low frequencies but that a greater number of receptors (hair cells or attached nerve fibers) underlying the low-frequency pattern would receive the increase in excitation because it is spread over a larger area. Hence, loudness would grow more rapidly for the low-frequency sound once threshold was exceeded.

Another scale of loudness that has been developed, aside from loudness level in phons, is the sone scale. The sone scale is derived by first defining the loudness of a 1000-Hz 40-dB SPL puretone as 1 sone. Next, the listener is asked to set the intensity of a second comparison stimulus to an intensity that produces a loudness sensation either one-half or twice that of the 1-sone standard stimulus. These intensities define the sound levels associated with 1/2 and 2 sones, respectively. This procedure is then repeated with the sounds having a loudness of either 1/2 or 2 sones serving as the new standard signals. Figure 5.11 illustrates the growth of loudness in sones with increase in sound intensity. Consistent with Steven's law described previously, we find that the loudness-growth function is a straight line when plotted on log-log coordinates with the exception of intensities near threshold. The slope of this line at higher intensities is 0.6, indicating that Steven's law for loudness is: $L = kP^{0.6}$, where L is loudness, k is a constant and P is sound pressure. Note that over the linear range of the function in Figure 5.11 a 10-dB increase in sound level yields a doubling of loudness.

The *dashed line* in Figure 5.11 illustrates a loudness-growth function obtained at 1000 Hz in the presence of a broad-band masking noise. The intersection of the x-axis and the *dashed line* at 40 dB SPL indicates that threshold has been elevated 40 dB (from 0 to 40 dB SPL) due to

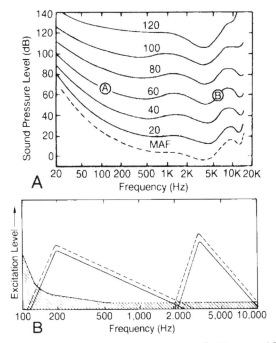

A

B

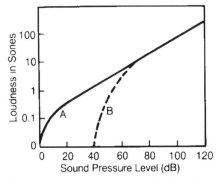

Figure 5.10. A, Equal-loudness contours from Robinson and Dadson (1956). The number above each curve corresponds to the loudness level in phons of all tones along the labeled contour. See the text for explanation of *points* labeled *A* and *B* and the 60-phon contour. B, Explanation of equal-loudness contours using the excitation pattern concept advanced by Moore (1982). Two sets of excitation patterns are shown at a low frequency and a high frequency. The *dashed excitation patterns* represent a comparable increase in signal intensity at each frequency.

Figure 5.11. Loudness-growth functions obtained from normal hearers in quiet (**A**) and in the presence of a broad-band masking noise (**B**). Note that loudness is reduced near masked threshold but is the same as in quiet at high intensities. (Adapted from Yost and Nielsen, 1977.)

the masking noise. As intensity is increased slightly above threshold, comparison of the two functions indicates that the loudness of a 45-dB SPL tone is greater in the quiet condition (about 1.5 sones) versus the masked condition (about 0.2 sone). At higher intensities, however, the two functions merge so that an 80-dB SPL tone has a loudness of 16 sones in both cases. Thus, in the masked condition, loudness grows very rapidly to "catch up" with the loudness perceived in the unmasked ear. This rapid growth of loudness is also a characteristic of ears that have a type of hearing loss affecting the hair cells within the cochlea known as sensory-neural hearing loss. The rapid growth of loudness in ears with cochlear hearing loss is known as loudness recruitment (see Chapter 11).

Pitch

The perception of pitch for puretones can also be explained, at least in part, through excitation patterns. We have seen that excitation patterns for different frequencies have their peaks located at different places along the basilar membrane. Excitation patterns of high-frequency puretones have their peaks located in the base, while those for low-frequency puretones are located in the apical region of the cochlea. For puretones, there is a monotonic relationship between pitch and frequency. That is, as frequency increases, pitch increases. Thus, we could say that puretones having high pitch are associated with excitation patterns having their peaks in the base, while low pitches are perceived when the excitation pattern indicates maximum excitation in the apex. This is known as the place theory of pitch perception. Each place along the basilar membrane is associated with a different pitch, with pitch decreasing from base to apex. This place information, moreover, is preserved throughout the pathways of the auditory system in the form of tonotopic organization.

As was the case for loudness, direct-scaling procedures have been used to construct a scale of pitch. This scale is known as the mel scale. The reference or standard for this scale is a 1000-Hz 40-dB SPL puretone that is said to have a pitch of 1000 mels. (Notice that a 40-dB SPL 1000-Hz puretone has a loudness of 1 sone, a loudness level of 40 phons, and a pitch of 1000 mels.) The listener is then asked to adjust the frequency of the puretone until its pitch is either twice that or half that of the standard. These values then become new standards and the procedure is repeated. An example of the resulting mel scale obtained from such a procedure is shown as the *solid function* in Figure 5.12. Note that as the frequency of the puretone signal increases, the pitch in mels also increases. The *dashed function* indicates the mapping of frequency to place of maximum displacement along the basilar membrane (tonotopic organiza-

tion). The close correspondence between these two functions suggests that the psychologic separation between the pitch of two tones corresponds roughly to the physical separation of the peak activity produced along the basilar membrane by the same two tones. These data are supportive of a place theory of pitch perception.

The place theory of pitch perception, however, is not the only theory that can explain the pitch perception of puretones. Another viable possibility is that the phase-locked firing pattern of neural discharges that encodes the period of the waveform is responsible for the perceived pitch. For puretones, the period (T) and frequency (f) are inversely related ($T = 1/f$). The mel scale indicates that pitch increases with frequency or the reciprocal of the period. Thus, it may be the coding of the period that is mediating the perception of pitch for puretones. This is generally referred to as the periodicity theory or temporal theory of pitch perception. Physiologic data from auditory nerve fibers indicate that the maximum puretone frequency for which the nerve fibers can preserve the period via phase locking is approximately 5000 Hz. Periodicity, therefore, cannot account for the perception of pitch for puretones having frequencies greater than 5000 Hz.

Evidence can be gathered to support either the place theory or the periodicity theory regarding the perceived pitch of puretones. Perhaps the strongest evidence that timing information or periodicity can be utilized to code pitch comes from a series of experiments with a phenomenon known as the "missing fundamental." An example of the stimulus used to produce the missing fundamental is shown in Figure 5.13. Figure 5.13A displays the amplitude spectrum. Four puretones separated in frequency by 100-Hz intervals (700, 800, 900, and 1000 Hz), but of the same starting phase and same amplitude are presented to the listener. These four puretones are the seventh, eighth, ninth, and tenth harmonics of a

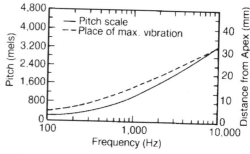

Figure 5.12. Illustration of the close correspondence between pitch and point of maximum vibration of the basilar membrane. The *solid line* represents direct scaling of pitch of puretones (mel scale), while the *dashed line* represents the basilar membrane data. Note that as the peak displacement moves from the apex to the base of the cochlea with increase in frequency, the pitch sensation evoked by the same frequencies changes in a similar manner.

fundamental frequency of 100 Hz. The fundamental it-self, however, is *not* present in the stimulus. Yet, the pitch perceived in this situation is one corresponding to the fundamental (100 Hz). Figure 5.13**B** illustrates the wave-form that results from the addition of these four pure-tones. Note that the waveform has a period of 10 msec. That is, it repeats itself every 10 msec. The reciprocal of a 10-msec period is 100 Hz. This corresponds to the pitch perceived by the listener when presented with this com-plex sound. The addition of a low-frequency masking noise, moreover, does not mask the 100-Hz pitch. This is further evidence that the place in the inner ear associ-ated with a frequency of 100 Hz is not responsible for this low pitch. Although the explanation of the situation de-picted in Figure 5.13 is somewhat oversimplified (Patter-son, 1973), it still remains true that the place theory cannot explain the missing fundamental.

The case of the missing fundamental just described demonstrates that timing information can be used to en-code pitch. There are other examples, however, that support a place theory of pitch perception. Current thinking about pitch perception suggests that only the temporal mechanism holds for frequencies below 50 Hz and only the place theory can describe pitch perception for frequencies above 5000 Hz. For frequencies between 50 and 5000 Hz, both mechanisms probably play a role (Moore, 1982; Warren, 1982).

Frequency and Intensity Discrimination

Another psychoacoustic phenomenon that has been studied in considerable detail and can be explained, al-though not entirely (see Moore, 1982), via excitation patterns is the ability of the ear to detect changes in ei-ther the intensity or frequency of a puretone. These tasks are often referred to as intensity and frequency dis-crimination tasks. Figure 5.14**A** depicts excitation pat-terns for a frequency discrimination task in which two puretones differing in frequency by a certain amount (Δf) are presented separately to the listener. The differ-ence in frequency (Δf) is adjusted until the change in ex-citation (ΔE) at a certain place exceeds some minimally detectable value. The data obtained from such an exper-iment are depicted in Figure 5.14**B** (Weir et al., 1977). Note that Δf increases with frequency and decreases with intensity. Thus, the smallest Δf values are obtained at high intensities for low frequencies while the largest δf values occur in the high frequencies at low intensities. For example, although two tones 80 dB above threshold with frequencies of 500 and 501 Hz could be discrimi-nated, frequencies of 8000 and 8083 Hz would be re-quired for discrimination at these same levels.

The case for intensity discrimination is depicted in the *lower portion* of Figure 5.14. The excitation patterns underlying the intensity discrimination task are shown in Figure 5.14**C.** Note that the patterns are located at the same place, indicating that they have the same fre-quency. They differ only in intensity as reflected by the height of the patterns. When the change in intensity (ΔI) produces a sufficient change in the underlying exci-tation (ΔE), the two tones can be discriminated. Results from a detailed study of intensity discrimination are pro-vided in Figure 5.14**D** (Jesteadt et al., 1977). Note that ΔI decreases with intensity, indicating, for example, that two puretones of 80 and 80.5 dB SPL could be discrimi-nated, but two at 20 and 20.5 dB SPL could not. At this lower intensity a difference of 1.3 dB would be required (20 versus 21.3 dB SPL). Intensity discrimination does

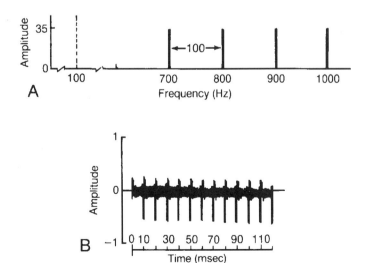

Figure 5.13. Amplitude spectrum (**A**) and waveform (**B**) of a com-plex sound consisting of four puretones of frequencies 700, 800, 900, and 1000 Hz presented simultaneously to the listener. See the text for explanation. (From Yost WA, and Nielsen DW. Fundamentals of Hearing: an Introduction. New York: Holt, Rinehart and Winston, 1977.)

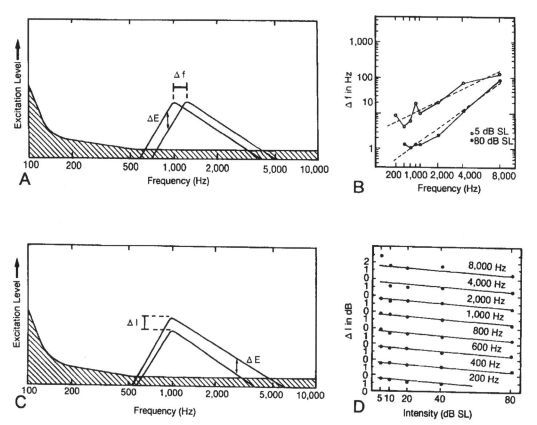

Figure 5.14. A, Explanation of frequency discrimination task using excitation patterns for two puretones of equal intensity but separated in frequency by Δ*f* Hz. Δ*E* refers to the change in excitation that occurs with the change in signals. For frequency discrimination, the change is greatest in the region indicated by Δ*E*. **B,** Frequency discrimination thresholds (Δ*f*) obtained by Wier et al. (1977). **C,** Excitation patterns for intensity discrimination of two puretones of the same frequency but differing in intensity by Δ*I* dB. Δ*E* again refers to change in excitation associated with the change in intensity. For intensity discrimination, the change is greatest in the region indicated by Δ*E*. **D,** Δ*I* in dB as a function of stimulus level and stimulus frequency. (From Jesteadt W, Wier CC, and Green DM. Intensity discrimination as a function of frequency and sensation level. J Acoust Soc Am 1977; 61:169–177.)

not appear to vary with signal frequency. The decrease in Δ*I* with increase in intensity can also be explained through the changes in the shapes of the excitation patterns as intensity is increased. Florentine and Buus (1982) have provided a detailed description of an excitation pattern model of intensity discrimination.

In summary, we have seen that the excitation-pattern concept can explain, in a fairly simple manner, a wide variety of psychoacoustic phenomena. All psychoacoustic phenomena reviewed thus far have been monaural phenomena. That is, all stimuli were delivered to one ear. The next section of this chapter deals with the manner in which the information encoded by one ear interacts with that encoded by the other ear. The processing of sound by two ears is referred to as binaural hearing.

Binaural Hearing

Regarding absolute hearing threshold and difference thresholds for frequency and intensity (Δ*f* and Δ*I*), two ears are generally more sensitive than one. Hearing thresholds, for example, are approximately 2 to 3 dB better when both ears receive the signal than when it is delivered to just one ear. Similarly, difference thresholds for frequency (Δ*f*) and intensity (Δ*I*) obtained binaurally are about two-thirds the size of those obtained monaurally (Jesteadt and Weir, 1977).

Sound Localization

Aside from enhanced sensitivity associated with the use of two ears, however, there are some tasks that can only be performed with reasonable accuracy by using two ears. The localization of sound in space, for intance, is largely a binaural phenomenon. A sound originating from the right side of a listener, for example, will result in the sound arriving first to the right ear because it is closer to the sound source. A brief time later the sound will reach the more distant left ear. This produces an interaural difference in time of arrival of the sound at the two ears. The ear being stimulated first will signal the direction from which the sound arose. As might be expected, the magnitude of this interaural time difference will decrease as the sound source changes from straight out to the side (90- or 270-degree azimuth) to straight ahead (0-degree azimuth). That is, when the sound originates directly in front of the listener the length of the path to both ears is the same and there is no interaural difference in time of arrival of the sound. At the extreme right or left, however, the difference in the length of the paths to the near ear and the far ear is greatest (corresponds to the width of the head). This then will produce the maximum interaural time difference. This situation is depicted in Figure 5.15.

For frequencies below approximately 1500 Hz, the interaural time difference could also be encoded meaningfully into an interaural phase difference. From Figure 5.15**B**, for example, we see that at 60-degree azimuth an interaural time difference of approximately 0.5 msec results. This would occur for all frequencies. For a puretone that completes one cycle in 1 msec (frequency =

1000 Hz), this means the signal to the far ear would be starting one-half cycle after the signal to the near ear. The two signals, therefore, would have a 180-degree phase difference between the two ears. A puretone of 500 Hz having a 2-msec period and also originating from 60-degree azimuth, however, would only be delayed one-fourth of the period (0.5 msec/2.0 msec), corresponding to a 90-degree interaural phase difference. Thus, although interaural time differences are the same for all frequencies, interaural phase differences resulting from these time differences vary with frequency.

Interaural intensity differences are also produced when a sound originates from a location in space. These differences result from a sound shadow being cast by the head. When the wavelength of the sound is small relative to the dimensions of the head, a sound shadow is produced. The magnitude of the sound shadow effect created by the head increases with frequency above 500 Hz (Shaw, 1974). It produces interaural intensity differences of 20 dB at 6000 Hz for 90- or 270-degree azimuth. That is, the intensity of a 6000-Hz puretone at the near ear is 20 dB greater than that measured at the far ear when the sound originates straight to the side of the listener (90- or 270-degree azimuth). At 500 Hz, the maximum interaural intensity difference is less than 4 dB. The interaural intensity difference decreases to 0 dB at all frequencies for 0-degree azimuth (straight ahead).

Thus, there are two primary acoustical cues for the localization of sound in space (specifically, in the horizontal plane): interaural time differences and interaural intensity differences. The duplex theory of sound localization (Stevens and Newman, 1936) maintains that both cues may be utilized over a wide range of frequencies by the listener in identifying the location of a sound source, but that interaural time differences predominate at low frequencies and interaural intensity differences at high frequencies.

Masking Level Difference

Masking is a topic that has also been explored in considerable detail in the binaural system. Experiments conducted over three decades ago indicated that certain combinations of binaural signals and maskers could make the signal more detectable than others (Hirsh, 1948; Licklider, 1948). Consider the following example. A noise masker and puretone signal are presented equally and identically to both ears. The signal threshold is then determined. Then the puretone signal is removed from one ear and the signal becomes easier to detect. This release from masking has been named the masking level difference (MLD) and corresponds to the change in threshold between the two test conditions. The initial or reference threshold is usually determined

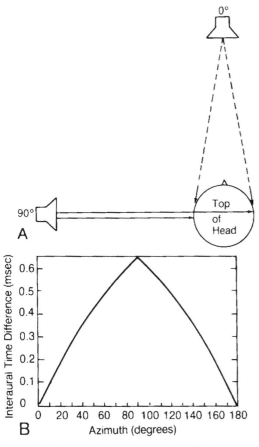

Figure 5.15. A, Schematic illustration of length of sound path to each ear for 0° and 90° azimuth. The sound would arrive to both ears simultaneously for 0° azimuth, while 90° azimuth would produce a difference in time of sound arrival between the two ears. **B,** Data from Feddersen et al. (1957) on variation of interaural time difference with azimuth of the sound source.

for identical maskers and signals delivered to both ears. This is referred to as a diotic condition. Diotic stimulus presentations are those that deliver identical stimuli to both ears. Sometimes the reference threshold involves a masker and signal delivered to only one ear. This is called a monotic condition. After establishing masked threshold in one of these reference conditions, signal threshold is measured again under any of several dichotic conditions. A dichotic test condition is one in which different stimuli are presented to the two ears. In the example described above in which the signal was removed from one ear, the removal of the signal made that condition a dichotic one. That is, one ear received the noise masker and puretone signal while the other received only the noise masker. In general, a signal is detected more readily under dichotic masking conditions than under diotic or monotic masking conditions. For a given dichotic condition, the MLD is greatest at low frequencies (100 to 500 Hz), increases with the intensity of the masker and is typically <15 dB under optimal stimulus conditions. Reviews of binaural hearing have been provided by Jeffress (1975) for sound localization and by Green and Yost (1975) for binaural masking. Clinical applications of the MLD are reviewed in Chapter 15.

APPLICATION TO HEARING-IMPAIRED LISTENERS

The excitation-pattern concept can also be applied to results obtained from psychoacoustic studies of hearing-impaired ears to assist in their interpretation. Unless otherwise specified, the term "hearing-impaired" will imply a sensory-neural hearing loss. Many basic issues regarding the perception of sound by hearing-impaired listeners are as yet unresolved. For recent reviews of the effects of sensory-neural hearing loss on sound perception, the reader is referred to Humes, Espinoza-Varas and Watson (1988), Glasberg and Moore (1989), and Humes and Jestcadt (1991).

Durlach et al. (1981) provide an excellent review of the results obtained from studies of binaural hearing in listeners having sensory-neural hearing loss. Also, much work in this area has been conducted with laboratory animals in which the hearing loss and other perceptual deficits can be correlated directly to the extent of damage observed anatomically. This literature has been reviewed by Humes and Konkle (1980).

In cochlear cases, it is usually assumed that the puretone hearing thresholds accurately reflect the underlying pathology at the various frequencies. This basic tenet of puretone audiometric testing has been challenged along several lines in recent years. Results obtained by Thornton and Abbas (1980) in a study of four listeners with low-frequency sensory-neural hearing losses, for example, indicated that the severity of low-frequency hearing loss may be underestimated by as much as 30 dB in some

cases. In their study, results from two of the four listeners indicated that individuals manifesting moderate low-frequency hearing loss may not be detecting the low-frequency puretone signal in the low-frequency region of the cochlea. Rather, as a consequence of upward spread of excitation, these listeners may be detecting it in their normal-hearing high-frequency region. This situation is depicted schematically in Figure 5.16. The *shaded rectangular region* is a schematic representation of a low-frequency hearing loss. The two *triangular patterns* represent the patterns of excitation generated within the auditory system for two tones of frequency F_1 and F_2 at threshold. Notice that the lower frequency signal, F_1, is detected at the place corresponding to a frequency of $F1$ and therefore provides an accurate reflection of the severity of the underlying lesion at the F_1 site. A higher frequency tone located nearer to the edge of the lesion, such as F_2 in Figure 5.16, on the other hand, is not detected at the place corresponding to F_2. Rather, it is detected in the high-frequency region where hearing is normal.

Thornton and Abbas (1980), measuring psychophysical tuning curves and masking patterns, demonstrated that some listeners detect remote portions of the excitation patterns of low-frequency tones. In the case of the masking pattern, for example, threshold was measured at several frequencies in the presence of a high-intensity (70 to 100 dB SPL) high-frequency puretone masker. The masker frequency was positioned along the rising portion of the audiogram. Results from a single normal listener indicated, as expected, that masking did not spread in a downward direction more than one octave for the range of masker levels employed. Comparable masked thresholds from the hearing-impaired subjects, however, revealed substantial threshold elevations for low-frequency signals that were several octaves below the

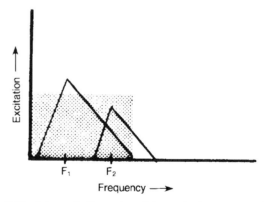

Figure 5.16. Schematic illustration of the excitation patterns of two tones of differing frequency (F_1 and F_2) at threshold in an individual with low-frequency sensory-neural hearing loss. The *shaded area* represents the low-frequency hearing loss. Notice that the presence of the higher frequency tone (F_2) is detected within the listener's region of normal hearing and not at F_2.

masker. Thornton and Abbas (1980) argued that this unusual masking behavior resulted from the low-frequency puretone signal being detected in quiet at a more remote high-frequency region in the manner described above Fig. 5.16. The introduction of a puretone masker in this same high-frequency region, however, eliminated this remote cue and forced the detection of the signal to take place in the low-frequency region of the cochlea. Thus, the masked low-frequency thresholds provided a more accurate indication of the severity of damage in the low-frequency region of the cochlea. The results from the tuning curve experiments, and some data obtained on the perception of filtered speech, also supported this basic conclusion.

The results of Thornton and Abbas (1980) have been confirmed, at least in part, by Turner and Nelson (1982), Florentine (1982), Goldstein et al. (1983) and Humes et al. (1984). In the latter study, it was demonstrated that hearing-impaired listeners with low-frequency hearing losses could detect a tone placed within their region of normal hearing sensitivity (situation suggested by the tone at F_2 in Fig. 5.16). This only occurred, however, when the tone frequency was less than an octave below the edge of the hearing loss and only when the slope of the loss was greater than 25 dB per octave.

SUMMARY

This chapter has provided a brief review of psychoacoustics from general psychophysical methods to specific psychoacoustic phenomena, such as pitch and loudness. The excitation-pattern concept comprised the framework around which the review of psychoacoustic phenomena was formulated. Although this concept can provide insight into may psychoacoustic phenomena, some difficulties arise when it is used to explain all details of some phenomena. Our understanding of the perceptual deficits experienced by listeners having sensory-neural hearing loss can be understood, to some extent, with the assistance of the excitation-pattern concept. Much more data from impaired ears are needed, however, before the excitation-pattern concept can be applied to sound perception in hearing-impaired listeners.

REFERENCES

Barry SJ, and Kidd GJ. Psychophysical scaling of distorted speech. J Speech Hear Res 1981;24:44–47

Durlach NI, Thompson CL, and Colburn HS. 1981. Binaural interaction in impaired listeners: a review of past research. Audiology 1981;20:181–211.

Fechner GT. Element der Psychophysik. Leipzig: Breitkopf & Harterl, 1860.

Fedderson WE, Sandel TT, Teas DC, and Jeffress LA. Localization of high-frequency tones. J Acoust Soc Am 1957;29:988–991.

Fletcher H. Auditory patterns. Rev Mod Phys 1940;12:47–65.

Florentine M. Tuning curves and pitch matches in unilateral, low-frequency hearing loss: a case study. Paper presented at the Acoustical Society of America, Orlando, FL, 1982.

Florentine M, and Buus S. 1981. An excitation-pattern model for intensity discrimination. J Acoust Soc Am 1981;70:1646–1654

Gescheider GA. Psychophysics: Method and Theory. Hillsdale, NJ: Lawrence Erlbaum Associates, 1976.

Glasberg BR, and Moore BCJ. Psychoacoustic abilities of subjects with unilateral and bilateral cochlear hearing impairments and their relationship to the ability to understand speech. Scand Audiol 1989;32(Suppl):1–25.

Goldstein R, Karlovich RS, Tweed TS, and Kile JE. Psychoacoustic tuning curves and averaged electroencephalic responses in a patient with low-frequency sensory-neural hearing loss. J Speech Hear Disord 1983;48:70–75.

Green DM, and Swets JA. Signal Detection Theory and Psychophysics. Huntington, NY: R.E. Krieger, 1974.

Green DM, and Yost WA. Binaural analysis. In Keidel WD, and Neff WD, Eds. Handbook of Sensory Physiology, Vol. 2. New York: Springer, 1975.

Harris RW, and Goldstein DP. Hearing aid quality judgements by magnitude estimation. Paper presented at the American Speech-Language-Hearing Association, Detroit, MI, 1980.

Hawkins JE, and Stevens SS. The masking of pure tones and of speech by white noise. J Acoust Soc Am 1950;22:6–13.

Hirsh IIJ. The influence of interaural phase on interaural summation and inhibition. J Acoust Soc Am 1948;20:536–544.

Humes LE. Spectral and temporal resolution by the hearing impaired. In Studebaker GA, and Bess FH, Eds. The Vanderbilt Hearing-Aid Report. Upper Darby, PA: Monographs in Contemporary Audiology, 1982.

Humes LE, Tharpe AM, and Bratt GW. The validity of hearing thresholds obtained from the rising portion of the audiogram in sensorineural hearing loss. J Speech Hear Res 1984;27:206–211.

Humes LE, Espinoza-Varas B, and Watson CS. Modeling sensorineural hearing loss, I. Model and retrospective evaluation. J Acoust Soc Am 1988;83:188–202.

Jeffress LA. Sound localization. In Keidel WD, and Neff WD, Eds. Handbook of Sensory Psy[?]iology. Vol. 2. New York: Springer, 1975.

Jesteadt W, and Weir CC. Comparison of monaural and binaural discrimination of intensity and frequency. J Acoust Soc Am 1977;61:1599–1603.

Jesteadt W, and Wier CC, and Green DM. Intensity discrimination as a function of frequency and sensation level. J Acoust Soc Am 1977;61:169–177.

Knight KK and Margolis RH. Magnitude estimation of loudness, II: Loudness perception in presbycusic listeners. J Speech Hear Res 1984;27:28–32.

Lawson GD, and Chial MR. Magnitude estimation of degraded speech quality by normal and impaired-hearing listeners. J Acoust Soc Am 1982;72:1781–1787.

Levitt H. Transformed up-down methods in psychoacoustics. J Acoust Soc Am 1971;49:467–477.

Licklider JCR. Influence of interaural phase relations upon the masking of speech by white noise. J Acoust Soc Am 1948;20:150–159.

Moore BC. An Introduction to the Psychology of Hearing. London: Academic Press, 1982.

Patterson RD. The effects of relative phase and the number of components on residue pitch. J Acoust Soc Am 1973;53:1565–1572.

Robinson DW, and Dadson RS. A redetermination of the equal loudness relations for puretones. Br J Appl Phys 1956;7:166–181.

Scharf B, and Florentine M. Psychoacoustics of elementary sounds. In Studebaker GA, and Bess FH, Eds. The Vanderbilt Hearing-aid Report. Upper Darby, PA: Monographs in Contemporary Audiology, 1982.

Shaw EAG. The external ear. In Keidel WD and Neff WD, Eds. Handbook of Sensory Physiology, Vol. 1. New York: Springer, 1974.

Sivian LJ, and White SD. On minimum audible fields. J Acoust Soc Am 1933;4:288–321.

Stevens SS. Psychophysics. New York: John Wiley & Sons, 1975.

Stevens SS, and Newman EB. The localization of actual sources of sound. Am J Acoust Soc Am 1936;73:297–306.

Thalmann R. Cross-modality matching in the study of abnormal loudness functions. J Acoust Soc Am 1965;73:297–311.

Thornton AR, and Abbas PJ. Low-frequency hearing loss: perception of filtered speech, psychophysical tuning curves, and masking. J Acoust Soc Am 1980;67:638–743.

Turner CW, and Nelson DA. Pitch perception in low-frequency hearing-loss listeners. Paper presented at the Acoustical Society of America, Chicago, IL, 1982.

Warren RM. Auditory Perception: A New Synthesis. New York: Pergamon Press, 1982.

Weir CC, Jesteadt W, and Green DM. Frequency discrimination as a function of frequency and sensation level. J Acoust Soc Am 1977;61:178–184.

Yost WA, and Nielsen DW. Fundamentals of Hearing: An Introduction. New York: Holt, Rinehart and Winston, 1977.

Zwicker E. Masking and psychological excitation as consequences of the ear's frequency analysis. In Plomp R, and Smoorenburg GF, Eds. Frequency Analysis and Periodicity Detection in Hearing. Leiden: A.W. Sijthoff, 1970.

Zwicker E, and Scharf B. A model of loudness summation. Psychol Rev 1965;72:3–26.

Zwislocki J, Maire R, Feldman A, and Ruben A. On the effect of practice and motivation on the threshold of audibility. J Acoust Soc Am 1958;30:254–262

CHAPTER 6

Calibration, Puretone, Speech and Noise Signals

Laura Ann Wilber

WHY CALIBRATE

In the first edition of this handbook, when the question "Why Calibrate?" was first asked, it was apparent that many clinicians believed that calibration was something that researchers did, and that such procedures did not seem to be necessary in the clinic. Today that attitude has changed dramatically. For example, the Professional Service Board (PSB) of the American Speech-Language-Hearing Association (ASHA) now requires regular calibration checks of clinic equipment (ASHA, 1984). The Occupational Safety and Health (OSHA) regulations (1983) also require that screening equipment be regularly checked. Some state regulations for hearing aid dispensers or for audiologists require that equipment calibration be maintained. Further, many state health departments concerned with school screening also insist on having calibration checked on a routine basis. Thus, we have learned, if nothing else, that we must calibrate if we are to meet the current regulations.

Most clinicians recognize that the initial audiometric calibration provided by the manufacturer is insufficient to guarantee that the audiometer will remain that way over time. In various clinics and laboratories we have found audiometers that emitted no frequencies above 1500 Hz although the dial continued to rotate normally. Other new audiometers were found to have differences of as much as 20 dB between air-conduction and bone-conduction hearing levels. One audiometer that we checked had no output below 25 dB. Thomas et al. (1969) described an audiometer that would not attenuate below 50 dB (thus all mild and many moderate hearing losses would have been missed.) Therefore, it can be seen that new audiometers that just arrived from the factory, as well as audiometers that were in perfect calibration when they were new can show variations in intensity, frequency, distortion, etc. Regardless of whether the audiometer is new or has been in use for some time, it is the responsibility of the user to either check its calibration personally, or to arrange for regular calibration of the equipment by outside services.

Checking calibration is necessary to be sure that an audiometer produces a puretone at the specified level and frequency, that the signal is present only in the transducer to which it is directed, and that the signal is free from distortion or unwanted noise interference. The audiologist who has demonstrated that the clinic equipment is "in calibration" can then be confident in reporting the obtained results. Calibration checks of can determine if an audiometer meets appropriate standards and also whether the instrument has changed over time.

It is the purpose of this chapter to show the audiologist who does not have an extensive electronic background how to check audiometers to see if they meet current national standards. Finally, there will be a brief discussion of the equipment that this author believes should be available in audiology facilities.

A chapter on the topic of calibration seems to be a necessary ingredient in a book on audiology. Because we generally cannot control the error of measurement produced by the client, we must put our efforts into controlling the other major sources of error to ensure the best possible results: (*a*) calibrating—educating the audiologist; and (*b*) calibrating—checking the audiometer. The other chapters in this book are devoted to educating (or calibrating) the audiologist. This chapter is devoted to calibrating the audiometer.

PARAMETERS OF CALIBRATION

Much "how to calibrate" information is available in the manuals that accompany audiometers, acoustic immittance devices, as well as the pieces of equipment used in checking or calibrating equipment. Although many of us seem to live by the slogan "When all else fails, read the manual," the first step in learning how to check calibration should always be to read the appropriate manual. Additional resources include electronic parts stores that often have basic manuals on test equipment. ASHA has a publication on earphone calibration for audiometers (ASHA, 1983). A number of recent books have also discussed procedures for acoustic measurements and equipment that might be used in such measurements (Decker, 1990; Beranek, 1988). The United States Government Printing Office is also a good source of information on basic test procedures. The specific parameters that must be checked in an audiometer are outlined in standards provided by the American National Standards Institute (ANSI) and the International Electrotechnical Commission (IEC). (see Table 6.1 for a listing of applicable standards). Some standards can also be obtained through the Acoustical Society of America (ASA) which prints copies of most of the acoustics standards that are adopted by ANSI. There is an IEC standard for audiometers (1988) and the ANSI has recently adopted a major revision of S3.6, the American National Standard Specification for Audiometers (ANSI, 1989b). The currently applicable standards may be obtained by contacting the American National Standards Institute (1430 North Broadway, New York, NY 10018) or the Standards Secretariat of the Acoustical Society of America (335 East 45th Street, New York, NY 10017). Generally the ANSI and IEC standards are in close agreement. When differences do exist (e.g., ANSI has more specific requirements for speech audiometers than does the current IEC standard), it is wise to use the ANSI standard when in the United States. The IEC standard is normally used by the rest of the world. In addition to the audiometer standard, ANSI has also approved a standard for acoustic impedance and admittance devices (ANSI, 1987b). It is beyond the scope of this chapter to discuss each area of calibration in detail. Therefore, it behooves the reader to obtain copies of the latest standards to verify the exact parameters and their permissible variability.

To better understand the procedures for checking calibration, one must first understand the parameters that need to be checked. For puretone and speech audiometers the three parameters are: (*a*) frequency, (*b*) intensity, and (*c*) time (both phase and signal duration). These parameters apply whether one is using a portable audiometer, a standard diagnostic audiometer, or a computer-based audiometric system. Standards for some parameters do not yet exist (e.g., characteristics of the acoustic stimulus used for ABR), but they should be measured nevertheless, so that one can determine if the equipment has changed over time. If or when such standards are developed, one can ascertain if past tests are likely to have been valid. Table 6.2 lists some equipment that can be used to check each of the above parameters. Although not discussed here, appropriately programmed and interfaced computers also may be used to check audiometric equipment.

Some organizations such as ASHA and OSHA specify time intervals at which calibration checks should be made in order to adhere to their standards. It is this author's opinion that with current electronic circuitry (printed circuit boards, transistors, etc. as opposed to vacuum tubes) frequency and time parameters should be checked when the audiometer is first acquired and at yearly intervals thereafter. Older equipment, especially equipment with vacuum tubes should be checked at least biannually. The output levels of all transducers (for both current and older audiometers) should be checked at trimonthly intervals or sooner if there is reason to suspect the audiometer output has changed. Research facilities generally check calibration weekly, or in some cases daily, during the running of an experiment. In addition to regularly scheduled checks, audiometers should be tested *whenever* the clinician notices anything unusual in their performance. Sometimes test results themselves reveal the need for an immediate check (e.g., obtaining the exact same hearing thresholds for two successive patients. It is always better to check the audiometer first rather than assume the problem lies with the client or clinician. A quick biologic check (described later) can always be performed and if this confirms the probability of an equipment problem, then a more elaborate electronic check should be carried out.

If the audiologist discovers that the frequency or time components of the audiometer are out of calibration, the manufacturer or representative should be contacted for immediate repair and proper calibration of the instrument. Only a qualified electronics technician should attempt to take the machine apart to rectify the problem. However, if there is a stable deviation in output level at a given frequency, calibration corrections can be made either by adjusting the trim pots (potentiometers) on the audiometer (if applicable), by using the audiometer's self-calibrating mechanism or by posting a note on the front of the audiometer indicating the corrections. The adjustment in decibels (plus or minus) that should be made at the various frequency(ies) should be shown. Most modern audiometers provide some sort of internal calibration system for air-conduction and many also provide this for bone conduction. If one plans to use bone vibrators for both mastoid and frontal bone testing, or two sets of earphones with the same audiometer (e.g., supra-aural earphones and insert receivers), it probably is advisable to use "paper corrections" rather than trying to adjust trim-pots between the use of each transducer. Unstable sound pressure level (SPL) variations or lack of attenuator linearity may require further investigation by a qualified technician. Further, if the trim-pots seem to need frequent adjustment it is probably wise to check with a qualified technician.

BASIC EQUIPMENT

The basic calibration equipment for checking output levels should include: (*a*) a voltmeter, or voltohmeter, (*b*) a condenser microphone (both pressure and free-field types), (*c*) a 6-cc coupler (ANSI requires the National Bureau of Standards [NBS] 9-A whereas IEC uses

Table 6.1
Current ANSI, IEC, and ISO Standards for Audiometers and Audiometric Testing[a]

Number	Title
ANSI S3.1-1991[b]	Maximum Permissible Ambient Noise for Audiometric Test Rooms
ANSI S3.2-1989	American National Standard Method for Measuring the Intelligibility of Speech over Communication Systems
ANSI S3.6-1989	American National Standard Specification for Audiometer
ANSI S3.7-1973[b] (R86)	American National Standard Method for Couple Calibration of Earphones
ANSI S3.13-1987	American National Standard Mechanical Coupler for Measurement of Bone Vibrators
ANSI S3.20-1973[b] (R86)	American National Standard Psychoacoustical Terminology
ANSI S3.21-1978 (R86)	American National Standard Method for Manual Puretone* Threshold Audiometry
ANSI S3.25-1989[b]	American National Standard for an Occluded Ear Simulator
ANSI S3.26-1981[b] (R 1990)	American National Standard Reference Equivalent Threshold Force Levels for Audiometric Bone Vibrators
ANSI S3.39-1987	American National Standard Specifications for Instruments to Measure Aural Acoustic Impedance and Admittance (Aural Acoustic Immittance)
ANSI S3.43-1992	Standard Reference Zero for the Calibration of Pure-Tone Bone-Conduction Audiometers
ANSI S1.5-1963 (R71)	Recommended Practices for Audio and Electro-acoustics: Loudspeaker Measurements.
ANSI S1.4-1983	American National Standard Specifications for Sound Level Meters.
ANSI S1.4A-1985	Amendment to ANSI S1.4, 1983.
ANSI C.5-1954 (R1971)	Volume measurements of electrical speech and program waves.
ANSI S4.14-1976	Magnetic Tape Recording and Reproducing (Reel-to-Reel)
ANSI S4.15-1976	Audio Cassette Recording and Reproducing
IEC 645, 1982[bc]	Part 1 - Pure-tone* Audiometers
IEC 318, 1970	An IEC artificial ear, of the wide band type, for the calibration of earphones used in audiometry.
IEC #, 1988[c]	Instrument for Measurement of Aural Acoustic Impedance/Admittance
IEC, 373, 1971	An IEC mechanical coupler for the calibration of bone vibrators having a specified contact area and being applied with a specified static force.
IEC 94-3, 1980	Magnetic tape recording and reproducing systems: Part III Methods of Measuring the characteristics of recording and reproducing equipment for sound on magnetic tape.
IEC 268-5A, 1980	Sound System Equipment Part 5: Loudspeakers.
ISO 6189, 1983.	Acoustics—pure-tone air-conduction threshold audiometry for hearing conservation purposes.
ISO 8253-1, 1989	Acoustics—audiometric test methods—Part 1: Basic pure-tone and bone conduction threshold audiometry.
ISO 389, 1964[b]	Acoustics—standard reference zero for the calibration of pure-tone audiometers
ISO 389 Addendum 1-ISO DAD-1, 1981	Acoustics—standard reference zero for the calibration of pure-tone audiometers.
ISO/DIS 7566, 1987	Acoustics—standard reference zero for the calibration of pure-tone bone-conducted audiometers and guidelines for its practical application.

*(note: The title of the standard does hyphenate pure-tone)
[a]ANSI, American National Standards Institute; ASHA, American Speech-Language-Hearing Association; IEC, International Electrotechnical Commission; ISO, International Standards Organization; ISO/DIS, Draft International Standard.
[b]Currently being revised.
[c]In press.

Table 6.2
Equipment Useful for Checking Various
Parameters of Audiometer Calibration

Parameter	Suggested Equipment
Intensity	Oscilloscope
	Voltmeter
	Condensor microphone
	Spectrometer
	Graphic level recorder
	Sound level meter
	Acoustic coupler (NBS 9-A)
	Mechanical coupler (artifical mastoid)
Frequency	Oscilloscope
	Electronic counter
	Frequency analyzer
	Distortion meter
	Spectrum analyzer
Time	Oscilloscope
	Electronic counter
	Graphic level recorder

the IEC 318 coupler), (*d*) a 500 g weight, (*e*) a mechanical coupler for bone vibrator measurements (artificial mastoid) and (*f*) a sound level meter or spectrum analyzer (or equivalent piece of equipment that allows one to read the output from an attached microphone in SPL). When purchasing any of the above components it is wise to check with others who use similar types of equipment to find the best specific brands available locally.

Although the IEC Publication 318 (1970) describes an international standard for a "true" artificial ear this has not been approved by ANSI as the appropriate device for checking calibration of audiometers. The ANSI standard currently accepts only the NBS 9-A coupler that is described in detail in the ANSI standards dealing with audiometers (ANSI S3.6-1989). Although ISO documents list other earphones, the current ANSI standard does give values for the TDH-39, TDH-49, TDH-50 and Telex 1470A as well as the WE-705 (ANSI, 1989b). It also gives values for insert receivers in its appendix.

In addition to the acoustic coupler, the mechanical coupler (artificial mastoid) should be an approved type. ANSI S3.13 "Mechanical Coupler for Measurement of Bone Vibrators" (ANSI, 1987a) describes this device.

Other equipment such as an oscilloscope (preferably a storage type), a graphic level recorder, an electronic counter, a frequency analyzer, and/ or a distortion meter will also prove to be invaluable in checking the acoustic parameters of audiometers. In many instances this latter equipment can be shared by more than one facility. Certainly their expense is such that a single-person facility is unlikely to want to bear the cost of this less frequently used electronic equipment. A rule of thumb

is that if one has only one audiometer, a service contract is most sensible. If one has two to five pieces of audiometric test equipment an "artificial ear" setup, a sound level meter, and a voltmeter are needed. With more than five pieces of audiometric equipment, a more elaborate array of electronic equipment is probably desirable. If the accuracy of the audiometer is questioned it necessitates shutting down the equipment or retesting patients at a later date. This translates into a time and financial loss, not to mention more serious consequences in surgical or medicolegal cases. Such a loss would surely be equivalent to the cost of one or more pieces of electronic test equipment that would prevent this problem.

CHECKING THE CALIBRATION OF PURETONE AUDIOMETERS

As soon as one obtains a new audiometer, the manual should be read and calibration instructions, if any, followed. Be as thorough as possible. These instructions describe the most effective way to check the performance of the audiometer. Perhaps one of the most common mistakes made by the audiologist is to assume that the audiometer is so simple that it is not necessary to read the instructions. Although that may be true for the operation of the machine, it is not necessarily true for its initial setup.

Biologic Check

After the audiometer has been installed, plugged in, turned on, and allowed to warm up, the operator should listen to the signal at different dial settings through each transducer (earphone, loudspeaker, and bone vibrator). Although few audiologists are equipped with "golden ears," with a little practice one can hear basic faults in the equipment. A vague complaint to the audiometer technician or distributor that it "sounds funny" is as futile as telling an auto repair person the same thing. However, a specific description of the sound and circumstances under which it occurs can help determine the source of the trouble. If the technician is given a detailed description of the problem the fault may be found immediately without wasting their time and your money.

A great deal of information on the source of the problem may also be obtained by inspecting the audiometer. Some areas of potential malfunctions that the audiologist should check periodically (normally on a daily basis) are listed below.

    a. Check the power, attenuator, earphone, and vibrator cords for signs of wearing or cracking. One way to determine if the transducer cord is defective is to listen to the tone through the transducer at a comfortable level while twisting and jiggling the cords. A defective cord will usually produce static or will cause the tone to be intermittent. Sometimes tightening the earphone screws, or resoldering the phone plug connections, is all that is necessary. If this does not alleviate the problem, it is wise to replace the cord.

b. Check the audiometer for loose dials or for dials that are out of alignment. If such faults exist the dial readings will be inaccurate. Defective dials should be repaired immediately (sometimes this simply requires tightening the screws holding the dial to the audiometer), and the audiometer should be recalibrated to determine outputs at the "new" dial settings.

c. The audiologist should listen for audible mechanical clicks through the earphone when the dials or switches are manipulated. The ANSI standard suggests that two normal hearing listeners should listen at a distance of 1 meter from the audiometer with the earphones in place but disconnected and with a proper resistive load (coinciding with the impedance of the earphone at 1000 Hz-usually 8 or 10 ohm) across the circuit while manipulating the presenter/interrupter switch, etc. to make sure that there are no audible signals that would clue the subject to the presence of the test signal. A mechanical click can often be detected more easily by listening than through the use of electronic equipment.

d. To determine if electronic clicks are audible it is wise to listen to the output at both a moderate, e.g., 60 dB hearing level (HL), and below the threshold of hearing. Electronic clicks will show up on an oscilloscope as an irregularity when the problem switch or dial is manipulated. The danger of an audible click, whether mechanical or electronic, is that the patient may respond to the click rather than the stimulus tone. Sometimes an antistatic or contact cleaner spray can alleviate the problem of electronic clicks.

e. The audiologist should listen for hum or static at high dial intensity levels both when a stimulus signal is present and when it is absent. One should not hear static or hum at levels below 60 dB on the dial; here again contact cleaner may help.

f. "Cross-talk" may occur between earphones; e.g., the signal that is sent to one earphone may be heard in the contralateral earphone. Such a problem could greatly affect the measurements obtained on that audiometer, especially for cases with unilateral hearing loss. Cross-talk may be detected by disconnecting a phone jack and

sending a signal to that phone. As before, when removing the earphone a proper resistive load must be put in its place. The signal at a suprathreshold dial setting (e.g., 70 dB HL) should not be heard in the opposite phone when a signal is presented in the normal manner. Cross-talk may be caused by external faulty wiring between the examiner's booth and that of the test subject or within the audiometer itself. Cross-talk must be corrected before any testing is carried out.

g. The clinician should listen to the signal while the attenuation dial is rotated from maximum to minimum levels. Sometimes a break in the wiring of the attenuator may cause lack of attenuation below a certain level. For instance, a proper tone may be heard at 20 dB on the dial although *no* tone occurs at 15 dB. In some cases, the tone stays at the same intensity level from 20 to 10dB HL on the dial. These problems are easily detected by listening to the audiometer.

h. Finally, the threshold of the clinician (or a person with known hearing thresholds) should be checked with the earphones and bone vibrators to make sure that the output is approximately correct. If the levels are not within ±10 dB of the previous threshold values, the output levels should be checked electronically.

Aside from these gross problems that can be detected by looking or listening (see Fig. 6.1 for an example of a form that may be used to aid the clinician in carrying out the listening check), the precise accuracy of the output levels must be evaluated when the audiometer is first purchased and at regular intervals thereafter. Frequency, output level, linearity of attenuation, and percentage of distortion should all be checked electronically in addition to the biologic check. Section 7.4 of ANSI S3.6 also describes some electronic procedures for checking for cross-talk and unwanted sound from the transducer.

Frequency Check

The frequency output from the audiometer is best checked by using an electronic counter. This instrument will tell the exact frequency of the output signal. In the absence of a frequency counter an oscilloscope can be used to check the frequency; however it is extremely difficult to be sure within the required ±3% accuracy using this procedure. Fortunately, the cost of adequate frequency counters has been reduced significantly since the first edition of this book. Thus, it is not really necessary to rely on other less precise procedures. The output from the audiometer may be sent directly to the instrument

Audiometer Serial # Date Time Checked By	Power Cord	Attenuator Cord	Earphone Cords	Bone Vibrator Cord	Hum	Dials/Indicators	Frequency	Attenuation	Right Phone	Left Phone	Bone Vibrator	Tone Interrupter	Cross-Talk	Acoustic Radiation	Loudspeaker(s)

Figure 6.1. Biologic check form.

because the frequency is determined by the audiometer rather than the transducer. By using an electronic counter one can easily determine if the output from the audiometer corresponds to the dial reading or electronically displayed number. The standard for audiometers allows a tolerance of ±3% of the indicated frequency value. For example, if the audiometer dial reads 500 Hz the actual output must be between 485 and 515 Hz and at 1000 Hz between 970 and 1030 Hz. Frequency needs to be checked on initial receipt of the audiometer and at yearly intervals thereafter. Nevertheless, it is appropriate to listen to the audiometer each day to judge whether the frequencies are maintaining reasonably good accuracy.

Linearity Check

Linearity of attenuation may be checked either electronically directly from the audiometer or acoustically through its transducer (earphone or bone vibrator). If measurements are to be made electronically, the earphone should be in the line, or a dummy load that electrically simulates the earphone should be inserted in the line. To check linearity the audiometer should be turned to its maximum output and then attenuated in 5 dB steps until the output can no longer be read. Each attenuator on the audiometer should be checked separately. To meet the ANSI S3.6 standard the attenuator should be linear within 0.3 of the interval step or by 1 dB, whichever is smaller. That is, if the dial indicates an attenuation of 5 dB, the audiometer must attenuate between 4 and 6 dB per step. If the step is 2 dB, the reading should be between 1.4 and 2.6 dB per step.

Attenuator linearity should be checked regularly. If a "fixed loss pad" (i.e., a device that automatically attenuates the signal by a set amount, e.g., 20 dB) is present in the audiometer, its attenuation must also be checked. If the audiometer attenuates in 1 or 2 dB steps, these smaller attenuation steps should be checked if they are used clinically. Unfortunately, most calibration equipment is simply not accurate enough to allow one to check intervals of less than 1 dB with confidence. Therefore, special equipment might be required if finer accuracy is necessary.

Distortion Check

Linearity measurements may also help detect distortion in a transducer or in the audiometer itself. Distortion will appear as a lack of linear attenuation especially at high output levels (90 dB dial and above). Harmonic distortion must be checked through the transducer itself. Harmonic distortion is rarely caused by the audiometer, but occurs not infrequently in the various transducers. The maximum permissible total harmonic distortion in the current standard is 3% for earphones and 5% for bone vibrators. The standard also presents values of permissible distortion for the second, third, fourth, and higher harmonics as well as the subharmonics. More detailed information on checking the transducers will be discussed in the "how to" check the output of transducers sections that follow.

Rise-Fall Time

The rise-fall time of the tone is a basic parameter of the audiometer that may be checked by taking the output directly from the audiometer and introducing it into a storage oscilloscope. Rise time is the length of time after the interrupter switch is activated and when the signal is between -20 and -1 dB of its final steady state value. The fall time is the converse, or the length of time between -1 and -20 dB relative to its steady state value at this frequency and dial setting. This is usually checked at a hearing level of 60 dB or more. The ANSI standard specifies a rise time as well as a fall time of not less than 20 msec and not more than 50 msec. A detailed description of the rise and fall characteristics is given in section 9.5 of ANSI S3.6-1989.

EARPHONE CALIBRATION

Real Ear Methods

There are two basic approaches for the calibration of earphones. One is the "real-ear" method and the other is the "artificial ear" or coupler method. With the original real ear method one simply tested the hearing of a group of normal hearing persons, averaged the results, and checked to see that the average hearing of this group was at zero on the dial for each frequency. Although this is theoretically feasible with a large population sample it is not a recommended procedure. To do the procedure properly the sample should consist of *at least* 10 young (18-25 years of age) otologically normal hearing adults and the procedure should follow one of the methods described for transfer of reference equivalent threshold values (see ANSI S3.6-1989, Appendix C). (Table 6.3.) Clearly this procedure is possible but quite unwieldy, especially if it is to be followed weekly or monthly. Further, this approach may be technically incorrect because the International Standards Organization (ISO) reference (which is also used in the ANSI standard) is no longer tied to normal hearing per se, but simply refers to an arbitrarily accepted level. If the audi-

Table 6.3
Reference Threshold Levels re 20 µPa for Audiometric Earphones

Frequency (Hz)	ANSI		ISO	
	TDH-49[a]	Telex 1470[a]	ER 3-A[b]	389-AD[c]
125	47.5	47.0	27.5	45.0
250	26.5	27.5	15.5	27.0
500	13.5	13.0	8.5	13.5
1000	7.5	6.5	3.5	7.5
2000	11.0	8.0	6.5	9.0
3000	9.5	7.5	5.5	11.5
4000	10.5	9.0	1.5	12.0
6000	13.5	17.5	-1.5	16.0
8000	13.0	17.5	-4.0	15.5

[a]Uses NBS 9-A type couple (ANSI S3.6-1989).
[b]Using HA-1 type coupler (ANSI S3.6-1989).
[c]Using IEC 318 coupler (ISO 389, ADD-1).

ologist wishes to use a new earphone (i.e., not listed in the ANSI standard or its appendix) a real ear procedure might be the only way to check calibration, but if generally accepted earphones are used, it is much easier to use an artificial ear/coupler method.

Artificial Ear (Coupler) Methods

The most commonly used procedure today is that of the artificial ear, which consists of a condenser microphone and a 6-cc coupler. The 6-cc coupler was originally chosen because it was thought that the enclosed volume was approximately the same as the volume under an earphone for a human ear (Corliss and Burkhard, 1953). However, because volume displacement is only one component of acoustic impedance it cannot be assumed that the coupler actually represents a human ear. Burkhard and Corliss (1954) pointed out that the impedance characteristics of a 6-cc coupler probably simulate the impedance of the human ear over only a small part of the frequency range. Because the 6-cc coupler does not replicate the impedance of the human ear, it cannot be considered a true artificial ear. Subsequent work by Zwislocki (1970, 1971), Killion (1978), Cox (1986), and Hawkins et al. (1990) have demonstrated the differences between real-ear and coupler values. In an attempt to solve this problem the IEC 318 coupler was developed. However, there is still some disagreement as to the accuracy of this "artificial ear" because its impedance characteristics are also not exactly those of a real human ear. It is clearly more accurate than the present NBS 9-A coupler, but may not be sufficiently better to warrant a shift in the standard.

In addition to the problem of acoustic impedance characteristics, the present 6-cc coupler (NBS 9-A) is known to have a natural resonance at 6000 Hz (Rudmose, 1964). This interferes with the measurement of the output of an audiometer earphone around that frequency. Other problems are the size of the coupler, its shape, and the hard walls that permit the possibility of standing waves at frequencies above 6000 Hz. Despite these difficulties the 6-cc coupler remains as the ANSI accepted device for measuring the acoustic output from the audiometer through an earphone. A coupler, developed by Zwislocki (1970, 1971, 1980) appears to very closely approximate the acoustic impedance of the human ear. It is used in KEMAR (a manikin that has a pinna and an ear canal, as well as an embedded coupler and microphone) (Burkhard and Sachs, 1975; Burkhard, 1978).

The procedure for using an artificial ear is simple. The earphone is placed on the coupler and a 500-g weight is placed on top of it. The output is read in voltage and then transformed to dB (or read directly in dB SPL) *re*20 micro Pascals (μPa). This is equivalent to the previously used 0 dB SPL references of 0.0002 dynes/cm^2 and 0.0002 microbar. After the earphone is placed on the coupler, a low frequency tone (125 or 250 Hz) is introduced and the earphone is readjusted on the coupler until the highest output intensity is read. This helps assure best placement on the coupler. The output from the earphone may then be compared to the ex-

pected values at each frequency. The standard SPL values that are used are given in (*a*) ISO Recommendation R 389 (1981), (this is often referred to as ISO-1964 because of its initial publication date) and (*b*) ANSI S3.6-1989. These values were evolved through a "round robin" in which several earphones were measured on various couplers at a group of laboratories throughout the world (Weissler, l968).

The ANSI standard as well as previous audiometer standards all reference the Western Electric (WE) 705-A earphone. However, that earphone has not been commercially available for many years. As mentioned above, the ANSI standard now gives reference equivalent threshold sound pressure levels for the Telephonics TDH-39, TDH-49, TDH-50, and the Telex-1470A earphones as measured using the NBS 9-A coupler. It also provides values in its appendix for the ER- 3A insert earphone using either an HA-1 coupler or an occluded ear simulator (ANSI S3.25-1989). Figure 6.2 shows an audiometer earphone calibration worksheet that contains the expected values at each frequency with TDH-49 earphones in Telephonics type 51 cushions on an NBS 9-A coupler. ANSI allows a tolerance of ±3 dB from 500 to 4000 Hz and ±5 dB for other frequencies.

Audiometer: _____ _____ S # _____ Earphone: _____ Channel: _____ Room: _____

Calibrated By: _____ Date: _____ Equpment: _____

FREQUENCY	125	250	500	750	1000	1500	2000	3000	4000	6000	8000
1. SPL*											
2. Audiometer Dial Setting											
3. Nominal Ref. SPL (Line 1 - Line 2)											
4. Equipment & Mike Correction											
5. Corrected Ref. SPL (Line 3 - Line 4)											
6. TDH - 49 Earphones**	47.5	26.5	13.5	8.5	7.5	7.5	11.0	9.5	10.5	13.5	13.0
ER 3-A Earphones***	27.5	15.5	8.5		3.5		6.5	5.5	1.5	-1.5	-4.0
7. Calibration Error (Line 5 - Line 6)											
8. Corrections @											

```
 * SPL = Sound Pressure Level in dB re 20 μPA
 ** TDH-49 values from ANSI S3.6-1989, p. 15 (see standard for coupler, and cushions)
*** ER 3-A values from ANSI S3.6-1989, App. G, p.20 (see standard for coupler)
  @ Correction - Rounded to the nearest 5 dB;  - = audiometer weak, make threshold better
                                               + = audiometer strong, make threshold poorer
```

Figure 6.2. Audiometer earphone calibration worksheet.

The output measurements referred to above are only valid when a supra-aural type earphone cushion (which touches the pinna) such as the Telephonics 51 is used and *not* when a circumaural cushion (which encircles the pinna) is used. The lack of an approved reference threshold for circumaural earphone cushions has been pointed out by Benson et al. (1967) and by Zwislocki et al. (1988). It is hoped that the Zwislocki coupler (especially when used in a device such as KEMAR) will permit the calibration of circumaural earphones for use in noisy environments. A reasonable estimate of the output differences between circumaural and supraaural earphones can be found by using the loudness balance procedure or a probe tube procedure described in the audiometer standard appendix (ANSI, 1989b) Although it is possible to place the earphone receiver on a coupler this does not ensure that the SPL at the ear drum will be the same when the earphone is placed in a circumaural cushion. Readings can also be obtained with a flat-plate coupler between the earphone and microphone. The above procedures and the outcome of the measurements have been described by Shaw and Thiessen (1962), Stein and Zerlin (1963), and Tillman and Gish (1964). Vilchur (1970) has also described a circumaural earphone and a procedure for calibration. However, until these problems are solved and a standard calibration procedure is devised for circumaural cushions, any audiometer using these earphones does *not* conform to the ANSI standard for audiometers.

When the output of the earphone has been established it is compared to a standard to determine if it is in calibration or not. If possible the audiometer trim-pots should be used to bring the audiometer into calibration. However, when this is not possible, or when different earphones will be used with the same audiometer, and when corrections are less than 15 dB, a calibration correction card may be placed on the audiometer showing the discrepancy from the established norm. Such corrections must then be taken into consideration when an audiogram is plotted. If an audiometer is off by more than 15 dB at any frequency or by 10 dB at three or more frequencies, it is advisable to have the audiometer put into calibration by the audiometer manufacturer or their representative. If the audiometer is new it should meet the ANSI tolerances cited above. With digital audiometers, the change in output is normally due to the transducer rather than the audiometer, so sometimes it is better to simply replace the earphones.

BONE VIBRATOR CALIBRATION

Real Ear Procedures

Checking the calibration of a bone vibrator presents a different problem than that of an earphone. Although earphones can be checked easily using a microphone as a pickup, bone vibrators cannot. The original technique for checking bone vibrator calibration was a real ear procedure (AMA, 1951), somewhat different than that used for earphones. The method assumes that air- and bone-conduction thresholds are equivalent; therefore, if 6 to 10 normal hearing subjects are tested for both air and bone conduction with an audiometer whose air-conduction system is in proper calibration, bone-conduction corrections for the audiometer, if any, can be determined by using the difference obtained between air- and bone-conduction thresholds. This procedure makes a few assumptions that are not always met. For example, it presupposes that true thresholds can be obtained for all the normal hearing subjects using the given audiometer. Because (*a*) many audiometers do not go below "0" dB HL, and (*b*) the ambient noise in test booths usually does not allow assessment below 0 dB HL often it is not possible to determine the true threshold. To avoid these problems, Roach and Carhart (1956) suggested using individuals with pure sensory-neural losses for subjects in the real ear procedure. Such an approach eliminates the problems of ambient noise and lack of audiometric sensitivity, thus increasing the probability that one will obtain "true" thresholds. A problem arises when trying to find a group of subjects with "pure sensory-neural" losses who have no conductive component and who have thresholds that do not extend beyond the bone-conduction limits of the audiometer. However, the more basic problem with real ear bone vibrator calibration is the supposition that air- and bone-conduction thresholds are equivalent in the absence of conductive pathology. Although this is certainly true for a large group of people it cannot be expected to be true for any individual or for small groups (Studebaker, 1967; Wilber and Goodhill, 1967).

Artificial Mastoid Procedure

The preferred procedure for calibrating bone vibrators involves the use of a mechanical coupler, often referred to as an artificial mastoid. Artificial mastoids were proposed as early as 1939 by Hawley. However, it was not until Weiss (1960) developed his artificial mastoid that they became commercially available. Just as replication of the acoustic impedance of the human ear is difficult with a coupler, replication of the mechanical impedance of the head is difficult with an artificial mastoid. Because no commercially available mastoid met the mechanical impedance requirements of the ANSI (S3.13-1972), or IEC (IEC 373-1971) standards (Dirks et al, 1979) both the ANSI and IEC standards were revised to conform more closely to an artificial mastoid that is available. (ANSI S3.13-1987). ANSI S3.43-1992 gives threshold values that are appropriate for a B-71 bone vibrator used with a P-3333 headband. The ISO has developed a draft standard for bone conduction thresholds (ISO/DIS 7566 [1987]) that gives one set of values that are to be used for all bone-vibrators having the circular tip described in the ANSI and IEC documents (see Table 6.4). It is important to recognize that both the ANSI and the ISO values are based on unoccluded ears using contralateral masking. Thus, the values presuppose that

masking will be used in the contralateral ear when obtaining threshold. Figure 6.3 shows a sample calibration worksheet for bone vibrators incorporating the ANSI values. In both earphone and bone vibrator calibration it is important to check distortion as well as overall intensity through the transducer. Distortion may be measured directly with (*a*) a distortion meter (connected to the output from the artificial mastoid), or (*b*) a frequency analyzer. An oscilloscope provides a visual picture of the distorted wave but it is difficult to determine the exact percent of distortion this way. As mentioned earlier, allowable distortion values for bone vibrators are slightly more lenient than for earphones. In addition to the above physical measurement procedures, the importance of just listening to the audiometer cannot be overly stressed. The normal sophisticated ear should be able to perceive gross attenuation and distortion problems. However, the electronic procedures serve to precisely describe the problems that the human ear only approximates. Because it cannot be assumed that any

Table 6.4
Recommended Root Mean Square Force Values (in dB re 1 µN) for "0" dB Hearing Levels for B-71 Bone Vibrators

Frequency (Hz)	ANSI S3.43-1992	ISO 7566-1987
250	67.0	67.0
500	58.0	58.0
1000	42.5	42.5
2000	31.0	31.0
3000	30.0	30.0
4000	35.5	35.5

Audiometer: _____ Channel: _____ Vibrator: _____

Room: _____ Calibrated by: _____ Date: _____

Equipment Used: _____

FREQUENCY	250	500	750	1000	1500	2000	3000	4000
1. dB re 1 dyne								
2. Mechanical Coupler Corrections*								
3. Line 1 + Line 2								
4. Audiometer Dial Setting								
5. Line 3 – Line 4								
6. B-71 (Mastoid)**	41.0	29.0		19.0		12.5	8.0	11.0
7. Line 5 – Line 6								
8. Corrections @								
9. FBC-MBC Difference	13.5	15.0	12.5	10.0	9.0	8.5	7.5	6.5
10. Frontal Bone Correction								

* for Mechanical Coupler _____ S #: _____

** Threshold for Mastoid Placement for B-71 vibrator re ANSI S3.26-1981

@ Correctons Rounded to Nearest 5 dB: + = Strong, make threshold poorer
                                      – = Weak, make threshold better

Figure 6.3. Audiometer bone conduction calibration worksheet.

two audiologists have the same ears, clearly the electronic procedures must serve as the final arbitrator.

The basic parameters of intensity, frequency and time should be checked at regular intervals using electronic equipment. Worksheets that may be used to record the output of the audiometer are shown in Figures 6.4 and 6.5.

SPEECH AUDIOMETERS

The speech audiometer or speech circuit of the diagnostic audiometer presents some of the same problems encountered with puretone audiometers. For example, the level and the linearity of attenuation should be checked. Because running speech fluctuates in SPL (as well as frequency and time) the preferred method is to introduce a puretone (1000 Hz) into the microphone, phonograph,

or tape input of the speech audiometer. For purposes of calibration, when an electronic signal is introduced the input impedance of the audiometer must be matched by the output impedance of the oscillator. The input intensity should be adjusted so that the volume unit (VU) meter on the face of the audiometer may be monitored at a suitable level, usually zero. The output from the transducer is then measured. The attenuator linearity should be checked in the same way as described above for puretone audiometers. With our audiometers we use a separate puretone oscillator whose output is fed into the speech audiometer input. If an oscillator is not available, one may use the 1000 Hz tone that precedes the test words on most commercially available speech material recordings for checking the phono and tape circuits. A tone from another audiometer might be used to check the microphone circuit.

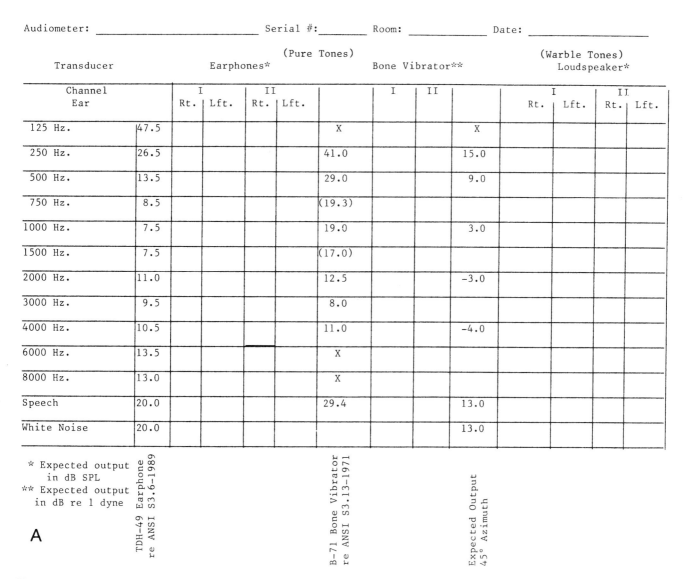

Audiometer: _____ Serial #: _____ Room: _____ Date: _____

| Transducer | Channel Ear | (Pure Tones) Earphones* | | | | | Bone Vibrator** | | | | (Warble Tones) Loudspeaker* | | | |
		I Rt.	Lft.	II Rt.	Lft.		I	II			I Rt.	Lft.	II Rt.	Lft.
125 Hz.	47.5					X			X					
250 Hz.	26.5					41.0			15.0					
500 Hz.	13.5					29.0			9.0					
750 Hz.	8.5					(19.3)								
1000 Hz.	7.5					19.0			3.0					
1500 Hz.	7.5					(17.0)								
2000 Hz.	11.0					12.5			-3.0					
3000 Hz.	9.5					8.0								
4000 Hz.	10.5					11.0			-4.0					
6000 Hz.	13.5					X								
8000 Hz.	13.0					X								
Speech	20.0					29.4			13.0					
White Noise	20.0								13.0					

* Expected output in dB SPL

** Expected output in dB re 1 dyne

TDH-49 Earphone re ANSI S3.6-1989

B-71 Bone Vibrator re ANSI S3.13-1971

Expected Output 45° Azimuth

A

Figure 6.4. Trimonthly calibration check worksheet.

Masking (Narrow Band) Noise Calibration

| Transducer | Earphones* | | | | | Loudspeaker* | | | | Attenuation | |

Channel Ear	I Rt.	I Lft.	II Rt.	II Lft.		I Rt.	I Lft.	II Rt.	II Lft.	(1k Rt. Ph) I	II
125 Hz.	47.5				X					110 / 105	
250 Hz.	26.5				15.0					100 / 95	
500 Hz.	13.5				9.0					90 / 85	
750 Hz.	8.5									80 / 75	
1000 Hz.	7.5				3.0					70 / 65	
1500 Hz.	7.5									60 / 55	
2000 Hz.	11.0				-3.0					50 / 45	
3000 Hz.	9.5									40 / 35	
4000 Hz.	10.5				-4.0					30 / 25	
6000 Hz.	13.5									20 / 15	
8000 Hz.	13.0									10 / 5 / 0	

Biologic Check
Mechanical Click: Yes: _____ (Where) _____   No: _____
Attenuation Complete: Ch. I Yes _____ No _____   Ch. II Yes _____ No _____
CrossTalk: Yes: _____ (Where) _____   No: _____
Earphone Cords: OK _____ Worn _____ Crackle _____ Needs Replacing _____
Bone Vibrator Cord: OK _____ Worn _____ Crackle _____ Needs Replacing _____
Power Cord: OK _____ Worn _____ Needs Replacing _____

B   Examiner: _____

Figure 6.4. *continued*

The standard for speech audiometers indicates that the output for the 1000 Hz tone at 0 dB HL should be 20 dB SPL using a TDH-49 earphone or 19 dB using a Telex 1470A earphone (i.e., 12.5 dB above the standard for the earphone at 1000 Hz). Bone vibrators should be calibrated separately. Presumably if one uses a Radioear B-71 vibrator the value should be 51.5 dB re 1 Newton. The values for the B-72 vibrator should also be 12.5 dB above its reference level for 1000 Hz. The 1000 Hz tone should be introduced into the audiometer as described above and the output measured at 60 dB HL to preclude measurement of ambient room noise. All subsequent speech testing must be carried out with the VU meter peaking at the same point as during the calibration check. If, for example, one prefers -3 on the VU meter rather than 0, then calibration of the 1000 Hz tone must be peaked at -3 or an appropriate correction made in reporting measurements.

The flatness of the frequency response of the speech audiometer is defined as ±5 dB from 1000 Hz for the frequencies 250 to 4000 Hz and not greater than 10 dB dif-ferent from the 1000 Hz signal for frequencies lower than 250 Hz or higher than 4000 Hz. The ANSI standard (ANSI 3.6-1989) gives specific requirements for checking the microphone circuit as well as the recording circuits. If the puretone and speech audiometers are separate machines, the speech audiometer must also be checked for cross-talk, internal noise, and attenuator linearity as described above.

VOLUME UNIT METER

VU meters are indicators of intensity and are found on the face of most audiometers. The VU meter is calibrated relative to the input signal that it monitors and should not be interpreted as yielding any absolute values such as 0 dB SPL. On a speech audiometer the VU meter is used to monitor the speech signal, or to aid the audiologist in adjusting the input calibration tone that precedes the recorded speech materials. The exact specifications for VU meters may be found in ANSI Cl6.5-1954 (R 1971) specifications for a VU meter, sections 3.2

to 3.5. In general it is important that the VU meter be stable, that there is no undershoot or overshoot of the needle indicator relative to the actual signal and that any dB change is accurately represented on the meter. It is possible to either remove the VU meter from the audiometer or to remove the front panel along with the VU meter from its casing to accurately check its characteristics. However, if this is impractical, the audiologist may check the VU meter and its entire accompanying input system as described below.

A puretone should be fed from an oscillator through an electronic switch to the input of the audiometer. The tone should be monitored by a voltmeter. By activating the electronic switch to produce a rapidly interrupted signal one can watch the VU meter to ascertain if there is any overshoot or undershoot relative to the signal in its steady state. One must also check the response time of the needle on the VU meter. A computer generated or tape recorded 270, 300 and 330 msec tone may be used to ensure that the needle reaches its 99% state deflection in 300 msec ±10%. This may be done by feeding the signal through the tape input and watching the deflection of the VU meter. To be certain of the nature of the input signal itself, it is recommended that an electronic switch with known characteristics be used. To check the relative accuracy of the VU meter's dB scale, one may insert a linear attenuator in the line between the oscillator and the audiometer input, or one may reduce the output from the oscillator and the audiometer input, or one may reduce the output from the oscillator by a known amount (as monitored by a voltmeter or oscilloscope). The change in input should be accurately reflected by a corresponding change on the VU meter. When inserting an electronic switch or attenuator in the line it is, of course, important that all electrical impedances are properly matched.

Audiometer: _____ Serial #: _____ Room: _____ Date: _____

Frequency Accuracy Transducer					Total Harmonic Distortion Earphones*						Bone Vibrator**	
Channel Ear		I	II		I Rt. | Lft.		II Rt. | Lft.				I	II
125 Hz.	3.75*			3%**	75@								
250 Hz.	7.50			3%	90					5%*	20@		
500 Hz.	15.00			3%	110					5%	50		
750 Hz.	22.50			3%	110					5%	50		
1000 Hz.	30.00			3%	110					5%	60		
1500 Hz.	45.00			3%	110					5%	60		
2000 Hz.	60.00			3%	110					5%	60		
3000 Hz.	90.00			3%	110					5%	60		
4000 Hz.	120.00			3%	110					5%	60		
6000 Hz.	180.00			3%	90								
8000 Hz.	240.00			3%	90								

* Allowable Variation in Hz.
** Allowable total harmonic distortion in percent
@ Hearing Level in dB for checking harmonic distortion

Rise/Fall – (Allowable 20 to 200 msec.) Channel I _____ Channel II _____

Masking Bandwidth Frequency: 125   250   500   750   1000   1500   2000   3000   4000   6000   8000
  Channel 1 Minimum   _____
    "   1 Maximum   _____
  Channel 2 Minimum   _____
    "   1 Maximum   _____

A

Figure 6.5. Annual calibration check worksheet.

Transducer	Earphones					Loudspeaker					Bone Vibrator	
Channel Ear	I		II				I		II		I	II
ON/OFF	Rt.	Lft.	Rt.	Lft.	ON/OFF		Rt.	Lft.	Rt.	Lft.		
125 Hz. 47.5/37.5					32.0/22.0							
250 Hz. 26.5/16.5					16.0/ 6.0							
500 Hz. 13.5/ 3.5					9.5/-0.5						−10 dB HL*	
750 Hz. 8.5/-1.5					5.5/-4.5						−10 dB HL*	
1000 Hz. 7.5/-2.5					5.5/-4.5						−10 dB HL*	
1500 Hz. 7.5/-2.5					4.5/-5.5						−10 dB HL*	
2000 Hz. 11.0/ 1.0					2.5/-7.5						−10 dB HL*	
3000 Hz. 9.5/ -.5					0.5/-9.5						−10 dB HL*	
4000 Hz. 10.5/ .5					1.5/-8.5						−10 dB HL*	
6000 Hz. 13.5/ 3.5					7.5/-2.5						−10 dB HL*	
8000 Hz. 13.0/ 3.0					13.0/ 3.0							
Speech 20.0/10.0					16.5/ 6.5							

On – Audiometer set at "On" with HL attenuator at 70 in non-test earphone
Off – Audiometer set at "Off" with attenuator set at 60 dB HL for test phone
(Levels may vary with loudspeakers – levels depend on HL values and azimuth used)

 * Use biologic check (10 dB below HL threshold – yes or no)

Frequency   125 250 500 750 1000 1500 2000 3000 4000 6000 8000
(Percent Warble)
Channel I (Right) _____
Channel II   "   _____

Modulation Rate: Channel I _____ Channel II _____

Automatic Pulse Duration Channel I _____ Channel II _____
Automatic Pulse Rise/Fall Time: Channel I Rise_____ Fall_____ Channel II Rise _____ Fall _____

Shock Hazard: OK _____

B

Figure 6.5. *continued*

LOUDSPEAKERS

If at all possible the calibration of the loudspeakers should be checked initially in an anechoic chamber so that precise frequency response characteristics can be obtained. It is often impossible to check the spectral characteristics of a loudspeaker in a standard test booth because the characteristics of the test booth, as well as the objects in them, may create standing waves, signal reverberation or absorption in the room, thus invalidating the results from the speaker. It should be remembered that even within an anechoic chamber, introduction of any object (such as a chair) can change the apparent response characteristics of the speaker by as much as 5 to 10 dB. Ideally a sweep frequency oscillator and a microphone attached to a graphic level recorder are used to check the frequency response curve of a loudspeaker. The output from the oscillator is fed directly into the loudspeaker. A condenser microphone is placed 1 meter in front of the face of the loudspeaker, taking care to account for the angle of incidence of the signal from the speaker to conform to the characteristics of the measuring microphone. The signal from the microphone is led through the necessary equipment to the graphic level recorder. A complete frequency response curve can be obtained quite rapidly and accurately in this manner. If, however, the above equipment is not available, the audiologist may introduce discrete tones into the loudspeaker and record the output through the condenser microphone from a spectrometer or voltmeter. In general, the loudspeaker should be relatively flat within its entire range. The necessary frequency response will depend on the use. If the speakers are used with a speech audiometer for production of speech signals they should at least be flat (±10 dB) within the range of 250 to 4000 Hz and should not vary by more than ±15 dB outside that range. If it is not possible to measure the output of the loudspeaker in an anechoic chamber, one may use very narrow bands of noise to make the measurements. The microphone should be placed where the listener's head would be. Although this procedure is not as precise as using puretones in an anechoic chamber, it will indicate the approximate frequency response of the loudspeaker in the test room.

Harmonic distortion measurements of the loudspeakers should also be carried out in an anechoic chamber as described above. In this instance a distortion meter or other device, as discussed in conjunction with earphone calibration, should be used. If an anechoic chamber is not available, it is theoretically possible to carry out the measurements in an open field free of reflecting surfaces. At the present time there is no standard for harmonic distortion of loudspeakers used with audiometers, but at the very least they should adhere to the manufacturer's specifications. However, it seems reasonable to expect that the requirements for distortion should be as stringent as those mentioned above for earphones (3%). General information about loudspeaker calibration may be found in IEC 268-5A 1980.

The standard for audiometers (ANSI, 1989b) describes some of the characteristics of sound field testing in its Appendix A, such as the test room, frequency response, method for describing the intensity of the speech signal, and the location of the speakers. The standard does not give specific values for puretones, warble tones, or narrow bands of noise in the sound field. An ASHA working group has written a tutorial for sound field testing that includes recommended interim values (ASHA, 1991). Work by Morgan, et al, (1979), Wilber (1991) and Walker et al. (1984) have provided specific values that may be used until an official standard is adopted.

Because the use of puretones is not recommended except in an anechoic chamber, it is suggested that white noise, or preferably, speech spectrum noise, be used to check the calibration for sound field speech testing. Speech spectrum noise has equal energy from 250 to 1000 Hz and a 12 dB/octave fall-off from 1000 to 4000 Hz. In this calibration procedure the noise is sent through the loudspeaker and is picked up by a condenser microphone placed where the center of the subject's head will be during the test conditions. A distance of 1 meter to 6 feet from the loudspeaker face has been recommended. The output from the audiometer to the loudspeaker is monitored to 0 on the VU meter and is read on the linear scale of the spectrometer or sound level meter. The examiner must be careful to use a signal that is loud enough to avoid contamination of output measurements by ambient room noise. Usually a signal of about 80 dB will eliminate this problem. Even when white noise is used it is essential that no object be present between the loudspeaker and the microphone. If possible, the examiner should be in another room to avoid further reflection or absorption. Obviously when testing a young child an examiner or parent may be present. This will contaminate the measurements somewhat, but currently there is no *standards* solution to that problem.

The amplifier hum or internal noise of the loudspeaker system should be checked. This may be done by adjusting the attenuator dial to some intense setting (between 80 and 90 dB HL) and then measuring the output from the loudspeaker when no signal is present. That is, everything is in normal position for testing except that there is no direct input signal (warble tone, white noise, etc.) to the speaker. The equipment noise should be at least 50 dB below the dial setting (i.e., if the dial reads 80 dB, the equipment noise should be less than 30 dB).

Figure 6.6 shows a worksheet that may be used to *monitor* the output intensity from the loudspeakers. As mentioned above, the frequency specific intensity values for warble tones are not currently part of either an ANSI or ISO standard.

CALIBRATION OF ANCILLARY EQUIPMENT

Masking Generator

One of the major differences between the ANSI-1969 standard and its 1989 revision is the greatly increased attention given to the masking stimulus. The 1989 standard defines white noise (broad-band noise), weighted random noise for puretones, weighted random noise for speech, and narrow-band noise. The band widths for narrow bands are recommended to be approximately one-third octave minimum and one-half octave maximum. Cut-off values are given in the ANSI 1989 standard for audiometers. When checking the calibration of the narrow-band noise it will be necessary to have a frequency analyzer or spectrum analyzer (or a computer program that allows one to produce a Fourier analysis of the noise) to determine if the band widths from the audiometer conform to specifications. The same transducer that will be used when delivering the masking source should be used to make final calibration measurements. However, because the characteristics of various transducers are quite different from one another, it is sensible to first do an electronic check directly from the audiometer to verify that any variation from the bandwidth is due to the transducer rather than the audiometer itself.

The masking sound should be checked periodically through the earphones that are used to present it. The SPL of the masking signal may be checked in the same way as puretones by presenting the noise through an earphone that is in place on an artificial ear. The examiner should be careful to use a signal that is intense enough to avoid interference by extraneous room noise (generally about 80 dB HL). In the case of narrow-band noise the SPL values measured (after correcting for any bandwidth variation) should be within ±3 dB at the frequency around which that band is centered. If white noise (see Chapter 8 on masking for a description of this

Audiometer: _____ S # _____ Loudspeaker: _____ Channel: _____ Room: _____

Calibrated By: _____ Date: _____ Equpment: _____

FREQUENCY	125	250	500	1000	1500	2000	3000	4000	6000	8000	Speech
1. SPL*											
2. Audiometer Dial Setting											
3. Nominal Ref. SPL (Line 1 - Line 2)											
4. Equipment & Mike Correction											
5. Corrected Ref. SPL (Line 3 - Line 4)											
6. 45 degree azimuth**		15.0	9.0	3.0		-3.0		-3.0			13.0
0 degree azimuth***	32.0	16.0	9.5	5.5	4.5	2.5	0.5	1.5	7.5	13.0	16.5@
7. Calibration Error (Line 5 - Line 6)											
8. Corrections @@											

```
 *  SPL = Sound Pressure Level in dB re 20 μPA
 ** 45 degrees azimuth from Wilber (1979)
*** 0  degrees azimuth from Walker, et al (1984)
  @  Speech values at 0 degrees azimuth from Dirks, et al. (1972)
 @@  Correction - Rounded to the nearest 5 dB;  - = audiometer weak, make threshold better
                                                + = audiometer strong, make threshold poorer
```

Figure 6.6. Sound field calibration worksheet.

and related terms) is the only masking signal on the audiometer, one need only check the output through the ear phone with a linear setting (no filter). The overall output and attenuation characteristics should be checked in the same basic manner as described for puretones using an artificial ear.

The audiologist should be aware that when making noise measurements, the characteristics of the measuring equipment are critical. Inasmuch as noise is not a "clean" (i.e., uniform and unvarying) signal it is highly susceptible to errors of overshoot and undershoot on a VU meter and to damping on a graphic level recorder. A spectrum analyzer with storage capabilities seems to present the best procedure for checking calibration of noise, but unfortunately, most clinics are not equipped with equipment of that sophistication.

Tape Players and Phonographs

Tape players that are used in a clinic for reproducing speech signals, filtered environmental sounds, or other test stimuli, should be checked at least once every 6 months. However, if the tape player is in regular use, weekly maintenance should be carried out, such as cleaning and demagnetizing the heads. The instruction manuals normally outline the procedures to be used with the particular tape player. If not, any good audio-equipment dealer can explain the procedure. In addition, the frequency response and time characteristics of the tape player should be checked.

At present there are no standards for tape players used with audiometers per se, but there is a very comprehensive document dealing with tape recording and reproducing systems. This document (IEC-94.3, 1980) may be obtained through the American National Standards Institute. In addition, several ANSI and National Association of Broadcasters (NAB) documents deal with specific problem areas. ANSI S4.14-1976, for example, is a standard for reel-to-reel magnetic tape recorders and players and ANSI S4.15 is a standard for audio cassette recording and reproducing.

The frequency response and time characteristics of the tape player may be checked by using a standard commercial tape recording of puretones of various frequencies. The ANSI standard recommends that such a recording be supplied with each speech audiometer. By checking the exact frequency of the tone with an electronic counter, it can be ascertained whether the tape player is operating at the proper speed. By checking the output from the tape player the flatness of the response curve can be determined. If you do not have access to such a tape it is possible to make one by introducing puretones from an audio oscillator into the machine, recording them, and playing them back. This enables the operator to check both the record and playback sections of the tape recorder. If both the record and playback are equally reduced (or increased) in intensity the output will appear normal. The output from the oscillator should be monitored with a voltmeter to make certain that a constant SPL signal is used. Distortion of the puretone from the tape player should also be checked. If none of the above is possible, the speed of the tape player can be checked grossly by marking a tape and then, after timing a segment as it goes across the tape head, measuring to see how many inches passed over the heads per second. Also if the machine is badly out of calibration, it will be audible as a pitch change in the recorded speech (higher if too fast, lower if too slow).

Phonographs also require weekly and daily maintenance such as cleaning the turntable and stylus. The frequency response and time characteristics of phonographs should also be checked at periodic intervals (usually when the equipment is new and at 3- or 6-month intervals thereafter). If it is not possible to procure a phonograph record of puretones, one may check the turntable speed by using a time disc and stroboscopic light. Although compact discs are not mentioned specifically in the standard, if compact disk players are used the manufacturer should state its characteristics. Generally, the problems described for other types of play-back devices do not occur with this type of player (e.g., it does not have heads that have to be cleaned).

It must be remembered that the tape recorder or phonograph used to reproduce speech materials is an integral part of the audiometer system. Thus, it should not be ignored when checking calibration.

Automatic Audiometers

A calibration check of automatic (or Bekesy) audiometers begins with frequency, intensity, cross-talk, and other aspects described for manual puretone audiometers. In addition, the attenuation rate and interruption rate for pulsed signals should be checked. The standard requires that a rate of change of 2.5 dB/sec be provided, as well as other rates if desired. As in manual audiometers, the permissible variance in intensity per step is 1 dB or 0.3 of the indicated difference, whichever is smaller.

The attenuation rate may be measured quite easily with a stopwatch. After starting the motor, a pen marking on the chart is begun and at the same instant as a stopwatch. One reads the chart to determine how far the signal was attenuated, or conversely increased, during the measured time interval. By dividing the time duration into the dB change in intensity one can find the dB per second attenuation rate. The audiometer should be checked for both increasing and decreasing signals.

The preferred repetition rate is 2.5/sec, however, a value of 2/sec is permissible. To check the pulsed stimulus duration one may go from the "scope sync" position on the back of the audiometer (if such exists) to an electronic counter, or if that is not available one may bridge across the terminals of the timing mechanism inside the audiometer. It is difficult to check the pulse speed on a graphic level recorder because of pen damping, but it is possible to check it on a storage oscilloscope. It is not difficult to estimate if there is roughly a 50% duty cycle (on half the time and off half the time), but it is quite difficult to judge whether the signal is on for 200 msec versus 210 msec. The standard recommends 200 msec on and off. The rise-fall times are those described above for manual audiometers.

If both pulsed and continuous signals are used, it is important to check the relative intensity of the pulsed and continuous signals. If they are not equal this should be corrected. The relative intensities can be compared by observing the envelope of the wave form on an oscilloscope or by recording the output with a graphic level recorder if there is no damping problem. The attenuation rate and pulse rate should be checked annually unless there is a reason to suspect a problem earlier.

AUDITORY BRAINSTEM RESPONSE (ABR) UNITS

There are no standards for Auditory Brainstem Response (ABR) equipment. However, an ANSI working group is trying to develop such a standard. In the absence of an accepted "HL" for ABR units most investigators recommend the determination of a normal hearing level "nHL" for one's own unit. The equipment should be checked to make sure that it does not change over time as well as to obtain data to allow comparison of results obtained on equipment in various centers.

The basic parameters of ABR are the same as for conventional audiometry. One must check output level, frequency, and time. In the case of ABR some of the instrumentation that was perfectly appropriate for checking these parameters in conventional audiometers is inappropriate for the briefer ABR signal. It is especially important to check the output from the ABR unit *acoustically* as well as *electronically*. It is easy to display the wave form from the ABR unit on an oscilloscope, but to analyze that display one needs to repeat it very rapidly, or, preferably use a storage oscilloscope. The overall SPL of the click (or tone pip) should be checked electronically by determining the peak equivalent voltage of the signal with a voltmeter or oscilloscope.

Even more importantly, the acoustic response should be checked by connecting the earphone to the coupler in the usual manner and then feeding the output through the condenser microphone to a sound level meter capable of handling impulse sounds and recording the maximum intensity of each signal. One might also use a storage oscilloscope or other device for this purpose, or ideally, use an analog to digital (A to D) converter to store the wave form information in a computer to be converted and read out in voltage or dB SPL. Clearly these SPL readings *cannot* be converted to HL readings, but they will give a basis for quantifying the nHL for one's own equipment. The acquisition of this data base may eliminate the need to *periodically* test a group of normals to determine the 0 nHL level for clicks, filtered clicks, and pips.

In addition to the overall intensity it is important to determine the frequency characteristics of the signal, i.e., its spectrum, *as it is played through the transducer.* One can never assume that an electronic representation of the frequency characteristics of this brief signal has more than a passing resemblance to the signal after it has been passed through a transducer. The spectrum of the signal can be measured by routing the acoustic signal through the condenser microphone and then to a spectrum analyzer with storage capabilities, or via an A to D converter to a computer that would do a Fourier analysis of the signal. In each case a picture of the spectrum of each signal type can be obtained. For completeness, also obtain the spectrum directly from the ABR unit (bypassing the transducer) so that if a change occurs you can determine whether the ABR unit or the transducer has changed.

The third dimension, time, can be checked directly from the ABR unit by feeding the signal into a storage oscilloscope, or through an A to D converter into the computer. One should determine the duration of the individual signal (i.e., click, pip), its repetition rate and the interval between stimuli. Next, determine the accuracy of the signal analysis system of the ABR unit itself by introducing a fixed signal with a specified temporal/amplitude pattern. Eventually we will probably be able to simulate a "typical" ABR response pattern with known time/intensity relationships to see if the unit correctly assesses (in time) where each simulated peak occurs. Such simulated ABR responses can be constructed today if a computer is available. Unfortunately no "standard ABR wave" exists yet, but clinicians can construct them for their own equipment to cleanly describe the ampli-

tude at specific points and thus serve as a standard laboratory (or clinic) reference.

Eventually other parameters of the ABR stimulus and the response measurement will, no doubt, be specified, and a standard developed. Until that time the above suggestions should at least allow one to determine the *consistency* of the ABR equipment and perhaps facilitate exchange of data among clinicians and researchers. One should not be so overwhelmed by the complexity of the equipment that one fails to make any attempt to check it.

ACOUSTIC IMMITTANCE DEVICES

The standard for acoustic immittance (impedance/otoadmittance) devices is ANSI S3.39-1987. It describes four types of units for measuring acoustic immittance (listed simply as Type 1, 2, 3, and 4) (ANSI, 1987b). The specific minimum mandatory requirements are given for Types 1, 2, and 3. There are no minimum requirements for the Type 4 device. Types 1, 2, and 3 must have at least a 256 Hz probe signal, a pneumatic system (manual or automatic) and a way of measuring static acoustic immittance, tympanometry, and the acoustic reflex. Thus to check the acoustic immittance device one may begin by using a frequency counter to determine the frequency of the probe signal(s). The frequency should be accurate within ±3% of the nominal value. The total harmonic distortion shall not exceed 5% of the fundamental when measured in an HA-1 type coupler (this is commonly called a 2-cc coupler). The probe signal shall not exceed 90 dB as measured in that coupler. The range of acoustic-admittance and acoustic-impedance values that should be measurable varies by instrument type. The accuracy of the acoustic-immittance measurements should be within ±5% of the indicated value, or $±10^9$ cm^3/Pa (±0.1 acoustic mmho) whichever is greater. The accuracy of the acoustic immittance measurement can be determined by connecting the probe to the test cavities and checking the accuracy of the output at specified temperatures and ambient barometric pressures. A procedure for checking the temporal characteristics of the acoustic-immittance instrument is described by Popelka and Dubno (1978) and by Lilly (1984).

Air pressure may be measured by connecting the probe to a manometer or "U" tube and then determining the water displacement as the immittance device air pressure dial is rotated. If the Systeme International (S.I.) unit of deca-Pascals (daPa) is used an appropriate measuring device must also be used. The air pressure should not differ from that stated on the device (i.e., 200 daPa) by more than ±10 daPa or ±15% of the reading, whichever is greater. The standard states that the air-pressure should be measured in cavities of 0.5 to 2 cm3.

Finally, one should check the reflex activating system. In checking the activation of a contralateral reflex, normally a supra-aural earphone will be used that may be measured on a standard NBS 9-A coupler. When measuring the ipsilateral reflex activator, normally a probe is used and it should be measured with an HA-1 type coupler. The frequency of the activator may be measured electronically directly from the acoustic immittance device. In this case one uses a frequency counter as described earlier for audiometers. Frequency, harmonic distortion, and intensity should have the same tolerances that one expects from an audiometer. That is, frequency should be ±3% of the stated value, harmonic distortion should be less than 3% at specified frequencies for earphones and 5% or less for the probe tube transducer or insert receiver. Noise bands should also be checked if they are to be an activating stimulus. Broadband noises should be uniform within ±5 dB for the range between 250 to 6000 Hz for supra-aural earphones. This can be checked by sending the output through the transducer connected to a coupler, a microphone, and thence to a graphic level recorder. The sound pressure level of tonal activators should be within ±3 dB of the stated value for frequencies from 250 to 4000 Hz and within ±5 dB for frequencies of 6000 and 8000 Hz and for noise. The rise and fall time should be the same as that described for audiometers and may be measured in the same way. One should have daily listening checks as well as periodic tests of one or two persons with known acoustic immittance to check immittance, tympanogram, and acoustic reflex levels to catch any gross problems.

In summary, acoustic immittance devices should be checked as carefully as one's puretone audiometer. Failure to do so may lead to variability in measurement which may invalidate the immittance measurement.

TEST ROOM STANDARDS

It is insufficient to limit the checks to the equipment. The environment in which the test is to be carried out must also be evaluated. ANSI S3.1-1991 provides criteria for permissible ambient noise during audiometric testing. Table 6.5 gives the values which should not be exceeded by the ambient noise when one wishes to test to levels of 0 dB HL. Table 6.6 compares the values in the ANSI standard for ears covered with an earphone to those of the ISO standard for industrial testing (ISO 6189.2, 1983) and the ISO standard (ISO 8253) that deals with threshold testing in clinical situations (ISO 8253, Part 1 - 1989). Although the levels are not exactly the same, there is general agreement between the ISO and ANSI standards. The ambient level in the test room is checked by using a sound level meter (SLM) that is

Table 6.5
Acceptable Noise Levels (in dB SPL for Octave Bands) in Audiometric Test Rooms when Testing Is Expected to Reach "0" dB HL (ANSI, 1991)

Frequency (Hz)	Under Earphones Only (in dB SPL)	Sound Field or Bone Conduction (in dB SPL)
125	34.0	28.0
250	22.5	18.5
500	19.5	14.5
1000	26.5	14.0
2000	28.5	8.5
4000	34.5	9.0
8000	43.5	20.5

Table 6.6
Comparison of Acceptable Noise Levels (in dB SPL for One-Third Octave Bands) for ANSI and ISO Standards in Audiometric Test Rooms when Testing is Expected to Reach "0" dB HL for Uncovered Ears (e.g., Bone Conduction or Sound Field).

Frequency (Hz)	ANSI S3.1-1991	ISO 8253-Part 1, 1989 (Assumes Testing Starts at 125 Hz)
125	23.0	20.0
250	13.5	13.0
500	9.5	8.0
1000	9.0	7.0
2000	3.5	8.0
4000	4.0	2.0
8000	15.5	15.0

sensitive enough to allow testing to levels of 8 dB SPL. Most current digital SLM devices can measure to levels of 5 dB. However, if the SLM is not that sensitive, an additive procedure of combining dB allows one to check how much sound is added in the ambient noise condition. Appendix B of the standard describes the technique.

Figure 6.7 provides a worksheet that may be used for checking the ambient noise in the test room. The ambient noise levels should be checked about every 6 months unless something has happened to the external environment, or unless noises are heard in the test booth.

SELECTING YOUR EQUIPMENT

One of the questions that I am asked most often, and am least able to answer, is "What equipment should I buy?" The selection of appropriate test and measurement equipment must necessarily be a personal decision influenced by factors such as: (a) expected uses of the equipment, (b) anticipated case load, (c) repair facilities in the area, and (d) financial resources. These, and other appropriate questions, can only be addressed by the user. Frankly, there are no absolute rules in this area. Some of

Place: _____ Room: _____ Date: _____

Calibrated By: _____ Equpment: _____

FREQUENCY	125	250	500	750	1000	1500	2000	3000	4000	6000	8000
1. Obtained Levels dB* Control Room											
2. Obtained Levels dB* Exam Room											
3a. Octave Levels** Earphone Testing	34.5	23.0	21.5	22.5	29.5	29.0	34.5	39.0	42.0	42.0	45.0
3b. Octave Levels*** Bone Cond. & Field	28.0	18.5	14.5	12.5	14.0	10.5	8.5	8.5	9.0	14.0	20.5
4. Difference Exam Room Phones											
5. Difference Exam Room Field & BC											

* dB = Sound Pressure Level in dB re 20 PA
** Permissible Octave levels in audiometeric test booth re ANSI S3.1-1977 for earphone testing
*** Permissible Octave levels in audiometeric test booth re ANSI S3.1-1977 for bone conduction and Sound Field Testing

Figure 6.7. Worksheet for audiometric test booth ambient noise levels.

us tend to use certain brands with which we have had success in the past (and which have provided stable and reliable measurements), although others of us choose to constantly try the latest available equipment. Because I have driven the same make of automobile for 30 years, I probably fall in the first group. First, sit down and think why you want a particular piece of equipment. Consider the uses to which you will put it. Second, ask other audiologists in the community about the reliability of the local distributors. Very complex equipment should not be purchased unless (a) one knows how to use it already and/or (b) one intends to take the time to take an appropriate short course or be taught its use. It is very tempting to buy the latest audiometric equipment—but decisions should be based on need, considering the particular patient population. It may make sense to lease equipment rather than purchase it if one has qualms about its use or usefulness.

A personal rule of thumb (except in my purchase of automobiles) is not to be the first, nor the last, to try a piece of equipment. Another guiding rule is to go for flexibility rather than innate complexity. Many of us were burned some years ago when we purchased evoked response units that were designed to look only at evoked response wave forms after 100 msec.

Some decisions will be based simply on one's training and experience. For example, should acoustic impedance or otoadmittance be tested? There seems to be no compelling evidence at this time for one or the other, but if the terminology is more familiar in one mode, that

is probably the way to go. Other decisions should be based on the current and immediately feasible state of the art. Although there are no standards for computerized audiometry, such standards are being developed and so this approach may provide more flexibility than hard-wired equipment. However, we are using some vacuum tube audiometers that are still quite reliable.

Other decisions may be based on financial considerations, e.g., today ABR units are quite expensive. If one does not have a large practice, or if one is testing mostly conductive hearing loss, or geriatric sensory-neural hearing loss clients, or doing mostly hearing aid selection and fitting, it is probably not cost-effective to purchase an ABR unit. On the other hand, with a large special-test population, or neonatal case load testing, such a purchase would make sense. The place where the equipment will be used can help determine what kind to buy. If the equipment is to be used in more than one facility, clearly portable equipment is preferable, but if a single test site is always used the portability is not an important consideration. Before the end of this century most of us will probably be using computers for most audiometric and acoustic immittance testing. We should, however, remember that although they are more flexible, computers are not inherently more accurate than other types of audiometric equipment. They are generally more *reliable* than most vacuum tube equipment. Even when using computers, one still must be concerned about the transducers that carry the signals from the computer to the patient.

When purchasing measurement equipment one may prefer to acquire only the basics and then share use of additional equipment with other audiologists in the area. The same approach may be used in testing as well. It is important that someone in the community has a spectrum analyzer; it is important that someone has an ABR unit. It is not important that each facility, regardless of size, has each piece of equipment.

Finally although one may say: "A rose is a rose is a rose...", one may *not* say a "voltmeter is a voltmeter is a voltmeter." In the case of sound level meters, a Type I instrument as described in ANSI S1.4-1983 should be used. The characteristics of the voltmeters, oscilloscopes and other instruments should be evaluated to make sure they are capable of measuring the output levels one will use. This is also true of electronic counters, graphic level recorders, etc. Some of the standards will describe the characteristics of the measurement equipment, others will not. The manuals of the measuring equipment should be read in advance to learn their input impedances to make sure that one matches these when inputting from the audiometric device. When reading the manual, and the accompanying material it is also important to note if correction factors should be considered. For example, both microphones and artificial mastoids normally are supplied with correction factors that must be incorporated to achieve accurate measurements. The tolerances of the measuring equipment should be known (if an audiometric standard requires a tolerance of less than 1 dB, then the measuring equipment must have an even more stringent requirement).

If one adheres to certain basic rules one should be able to select appropriate equipment: (*a*) the equipment should adhere to published standards, (*b*) the sensitivity of the equipment should be greater than the standard for the audiometric equipment that one wishes to measure, (*c*) the tolerance of the equipment should be tighter than the tolerance stated in the standard, and (*e*) the equipment should be compatible with the audiometric test equipment (in terms of impedance) and with other equipment in ones clinic.

In short, there are no easy answers to the decisions about which equipment to acquire, but by carefully considering what the equipment will be used for and what it can and cannot do, one will seldom be led astray.

CONCLUSION

This chapter has emphasized that the first responsibility of the audiologist is to listen to the output of the equipment and to test oneself with it. There are many problems that can be detected by a trained human ear. However, the listener is simply not good enough to check the auditory equipment with the precision that is needed to ensure its proper working. Thus, it has been stressed that to determine the precise characteristics of the equipment, that routine electronic checks must be carried out. Because the test results that one obtains are no more accurate than the equipment on which they are performed, both clinical and calibration equipment must be chosen and maintained with care. The ultimate responsibility for the accuracy of the test results lies with the audiologist. Therefore, the audiologist must make sure that the equipment is working properly by carrying out routine calibration checks.

REFERENCES

American Medical Association. Specifications of the council of physical medicine and rehabilitation of the American Medical Association. JAMA 1951;146:255–257.

American National Standards Institute. Volume Measurements of Electrical Speech and Program Waves. ANSI C16.5–1954 (R 1971). New York: American National Standards Institute, 1971.

American National Standards Institute. American National Standard Method for Coupler Calibration of Earphones. ANSI S3.7–1973. New York: American National Standards Institute, 1973.

American National Standards Institute. Audio Cassette Recording and Reproducing. ANSI S4.15–1976. New York: American National Standards Institute, 1976a.

American National Standards Institute. Magnetic Tape Recording and Reproducing (Reel-to-Reel), ANSI S4.14–1976. New York: American National Standards Institute, 1976b.

American National Standards Institute. American National Standard Criteria for Permissible Ambient Noise during Audiometric Testing. ANSI S3.1–1977. New York: American National Standards Institute, 1977.

American National Standards Institute. American National Standard Reference Equivalent Threshold Force Levels for Audiometric Bone Vibrators. ANSI S3.26–1981. New York: American National Standards Institute, 1981.

American National Standards Institute. American National Standard Specifications for Sound Level Meters. ANSI S1.4–1983 New York: American National Standards Institute, 1983.

American National Standards Institute. American National Standard Mechanical Coupler for Measurement of Bone Vibrators. ANSI S3.13–1987. New York: American National Standards Institute, 1987a.

American National Standards Institute. American National Standard Specifications for Instruments to Measure Aural Acoustic Impedance and Admittance (Aural Acoustic Immittance) ANSI S3.39–1987. New York: American National Standards Institute, 1987b.

American National Standards Institute. American Natifonal Standard for an Occluded Ear Simulator. ANSI S3.25–1989. New York: American National Standards Institute, 1989a.

American National Standards Institute. American National Standard Specifications for Audiometers. ANSI S3.6, 1989. New York: American National Standards Institute, 1989b.

American National Standards Institute. Maximum permissable ambient noise for audiometric testing. S3.1, 1991. New York: American National Standards Institute, 1991.

American National Standards Institute. Standard reference for the calibration of pure-tone bone-conduction audiometers. ANSI S3.43, 1992. New York: American National Standards Institute, 1992.

American Speech-Language-Hearing Association. Members of Working Group on Electroacoustic Characteristics of the Committee on

Audiometric Evaluation, Eds. Calibration of pure tone air-conducted signals delivered via earphones. Rockville, MD: American Speech-Language-Hearing Association, 1983.

American Speech-Language-Hearing Association. Professional Service Board Standards for Accreditation of Professional Service Programs in Speech-Language Pathology and Audiology. Rockville, MD: American Speech-Language-Hearing Association, 1984.

Benson R, Charan K, Day J, Harris J, Niemoller J, Rudmose W, Shaw E, and Weissler P. Limitations on the use of circumaural earphones. J Acoust Soc Am 1967;41:713–714.

Beranek LL. Acoustical Measurements. New York: American Institute of Physics, 1988.

Burkhard MD. Manikin Measurements-Conference Proceedings. Elk Grove Village, IL: Industrial Research Products, 1978.

Burkhard MD, and Corliss ELR. The response of ear phones in ears and couplers. J Acoust Soc Am 1954;26:679–685.

Burkhard MD, and Sachs RM. Anthropometric manikin for Acoustic Research. J Acoust Soc Am 1975;58:214–222.

Corliss ELR, and Burkhard MD. A probe tube method for the transfer of threshold standard between audiometer earphones. J Acoust Soc Am 1953;25:990–993.

Cox R. NBS-9A coupler-to-eardrum transformation: TDH-39 and TDH-49 earphones. J Acoust Soc Am 1986;79:120–123.

Decker TN. Instrumentation: An Introduction for Students in the Speech and Hearing Sciences. New York: Longman, 1990.

Dirks DD, Lybarger SF, Olsen WO, and Billings BL. Bone conduction calibration: current status. Speech Hear Disord 1979;44:143–155.

Hawkins DB, Cooper WA, and Thompson DJ. Comparisons among SPLs in real ears, 2 cm^3 and 6 cm^3 couplers. J Am Acad Aud 1990;1:154–161.

Hawley MS. An articial mastoid for audiophone measure ments. Bell Lab Rec 1939;18:73–75.

International Electrotechnical Commission. An IEC Artificial Ear, of the Wide Band Type, for the Calibration of Earphones Used in Audiometry. IEC-318 1970. Geneva, Switzerland: International Electrotechnical Commission, 1970.

International Electrotechnical Commission. An IEC Mechanical Coupler for the Calibration of Bone Vibrators having a Specified Contact Area and Being Applied with a Specified Static Force. IEC-373 1971. Geneva, Switzerland: International Electrotechnical Commission, 1971.

International Electrotechnical Commission. Magnetic Tape Recording and Reproducing Systems: Part III Methods of Measuring the Characteristics of Recording and Reproducing Equipment for Sound on Magnetic Tape. IEC 94-3 1980. Geneva, Switzerland: International Electrotechnical Commission, 1980a.

International Electrotechnical Commission. Sound System Equipment. Part 5: Loudspeakers. IEC 268-5A 1980. Geneva, Switzerland: International Electrotechnical Commission, 1980b.

International Electrotechnical Commission. Audiometers. IEC-645 1986. Geneva, Switzerland: International Electrotechnical Commission, 1986.

International Standards Organization. Acoustics—Pure Tone Air-Conduction Threshold Audiometry for Hearing Conservation Purposes. ISO/DIS 6189.2. Geneva, Switzerland: International Electrotechnical Commission, 1983.

International Standards Organization. Acoustics—Standard Reference Zero for the Calibration of Pure-Tone Audiometers. ISO 389 1975. Geneva, Switzerland: International Electrotechnical Commission, ADDENDUM 1- ISO DAD-1, 1981.

International Standards Organization. Acoustics—Standard Reference Zero for the Calibration of Pure-Tone Bone-Conducted Audiometers and Guidelines for Its Practical Application . ISO 7566. Geneva, Switzerland: International Electrotechnical Commission, 1987.

International Standards Organization. Acoustics—Audiometric Test Methods. Part 1: Basic Pure Tone Air and Bone Conduction Threshold Audiometry. ISO 8253 1989. Geneva, Switzerland: International Electrotechnical Commission, 1989.

Killion MC. Revised estimate of minimum audible pressure: Where is the "missing 6 dB"? J Acoust Soc Am 1978;63:1501–1508.

Lilly DJ. Evaluation of the response time of acoustic-immittance instruments. In Silman S, Ed. The Acoustic Reflex, New York: Academic Press, 1984.

Morgan DE, Dirks DD, and Bower DR. Suggested sound pressure levels of frequency modulated (warble) tones in the sound field. J Speech Hear Disord 1979;44:37–54.

Occupational Safety and Health Administration. Occupational Noise Exposure, Hearing Conservation Amendment. Rule and Proposed Regulation. Washington, DC: Fed Reg, United States Government Printing Office, 1983.

Popelka GR, and Dubno JR. Comments on the acoustic-reflex response for bone-conducted signals. Acta Otolaryngol (Stockh) 1978;86:64–70.

Roach R, and Carhart R. A clinical method for calibrating the bone-conduction audiometer. Arch Otolaryngol 1956;63:270–278

Rudmose W. Concerning the problem of calibrating TDH-39 earphones at 6kHz with a 9 A coupler. J Acoust Soc Am 1964;36:1049(A).

Shaw EAG, and Thiessen GJ. Acoustics of circumaural earphones. Acoust Soc Am 1962;34:1233–1246.

Stein L, and Zerlin S. Effect of circumaural earphones and earphone cushions on auditory threshold. J Acoust Soc Am 1963;35:1744–1745.

Studebaker G. Intertest variability and the air-bone gap. J Speech Hear Disord 1967;32:82–86.

Thomas WG, Presslar MJ, Summers R, and Stewart JL. Calibration and working condition of 100 audiometers. Public Health Rep 1969;84:311–327.

Tillman TW, and Gish KD. Comments on the effect of circumaural earphones on auditory threshold. J Acoust Soc Am 1964;36:969–970.

Villchur E. Audiometer-earphone mounting to improve inter-subject and cushion-fit reliability. J Acoust Soc Am 1970;48:1387–1396.

Walker G, Dillon H, and Byrne D. Sound field audiometry: recommended stimuli and procedures. Ear Hear 1984;5:13–21.

Weiss E. An air-damped artificial mastoid. J Acoust Soc Am 1960;32:1582–1588.

Weissler P. International standard reference zero for audiometers. J Acoust Soc Am 1968;44:264–275.

Wilber LA, and Goodhill V. Real ear versus artificial mastoid methods of calibration of bone-conduction vibrators. J Speech Hear Res 1967;10:405–416.

Wilber LA. Pure tone audiometry: air and bone conduction. In Rintlemann WF, Ed. Hearing Assessment. Baltimore: University Park Press, 1979.

Zwislocki JJ. An Acoustic Coupler for Earphone Calibration. Rep LSC-S-7. Syracuse, New York: Lab Sensory Commun, Syracuse University, 1970.

Zwislocki JJ. An Ear-Like Coupler for Earphone Calibration. Rep LSC-S-9. Syracuse, New York: Lab Sensory Commun, Syracuse University, 1971.

Zwislocki JJ. An ear simulator for acoustic measurements. Rationale, principles, and limitations. In Studebaker G, and Hochberg ?, Eds. Acoustical Factors Affecting Hearing Aid Performance, Baltimore: University Park Press, 1980.

Zwislocki J, Kruger B, Miller JD, Niemoeller AF, Shaw EA, and Studebaker G. Earphones in audiometry. J Acoust Soc Am 1988: 83:1688–1689.

Behavioral Evaluation
Peripheral Hearing Functions

CHAPTER 7

Puretone Air-Conduction Threshold Testing

Phillip A. Yantis

Puretone threshold audiometry is the standard behavioral procedure for describing auditory sensitivity. The comparison of air- and bone-conduction thresholds provides a fundamental index of auditory function for otologic diagnosis (see Chapter 2). Puretone thresholds are an important component of diagnostic procedures, in the evaluation of hearing aids and in rehabilitation planning. State and federal statutes regarding hearing dysfunction often require air-conduction threshold information, as do standards for defining hearing "impairment" and "handicap." It is important, therefore, that the auditory behaviors observed in threshold audiometry are obtained reliably, and are of defensible validity.

This chapter explores factors that may influence audiometric reliability and accuracy. Strategies for reducing test variability are reviewed, and applications of hearing threshold testing are discussed. Two basic aspects of threshold audiometry, test ear isolation by contralateral masking and stimulation by bone conduction, are covered in the following chapters. Although the focus here is on the evaluation of hearing at minimum sensation levels, certain aspects of the discussion relate just as well to other audiologic procedures.

DETERMINING AUDITORY THRESHOLD

Many strategies can be used to find auditory sensitivity by studying the listener's motor response. Decisions must be made about the test environment, the test signal, instrumental hardware, characteristics of the listener, and the evaluation procedures themselves. It is vital to use test conditions that are most conducive to valid and reliable results. Different levels of stringency are required depending on the type of threshold information desired. For example, is the intent (*a*) to establish minimum audible pressures to which a person is capable of responding under ideal laboratory circumstances, or (*b*) to compare an individual's sensitivity with that of the "normal" population when tested under clinical conditions? Answers to these questions dictate variations in the test strategy and determine the degree to which significant variables must be controlled.

Threshold of Audibility

The minimum effective sound pressure level of an acoustic signal producing an auditory sensation "in a specified fraction of the trials" is defined in American National Standards Institute (ANSI) S3.20-1973 (R 1986) as the "*threshold of audibility.*" Attempts to discover a specific signal level below which no sensation consistently occurs have been generally unsuccessful, even under ideal laboratory conditions. Because minimum auditory sensation is variable, threshold must be described in terms of a probability statement. A threshold level is commonly defined as the lowest signal intensity at which multiple presentations are detected 50% of the time.

Threshold variability is often due to factors other than the person's hearing sensitivity per se. Those influencing *extrinsic* variability generally can be reasonably controlled under laboratory conditions. The physical environment (temperature, humidity, light, ambient noise level) also must be considered. Measuring instruments must be accurately calibrated and operate reliably. The test methodology and listener instructions should be carefully selected.

Intrinsic variables affecting auditory sensitivity include (*a*) neurophysiologic factors governing organic sensation and (*b*) subjective considerations, such as motivation, intelligence, attention, familiarity with the listening task, and variations in how listeners interpret the same test instructions. Under laboratory conditions, experimental control over these variables is attempted by adopting stringent subject selection criteria and by ensuring that subjects are experienced in the listening task.

A major intrinsic variable in detecting minimally audible signals is associated with internal noise. Physiologic activity linked with vascular, digestive, and respiratory functions can establish a "masking floor" below which signal detection is absent even though the organism may be *capable* of sensation. Random acoustic or neural energy generated within the system, including tinnitus, can contribute to this result. It is for these reasons that some modern psychophysicists question whether a single level of threshold performance can be specified experimentally. Research designed to explore human performance in detecting acoustic signals has used procedures requiring forced choices involving multiple response criteria (Green and Swets, 1966; Clarke and Bilger, 1973). A number of trials is usually required at each of several values of the signal parameter. When compared to more conventional clinical methods used in threshold audiometry, such approaches have shown increased sensitivity averaging almost 5 dB in normals (Barr-Hamilton et al., 1969) and have reduced threshold variability by 20 to 30% (Bryan and Tempest, 1967). However, the excessive time required for data collection and the need for specialized techniques of test administration have limited the clinical application of these procedures.

Audiometric Threshold

To determine audibility thresholds of clinical cases in a relatively short period of time, compromises must be made in managing the variables described above. Clinical tests are not usually conducted in anechoic environments. Under clinical conditions there is often variation due to subjective factors that affect behavioral responses. Unlike the subject in a psychoacoustic experiment, the responses of a client or patient in the audiology clinic are often inconsistent because these listeners are not ordinarily trained to be highly competent and reliable observers. Indeed, they may be quite naive at the task. They commonly represent wide ranges of innate intelligence, motivation, and experience.

The equipment and technique must conform to practical requirements of cost effectiveness. The time necessary for test administration is an important factor. The procedure must be a reasonably simple task for the examiner who must work quickly and consistently. Threshold response criteria may vary between 50 and 75% or higher, depending on the test technique and the listener's responses.

Because administration time is often limited, attenuator steps of 5 dB are used. This introduces a minimum SE of ±5 dB. Inasmuch as tolerances contained in ANSI standards are from ±3 to 5 dB of designated sound pressure levels (SPL), the SE can potentially expand to ±10 or 15 dB depending on the listener's actual physiologic sensitivity. It is therefore questionable whether true audibility thresholds are observed in conventional audiometry (Harris, 1978).

Clinically, audiometric threshold levels are likely to be elevated over what they might be under laboratory conditions. Even so, the validity of clinical data is acceptable for most purposes. Hearing levels on the audiometer are calibrated to referent sound pressures (ANSI S3.6-1989) that describe the typical (modal) sensitivity of normal, young adults when tested under reasonably quiet test conditions. The resultant dB levels offer a convenient means of describing a listener's threshold performance on a comparative scale.

One might question the logic of quantifying threshold levels in older listeners using standards based on the sensitivity of young adults. Because auditory sensitivity in otologically normal listeners decreases with age (Corso, 1963), especially for higher frequencies, correction formulas have been suggested to estimate central threshold values by age and sex (see Chapter 35). Robinson and Sutton (1979), for example, have reviewed 14 data sets from eight studies. They derived a formula for predicting age effect of otologically screened groups across a frequency range from 0.125 to 12 kHz. Certainly there is merit in peer comparisons when describing "normal" audibility, especially in counseling older individuals regarding their hearing status. For the present, however, criteria for threshold normality are restricted to those of the comparatively young ear.

Approaches to audiometric threshold testing by air conduction have followed two developmental paths. *Manual* audiometry uses a modified method of limits in which the examiner controls the signal parameters. *Automatic* (tracking) audiometry requires listener control of signal amplitude and is a variant of the classical method of adjustment.

MANUAL AUDIOMETRY

Conventional threshold audiometry involves manual control of the signal parameters by the examiner. Tones are presented in a way that is likely to result in a consistent response observed from the listener. Typically, thresholds are obtained for signals that are presented through headworn earphones, although threshold can also be established using loudspeakers in a sound field.

Various commercial instruments are available for manual puretone audiometry. All "wide range" audiometers provide at least the frequencies in octave multiples between 0.25 and 8 kHz, as well as the intermediate frequencies of 1.5, 3, and 6 kHz. Maximum hearing levels (HL) range from 70 to 120 dB depending on the specific frequency and type of audiometer.

Screening audiometers may be used for identifying individuals in large populations who are likely to have significant hearing impairments. All signals across a specified frequency range are usually presented at a single criterion hearing level. Threshold audiometry is then conducted on those not responding to one or more signals in each ear. Screening procedures are discussed elsewhere as they relate to specific populations of children (Chapter 30) and adults (Chapter 33). Although the maximum HL and frequency range of screening audiometers may be limited compared to those used for threshold testing, ANSI S3.6-1989 standards for the accuracy and tonal purity of the frequencies and the SPL at each decibel step apply to *all* instruments.

Threshold Testing Procedures

Shortly after the commercial introduction of vacuum-tube audiometers in the 1920s, various methods were suggested for obtaining puretone thresholds. There was considerable disparity in the suggested approaches (Bunch, 1943; Watson and Tolan, 1949; Curry and Kurtzrock, 1951; Corso and Cohen, 1958). No "standard" strategies for threshold exploration were adopted until 1944, when the Committee on Conservation of Hearing of the American Academy of Ophthalmology and Otolaryngology formally recommended the Hughson-Westlake "ascending method" (Newhart and Reger, 1945).

Guidelines for test administration have been proposed only recently within national organizations representing professional audiology, such as the American Speech-Language-Hearing Association's (ASHA) Committee on Audiometric Evaluation (1978) and the British Society of Audiology's Education Committee (1978). The first ANSI standard on manual audiometry (S3.21), which was approved in 1978 and reaffirmed in 1986, closely parallels the ASHA guidelines.

One might question whether a standardized technique is really appropriate in manual audiometry. Some experienced clinicians believe that the rigidity inherent in standard approaches may preclude procedural variations that could improve listener interest and motivation, and thus enhance reliability.

However, a "conventional" approach often improves face validity among those learning audiometric procedures. It provides an initial foundation for obtaining clinical experience. Such standards are also convenient methods for exploring research questions that require careful methodologic control. Certainly there are times when "standard" protocols must be abandoned by the clinician, as when testing children and individuals having physical and cognitive disabilities. Whenever such alternative strategies are used, however, they should be fully described to reduce possible confusion regarding the techniques used.

The following are factors worthy of consideration in maintaining optimum levels of validity and reliability during threshold testing with cooperative listeners. Some are found in the guidelines and standards mentioned above. Others are based on personal experience and on information reported in the literature.

Preliminary Considerations

Calibration Check. As in all audiometric applications, the examiner must be satisfied that (*a*) instrumental procedures are conducted periodically to verify that the audiometer and associated transducers produce signals meeting current ANSI calibration standards, (*b*) a listening check has confirmed that signals are reaching the earphones to which they are directed, and (*c*) the environmental conditions conform to permissible ambient noise levels as defined in ANSI S3.1-1977 (R 1986) for the levels anticipated during audiometric testing. These matters are discussed in Chapter 6. Their importance to audiometric accuracy cannot be overstressed.

Listener Information. The examiner should spend a short period becoming acquainted with the client or patient before the test begins. In addition to obtaining pertinent case history information, rapport must be established. Demonstration of personal interest in the listener's welfare promotes a cooperative relationship and helps to reduce apprehension. The examiner also has an opportunity to study the listener's communicative behavior. The importance of visual cues to comprehension can be observed if the examiner's mouth or face is temporarily obstructed from time to time during the interview. General estimates of overall impairment levels can be made by varying vocal intensity during questioning. Specific answers to the following questions have significance in threshold testing: In which ear does hearing seem best? Which ear is preferred when using the telephone? Is there any tinnitus, and what does it sound like? Is there intolerance to loud sounds, and of what types? What sounds seem the most difficult to hear?

Ear Canal Examination. It is important that the ear canals are not occluded with debris such as cerumen or cotton. This should be confirmed by the examiner, using either an otoscope or a speculum and a bright external light source. Clearly, the examiner should be trained in this procedure so that the tympanic membrane can be visualized easily and quickly. The intent is *not* to determine the presence of drum abnormality, but simply to confirm that the canal is unoccluded. The helix of the pinna should be firmly grasped and moved in a posterior-superior direction to straighten the canal. If it is impossible to visualize the drum, or if considerable material such as cerumen is observed, this finding must appear on any audiogram or written report should the test proceed. The listener must be retested after removal of obstructive material.

While examining the canal, pressure should be exerted on portions of the pinna cartilage around the opening to observe the potential for collapse of the canal walls when standard supraaural earphone cushions are placed on the head. This problem may be more prevalent in audiometric testing than is realized, especially among young children and in the elderly. For example, Creston (1965) found collapsed canals to be responsible for screening failures in 24% of 41 children between six and nine years of age. Schow and Goldbaum (1980) discovered elevated thresholds due to this obstruction in 41% of 104 nursing home residents. A quick way to confirm whether a potential problem exists is to retest with the earphone elevated slightly from the pinna. If threshold improves, canal wall collapse must be seriously considered.

Various management techniques have been suggested when a patient demonstrates a collapsed canal. One is to place pads of gauze or tissue behind the pinna so that it and the posterior canal wall are forced backward when the earphones are replaced. Others have recommended inserting into the canal a thick-walled plastic tube, ear stopple, stock earmold, or probe tip like those used in immittance audiometry. These procedures might result in the attenuation of high-frequency sensitivity (Bryde and Feldman, 1980). However, these measures usually work well. Other suggestions include open-ear retests in calibrated sound field, and substitution of circumaural for conventional supraaural cushions. The latter alternative has clear advantages over inserts and postpinna pads (Marshall and Gossman, 1982), although necessary adjustments in calibration levels must be considered. Perhaps the best alternative in such cases, of course, is to use insert earphones (see below).

Instructions. The directions to the listener should be as short and uncomplicated as possible. However, certain critical facts *must* be understood. If linguistic differences occur between examiner and listener, a family member or friend should be available for interpretation. Whenever possible, instructions should be given in the immediate physical presence of the listener. Gestures depicting "smallness" and mimicking response patterns are often helpful.

The examiner must be sure that the following points are clearly understood by the listener: (*a*) that the object of the test is to find the faintest tones the listener can hear; (*b*) that different tone pitches will be heard in only one ear at a time; (*c*) that an immediate physical response should be made *each time* a tone is heard, even when very faint and the listener has to guess; and (*d*) that the motoric response should cease immediately after tone cessation. The listener should repeat the instructions, if necessary, and should be asked if there are any questions before the test begins.

Response Strategy. No specific response pattern has become an accepted standard in manual audiometry.

Usually a method is selected that is familiar to the examiner, is easily understood by the listener, and requires a distinct motor response. Most clinicians prefer that the listener raise and lower the forearm, hand, or finger, reasoning that subtle cues may be observed in such movements that are helpful to the examiner (Green, 1978). Others use a hand-held switch that activates a light visible to the examiner. However, it is possible that some responses may be missed with these devices. This is especially true for signal levels near threshold. The listener may unconsciously reduce the physical pressure on the switch, and the desired electrical contact may not occur.

The response mode should result in a clear and reliable indication of the listener's "on" signal to the examiner when the tone starts and, when possible, an "off" response when the stimulus ceases. Although response latency may be slightly increased at levels close to threshold, it should be brief at suprathreshold levels. If latency is protracted, the listener should be reinstructed and presented with comfortably loud stimuli until the latency period becomes acceptably short.

Earphone Placement. Earphones used in audiometry may be coupled to the ear with supraaural or circumaural cushions, or by insertion into the ear canal using foam earplugs. Supraaural cushions, such as the MX-41/AR, have been used for many years as the standard means for earphone coupling. Cushions encircling the pinna may offer greater comfort to the subject, because pressure is displaced to the skull rather than to the pinna. Insert earphones that are surrounded by foam earplugs, a rather recent development, offer significantly greater attenuation in the low frequencies than either the supraaural or circumaural cushion (Frank and Wright, 1990). Other advantages of circumaural and insert earphones have been described by Killion and Villchur (1989). The reliability of threshold testing is improved with insert earphones (Wilber et al., 1988), and they reduce the potential of collapsed ear canals (Chaiklin and McClelland, 1971; Riedner, 1980; Marshall and Gossman, 1982). Even so, present ANSI standards (S3.6-1989) still call for the use of supraaural cushions in audiometry.

Although procedures for transferring reference equivalent threshold values to nonstandard earphones and couplers are provided in S3.6-1989, and interim levels for a specific type of insert earphone (the ER-3A) are designated, most threshold audiometers in use today employ supraaural earphones. The primary reasons include the lack of standard calibration procedures for other types of earphones and cushions, and concerns about hygiene and controlling the position of insert phones in the ear canal (Zwislocki et al., 1988; Zwislocki, 1989). Our discussion will therefore be limited to the use of earphones in supraaural cushions.

The listener should be asked to remove any eyeglasses, ear jewelry, hearing aid(s), or chewing gum. The position of the two earphones should be maximally extended on the headband before placement to provide adequate room for the client's head. Earphones should not be hand held during the test; pressure and position can easily vary over time, and undesirable low frequency energy can be transmitted to the ear canal through contact with the hand. Any hair covering the pinna should be displaced.

The earphones should be placed simultaneously over the ears, being sure that the earphone for the right (or left) channel is on the proper side of the head. The headband is then tightened with the examiner's thumbs as the earphones are held in place. Final observation of earphone position should then be carefully made to see if further adjustment is needed. *It is extremely important that the center of the earphone diaphragm is directly opposite the opening of the ear canal on each side.* The listener should be specifically asked if the earphones are comfortable, and they should be adjusted again if they are not.

Test/retest consistency is particularly difficult to maintain for low frequencies due to leakage and for the higher frequencies because of subtle changes in canal resonance effects (Harris, 1954; Hempstock et al., 1966; Shaw, 1966). Intertest reliability improves significantly for these frequencies when earphones either remain in place between tests (Hickling, 1966), or are replaced in the same position (Atherly and Lord, 1965). But these strategies are often impractical in clinical applications. Richards et al. (1979) discovered various sized diameters in the openings of MX-41/AR cushions that can lead to variations in high frequency output for the same earphone. A thorough discussion of circumaural cushions is found in Chapter 6.

Cushion Contamination. In certain clinical settings, earphone cushions may be used with listeners who have outer or middle ear infections. This raises obvious questions regarding possible bacterial contamination. Ultraviolet irradiation of cushions has been suggested in such cases (Talbott, 1969; Wolff and Borchardt, 1975), as has use of an antibacterial solution such as Zephiran chloride (Hodgson, 1980).

Ear Selection. Normally the test should begin with the ear that appears more sensitive. This determination may be a "best guess," of course, because it depends on the extent and accuracy of pretest information about the listener. The presumption is that the better ear will not need retesting in the event masking must be used after the poorer ear is evaluated. Such an expectation may not always be accurate, of course, especially after testing by bone conduction. Appropriate strategies for masking are mandatory to ensure that cross-head stimulation does not occur. Whenever the AC threshold in the test ear exceeds the BC threshold in the nontest ear by at least 40 to 50 dB, depending on frequency, masking must be seriously considered (see Chapter 8).

Frequency Sequencing. Threshold testing usually begins at 1000 Hz. There are two primary reasons: (*a*) 1000 Hz is identified perceptually as a pitch familiar to most listeners, and (*b*) threshold levels obtained at this frequency tend to be more reliable (Harris, 1945; Dadson and King, 1952). Once the threshold is found at 1000 Hz, similar searches are normally undertaken at 2000, 4000, and 8000 Hz. Threshold finding at 1000 Hz is repeated as a reliability check, followed by testing at 500 and 250 Hz; 125 Hz is rarely used as a test signal.

Abrupt changes (20 dB) in threshold sensitivity occurring between standard test frequencies should be explored with half-octave signals, if available (0.75, 1.5, 3, and 6 kHz). Such information could have value in medical diagnosis; it also may be helpful in rehabilitative planning, especially in relationship to decisions about hearing aid amplification.

Listener Position. If threshold tests are conducted in a single room, the listener must be seated so that movements of the examiner cannot be directly observed but those of the listener are visible to the examiner. It is also important that acoustic radiation does not emanate from the chassis of the audiometer.

Both of these factors become minimal considerations when audiometric instrumentation is outside the examining room. The listener can be observed almost in full face if instructed to gaze at a 30° angle, for example. In addition, the two-way talkback system normally available in such arrangements allows the examiner to reinstruct without removing the earphones.

Signal Presentation

The ascending method suggested by Hughson and Westlake in 1944 was to be initiated after the presentation of a continuous tone as a "reasonably loud signal" for recognition by the listener. After attenuation to inaudibility in 5- to 10-dB steps, they recommended that the signal be increased "until the tone is heard." This procedure was then repeated. Threshold for a specific frequency was defined as the level at which a "uniform response" was obtained at least three times.

Carhart and Jerger (1959) modified the above procedure by suggesting that (*a*) initial signal presentations should be at clearly perceived amplitudes; (*b*) the signal should be decreased in 10- to 15-dB steps to inaudibility; and (*c*) the Hughson-Westlake paradigm should then be instituted using short presentations in an "up 5 dB-down 10 dB" approach to find the lowest hearing level at which a response is obtained on at least three trials. They found that using a descending method resulted in threshold values slightly less than those found with ascending or ascending-descending techniques. Even so, they believed the ascending method was still preferable. It minimizes the potential for perstimulatory adaptation and reduces the possibility that the examiner may provide inappropriate cues by using rhythmical patterns of signal presentation.

Stimulus on-time was from 1 to 2 sec, separated by toneless intervals of at least 3 sec. Short tones were preferred over continuous signals to take advantage of neural on-effects and to reduce the potential of auditory adaptation.

Manual presentation of puretones involve the following distinct phases:

Listener Familiarization. Two popular approaches have been used for making initial tone presentations. The intent is to select a clearly audible signal to confirm that the response instructions are understood. It is important, however, that the initial sensation level is sufficiently low to prevent listener discomfort.

One technique contained in the ANSI S3.21-1978 (R 1986) standard is to make the initial presentation at 30 dB HL for every listener. If the tone is heard, the test is then begun; if not, the tone is presented again 20 dB higher. If still inaudible, 10-dB increases are recommended until a response is obtained.

A second approach, also endorsed in the ANSI standard, begins at the minimum audiometer hearing level. The level of a continuous signal is gradually increased until a response is first detected. The tone is then turned off for a minimum of 2 sec and presented again at the same level. If a response occurs, the test can begin at that intensity. If there is no response, the familiarization procedure should be repeated. Many audiologists prefer this technique for several reasons: (*a*) it often reduces administration time; (*b*) the amplitude range around threshold is narrowed more efficiently; and (*c*) behavioral characteristics associated with pseudohypacusis and loudness recruitment may often be elicited.

Threshold Determination. The first tonal presentation should be made 10 dB below the minimal response level found during the familiarization stage. The duration of each tone need be no longer than 1 sec with most listeners. Signals should be presented in an irregular temporal pattern, with the interval between tones being no shorter than 1 sec.

Following each lack of response the presentation level should be increased 5 dB until one occurs. After noting the hearing level, the intensity is then decreased 10 dB and another series of 5-dB ascending levels is begun. This sequence is repeated until a threshold level is determined. The ANSI S3.21 threshold criterion is "the lowest hearing level at which responses occur in at least one-half of a series of ascending trials, with a minimum of two responses out of three required at a single level."

The ANSI criterion varies slightly from the ASHA guideline, which recommends a minimum of *three* responses at a single level. This might require as many as four or five ascending series, compared to two or three for the ANSI criterion. Using computerized versions of the modified Hughson-Westlake technique, Harris (1979) found that hearing levels using the ANSI requirement were as reliable as those obtained with the ASHA model, yielded similar means, and saved nearly 5 min of test time for each subject. These conclusions were supported in 1980 by Tyler and Wood, using manual techniques.

Audiogram and Symbolization

Audiometric threshold data may be recorded in tabular form (numerical hearing level in dB for each test frequency) or by graphic representation on an audiogram. The tabular technique is especially useful when an individual is to have several retests over a period of time. For example, when hearing is being monitored as in industry or the schools, many retests can be shown on a single page for comparative purposes. Audiograms, using a standard symbol system, provide a convenient way to visualize AC and BC threshold levels (with or without masking) on a scale related to the "normal" range of hearing. This approach has clear advantages in explaining to the listener the implications of the hearing impairment.

A graphic form and a symbol system were recommended by ASHA in 1974 and by ANSI S3.21-1978 (R 1986). The guidelines recommended by ASHA were revised (1990) and appear in Figures 7.1 and 7.2. Note that frequency on the abscissa is expressed on a log scale and that amplitude is on a linear scale; the space for one octave on the abscissa is meant to be equal to that for 20 dB on the ordinate. Data for the right ear are traditionally recorded in red, and in blue for the left ear.

Jerger (1976) pointed out that graphic portrayal of threshold data can sometimes become confusing to the reader (*a*) when represented without color differentiation in texts and scholarly publications, and (*b*) when obtained by both air and bone conduction, with and without masking, and presented for both ears on the same audiogram form. He suggested a separate audiogram for each ear, using only open/solid circles to symbolize unmasked/masked air conduction threshold and open/solid triangles for bone conduction levels without/with masking of the nontest ear.

Subject Variability

As careful as one might be in following the suggestions described above, intrinsic factors associated with the listener's emotional motivation, general physical condition, and auditory pathology can significantly influence test accuracy and the consistency of repeated examinations. The presence of physical discomfort or antagonism about the test process can easily lead to inconsistent response behavior. Certain types of hearing impairment, such as middle-ear infections, Meniere's

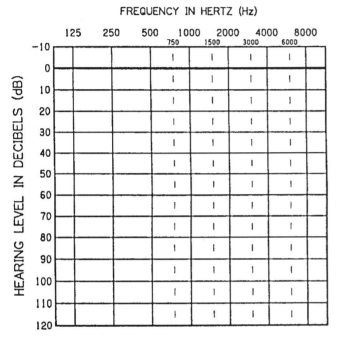

Figure 7.1. Audiogram form recommended by ASHA. (1990).

disease, ototoxicity, vascular insufficiency, and temporary threshold shifts due to noise exposure can lead to significant sensitivity changes in a matter of hours or days. The examiner must always be alert to these eventualities so that appropriate modifications in procedure are used or further testing is scheduled at another time. Certain individuals, such as young children and those with intellectual impairments, may require unusual strategies in finding sensitivity thresholds using behavioral techniques. Specialized protocols and instrumentation, together with the expertise of trained examiners, can result in reasonably reliable and valid threshold data in such listeners (see Chapters 29, 32, 34, and 35).

Two kinds of false responses can occur in threshold audiometry: (*a*) a false *negative,* when no response follows an audible stimulus, and (*b*) a false *positive,* when a response is given without the presence of a signal. False negatives occur less often than do false positives. They may simply reflect lack of attention to the task, in which case reinstruction and positive verbal reinforcement for correct responses may be all that are needed. A second possibility is associated with pseudohypacusis; an individual who is feigning a loss may have difficulty maintaining a consistent "threshold" level and thus, appear to have occasional false negative responses (when in fact, all of the behaviors near threshold levels are false negative).

False positive responses are often noted when the listener has tinnitus. Such an individual may respond consistently but show a sudden change in behavior for a frequency at which tinnitus interference occurs. If this eventuality is suspected, the examiner should switch to

MODALITY	Response EAR			No Response EAR		
	LEFT	UNSPECIFIED	RIGHT	LEFT	UNSPECIFIED	RIGHT
AIR CONDUCTION–EARPHONES						
UNMASKED	✗		○	✗		○
MASKED	□		△	□		△
BONE CONDUCTION–MASTOID						
UNMASKED	>	↑	<	>	↑	<
MASKED	]		[	]		[
BONE CONDUCTION–FOREHEAD						
UNMASKED		⌄			⌄	
MASKED	⌐		⌐	⌐		⌐
AIR CONDUCTION–SOUND FIELD	✶	$	∅	✶	$	∅
ACOUSTIC–REFLEX THRESHOLD						
CONTRALATERAL	⊃		⊂	⊃		⊂
IPSILATERAL	⊢		⊣	⊢		⊣

Figure 7.2. Autometric symbols recommended by ASHA (1990).

either an automatically pulsed signal of no less than 200 msec on/off time or a distinctive warble (frequency-modulated) tone. The listener is usually able to distinguish the test signal from intrinsic tinnitus under these circumstances.

If simple reinstruction or changes in presentation time are not successful in reducing false responses, the examiner should abandon the conventional ascending approach and use either a descending or a combination of descending-ascending signal presentations. If all attempts fail, and the examiner has little confidence in response validity, it is mandatory that this impression be stated clearly on the examination report. Any attempts to overcome unreliable response behavior should be detailed.

Sound Field Audiometry

Audiometry conducted by loudspeaker in a quiet sound field is often used in evaluating infants and young children and in assessing the functional gain of hearing aids. Because tests are rarely conducted in anechoic (absence of reverberation) environments, tonal stimuli are usually frequency-modulated to reduce the possibility of standing waves. Narrow-band noises are sometimes used for the same reason, but it appears that warble tones are preferable in evaluating normal-hearing children (Orchik and Rintelmann, 1978) as well as hypacusic adults (Stephens and Rintelmann, 1978).

Because SPL standards for warble tones do not exist at present, those using this approach must develop their own normative data for the specific environment and equipment under consideration. After studying many frequency variations and modulation ratios with experienced listeners, Staab and Rintelmann (1972) found similar thresholds using either pure tones or warble tones having modulation rates as great as 32/sec and frequency deviations as high as ±10%.

One should remember that the threshold levels obtained in sound field refer essentially to the sensitivity of the better ear. Efficient occlusion of the nontest ear must be accomplished, preferably with effective masking, before separate levels can be established for each ear.

Implications of Audiometric Results

Describing Impairment/Handicap

An impairment refers to structural or functional abnormality, an anatomic or physiologic condition that is outside "the range of normal." A handicap is the disadvantage imposed by an impairment. A handicap occurs when "one's personal efficiency in the activities of daily living" is affected by an impairment (American

Academy of Otolaryngology and the American Council of Otolaryngology (AAO-ACO, 1979). A handicap imposed by an auditory impairment could be defined in terms of the social, emotional, intellectual, and occupational consequences imposed by the functional loss of hearing.

Systems for classifying degree of "impairment" or "handicap" began appearing more than 60 years ago (Fletcher, 1929). They have been designed to provide more descriptive information than the audiogram, using familiar terminology. Classification systems are used in interpreting audiometric information to others in clinical and educational settings, for medicolegal and compensation purposes, and in research. In general, these systems are simple refinements of the threshold information provided by air-conduction audiometry under earphones.

Two general approaches have been used to describe impairment and handicap. The first provides a means for converting hearing levels into a rating scale based on percentage. Various formulas have been recommended within the medical profession since 1942 (American Medical Association) and have been accepted widely as statutory definitions. A revision of this approach was adopted by the (AAO-ACO) in 1979. The primary change was a widening of the frequency range included in the formula. In recognition of the importance of high-frequency information to speech intelligibility, the inclusive threshold hearing levels that had previously been limited to 0.5, 1, and 2 kHz were expanded to include 3 kHz.

This system is based on several assumptions (AAO-ACO, 1979). The following are most relevant: (a) impaired hearing function begins at an average hearing level of 25 dB (the low fence) for the selected frequencies and is complete at 92 dB HL (the high fence); (b) the resultant range of hearing impairment (about 66 dB) allows each dB unit to be assigned a value of 1.5% on a linear scale; (c) better ear sensitivity contributes to binaural audibility by a factor of 5:1; and (d) average sensitivity for puretones at the four selected frequencies is a valid indicator of a person's ability to hear speech in a "variety of everyday listening conditions." Based on these factors, the percentages of hearing impairment for each ear and of binaural handicap are calculated as follows:

(a) Find the puretone threshold average (PTA) for 0.5, 1, 2 and 3 kHz for each ear, air conduction only; (b) subtract 25 dB from the PTA; (c) multiply by 1.5% to find "percentage of hearing impairment" for each ear; (d) multiply the smaller of the two percentages (better ear) by 5; (e) add the percentage impairment for the poorer ear; and (f) divide by six to find the combined "percentage of hearing handicap."

The assumptions on which the above scale is based are highly argumentative. They are not adequately supported experimentally or pragmatically, especially as they relate to a description of hearing handicap (Noble, 1978). Certainly any ideal definition of handicap must consider such factors as age at onset, anatomic site of pathology, presence of tinnitus, degree of speech distortion in quiet and noise, specific communicative needs in the listener's life, relation to impairment of other sensory or motor systems, success or failure of past rehabilitative measures, family support, intellectual status, etc. There is little disagreement that direct measures of speech intelligibility would be of greater relevance, but lack of procedural standardization has impeded general acceptance of these data. Considerable disagreement still exists regarding the low and high fence values, and the frequencies selected for consideration (Clark, 1981). A review of these factors (ASHA Task Force on the Definition of Hearing Handicap, 1981) led to their recommendation that percentage formulas should include hearing thresholds for 1, 2, 3, and 4 kHz, and low-high fences of 25 and 75 dB HL, respectively. This would assume a 2% per dB linear growth. The 5:1 weighting concept for better ear-poorer ear combinations was retained in this recommendation.

A second approach for describing impaired hearing also uses monaural PTA in the speech frequencies but attaches adjective descriptors to the resultant levels. These suggestions are summarized by Clark (1980). Although not yet standardized, modifications of Goodman's proposal (1965) are popular among some audiologists (Table 7.1). Certainly such descriptors applied to either PTA or spondaic thresholds, although convenient and useful in clinical practice, provide limited information about the true degree of communicative dysfunction exhibited by a specific listener. They do not consider high frequency sensitivity, and they suffer from the same failings as those applied to percentage scales. Whenever such labels are used, they should always be supplemented with further information describing communicative behavior.

More detailed information regarding the listener's auditory experiences can be obtained by using one of a variety of self-assessment questionnaires that have been developed for the purpose (see Schow and Gatehouse, 1990, for a review of these instruments). Self-assessment data offer significantly more information about the implications of hearing impairment in a person's life than can be deduced from a complete audiometric evaluation, much less audiometry limited to air-conduction thresholds. Although this approach has been adopted in New Zealand for compensation assessment (Noble, 1978), legal definitions of handicap in other jurisdictions are still restricted to calculations based on threshold hearing levels obtained by AC audiometry.

Diagnostic Implications

Puretone thresholds obtained solely by air conduction have limited value for diagnostic purposes. Certain patterns of impairment across frequency are often noted clinically, but relationships to specific pathology must be made with considerable caution. For example, middle ear pathology often produces impairments at all frequencies (a "flat" audiogram), as does Meniere's disease. Intra- and interaural threshold comparisons, coupled with hearing levels in the speech frequencies, provide useful information for describing a person's sensitivity. Such data are often helpful for setting appropriate presentation levels and for interpreting other audiometric tests, as well as being widely used in hearing conservation programs. These applications are well documented throughout this text. But information limited to AC sensitivity is insufficient to make valid judgments regarding site of lesion.

High Frequency Audiometry

Increasing interest has been shown recently in sensitivity studies at signal frequencies above 8 kHz. Such information may have both diagnostic and rehabilitative value (Fausti et al., 1979b; Berlin, 1982; Fausti and Rappaport, 1985). Specialized equipment and unique calibration procedures are required for high-frequency audiometry. Once these hardware requirements are met, signals transduced under MX-41/AR cushions by wide response earphones have produced reliable audibility thresholds up to 20 kHz using standard manual techniques in children (Zislis and Fletcher, 1966; Harris and Ward, 1967) and adults (Beiter and Rupp, 1972; Beiter and Talley, 1976; Fausti et al., 1979a). Acceptable reliability has also been reported using automatic

Table 7.1
Scale of Hearing Impairment[a]

Average Threshold Level (dB)[b]	Suggested Description
-10 to 15[c]	Normal hearing
16 to 25[c]	Slight hearing loss
26 to 40	Mild hearing loss
41 to 55	Moderately severe hearing loss
56 to 70	Severe hearing loss
71 to 90	Profound hearing loss
91 plus	

[a]Modified from Goodman, A. 1965. Reference zero levels for puretone audiometer, Asha 7, 262-263.
[b]Average threshold level re ANSI-1989 for 0.5, 1 and 2 kHz.
[c]Modified by Clark (1981); Goodman recommended normal hearing from -10 to 25 dB.

tracking under earphones (Fletcher, 1965; Harris and Myers, 1971; Northern et al., 1972), and by conventional testing in sound field (Osterhammel, 1978). Myers and Harris (1970) compared threshold reliability in seven systems encompassing both sound field and earphone presentation of tones and noise. They concluded that each of the techniques yielded acceptably reliable data. Fausti et al. (1982) constructed release-from-masking functions for frequencies between 8 and 14 kHz in normal ears. The findings suggested that listeners were not responding to distortion products involving the lower frequencies, but were validly perceiving high frequency stimuli.

Threshold audiometry at frequencies above 8 kHz is instrumentally feasible, clinically reliable, and appears to be a valid indication of auditory sensitivity. The increased knowledge gained by expanding the test frequency range in threshold audiometry may be significant and deserves further exploration.

AUTOMATIC AUDIOMETRY

An alternative approach to manual threshold audiometry involves listener control of signal intensity. A technique was described by Bekesy in 1947 that automatically increased tonal frequency from 100 to 10,000 Hz at a set speed. The intensity of the signal was decreased or increased by the listener manipulating a switch when the tone became audible or inaudible. A graphic representation of amplitude change versus frequency was recorded simultaneously.

Various instruments became available in ensuing years that allow listener tracking of pulsed and continuous signals presented at either discrete or changing frequencies. Comparisons of tracking results in hearing-impaired individuals led to a number of response patterns that have become useful in the differential evaluation of auditory function (see Chapter 11). In addition, automatic audiometry is being used in making functional gain measurements with hearing aids in sound field.

Tracking audiometry has become increasingly popular for determining threshold because (*a*) one examiner can evaluate two or more individuals simultaneously and (*b*) the technique lends itself well to microprocessor control and recording (see Chapter 33). Increased cost efficiency and potential improvements in test accuracy have enhanced interest in techniques involving self-recorded responses.

CONCLUSION

Threshold audiometry by air conduction is a widely applied procedure. The apparent simplicity of the test procedures, however, may mask the importance of proper

caution in test administration and interpretation to ensure maximum validity and reliability.

Several areas have been emphasized in which the application of present knowledge and technology can potentially improve the accuracy and consistency of clinical threshold measurement. Recent developments in standards governing test environment, calibration procedures, and manual testing protocols have been helpful. Engineering of solid-state instrumentation has significantly improved the reliability of hardware used in audiometric evaluation.

But there is still much to be done. Future adoption of new earphone configurations should substantially reduce test variability in most audiometric applications. Computer-assisted protocols offer many opportunities to improve test validity. True psychometric methodology, combined with forced-choice responses, might be applied within time constraints acceptable for both group and individual testing. Calibration inconsistencies could be practically eliminated by using a probe tube in the ear canal that could constantly monitor SPL and make instantaneous adjustments of audiometric levels relative to ANSI standards (Harris, 1978). Deficiencies in electric or acoustic operating status could be immediately conveyed to the operator with such an apparatus.

Finally, alternatives to the use of AC thresholds as the sole indicator of hearing handicap must be adopted. The "model of convenience" embodied in percentage scales is grossly inadequate as a valid descriptor in this context. Supplementary information must be given greater attention, including better insights into speech-processing skills. Tonal sensitivity is a helpful index in many applications, as discussed in this chapter. But a complete understanding of a person's hearing handicap cannot be had without adequate consideration of how speech is heard under noise interference conditions as well as in quiet.

REFERENCES

AAO-ACO (American Academy of Otolaryngology and American Council of Otolaryngology). Guide for evaluation of hearing handicap. JAMA 1979;241:2055–2059.

American Medical Association. Tentative standard procedure for evaluating the percentage of useful hearing loss in medicolegal cases. JAMA 1942;119:1108–1109.

American National Standards Institute. American National Standard Specifications for Audiometers. ANSI S3.6-1989, New York.

American National Standards Institute. American National Standard Psychoacoustical Terminology. ANSI S3.20-1973 (R 1986), New York.

American National Standards Institute. Criteria for Permissible Ambient Noise during Audiometric Testing. ANSI S3.1-1977 (R 1986), New York.

American National Standards Institute. Methods for Manual Pure-Tone Threshold Audiometry. ANSI S3.21-1978 (R 1986), New York.

American Speech and Hearing Association, Committee on Audiometric Evaluation. Guidelines for audiometric symbols. ASHA 1974;17:260–264.

American Speech and Hearing Association, Committee on Audiometric Evaluation. Guidelines for manual pure-tone threshold audiometry. ASHA 1978;20:297–301.

American Speech-Language-Hearing Association, Task Force on the Definition of Hearing Handicap. On the definition of hearing handicap. ASHA 1981;23:293–297.

American Speech-Language-Hearing Association. Guidelines for audiometric symbols. ASHA 1990;20(Suppl 2):25–30.

Atherley GRC, and Lord P. A preliminary study of the effect of earphone position on the reliability of repeated auditory threshold determination. Int Audiol 1965;4:161–166.

Barr-Hamilton RM, Bryan ME, and Tempest W. Applications of signal detection theory to audiometry. Int Audiol 1969;8:138–146.

Beiter RC, and Rupp RR. Standard audiometric procedures for thresholds above 8 kc/s: a normative study. J Aud Res 1972;12:199–202.

Beiter RC, and Talley JN. High-frequency audiometry above 8000 Hz. Audiology 1976;;15:207–214.

Bekesy Gv. A new audiometer. Acta Otolaryngol (Stockh) 1947;35:411–422.

Berlin CI. Ultra-audiometric hearing in the hearing impaired and the use of upward-shifting translating hearing aids. Volta Rev 1982;84:352–363.

British Society of Audiology, Education Committee. Recommended procedure for pure-tone audiometry using a manually-operated instrument. Br Soc Audiol Newslett 1978;April, 9–13.

Bryan ME, and Tempest W. Precision audiometry. Acta Otolaryngol (Stockh) 1967;64:205–212.

Bryde RL, and Feldman AS. An approach to the management of collapsing ear canals. ASHA 1980;22:734.

Bunch CC. 1943. Clinical Audiometry. St Louis: CV Mosby.

Carhart R, and Jerger JF. Preferred method for clinical determination of pure-tone thresholds. J Speech Hear Disord 1959;24:330–345.

Chaiklin JB, and McClelland ME. Audiometric management of collapsible ear canals. Arch Otolaryngol 1071;93:397–407.

Clark JG. 1980. Audiology for the School Speech-Language Clinician. Springfield, IL: Charles C Thomas.

Clark JG. Uses and abuses of hearing loss classification. ASHA 1981;23:493–500.

Clarke FR, and Bilger RC. The theory of signal detectability and the measurement of hearing. In Jerger, J., Ed. Modern Developments in Audiology, Ed. 2. New York: Academic Press, 1973:437–467.

Corso JF. Age and sex differences in pure-tone thresholds. Arch Otolaryngol 1963;77:385–405.

Corso JF, and Cohen A. Methodological aspects of auditory threshold measurements. J Exp Psychol (Gen) 1958;55:8–12.

Creston JE. Collapse of the ear canal during routine audiometry. J Laryngol Otol 1965;79:893–901.

Curry ET, and Kurtzrock GH. A preliminary investigation of the ear-choice technique in threshold audiometry. J Speech Hear Disord 1951;16:340–345.

Dadson RS, and King JH. A determination of normal threshold of hearing and its relation to the standardization of audiometers. J Laryngol Otol 1952;66:366–378.

Fausti SA, Rappaport BZ, Schechter MA, and Frey RH. An investigation of the validity of high-frequency audition. J Acoust Soc Am 1982;71:646–649.

Fausti SA, and Rappaport BC, Eds. High-Frequency Audiometry. Semin Hearing 1985;6:369–386, 397–404.

Fausti SA, Frey RH, Erickson DA, and Rappaport BZ. 2AFC versus standard clinical measurement of high frequency auditory sensitivity (8-20 kc/s). J Aud Res 1979a;19:151–157.

Fausti SA, Frey RH, Erickson DA, Rappaport Bz, and Cleary ej. A system for evaluating auditory function from 8000-20000 Hz. J Acoust Soc Am 1979b; 69:1343–1349.

Fletcher H. 1929. Speech and Hearing. New York: Van Nostrand.

Fletcher JL. Reliability of high-frequency thresholds. J Aud Res 1965;5:133–137.

Frank T, and Wright BC. Attenuation provided by four different audiometric earphone systems. Ear Hear 1990;11:70–78.

Goodman A. Reference zero levels for pure-tone audiometer. ASHA 1965;7:262–263.

Green DM, and Swets JA. 1966. Signal Detection Theory and Psychophysics. New York: John Wiley and Sons.

Green DS. 1978. Pure tone air-conduction testing. In Katz J, Ed. Handbook of Clinical Audiology, Ed. 2. Baltimore: Williams & Wilkins, 1978:90–109.

Harris JD. Group audiometry. J Acoust Soc Am 1945;17:73–76.

Harris JD. Normal hearing and its relation to audiometry. Laryngoscope 1954;64:928–957.

Harris JD. Proem to a quantum leap in audiometric data collection and management. J Aud Res 1978;18:1–29.

Harris JD. Optimum threshold crossings and time window validation in threshold pure-tone computerized audiometry. J Acoust Soc Am 1979;66:1545–1547.

Harris JD, and Myers CK. Tentative audiometric threshold-level standards from 8 through 18 kHz. J Acoust Soc Am 1971;49:600–601.

Harris JD, and Ward MD. High-frequency audiometry to 20 kc/s in children of age 10-12 years. J Aud Res 1967;7:241–252.

Hempstock TI, Bryan ME, and Webster W. Free-field threshold variance. J. Sound Vib 1966;4:33–44.

Hickling S. Studies on the reliability of auditory threshold values. J Aud Res 1966;6:39–46.

Hodgson WR. 1980. Basic Audiologic Evaluation. Baltimore: Williams & Wilkins.

Hughson W, and Westlake H. Manual for program outline for rehabilitation of aural casualties both military and civilian. Trans Am Acad Ophthalmol Otolaryngol 1944; (Suppl 48):1–15.

Jerger J. A proposed audiometric symbol system for scholarly publications. Arch Otolaryngol 1976;102:33–36.

Killion MC, and Villchur E. Comments on "Earphones in audiometry" (Zwislocki et al., J Acoust Soc Am 1989;83:1688–1689 (1988)). J Acoust Soc Am 1989;85:1775–1778.

Marshall L, and Gossman MA. Management of ear-canal collapse. Arch. Otolaryngol 1982;108:357–361.

Myers CK, and Harris JD. Comparison of seven systems for high-frequency air-conduction audiometry. J Speech Hear Res 1970;13:254–270.

Newhart H, and Reger SN, Eds. Syllabus of audiometric procedures in administration of a program for the conservation of hearing of school children. Trans Am Acad Opthalmol Otolaryngol 1945;(Suppl)April, 1-28.

Noble WG. 1978. Assessment of Impaired Hearing. New York: Academic Press.

Northern J, Davis MP, Rudmose W, Glorig A, and Fletcher JL. Recommended high frequency audiometric threshold levels (8000-18000 Hz). J Acoust Soc Am 1972;52:585–595.

Orchick DJ, and Rintelmann WF. Comparison of pure-tone, warble-tone and narrow band threshold of young normal-hearing children. J Am Aud Soc 1978;3:314–320.

Osterhammel D. High-frequency thresholds using a quasi-free-field technique. Scand Audiol 1978;7:27–30.

Richards WD, Frank TA, and Prout JH. Influence of earphone-cushion center-hole diameter on the acoustic output of audiometric earphones. J Acoust Soc Am 1979;65:257–259.

Riedner ED. Collapsing ears and the use of circumaural ear cushions at 3000 Hz. Ear Hear 1980;1:117–118.

Robinson DW, and Sutton GJ. Age effect in hearing—a comparative analysis of published threshold data. Audiology 1979;18:320–334.

Schow RL, and Gatehouse S. Fundamental issues in self-assessment of hearing. Ear Hear 1990;11(Suppl):6S–16S.

Schow RL, and Goldbaum DE. Collapsed ear canals in the elderly nursing home population. J Speech Hear Disord 1980;45:259–267.

Shaw E. Ear canal pressure generated by circumaural and supraaural earphones. J Acoust Soc Am 1966;39:471–479.

Staab WJ, and Rintelmann WF. Status of warble-tone in audiometers. Audiology 1972;11:244–255.

Stephens MW, and Rintelmann WF. The influence of audiometric configuration on pure-tone, warble-tone and narrow-band noise thresholds of adults with sensorineural hearing losses. J Am Aud Soc 1978;3:221–226.

Talbott RE. Bacteriology of earphone contamination. J Speech Hear Res 1969;12:326–329.

Tyler RS, and Wood EJ. A comparison of manual methods for measuring hearing levels. Audiology 1980;19:316–329.

Watson LA, and Tolan T. 1949. Hearing Tests and Hearing Instruments. Baltimore: Williams & Wilkins.

Wilber A, Kruger B, and Killion MC. Reference thresholds for the ER-3A insert earphone. J Acoust Soc Am 1988;83:669–676.

Wolff DA, and Borchardt KA. Two methods of controlling bacterial contamination of audiometer earphones. Milit Med 1975;140:329–330.

Zislis T, and Fletcher JL. Relation of high frequency thresholds to age and sex. J Aud Res 1966;6:189–198.

Zwislocki J. Reply to "Comments on 'Earphones in audiometry'" (Killion MC, and Villchur E. J Acoust Soc Am 1989;85:1775–1778. J Acoust Soc Am 1989;85:1778–1779.

Zwislocki J, Keuger B, Miller JC, Niemoller AF, Shaw EA, and Studebaker G. 1988. Earphones in audiometry. J Acoust Soc Am 83:1688–1689.

CHAPTER 8

Clinical Masking: A Decision-Making Process

Beverly A. Goldstein and Craig W. Newman

The application of clinical masking is often essential during audiometric testing. The need to mask arises when an individual being tested demonstrates substantial threshold differences in air conduction for the test ear and bone conduction for the nontest ear and/or demonstrates the presence of an air-bone gap. Because the goal in audiologic measurements is to obtain valid and reliable results, audiologists must gain skills in clinical masking procedures to evaluate accurately each ear independently.

Masking is a complex and somewhat variable phenomenon. Therefore clinicians, especially the less experienced ones, may have difficulty in making appropriate masking decisions and correctly interpreting the results. In order to deal with masking more effectively, it is best to view the task as a continual decision-making process. Thus, the overall task that may be difficult to conceptualize can be broken down into simple steps which the clinician can follow. Eventually, masking decisions become rather automatic and conceptualization is crystalized. This chapter will focus on a series of clinical questions and decisions, such as what is an appropriate masking signal, when to employ masking, and what are adequate levels to use. In addition, masking problems shall be presented, solutions discussed, and the vital question of how to calibrate the masking signal reviewed.

Appropriate procedural decisions depend upon an understanding of the psychoacoustic principles underlying clinical masking. While the important concepts will be reviewed here, clinicians should familiarize themselves with publications regarding theoretical aspects of masking (Hawkins and Stevens, 1950; Bilger and Hirsh, 1956; Dirks and Malmquist, 1964; Chaiklin, 1967; among others) for greater detail. Based on knowledge of these psychoacoustic concepts, clinical masking procedures have been developed and employed successfully with appropriate populations (Hood, 1960; Studebaker, 1967; Martin, 1972; Staab, 1974; Goldstein, 1979).

The purposes of this chapter are to: (*a*) identify decisions that need to be made during clinical masking; (*b*) describe the rationales which form the basis for procedural decisions; (*c*) present sets of recommended rules on which to base decisions; and (*d*) assist clinicians in developing clinical masking skills. A hierarchy of masking operations is presented in this chapter to promote a logical decision-making model.

PRELIMINARY CONSIDERATIONS

What Is Masking?

Almost all authors who discuss clinical masking present definitions at the outset. The American National Standards Institute (ANSI) specification for audiometers (S3.6-1989) defines masking as ". . . The process by which the threshold of audibility for one sound is raised by the presence of another (masking) sound" (p. 3). In an excellent review of auditory masking, Studebaker (1973) provided additional definitions by Meyer (1959), Carter and Kryter (1962), and Deatherage and Evans (1969). These definitions are concerned basically with the concepts of interference with the primary signal by a secondary source and the elevation or shift in threshold.

In the clinical setting, audiologists rely on the use of a masking noise to elevate the nontest ear (NTE) threshold without interfering with or influencing the audiometric results of the test ear (TE). Because the separate evaluation of each ear is important for diagnostic and rehabilitative decisions, clinical supervisors often tell beginning students that masking is used to keep the NTE "busy" while evaluating the TE.

Both ipsilateral and contralateral masking functions can be generated. Ipsilateral masking functions refer to mixing the test signal and masking noise in the *same* ear. For clinical purposes, ipsilateral masking is used to determine the amount of threshold shift that is produced by a particular masking noise. This shift is dependent on the intensity/bandwidth relationship of the test signal and masking noise. Ipsilateral masking can be used for calibrating the masking noise. In contrast, contralateral masking refers to the presentation of the test signal to one ear and the masking noise to the *opposite ear*. For clinical purposes, contralateral masking is used to elevate the threshold in the NTE so that it cannot respond to the signal being presented to the TE. Unless specified otherwise, the use of the term *masking* in the remaining portions of this chapter will refer to contralateral masking.

When the audiometric configurations of an individual's two ears differ greatly, masking becomes necessary for both threshold procedures (e.g., puretones, spondees) and suprathreshold procedures (e.g., speech discrimination testing). Slight differences between ears typically require masking for suprathreshold procedures only. This occurs because presentation levels for such procedures may create artificially large differences between ears, allowing the NTE to perceive the more intense test signal.

Why Is Masking Necessary?

As suggested above, clinical masking is used to eliminate participation of the NTE when evaluating the TE. More specifically, a second sound source (usually some type of *noise presented via the air-conduction mode* through an earphone) is employed to shift the *sensitivity of the nontest cochlea* to prevent the NTE from responding when presenting a signal to the TE. Masking must be used during an audiologic assessment when the patient presents air- and/or bone-conduction thresholds that are not similar bilaterally. Thus, masking is typically used in the cases of unilateral or asymmetric bilateral hearing loss.

When a signal is presented to the poorer ear (TE) at a sufficiently loud intensity level, it may pass across the skull and be perceived by the opposite, better ear (NTE). Without using masking for the NTE, patients will respond to the signal in the better ear. Responses to air-conducted puretones that have crossed over from the poorer ear will actually shadow the thresholds of the better ear. These "shadow" responses on the audiogram mimic the threshold levels of the better ear, elevated by the amount of the interaural attenuation at each frequency. When crossover occurs, the obtained thresholds for the poorer ear (TE) are better than the "true" thresholds.

The above example illustrates the necessity to mask. Without application of appropriate masking procedures, validity of test findings is in question. Clinicians must, therefore, examine the obtained results to determine whether they represent the actual hearing levels or may be due to cross hearing. The consequences of failing to mask, or the inappropriate use of masking, have potentially serious negative ramifications on both medical and audiologic management.

Variables Affecting Masking

Masking is often a difficult task for the inexperienced tester because many variables must be considered and manipulated (Studebaker, 1967, 1979; Sanders, 1972, 1978). Studebaker (1979) pointed out that it is inappropriate simply to select a single masking level that is used with a variety of cases as this frequently results in over- or undermasking. Also, one cannot depend on the listener's judgment of which ear is being stimulated.

Studebaker further indicated that clinicians must learn to deal with the following: (*a*) the presentation level of the test signal, (*b*) the air-bone gaps in each ear, (*c*) the occlusion effect, if present, (*d*) the interaural attenuation for both air- and bone-conducted signals and masker, and (*e*) the effective masking level of the masker. To help the reader approach the task in an organized manner, seven variables and their definitions are presented below. A clear understanding of these concepts is requisite to mastering clinical masking skills.

Test Ear (TE)

During audiometric procedures that require masking, the TE, the ear to which the test signal is being directed, is always the poorer ear. Masking levels chosen during testing are *not* based on the unmasked threshold response of the TE.

Nontest Ear (NTE)

During audiometric procedures that require masking, the NTE receiving the masking is the better ear. Masking levels chosen during testing are based on the air-conduction threshold(s) of the NTE.

Sensory-Neural Level of the NTE

Whether there is or is not an air-bone gap, the bone-conduction threshold of the NTE will shift the same amount as the air-conduction threshold of the same ear when masking is applied. Cross-over of the signal from the TE can be received by the better bone-conduction sensitivity of the NTE if an air-bone gap is present. Therefore, sufficient air-conducted masking must be directed to the NTE to assure that the test signal is not picked up by bone conduction. A "shadow response" of the NTE will be obtained if the masking level is not sufficient to remove the NTE from participation.

Sensory-Neural Level of the TE

When masking is directed to the NTE, masking levels must remain less than bone-conduction thresholds of the TE in order to avoid "overmasking." This points out that masking from the NTE can be received at the TE by bone conduction, just as signals from the TE can crossover to interfere with bone conduction of the NTE.

Accurate Masking Level

Neither too much nor too little masking is desirable. Many clinicians in the early stages of training believe that a substantial amount of masking to the NTE is appropriate for eliminating a "shadow response." Clinical masking can be annoying, distracting or occasionally painful. Thus, excessive use of masking can interfere with measurement of the TE. It is recommended that the audiologist use accurate rather than excessive masking levels to obtain valid results.

Selection of Starting Level for Masking

Selection of appropriate levels is based on the air-conduction thresholds of the NTE and the bone-conduction thresholds of the TE. These procedures will be discussed in a later section.

Occlusion Effect (OE)

Special consideration is necessary for masking in bone-conduction testing. When an earphone is placed on the NTE to present the masking signal, the earphone itself produces an artificial improvement in the bone-conduction response, known as the OE. Sanders (1978, p 136) points out, "The improved responses are a result of sound pressure generated in the closed external auditory canal and transmitted through the conductive mechanism." It is associated with additional energy reaching the cochlea rather than any change in true sensitivity. The OE will occur when occluding a normal ear or one with a sensory-neural loss and therefore should be considered in the masking calculations. In contrast, no additional improvement is noted in bone conduction when an earphone is placed on an ear with a middle ear disorder. Conductive pathology produces an improvement in bone-conducted responses equal to the OE regardless of ear canal occlusion. Therefore, no correction for the OE is made in cases with conductive losses.

Effective Masking and the Critical Bandwidth Concept

Masking signals of given intensities do not necessarily produce shifts in threshold equal to the audiometric dial reading. ANSI S3.6-1989 defines effective masking (EM) as the level to which a tonal threshold (using a 50% criterion) is shifted by a particular noise whose center frequency is the same as the test tone. The EM level of the masker is equal to the hearing level of the *shifted puretone threshold*. This emphasizes that EM is defined according to the effect a noise will have on the threshold of the signal in the TE rather than according to the dial reading of the masker. EM levels can be expressed in the same unit of measurement as the test signal (HL). The application of EM in clinical audiometry has simplified the use of masking procedures. It permits the clinician to know the masking efficiency for a particular noise, thereby specifying the threshold (in HL) to which the signal will be shifted by the masker when presented to the NTE. The procedure for calibrating masking noises to effective masking levels will be presented in a subsequent section.

A fundamental understanding of the *critical bandwidth* (CBW) concept is essential to clinical application of EM. It forms the basis for decision making regarding both the selection of masking signals as well as their calibration. A brief summary of three germinal studies investigating the CBW concept is presented to highlight the relationship between masking noises and test signals.

Fletcher (1940) hypothesized that a restricted bandwidth of frequencies contained within a given broadband noise was sufficient to mask effectively a puretone signal. This narrow "critical band" had at its center the same frequency as the test signal. Further, Fletcher suggested that widening this bandwidth would not enhance the efficiency of the masking signal. Since 1940, the literature has supported the use of narrow-band noises to mask single frequency test signals.

Hawkins and Stevens (1950) documented critical bandwidths for monaural masking of puretones by white noise at eight sensation levels (20–90 dB) at 16 selected frequencies (100–9000 Hz). Their findings embodied both dimensions of the CBW concept: frequency bandwidth (Hz) and intensity level (dB). They concluded that for a flat broad-band masking noise, a critical bandwidth calculation will accurately determine the band of frequencies necessary to achieve effective masking of a given puretone whose frequency is located at the center of the masking band. They further indicated that ". . . when a critical band of frequencies is at a just audible level, the total energy in the band [[dB]] is the same as the threshold energy of the pure tone whose frequency lies at the center of the band" (Hawkins and Stevens, 1950, pp 10–11).

Through use of a modified Bekesy procedure, tabulated for 39 frequencies (150–6000 Hz) at intensity levels varying from 40 to 120 dB sound pressure level (SPL), Bilger and Hirsh (1956) confirmed the linear relationship between the extent of masking and the intensity level of the critical band. This finding became important for clinical application because it provided the basis for predicting reliable threshold shifts with specific masker intensities. They summarized their findings as follows (p 623):

First, and most directly connected with the original definition, the critical band is defined as that band of frequencies in a noise beyond which broadening the band will not further increase the masking of a pure tone in the center of the band. Second, a critical band may also be defined as that band width of noise whose over-all energy is equal to the energy of a pure tone in the center of the band when the tone is just barely masked by the noise. Third, and as a corollary of the second, the critical band of noise is that band width whose absolute threshold is equal to the threshold of a pure tone in the center of the band.

Description of Masking Signals

Discussion of CBW has pointed out that the extent of threshold shift produced by a masking signal results from both the masker's intensity and its frequency composition. The key issue in selection of type of masking noise is that of "relative masking efficiency," the ratio of the shift in threshold relative to the overall intensity of the noise (Sanders, 1978). The objective is to achieve the largest shift in threshold with the least overall noise intensity. All masking signals have limited effectiveness in the lower frequencies because the human auditory system requires a greater amount of SPL to reach threshold in that region. The relationship between the masking effect and any given noise level is linear once EM has been established (Bilger and Hirsh, 1956).

Broad-Band White Noise

A masking signal composed of random energy at all frequencies with approximately equal intensity has been termed thermal or white noise. Audiometric transducers limit the bandwidth and frequency response of white noise, as the noise assumes the spectral characteristics of the earphone or speaker.

There are numerous methods available to produce white noise and each is based on the requirements of the audiometer design. The noise is selectively filtered via electronic band-pass active filters to create the required noise spectra.

Speech by nature is broad frequency, and the speech noise needed for masking during speech audiometry is filtered to mimic the long term spectrum of speech. A description of ANSI's requirement for "masking for speech tests" is presented in the next section, and a frequency response of such a noise is presented in Figure 8.1. Speech noise for audiometers is produced by filtering white noise using a "two-pole" low pass active filter having a corner frequency of 1000 Hz and a rejection rate of 12 dB/octave above the corner.

Narrow-Band/Filtered White Noise

Narrow-band noise is created by passing a broad-band white noise source masking signal through a series of narrow-band electronic active filters, each having its pass band centered at the test tone frequency. (Narrow-band noise can also be produced by a narrow-band noise masking generator that creates a different noise for each bandwidth. This method is not commonly used in audiometers today.) A narrow-band signal is defined by three features: (a) the center frequency, (b) the bandwidth in Hz at 3 dB below the intensity of the peak component, and (c) the filter rejection rate or decrease in intensity per octave above and below the bandwidth.

The wave envelope (spectrum) intensity levels of CBWs produce the most efficient masking for puretone signals (Hawkins and Stevens, 1950); however, critical bands tend to have considerable tonality and may be confused with TE test frequencies. To overcome this problem, bandwidths greater than CB have been manufactured (J. W. Ward, personal communication 1984); four-tenths octave has been commonly used. According

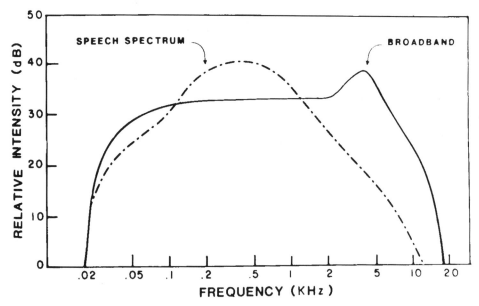

Figure 8.1. Acoustic amplitude spectra for speech spectrum and broad-band noise typically used for masking the contralateral ear in speech audiometry . . . representative of these stimuli when they are transduced by a TDH-39 earphone. (From Konkle DF, and Rintelmann WF. Principles of Speech Audiometry. Baltimore: University Park Press, 1983.

to ANSI S3.6-1989, audiometers with narrow band stimuli have leeway in producing both lower and upper cut-off frequencies. The bands of noise should be at a minimum one-third of an octave and one-half octave as a maximum. Masking bands, which are either smaller or larger than CBW (in Hz), are less efficient maskers of test signals. Thus, more intensity is required to produce equivalent masking. This is because only the intensity in the CB accomplishes the masking, not the overall intensity level of the signal. "For center frequencies of 500 Hz and above, these bands are wider than the critical masking bands and require a sound pressure level approximately 3 dB greater than critical bands for effective masking (ANSI S3.6-1989, p. 9)."

Narrow-band noises are preferred for puretone test procedures because of their masking efficiency. How to compare intensity levels of masking noises to tones and "calibrate" the hearing level dial electronically or biologically will be presented in a subsequent section.

ANSI Requirements for Masking Signals and Use of Masking

The ANSI S3.6-1989 standard provides specifications for audiometers, including recommendations for masking signals[a]. The measurements of air-conducted masking sounds should be made in an acoustic coupler or artificial ear. The measurements, in general, are to be ± 5 dB of the target value.

The standard states that: (a) the frequency range of narrow band noise should be centered around the test tone, (b) if a weighted random noise is used for masking of puretones, the SPL, in one-third octave bands (from 250–4000 Hz), should be equal to that of the specific puretone, (c) broad-band (white) noise should contain the same energy at frequencies in the range from 250 to 6000 Hz as at 1000 Hz, and (d) noise for masking speech should have a spectrum density (energy per Hz) that is constant from 250 to 1000 Hz, with a reduction in the energy level of 12 dB/octave from 1000 Hz to 4000 Hz.

Other specifications dealing with masking include the designation of masking increments of 5 dB or less and that the dial should specify decibels of effective masking. The NB masker should have the same dB specification +3 dB as the tone around which it is centered. For other masking signals, the control dial should read either SPL or EM. The masking sound through earphones shall be from +5 to -3 dB of the specified values and the output at successive steps on the attenuator must deviate no more than three-tenths of the indicator increments, or 1 dB, if this value is smaller. The masking should be sufficient to

mask tones of 60 dB HL at 250 Hz, 75 at 500 Hz, and 80 dB from 1000 to 4000 Hz. The masking output is not to exceed 125 dB at any frequency.

Although the requirement of masking generators is specified in ANSI Standard S3.6-1989, the decision to mask rests with the tester. This, however, is not the case for ANSI Standard S3.26-1981, "Reference Equivalent Threshold Force Levels for Audiometric Bone Vibrators." This standard includes force values representing normal bone-conduction thresholds, the validity of which is based on the requisite use of 30 to 35 dB of effective masking presented to the nontest ear. Ideally, to conform to the standard, masking must be used for all clients during bone-conduction audiometry, or a central masking threshold correction (discussed in a subsequent section) should be made. In daily clinical practice, when there is no significant air-bone gap, additional time-consuming masking procedures are frequently omitted. The use of masking for bone conduction in this situation provides no additional clinical information. There is support in the literature to use masking judiciously: "The better approach for threshold testing is the one used now, that is, first obtaining unmasked thresholds and then masked thresholds as necessary" (Studebaker, 1979, p 88).

Methods of Calibrating Masking Signals

The initial step in clinical masking is to develop an understanding of masking signal intensity level as compared to test signal intensity level. Relationships between effects of masking and HL dial settings are inconsistent and vary across manufacturers. The goal in using any of the noises described above is to achieve the status of EM defined operationally as the ability of a given increase in a masking signal to shift linearly a given test signal an equivalent and predictable amount. Changing an SPL masking level to an EM level requires one to identify the effective level of the noise. Knowledge of EM levels permits the tester to predict shifts in threshold produced by specific HLs of masking. EM calibration can be accomplished for narrow-band noise through internal equipment modification in which masking signal SPLs are set to equal test signal SPLs plus 3 dB. Once internal calibration is completed, dial readings of the audiometer are accurate in producing EM. This provides for simplicity of operation, because it is known that a 40-dB dial reading will produce approximately 40 dB of EM.

Internal calibration is not feasible for broad-band noises because SPL threshold levels differ across frequency. Therefore, one overall level of noise produces different amounts of masking at different frequencies. The masking effect for each frequency can be determined through formula computation/electroacoustic analysis or biologic calibration methods. These proce-

[a]Copies of this standard may be obtained from the Standards Secretariat, in care of the Acoustical Society of America, 335 E. Street, New York, NY 10017-3483.

dures will provide the masking dial reading value equal to 0 dB HL at each test frequency. These correction factors for the broad-band noise should be recorded on an EM table, posted on the audiometer, and must be taken into account when determining how much masking to use in any given masking situation. The two basic calibration methods used to arrive at EM are presented below. Clinicians must decide which method best suits their clinical site.

Biologic (Real Ear)

Calibration through the use of human hearing is most commonly used when more objective measurements are unavailable. The most typical biologic approach is to mix electronically the test tones or speech, and the masking noise into one earphone and then measure threshold shifts at three hearing levels (50-, 70-, and 90-dB dial settings) for 10 normal-hearing subjects (Sanders and Rintelmann, 1964). The average threshold produced by the masking noise is the EM value for the specific frequency and hearing level. An average effective masking level can then be determined per frequency from information obtained at the various hearing levels. A simple correction factor can be designated, or the masking curves can be used to provide the desired shift.

Veniar (1965) suggested an alternative biologic approach. She does not recommend basing masking decisions on mean threshold values of a normal population, because pathologic ears may well respond differently to masking. Veniar determines a minimum effective masking level (MEML) for each client at each frequency that requires masking. With this procedure, the masking noise is introduced (mixed) into the same earphone that is receiving the puretone at threshold intensity. The noise is raised in 10-dB steps until it just masks the test signal. The amount of masking needed to eliminate the test tone is then considered 0 dB MEML. The values obtained for each frequency can also be employed when masking is used in bone-conduction audiometry.

Coles and Priede (1975) briefly described a biologic masking calibration procedure that would be effective in speech audiometry. They defined effective masking as the difference between the speech and noise levels that reduce a 95% or better intelligibility score to 10% or below in normal listeners. This effective masking correction would then be determined for each dial reading of that speech audiometer.

All of the biologic methods require signal mixing potential. The second method requires mixing equipment on a daily basis. The mixing of outputs from two amplifiers into a single transducer causes an equal intensity drop in both signal levels in some cases. Thus, the intensity relationships between the test signal and the masking remain the same, but both occur at reduced levels. Although appropriate mixing equipment may be needed (e.g., for portable audiometers that do not permit internal mixing), it is less costly than electroacoustic instrumentation necessary for the methods described below.

Formula Computation/Electroacoustic Analysis

One method of calibrating EM by formula computation/electroacoustic analysis is presented by Sanders (1972, pp 125–127). This approach allows for accurate calibration for either broad-band or narrow-band noise. Effective masking levels can be determined through the use of three successive formulas:

(a) LPC = OA SPL – 10 log BW in Hz
(b) E in CB = LPC + 10 log CBW
(10 log CBW in Hz = CBW in dB)
(c) Z [EM] = E in CB – threshold in quiet

As seen above, level per cycle (LPC) is equal to the overall sound pressure level (OA SPL) minus 10 times the log of the bandwidth (BW) in Hz. Bandwidth is based on the frequency component of the employed signal, broad or narrow band, and is modified by the earphone's frequency response. The computation of energy in the critical band (E in CB) is based on accurate determination of LPC and knowledge of the width of the critical band (CBW) based on Fletcher (1940) and Hawkins and Stevens (1950). The LPC is added to 10 times the log of the CBW in Hz, and the normal threshold in quiet (expressed in dB SPL) at that frequency is subtracted out. The remaining value is the effective masking level (Z) for that narrow- or broad-band noise.

The effective masking values calculated for puretones can be applied to calculation of EM for speech audiometry. Sanders (1972, p 139) recommended "averaging the effective levels at 500, 1000, and 2000 Hz for each dial setting." This calibration by formula procedure requires electroacoustic equipment to determine the OA SPL, the frequency response of the earphone and the number of cycles present in the generated broad and narrow bands. Manufacturer's specification sheets should provide some of this information.

Another method of calibrating the HL dial of the audiometer to EM by formula computation/electroacoustic analysis is presented below (see Table 8.1) (J. W. Ward, personal communication, 1984):

(a) Masking band (MB) expressed in Hz. MB must be one-third to one-half octave bandwidths per ANSI revised audiometer specification. For the example given, the geometric mean bandwidth, 0.4 octave, is used. If the audiometer masking BW is known or specified, then SPLs would be measured using a 1 octave or wider filter set. The filter network meter BW must be wider

Table 8.1
Necessary Electroacoustic Measurements of Masking Signals Compared with Computed Expected EM Values Using Example of MB = 0.4 Octave

Frequency in Hz	MB in Hz[a] (0.4 Octave)	CB in Hz[b]	Log MB	Log CB	Log MB—log CB	E10(Log MB - Log CB)	HL	Expected Masking Levels in HL	SPL = 0 dB HL ANSI S3.6-1969; TDH-50 Earphone	Expected EM Level in SPL	Obtained Noise Measured in dB SPL for Broad-Band Signal[c]	EM Table Difference in dB Rounded[d]	Obtained Noise Measured in dB SPL for Narrow-Band Signals	EM Table Difference in dB Rounded[d]
125	34.8	70.8	1.54	1.85	-0.31	-3.1	70	66.9	26.7	98.1	78	20	101	-3
250	69.5	50.0	1.84	1.70	0.14	1.4	70	71.4	13.5	87.9	81	7	85	3
500	139.1	50.0	2.14	1.70	0.44	4.4	70	74.4						
750	208.6	56.2	2.32	1.75	0.57	5.7	70	75.7						
1000	278.1	64.0	2.44	1.81	0.63	6.3	70	76.3	7.4	83.7	84	0	78.5	5
1500	417.2	79.4	2.62	1.90	0.72	7.2	70	77.2						
2000	556.3	100.0	2.75	2.00	0.75	7.5	70	77.5	11.1	88.6	84	5	82	7
3000	834.4	158.0	2.92	2.20	0.72	7.2	70	77.2						
4000	1113.0	200.0	3.05	2.30	0.75	7.5	70	77.5	10.7	88.2	84	4	83.5	5
6000	1869.0	376.0	3.27	2.58	0.69	6.9	70	76.9						
8000	2225.0	501.0	3.35	2.70	0.65	6.5	70	76.5	13	89.5	79	11	81	9

[a]Ward JW, personal communication, 1984.
[b]Hawkins and Stevens, 1950.
[c]Broad-band signal using a 70-dB HL dial setting and a linear coupler reading of 89.5 dB SPL.
[d]See Table 8.2.

than the masking BW or false, low SPLs will be recorded.

(b) Critical band (CB) (re Hawkins and Stevens, 1950) is expressed in Hz.

(c) Compute log MB in Hz.

(d) Compute log CB in Hz.

(e) Effective masking level (EML)

EML (in dB SPL) = HL (dial setting) + 10(log MB – log CB) + ANSI HL value.

Using a one-third or one-half octave filter set and an artificial ear assembly, measurements of the masking noise are taken at a 70-dB HL setting at the specified frequencies (Townsend and Schwartz, 1976). The obtained measurements (in dB SPL) and the calculated EML (in dB SPL) are then compared at each individual frequency. Differences are obtained. These differences represent the HL dial reading necessary to reach 0 dB EM. An effective masking table derived from Table 8.1 should be charted (see Table 8.2) and posted prominently on the face of the audiometer. This procedure also requires electroacoustic analysis equipment to obtain the SPL output of the noise for each test frequency.

The values obtained through the use of the above procedures define the EM values or the correction factors to be applied to the dial reading to get the desired EM levels. A value of 40 dB EM indicates that a given amount of narrow-band or broad-band noise (masking) is sufficient to just mask a 35-dB HL test signal. The threshold should therefore be shifted to 40 dB HL. Once the masking signals are calibrated, the clinician can then move on to the next sections of this chapter, "when" and "how" to mask.

ESSENTIAL MASKING DECISION: WHEN TO MASK

Masking may be necessary when the air- and/or bone-conduction thresholds are not similar bilaterally or air and bone responses are not interweaving. Under such circumstances, the phenomena of *cross-over* and *interaural attenuation* (IA) serve as the bases for determining when to mask. With an asymmetric audiometric configuration (i.e., more of a hearing loss in one ear), signals presented to the poorer ear (TE) may reach sufficient

intensity levels to cross over to the opposite ear (NTE). In this case, masking must be employed to prevent the NTE from responding for the TE, because a goal of audiometry is to evaluate each ear independently. Synonymous terms for cross-over include "cross-hearing," "transcranial hearing," and "shadow hearing" (Chaiklin, 1967).

It is important to recognize that air-conducted signals (puretones and speech), are transmitted to the opposite side of the skull primarily by bone conduction (Chaiklin, 1967). This has ramifications for making decisions regarding when to use masking. That is, clinicians must determine if the air-conduction responses obtained at the TE are valid, or simply a shadow response of the cochlear sensitivity of the NTE. Recommended guidelines for making such judgments will be presented in a subsequent section.

Cross-over refers to the actual transmission of sound (introduced either by headphone or bone oscillator) emanating at the TE and arriving at the cochlea of the NTE. In contrast, *interaural attenuation* is the drop in intensity (dB) of an acoustic signal from the TE audiometric transducer to the NTE cochlea. For example, if a 1000-Hz air-conducted puretone is presented to the TE at 60 dB HL, and IA (transmission loss of the signal) is 40 dB, the puretone will reach the nontest cochlea at a level of 20 dB (60 dB (TE) – 40 dB (IA) = 20 dB (NTE)). Using this illustration, consider a client with an actual air-conduction threshold of 80 dB HL in the TE and a bone-conduction threshold of 15 dB HL in the NTE. When the puretone is presented through an earphone to the TE at 60 dB HL during the threshold search procedure, it is likely that the client will respond positively to the signal. This is because the 1000-Hz puretone in the TE exceeds the 40-dB IA by 20 dB, and these 20 dB are more intense than the 15-dB HL bone-conduction level in the NTE. In this case, masking must be applied to the NTE to shift the bone-conduction threshold so that the actual air-conduction threshold of 80 dB HL can be obtained in the TE.

Many variables account for differences in IA values. These include the type of earphone/receiver and cushion, the frequency being examined and the ear canal volume and condition. All of these variables interact; for any particular set of conditions, the range of IA values for air-conduction can be determined.

Table 8.3 shows the ranges of IA results that have been obtained in three different studies at various audiometric frequencies. There is a slight trend toward greater IA at the higher frequencies. In each study, the least IA at 2000 Hz and above was 45 dB while between 250 and 1000 Hz the range went as low as 40 dB. Generally speaking, the most common low was 45 dB, and the most common high was 70 dB, with most subjects falling in between.

Table 8.2
Effective Masking Table—Levels at which Audiometer HL Dial Needs To Be Set To Equal 0 dB EM at Specific Test Frequencies (Based on Computation from Table 8.1)

Type of Noise	Frequency (Hz)					
	250	500	1000	2000	4000	8000
				dB		
Broad-band	20	7	0	5	4	11
Narrow-band	-3	3	5	7	5	9

Table 8.3
Range of Interaural Attenuation Values for Air-Conducted Signals under Supraural Earphones

Study	Frequency (Hz)						
	125	250	500	1000	2000	4000	8000
Coles and Priede (1968)		50–80	45–80	40–80	45–75	50–85	
Liden et al. (1959a)	40–75	45–75	50–70	45–70	45–75	45–75	45–80
Chaiklin (1967)	32–45	44–58	54–65	57–66	55–72	61–85	51–69

According to Chaiklin (1967), average IA values (average HLs at which cross-hearing occurs) are less useful clinically than knowledge and employment of the lowest levels. Basing masking decisions on the lowest values frequently causes clinicians to mask when masking is unnecessary. This, however, should prevent audiologists from failing to mask when it is needed. Table 8.4 presents the recommended IA values to use when deciding on the need to mask during air-conduction testing.

In contrast to the air-conduction, the lower limit of *interaural attenuation* for bone-conduction is essentially 0 dB across frequencies (Liden et al, 1959a; Hood, 1960). Regardless of the bone oscillator placement, either forehead or mastoid, both cochleas may be assumed to be stimulated equally and simultaneously. Under this assumption, the better cochlea will prompt a response. This supports the routine use of masking for bone-conduction when threshold levels between ears are asymmetric.

Masking Rationale and Recommended Rules

Listed below are the rules for when to mask during various test procedures. The basic use of IA is to compare the air-conduction response obtained in the TE and the bone-conduction threshold in the NTE. If the difference is greater than IA, it is appropriate to mask. The audiologist, however, typically does not know the bone-conduction thresholds until after the air-conduction information is obtained. Therefore, in most situations, it is necessary to make an initial determination based on the air-conduction thresholds of the two ears. When bone-conduction responses are available, the need for masking should be reevaluated. Some of the rules shown below have subsections (*a*) and (*b*). Subsection (*a*) refers to the initial consideration based on the air-conduction comparisons. The (*b*) subsection should be considered when masking was not used in the (*a*) subsection. Rule 2, masking for bone conduction, is predicated on the assumption that IA for bone-conducted signals is theoretically 0 dB (Sanders, 1978). If none of the conditions is met, masking is unnecessary.

Table 8.4
Recommended Values for Interaural Attenuation for Air-Conducted Signals[a]

	Frequency (Hz)						
	125	250	500	1000	2000	4000	8000
dB difference between ears	35	40	40	40	45	50	50

[a]It should be noted that these values are slightly more conservative than those suggested by Martin (1972) based on the work of Coles and Priede (1968) but are similar to those suggested by R. K. Beedle (unpublished manuscript, 1971) based on the work of Liden et al. (1959a) (See Table 8.3). Using these values would allow for appropriate decision making on the part of the clinician.

(*a*) When the air-conduction threshold of the TE and the air-conduction threshold of the NTE differ by IA for the test frequency or more, use masking.

(*b*) When the air-conduction threshold of the TE and the bone-conduction threshold of the NTE differ by IA or more, use masking.

Rule 2: Puretone bone-conduction audiometry
When the air-conduction threshold of the TE and the bone-conduction threshold of that same ear differ by more than 10 dB, use masking.

Rule 3: Spondee threshold (ST) audiometry
(*a*) When the ST of the TE and the ST or puretone average of the NTE differ by 45 dB or more, use masking.

(*b*) When the ST of the TE and the puretone bone-conduction threshold average of the speech frequencies (500, 1000, and 2000 Hz) of the NTE differ by 45 dB or more, use masking.

Rule 4: Speech discrimination audiometry
(*a*) When the presentation level (PL) to the TE and the ST or puretone average of the NTE differ by 45 dB or more, use masking.

(*b*) When the PL to the TE and the puretone bone-conduction threshold average of the speech frequencies of the NTE differ by 45 dB or more, use masking.

Rule 5: Short Increment Sensitivity Index (SISI) and tone decay audiometry
(*a*) When the PL to the TE and the air-conduction threshold of the NTE differ by IA for the test frequency or more, use masking.

(*b*) When the PL to the TE and the bone-conduction threshold of the NTE differ by IA for the test frequency or more, use masking (Goldstein, 1979).

The preceding rules form the foundation for the initial step in the clinical decision-making process of "when to mask." The next section describes the bases for "how to mask," employing both psychophysical and formula approaches.

ESSENTIAL MASKING DECISION: HOW TO MASK

There has been considerable discussion in the literature regarding how to proceed with masking the NTE (Liden et al., 1959b; Hood, 1960; Studebaker, 1962, 1967, 1979; Martin, 1967, 1972, 1974). Each of the publications provided information on how to determine when a minimum amount, a sufficient amount and an excessive amount of EM had been reached. The terms "minimum effective masking level" (Liden et al., 1959b), "minimum effective masking" (Lloyd and Kaplan, 1978) or "minimum masking level" (Studebaker, 1962) refers to the minimum amount of masking signal needed to prevent the NTE from hearing a crossed-over test signal. In contrast, "maximum effective masking level" is the masking signal intensity just sufficient to cross-over and mask the test signal in the TE. Several alternative methods of masking are presented below.

Psychoacoustic Method

Three terms have been used to describe psychoacoustic masking procedures, including plateau searching, NTE threshold shifting and shadowing (Sanders, 1978). Studebaker (1979, p 82) has indicated that such psychoacoustically founded procedures "... are those based upon observed shifts in the measured threshold as a function of suprathreshold masker effective levels in the nontest ear."

Hood (1960) introduced a psychoacoustic procedure for masking during bone-conduction testing in which (*a*) masking is presented to the NTE when the TE unmasked threshold demonstrates an air-bone gap, (*b*) threshold is then reestablished in the presence of masking in the NTE and, in the event of a shift, (*c*) both threshold (in 5-dB steps) and masking (in 10-dB steps) are increased until further increases in masking do not produce further increases in threshold level. At this point, the plateau has been reached. Hood recommended that the initial level should be based on selecting a noise intensity equal to the air-conduction threshold of the NTE + 10 dB; Martin (1972) concurred but reminded clinicians to account for the OE.

Sufficient masking has been discussed by both Martin (1972) and R. K. Beedle (unpublished manuscript, 1971) and is generally thought to be 30 dB of masking above threshold for the NTE. Martin supports a value as low as 10 dB SL, although Beedle supports 30 dB SL. One successful method of plateau searching is to begin

by choosing a masking level in the *nontest ear* based upon the air-conduction threshold of that ear plus 15 dB, plus the occlusion effect value for that frequency in the case of testing for bone-conduction thresholds where the masked ear is either normal or sensory-neural. The benefit of initially using threshold plus 15 dB SL is that this amount is generally enough to begin to cause a TE threshold shift if true threshold has not been reached in the unmasked test condition. Plateau searching is then initiated. After the response in the TE is reestablished, the masking level of the NTE should be raised 5 dB three consecutive times to obtain the acceptable plateau (Goldstein, 1979).

Psychoacoustic masking procedures have been widely accepted in clinical audiometry (Studebaker, 1979). There are, however, other recommended procedures which call for the use of formula computation to determine how much masking to use. The next section discusses the values and drawbacks of this alternative approach.

Pros and Cons of Masking Formulas

Several authoritative sources have presented masking formulas for puretone and speech audiometry that can be used to: (*a*) determine when to mask (Martin, 1974, 1975); (*b*) calculate minimum and maximum masking levels (Liden et al., 1959b; Studebaker, 1962, 1964; Martin, 1967, 1974, 1975; Konkle and Berry, 1983); and (*c*) establish guidelines for identifying overmasking (Studebaker, 1962; Martin, 1975). Studebaker (1979) has termed such approaches to masking the "acoustic method" because the determination of masking is based on calculation of "... the approximate acoustic levels of the test and masker signals in the two ears" (p 82). An example of a masking formula to determine appropriate masking levels during speech audiometry was presented by Konkle and Berry (1983, pp 315–316).

$$EML = PL_{ts} + \left(\frac{ABG_n - ABG_t}{2} \right)$$

"... EML is the amount of effective masking in dB HL necessary to reach the mid-plateau point of the contralateral masking function; PL_{ts} = the presentation level in dB HL of the test signal; ABG_n, the air/bone gap of the nontest ear; and ABG_t, the air/bone gap of the test ear."

For the beginning student, an understanding of such formulas may facilitate the grasp of theoretical concepts underlying masking. In the clinical setting, however, formula application is problematic. First, calculations based on formulas are time consuming, and it is typically prohibitive for a clinician to work out a series of formulas while the patient is made to wait. For example, if masking is required for air and bone conduction from 250 to 8000 Hz, for the poorer ear, approximately 11 formulas calculations would be necessary. Second, information required to complete a computation may not be available at any given time during an evaluation. When assessing the hearing of difficult-to-test individuals, speech audiometry may be performed prior to puretone testing, and the needed information for computation of the above formula (ABG) would not yet have been determined. Recognizing the limitations of this approach, Studebaker (1964) suggested that formulas were not practical tools for routine clinical application. It is therefore recommended that clinicians acquire a set of general rules which provide a foundation for making appropriate decisions regarding "how to mask." Presented below are masking procedures and descriptive examples for the basic audiologic test battery.

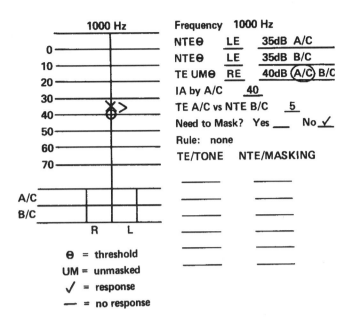

Figure 8.2. Example of test results that do not require masking for air-conduction testing.

Recommended Masking Procedures

Threshold Procedures: Air Conduction

(a) Obtain and record the TE air-conduction threshold unmasked.

(b) Compare the obtained unmasked threshold with the air- and bone-conduction thresholds of the NTE and determine if rules 1(a) or 1(b) apply. If the difference is equal to or greater than IA, the decision to mask is affirmative when testing the poorer ear.

(c) Select the initial amount of masking for the NTE: NTE air-conduction threshold plus 15 dB EM (R. K. Beedle, unpublished manuscript, 1971).

(d) Reestablish threshold in the TE with this initial amount of masking in the NTE.

(e) Each time the client responds to the puretone signal presented to the TE, increase the masking presented to the NTE by 5 dB.

(f) Each time the client does not respond to the tone presented to the TE, increase the signal in 5-dB steps until the client again responds.

(g) Continue the procedure until the masking can be increased three consecutive 5-dB steps without producing a shift in the threshold level of the TE. When this is accomplished, a "plateau" in threshold response has been reached (R. K. Beedle, unpublished manuscript, 1971).

(h) At this point, record both the threshold (on an audiogram using the correct masking symbol) and the final masking level.

Examples: Air Conduction

Figure 8.2. The case presented for 1000 Hz shows air-conduction thresholds that are within 5 dB of one another and no air-bone gap. There is no need to mask for air-conduction because differences between ears do not equal or exceed IA.

Figure 8.3. The case presented for 250 Hz shows a 50-dB difference between air-conduction thresholds. This

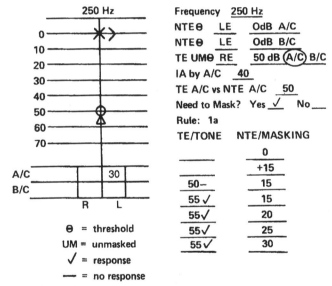

Figure 8.3. Example of test results that require masking for air-conduction testing according to rule 1(a).

difference exceeds IA at 250 Hz (40 dB) by 10 dB, and therefore, according to rule 1(a) masking is necessary when testing the right ear. The initial masking level in the left ear is 0 dB HL (threshold) + 15 dB EM = 15 dB HL. The plateau searching procedure is complete with a 55-dB HL masked threshold and 30 dB HL masking to the NTE.

Figure 8.4. The case presented for 500 Hz shows a 25-dB difference between air-conduction thresholds. This

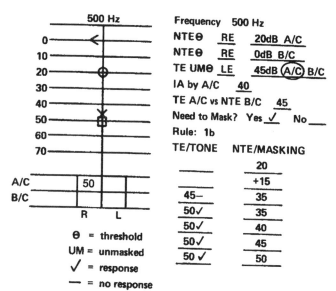

Figure 8.4. Example of test results that require masking for air-conduction testing according to rule 1(b).

Table 8.5
Average Occlusion Effect Values of Four Studies and Recommended Values for Clinical Use

Study	Frequency (Hz)			
	250	500	1000	2000
			dB	
Huizing (1960)	13.0	15.0	8.0	1.0
Elpern and Naunton (1963)	28.0	20.0	9.0	0.0 (TDH 39 with firm rubber cushion)
Goldstein and Hayes (1965)	19.4	12.6	5.7	1.1
Dirks and Swindeman (1967)	22.9	20.2	8.8	0.5 (MX41/AR cushion)
Recommended	15	15	10	0

difference does not exceed IA at 500 Hz. After obtaining an unmasked right mastoid bone-conduction threshold of 0 dB HL, it becomes apparent that masking is necessary. The difference between the air response of the TE and the bone response of the NTE exceeds IA by 5 dB, and masking is necessary according to rule 1(b). The initial masking level in the right ear is 20 dB HL (threshold) + 15 dB EM = 35 dB HL. The plateau searching procedure is complete with a 50-dB HL masked threshold and 50 dB HL masking to the NTE.

Threshold Procedures: Bone Conduction

(a) Obtain and record the TE bone-conduction threshold unmasked with the NTE unoccluded.

(b) Compare the bone-conduction threshold of the TE to the air-conduction threshold of the TE. If the difference is greater than 10 dB (bone better than air), rule 2 applies and masking is indicated.

(c) Select the initial amount of masking for the NTE: NTE air-conduction threshold, plus the occlusion effect (OE) value for the test frequency, plus 15 dB EM (R. K. Beedle, unpublished manuscript, 1971). Table 8.5 presents average OE data from the literature as well as recommended OE values.

(d) Clinicians should not account for the OE when employing masking procedures with conductive hearing losses.

(e) Continue and conclude the masking process following steps d to h presented for air-conduction procedures.

Examples: Bone Conduction

Figure 8.5. The case presented for 500 Hz shows air-conduction thresholds that differ by 10 dB. Unmasked bone-conduction at both mastoid placements does not demonstrate an air-bone gap for either ear exceeding

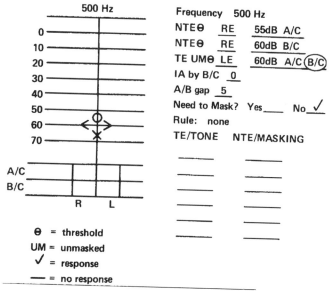

Figure 8.5. Example of test results that do not require masking for bone-conduction testing.

10 dB. Masking for bone conduction is therefore unnecessary.

Figure 8.6. The case presented for 1000 Hz shows an unmasked left mastoid bone-conduction response at 5 dB consistent with the response of the better cochlea. The air-conduction response, however, is at 35 dB HL, presenting an apparent air-bone gap of 30 dB. According to rule 2, masking is indicated. The initial masking level in the right ear is 5 dB HL (threshold) + 10 dB (occlusion effect at 1000 Hz) + 15 dB EM = 30 dB HL. The plateau searching procedure is complete with a 35-dB HL masked threshold and 45 dB HL masking to the NTE.

Threshold Procedures: Spondee Threshold

(a) Obtain and record the TE spondee threshold (ST) unmasked.

(b) Compare the obtained unmasked ST with (a) the ST and (b) bone-conduction puretone average (PTA) of the NTE and determine if rules 3(a) or 3(b) apply. If the difference is equal to or greater than interaural attenuation for speech (45 dB), the decision to mask is affirmative when testing the poorer ear.

(c) When masking for speech audiometry, it is better to choose one adequate level of masking at the outset, so that the masking remains constant for the entire test. The recommended rule is to use a masking level in the NTE which is no less than 30 dB below the ST of the TE. In unilateral conductive hearing losses, where the TE is both sensory-neural and poorer in threshold, the amount of masking needed in the conductive (NTE) is equal to 30 dB below TE + the air-bone gap. Refer to a later section, "Problems Encountered in Masking," to determine masking levels in bilateral conductive cases.

(d) If ST in the TE shifts sufficiently to recreate a crossover condition, additional masking will be necessary.

Examples: Spondee Threshold

Figure 8.7. The first case presented for spondee threshold shows differences between ears which do not exceed IA for speech between the air-conduction response in the TE and the bone-conduction response in the NTE. Masking is therefore unnecessary.

Figure 8.8. The second case presented for spondee threshold shows a 46-dB difference between the unmasked ST of the TE and ST of NTE. This difference exceeds IA, and thus according to rule 3(a), masking is necessary when testing the right ear. The masking level is selected by taking the unmasked TE ST in dB HL and subtracting 30 dB. In the example presented, the minimum amount of masking to be used is 28 dB HL, although some additional masking would not negatively affect the results. The procedure must account for shifts in ST.

Figure 8.9. The third example presents an interesting computation situation. There is a 48-dB difference between the unmasked ST of the TE and the bone-conduction PTA of the NTE. Rule 3(b) requires the use of masking in this case. The minimum masking level is identified initially by taking the unmasked TE ST in dB HL and subtracting 30 dB. This would require the use of 38 dB HL of masking to the left NTE. Such an amount of broad-band masking, however, would shift the NTE ST only 2 dB and the NTE bone-conduction PTA also 2 dB. Shifting the bone-conduction PTA only 2 dB is not adequate to close the IA gap between the TE ST and the shifted NTE bone-conduction PTA (68 − (20 + 2) = 46-dB difference). In this example, an additional 15 dB (53 dB HL) are employed to reduce this TE ST vs NTE bone-conduction PTA gap to approximately 31 dB (68 − (20 + 2 + 15) = 31).

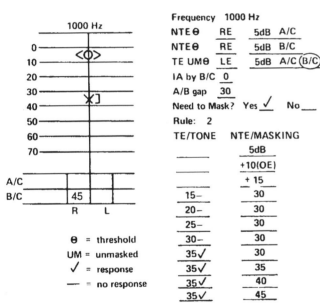

Figure 8.6. Example of test results that require masking for bone-conduction testing according to rule 2.

SPONDEE THRESHOLD/BROADBAND

	NTE RE	TE LE
A/C PTA	40	55
B/C PTA	40	55
UM ST (A/C)	38	52
IA for speech by A/C		45dB
TE UM ST vs NTE B/C PTA		12
Need to Mask?	yes ___	no ✔ Rule: none
UM TE/SPEECH	NTE/MINIMUM MASKING	

Figure 8.7. Example of test results that do not require masking for spondee threshold testing.

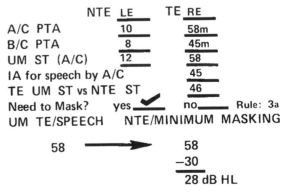

SPONDEE THRESHOLD/BROADBAND

	NTE LE	TE RE
A/C PTA	10	58m
B/C PTA	8	45m
UM ST (A/C)	12	58
IA for speech by A/C		45
TE UM ST vs NTE ST		46
Need to Mask?	yes ✔	no ___ Rule: 3a
UM TE/SPEECH	NTE/MINIMUM MASKING	

58 ⟶ 58
         −30
        ─────
        28 dB HL

Figure 8.8. Example of test results that require masking for spondee threshold according to rule 3(a).

SPONDEE THRESHOLD/BROADBAND

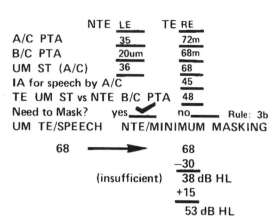

Figure 8.9. Example of test results that require masking for spondee threshold according to rule 3(b).

Suprathreshold Procedures: Speech Discrimination

(a) Determine the PL in dB HL at which the procedure will be administered in the poorer TE. (If masking was necessary for ST, it will again be necessary for speech discrimination. If it was unnecessary in ST, it may or may not be required here.)

(b) Compare the PL of the TE to the ST and the bone-conduction PTA of the NTE and determine if rules 4 (a) or 4(b) apply. If the difference is equal to or greater IA for speech (45 dB), masking should be used.

(c) One adequate level of masking is chosen at the outset. Which level is relatively easy to determine because the procedure is completed at a constant HL. As in masking for ST, the recommended rule is to use a masking level in the NTE which is no less than 30 dB below the PL of the TE. When a conductive hearing loss is present in the NTE, add the air-bone gap to this level for adequate masking.

Examples: Speech Discrimination

Figure 8.10. The first case presented for speech discrimination shows differences between the speech PL of the TE and the bone-conduction response in the NTE which do not exceed IA for speech. Masking is unnecessary.

Figure 8.11. The second case shows a 64-dB difference between the PL of the TE and the ST of the NTE. This difference exceeds IA, and thus according to rule 4(a), masking is necessary when testing the left ear. The masking level is selected by taking the TE PL in dB HL and subtracting 30 dB. In the example presented, the minimum amount of masking to be used is 40 dB HL, although some additional masking would not negatively affect the results.

Figure 8.12. The third example presents a case in which the original calculation may result in an insuffi-

SPEECH DISCRIMINATION/BROADBAND

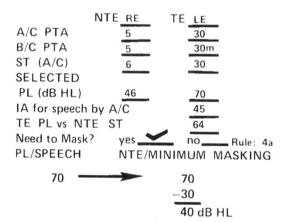

Figure 8.10. Example of test results that do not require masking for speech discrimination testing.

SPEECH DISCRIMINATION/BROADBAND

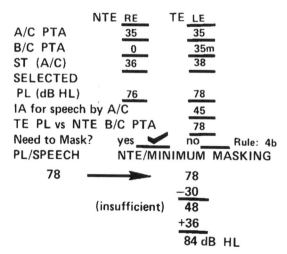

Figure 8.11. Example of test results that require masking for speech discrimination testing according to rule 4(a).

SPEECH DISCRIMINATION/BROADBAND

Figure 8.12. Example of test results that require masking for speech discrimination testing according to rule 4(b).

cient amount of masking. There is only a 42-dB difference between the PL of the TE and the ST of the NTE, but there is a 78-dB difference between the TE PL and the bone-conduction PTA of the NTE. Rule 4(b) requires the use of masking in this case. The minimum masking level is identified initially by taking the PL in the TE in dB HL and subtracting 30 dB. This would require the use of 48 dB HL of masking to the right ear. Such an amount of broad-band masking, however, would shift the NTE ST only 12 dB and the NTE bone-conduction PTA also 12 dB. Shifting the bone-conduction PTA only 12 dB is not adequate to close the IA gap between the TE PL and the shifted NTE bone-conduction PTA (78 − (0 + 12) = 66-dB difference). In this example, an additional 36 dB of masking (84 dB HL) were selected to reduce this TE vs NTE gap to approximately 30 dB (78 − (0 + 12 + 36) = 30).

Suprathreshold Procedures: Special Tests

(a) Determine the PL in dB HL at which the procedure will be administered in the poorer TE.

(b) Compare the PL of the TE to the air- and bone-conduction PTAs of the NTE and determine if rules 5(a) or 5(b) apply. If the difference is equal to or greater than IA for each individual frequency tested, masking must be used.

(c) One adequate level of masking is chosen at the outset because the masked puretone air-conduction threshold for each frequency has already been determined. The recommended rule is to use a masking level in the NTE of 40 dB below the PL of the TE. Conductive hearing loss will require additional masking.

(d) When greater than 40 dB HL of masking is necessary, the procedure should not be completed or positive test results should be evaluated with caution (consult section on "Central Masking").

Procedure for Recording Masked Test Results and Masking Levels

When completing the masking procedures selected, puretone results should be recorded with masked symbols according to the Guidelines for Audiometric Symbols (ASHA, 1990) (See Fig. 7.2 in the previous chapter). Masked speech tests should be identified by the letter "m" following the threshold value or percent correct score.

Considerable confusion has existed regarding identification of correct procedures for recording *final masking level* on the audiogram. According to the Guidelines for Audiometric Symbols (ASHA, 1990), the following recommendation is made: "While entirely optional, effective masking levels could be recorded on the audiogram for both air conduction and bone conduction thresholds, depending upon individual preference. When this policy is followed, the maximum effective masking level used to obtain threshold at each fre-

quency should be recorded. This level should be reported for the nontest ear, because this is the ear to which the masking stimulus is being delivered (pp 29—30)." Final masking levels for speech audiometry should be recorded along with the test results on a line designated "dBWN" (or dBBB; dBSN; masking). Refer to the audiometric results of Figures 8.15 and 8.16 for examples of recorded final masking levels.

SECONDARY CONSIDERATIONS

Too Much or Too Little Masking?

Another important decision the audiologist must make is whether too much or too little masking has been used. Therefore, the masking procedure is not complete until the clinician has determined that neither *overmasking* nor *undermasking* has occurred.

Overmasking

The concept of overmasking is based on interaural attenuation. If masking is introduced to the NTE and increased in intensity to the level of IA and beyond, it will eventually cross over to reach and mask the test cochlea. This creates a false shift in threshold. This actually produces an ipsilateral masking condition in the TE in which the noise obliterates the test signal. In order to avoid overmasking, clinicians can use only as much masking as IA will allow.

Figure 8.13 presents interweaving air- and bone-conduction thresholds at 25 dB HL for the left ear, with a right ear air-conduction response at 40 dB HL. The following masking decisions can be made. Masking is unnecessary when testing air conduction for the poorer right ear because neither section of rule 1 applies. It is also unnecessary to mask when testing bone conduction at the left mastoid because rule 2 is not applicable. However, when testing bone conduction at the right mastoid, it can be assumed that the initial response will be 25 dB HL because IA for bone conduction is theoretically 0 dB, and the better cochlea will respond irrespective of vibrator placement. A response at 25 dB HL suggests the presence of an air-bone gap, requiring masking.

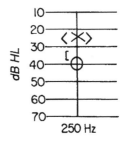

Figure 8.13. Example of bone-conduction threshold for the right cochlea which, when masked, will not result in overmasking.

With the decision to mask already made, the clinician must select the starting level and proceed with the procedure. The masking is initially presented to the NTE (left) at 55 dB HL: (threshold = 25 dB HL, plus OE at 250 Hz = 15 dB, plus 15 dB). With 55 dB HL of masking, the bone-conduction threshold shifts to 35 dB HL and is maintained at this level following the three 5-dB additional increments of masking. The masking procedure is then concluded with a 35 dB HL threshold at the right mastoid with 70 dB HL masking in the left ear.

The next decision: Has overmasking occurred? No, it has not, as can be readily ascertained by application of the following procedure. The 70 dB HL of masking at 250 Hz crossed over to the test cochlea at 30 dB HL considering a minimum of 40 dB of IA. This 30 dB HL of masking at the right cochlea is 5 dB softer than the masked bone-conduction threshold for that ear (35 dB HL) and therefore was not intense enough to create overmasking. Overmasking does not occur until the crossed-over masking signal (in EM or HL) equals or exceeds the bone-conduction threshold of the TE.

Figure 8.14 presents a condition of bilaterally symmetrical air-conduction thresholds at a level of 35 dB HL. The unmasked bone-conduction response at the left mastoid is 15 dB HL. Masking is unnecessary in this case when testing air conduction for either ear because neither rule 1(a) nor rule 1(b) applies. However, when testing bone conduction at the left or right mastoid, following an unmasked response of 15 dB HL, the decision to mask is affirmative. This need for masking is based on rule 2, an air-bone gap greater than 10 dB.

Having decided to mask, the clinician will select the starting level and proceed. In testing for the response of the left cochlea, the masking is initially presented to the NTE (right) at 50 dB HL: (threshold = 35 dB HL, plus 15 dB). Inasmuch as the right ear may also have a conductive loss (based on the case history), the OE will not be taken into account in this calculation. When presenting the 50 dB HL of masking to the right ear, the left ear bone-conduction response remains at 15 dB HL, and so the masking is then raised to 55 dB HL. At 55 dB HL, no

change is noted in the bone-conduction threshold. Masking is then increased to the level of 60 dB HL, and this time the bone-conduction threshold shifts to 20 dB HL. Masking is once again raised to 65 dB HL, and the bone-conduction threshold shifts to 25 dB HL.

The goal is generally to use threshold plus 30 dB EM which in this case is 65 dB HL. As threshold shifts begin to occur, it is time for the clinician to suspect overmasking. The initial 50 dB HL of masking at 1000 Hz crossed over to the test cochlea at 10 dB HL due to presumed 40 dB of IA. However, this is 5 dB softer than the bone-conduction threshold of that ear, and, at this level, the masking has not begun to shift or overmask the test cochlea. With an increase to 55 dB HL of masking, cross-over to the test cochlea occurs and would be heard at a level of 15 dB HL in the test cochlea. At this point, the crossed-over masking and the bone-conduction threshold of the TE are essentially equal, 15 dB HL. With equal intensities reaching the TE, it is possible to hear the tone through the masking 50% of the time. However, once the masking is increased beyond 55 dB HL, shifts in the bone-conduction response will occur due to overmasking and begin to confound threshold interpretation.

Interaural attenuation is the guideline for overmasking judgments. The clinician must determine if and when overmasking has occurred and subsequently terminate plateau searching. In suprathreshold testing, masking cannot exceed the TE bone-conduction threshold plus the SL of the test material. Once masking is intense enough to cross, reach or exceed the cochlear level (plus SL) of the TE, conclude the procedure and record both the unmasked and masked thresholds and the masking. In the case above, record unmasked and masked thresholds of 15 dB HL with 55 dB HL of masking. Indicate under the remarks section that "a plateau could not be reached due to overmasking."

Undermasking

The concept of undermasking is also based on IA values. It refers to insufficient masking to produce the needed threshold shift. Undermasking can occur when (*a*) the level of the noise is overestimated (due to a calibration error) or (*b*) an insufficient level is delivered to the NTE because of calculation error or underestimating the extent of the crossover signal. The latter is possible with threshold measures but is more apt to occur with suprathreshold procedures. This situation could occur when both minimal or large differences exist between ears and a high signal presentation level in the TE is required. The clinician must select enough masking in the NTE to prevent it from responding for the TE. If undermasking goes unnoticed, the validity of obtained results in the test ear is questionable.

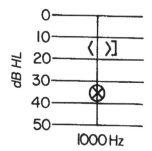

Figure 8.14. Example of a bone-conduction threshold for the left cochlea which, when masked, could result in overmasking.

Masking for ST is generally a straight-forward procedure. Figure 8.15 presents a normal-hearing configuration in the right ear; air- and bone-conduction thresholds are interweaving. The left ear demonstrates a masked air conduction PTA of 50 dB HL. A decision to mask was made in this case when testing air and bone for the left ear because both rules 1(a) and 1(b) (difference between ears) and 2 (air-bone gap) applied. A small amount of masking, 18 dB HL, which amounted to 14 dB of EM for the right ear (18 dB HL – 4 dB HL) (right ear ST)), was used when obtaining the left ear ST. This amount was adequate because it reduced the IA for speech between the two ears to 30 dB (48 dB HL (ST) – 18 dB HL (EM)).

Figure 8.16 presents a left ear configuration sloping from normal thresholds through 1000 Hz to a moderate sensory-neural loss in the higher frequencies; air- and bone-conduction thresholds are interweaving. The right ear demonstrates a masked air-conduction two-frequency (Fletcher) PTA of 62 dB HL. A decision to mask was made in this case when testing air and bone conduction for the right ear because rules 1(a) and 1(b) and 2 applied. ST for the right ear was obtained employing 48 dB HL of masking, which amounted to 33 dB of EM for the left ear in the low frequencies (48 dB HL – 15 dB HL (left ear ST)). This amount was adequate because it reduced IA for speech between the two ears to 30 dB (78 dB HL (ST) – 48 dB HL (EM)).

Speech discrimination testing appears to be more susceptible to the problem of undermasking because of

it being a suprathreshold measurement procedure. In Figure 8.15 the PL for the left ear is 48 dB (ST) + 40 dB SL, or 88 dB HL. If the clinician would chose to employ only 30 dB of EM in the NTE, which is the amount frequently considered sufficient for accurate measurement, undermasking could occur because the selected IA value for speech audiometry (45 dB) has been exceeded. To test for undermasking, take the PL of 88 dB HL and subtract from it the initially chosen masking level of 34 dB HL (4 dB HL (ST) + 30 dB HL (EM) + 34 dB HL), and a difference of 54 dB will result. A 54-dB difference exceeds allowable interaural attenuation by 9 dB. Therefore, at least an added 10 to 15 dB of EM are necessary to close the interaural attenuation gap and provide sufficient masking. One correct masking level would be 58 dB HL (88 dB HL (PL) – 30 dB) and the IA gap would then be reduced to 30 dB, within acceptable limits. In Figure 8.16, the PL for the right ear is 78 dB (ST) + 22 dB SL, or 100 dB HL. To reduce the existing 85-dB IA gap (100 dB HL (PL) – 15 dB HL (ST NTE)) to an acceptable level, 70 dB HL (100 dB HL (PL) – 30 dB) of broad-band/white noise should be used to prevent undermasking.

Once clinicians have determined that with added masking undermasking is not occurring, they must then remember to go back and check for overmasking before the presentation of the test. Individuals who have conductive hearing losses which prompt undermasking at one PL and go to overmasking at the next masking level present unresolvable masking dilemmas. The next section will elaborate on this problem.

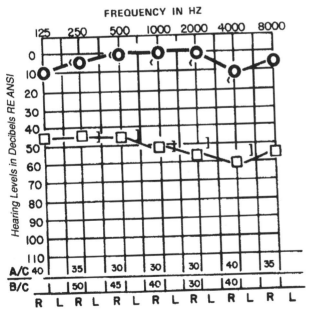

Figure 8.15. Example of masking for air-conduction, bone-conduction, spondee threshold, and speech discrimination testing where undermasking could occur during speech discrimination testing (normal hearing, right ear).

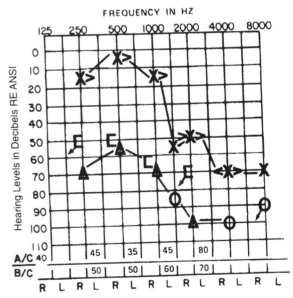

Figure 8.16. Example of masking for air-conduction, bone-conduction, spondee threshold, and speech discrimintion testing where undermasking could occur during speech discrimination testing (left ear).

PROBLEMS ENCOUNTERED IN MASKING

Special problems may be encountered during masking that will require different strategies and approaches by the audiologist. One such problem is adequately masking for bilateral conductive pathology, while avoiding overmasking. A second problem is central masking (as differentiated from peripheral masking) that may occur during puretone and speech testing, tests of differential intensity discrimination, tone decay and Bekesy audiometry.

Conductive Pathology

According to Naunton (1960, p 757),

> There are theoretical grounds for believing that in some subjects with bilateral middle ear deafness it is impossible adequately to mask the hearing of the untested ear without at the same time masking the hearing of the tested ear. Measurements of the masking effect of white noise made on a series of 20 listeners with bilateral otosclerosis have indicated that the problem is encountered in practice and is therefore more than a theoretical concept without foundation in fact.

The need to mask for bilateral conductive pathology is generally suspected first (with adequate case history information) during air-conduction testing. If the air-conduction thresholds of either ear equal or exceed the level of interaural attenuation, an immediate assessment of the cochlear reserve (bone conduction) should be obtained. If the bone-conduction thresholds are within normal limits and the air-conduction thresholds equal or exceed interaural attenuation, then masking is necessary (rule 1(b)). However, if bone conduction is in the normal range and air-conduction thresholds exceed IA, then it will not be possible to obtain valid results employing standard audiologic procedures if masking is used. Konkle and Berry (1983, pp 301—302) provide a good rule of thumb, ". . . when the sum of the conductive components is greater than twice the interaural attenuation value, the ipsilateral function for the non-test ear will merge with that of the test ear." In the unmasked air-conduction condition, the obtained thresholds may reflect responses of the NTE. In the masked condition, the obtained hearing levels will most likely appear worse than actual thresholds due to overmasking whether using puretone or speech signals.

The next level in the decision-making process will affect bone-conduction threshold test procedures. The clinician has already determined that for air conduction the undermasking/overmasking dilemma exists bilaterally. Although masking for bone conduction in conductive hearing loss is generally necessary (rule 2), valid bone-conduction thresholds will also be impossible to obtain due to effects of overmasking. Therefore, bone-conduction procedures cannot be completed.

Sensorineural Acuity Level (SAL)

The problem of overmasking in bilateral conductive pathology prompted Jerger and Tillman's (1960) development of the SAL procedure which was later subjected to independent evaluations by Tillman (1963) and Jerger and Jerger (1965). The clinical result obtained from the SAL test indicated "the amount by which a bone conducted thermal noise shifts the air-conduction threshold of a subject with impaired hearing at a given frequency [as] compared to the shift produced at that frequency in normal ears by the same noise" (Tillman, 1963, p 20). Tillman (1963) indicated that SAL was developed to be considered a substitute for conventional bone-conduction audiometry, but found it inadequate for such a purpose. Although SAL eliminated the masking decision-making procedure in bone-conduction audiometry, Tillman found that bone conduction and SAL did not yield the same estimates of sensory-neural sensitivity for otosclerotic patients in the low frequencies. This was a disturbing finding considering that the test was initially developed to facilitate the evaluation of cochlear reserve in those with bilateral conductive pathology.

Jerger and Jerger (1965) performed extensive experiments to verify the clinical usefulness of the SAL. They determined that the procedures underlying SAL audiometry were sound. The discrepancy noted in the above study for otosclerotic individuals in the low frequencies was found to be a calibration problem. "If the conventional bone-conduction system of the audiometer has been calibrated on open or unoccluded ears, then this system will measure relative bone-conduction. SAL and BC will then differ in the low frequency region on conductive losses simply because the built-in occlusion effect of the patient with conductive loss gives him an artificial advantage relative to the normals . . ." (p 126). Jerger and Jerger found that SAL and bone-conduction audiometry are equivalent for both pathologic populations if both tests are performed unoccluded. The SAL procedure, however, has not been widely adopted for clinical use.

Insert Receiver

When using a standard earphone receiver, it has been shown that true masked thresholds poorer than 35 to 50 dB HL (depending on frequency) for individuals with bilateral conductive pathology cannot be adequately determined (Naunton, 1960). Through use of an insert receiver, overmasking problems can be reduced by increasing IA. An insert receiver is an earphone that is placed and sealed at the opening of the external auditory meatus and is designed to reduce the area of the head exposed to the tone or masking signal. The effects of reduction in earphone size and cushion exposure area to a small opening close to the eardrum reduce the amount of energy that needs to be generated. Because less energy strikes the skull, more EM can be produced without masking the opposite cochlea. Thus the IA values are larger than displayed in Table 8.4, creating a greater range of permissible masking (Studebaker, 1962). Insert receivers also cause reduction of the OE in the low frequencies for normals and sensory-neurals, stabilizing bone-conduction threshold responses (Chaiklin, 1967). Zwislocki (1953) found increases of 30 to 40 dB in IA when employing an insert receiver. Table 8.6 provides additional IA data for insert receivers *re* Studebaker (1962), Konig (1962), Larson et al. (1983), and Killion et al. (1985)

Chaiklin (1967) investigated the effects on IA while deep plugging the NTE (as would be the case with an insert receiver). It was noted that IA varied with frequency and test conditions. The mean IA value in the plugged condition was 5 to 19 dB higher than without the plug. Chaiklin suggested that these findings support the disputed belief that cross-hearing in the plugged condition is clearly via bone conduction. Further, he pointed out than an awareness of the problems associated with employing insert receivers is critical. These include (*a*) individual calibration is necessary, and a 2-cc coupler is needed to perform this calibration; (*b*) the frequency responses of insert receivers can vary with manufacturers; (*c*) precise IA values are difficult to obtain and may vary with receiver; (*d*) ear canal sizes vary, and an adequate seal may be difficult to obtain; and (*e*) the inserts must be cleaned following each use. This unique set of problems has previously discouraged the widespread use of insert receivers.

Recently, Killion and Villchur (1989) reported on the advantages of state-of-the-art insert phones which include: (*a*) unsurpassed accuracy in frequency response; (*b*) linear measurements at output levels well below 0 dB SPL while able to produce stimuli at 110 dB

HL from 500 to 4000 Hz; (*c*) smaller standard deviations across subjects at all frequencies except 1000 Hz; (*d*) satisfactory hygiene is achievable with disposable eartips; (*e*) more valid results in populations having bilateral conductive hearing loss, "left-corner audiograms" and collapsable ear canals, in non-sound-treated test environments and for hearing aid fitting purposes.

Central Masking

Peripheral masking refers to either the shifting of threshold in an ear by a second signal presented to it, or by a signal that is presented to the NTE which crosses over and shifts the TE threshold. Central masking is neither of the above. Central masking, a term coined by Wegel and Lane (1924), refers to a shift or worsening in threshold of the TE due to the introduction of masking in the NTE at masking intensities below the level of cross-over. The central masking shift begins to occur at low masking intensities and appears to increase with increased masking (Studebaker, 1962; Martin and DiGiovanni, 1979).

According to Liden et al. (1959b, p 133), central masking implies that the shifts in threshold are mediated through the central nervous system. "The efferent fibers interconnect the superior olivary nucleus, on each side, and the contralateral cochlea; . . . stimulation of the superior olivary area weakens the afferent impulses from the opposite cochlea" and more signal intensity is required to override this attenuation of neural activity. Therefore, an increase in the test signal may be necessary to obtain a response.

Effects on Puretone Thresholds

Several studies have noted puretone threshold shifts in the presence of low levels of masking. Central masking shifts for pulsed air-conduction stimuli were noted to be 1 to 3 dB (Dirks and Malmquist, 1964). Dirks (1964) found bone-conduction thresholds at the mastoid to be 4 to 5 dB worse and 7 to 8 dB worse at the frontal bone with the introduction of low level masking. Liden et al. (1959b) found air- and bone-conduction puretone central masking shifts from 5 to 15 dB; Studebaker (1962) found that the greatest shifts for bone conduction fell between 7 and 12 dB at 2000 Hz. Central masking shifts are generally overlooked in plotting masked puretone thresholds in the clinical setting. One problem in attempting to account for central masking is to determine the exact threshold correction, as researchers have obtained variable results.

Effects on Speech Audiometry

Central masking has also been found to affect speech audiometry. Martin et al. (1965) found that contralat-

Table 8.6
Interaural attenuation differences noted between standard and insert receivers

Study	Frequency (Hz)						
	250	500	1000	2000	3000	4000	6000
				dB			
Studebaker (1962)		14	12	14.5		10.5	
Konig (1962)[a]	28	25	24	18	22	28	17
Larson et al. (1983)[b]	31	26	15	8		13	
Killion et al. (1985)[c]	40	38	22	10	18	18	

[a]Figure 3 (Konig).
[b]Data average from Figure 3 (Larson et al.).
[c]Figure 1 (Killion et al.).

eral thermal noise presented below the level of cross-over shifted speech thresholds in normal-hearing subjects. They recommended the use of a 4- to 8-dB correction factor for masked ST scores. In 1966, Martin found that "high-level masking produces a 5-dB modal threshold shift (central masking) in the opposite ear for spondee words, where cross-conduction masking is ruled out" (p 203). He further found that intense masking at appropriate levels did not affect speech discrimination ability of individuals with bilaterally asymmetric sensory-neural hearing losses. A formula to compute effective masking for speech discrimination testing was presented.

Martin and DiGiovanni (1979) assessed the effect of central masking for ST on both normal subjects and those with sensory-neural hearing loss. They found limited improvement in ST at low sensation levels (SLs) of noise, but that thresholds increased as the noise presented to the NTE was increased. Considerable intersubject variability was seen. Normal and hearing-impaired subjects demonstrated similar shifts for masker SLs but differing extents in shifts of ST. The researchers indicated that central masking for spondees is a function of SL and not masker SPL. They recommended that if a masked ST shifts less than 5 dB, no correction should be made and the nonmasked threshold should be recorded. If the shift equals or is greater than 5 dB, record the masked threshold.

Coles and Priede (1975) suggested that a single-level-of-masking technique is commonly used for speech testing. They reported results on masking for speech discrimination which were basically in conflict with those of Martin (1966). They found that "central masking effects of up to 1% intelligibility decrement for every 3 dB sensation level (SL) of wide-band contralateral noise may occur in a small percentage of normal hearing persons" (pp 218—219). Based on these two studies, it is presently difficult to understand the effect which central masking has on speech discrimination test scores.

Effects on Special Audiometric Tests

Studies have been carried out to determine the effects of masking noise on the results of special auditory tests. They suggest that use of masking for these procedures can alter the test results even if the masking is of insufficient intensity to cause overmasking. Central masking has been found to cause slight increases in SISI scores at 1000 Hz and significant changes at 4000 Hz (Blegvad and Terkildsen, 1967). The intensity of the tone used, as compared with the intensity of the masking (signal to noise ratio), has been proven to affect results (Swisher et al., 1969). Both normal-hearing subjects and those with conductive pathologies were seen to shift from negative

unmasked SISI scores to questionable and positive masked scores (Shimizu, 1969). Subjects were also seen to demonstrate slight to significant apparent tone decay at 1000 Hz and above when masking was used (Shimizu, 1969; Priede and Coles, 1975). Bekesy audiometry was also affected by masking, especially when the tone and masking were either both pulsed or both continuous (Dirks and Norris, 1966). With increased frequencies, greater threshold shifts, separation of tracings, and narrowed excursions appeared to occur due to central masking (Blegvad, 1967). Type tracings were seen to shift from Type I to II, from Type I to IV, and from Type II to IV. None shifted to a Type III (Blegvad, 1968).

Although the rules presented in this chapter have included information on when and how to mask for special auditory tests, the literature suggests that masking will sometimes cause a significant alteration of the true audiometric results. The decision to proceed with masking during special auditory testing presents a dilemma to the clinician. If masking is necessary, based on the previous rules, it may not be possible to rule out participation by the NTE. If masking is used, then the central masking artifact is inherent in the test results and cannot be subtracted out. This then leaves the options of (a) increasing the IA, (b) not performing the test, or (c) using less than 40 dB EM because most of the researchers began to note changes in their test results when the masking levels reached 40 dB HL.

CASE PRESENTATIONS

Through a decision-making approach, this chapter has taught the student clinician to (a) comprehend the definitions and purposes of masking, (b) understand the types of masking signals, (c) determine the need for masking and (d) use correct procedures and levels of masking. Development of masking skills is one of the immediate goals of novice clinicians; however, the ultimate goals must be precise differential diagnosis of site of lesion and quality rehabilitative management. The two cases presented below demonstrate why appropriate masking techniques are necessary for obtaining accurate test results.

Case I (See Fig. 8.15)

Male, age 57 years

Significant Case History:

  Left ear hearing loss
  Business executive
  No difficulty with tinnitus or vertigo
  Occasional headaches with left side pressure
  Serious car accident at age 22 years
  No medical problems

Medical Test Results:

MRI of internal auditory canals were normal

Ear-nose-throat examination was unremarkable

Audiologic test results:

Cochlear site of lesion

Right ear:

Normal audiometric and immittance results

Left ear:

Masked thresholds reveal moderate sensory-neural loss

Masked spondee threshold is in good agreement with PTA

Speech discrimination score is 72%

Negative tone decay

Normal tympanogram

Reduced reflex sensation levels

Overall Case Management:

Medical clearance for a hearing aid was obtained

A monaural in-the-ear hearing aid was fit at the left ear which improved thresholds to borderline-normal levels

The individual participated in aural rehabilitation education sessions

Value of masking:

Type of loss confirmed—cochlear pathology

All left ear thresholds (except air conduction for 2000 and 4000 Hz) would not have been valid without masking

Left ear spondee threshold would not have been valid without masking

Masking for left ear speech discrimination testing allowed identification of good word recognition ability for that ear

Tone decay results would have reflected the response of the better ear without masking

Case II (See Fig. 8.16)

Male, age 64 years

Significant Case History:

Right ear hearing loss

Unusual temperature sensations in both legs

History of neuropsychiatric problems and treatment

No perception of vertigo or lightheadedness

Unable to stand without swaying

Medical test results:

Left ear tomography shows diameter of internal auditory canal within normal limits

Right ear tomography shows markedly dilated canal with obvious bony destruction (acoustic tumor of the right cerebellar-pontine angle)

Positive signs on neurologic examination consistent with cerebellar dysfunction

Audiologic test results:

Retrocochlear site of lesion

Left ear:

Hearing within normal limits sloping to a moderate sensory-neural loss

Spondee threshold agrees with two-frequency average

Fair speech discrimination (72%)

Negative tone decay

Normal tympanogram

Ipsilateral reflex thresholds within normal limits; contralateral reflex thresholds absent

Negative electronystagmography findings

Right ear:

Masked thresholds show severe to profound sensory-neural loss

Masked spondee threshold is 16 dB poorer than masked puretone average

Masked speech discrimination score is 0%

Masked tone decay at 500 Hz is positive

Normal tympanogram

Ipsilateral reflex thresholds absent; contralateral reflex thresholds present at normal sensation levels (consistent with left ear thresholds)

Electronystagmography identified a unilateral weakness and failure of fixation suppression

Overall case management:

The medical staff recommended surgery to remove the acoustic neurinoma

The patient declined surgery

The original audiologic recommendations included postoperative assessments

Because surgery was declined, the recommendations were altered to quarterly monitoring and a contralateral routing of signals (CROS) hearing aid fitting including orientation and counseling

Further decreases in hearing have been documented

Value of masking:

Type of loss confirmed—retrocochlear pathology

Low frequency air- and bone-conduction thresholds for the right ear would not have been valid without masking

Right ear spondee threshold would not have been a valid measurement without masking and would not have emphasized the severe word recognition disability present

Absence of speech discrimination in the right ear would not have been observed without masking

Tone decay would have been negative without masking once IA had been exceeded

The above cases differ dramatically in terms of patient management. Case I had a moderate sensory-neural loss in the left ear with speech discrimination adequate to fit a hearing aid at the poorer ear. Case II had an asymmetrical markedly sloping hearing loss, with the better ear speech discrimination adequate for a CROS, BiCROS or other creative hearing aid fittings. This second client, however, demonstrated audiologic signs consistent with retrocochlear pathology. Without *adequate* masking, differential audiologic diagnosis would not have been accurate.

CONCLUSION

The objectives of this chapter were to summarize the extensive literature available on the subject of masking, and to convey this information to clinicians in a logical format. The material provides a foundation upon which appropriate masking decisions can be made for any given set of audiologic circumstances. The subject of masking is complex, and extensive study and actual experience are necessary to become clinically proficient. The validity of all audiologic test procedures, and their resulting differential diagnosis and management, are at risk if masking is necessary but overlooked or inappropriately used. The correct use of masking ensures that each ear is assessed independently.

REFERENCES

American National Standards Institute. Criteria for Background Noise in Audiometer Rooms. ANSI S3.1-1960, New York, 1960.

American National Standards Institute. Specifications for Audiometers. ANSI S3.6-1989, New York, 1989.

American National Standards Institute. 1981. Reference Equivalent Threshold Force Levels for Audiometric Bone Vibrators. ANSI S3.26-1981, New York.

American Speech and Hearing Association, Committee on Audiometric Evaluation. Guidelines for audiometric symbols. Asha 1990;(Suppl.)32:25—30.

Bilger RC, and Hirsh LJ. Masking of tones by bands of noise. J Acoust Soc Am 1956;28:623—630.

Blegvad B. Contralateral masking and Bekesy audiometry in normal listeners. Acta Otolaryngol 1967;64:157—165.

Blegvad B. Bekesy audiometry and clinical masking. Acta Otolaryngol 1968;66:229—240.

Blegvad B, and Terkildsen K. 1967. Contralateral masking and the SISI-test in normal listeners. Acta Otolaryngol 1967;63:556—563.

Carter NL, and Kryter KD. Masking of pure tones and speech. J Aud Res 1962;2:66—98.

Chaiklin JB. Interaural attenuation and cross-hearing in air conduction audiometry. J Aud Res 1967;7:413—424.

Coles RRA, and Priede VM. Problems in Crosshearing and Masking. Institute of Sound and Vibration Research, Annual Report, 26, South Hampton, England, 1968.

Coles RRA, and Priede VM. Masking of the non-test ear in speech audiometry. J Laryngol Otol 1975;89:217—226.

Deatherage BH, and Evans TR. Binaural masking: backward, forward, and simultaneous effects. J Acoust Soc Am 1969;46:362—371.

Dirks DD. Factors related to bone conduction reliability. Arch Otolaryngol 1964;79:55—558.

Dirks DD, and Malmquist CW. Changes in bone-conduction thresholds produced by masking in the non-test ear. J Speech Hear Res 1964;7:271—278.

Dirks DD, and Norris JN. Shifts in auditory thresholds produced by ipsilateral and contralateral maskers at low intensity levels. J Acoust Soc Am 1966;40:12—19.

Dirks DD, and Swindeman JG. The variability of occluded and unoccluded bone-conduction thresholds. J Speech Hear Res 1967;10:232—249.

Elpern B, and Naunton RF. The stability of the occlusion effect. Arch Otolaryngol 1963;77:376—384.

Fletcher H. Auditory patterns. Rev Mod Physics 1940;12:47—65.

Goldstein BA. To mask, and how to mask: teaching masking to students. Audiol Hear Educ 1979;5(1):5—7, 16; 5(2):8—10; 5(3):7—10.

Goldstein DP, and Hayes CS. The occlusion effect in bone-conduction hearing. J Speech Hear Res 1965; 8:137—148.

Hawkins JE Jr, and Stevens SS. The masking of pure tones and of speech by white noise. J Acoust Soc Am 1950;22:6—13.

Hood JD. The principles and practice of bone conduction audiometry. Laryngoscope 1960;70:1211—1228.

Huizing EH. Bone conduction, the influence of the middle ear. Acta Otolaryngol 1960;(Suppl.):155.

Jerger JF, and Jerger S. Critical evaluation of SAL audiometry. J Speech Hear Res 1965;8:103—128.

Jerger J, and Tillman T. A new method for the clinical determination of sensorineural acuity level (SAL). Arch Otolaryngol 1960;71:948—953.

Killion MC, and Villchur E. Comments on "Earphones in audiometry" (Zwislocki et al. J Acoust Soc Am 1988;83:1688—1689). J Acoust Soc Am 1989;85:1775—1778.

Killion MC, Wilber LA, and Gudmundsen GI. Insert earphones for more interaural attenuation. Hear Instr 1985;36:34—36.

Konig E. On the use of hearing-aid type earphones in clinical audiometry. Acta Otolaryngol 1962;55:331—341.

Konkle DF, and Berry GA. Masking in speech audiometry. In Konkle DF, and Rintelmann WF, Eds. Principles of Speech Audiometry. Baltimore: University Park Press, 1983:285—319.

Larson VD, Talbott RE, and Harrell DA. Insert transducers: hearing level and interaural attenuation data. Presented at American Speech-Language-Hearing Association Convention, Cincinnati, OH, 1983.

Liden G, Nilsson G, and Anderson H. 1959a. Narrow band masking with white noise. Acta Otolaryngol 1959a;50:116—124.

Liden G, Nilsson G, and Anderson H. Masking in clinical audiometry. Acta Otolaryngol 1959b;50:125—136.

Lloyd LL, and Kaplan H. 1978. Audiometric Interpretation: A Manual of Basic Audiometry. Baltimore: University Park Press, 1978:151—159.

Martin FN. Speech audiometry and clinical masking. J Aud Res 1966;6:199—203.

Martin FN. A simplified method for clinical masking. J Aud Res 1967;7:59—62.

Martin FN. Clinical Audiometry and Masking. Bobbs-Merrill, Indianapolis, IN, 1972.

Martin FN. Minimum effective masking levels in threshold audiometry. J Speech Hear Disord 1974;39:280—285.

Martin FN. Introduction to Audiology. Prentice-Hall, Englewood Cliffs, NJ, 1975.

Martin FN, and DiGiovanni D. Central masking effects on spondee threshold as a function of masker sensation level and masker sound pressure level. J Am Aud Soc 1979;4:141—146.

Martin FN, Bailey HAT, and Pappas JJ. The effect of central masking on threshold for speech. J Aud Res 1965;5:293—296.

Meyer MF. Masking: why restrict it to the threshold level? J Acoust Soc Am 1959;31:243.

Naunton RF. A masking dilemma in bilateral conductive deafness. Arch Otolaryngol 1960;72:753—757.

Priede VM, and Coles RRA. Masking of the non-test ear in tone decay. Beskesy audiometry, and SISI tests. J Laryngol Otol 1975;89:227—236.

Sanders JW. Masking. In Katz J, Ed. Handbook of Clinical Audiology, Ed. 1. Baltimore: Williams & Wilkins, 1972:111—142.

Sanders JW. Masking. In Katz J, Ed. Handbook of Clinical Audiology. Ed. 2. Baltimore: Williams & Wilkins, 1978:124—140.

Sanders JW, and Rintelmann WF. 1964. Masking in audiometry. Arch Otolaryngol 1964;80:541—556.

Shimizu H. 1969. Influence of contralateral noise stimulation on tone decay and SISI test. Laryngoscope 1969;79:2155—2164.

Staab WJ. 1974. Masking in pure-tone audiometric testing. Hear Aid J 1974;27:10—11, 34—35, 37—38.

Studebaker GA. On masking in bone-conduction testing. J Speech Hear Res 1962;5:215—227.

Studebaker GA. 1964. Clinical masking of air- and bone-conducted stimuli. J Speech Hear Res 1964;29:23—35.

Studebaker GA. 1967. Clinical masking of the non-test ear. J Speech Hear Disord 1967;32:360—371.

Studebaker GA. Auditory masking. In Jerger J, Ed. Modern Developments in Audiology, Ed. 2. New York: Academic Press, 1973:117—154.

Studebaker GA. Clinical masking. In Rintelmann WF, Ed. Hearing Assessment. Baltimore: University Park Press, 1979:51—100.

Swisher LP, Dudley JG, and Doehring DG. Influence of contralateral noise on auditory intensity discrimination. J Acoust Soc Am 1969;45:1532—1536.

Tillman TW. Clinical applicability of the SAL test. Arch Otolaryngol 1963;78:20—32.

Townsend TH, and Schwartz DM. 1976. Calculation of effective masking using one octave and one-third octave analysis. Audiol Hear Educ 1976;2:27—28, 30—31, 34.

Veniar FA. Individual masking levels in pure-tone audiometry. Arch Otolaryngol 1965;82:518—521.

Wegel RL, and Lane CE. The auditory masking of one pure tone by another and its probable relations to the dynamics of the inner ear. Physics Rev 1924;23:266—285.

Zwislocki J. 1953. Acoustic attenuation between ears. J Acoust Soc Am 1953;25:752—759.

CHAPTER 9

Bone-Conduction Threshold Testing

Donald D. Dirks

As Hood (1962) observed, no specific physiologically useful purpose has been attributed to the bone-conduction system in man. According to Barany (1938) and Bekesy (1939) the ossicular chain in man appears to be balanced to diminish bone conduction by the development of relatively substantial masses above the chain's axis of rotation. Although this design is not optimal for air-conduction transmission, it does minimize the effect of bone conduction. Thus the potential annoyance from body noises such as breathing, chewing, blood flow, and creaking of joints is reduced.

With the exception of certain theoretical considerations, the interest in bone conduction has been its usefulness as a diagnostic tool. It is applied especially to determine the presence of conductive loss or middle ear pathology. In the range of hearing encompassing frequencies necessary for speech reception, bone-conduction thresholds from airborne sound are not obtained until the sound pressure level is approximately 60 dB above the air-conduction threshold. This relatively poor threshold is a result of the impedance mismatch between the skull and the surrounding air. Bekesy (1932) was the first investigator to demonstrate clearly that the mode of excitation of the cochlear receptors was identical for both air- and bone-conducted signals. He applied a 400-Hz bone-conducted tone at a level of 57 dB above threshold to the forehead simultaneously with an air-conducted tone of the same frequency. By adjusting the intensity and phase of the air-conducted signal he was able to cancel the bone-conducted signal. Bekesy concluded that the vibrations of the basilar membrane are produced by movements of the fluid near the stapes and thus the two modes of transmission must excite the sensory cells in the same manner. This experiment was a key contribution to bone-conduction theory. It also provided fundamental information for the clinical use of bone-conduction thresholds to estimate the integrity of the sonsory-neural system.

Despite the importance and extensive use of bone-conduction measurements, the clinical assessment has many inherent problems. These difficulties are related to (*a*) the participation of the middle ear in the total bone-conduction response, (*b*) the lack of a reliable and valid method of specifying the vibrational output of a bone-conduction testing system, (*c*) difficulties and limitation of masking the non-test ear, and (*d*) other equipment and procedural variables that substantially influence the outcome of the test such as the type of vibrator, the placement of the vibrator, and the force of vibrator application. Before discussing some of the problems associated with the clinical measurement of bone conduction, a brief review of the mechanism of bone conduction is provided.

MECHANISM OF BONE

Most of the currently accepted concepts regarding bone conduction have evolved from the investigations and theoretical explanations of Herzog and Krainz (1926), Bekesy (1932), Barany (1938), Kirikae (1959), Huizing (1960), and Groen (1962). Although each of the mechanisms stressed by the various investigators plays a major or minor role depending on the conditions of the experiment, two modes of stimulation, compression and inertia, are the most commonly accepted concepts among the early theorists.

According to Herzog and Krainz (1926), in compression bone conduction, the vibratory energy reaching the cochlea causes alternate compressions and expansions of the cochlear shell. The incompressible cochlear fluid must yield under the influence of these opposite movements and produce a displacement of the basilar membrane. If the elastic characteristics of the cochlear scalae were equal, then a compression of the cochlea would not prodece fluid displacement. This condition is illustrated in Figure 9.1**A**. A compensatory mechanism, as shown in Figure 9.1**B**, would be required to produce volume changes of the cochlear spaces. Such a mechanism is possible because the round window is more compliant than the oval window. In addition, the presence of semicircular canals and vestibules in the region of the stapes (Fig. 9.1**C**) enhances further a displacement of the fluid from scala vestibuli to scala tympani. The contribution of compressional bone conduction is greatest at high frequencies where the skull no longer moves as a rigid body but rather is compressed and expanded segmentally in response to an alternating vibration (Bekesy, 1932).

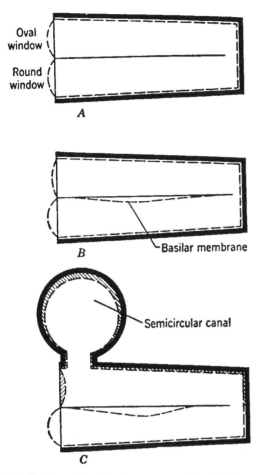

Figure 9.1. Compression of the inner ear and the displacement of the basilar membrane. *The broken lines* indicate the position of the various membranes during compression. **A** shows a hypothetical case of equal yielding at both windows, symmetrical compression and no movement of the basilar membrane. The round window actually yields more than the oval window (**B**), and the compression is nonsymmetrical, leading to a downward displacement of the basilar membrane. Inasmuch as the semicircular canals are also compressed (**C**), more fluid is forced into the upper canal, and the basilar membrane is forced downward even more. (From Bekesy G, and Rosenblith WA. In Stevens SS, Ed. *Handbook of Experimental Psychology,* John Wiley & Sons, New York; 1951:1110.

The second mode is referred to as inertial bone conduction because it arises from the inertia of the ossicular chain. According to Bekesy (1932) and Barany (1938), the inertia of the ossicles during forced vibrations of the skull sets up a relative motion between the stapes and the oval window. This motion leads to cochlear stimulation in the same manner as that produced by an air-conducted signal.

The most significant contributions to the theory of bone conduction are by Tonndorf (1966, 1972) who stressed the futility of accounting for all bone-conduction phenomena by a single mechanism. Among the factors contributing to the total bone-conduction responses are three major mechanisms: (*a*) the reception of sound energy radiated into the external canal, (*b*) the inertial response of the middle ear ossicles and inner ear fluid, and (*c*) the compressional response of the inner ear spaces.

Tonndorf observed that when a vibrating signal is applied to the skull, energy is produced by the walls of the external canal and transmitted to the tympanic membrane. This mode may be increased or decreased by closing or opening the external canal, or by changing the canal resonance or the impedance of the tympanic membrane. An impairment of the middle ear may eliminate or reduce the transmission of the sound energy developed in the external canal.

The inertial response, according to Tonndorf, is primarily a result of the impedance of the middle ear ossicles and the inertia of the ossicular chain can be modified by the air column within the external canal and by the air enclosed in the middle ear.

The compressional response is a product of the distortional vibrations of the cochlear shell and may be independent of the cochlear openings. The response, however, is modified by the oval and round window release as well as by the "third" window release of the cochlear aqueduct. The normal ear integrates these components according to their amplitude and phase relationships. The clinical orientation of this chapter does not permit further formal discussion of theory, but the interested reader will find ample references throughout the chapter. Tonndorf's (1972) contribution is of considerable importance in understanding the basic mechanisms involved in bone conduction.

EFFECT OF MIDDLE EAR ON BONE-CONDUCTION RESPONSE

Clinical bone-conduction thresholds are used primarily to ascertain the presence or absence of an external or middle ear lesion and to determine quantitatively the magnitude of the conductive hearing impairment. The usefulness of the difference between the air- and bone-conduction threshold (air-bone gap) is based on two assumptions: first, that the threshold for bone-conducted signals is a measure of the integrity of the sensory-neural system and, second, that the air-conduction threshold reflects the function of the total hearing system both conductive and sensory-neural. As a result, the discrepancy between the air- and bone-conduction thresholds is often assumed to indicate the magnitude of the conductive component. Theoretically, in a purely conductive loss, the bone-conduction thresholds should be normal. However, the fact that bone-conduction sensitivity is not independent of the state of the middle ear has been repeatedly demonstrated in both animal and human experiments. It is instructive to review some of the literature on this problem.

Experimental Results in Animals

Various investigators have demonstrated both increased and decreased bone-conduction responses in animals after alterations of the external middle ear systems. Particularly good examples can be found in experiments in which the tympanic membrane was weighted down (loaded) or various middle ear structures were selectively removed or fixated.

Most experimenters report improvements in bone-conduction response after loading the eardrum with water, mercury, pieces of metal, or other materials (Barany, 1938; Rytzner, 1954; Kirikae, 1959; Legouix and Tarab, 1959; Allen and Fernandez, 1960; Abu-Jaudeh, 1964; Brinkmann et al., 1965). Tonndorf (1966) demonstrated that a loaded tympanic membrane caused the resonant frequency of the ossicular system to shift downward. Thus, the bone-conduction responses were elevated at frequencies above the newly established resonant point but improved at frequencies below this resonant point.

Tonndorf has also reported changes in bone-conduction responses (as determined from changes in the amplitude and phase of cochlear microphonics) after certain alterations of the middle ear system, such as disarticulation of the incudostapedial joint, severing of the stapedial tendon, removal of the stapes superstructure, stapedectomy, occlusion of the oval or round window, and fixation of the stapes. Among seven specific components that Tonndorf identified as contributing to the total bone-conduction response, four (middle eare interia, middle ear cavity compliance, and round window and oval window pressure release) were directly related to participation of the middle ear.

Smith (1943) fixated the stapes in cats by means of a thread attached to one stapedial crus. Essentially, no mass was added to the stapes by this method, although the fixation was probable not very firm. The results indicated poorer bone-conduction response, especially in the frequency range around 500 to 1000 Hz. In other experiments of stapes fixation, amplitude losses centering around 500 Hz were reported by Tonndorf and Tabor (1962) and Tonndorf (1966). The magnitude of the loss depended on the degree of fixation.

Tonndorf further demonstrated elevation in the bone-conduction responses in various species of animals after removal of the middle ear structures or immobilization of the tympanic membrane. In these instances the loss was due to the total or partial elimination of the ossicular inertial component, and the frequency region of maximal loss was related to the ossicular resonant frequency characteristics of the particular animal species examined.

Clinical Observations

Numerous examples of changes in bone-conduction thresholds have been reported in humans with various middle ear lesions. Clinical patients with otosclerosis often show a loss in bone-conduction thresholds in the frequency region around 2000 Hz. This notch in the bone-conduction audiogram was described originally by Carhart (1950) and now bears his name. In Figure 9.2A is an example of the bone-conduction loss resulting from stapedial fixation. The Carhart notch is present with the maximum bone-conduction loss at 2000 Hz. **B** shows bone-conduction levels for the same patient 8 months after successful stapedial mobilization with almost perfect restoration of hearing. The postoperative bone-conduction levels have improved by 5 dB at 500 Hz, 10 dB at 1000 Hz, 15 dB at 2000 Hz, and 5 db at 4000 Hz. These improvements in the postoperative bone-conduction levels correspond closely to the average shifts in the bone-conduction responses due to stapedial fixatin as described by Carhart. Obviously the improvement is due to mechanical changes in the ossicular system and not to cochlear modification.

Fournier (1954), Hirsh (1952), and Carhart (1962) have commented on the incompatibility of the bone-conduction loss due to stapedial fixation with the theory of inertial bone conduction. They suggest that because the head moves as a whole with no compression waves at low frequencies, the middle ear inertia factor is the dominant mode of bone conduction, although compression bone conduction is the dominant feature at high frequenies. It might be anticipated from classical theory that

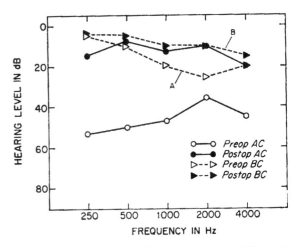

Figure 9.2. Pre- and postoperative air-conduction (**AC**) and bone-conduction (**BC**) audiogram for a patient with otosclerosis.

stapedial fixation should impair interial bone conduc-tion with a loss primarily in the low and not the high frequencies. Tonndorf (1966) explained and demon-strated that it is essentially the missing ossicular inertial componant that determines the frequency value of the maximal loss by bone conduction due to stapedial fixa-tion. He suggests that the middle ear contribution is not confined to low frequencies as classical theory sug-gested. Rather the ossicular vibrating system has a reso-nant frequency that varies from species to species. When responding to vibratory stimulation, the resonant frequency of the ossicular chain in man is found at 1500 to 2000 H3. If the participation of the ossicular chain is eliminated or reduced due to stapedial fixation, the maximan bone-conduction loss should also correspond closely to this frequency area.

Other types of middle ear impairment, that influence the bone-conduction thresholds have been reported among clinical cases. Bekesy (1939) and Tonndorf (1966) have each described a case in which bone-con-duction thresholds were altered after radical mastoidec-tomy. Reduction in hearing by bone conduction was noted especially in the frequencies around 2000 Hz, the frequency area of ossicular resonance in man. Goodhill (1965) reported a Carhart type notch extending into the higher frequencies for a patient with surgically con-firmed mallear fixation. Subsequently, a patient with surgically confirmed mallear fixation was reported by Dirks and Malmquist (1969). Figure 9.3 shows the re-sults of air-conduction, pre- and postoperatively, and preoperative bone-conduction thresholds at the mastoid process and frontal bone.

The audiometric results in Figure 9.3 must be re-viewed rather carefully because there is also a sensory-neural component. The question is, how large is the

sensory-neural component? The bone-conduction thres-holds obtained at the frontal bone suggest considerably less sensory-neural involvement than do the measure-ments at the mastoid process. The largest difference be-tween the measurements is 20 dB at 2000 Hz. Large differences are also present at 1000 and 4000 Hz. The difference is gradualy reduced as the test frequency is lowered and becomes nonexistent at 250 Hz. The dis-crimination score for phonetically balanced (PB-40) words was 80%. It is important to note that the postop-erative air-conduction curve interweaves with the preop-erative frontal, but not the mastoid measurements. Although there was an overclosure of the air-bone gap relative to bone-conduction measurements at the mas-toid process, it would appear that bone-conduction thresholds at the frontal bone were the better predictor of surgical gain in this case. These results are instructive for two reasons: first, they demonstrate clearly the sub-stantial effect that a middle ear lesion may have on bone-conduction responses and, second, they illustrate that bone-conduction thresolds may be affected differ-ently depending on the location of vibrator placement.

Hulka (1941) described a gain in the low and a loss in the high frequency areas for patients with otitis media. However, Palva and Ojala (1955), did not find a shift in bone-conduction thresholds in similarly diagnosed cases. Naunton and Fernandez (1961) reported results of bone-conduction tests at the forehead for three indi-viduals during and after attacks of bilateral secretory oti-tis. When fluid was present in the middle ears of these patients, there was an improvement in bone-conduction responses at the low frequencies, and a slight loss in the high frequencies. Huizing (1960) has also reported bone-conduction threshold changes in patients with oti-tis media, tubotympanitis, and chronic inflammatory processes. One patient with secretory otitis media was followed in our laboratory over a period of 7 months. Figure 9.4 illustrates the pre- and posttreatment air- and bone-conduction audiograms. Notice the depression in the bone-conduction thresholds especially around 2000 Hz when the patient was initially tested. After medical treatment there was no air-bone gap and the thresholds returned to normal levels.

The results of numerous investigations, primarily in-volving individuals with normal auditory systems, have demonstrated that bone-conduction responses can be al-tered experimentally by (a) air pressure changes in the external auditory canal (Fowler, 1920; Loch, 1942; Barany, 1938; Kirikae, 1959; Allen and Fernandez, 1960; Huizing, 1960); (b) loading of the tympanic membrane (Barany, 1938; Kirikae, 1959; Allen and Fernandez, 1960); and (c) the occlusion of the external auditory canal (Pohlman and Kranz, 1926; Bekesy, 1932; Kelley and Reger, 1937; Watson and Gales, 1943; Sullivan et al.,

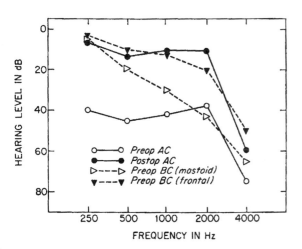

Figure 9.3. Pre- and postoperative air-conduction (**AC**) and preop-erative bone-conduction (**BC**) audiogram for a patient with mallear fixation.

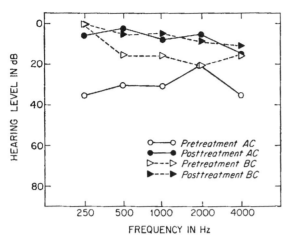

Figure 9.4. Pre- and posttreatment air- (**AC**) and bone-conduction (**BC**) audiogram for a patient with secretory otitis media.

1947; Onchi, 1954; Allen and Fernandez, 1960; Huizing, 1960; Elpern and Nauton, 1963; Goldstein and Hayes, 1965; Hodgson and Tillman, 1966; Dirks and Swindeman, 1967). Details of the specific gains or elevation of the bone-conduction thresholds under these conditions are given in the literature. In these experiments modification of either the external or middle ear system produced changes in the bone-conduction response.

Substantial data have accumulated demonstrating that bone-conduction thresholds do not represent a pure estimate of "cochlear reserve." Surely this is a serious shortcoming when bone-conduction audiometry is used as a quantitative measure of sensory-neural sensitivity. Such a limitation is not reported to discourage the clinician from attempting to estimate the magnitude of the conductive hearing loss with bone-conduction tests. Rather, it is mentioned to impress on the clinician the practical limitations of bone-conduction thresholds, so that they may be used more realistically.

CALIBRATION OF THE BONE-CONDUCTION TESTING SYSTEM

The physical calibration of bone vibrators supplied with audiometers has been enhanced greatly with the development of standardization of a mechanical coupler, more commonly known as an artificial mastoid. The specifications for this coupler can be reviewed in the United States standard entitled "Mechanical Coupler for Measurement of Bone Vibrators (ANSI S3.13-1987)." This standard, in general, corresponds closely with an international standard (International Electrotechnical Committee Publication 373) on the same topic. In addition, the International Organization for Standardization has issued a document (International Standard, ISO/DIS 7566) that recommends reference equivalent threshold force levels that correspond to the threshold

for hearing for young otologically normal persons by bone conduction. A standard (ANSI 53, 43, 1992) that corresponds closely to the ISO recommendations for threshold force levels for normal listeners was recently approved in the United States. A more complete discussion of bone conduction standardization can be found in Chapter 6.

MASKING

When earphones encased in supraaural cushions are used, the mass of the head provides an average interaural attenuation factor of about 60 dB for air-conduction measurements. Unfortunately for bone conduction, the interaural attenuation factor is almost negligible regardless of the position of the vibrator on the skull. Hence, it is necessary to exclude the non-test ear by an adequate air-conducted masker when obtaining bone-conduction thresholds. There are instances such as bilaterally symmetrical sensory-neural losses when masking may not be necessary (Naunton, 1963), but these cases should be the exception and not the general rule. Studebaker (1964) suggested that a more efficient rule is to apply a masker to the non-test ear whenever an air-bone gap appears.

The specific procedure for masking when testing for bone-conduction thresholds is described in Chapter 8. However, a few brief statements concerning masking are appropriate. Although masking theoretically may be accomplished by almost any sound, it is generally accepted that narrow bands of noise centered around the test frequency provide the greatest shift in the non-test ear threshold with a minimum of sound energy (Fletcher, 1940; Zwislocki, 1951; Denes and Naunton, 1952; Hood, 1957; Liden et al., 1959; Hood, 1962; Konig, 1963; Sanders and Rintelmann, 1964; Studebaker, 1964).

The results of Zwislocki (1953), Littler et al. (1952), and Strdebaker (1962) have demonstrated that the interaural attenuation factor can be increased as the area of the head exposed to the transducer is decreased. This may be accomplished by introducing the masking signal via an insert receiver rather than by the standard earphone encased in either a supraaural or circumaural cushion. There are still some calibration problems associated with the use of insert receivers and their coupling to the ear. Nevertheless, the introduction of narrow bands of noise delivered to the nontest ear via an insert receiver is highly desirable when measuring bone-conduction thresholds.

The least complex and most accurate method for masking in bone-conduction testing has been detailed by Hood (1962). A recent and useful discussion of the basic and practical aspects of clinical masking during bone-conduction thresholds testing can be found in the work of Studebaker (1979). Chapter 8 also provides more details concerning clinical masking procedures used for both air- and bone-conduction audiometry.

Regardless of the method, there are numerous instances in which sufficient masking is unavailable, and therefore the responses obtained cannot be assumed to be a measure of the desired test ear. The limitations of masking in clinical audiometry have recieved a rigorous appraisal by Konig (1963). These difficulties and limitations should encourage the clinician to perform additional auditory tests to determine the presence or absence of a conductive component when problems of insufficient masking or overmasking arise.

EQUIPMENT AND PROCEDURAL VARIABLES

Bone-Conduction Vibrators

The requirements for the physical characteristics of an idealized bone receiver were generally well described by Lierle and Reger (1946). They suggested a "mechanical design that will stand up under continued and rough usage without change in calibration, extension of the frequency range to values near or coincident with the normal upper limits of audibility, freedom from overtones, freedom from the effects of differences in pressure when the vibrator is held against the head and a wide a.c.-b.c. differential" (p. 221).

In the early days of clinical bone-conduction audiometry, bone vibrators were often held by hand against the mastoid process. It was important, therefore, that the housing of the vibrator be isolated from the vibration system itself. Such units were large and cumbersome and are not in general use today. Grossman and Malloy (1943) compared the physical characteristics of vibrators commonly designed as hearing aids with some of the older bone-conduction receivers composed of a rod connected to an electrmagnetically excited driving system. They concluded that the older bone vibrators were probably more advantageous from a physical point of view than the hearing aid type vibrators. In particular, the investigators reported more variability in the response of the hearing aid type receiver than in the older grenade type vibrators. Furthermore, the harmonic distortion of the X modern hearing aid-type vibrator was found to be large, especially at low frequencies.

Sanders and Olsen (1964) have also reported undesirable harmonic distortion at low frequencies for a hearing aid-type vibrator. Their results were obtained from measurements of the vibrational output of a vibrator with the receiver placed on the mass of an artificial mastoid. In addition, the data of Sanders and Olsen (1964) indicated that the intensity output of the second and third harmonics grows disproportionately to the input.

Another practical problem with the hearing aid-type vibrator is that the entire case vibrates. As a result, there is always the unfortunate possibility that some part of the vibrator mechanism, when located on the mastoid process, might touch the pinna and transmit sound into the external auditory canal. In addition, any holding device must grip the hearing aid-type vibrator at some location on its vibrating case, thereby increasing the possiblity of a change in the frequency response characteristics of the vibrator.

Both national and international standards recommend that bone vibrators used in audiometry have a plane circular contact tip area of 1.75 cm. In the United States many clinics still use audiometers that were supplied with the old Radioear B-70 series vibrators. These vibrators have a contact tip area larger than recommended by current standards. The newer Radioear B-71 and B-72 vibrators contain contact tips corresponding to the current standards on bone-conduction audiometry. The physical output of the B-71 vibrator is similar to the older B-70AA, whereas the output of the B-72 has a significantly greater output at 250 Hz than the other bone-conduction transducers. Figure 9.5 shows examples of the frequency responses of two bone-conduction vibrators with contact tip areas conforming to size recommended by the standards. Both responses were obtained on a Bruel and Kjaer 4930 artificial mastoid.

The resonance of the B-72 vibrator is found at a lower frequency (~250 Hz) than for the B-71 vibrator. Thus the output is greater for the B-72 vibrator at 250 Hz, increasing the potential dynamic range for testing and reducing the harmonic distortion. These advantages initially seemed to be positive features of the new B-72 units and suggested that they might become the desired vibrator for clinical use. Subsequently, it was observed (Frank and Holmes, 1981) that the B-72 vibrator radiated aerial sound waves at sufficiently high levels so that

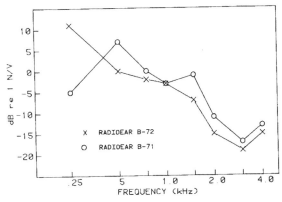

Figure 9.5. Frequency response of Radioear B-71 and B-72 bone vibrators in dB *re* 1 N/V as measured on a Bruel and Kjaer 4930 artificial mastoid.

thresholds obtained from bone vibrator signals at 2000 Hz and higher became suspect. If the B-72 vibrator is used at high test frequencies, the test ear would have to be occluded to obtain valid bone-conduction thresholds unaffected by radiated aerial sound. Especially, for this reason, the Radioear B-72 may not be the vibrator of choice for clinical use.

According to data supplied by Shipton et al. (1980) and Haughton (1982), the mechanical behavior of the B-71 vibrator may also lead to unsatisfactory acoustic radiations at the high frequencies (3000 and 4000 Hz). These authors have suggested that the test ear of the patient be occluded by a small earplug when bone-conduction testing is conducted at these frequencies. Thus, the air-conducted signal will be attenuated in the ear canal and eliminate the influence of air radiations of the bone-conduction thresholds. This suggestion is reasonable because the occlusion effect for bone-conduction is minimal or absent at these high frequencies. However, the results of Frank and Holmes (1981) suggested that the acoustic radiations for the B-71 vibrator were minimal at these frequencies although sufficient in 3 of 10 of the experimental subjects to influence bone-conduction thresholds. Haughton (1982) observed that acoustic radiations for the B-71 vibrator could be reduced by enclosing the vibrator in a more rigid case. There is obviously a need to recognize the possible influence of acoustic radiations on bone-conduction thresholds at high test frequencies when a vibrator such as the B-71 is used. Although the effects of acoustic radiations are generally minimal with this vibrator, elimination of the problem can be accomplished by occluding the test ear with an ear plug. This procedure will probably be an annoyance for the tester and hopefully suggestions, similar to those of Haughton, may result in the development of vibrators in which acoustic radiations are not a significant problem.

In summary, the commonly used hearing aid-type vibrator is, no doubt, more convenient to use than older grenade-shaped bone receiver containing a vibrating rod. However, the convenience of adjusting the modern vibrator to the skull may not outweigh the loss of certain desirable physical characteristics found in some of the older bone vibrators.

Vibrator Placement

Traditionally, clinical bone-conduction measurements have been performed with the vibrator or the tuning fork located on the mastoid process. The preference of the site on the skull was perhaps based on the erroneous assumption that the ear under examination could be tested more or less independently of the non-test ear. Unfortunately there is generally little interaural isolation by bone conduction and, hence, both cochleas may participate in the response regardless of the bone vibrator location on the skull.

The question of the placement of the bone vibrator for the clinical determination of the bone-conduction threshold has not as yet been completely resolved. Although the vertex (Barany, 1938; Studebaker, 1962) of the skull and the teeth have been considered, the mastoid process and frontal bone have received the most attention. Three major arguments have been advanced in favor of placement of the vibrator on the frontal bone rather than on the mastoid process.

First, it has been suggested that there is an increase in the test-retest reliability of bone-conduction measurements at the frontal bone. These observations were based originally on the report by Bekesy (1932) that the displacement of the vibrator away from the middle of the forehead gives rise only to relatively small fluctuations in bone conduction thresholds, whereas similar variations in placement at the mastoid process result in changes of 10 dB or more. Results of five repeated measurements by Hart and Haunton (1961) indicated that there was less variation when tests were performed on the frontal bone as compared to the mastoid process. It may be noteworthy that these observations were made with vibrators containing vibrating tips covering only a small contact area. The comparative results of more recent investigations (Studebaker, 1962; Dirks, 1964) using hearing aid-type vibrators with large contact areas have not demonstrated test-retest differences between mastoid and frontal bone placement that were of great practical advantage.

The second argument favoring frontal bone placement is concerned with intersubject variability. At the frontal bone, the tissues seem to be more homogeneous over the general test area than at the mastoid process, and, thus, the difference in bone-conduction thresholds among the individuals should be reduced. The results of Studebaker (1962) and Dirks (1964) seem to verify this contention. The differences in intersubject variability between the two sites, however, were small.

A third advantage of forehead placement was evolved primarily from the classical investigation by Barany in 1938. He suggested that bone-conduction tests at the frontal bone reduce the participation of the middle ear more effectively than those performed at the mastoid process. Experimental results by Link and Zwislocki (1951) on patients with otitis media demonstrated less hearing loss from measurements at the frontal bone than at the mastoid process. Studebaker (1962) and Dirks and Malmquist (1969) made similar comparisons on individuals with middle ear impairments and observed less hearing loss (re normal hearing at each placement site) when measurements were obtained at the forehead than at the mastoid process. However, the average threshold difference at the test frequencies was only about 5 dB. In the Dirks and Malmquist data, however, average threshold differences of over 10 dB favoring the frontal bone were observed in a selected group of clients with middle ear impairments.

The principal and probable overriding disadvantage of testing bone-conduction thresholds at the frontal bone is the reduced sensitivity at this site as compared to measurements at the mastoid. Thus, the dynamic range for threshold is reduced when tests are conducted with the vibrator located on the forehead.

Standards for normal hearing with the vibrator coupled to the frontal bone are established either by reporting a separate set of normal bone-conduction threshold values for forehead application or by producing a standard forehead-mastoid difference to use together with the standard established for mastoid placement. The latter has often been used because audiometers are almost always calibrated for mastoid applications and the user can simply adjust bone-conduction thresholds obtained at the forehead with this information. The decibel differences between thresholds obtained at the frontal bone and those at the mastoid are summarized in Table 9.1 which shows the differences recommended in ANSI S3.43-1992 together with the results from several recent investigations. The overall forehead-mastoid differences suggested in the standard appear to be in close agreement with the other studies cited.

Vibrator Application Force and Surface Area

Another source of variability in bone-conduction measurement is the force of application of the bone vibrator on the skull. In general, as vibrator application force is increased, less energy is required to reach threshold by bone conduction. However, there are certain limitations and modifications to this general principle. Bekesy (1939) and Konig (1955) investigated the variation of bone-conduction thresholds over a wide range of static forces. Their findings suggested that the largest changes in bone-conduction thresholds are observed at forces below 750 gm. Although some changes could still be observed between 1000 and 1500 gm in Konig's results, they were small. Konig suggested that it would be desirable to use a coupling force of approximately 1000 gm in clinical audiometry so the variability would be minimal.

Harris et al. (1953) investigated the effects of increased application force from 100 to 400 gm at the test frequencies of 250, 1000, and 8000 Hz. The greatest change in threshold was found at 250 Hz although little change was observed at 1000 and 8000 Hz. They suggested that bone-conduction receiver application force be standardized somewhere between 200 and 400 gm. In the ranges of application force where the measurements of Harris et al. and Konig overlap, the results indicated that thresholds continue to change as force is increased above 400 gm, whereas the results of Harris et al. suggested that thresholds do not change substantially once 400 gm is reached.

Goodhill and Holcomb (1955) studied the changes in cochlear microphonics produced by bone-conducted signals with the vibrator placed on the skull of cats. Erratic responses were reported when the force was less than 200 gm, but little change was observed as force was modified between 300 and 600 gm.

Whittle (1965) recorded bone-conduction thresholds on normal listeners at forces of 250, 350, and 750 gm. For two bone vibrators, thresholds were compared at forces of 350 and 750 gm. Although there was a tendency for average thresholds to be better with the greater force, intersubject variations were as large at a force of 750 gm as the lowest application forces used.

The surface area under the vibrator may constitute another source of variability, but its influence on bone-conduction thresholds has not been studied in depth. Watson (1938) reported that thresholds varied only negligibly at low frequencies but inproved with larger surface areas for frequencies between 3000 and 7000 Hz. However, Goodhill and Halcomb (1955) suggest that bone-conduction thresholds were more consistent with a vibrator surface area of 1 cm than for a comparative vibrator with a surface area of 3.2 cm. Nilo (1968) observed that vibrator surface area had no influence on bone-conduction thresholds at frequencies up to 2000 Hz. At 2000 Hz, the bone-conduction thresholds improved as the surface increased from 1.125 to 4.5 cm. The investigator noted that in a subsequent study threshold levels were improved at 4000 Hz as the vibrator surface area increased.

A more recent comprehensive investigation of the effects of vibrator contact area on bone-conduction thresholds has been reported by Queller and Khanna

Table 9.1.
Differences between Mean Thresholds Measured at Forehead and Mastoid as Recommended by ANSI S3.43-1992 and from other Laboratories that Used B-71 Bone Vibrator

	Frequency in Hz					
	250	500	1000	2000	3000	4000
	Forehead—Mastoid in dB					
ANSI S3.43-1992	12.0	14.0	8.5	11.5	12.0	8.0
Haughton and Pardoe (1981)	10.7	11.0	8.5	10.8	9.9	7.4
Frank (1982)	14.3	14.7	8.7	12.0	12.4	13.5

(1982). They measured the physical force and acceleration at threshold on six subjects over a frequency range of 150 to 6000 Hz with a vibrator having a contact area range from 1.6 to 3.8 cm in diameter. They observed that variations in force of threshold with contact area were smaller for their group of listeners than comparative variations in acceleration at threshold. Practically the investigators point out the changes in contact area between the vibrator and the skull cannot be avoided when testing bone-conduction thresholds. This is due to the variations in curvature of the skull from person to person. Inasmuch as the force thresholds were relatively insensitive to variations in contact area and skin impedance, they recommend that bone-conduction threshold be specified in force units. That recommendation is followed in ANSI S3.43-1992.

Even though it might be desirable to test bone-conduction thresholds with a force of 750 to 1000 gm, this application force is not practical. Static force application of this magnitude causes severe discomfort for the patient. As a consequence standard recommendations call for an application force of 5.4 Newtons or approximately 550 gm.

Other Clinical Procedures

Occlusion of the External Auditory Canal

There are several other auxiliary diagnostic procedures involving bone conduction which have received both substantial audiologic and otologic considerations. The first of these is modifying bone-conduction thresholds by occluding the external auditory meatus. It has been well established that the occlusion of the external auditory canal produces low frequency enhancement for bone-conducted signals. Numerous references on the effects of occlusion have been listed previously.

Clinical interest in the occlusion effect stems from the observation that, in general, the effect is absent in almost all impairments located anywhere along the conductive pathway. Bing, in 1891, was probably the first to use the occlusion of the auditory canal as a method of clinical examination. Briefly, the audiologist can perform the test by obtaining bone-conduction thresholds for low frequency signals with the test ear open and then occluded by an earphone and the supraaural cushion (MX41/AR) customarily used in clinical testing. If there is no difference in these thresholds, this suggests the presence of a lesion in the conductive mechanism. If the threshold improves under occluded conditions, it is an indication that the hearing loss is due to a sensory-neural lesion. Especially for the patient with a small air-bone gap, the absence of an occlusion effect will help to assure the clinician that the measured difference between air and bone conduction

is not due to variability in the test measurement or patient unreliability, but is, in fact, indicating the presence of a conductive component.

The question often arises of whether bone-conduction tests should be performed routinely with the test ear occluded or open. According to Huizing (1960), some authors formerly recommended that the external auditory canal be closed for bone-conduction audiometry. This advice was given to eliminate the masking effect due to ambient room noise and thereby the supposed real or "absolute" threshold could be measured. Subsequent observations have shown that the presence of the occlusion effect is not based on the elimination of masking. According to Tonndorf (1966), the occlusion effect is more likely due to the elimination of the high pass effect of an open ear canal when the external auditory meatus is occluded.

The clinical use of performing bone-conduction thresholds under occluded or unoccluded conditions also rests on the reliability and consistency of the occlusion effect. Elpern and Naunton (1963) reported that the reliability of the occlusion effect was poor from subject to subject and from test to retest. Earlier results (Carhart and Hayes, 1949; Roach, 1951; Studebaker, 1962; Dirks, 1964) demonstrated that unoccluded bone-conductin thresholds may be highly consistent from test to retest when sufficient controls are used. Thus, it might be conjectured that the prime source of variability in the Elpern and Naunton data was a result of the introduction of the occluding device. However, Malmquist and Jerger (1966) and Dirks and Swindeman (1967) found that bone-conduction thresholds obtained during occluded conditions were as reliable as those obtained with the ear open. Hodgson and Tillman (1966) observed a positive correlation between the application force of an occluding earphone and magnitude of the occlusion effect. They suggested that the common failure to control the force of the earphones against the head adds an important source of variability to occluded bone-conduction measurements.

The basis for deciding whether the clinician should perform bone-conduction tests with the ear open or occluded will probably depend on the final and complete explanation of the effect. Practically, it will also depend on whether the clinician performs bone-conduction tests at the forehead or at the mastoid process; it is difficult to occlude the test ear properly without the earphone and cushion touching the bone vibrator when tests are conducted at the mastoid process. For all clinical purposes, standard organizations recommend testing bone conduction with the ear open.

It is also important to remember that the masking signal is delivered to the nontest ear through an earphone and cushion which also produce an occlusion effect. Care must be taken to ensure that the intensity level of the masker is sufficient to eliminate the resultant improved bone-conduction threshold in the non-test ear.

Weber Test

Clinical interest in the Weber test stems from the general observation that various impairments of the middle ear produce lateralization of a bone-conducted signal to the involved ear or to the ear with the greater conductive component. The patient is asked to determine the location of the sound after stimulation by a bone-conducted tone with the vibrator located at the forehead.

Various explanations have been offered for the lateralization of the sound during the Weber test. These explanations fall into two general categories. It has been suggested, first, that the tone lateralizes to the conductively impaired ear because the effective amplitude in the cochlea is greater on that side and, second, that the lateralization is based on a phase lead at the ear with a conductive loss.

Several investigators (Christian and Roser, 1957; Legouix and Tarab, 1959; Allen and Fernandez, 1960) reported findings favoring the phase lead explanation. Others (Spoor et al., 1957; Groen and Hoogland, 1958; Naunton and Elpern, 1964) presented evidence that suggests that interaural intensity differences play a relatively major role in the lateralization of the signal in the Weber test.

Groen (1962) presented an extensive review of the Weber test. He reported that the Weber test is a reliable procedure in frequency areas below 1000 Hz and above 3000 Hz. Somewhat unreliable results appeared in the area around 2000 Hz. The investigator suggested that around 2000 Hz, lateralization frequently occurred toward the side of the uninvolved ear. Tonndorf (1966) reported that the lateralization toward the involved ear depends on the particular middle ear problem; in some instances, interaural intensity differences play the major role, and, in others, interaural phase differences account for the lateralization.

Sensorineural Acuity Level (SAL) Test

In 1959, Rainville introduced an attractive technique as an alternative for bone-conduction audiometry. Instead of measuring the threshold for bone-conducted tones with air-conducted masking noise, she obtained air-conduction thresholds in the presence of bone-conducted thresholds masking noise. Jerger and Tillman (1960) modified and popularized this technique. In their modified procedure, air-conduction thresholds are obtained with masking presented at a fixed level via the bone vi-

brator. These thresholds are compared with the individual's unmasked air-conduction thresholds. The difference between the two sets of air-conduction thresholds is then compared to the average shift obtained under the same conditions as obtained on a group of normal-hearing listeners. A conductive hearing loss will produce a major shift in thresholds similar to that obtained on persons with a normal auditory system. In contrast, a sensory-neural hearing loss will produce smaller or no shift in threshold because both the threshold signal and masker are limited by the hearing loss.

The SAL procedure was especially attractive in contrast to bone-conduction measurements because it required no special considerations concerning minimum or maximum masking levels. Masking was always used and the level was predetermined during the biologic calibration that was conducted on normal-hearing subjects. It became apparent (Goldstein et al., 1962; Tillman, 1963) that the SAL level did not compare favorably at low and mid-frequencies to bone-conduction thresholds of patients with conductive hearing loss. The problem is that the SAL technique fails to compensate for the occlusion effect that is present in the standard threshold values obtained on normal-hearing listeners but absent in patients with conductive hearing loss (Tillman, 1963). In addition, the occlusion effect is somewhat variable among subjects, and therefore any correction factor that is applied effectively to group data may be somewhat in error for an individual result.

The SAL procedure received much attention in the decade after its original description. Subsequently interest in the test has been markedly reduced. Jerger and Jerger (1965) observed that the SAL and bone-conduction thresholds could be equivalent if earphones were used that did not cause an "occlustion effect." Eliminating the "occlusion effect" requires the use of earphones that enclose a large volume of air. Earphones, such as the Pederson type B-228 A, which consist of a loudspeaker mounted in a 7-inch spherical enclosure, were considered for such a purpose. However, physical calibration of these earphones has not been standardized, and they are quite cumbersome for routine clinical testing. Possibly interest in the SAL also diminished with the advent of the artificial mastoid for convenient physical calibration of bone vibrators, the more efficient use of maskers with narrow bands of noise and a more practical understanding of masking.

Immittance Measurements

Immittance studies, including tympanometry and the measurement of the acoustic reflex, have become routine diagnostic tests for identifying middle ear lesions. These procedures are especially powerful for this purpose because of their objectivity and sensitivity to almost all forms of middle ear impairments. Some investigators and clinicians suggest that these objective tests for identifying middle ear disorders have reduced the need for bone-conduction audiometry. In most hearing clinics, immittance measurements have certainly become the major test for determining the presence or absence of a middle ear lesion. However, as Wilber and Feldman (1976) have pointed out, bone-conduction testing can only be eliminated when the clinician is "uninterested in quantification of the magnitude of the conductive loss, or when the impedance measurement clearly and consistently demonstrates normal middle ear function." Even though bone-conduction thresholds cannot be accepted without qualification as a pure measure of "cochlear reserve," the measurement of bone-conduction audiometry provides the only quanititative information concerning the magnitude of the conductive loss. Assessment of the magnitude of the conductive loss continues to be essential in decisions regarding the medical management of most cases with conductive le-

sions. As an example, Figure 9.6 shows the air- and bone-conduction thresholds together with immittance results from ears of two patients with the clinical diagnosis of otosclerosis. Patient 2 suffered several attacks of Ménière's disease before the appearance of the otosclerosis. Notice that in both patients tympanometry and the absent reflex (not shown Figure 9.6) suggest the presence of a conductive loss. However, in patient A a large air-bone gap is present with nearly normal bone-conduction thresholds. In patient B, an air-bone gap is present but the bone-conduction thresholds are severly reduced, indicating the presence of a substantial sensory-neural component. In the first patient, the surgeon decided to perform surgery because of the good potential for improving hearing to near normal levels. This decision was based primarily on the normal bone-conduction results. The immittance results simply indicated the presence of a middle ear lesion. In the second patient, the surgeon decided not to perform surgery because of the poor bone-conduction thresholds and small air-bone gap. The potential for improvement was

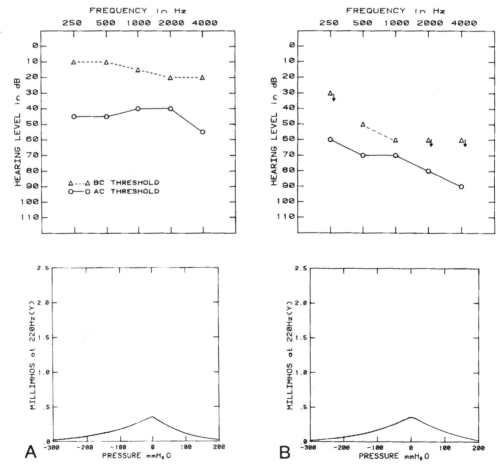

Figure 9.6. Air- and bone-conduction thresholds (**top panels**) for two patients with otosclerosis (**A**) and otosclerosis and accompanying sensory-neural hearing loss (**B**). The **bottom panels** show the tympanograms for each patient.

minimal, based on the air- and bone-conduction results, and the risks seemed to outweigh the possible improvement from surgery. In both instances the magnitude of the air- and bone-conduction thresholds played an important role in the final decision regarding medical or surgical therapy. These decisions cannot be made with sufficient insight if based merely on immittance results.

There are also patients in whom the immittance measurements present paradoxical results and bone-conduction thresholds become particularly useful in arriving at a diagnosis. An example of such a patient was reported by Jenkins et al. (1980). The preoperative air- and bone-conduction thresholds of this patient are shown in Figure 9.7 with acoustic reflex and immittance test results obtained with a probe tone at 220 Hz. Acoustic immittance tests were also conducted with a probe tone of 660 Hz (not shown). A "W-shape" tympanogram was observed at 660 Hz, reflecting a mass-controlled middle ear system that might be found in either ossicular discontinuity or a tympanic membrane anomaly. To confound the diagnosis, an acoustic reflex was observed in both ears. Thus, the tympanogram was abnormal but the reflex was present. A bilateral disruption of the stapes crura, central to the stapedial tendon insertion, was confirmed surgically. The investigation concluded that for diagnostic purposes "eliminating bone-conduction audiometry is applicable only in those situations in which the impedance studies unequivocally rule out a middle ear site of lesion" (p 272). In this context it should be remembered that it is not uncommon to observe immittance studies implying a low impedance system resulting from a tympanic membrane abnormality. Inasmuch as such abnormalities often do not require treatment, there is a tendency to disregard these tympanometric findings. In such cases the presence of a reflex would ordinarily confirm a normal middle ear. The case described with a large air-bone gap and the presence of reflex suggests that the

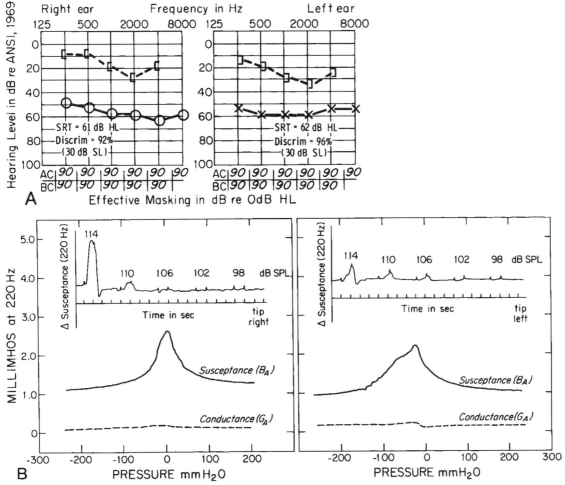

Figure 9.7. Preoperative audiogram showing puretone air- (O-X) and bone- ([—]) conduction results and speech test results (**A**) and susceptance (**B**$_A$) and conductance (**G**$_A$) tympanograms for a 220-Hz probe tone; results from a reflex-inducing stimulus are included (**B**) for patient with osteogenesis imperfecta, with bilateral ossicular discontinuity and intact acoustic reflexes.

best approach to diagnosis is the use of a complete battery of tests including bone-conduction audiometry.

CONCLUSION

Important features of this chapter are summarized by the following statements.

(a) Regardless of whether bone-conductin measurements are made at the forehead or mastoid process, the result will be influenced by the status of the external and middle ear. As a result, the clinician must use considerable restraint in the acceptance of any bone-conduction threshold as a pure measure of "cochlear reserve." There are sufficient examples of changes in bone-conduction thresholds due to middle ear impairments, and this limitation should be well understood.

(b) In bone-conduction audiometry, the sound applied to one mastoid will pass to the other mastoid process with little or no attenuation. As a result, a masking signal must be carefully used to exclude participation of the non-test ear. Although there may be instances in which the clinician may dispense with masking, the more conservative general rule is to use masking routinely for bone-conduction measurements. There is no shortcut to masking procedures, and it is incumbent upon the clinician to understand the physical characteristics of the noise, the procedure, and the limitations of the masker. This requires study and additional clinical time; however, for the sake of accuracy the effort is well spent.

(c) International and national standards have been issued recommending the mechanical impedance characteristics for a mechanical coupler used in calibrating bone vibrators. In addition, both a national and an international standard recommending the force threshold levels for normal hearing by bone conduction have finally been approved and provide needed guidance for both clinicians and manufacturers of audiometers.

(d) Various locations for application of the vibrator on the skull have certain assets and limitations. The frontal bone has often been advocated because thresholds obtained with the vibrator at this site appear to offer slightly greater reliability than mastoid or vertex placements. Unfortunately the sensitivity of the ear to bone-conduction energy is lower when the vibrator is located at the forehead than when coupled to the mastoid process. The mastoid process is usually chosen as the site for bone-conduction measurements because of the greater dynamic range and practically because of the absence of a commercially available headband arrangement which will accommodate the vibrator to the forehead at the static force recommended by standards.

(e) Acoustic radiations emitted by commercially available bone vibrators have received some investigative attention but the problem has not been eliminated. The problem is greatest at the high test frequencies, above 2000 Hz. Some investigators have suggested that the test ear be occluded by an earplug that has sufficient attenuation to eliminate the influence of acoustic radiations.

(d) Modern auditory diagnostic testing procedures include the use of acoustic immittance measurements to determine the presence or absence of a conductive lesion. Greater dependence is correctly being placed on these objective tests for diagnosing the presence of a middle ear lesion. However, bone-conduction thresholds continue to present important clinical information when the immittance studies are not clear-cut and for making therapeutic decisions, especially regarding the potential effects of surgical intervention.

REFERENCES

Abu-Jaudeh CN. The effect of simultanious loading of the tympanic membrane of the external auditory canal of bone conduction sensitivity of the normal ear. Ann Otol 1964; 69:5–29.

Allen GW, and Fernandez C. The mechanism of bone conduction. Ann Otol 1960;69:5–29.

American Natinal Standards Institute. Specification for Artificial Head Bone. ANSI S3.13-1972, New York, 1972.

American National Standards Institute. 1992. Standard Reference Zero for the Calibration of Pure-tone Bone Conduction Audiometers. ANSI S3.43-1992, New York.

American National Standards Institute. Mechanical Coupler for Measurement of Bone Vibrators. ANSI S3.13-1987, New York, 1987.

Barany E. A contribution to the physiology of bone conduction. Acta Otolaryngol 1938;26(Suppl):1–223.

Bekesy Gv. Zur theorie des noren bei der schallaufnahme durch knochenleitung. Ann Physik 1932;13:111–136.

Bing A. 1891. Ein neuer stimmgabelversuch. Beitrag zur diffentialdiagnostik der Kranheiten des mechanischen schallleitungs und nervosen horapparates. Weiner med. Blatter German journal, No. 41. In Tonndorf J, Ed. Bone conduction. Acta Otolaryngol 1966;213(Suppl):24.

Brinkmann WFB, Marres EHAM, and Tolk J. The mechanism of bone conduction. Acta Otolaryngol 1965;59:109–115.

Carhart R. Clinical application of bone conduction. Arch Otolaryngol 1950;51:798–807.

Carhart R. 1962. Effect of stapes fixation on bone conduction. In Schuknecht F, Ed. International Symposium on Otosclerosis. Little, Brown & Co., Boston, 1962.

Carhart R, and Hayes C. The clinical reliability of bone conduction audiometry. Laryngoscope 1949;59:1084–1101.

Carlisle RW, and Mundel AB. Practical hearing aid measurements. J Acoust Soc Am 1944;16:45–51.

Christian W, and Roser D. Ein beitrag zum richtungshoren. Z Laryngol Rhinol Otol 1957;36, 432–445.

Corliss ELR, and Koidan W. Mechanical impedance of the forehead and mastoid. J Acoust Soc Am 1955;27:1164–1172.

Dadson RS. The normal threshold of hearing and other aspects of standardization in audiometry. Acustica 1954;4:151–154.

Denes P, and Naunton RR. Masking in puretone audiometry. Proc R Soc Med 1952;45:790–794.

Dirks D. Factors related to bone conduction reliability. Arch Otolaryngol 1964;79:551–558.

Dirks D, and Kamm C. Bone vibrator measurements; physical characteristics and behavioral thresholds. J Speech Hear Res 1975;18:242–260.

Dirks D, and Malmquist C. Comparison of frontal and mastoid bone conduction thresholds in various conduction lesions. J Speech Hear Res 1969;12:725–746.

Dirks D, and Swindeman J. The variability of occluded bone conduction thresholds. J Speech Hear Res 1967;10:232–249.

Dirks D, Malmquist C, and Bower D. Toward the specification of normal bone conduction threshold. J Acoust Soc Am 1968;43:1237–1242.

Elpern BS, and Naunton RF. The stability of the occlusion effect. Arch Otolaryngol 1963;77:376–384.

Fletcher H. Auditory patterns. Rev Mod Phys 1940;12:47–65.

Fournier JE. The "flase-Bing" phenomenon; some remarks on the theory of bone conducin. Laryngoscope 1954;64:29–34.

Fowler E Bl Sr. Drum tension and meddle ear pressure, their determination, significance and effect upon hearing. Ann Otol 1920;29:668–694.

Frank T. Forehead versus mastoid threshold differences with a circular tipped vibrator. Ear Hear 1982;3:91–92.

Frank T, and Holmes A. Acoustic radiation from bone vibrators. Ear Hear 1981;2:59–63.

Goldstein R, and Hayes C. The occlustion effect in bone conduction hearing. J Speech Hear Res 1965;8:137–148.

Goldstein DP, Hayes CS, and Peterson JL. A comparison of bone conduction thresholds by conventional and Rainville methods. J Speech Hear Res 1962;5:244–255.

Goodhill V. The fixed malleus syndrome: surgical and audiological considerations. Trans Am Acad Ophthalmol Otolaryngol 1965;69:797(Abstr).

Groen JJ. The value of the Weber test. In Schuknecht HF, Ed. International Synmposium on Otosclerosis. Little, Brown & Co., Boston, 1962.

Groen JJ, and Hoogland GA. Bone conduction and otosclerosis of the round window. Acta Otolaryngol 1958;49:206–212.

Grossman F, and Malloy C. Physical characteristic of some bone oscillators used with commercially available audiometers. Arch Otol 1943;40:2–17.

Harris JD, Haines HL, and Myers CK. A helmet-held bone conduction vibrator. Laryngoscope 1953;63:998–1007.

Hart C, and Naunton R. Frontal bone conduction tests in clinical audiometry. Laryngoscope 1961;71:24–29.

Haughton PM. A system for generating a valuable mechanical impednce and its use in an investigation of the electromechanical properties of the B-71 audiometric bone vibrator. Br J Aud 1982;16:1–7.

Haughton PM, and Pardoe K. Normal puretone thresholds for hearing by bone conduction. Br J Aud 1981;15:113–121.

Hawley MS. Artificial mastoid for audiophone measurements. Bell Lab Rec 1939;18:73–75.

Herzog H, and Krainz W. Das Knochenleitungsproblem. Z Hals Usw Heilk 15. 1926. Cited by Tonndorf J. Bone conduction. Acta Otolaryngol 1926;(Suppl):213.

Hirsh IJ. The Measurement of Hearing. McGraw-Hill, New York, 1952.

Hodgson WR, and Tillman T. Reliability of bone conduction occlusion effects in normals. J Aud Res 1966;6:141–153.

Hood J. The principles and practice of bone conduction audiometry: a review of the present position. Proc R Soc Med 1957;50:689–697.

Hood JD. 1962. Bone conduction: A review of the present position with special reference to the contributions of Dr. Georg von Bekesy. J Acoust Soc Am 1962;24:1325–1332.

Huizing EH. 1960. Bone conduction-the influence of the middle ear. Acta Otolaryngol 1960;(Suppl)155:1–99.

Hulka J. Bone conduction changes in acute otitis media. Arch Otolaryngol 1941;33:333–346.

International Electrotechnical Commission. An IEC mechanical coupler for the calibration of bone vibrators having a specified contact area and being applied with a specific static force. IEC 373, Geneva, Switzerland, 1971.

Internationl Organization for Standardization. Standard Reference Zero for the Calibration of Pure-Tone Bone Conduction Audiometers. ISO/DP 7566. Geneva, Switzerland, 1987.

Jenkins HA, Morgan DE, and Miller RH. Intact acoustic reflexes in the presence of ossicular disruption. Laryngoscope 1980;90:267–273.

Jerger J, and Jerger S. Critical evaluation of SAL audiometry. J Speech Hear Res 1965;8:103–127.

Jerger J, and Tillman T. A new method for the clinical determinatin of sensorineural acuity level (SAL). Arch Otolaryngol 1960;71:948–953.

Kelley NH, and Reger SN. The effect of binaural occlusion of the external auditory meati on the sensitivity of the normal ear for bone conducted sound. J Exp Psychol 1937;21:211–217.

Kirikae I. An experimental study on the fundamental mechanism of bone conduction. Acta Otolaryngol 1959;145(Suppl):1–111.

Konig E. 1955. Les variations de la conduction osseuse en fonction de la force de pression excercee sur le vibrateur. Societe International d'Audiologie, Paris, 1955. (Cited from its English translation edited by Beltone Institute for Hearing Research, no. 6, May 1957.)

Konig E. 1963. The use of masking noise and its limitations in clinical audiometry. Acta Otolaryngol 1963;(Suppl)180:1–64.

Legouix JP, and Tarab S. Experimental study of bone conduction in ears with mechanical impairment of the ossicles. J Acoust Soc Am 1959;31:1453–1457.

Liden G, Nelsson G, and Anderson H. Narrow band masking with white noise. Acta Otolaryngol 1959;50:116–124.

Lierle D, and Reger S. Correlations between bone and air conduction acuity measurements over wide frequency ranges in different types of hearing impairments. Laryngoscope 1946;5:187–224.

Link R, and Zwislocki J. Audiometrische knochenleitungsuntersuchungen. Arch Klin Exp Ohr Nas Kehkopfheik 1951;160:347–357.

Littler TS, Knight JJ, and Strange PH. Hearing by bone conduction hearing aids. Proc R Soc Med 1952;45:783–790.

Loch WE. Effect of experimentally altered air pressure in the middle ear on hearing acuity in man. Ann Otol 1942;51:995–1006.

Malmquist CW, and Jerger JR. Some aspects of the normal occlustion effect. Presented at the Annual Convention of the American Speech and Hearing Association. Washington, D.C., 1966.

Naunton RF. The measurement of hearing by bone conduction. In Jerger JF, Ed. Modern Developments in Audiology. Academic Press, New York, 1963.

Naunton RF, and Elpern BS. Interaural phase and intensity relationships; the Weber test. Laryngoscope 1964;75:55–63.

Naunton RF, and Fernandez C. Prolonged bone conduction; observations on man and animals. Laryngoscope 1961;71:306–318.

Nilo ER. 1968. The relation of vibrator surface area and static application force to the vibrator-to-head coupling. J Speech Hear Res 1968;11:805–810.

Onchi Y. The blocked bone conduction test for differential diagnosis. Ann Otol 1954;63:81–96.

Palva T, and Ojala L. Middle ear conduction deafness and bone conduction. Acta Otolaryngol 1955;45:135–142.

Pohlman AG, and Kranz FW. 1926. The influence of partial and compete occlusion of external auditory canals on air and bone transmitted sound. Ann Otol 1926;35:113–121.

Queller JE, and Khanna SM. Changes in bone conduction thresholds with vibrator contact area. J Acoust Soc Am 1982;71:1519–1526.

Rainville MJ. New method of masking for the determination of bone conduction curves. Trans Beltone Inst Res 1959;11.

Roach RE. A study of reliability and validity of bone conduction audiometry [Ph.D. dissertation]. Northwestern University, Chicago: School of Speech, 1951.

Rytzner C. 1954. Sound transmission in clinical otosclerosis. Acta Otolaryngol. 1954;117:(Suppl)1–137.

Sanders JW, and Olsen WO. An evolution of a new artificial mastoid as an instrument for the calibration of audiometer bone conduction systems. J Speech Hear Disor 1964;29:247–263.

Shipton MS, John AJ, and Robinson DW. Air-radiated sound from vibration transducers and its implication for bone conduction audiometry. Fr J Audiol 1980;14:86–99.

Smith KR. Bone conduction during experimental fixation of the stapes. J Exp Psychol 1943;33:96–107.

Spoor A, Schmidt PH, and Van Dishoeck HAE. The location on the skull of a bone conduction receiver and the lateralization of the sound impression. Acta Otolaryngol 1957;48:594–597.

Stisen B, and Dahm M. 1969. Sensitivity and mechanical impedance of artificial mastoid type 4930. Bruel & Kjaer Technical Information, Larsen and Sons; Soborg Denmark.

Studebaker GA. Placement of vibrator in bone conduction testing. J Speech Hear Res 1962;5:321–331.

Studebaker GA. Clinical masking of air and bone conducted stimuli. J Speech Hear Disord 1964;29:23–35.

Studebaker GA. Clinical Masking. In Rintelmann WF, Ed. Hearing Assessment. Baltimore: University Park Press, 1979.

Sullivan JA, Gotieb CC, and Hodge WE. Shift of bone conduction thresholds on occlusion of the external ear canal. Laryngoscope 1947;57:690–703.

Tillman TW. Clinical applicability of the SAL test. Arch Otolaryngol 1963;78:20–32.

Tonndorf J. Bone conductin; studies in experimental animals. Acta Otolaryngol 1966;213:(Suppl)1–132.

Tonndorf J. Bone conduction. In Tobias JV, Ed. Foundation of Modern Auditory Theory. New York: Academic Press, 1972.

Tonndorf J, and Tabor JR. Closure of the cochlear windows; its effect upon air and bone conduction. Ann Otol 1962;71:5–29.

Watson NA. Limits of audition for bone conduction. J Acoust Soc Am 1938;9:294–300.

Watson NA, and Gales RS. Bone conduction threshold measurements; effects of occlusion, enclosures and masking devices. J Acoust Soc Am 1943;14:207–215.

Weiss E. An air damped artificial mastoid. J Acoust Soc Am 1960;32:1582–1588.

Weston PB, Gengel RW, and Hirsh IJ. Effects of vibrator types and their placement on bone conduction threshold measurements. J Acoust Soc Am 1967;41:788–792.

Whittle LS. A determination of the normal threshold of hearing by bone conduction. J Sound Vibration 1965;2:227–248.

Wilber LA, and Feldman A. The middle ear measurement battery. In Feldman A, and Wilber L, Eds. Acoustic Impedance and Admittance—The Measurement of Middle Ear Function. Baltimore: Williams & Wilkins, 1976.

Wilber LA, and Goodhill V. Real ear versus artificial mastoid methods of calibration of bone conduction vibrators. J Speech Hear Res 1967;10:405–417.

Zwislocki J. Eine verbesserte vertaubungsmethode fur die sudiometrie. Acta Otolaryngol 1951;39:338–356.

Zwislocki J. Acoustic attenuation between the ears. J Acoust Soc Am 1953;25:752–759.

CHAPTER 10

Speech Threshold and Word Recognition/Discrimination Testing

John P. Penrod

The ability to understand speech must be considered the most important measurable aspect of human auditory function. It is fundamental for most of life's activities and a prerequisite for fully effective participation in our complex auditory world. Assessment of hearing for puretones provides valuable information regarding sensitivity, but only limited information concerning receptive auditory communication ability. Moreover, investigations of puretone sensitivity and speech understanding have shown no clear-cut relationship between these two measures. There appears to be no satisfactory means of accurately predicting speech understanding ability from puretone results (Solomon et al., 1960; Young and Gibbons, 1962; Elliot, 1963; Harris, 1965; Marshall and Bacon, 1981).

The use of a variety of speech stimuli to assess directly both the loss of hearing sensitivity for speech and discrimination of speech has come to be a fundamental part of a comprehensive audiologic evaluation. It has been repeatedly demonstrated that a strong relationship exists between certain puretone thresholds and the intensity necessary for speech understanding (Hughson and Thompson, 1942; Carhart, 1946a; Fletcher, 1950; Harris et al, 1956; Sieganthaler and Strand, 1964). An average for puretones in the speech frequencies (500, 1000, and 2000 Hz) is a relatively simple number to compute but it is restricted in its clinical use. Obviously, limitations in receptive speech understanding can only be reliably demonstrated using speech stimuli.

SPEECH THRESHOLDS

As in the case of puretones, one can determine a level representing the threshold for speech. There are well-established relationships that exist with respect to the intensity of the speech signal and a listener's ability to understand speech. It is important that the clinician be familiar with these relationships as a thorough understanding will prove clinically invaluable. The two most important factors are (a) that speech can be detected at intensity levels lower than that necessary for understanding and (b) the degree of understanding is related to the signal intensity and varies with respect to the type of speech signal (i.e., monosyllabic or polysyllabic words, sentences, etc.). The lowest hearing level at which speech can be detected is referred to as the speech detection threshold (SDT) or speech awareness threshold (SAT). Recognition or understanding of the speech stimuli does not occur until about 8 or 9 dB above the level of detection (Chaiklin, 1959). Hughson and Thompson (1942) first reported this correlation between certain puretone thresholds and speech understanding and labeled it the speech reception threshold. It is the purpose of this chapter to (a) provide information concerning the development of materials for assessing reception and understanding of speech; (b) describe some of the materials and tests currently in use; (c) discuss physical, linguistic, and test administration variables that may affect performance; and (d) discuss clinical applications and some commonly encountered modifications used with these tests.

In a basic audiologic evaluation, two tests using speech signals are routinely administered. The first is a threshold measure for speech understanding. Any of several speech materials may be used for this measure but two syllable words with a spondaic stress pattern are most commonly used. This is referred to as the speech reception threshold although sometimes labeled spondee threshold to denote the stimuli used. It is the intensity level at which the listener can repeat (or otherwise indicate recognition) 50% of the material presented. The other speech test is a suprathreshold measure that uses monosyllabic words to determine the listener's ability to understand speech under ideal listening conditions. Although there is not unanimous agreement, the score derived from this test is most frequently referred to as the speech discrimination or word recognition score.

The term speech reception threshold (SRT) will be used throughout this chapter when referring to measures of sensitivity for speech. With respect to speech understanding, many different terms have been used to describe an individual's comprehension of speech stimuli including articulation, intelligibility, discrimination, understanding, identification, perception, and recognition. Currently, speech intelligibility is generally used when referring to the reproduction of speech through a transmission system (e.g., a telephone) although speech discrimination is commonly used audiologically when referring to the clinical assessment of an individual's ability to understand speech (Owens and Schubert, 1968; Schubert and Owens, 1971). Although the term "speech recognition" has become more popular in recent years, "speech discrimination," which is the most common term, will be used here when referring to the clinical assessment of speech understanding.

HISTORY

Evaluation of speech understanding was carried out long before the advent of reception and discrimination tests and electronic audiometers. Informal testing of speech understanding was simply a matter of speaking to the person and making judgments about his ability to understand. By varying the level of the voice, whispering or increasing the distance between the talker and the listener, a skilled observer might obtain a general estimate of a person's speech understanding. Such a procedure provides valuable but limited information because there is inadequate control of signal parameters and quantification of responses is lacking.

Bryant (1904) recognized the difficulties inherent in testing speech understanding. The invention of the phonograph in 1877 by Edison made recorded presentation of materials possible and Bryant used this as part of a device he referred to as a phonographic acoumeter. This consisted of an Edison phonograph in a "sound-proof" box. Rubber tubing was led through the box wall to a valve that was used to regulate the sound presented to the listener, either monaurally or binaurally. Bryant's efforts are noteworthy as one of the earliest attempts to exercise control over the test stimuli. Before discussing the development of speech threshold and speech discrimination tests, it is necessary to recognize the relationship that exists between understanding and intensity. (Figure 10.1 illustrates this relationship.) Most early tests of speech understanding were used to evaluate communication transmission systems and were referred to as articulation tests. The values derived from the use of these tests were called articulation scores. By plotting a graph with percentage of correct responses on the ordinate and presentation level (intensity) on the abscissa, an articulation-gain function can be generated. Such a graph depicts the relationship of understanding to changes in intensity. Unquestionably, the relationship is a strong one. As intensity increases, the articulation score increases (Licklider and Miller, 1951). The steepness of the articulation-gain function will vary depending on the particular stimulus material used (Fletcher and Steinberg, 1930; Hudgins et al., 1947; Miller et al., 1951; Hirsh et al., 1952; Traul and Black, 1965).

In its contemporary usage, the term "articulation" has come to have a different meaning for most professionals in speech-language pathology and audiology. The relationship of understanding to changes in intensity is now more commonly referred to as a performance-intensity (PI) function (Speaks et al., 1966). Regardless of the

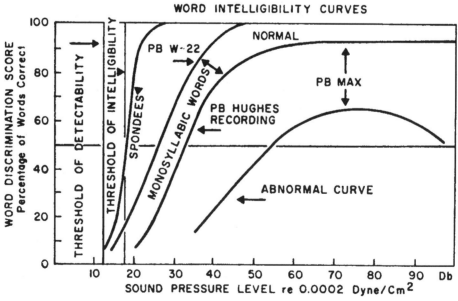

Figure 10.1. Articulation functions for the Rush Hughes, W-22, and spondee tests. Also shown is the articulation function as obtained for some pathological ears. Note that the curve passes through a maximum and the declines with increased intensity. The thresholds of detectability and intelligibility for spondaic words are indicated. (Modified from Davis and Silverman (1960) by Goetzinger CP, 1972. Word discrimination testing, In J. Katz, ed. Handbook of Clinical Audiology, Baltimore: Williams & Wilkins.)

nomenclature, a thorough knowledge of the PI functions of a broad variety of speech materials is essential for a proper understanding of speech audiometry.

SPEECH THRESHOLD MATERIALS

The first recorded auditory test was developed to determine an individual's threshold level for speech. This test was the Western Electric 4A developed at Bell Telephone Laboratories (BTL) by Fletcher (1929). Pairs of recorded digits served as the stimuli with 3 dB of attenuation from one pair to the next. The Western Electric 4A was subsequently revised and became the Western Electric 4C. It was used to screen hearing in the public schools and was the first widely accepted recorded auditory test. In this role, it set the stage for the development and acceptance of other recorded auditory speech tests.

Materials for establishing the SRT were developed at Harvard Psycho-Acoustic Laboratories (PAL) by Hudgins et al. (1947). Sentences were used by Hughson and Thompson (1942) but Hudgins and his coworkers, after studying the available speech materials, selected spondaic words (spondees) as the stimuli. Spondees are two syllable words with approximately equal stress on each syllable. The items selected had to meet four criteria: (a) familiarity; (b) phonetic dissimilarity; (c) normal sampling of English speech sounds; and (d) homogeneity with respect to audibility. Satisfying the last criterion is crucial because it ensures that the understanding for the group of words will increase rapidly with small changes in intensity. This increases the precision of the test because variability will be reduced and listener fatigue will be avoided because fewer items will be needed to establish threshold. It is readily apparent from Figure 10.1 that the articulation function for spondees is very steep. There is approximately a 10% increase in correct identification for each 1 dB change in intensity throughout the range from 20 to 80%. A total of 84 spondees was selected by Hudgins et al and divided into two lists of 42 words each. Both lists were used in PAL test recordings numbers 9 and 14. PAL number 9 consisted of six different scramblings of each list recorded with 4 dB of automatic attenuation after every group of six words. PAL number 14 used the same spondees but all of the stimulus items were recorded at the same intensity level. Hirsh et al. (1952) modified the original PAL spondaic word list by eliminating items that were considered too easy or too difficult. This reduced the number of spondees to 36. Additional modifications were made with respect to recording intensity. The more easily identified words were decreased in intensity by 2 dB and those considered more difficult were increased 2 dB on the final recordings. A carrier phrase "Say the word..." was recorded at a level 10 dB greater than the spondaic word that followed. This became Central Institute for the Deaf (CID) Auditory Tests W-1 in which spondees are recorded at a constant level. There is a 1000 Hz calibration tone recorded at the same level as the carrier phrase making it necessary to subtract 10 dB from the hearing level dial before recording the SRT. CID Auditory Test W-2 contains built in attenuation. The spondees are recorded in groups of three with each successive group 3 dB less intense than the preceding group. CID W-1 has been widely accepted and commonly used; W-2 is used infrequently.

Speech Reception Threshold Testing

Spondaic words are the most commonly used stimuli for establishing the SRT. These may be presented from records or tape recordings but it is more common for clinicians to use monitored live voice (MLV). Presentation by MLV offers greater flexibility and requires less test time to obtain the SRT. This is of particular importance when dealing with children with short attention spans and individuals who have limited vocabularies or have difficulty responding to recorded materials. The clinician should keep in mind that the SRT is also a discrimination task but one which is very simple due to the nature of the test. The listener should be given clear, concise instructions regarding what to be listening for and the required responses. This may be done face to face before placement of the headphones or through the microphone circuit. It is recommended that the better ear be tested first. In the event that masking will be necessary when testing the poorer ear, this permits some familiarity with the procedure and will often avoid confusion. Masking is necessary during SRT testing following the same general rules as in puretone air conduction testing (see Chapter 8). Usually a difference of 45 dB or more between the SRT in the test ear and bone conduction average for the speech frequencies in the nontest ear is considered great enough to require masking. Speech noise or white noise may be used to mask the nontest ear. Responses are usually verbal and monitored via a microphone or talkback circuit.

Clinically, determination of the SRT is not normally done in the presence of competing noise. However, recent research by Middelweerd et al. (1990) suggests that such a procedure may have clinical use with normally hearing patients who complain of difficulty hearing in noise.

Descending and Ascending Methods

In the descending method, the initial presentation is at a hearing level judged to be adequate for understanding. This can be estimated based on the three frequency speech average (Carhart, 1971) or the average of the two best of the three frequencies (Fletcher, 1950) when there is a sharply sloping audiometric contour involving the middle frequencies. A reasonable starting level is 25 dB above the speech average. If this information is not available, an initial presentation at 25 dB above the threshold at 1000 Hz may be used. In situations where that is unknown, a general idea of an initial presentation level may usually be determined based on the patient's responses to spoken conversation. If a patient does not attempt a response at 25 dB above the speech frequency average, the examiner should be alert to the possibility of nonorganic dysfunction. This is discussed in greater detail in Chapter 36. After the initial presentation, intensity can be reduced in relatively large steps (e.g., 10 dB) due to the steepness of the PI function. When threshold is approached, intensity steps are made smaller and more items are presented at each level. Although 2 dB steps are still advocated by some, 5 dB decrements are more commonly used. The differences in threshold between 2 and 5 dB steps are negligible (Chaiklin, 1959; Chaiklin and Ventry, 1964; Tillman and Olsen, 1973). The Committee on Audiometric Guidelines of the American Speech-Language-Hearing Association recommends a descending approach and provides detailed instructions regarding their recommended test procedure (ASHA, 1988). The SRT is the point at which the listener can respond correctly 50% of the time. In actual practice, there will be occasions when all items are correct at a particular presentation level and no items are correct at the next lower level. The true SRT lies somewhere between those two values. Assuming that intensity decrements are no greater than 5 dB, the higher value is accepted.

For the ascending method the initial presentation is at the lowest level of the audiometer and intensity is increased, usually in 10 dB steps, until a response is obtained. Intensity is then decreased to 15 dB below the level of the first correct response and two or three test items are presented in 5-dB increments. Additional ascending series are completed following this procedure and the threshold is defined as the lowest level at which at least half of the items are identified. A minimum of two ascending series is required. This method takes more time than the descending approach and experience has shown it to be more difficult for some listeners. It should be noted that in general the differences in SRT using ascending and descending methods are minimal. However, comparison of SRTs using both an ascending and a descending approach is recommended for medicolegal evaluations. A difference of 6 dB or greater between these methodologies should be considered suspicious. When differences of more than 6 dB are present, additional is needed to resolve this disparity. Many different methods exist for establishing a reliable SRT and it is not the intent of this chapter to advocate a par-

ticular methodology. It is strongly recommended that a systematic procedure be adopted that is comfortable for the examiner and capable of providing adequate controls for establishing the SRT in a reliable fashion.

Modifications of SRT Procedures

Basically, modifications in the usual SRT procedure may be necessary when any factor is present that prevents an understanding of the test procedure, affects the reception of the test stimuli or precludes the use of the usual verbal response. Frequently, adaptations in both presentation and response modality will be necessary. The astute clinician will anticipate the need for deviations from the usual test procedure and be prepared to make the necessary modifications.

The simplest variation in procedure usually involves the required response. Pointing to the printed word, pictorial representation or the object represented by the stimulus word offers viable alternatives to verbal responses. Response modifications are frequently necessary with stroke and cerebral palsy patients, laryngectomees, shy children, and in cases of severe articulation or stuttering problems.

Vocabulary limitations may make it necessary to restrict the items used during testing or to use stimuli other than spondees. With young children it is often possible to obtain an SRT using pictures or objects representing items within their vocabulary (see Chapter 30). In such instances, both receptive and expressive vocabulary are limited and modifications must be made for both the stimulus and the response. Having the child point to the picture or pick up the stimulus item is generally a practical alternative. Frequently children will be encountered who have adequate vocabulary but are shy or unwilling to talk during the evaluation. Consistent responses of pointing to pictures of the test items provide information equivalent to verbal responses. If linguistic skills do not permit the use of spondees or common items in the environment, often the child will be able to identify a number of body parts and those can be easily incorporated into the test as a game of "Show me_____".

With multiply handicapped persons and particularly those with mental, motor, and linguistic involvement, gross modifications from the usual procedure will be necessary. There will be times when an SRT cannot be established but important information might be gained by determining the SAT or SDT and whether *localization* of the signals was demonstrated. These responses coupled with case history, immittance, observations, and objective measures such as auditory evoked responses can provide useful information regarding auditory sensory input.

SPEECH DISCRIMINATION/RECOGNITION

Although there are currently numerous tests and a wide variety of materials available for assessing speech recognition, this has not always been the case. Historically, the first tests of speech recognition were neither developed nor used for assessing an individual's understanding of speech. The impetus for the development of such tests was the evaluation of communications systems, particularly the evaluation of telephone circuits. The development of clinical tests of speech understanding was a logical by-product of this research.

Speech Discrimination Materials

The earliest well controlled work concerning the measurement of speech intelligibility appears to be that of Campbell (1910). He used 10 lists of 100 common monosyllables using 20 common consonants followed by the vowel /i/. The purpose was to assess consonant intelligibility over the telephone. He compared telephonic intelligibility to open air transmission with the talker and listener in a quiet room. The percentage of consonants correctly identified was used to rate the effectiveness of the system. Crandall (1917), following the precedent of Campbell, used consonant-vowel (CV) and vowel-consonant (VC) syllables for the same purpose. The test materials were constructed to approximate the frequency of use in everyday written materials. Fletcher (1922) described a similar method used at BTL. These were lists comprised of 8700 syllables divided into groups of 50 items. Each group was composed of an equal number of the basic vowel and consonant sounds. These lists were known as the Standard Articulation Lists. The development of modern speech intelligibility tests is associated with the work of Fletcher and Steinberg (1930) at BTL. It was their assertion that the stimulus lists must be representative of speech and must be suitable for producing tests. They revised the Standard Articulation Lists and developed what was referred to as the New Standard Articulation Lists in which only consonant-vowel-consonant (CVC) syllables were used. Each sound was represented with approximately equal frequency on these lists rather than with the approximate frequency of occurrence in the language. It is also of interest to note that the CVC syllables were not spoken in isolation but were preceded by an introductory sentence. Identification of syllables was reportedly higher using an introductory sentence and this methodology was also believed to more closely approximate connected speech. In addition to the syllable articulation lists, Fletcher and Steinberg (1930) devised sentence intelligibility lists using interrogative and imperative sentences. Because their function was to test the listener's speech understanding

ability and not his intelligence, each sentence was designed to convey a single idea. Five lists of 50 items were compiled. A response was considered correct if the listener could either repeat the sentence or answer it correctly. Interestingly, the precedent of using 50 items per list has apparently been well received as virtually all subsequent tests of speech discrimination have used 50 items.

Description of Various Speech Discrimination Tests

PAL PB-50 Word Lists

A series of lists was devised at Harvard PAL and underwent numerous revisions. These were the revised monosyllabic (RM) word lists (Egan, 1948). From a core vocabulary of 1200 words, 24 lists of 50 words each were produced. Phonetic balance, the appearance of a sound in the list with respect to its proportion of occurrence in everyday speech, was confined to the first part of the word. These lists were considered reasonably satisfactory, but were revised to be more phonetically balanced (PB). As a result of this work at PAL the well known phonetically balanced (PB) word lists were created. The PB lists were devised to meet the following criteria: monosyllabic words, equal average difficulty, range of difficulty and phonetic composition for each list, as well as representative of English speech, using words in common usage. Egan reported that the spread of difficulty was approximately the same from list to list and that nearly the same average difficulty was present in each list. The criterion of monosyllabic structure was obviously one of the easiest to satisfy although phonetic balance presented certain difficulties. The phonetic composition of the lists was based on data reported by Dewey (1923) of the speech sounds in a sample of 100,000 words. Certain compromises were necessary, and therefore the phonetic balance of the lists was not exact. To meet the criterion of familiarity, unfamiliar or rarely used words were excluded from consideration. The remaining vocabulary was submitted to a panel of 23 judges for rating of familiarity. A rating of "familiar" was given a score of 1, "somewhat familiar" a 2, and "quite unfamiliar" a 3. Any word receiving a total rating equal to or exceeding 35 was considered to be too unfamiliar and was excluded as a test item. Recordings were made of eight of the PAL PB-50 lists (lists 5 to 12) at Central Institute for the Deaf (CID) in St. Louis, MO (Davis et al., 1949). These recordings were produced with the objective of obtaining standardized results because it was recognized that different talkers do not say words in exactly the same manner and a single talker produces different acoustic patterns repeating the same word (Eldert and Davis, 1951). The talker on these recordings is Rush Hughes.

CID W-22

Eldert and Davis (1951) reported on the clinical use of the PAL PB-50 recordings and indicated a number of problems with them. Chief among these were low reliability, a wide range of difficulty among individual test items and uneven distribution of difficulty among the eight recorded lists. Hirsh et al. (1952) also reported some clinical deficiencies in the PAL PB-50 lists. Specifically, the vocabulary was too unfamiliar for many patients, and the recordings were not suitably standardized. Even the articulation of the talker on these recordings has been criticized, noting that he "...clips his words so badly that some sounds are entirely missing by physical analysis..." (Davis and Silverman, 1978). Work was initiated at CID to overcome these weaknesses. The vocabulary of the PAL PB-50 lists was modified to include words meeting certain criteria of familiarity. An additional improvement resulted from the use of magnetic recording tape. By using tape recordings, a particular word had to be spoken only one time and could then be dubbed to any list as desired. This made possible the presentation of words with identical acoustical properties on each list. The modified PB lists became CID Auditory Test W-22. The criteria for the vocabulary of the revised lists were that all words be of one syllable, that none appear on more than one list, that all words be familiar, and that the phonetic composition of each list be representative of English. The vocabulary consisted of 120 words selected from the original 1000 words of the PAL PB-50 lists and 80 additional words. The entire 200 word vocabulary was rated by five judges for familiarity, and only one word was rated as being very unfamiliar. Of the 200 words, all except *ace* appear on the Thorndike list (1932), and 190 are among the 4000 most common English words according to Thorndike. Furthermore, 128 were among the 2000 most familiar, and each of these is on Dewey's (1923) list.

The requirement of phonetic balance was the most difficult to meet because no definitive study of spoken English existed. Hirsh et al. (1952), relied on Dewey's report of frequently occurring words in print and the report of French et al. (1930) of the most frequently occurring sounds in telephone conversations. The necessity of phonetic balance has been questioned, and there is no agreement on this point. Tobias (1964) indicated that phonetic balance is an interesting but unnecessary component. Carhart (1965) stated that "In general, as long as the test items are meaningful monosyllables for the patient and their phonetic distribution is appropriately diversified, one 50-word compilation is relatively equivalent to another." The final compilation of four lists of 50 words was tape recorded with the carrier phrase "You will say_____" preceding each word. The talker on these recordings is Ira Hirsh. The lists are numbered as 1, 2, 3, and 4, and the six scramblings of each list appear as the letters A through F. Subsequent research and clinical use demonstrated that the CID W-22 test was easier than the PAL PB-50 recordings. Clinical studies have verified that the W-22 recordings are rather easy, even for many individuals with sensory-neural hearing impairment (Silverman and Hirsh, 1955; Carhart, 1965; Linden, 1965; Geffner and Donovan, 1974). Additional criticisms were voiced by Campbell (1965) who used subjects with sensory-neural or mixed hearing impairments and concluded that the recordings of CID W-22 are not all equivalent with respect to word difficulty. He presented reconstructed lists that were purported to have greater homogeneity. However, Elpern (1960) and Ross and Huntington (1962) studied the equivalency of the W-22 recordings and concluded that the differences among lists are minimal and insignificant clinically. The broad acceptance of these lists by audiologists has been substantiated by surveys regarding their use in clinical practice (Martin and Pennington, 1971; Martin and Forbis, 1978).

Northwestern University Auditory Tests Numbers 4 and 6

The lack of phonetic balance of the PAL PB-50 list was the impetus for Lehiste and Peterson's (1959) development of a new monosyllabic word test for assessing speech discrimination. They pointed out that true phonetically balanced lists are not possible because a particular speech sound will vary depending on the sounds that precede and follow it. Rather than phonetic balance, they advanced the concept of "perceptual phonetics" or "phonemics" and strove to develop phonemically balanced lists. The materials used by Lehiste and Peterson (1959) were all of the consonant-vowel-consonant variety and were referred to as CNC words because they identified the vowel as the "syllable nucleus" in a word. Their CNC words were drawn from the Thorndike and Lorge (1944) lists and included all CNC words appearing at least once per million words. This provided a pool of 1263 CNC monosyllables. Phonemic balance was based on the composition of these words rather than on English as a whole.

Lehiste and Peterson (1959) constructed 10 lists of 50 words that conformed closely to the phonemic balance of the entire group of monosyllables. Later, these initial lists were revised in an effort to eliminate unfamiliar words (Peterson and Lehiste, 1962). Tillman et al. (1963) used 95 of the words from the original CNC list and added 5 additional words in developing two new 50-item lists. These were recorded and designated as Northwestern University Auditory Test number 4 (NU-4). Subsequently, Tillman and Carhart (1966) expanded this to four 50-item lists with 185 of the CNC words drawn from the parent list of 1263 words and 15 coming from other sources. These lists became Northwestern University Auditory Test number 6 (NU-6). Recordings of these lists by both male and female talkers are commercially available, and these materials currently enjoy relatively broad research and clinical applications.

Rhyme Tests

Not all discrimination tests are of the open set response type. Closed set discrimination tests have also been developed. The first of these was by Black (1957) who used a multiple choice format. Fairbanks (1958) used lists of rhyming monosyllabic words in his 50-item rhyme test. The listener's task was to identify the initial consonant and write it on the response form. Modifications of Fairbanks' rhyme test were made by House et al. (1965) and became known as the Modified Rhyme Test (MRT). Kreul et al. (1968) altered the MRT to make it more clinically useful. Adaptations were made in the areas of timing consistency, carrier phrase, test instructions, and forms used, with both male and female talkers. Further refinement of the MRT was reported by Griffiths (1967) who added new items to obtain response foils consisting of what he called "minimal rhyming contrasts." Schultz and Schubert (1969) used the monosyllables from CID W-22 to develop their Multiple Choice Discrimination Test (MCDT). McPherson and Pang-Ching (1979) reported on the development of a Distinctive Feature Discrimination test (DFDT) using items from the MRT. Their test uses a closed set scoring procedure with four foils per item. Each item is scored on the basis of whether it is one, two, or three features removed from the stimulus word. The authors indicate that the DFDT may provide more diagnostic information than conventional speech discrimination tests. Each of these tests requires identification of consonants in some form. Assessment of hearing-impaired individuals' vowel confusions has revealed very few items with sufficient difficulty for test purposes (Owens et al., 1971).

California Consonant Test (CCT)

Owens and Schubert (1977) reported on the development of the CCT. This is a closed set response discrimination test using 100 CVC items. The items selected for inclusion were based on the phoneme recognition errors of hearing-impaired subjects (Owens and Schubert, 1968; Owens et al., 1971; Sher and Owens, 1974). Each test item consists of four words, (the stimulus word and three foils,) which differ only in either the initial or final consonant position. The test has been shown to be sensitive to phoneme recognition errors that are prevalent in listeners with high frequency, sensory-neural hearing impairment (Schwartz and Surr, 1979). Error analysis of the CCT has resulted in the criticism that the CCT has

an imbalanced distribution of consonants for everyday speech with respect to manner of articulation (Townsend and Schwartz, 1981). It was believed that this might result in errors in estimation of word recognition ability for some listeners and possibly preclude the use of the CCT to predict listener difficulty for conversational speech.

Tape recorded versions of various monosyllabic word tests using different speakers are available from Auditec of St. Louis, 156 W. Argonne, Suite 2E, St. Louis, MO 63122.

Children's Materials

Various materials have been devised specifically for use with young children. Some of these are commercially available in recorded form, and normative data are provided. Other tests consist simply of printed lists which may be administered by monitored live voice or by self-recorded presentations. The available stimuli consist of monosyllabic words (Haskins, 1949; Sieganthaler and Haspiel, 1966; Ross and Lerman, 1970; Goldman et al., 1970; Katz and Elliott, 1978), sentences (Weber and Redell, 1976; Jerger et al., 1980), numbers (Erber, 1980), and environmental sounds (Finitzo-Hieber et al., 1980). Both open (no options given) and closed set (forced choice) response formats are used, and the response mode may be verbal or psychomotor (pointing). The materials are applicable to a wide age range, and the selection of which test or tests to use depends to a large degree on the linguistic sophistication of the patient. In general, with increased language development, there is a wider variety of applicable materials. A factor that must be considered when selecting materials for children is whether the patient has intelligible speech because its presence will permit the use of an open set response format and allow for more precise assessment. A more detailed discussion of the use of speech discrimination tests with children and some common adaptations and modifications is presented later in this chapter. The most popular materials currently used with children appear to be Haskins' (1949) 50-item phonetically balanced kindergarten word lists (PBK-50) and Ross and Lerman's (1970) Word Intelligibility by Picture Identification Test (WIPI). The WIPI uses a closed set response mode (pointing) and is of greatest use with 4- and 5-year old children. It consists of 25 sets of colored pictures. Each set of six pictures consists of four that rhyme and two others used as foils to decrease elevated scores due to guessing.

Sentence Tests

Speech discrimination ability may be assessed using sentence materials as well as monosyllabic words. Fletcher and Steinberg (1930) devised sentence intelligibility lists at BTL. These consisted of five lists of 50 items following the format of simple interrogative or imperative sentences. Egan (1948) and Hirsh (1952) had two major criticisms of the BTL sentence intelligibility lists. The questions often required specific knowledge of the New York City area and many of the items were inordinately difficult and beyond the abilities of many people to answer correctly. Because of this, they did not prove to be as clinically useful as anticipated (Hirsh, 1952). PAL Auditory Test number 12 (Hudgins et al., 1947), although designed for determining the threshold of speech with sentences, may be adapted to speech recognition testing. It offers the advantages of requiring little specific information, and items can be answered by a one-word response. Most of the items are so easy that a high level of intellectual functioning is not required. A set of everyday sentences was developed at CID (Davis and Silverman, 1978) which consists of 10 sets of 10 sentences with 50 key words contained within each set of sentences. Interrogative, declarative, and imperative sentences are used, and scoring is based on the number of key words identified.

A unique approach to the use of sentence materials was advanced by Speaks and Jerger (1965) with the introduction of their Synthetic Sentence Identification (SSI) test. The test materials are not real sentences in that they do not make sense, but they are in a sentence format. The words used to formulate the synthetic sentences were selected following specific syntactic rules. The SSI uses a closed set format and has gained widespread clinical acceptance (see Chapter 18). Dubno and Dirks (1983) have made suggestions for optimizing reliability on the SSI.

Kalikow et al. (1977) developed an open set response sentence test called the speech perception in noise (SPIN) test. It is comprised of 8 sets of 50 sentences. Half of the sentences contain items with high predictability, and half contain items with low predictability based on contextual, syntactic, and prosodic cues. Scoring is based on correct identification of the key words. The background noise consists of a babble of 12 talkers.

Factors Affecting Speech Discrimination Scores

The factors affecting speech discrimination scores are numerous. First, there are physical factors related to the test stimulus such as level of presentation, frequency composition, distortion, signal to noise ratio, and duration, to mention a few. Second, there are factors that are linguistic in nature. Most prominent among these are articulation and dialect, contextual cues, redundancy, and the familiarity of the words to the listener. Third, there are test administration variables that may produce undesired effects. Included under this heading are manner and rate of presentation, response mode, scoring, stimulus materials used, talker differences, and a host of variables related to the patient including hearing loss, motivation, experience, intelligence, instructions, and cooperation. These examples should serve to remind the reader of the complexity of a seemingly simple task and the need for adequate controls to assure reliable results. With few exceptions, alterations in performance due to these factors reduce the speech discrimination score rather than enhance it. Clearly, it is relatively simple to degrade performance but not to enhance it. Spuriously high scores can also occur. Inflated scores may occur due to procedural errors such as permitting visual cues along with the auditory signal, errors in scoring, or failure to mask the non-test ear.

Presentation Level

The effects of presentation level on understanding of speech can be determined by using the performance-intensity (PI) function method described previously. Figure 10.1, adapted from Davis and Silverman (1960), depicts the PI functions for normal-hearing listeners for spondees, recorded CID W-22 and PAL PB-50 monosyllables as well as an abnormal PI function. It can be seen that the 50% correct identification point occurs at a lower sound pressure level (SPL) for spondees (20 dB SPL) than for recorded CID W-22 monosyllables (27 dB SPL) or recorded PAL PB-50 monosyllables (33 dB SPL). The steepness of the PI functions also varies, showing a greater increase in correct identifications with changes in intensity for spondees as opposed to monosyllables. A third important feature is that with spondees and the CID W-22 monosyllables, 100% correct identification eventually occurs as presentation level is increased, but the Rush Hughes recordings of PAL PB-50 monosyllables peak at a maximum of 92% regardless of presentation level. Scores for any of these materials will remain at maximum levels with subsequent increases in presentation level with normal-hearing persons. With certain pathologic conditions, increases in the presentation level above the level at which the maximum score is obtained (PB Max) result in a marked decrease in speech discrimination. This systematic performance decrement has been termed "rollover" and has been shown to be diagnostically useful (Jerger and Jerger, 1971; Dirks et al., 1977; Bess et al., 1979; Shirinian and Arnst, 1980). Beattie and Zipp (1990a) have reported on the range of intensities yielding PB MAX for hearing-impaired listeners. They recommend that speech recognition scores be obtained at a minimum of two levels. They also reported that maximum scores were more likely to be obtained at the Loudness Discomfort Level rather than at the Most Comfortable Level. Beattie and Zipp (1990b) recommended generating word recognition functions and averaging the scores that fall on the plateau of the function. Their findings for elderly hearing-impaired subjects demonstrated reliability consistent with the binomial theorem using this procedure.

Signal to Noise Ratio and Type of Competing Noise

In general, the intelligibility of speech materials falls along a continuum of difficulty based on the meaningful information in the utterance. The more information there is, the steeper its PI function. Four-syllable words are more intelligible than three-syllable words. Three-syllable words are more intelligible than two-syllable words and so on. Monosyllabic words are more intelligible than nonsense syllables, and sentences are more intelligible than polysyllabic words. The number of sounds in a word, as well as the number of syllables, has been shown to affect intelligibility (Egan, 1948; Miller et al., 1951; Hirsh et al., 1954). A PI function plotted for single-syllable words will become steeper when the same words are heard in sentences (Miller et al., 1951). These same researchers demonstrated that the PI function varies depending on the signal to noise ratio. The variations occurring due to the presence of noise are also influenced by the type of hearing loss. As the signal to noise ratio becomes less favorable, the effects on speech discrimination scores are more pronounced for sensory-neural-impaired subjects than for normally hearing subjects (Olsen and Tillman, 1968). Not only will the signal to noise ratio be a factor, but the type of masking noise used has been shown to affect performance (Lovrinic et al., 1968; Williams and Hecker, 1968; Garstecki and Mulac, 1974). The performance of a single group of subjects was compared on five measures of speech discrimination by Lovrinic et al. (1968). Although the vocabulary for the two CID W-22 lists used in this study has been shown to be very similar with respect to difficulty (Elpern, 1960; Ross and Huntington, 1962), large differences in mean scores were seen for the material presented in the presence of masking noise at a +12 dB signal to noise ratio (speech 12 dB greater than noise). Lovrinic et al. (1968) observed not only markedly poorer performance but almost an absence of "easy" items in the presence of ipsilateral noise (i.e., background of speech babble). Loven and Hawkins (1983) also reported nonequivalency for lists presented in noise.

Findlay (1976) compared the performance of young normal hearing male subjects with that of subjects with noise-induced hearing loss on a number of auditory tasks. Among these were speech discrimination in the presence of speech spectrum noise and "cocktail party" noise (i.e., six-talker babble). Speech discrimination scores were more depressed for the hearing-impaired subjects under both conditions, but a larger separation in performance between the two groups was evident with CID W-22 in the presence of speech babble. The finding of poorer speech discrimination in the presence of competing speech has important clinical implications, particularly with respect to counseling hearing-impaired patients. Primarily, this is related to expected performance in noise either with or without amplification, and the importance of incorporating visual and situational cues to aid in understanding.

Word Familiarity

Various authors have indicated that word familiarity is an important variable in speech discrimination testing (Howse, 1957; Hutton and Weaver, 1959; Owens, 1961; Carhart, 1965; Epstein et al., 1968). There is no doubt that the use of items that are not within the vocabulary of the patient can have a marked effect on performance. This is certainly a critical variable for the clinician to be aware of, for it is the responsibility of the audiologist to select materials that are linguistically appropriate for the patient. The use of a test containing items that are not within the patient's vocabulary can result in spuriously low scores, leading to unnecessary testing, mismanagement, or misdiagnosis.

Closed Set Response

Performance may also be affected by the number of available alternative responses. The use of a closed set response (multiple choice) paradigm is an example of limited alternative response availability and can be expected to yield higher scores than an open set procedure. Consider the hypothetical case of a 50-item printed word or picture identification task consisting of 5 possible choices for each item. There is a one in five probability of correct identification by chance alone on each item. In actual clinical application, a greater probability will exist on some items if one of the foils can be eliminated by the listener. Tests of this nature tend to overestimate speech recognition ability. For this reason, it is important that the particular test used be noted on the patient's record. Closed set response tests such as the MRT, DFDT, MCDT, SSI, and CCT impose other physical (i.e., sensory and motor) and linguistic constraints because each requires adequate visual acuity and at least minimal reading skills, as well as a motoric response of some type. This precludes their use with individuals who do not possess the requisite sensory, motor, or linguistic skills.

Certain tests devised for use with young children, although not requiring reading ability, may not be applicable even in the presence of adequate language due to factors such as poor psychomotor skills or decreased visual acuity. Those that use a closed set response, such as the WIPI, may overestimate speech discrimination. The amount by which any score may be expected to deviate from the true score due to the effects of the closed set is a function of the number of foils per item and their acoustic similarities to the key word. The previous caveat regarding notation on the patient record of the particular test used also applies to children.

Response Mode

The response mode may also adversely affect speech discrimination scores. Write-down responses, for example, tap linguistic skills. Other factors to be considered are legibility of writing, eye-hand coordination, spelling ability, visual acuity, and the available time (written responses generally require more time). With either talkback or written responses, auditor error may affect the scores (Merrell and Atkinson, 1965). Nelson and Chaiklin (1970) found that even experienced examiners could make clinically significant scoring errors. Contributing factors include distortion within the talkback system and patient articulation, but examiner experience and monitoring level were identified as the critical factors contributing to auditor error. Auditory monitoring of patient responses is still widely practiced (Martin and Pennington, 1971; Martin and Forbis, 1978). Written responses have been advocated as a means of eliminating auditor error (Northern and Hattler, 1974). If written responses are not a viable alternative, there are certain steps that may be taken to keep auditor error to a minimum. A good quality monitoring system is essential, and adequate loudness is critical. The target words should be available to the examiner in printed form so that the presentations may be followed visually. The examiner should watch the patient so as to make use of lipreading cues for identification of phonemes such as /f/ and /-/. One should not hesitate to seek clarification from the patient regarding a response when any doubt exists. The patient should be asked to spell the word, use it in a sentence or tell what it means, whichever is appropriate, rather than simply to repeat the word.

Acoustic Frequency Composition

The frequency content of the speech signal is another factor capable of affecting speech discrimination performance. Early research by French and Steinberg (1947) using high and low pass filter conditions demonstrated the importance of the high frequencies for correct identification of CVC syllables. The disparity in scores between high and low pass filtered CVC syllables is illustrated in Figure 10.2. When all frequencies above 1000 Hz were passed, 90% of the syllables were recognized correctly. However, when only the frequencies

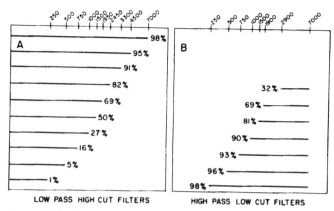

Figure 10.2. Maximum discrimination for syllable articulation for low and high pass filter conditions as related to the cut-off frequecy. The discrimination scores were derived from the curves of French and Steinberg (1947) at an orthotelephonic gain of +10 dB (75 dB SPL). (From Goetzinger CP, 1978. Word discrimination testing. In J. Katz, ed. Handbook of Clinical Audiology, Ed. 2. Baltimore: Williams & Wilkins.)

below 1000 Hz were presented, correct identification of the items declined to 27%. Similar findings were reported by Hirsh et al. (1954) using filtered CID W-22 monosyllables. Clinically, high frequency hearing impairment is a common entity, and speech discrimination scores may suffer due to the combined effects of filtering and distortion. The prominent role of high frequency energy with respect to speech understanding becomes even more conspicuous when one examines the relative phonetic power of individual speech sounds. It is the high frequency consonants that contain the least power, and yet these sounds provide the major contribution to intelligibility (Fletcher, 1953).

Half- Versus Full-List Presentation

In an effort to reduce clinical testing time and to avoid patient fatigue, it has become common practice for many audiologists to use only half of a 50-item speech discrimination list. This procedure has come under the scrutiny of a number of researchers using a variety of subjects. Investigations of half- list testing have been carried out for PAL PB-50 (Resnick, 1962; Shutts et al., 1964; Burke et al., 1965), CID W-22 (Elpern, 1961; Deutsch and Kruger, 1971; Margolis and Millin, 1971; Jirsa et al., 1975; Penrod, 1980; Beattie and Zipp, 1990b), NU-6 (Schumaier and Rintelmann, 1974; Jirsa et al. 1975; Schwartz et al., 1977; Beattie et al., 1978) and PBK-50 (Manning et al., 1975). Presently, no consensus exists regarding the clinical use of half-list testing. Some authors have advocated its use, others have advised against it and some have recommended its use but with certain cautions. Considerable savings of time can be realized with the half-list procedure, but not without risks.

There are two concerns: (a) whether the results are valid and (b) whether they are reliable. If 25 items are given and the speech discrimination score is high (e.g., 92% or better), there is a reasonable expectation that there is no significant artifact adversely affecting performance. In addition, from the standpoint of reliability, there is relatively little concern that the patient will suddenly drop in discrimination on the last 25 items (by chance finding the first items highly intelligible but many errors on the last 25).

If there is an artifact due to deficiency in the talkback system or the materials are inappropriate for the patient, then it is not likely that 25 more items will solve the problem. In addition, from the standpoint of reliability, scores at the very highest and lowest ends are least vulnerable when administering a half-list. Thornton and Raffin (1978) point out the tradeoff between measurement error and sample size. This is illustrated in Figure 10.3. As sample size is reduced, variability in scores increases, and the farther the score is from 100 or 0%, the less confidence one can have in the specific value. Thornton and Raffin (1978) have provided confidence intervals and expected ranges of scores based on evaluation of more than 4000 patients with CID W-22. For example, a patient who obtains a score of 92% may vary between 78 and 98% on a 50-item list and still be within expected variation (95% confidence interval). However, the expected range of variation for a 25-item list is even greater at 72 to 100%. For the patient with a discrimina-

tion score of 60%, the range of variation for 50 items is from 42 to 72%, and for 25 items it is 36 to 84%. Thus it can be seen that no single criterion value (e.g., 10%) can be specified for test-retest purposes.

Carrier Phrase Versus No Carrier Phrase

Another variable that may affect speech discrimination scores is the use or omission of a carrier phrase. Recall that Fletcher and Steinberg (1930) reported that identification of CVC syllables was higher when using an introductory sentence. Typically, during speech discrimination testing, a carrier phrase precedes the stimulus word. The most commonly used carrier phrases are "Say the word _____," "You will say _____," "Write the word _____" and "Show me _____." However, the use of the carrier phrase in clinical practice may be on the wane (Martin and Forbis, 1978). Martin et al. (1962) found no difference in performance when the carrier was omitted. Other authors have reported the opposite (Gladstone and Sieganthaler, 1971; Gelfand, 1975; Penrod, 1978).

Lynn and Brotman (1981) indicate that the carrier phrase "You will say _____" contains perceptual cues that may assist the listener in identifying some initial sounds of test words. McLennan and Knox (1975) also studied the effects of omission of the carrier phrase. They compared the performance of normal-hearing and sensory-neural-impaired listeners using a conventional presentation (carrier phrase-examiner controlled rate) and a free operant (FO) procedure in which the subject had control of the stimulus presentation and therefore was free to respond at his own rate. With this method the authors point out that standardization of presentation can be maintained using a full 50-item recorded list, but a savings in time can be realized due to the free operant procedure. The scores obtained by normal-hearing as well as sensory-neural-impaired listeners were unaffected by the omission of the carrier phrase using the FO procedure. In addition, there was a marked preference for the FO procedure by the subjects.

Lynn (1962) reported a modification of the usual discrimination test procedure that was designed to save time but still use the complete 50-item list. He referred to this as the "paired PB-50 discrimination test." The test items are presented in a paired format using a single carrier phrase (e.g., Say the words your-bin). Although it is true that the use of the entire list is maintained, this procedure introduces additional variables that may affect performance and scoring. There are not sufficient data available to recommend adopting this methodology.

Recorded Versus Monitored Live Voice Testing

Speech discrimination tests may be administered not only by means of phonographic or tape-recorded presenta-

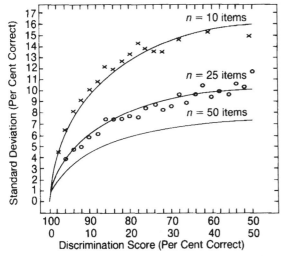

Figure 10.3. Within-subject standard deviations for 10- and 25-word tests grouped by estimated true scores (50 words). **Solid lines** show standard deviations of binominal distributions as a function of *n* (in percentage) for *n* = 10, *n* = 25, and *n* = 50. Measured standard deviations for *n* = 10 and *n* = 25 are shown by **X** and **O**, respectively. (From Thornton AR, and Raffinn MJM. Speech discrimonation scores modeled as a binominal variable. J Speech Hear Res 19788; 21:507–518.)

tions but by monitored live voice (MLV). The use of the latter has been prevalent due to its flexibility, rapidity, and ease of administration. A great deal of information is available, especially with respect to the talker variations (French and Steinberg, 1947; Hirsh et al., 1954; Palmer, 1955; Silverman and Hirsh, 1955; Asher, 1958; Carhart, 1965; Brandy, 1966; Kreul et al., 1969; Tillman and Olsen, 1973; Davis and Silverman, 1978; Penrod, 1979; Gengel and Kupperman, 1980). Carhart (1946a, p 349) indicated that "Phonographic presentation increases the stability of the condition but tends to reduce the flexibility of the technique" but was of the opinion that both procedures had clinical utility. Carhart (1965) also pointed out that test results obtained by different talkers are not readily comparable unless the equivalency of the talkers has been demonstrated. He did believe that valid comparisons could be made based on the results obtained by a single talker, but even the validity of that procedure is questionable. Brandy (1966) demonstrated that a single talker's presentations of the same words will vary at different times. Kreul et al. (1969) investigated a number of variables affecting the reliability of speech discrimination scores. One of the variables studied was the effects of different talkers. They reported that the scores for repeat testing for either of two talkers on different occasions were not significantly different. Their findings are not in agreement with those of Brandy (1966), but major procedural differences exist in the two studies. The recordings of Kreul et al. (1969) were carefully monitored, and intensity and articulation of the talker were closely controlled. The "live voice" presentations in the Brandy study underwent no acoustical corrections for intensity. Probably of greater importance is the fact that Kreul et al. (1969) used the MRT, a closed set response test, whereas Brandy used 25 selected monosyllables from list 3 of CID W-22. Tillman and Olsen (1973) have commented on the absence of a standardized test for speech discrimination, denoting that such a test is not possible unless recordings are used. Northern and Hattler (1974) have also called for a standardized recorded test or tests and specified that the answer does not lie in the development of new tests but with tests that are currently available.

Penrod (1979) investigated talker effects with CID W-22 and subjects with varying degrees of sensory-neural hearing impairment. Recordings were made of four talkers' clinical presentations that were then presented, unaltered, to listeners in randomized order. Although the mean scores obtained by the listeners for the four talkers were not significantly different statistically, there were excessive variations in scores for individual listeners when compared to the confidence intervals of Thornton and Raffin (1978). The distinction of individual as opposed to group variation is an important one, for it is after all, individual scores that are of concern clinically.

The primary factor responsible for the variations in scores was identified as talker-listener interaction. It was also determined that there is a greater probability of excessive variation in individuals with poor speech discrimination ability. Similar findings of increased variability for subjects whose scores fall within the middle range (30-70%) have also been reported by Beattie et al. (1978) and Thornton and Raffin (1978). The increase in variation in scores with regard to decreased speech discrimination ability should be duly noted because of the implications with respect to determining significant variations in patient scores. It is reiterated here that a single number criterion for significant variation is inadequate. One must be aware of the expected variation for the area of the range of measurement in which the patient falls and the number of items employed for testing.

Clinical Applications

Historically, speech discrimination testing has been used to (a) assist in the determination of the site of peripheral lesion, (b) evaluate social adequacy and effectiveness of communication, (c) determine candidacy for surgery, (d) plan and evaluate aural rehabilitation programs, (e) evaluate hearing aid candidacy and select appropriate amplification, and (f) to assess central auditory function. There are marked differences in the degree to which it has been successful in each of these areas. Before discussing the clinical applications of speech discrimination tests, it should be emphasized that decisions are not made solely on the basis of performance on tests of speech discrimination. Rather, speech discrimination test results constitute only one of many factors that are considered in the decision-making process. Some illustrative cases of the uses of speech discrimination testing may be seen in Figure 10.4.

Determination of Site of Lesion

The diagnostic value of speech discrimination testing alone for determination of site of lesion is limited, particularly if discrimination is assessed at only a single level. The primary factors limiting its usefulness are the wide range of variation in scores seen for a particular etiology and the tremendous overlap in scores associated with different pathologies. Factors contributing to overlap in scores include degree of loss, audiometric contour, or the so-called "shape" of the loss (Bess and Townsend, 1977), upward spread of masking (Jerger et al., 1960); Martin and Pickett, 1970; Danaher and Pickett, 1975) and the true speech recognition ability of the patient (Beattie et al., 1978; Thornton and Raffin, 1978; Penrod, 1979). The variation in scores associated with a single etiology is clearly evident in a report by Johnson (1968) regarding patients with confirmed acoustic neuromas. Speech dis-

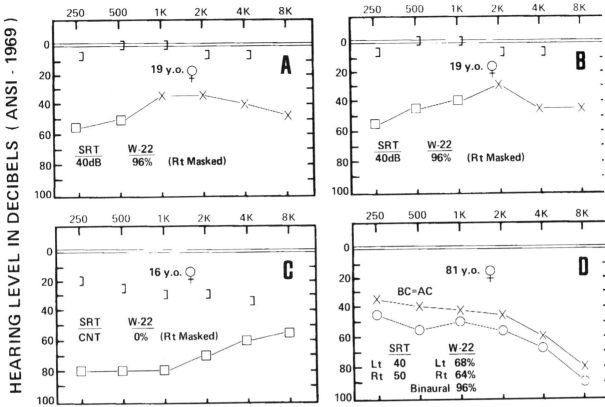

Figure 10.4. A Preoperative audiogram of a 19-year-old girl with a cholesteatoma that, at surgery, was found to have invaded the mastoid area and eustachian tube. Speech discriminationn was 96%. **B,** Postsurgically (radical mastoidectomy) there was no improvement in hearing thresholds and speech discrimination remained unchanged. A hearing aid was subsequently fitted with excellent results. **C,** Contrast this with a 16-year-old with a congenital mixed hearing loss. The lack of any measurable speech discrimination contraindicated surgical attempts to close the air-bone gap as well as amplification on that ear. **A,** CROS (contralateral routing of signals) hearing aid was recommended. **D,** This case illustrates substantial improvement in speech understanding with bilateral stimulation, suggesting maximum benefit from binaural amplification.

crimination scores ranged from 0 to 100%. The value of speech discrimination tests in differentiating cochlear from retrocochlear losses is strengthened somewhat if scores of 30% or less are accepted as an indicator of retrocochlear site of lesion. Although the finding of extremely reduced speech discrimination is a strong indicator of retrocochlear involvement it is not confirmatory. Neither do scores falling well above this level preclude a retrocochlear site of lesion.

The clinical use of speech discrimination tests in differentiating cochlear from retrocochlear lesions is enhanced by the use of a complete performance-intensity function using monosyllabic words (Jerger and Jerger, 1971; Dirks et al., 1977; Bess et al., 1979). This is discussed further in Chapter 12. For the use of speech tests with suspected pseudohypacusic patients see Chapter 36.

Adequacy and Effectiveness of Communication

Speech discrimination tests provide insight into an individual's social adequacy in hearing. However, when considered by themselves, they are by no means perfect indicators of receptive auditory communication ability. In most cases, clinicians may make valid assumptions regarding communication efficiency for those individuals who fall at the extremes of measurement. Presently, there is no way to equate a particular score with a given level of social functioning. A host of other factors contribute to communication performance, including intelligence, motivation, experience, communication set, closure ability, situational cues, expectation, redundancy, and linguistic sophistication, to mention a few. This is not meant to imply that one should not administer speech discrimination tests—quite the contrary. Valuable information is gained regarding the amount of difficulty and the types of errors made under relatively well controlled listening conditions for each ear. When these data are integrated with patient history, observation of communication performance throughout the clinical session and the clinician's knowledge of factors influencing speech understanding, a clearer picture emerges. Even though precise quantification is not possible, qualitative judgments can be made and impressions formed with respect to social adequacy and communication efficiency. Often, the inexperienced clinician relies too heavily on formal test results and virtually ignores valuable information that is readily acquired through interaction with the patient. Total reliance on formal test scores is an approach to be discouraged. Instead, one should rely on all available sources of information and integrate this knowledge to arrive at a decision. Ultimately, it is the audiologist's responsibility to counsel the patient regarding communication needs, and this can be done with confidence only when sufficient information has been acquired.

Determination of Candidacy for Surgery

Qualifying the existence of conductive pathology is a relatively straightforward task given the state of the art in air- and bone-conduction audiometry and impedance measurements. However, there is little to be gained from surgical correction of an air-bone gap to improve communication ability if usable understanding of speech is not present. On the other hand, there will be times when surgery is undertaken in the absence of measurable speech discrimination because of potentially life-threatening conditions. In either instance, it is imperative that the level of speech discrimination ability be documented before surgical intervention.

Postsurgical evaluation using speech recognition tests has also been shown to be a valuable clinical procedure. Significant improvements in speech understanding have been demonstrated after surgical removal of acoustic tumors (Cohen et al.; 1985: Shelton and House, 1990).

Because there is a relatively high probability of cross-hearing when using a suprathreshold test in the presence of a conductive loss or with unilateral sensory-neural losses, the examiner must be certain that the reported score is actually that of the ear under test. Masking must be used in speech discrimination testing to eliminate participation by the non-test ear. If masking is called for but cannot be used, a notation should be made on the audiogram.

Regarding the use of masking during speech discrimination testing, in Martin and Forbis' (1978) survey only 17% of the audiologists responded that they mask when there is a 40-dB difference between SRT/presentation level of the speech discrimination test and the best bone-conduction threshold of the nontest ear, and 10% responded that masking is never used during speech discrimination testing. The rationale for this latter approach is not stated. The 40-dB difference cited here appears overly conservative because, at most, only detection and not understanding of the speech stimulus could be expected. A general rule of thumb is to use masking during speech discrimination testing anytime

there is a difference of 50 dB or greater between the presentation level to the test ear and either the best bone-conduction threshold or the puretone bone-conduction average in the non-test ear.

Planning and Evaluation of Rehabilitation

Speech discrimination tests provide the audiologist specific information regarding the types of errors made as well as a general idea of communication difficulties experienced by the patient. When used to plan aural rehabilitation programs, additional testing is usually carried out, including assessment of communication performance using auditory, visual, and combined auditory-visual input. The selection of appropriate rehabilitative strategies is enhanced by determining to what extent visual cues are used by the patient (Erber, 1971, 1972). The results form the basis not only for counseling the patient regarding the effects of the hearing loss but also provide specific data that are used in the formulation of rehabilitation strategies. Speech discrimination testing alone or in conjunction with visual input (lipreading) is helpful throughout aural rehabilitation efforts as a means of evaluating progress. Giolas (1982) has offered some specific suggestions regarding how speech discrimination testing may be used to provide an indication of how well a patient will respond to auditory training.

Hearing Aid Selection/Evaluation/Fitting

Speech discrimination testing in some form is an integral part of most hearing aid selection procedures (Burney, 1972). This has been the case following Carhart's (1946b) description of an evaluation procedure comparing speech understanding with different hearing aids in quiet and noise. Still, there is far from complete agreement on what method is most efficient or which procedure discriminates best among hearing aids. However, it is clear that the patient's speech discrimination ability is one of the critical factors in determining which ear to fit and the prognosis for successful use of amplification. A variety of speech stimuli have also been used to assess patient performance with the newest type of auditory prosthetic device, the cochlear implant (Eddington, 1980: Dowel, et al.; 1987: Dorman, et al.; 1989).

Chapters 43 and 44 contain information on hearing aid selection/evaluation/dispensing and fitting philosophies. Cochlear implants are discussed in Chapter 46. The use of speech tests for evaluating central auditory function is discussed in Chapters 14 to 18.

Modifications

Testing Adults

Alterations in normal procedure are often necessary with certain adult patients. The need for modification is probably most apparent in patients who possess limited language skills. With these individuals, it is often more appropriate to use tests designed for children because of the reduced linguistic demands. In patients with severely reduced speech discrimination ability, monosyllabic word lists may be abandoned in favor of sentence tests. Although not easily quantifiable, they may actually be more meaningful than a percentage score on a monosyllabic word list. Sentences provide information regarding the patient's use of residual hearing when additional cues from semantic, syntactic, and prosodic features are present. In addition, for patients with extremely reduced speech discrimination ability, it is a far less frustrating procedure. Miller et al. (1951) demonstrated that even with very reduced speech discrimination there may be good ability to follow conversational speech.

Response mode modifications must be considered for patients who do not possess normal speech or who have unintelligible speech, including some retarded individuals, those with severe articulation disorders, stutterers, and laryngectomees. Altering both materials and response paradigms must be considered when testing aphasic patients and the multiply handicapped. Other complications, such as blindness, illiteracy, emotional disturbance, and motoric involvement, place similar limitations on speech discrimination testing, and the clinician must be alert to the need for modifications of test materials or procedures.

Testing Young Children

Speech discrimination testing of young children can be a challenging task. Of critical importance is the selection of materials that are within the receptive vocabulary of the child. Careful thought must also be given to selecting response modes and reinforcement strategies because of difficulties in scoring associated with articulation errors and the frequently encountered taciturn nature and uncooperative attitude some children demonstrate in the test situation.

With children who cannot or will not respond verbally, a psychomotor approach may be used showing either pictures or common objects selected for their interest and suitability to speech discrimination testing. A child can frequently be engaged in conversation or will willingly participate in activity games such as "Simon says..." using simple commands.

A frequent problem encountered with young children is their refusal to accept earphones. One alternative is to use the bone-conduction receiver to deliver the speech signals. This has been shown to be a usable approach with both children and adults (Edgerton et al., 1977; Valente and Stark, 1977; Johnson and Bordenick, 1978; Karlsen and Goetzinger, 1980). Despite the apparent incongruity, children will often accept the placement of the BC oscillator even though adamantly refusing earphones. Of course the procedure suffers from an inability to mask the non-test ear. Specific information regarding the evaluation of infants and young children may be found in Chapter 30.

SUMMARY

This chapter has reviewed the development of speech threshold and discrimination testing in the United States and provided a description of some of the most commonly encountered test materials. Factors that may influence performance on these tests were discussed, and the primary clinical applications were presented. Some frequently encountered procedural modifications were also mentioned.

REFERENCES

American Speech-Language-Hearing Association. Guidelines for determining threshold level for speech. ASHA 1988;30:85–90.

Asher JW. Intelligibility tests: a review of their standardization, some experiments, and a new test. Speech Monogr 1958;25:14–28.

Beattie RC, Svihovec DA, and Edgerton BJ. Comparison of speech detection and spondee thresholds and half- versus full-list intelligibility scores with MLV and taped presentations of NU-6. J Am Aud Soc 1978;3:267–272.

Beattie RC, and Zipp JA. Range of intensities yielding PB MAX and the threshold for monosyllabic words for hearing-impaired subjects. J Speech Hear Disord 1990a;55:417–426.

Beattie RC, and Zipp JA. Reliability of PB MAX for monosyllabic words using the plateau averaging procedure. Aust J Audiol 1990b;12:17–20.

Bess FH, and Townsend TH. Word discrimination for listeners with flat sensorineural hearing losses. J Speech Hear Disord 1977;42:232–237.

Bess FH, Josey AF, and Humes LE. Performance intensity functions in cochlear and eighth nerve disorders. Am J Otol 1979;1:27–31.

Black JW. Multiple choice intelligibility tests. J Speech Hear Disord 1957;22:213–235.

Brandy WT. Reliability of voice tests of speech discrimination. J Speech Hear Res 1966;9:461–465.

Bryant WS. A phonographic acoumeter. Arch Otolaryngol 1904;33:438–443.

Burke KS, Shutts RE, and King WP. Range of difficulty of four Harvard phonetically balanced word lists. Laryngoscope 1965;75:289–296.

Burney PA. A survey on hearing aid evaluation procedures. ASHA 1972;14:439–444.

Campbell GA. Telephonic intelligibility. Philo Mag J Sci 1910;19:152–159.

Campbell RA. Discrimination and word test difficulty. J Speech Hear Res 1965;8:13–22.

Carhart R. Monitored live-voice as a test of auditory acuity. J Acoust Soc Am 1946a;17:338–349.

Carhart R. Problems in the measurement of speech discrimination. Arch Otolaryngol 1946b;44:1–18.

Carhart R. Problems in the measurement of speech discrimination. Arch Otolaryngol 1965;82:253–260.

Carhart R. Observations on relations between thresholds for pure tones and for speech. J Speech Hear Disord 1971;36:476–483.

Chaiklin J. The relation among three selected auditory speech thresholds. J Speech Hear Res 1959;2:237–243.

Chaiklin J, and Ventry IM. Spondee threshold measurement; a comparison of 2- and 5-dB methods. J Speech Hear Disord 1964;2:47–59.

Cohen NL, Ransohoff J, and Jacobs J. Restoration of speech discrimination following suboccipital transmeatal excision of extracanalicular acoustic neuroma. Otolaryngol Head Neck Surg 1985;93: 126–131.

Crandall IB. The composition of speech. Phys Rev 1917;10:74–76.

Danaher EM, and Pickett JM. Some masking effects produced by low frequency vowel formants in persons with sensorineural hearing loss. J Speech Hear Res 1975;18:261–271.

Davis H, and Silverman SR. Hearing and Deafness. New York: Holt, Rinehart and Winston, 1960.

Davis H, and Silverman SR. Hearing and Deafness, 4th Ed. New York: Holt, Rinehart and Winston, 1978.

Davis H, Morrical KC, and Harrison CE. Memorandum on recording characteristics and monitoring of word and sentence tests distributed by Central Institute for the Deaf. J Acoust Soc Am 1949; 21:552–553.

Deutsch LJ, and Kruger B. The systematic selection of 25 monosyllables which predict the CID W-22 speech discrimination score. J Aud Res 1971;11:286–290.

Dewey G. Relative Frequency of English Speech Sounds. Cambridge, MA: Harvard University Press, 1923.

Dirks DD, Kamm C, Bower D, and Betsworth A. Use of performance-intensity functions for diagnosis. J Speech Hear Disord 1977;42: 408–415.

Dorman MF, Hannley M, Dankowsky K, Smith L, and McCandless G. Word recognition by 50 patients fitted with the Symbion multichannel cochlear implant. Ear Hear 1989;10:44–49.

Dowell RC, Seligman BE, Blaney PJ, and Clark GM. Speech perception using a two-formant 22-electrode cochlear prosthesis in quiet and noise. Acta Otolaryngol 1987;104:439–446.

Eddington D. Speech discrimination in deaf subjects with cochlear implants. J Acoust Soc Am 1980;68:885–891.

Edgerton BJ, Danhauer JL, and Beattie RC. Bone conducted speech audiometry in normal subjects. J Acoust Soc Am 1977;3:84–87.

Egan JP. Articulation testing methods. Laryngoscope 1948;58:955–991.

Eldert E, and Davis H. The articulation function of patients with conductive deafness. Laryngoscope 1951;61:896–909.

Elliot LL. Prediction of speech discrimination scores from other test information. J Aud Res 1963;3:35–45.

Elpern BS. Differences in difficulty among the CID W-22 auditory tests. Laryngoscope 1960;70:1560–1565.

Elpern BS. The relative stability of half-list and full-list discrimination tests. Laryngoscope 1961;71:30–36.

Epstein A, Giolas TC, and Owens E. Familiarity and intelligibility of monosyllabic word lists. J Speech Hear Res 1968;11:435–438.

Erber NP. Auditory and audiovisual reception of words in low frequency noise by children with normal hearing and children with impaired hearing. J Speech Hear Res 1971;14:496–512.

Erber NP. Auditory, visual, and auditory-visual recognition of consonants by children with normal and impaired hearing. J Speech Hear Res 1972;15:413–422.

Erber NP. Use of the auditory numbers test to evaluate speech perception abilities of hearing-impaired children. J Speech Hear Disord 1980;45:527–532.

Fairbanks G. Test of phonemic differentiation: the rhyme test. J Acoust Soc Am 1958;30:596–599.

Findlay RC. Auditory dysfunction accompanying noise-induced hearing loss. J Speech Hear Disord 1976;41:374–380.

Finitzo-Hieber T, Gerlin IJ, Matkin ND, and Cherow-Skalka E. A sound effects recognition test for the pediatric evaluation. Ear Hear 1980;1:271–276.

Fletcher H. The nature of speech and its interpretation. J Franklin Inst 1922;193:729–747.

Fletcher H. Speech and Hearing. Princeton, NJ: Van Nostrand, 1929.

Fletcher H. A method of calculating hearing loss for speech from the audiogram. Acta Otolaryngol Suppl 1950;90:26–37.

Fletcher H. Speech and Hearing in Communication. Princeton, NJ: Van Nostrand, 1953.

Fletcher H, and Steinberg JC. Articulation testing methods. J Acoust Soc Am 1930;1:1–97.

French NR, and Steinberg JC. Factors governing the intelligibility of speech sounds. J Acoust Soc Am 1947;19:90–119.

French NR, Carter CW, and Koenig W. The words and sounds of telephone conversations. Bell Sys Tech J 1930;9:290–324.

Garstecki DC, and Mulac A. Effects of test material and competing message on speech discrimination. J Aud Res 1974;3:171-178.

Geffner D, and Donovan N. Intelligibility functions of normal and sensorineural loss subjects on the W-2 lists. J Aud Red 1974;14: 82–86.

Gelfand SA. Use of the carrier phrase in live voice speech discrimination testing. J Aud Res 1975;15:107–110.

Gengel RW, and Kupperman GL. Word discrimination in noise: effect of different speakers. Ear Hear 1980;1:156–160.

Giolas TG. Hearing Handicapped Adults. Englewood Cliffs, NJ: Prentice-Hall, 1982.

Gladstone VS, and Sieganthaler BM. Carrier phrase and speech intelligibility test score. J Aud Res 1971;11:101–103.

Goldman R, Fristoe M, and Woodcock R. Test of Auditory Discrimination. Circle Pines, MN: American Guidance Services, 1970.

Griffiths JD. Rhyming minimal contrasts: a simplified diagnostic articulation test. J Acoust Soc Am 1967;42:236–241.

Harris JD. Puretone acuity and the intelligibility of everyday speech. J Acoust Soc Am 1965;37:824–830.

Harris JD, Haines HL, and Meyers CK. A new formula for using the audiogram to predict speech hearing loss. Arch Otolaryngol 1956;64:447.

Haskins HA. A phonetically balanced test of speech discrimination for children. [Master's thesis], Evanston, IL: Northwestern University, 1949.

Hirsh IJ. The Measurement of Hearing. New York: McGraw-Hill, 1952.

Hirsh IJ, Davis H, Silverman SR, Reynolds EG, Eldert E, and Benson RW. Development of materials for speech audiometry. J Speech Hear Disord 1952;17:321–337.

Hirsh IJ, Reynolds EG, and Joseph M. Intelligibility of different speech materials. J Acoust Soc Am 1954;26:530–538.

House AS, Williams CE, Necker MHL, and Kryter KD. Articulation testing methods. Consonantal differentiation in a closed response set. J Acoust Soc Am 1965;37:158–166.

Howse D. On the relation between the intelligibility and frequency of occurrence of English words. J Acoust Soc Am 1957;29: 296–305.

Hudgins CV, Hawkins JE, Karlin JE and Stevens SS. The development of recorded auditory tests for measuring hearing loss for speech. Laryngoscope 1947;57:52–89.

Hughson W, and Thompson E. Correlation of hearing acuity for speech with discrete frequency audiograms. Arch Otolaryngol 1942;36:526–540.

Hutton C, and Weaver SJ. PB intelligibility and familiarity. Laryngoscope 1959;67:1143–1150.

Jerger J, and Jerger S. Diagnostic significance of PB word functions. Arch Otolaryngol 1971;93:573–580.

Jerger JF, Tillman TW, and Peterson JL. Masking by octave bands of noise in normal and impaired ears. J Acoust Soc Am 1960; 32:385–390.

Jerger S, Lewis S, Hawkins J, and Jerger J. Pediatric speech intelligibility test. I. Generation of test materials. Int J Pediatr Otorhinolaryngol 1980;2:217–230.

Jirsa RF, Hodgson WR, and Goetzinger CP. Unreliability of half-list discrimination tests. J Am Aud Soc 1975;1:47–49.

Johnson CW, and Bordenick RM. Bone conduction speech reception thresholds with the mentally retarded. J Aud Res 1978;18:229–235.

Johnson EW. Auditory findings in 200 cases of acoustic neuromas. Arch Otolaryngol 1968;88:598–603.

Kalikow DN, Stevens KN, Elliot LL. Development of a test of speech intelligibility in noise using sentence materials with controlled word predictability. J Acoust Soc Am 1977;61:1337–1351.

Karlsen EA, and Goetzinger CP. An evaluation of speech audiometry by bone conduction in hearing impaired adults. J Aud Res 1980;20:89–95.

Katz DR, and Elliot LL. Development of a new children's speech discrimination test. Paper presented at American Speech-Language Hearing Association Convention, Chicago, 1978.

Kreul EJ, Nixon JC, Kryter, KD, Bell DW, Lang JS, and Schubert ED. A proposed clinical test of speech discrimination. J Speech Hear Res 1968;11:536–553.

Kruel EJ, Bell DW, and Nixon JC. Factors affecting speech discrimination test difficulty. J Speech Hear Res 1969;12:281–287.

Lehiste I, and Peterson GE. Linguistic considerations in the study of speech intelligibility. J Acoust Soc Am 1959;31:280–286.

Licklider JCR, and Miller GA. The perception of speech. In Stevens SS, Ed. Handbook of Experimental Psychology. New York: John Wiley & Sons, 1951.

Linden A. Undistorted speech audiometry. In Graham A, Ed. Sensorineural Hearing Processes and Disorders. Boston, MA: Little, Brown, & Co, 1965.

Loven FC, and Hawkins DB. Interlist equivalency of the CID W-22 word lists presented in quiet and in noise. Ear Hear 1983;4:91–97.

Lovrinic JH, Burgi EJ, and Curry ET. A comparative evaluation of five speech discrimination measures. J Speech Hear Res 1968;11:372–381.

Lynn G. Paired PB-50 discrimination test: a preliminary report. J Aud Res 1962;2:34–36.

Lynn JM, and Brotman SR. Perceptual significance of the CID W-22 carrier phrase. Ear Hear 1981;2:95–99.

Manning WH, Shaw CK, Maki JE, and Beasley DS. Analysis of half-list scores on the PBK-50 as a function of time compression and age. J Am Aud Soc 1975;3:109–111.

Margolis RH, and Millin JP. An item-difficulty based speech discrimination test. J Speech Hear Res 1971;14:865–873.

Marshall L, and Bacon SP. Prediction of speech discrimination scores from audiometric data. Ear Hear 1981;2:148–155.

Martin ES, and Pickett JM. Sensorineural hearing loss and upward spread of masking. J Speech Hear Res 1970;13:426–437

Martin FN, and Forbis NR. The present status of audiometric practice: a follow-up study. ASHA 1978;20:531–541.

Martin FN, and Pennington CD. Current trends in audiometric practices. ASHA 1971;13:671–677.

Martin FN, Hawkins RR, and Bailey HAT. The nonessentiality of the carrier phrase in phonetically balanced (PB) word testing. J Aud Res 1962;2:319–322.

McLennan RO Jr, and Knox AW. Patient-controlled delivery of monosyllabic words in a test of auditory discrimination. J Speech Hear Disord 1975;40:538–543.

McPherson DF, and Pang-Ching GK. Development of a distinctive feature discrimination test. J Aud Res 1979;19:235–246.

Merrell HB, and Atkinson CJ. The effect of selected variables upon discrimination scores. J Aud Res 1965;5:285–292.

Middelweerd MJ, Festen JM, and Plomp R. Difficulties with speech intelligibility in noise in spite of a normal pure-tone audiogram. Audiolology 1990;29:1–7.

Miller GA, Heise GA, and Lichten W. The intelligibility of speech as a function of the context of the test materials. J Exp Psychol 1951;41:329–335.

Nelson DA, and Chaiklin JB. Writedown versus talkback scoring and scoring bias in speech discrimination testing. J Speech Hear Res 1970;13:645–654.

Northern JL, and Hattler KW. Evaluation of four speech discrimination test procedures on hearing impaired patients. J Aud Res Suppl 1974;1:1–37.

Olsen WO, and Tillman TW. Hearing aids and sensorineural hearing loss. Ann Otol 1968;77:717–727.

Owens E. Intelligibility of words varying in familiarity. J Speech Hear Res 1961;4:113–129.

Owens E, and Schubert ED. The development of consonant items for speech discrimination testing. J Speech Hear Res 1968;11:656–667.

Owens E, Schubert ED. Development of the California Consonant Test. J Speech Hear Res 1977;20:463–474.

Owens E, Benedict M, and Schubert ED. Further investigation of vowel items in multiple-choice speech discrimination testing. J Speech Hear Res 1971;14:841–847.

Palmer JM. The effect of speaker differences on the intelligibility of phonetically balanced word lists. J Speech Hear Disord 1955;20:192–195.

Penrod JP. Discrimination performance on a carrier phrase vs a no carrier phrase speech discrimination task. Paper presented at the joint meeting of the Tennessee/Georgia Speech and Hearing Associations, Chattanooga, TN: 1978.

Penrod JP. Talker effects on word-discrimination scores of adults with sensorineural hearing impairment. J Speech Hear Disord 1979;44:340–349.

Penrod JP. A comparison of half- vs full-list speech discrimination scores in a hearing impaired geriatric population. J Aud Res 1980;20:181–186.

Peterson GE, and Lehiste I. Revised CNC lists for auditory tests. J Speech Hear Disord 1962;27:62–70.

Resnick DM. Reliability of the twenty-five word phonetically balanced lists. J Aud Res 1962;2:5–12.

Ross M and Huntington DA. Concerning the reliability and equivalency of the CID W-22 auditory tests. J Aud Res 1962;2:220–228.

Ross M, and Lerman J. A picture identification test for hearing impaired children. J Speech Hear Res 1970;13:44–53.

Schubert ED, Owens E. CVC words as test items. J Aud Res 1971;11:88–100.

Schultz MC, and Schubert ED. A multiple choice discrimination test (MCDT). Laryngoscope 1969;79:382–399.

Schumaier DR, and Rintelmann WI. Half-list vs full-list discrimination testing in a clinical setting. J Aud Res Suppl 1974;2:16–17.

Schwartz DM, and Surr RK. Three experiments on the California Consonant Test. J Speech Hear Disord 1979;44:61–72.

Schwartz DM, Bess FH, and Larson VD. Split-half reliability of two word discrimination tests as a function of primary-to-secondary ratio. J Speech Hear Disord 1977;42:440–445.

Shelton C, and House WF. Hearing improvement after acoustic tumor removal. Otolaryngol Head Neck Surg 1990;103:963–965.

Sher A, and Owens E. Consonant confusions associated with hearing loss above 2000 Hz. J Speech Hear Res 1974;17:669–681.

Shirinian MJ, and Arnst DJ. PI-PB rollover in a group of aged listeners. Ear Hear 1980;1:50–53.

Shutts RE, Burke KS, and Creston JE. Derivation of twenty-five word PB lists. J Speech Hear Disord 1964;29:442–447.

Siegenthaler BM, and Haspiel G. Development of two standardized measures of hearing for speech by children. US Department of Health, Education and Welfare. Project No. 2372, Contract OE-5-10-003.

Sieganthaler BM, and Strand R. Audiogram average methods and SRT scores. J Acoust Soc Am 1964;36:589–593.

Silverman SR, and Hirsh IJ. Problems related to the use of speech in clinical audiometry. Ann Otol Rhinol Laryngol 1955,64: 1234–1244.

Solomon LN, Webster JC, and Curtis JC. A factorial study of speech perception. J Speech Hear Disord 1960;3:101–107.

Speaks C, and Jerger J. Method for measurement of speech identification. J Speech Hear Res 1965;8:185–194.

Speaks C, Jerger J, and Jerger S. Performance-intensity characteristics of synthetic sentences. J Speech Hear Res 1966;9:305–312.

Thorndike EL. A Teacher's Word Book of the Twenty Thousand Words Found Most Frequently and Widely in General Reading for Children and Young People. New York: Teachers College, Columbia University, 1932.

Thorndike EL, and Lorge I. The Teacher's Word Book of 30,000 Words. New York: Columbia University Press, 1944.

Thornton AR, and Raffin MJM. Speech discrimination scores modeled as a binomial variable. J Speech Hear Res 1978;21:507–518.

Tillman TW, and Carhart R. An expanded test for speech discrimination utilizing CNC monosyllabic words: Northwestern University Auditory Test No. 6. Technical report no. SAM-TR-66-55. USAF School of Aerospace Medicine, Brooks Air Force Base, TX, 1966.

Tillman TW, Carhart R, and Wilber L. A test for speech discrimination composed of CNC monosyllabic words: Northwestern University

Test No. 4. Technical report no. SAM-TDR-62-135. USAF School of Aerospace Medicine, Brooks Air Force Base, TX, 1963.

Tillman TW, and Olsen WO. Speech audiometry. In Jerger J, Ed. Modern Developments in Audiology, 2nd Ed. New York: Academic Press, 1973.

Tobias JV. On phonemic analysis of speech discrimination tests. J Speech Hear Res 1964;7:102–104.

Townsend TH, and Schwartz DM. Error analysis of the California Consonant Test by manner of articulation. Ear Hear 1981;2:108–111.

Traul GN, and Black JW. The effect of content on aural perception of words. J Speech Hear Res 1965;8:363–369.

Valente MK, and Stark EW. Bone conducted speech audiometry with normal-hearing and hearing-impaired children. J Aud Res 1977;17: 105–108.

Weber S, and Redell RC. A sentence test for measuring speech discrimination in children. Audiol Hear Educ 1976;2:25–30, 40.

Williams C, and Hecker M. Relation between intelligibility scores for four test methods and three types of speech discrimination. J Acoust Soc Am 1968;44:1002–1006.

Young MA, and Gibbons EW. Speech discrimination scores and threshold measurements in a non-normal hearing population. J Aud Res 1962;2:21–33.

CHAPTER 11

Tests of Cochlear Function

Michael A. Brunt

Two procedures, sensitive to cochlear function, which have been used in diagnostic test batteries are loudness balance techniques and the short increment sensitivity index (SISI). Loudness balance techniques were first developed by Edmund Fowler (1936) for comparing loudness growth in a normal versus an abnormal ear. Reger (1936) is credited with the loudness balance procedure used to study symmetrical, binaural losses when there is normal hearing at some frequencies. Jerger et al. (1959) developed the SISI test as an outgrowth of studies of the difference limen for intensity (DLI) (Jerger, 1952, 1953).

Since the advent of these procedures, other behavioral and electrophysiologic tests have been developed for clinical use. In many cases tone decay, Bekesy audiometry, immittance, and auditory brainstem evoked response techniques have been used in conjunction with the loudness balance and SISI procedures in diagnostic test batteries. The purposes of this chapter are to review the loudness balance and SISI tests, to outline test administration and to consider their value in diagnostic audiology today.

LOUDNESS BALANCE PROCEDURES

There has been an interest in and research on presumed abnormal loudness growth for more than 60 years. Pohlman and Kranz (1924) and Fowler (1928) first commented on abnormal loudness growth in impaired ears, while Fowler provided the label "recruitment" in 1937. Recruitment is defined as an abnormal growth of loudness for signals at suprathreshold intensities. Consider an individual with a threshold at 1000 Hz of 5 dB hearing level (HL) in one ear and 45 dB HL in the other. At 5 and 45 dB, respectively, the tones are perceived as equally loud as both are at threshold. If the level was increased to 70 dB HL (65 dB SL) in the normal ear and a level of 70 dB HL (25 dB SL) in the poor ear was judged equally loud, then an abnormal growth of loudness or recruitment has been shown. Only a 25-dB increase in intensity over threshold was needed in the poor ear to sound equally loud as a 65 dB increase in intensity over the threshold in the normal ear. Thus, the poor ear showed a rapid rise in loudness growth.

General Principles and Procedures

The previous example illustrates one of the two most commonly used loudness balance procedures, the alternate binaural loudness balance or ABLB. Fowler's (1936) ABLB technique is for unilateral losses. Because most clients present with bilateral losses, Reger (1936) described the monaural loudness balance (MLB) technique which would be suitable for such cases.

The essence of either procedure requires loudness balancing between a frequency within normal limits (25 dB HL or better) and one showing a loss. If loudness balancing is done with both frequencies having a loss, the test results might be confounded (e.g., a finding of "no recruitment" might reflect recruitment in *both* ears).

ABLB compares loudness growth between the same frequencies for the two ears. MLB compares loudness growth between two different frequencies in the same ear. In this chapter when reference is made to two ears for ABLB the same would apply to the two different test frequencies in the MLB procedure.

For either procedure, a series of loudness judgments is made at different levels. For the ABLB, the intensity is held constant in one ear while intensity is varied in the other until the listener judges both signals to be of equal loudness. The ear with the constant or fixed intensity is termed the "reference ear" because loudness judgments are matched to this ear. The signals are rapidly alternated from ear to ear in ABLB and are alternated from frequency to frequency in MLB. Loudness balance judgments are made at several levels of fixed intensity in the reference ear.

The client's task is to state whether the variable tone is "softer than," "louder than," or "equal" in loudness to the reference ear. To assure that the client understands the task and to maximize validity and reliability of results, a bracketing procedure is used. Initial judgments should be based on a variable tone that is clearly perceived as "louder" than the reference tone, whereas the next judgment should be for a tone that is likely to be much "softer" than the reference. Further balances follow with intensity of the variable tone approaching the presumed equal loudness point.

The client is told that he will hear two tones, one constant in loudness and one variable. Judgments of loudness are to be made only from the variable ear (or tone) to the reference. It is suggested that the client listen to the constant signal in the reference ear at each test level for a few seconds before presenting the variable tone. This helps the listener to judge loudness because of a better sense of the reference signal as compared to the variable one. The client is cautioned to pay attention only to loudness changes and to ignore pitch differences. This would apply to MLB or to ABLB in which the same tone in each ear may sound different because of diplaucusis.

Procedural Considerations

Carver (1978) cites four variables to consider in loudness balance testing: (a) psychophysical method, (b) reference versus variable ear, (c) number of reference levels at which loudness balances are carried out, and (d) on-off duty cycle and switching rate of the signal. For three of these, there is no uniformity of procedure. Duty cycle and switching rate are somewhat uniform in clinical practice because of equipment similarities among manufacturers.

Method of Limits Versus Method of Adjustment

In the method of limits, the clinician controls both the reference and variable ear intensity settings. With the method of adjustment the clinician sets the levels in the reference ear whereas the client controls the variable tone intensity. Some individuals, such as Hood (1969), stress the importance of the clinician's control of all test stimuli. Others, such as Jerger (1962), advocate the method of adjustment. Client control of the variable stimulus has the advantage of reducing potential clinician bias. If the clinician controls the variable tone intensity, preconceived notions concerning the client's site of lesion might influence the accepted response and possibly could result in invalid or at least questionable results. The method of adjustment would seem preferable if the client is capable of the task and if the equipment allows client control. If the latter is not possible with a given audiometer, sometimes the equipment can be modified.

Reference Versus Variable Ear

There are two choices with regard to the reference versus variable ear. Some workers, such as Priede and Coles (1974), follow Jerger's suggestion of using the poor ear as the reference ear. Jerger (1962) noted that if clinical interest is in the presence or absence of recruitment, then a few fixed settings in the poor ear should be suffi-

cient. Originally, Fowler (1937) had described just the opposite, using the good ear as the reference. More recently, Hood (1969) also advocated the use of the good ear for reference with intensity variation in the poor. He stated that this procedure would result in less variability in response because the poor ear, if recruiting, will be more sensitive to changes in intensity. The reader is referred to articles by Hood (1969, 1977), Priede and Coles (1974), and Coles and Priede (1976) for further discussion.

If the audiologist is interested in plotting a loudness growth function as well as determining presence or absence of recruitment, Hood's method would be preferable. If the interest is primarily in the presence or absence of recruitment, then Jerger's procedure may prove more useful and quicker in clinical practice. Priede and Coles (1974) also remarked that the Jerger method was preferred by clients, because they found it less difficult than Hood's method. However, from the clinical point of view, validity of results is of prime importance as opposed to clients' subjective views. In this regard, Fritze (1978) noted that among 26 subjects with unilateral cochlear lesions, 23 evidenced complete recruitment by the Hood procedure versus 8 by the Jerger method. No procedural details were given.

Number of Loudness Balance Levels

To some degree the numbers of levels selected relates to (a) which ear is reference, (b) whether only the search for recruitment is of importance, and (c) whether determination of a loudness growth function is also desired. If the Jerger (1952) method is strictly adhered to, loudness balance would be done at 20 and 40 dB SL with the poor ear as reference. He noted that use of the good ear as reference would require more balances before presence or absence of recruitment can be made. However, if the good ear serves as reference (Hood, 1969; 1977) then a greater portion of the loudness function can be plotted while determining recruitment or its absence. It is obvious that, with the good ear as reference, intensity could be set at many 10 to 20 dB steps. The number of SLs would be significantly reduced with the poor ear as reference.

Duty Cycle and Alternation Rate

Jerger (1962) recommended a tone alternation rate of one per second with a duty cycle of 500 msec on and off per ear. These parameters or close approximations are available on most diagnostic audiometers. It appears that most are satisfied with such settings, although Hood (1969) stated that adaptation may occur with this format. Further comments on this issue are covered by Hood (1969) and Carver (1978).

PLOTTING RESULTS AND INTERPRETATION

Two primary methods have been used in plotting loudness balance results. One is the laddergram, often charted on the puretone audiogram. Examples are illustrated in Figures 11.1 and 11.2. Equal loudness judgments between the two ears are connected by straight lines. It is often convenient to connect the original "equal loudness" points (i.e., threshold per ear) by a dotted line. This distinguishes the threshold values from the formal loudness balance judgments. Inspection of the line pattern and intensity settings of equal loudness judgments determines presence or absence of recruitment.

Graphing of loudness balance results is illustrated in Figures 11.1 and 11.2. These graphs are plots of the

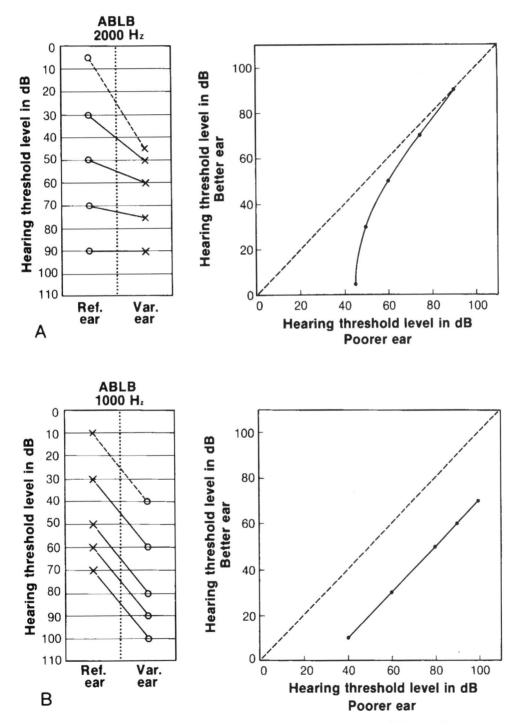

Figure 11.1. Plotting loudness balance results by laddergrams or graph. **A**, Complete recruitment. **B**, No recruitment.

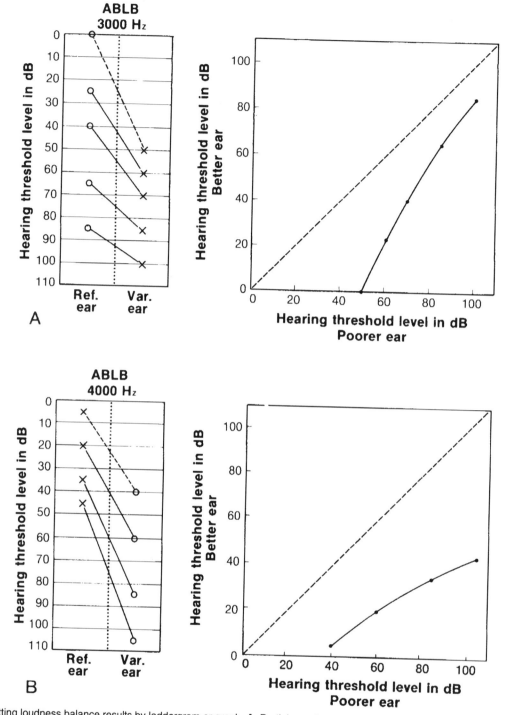

Figure 11.2. Plotting loudness balance results by laddergram or graph. **A**, Partial recruitment. **B**, Decruitment.

same data as the laddergrams. The good ear is plotted on the ordinate and the poor ear on the abscissa. The 45° diagonal represents the idealized result for loudness balance judgments between two normal ears. Comparison of the line connecting the equal loudness points to the idealized function determines presence or absence of recruitment. Interpretation generally has followed Jerger's (1962) suggestions. Four results are possible. Three discussed by Jerger are complete recruitment, partial recruitment, and no recruitment. A fourth pattern, decruitment, has been noted by some authors. The interpretation primarily is based on loudness judgments at the most intense level in the reference ear, whereas the overall pattern is of value in viewing the loudness growth function. Except for decruitment the following interpretations are those of Jerger (1962).

Complete recruitment is present when reference and variable ears are judged equally loud at equal HLs ± 10 dB (Fig. 11.1A). In this case, at threshold equal loudness was assumed at 5 and 45 dB HL for the good and poor ears, respectively, whereas signals were judged equally loud at 90 dB HL. Occasionally authors have cited "over-recruitment" as well. Overrecruitment would be demonstrated when equal loudness is achieved with the better ear HL generally over 10 dB more intense than the poorer.

If equal loudness judgments are made at equal SLs ±10 dB, then no recruitment is shown. As shown in Figure 11.1B even with intensity increases, equal loudness judgments remained at equal SLs. For example, at 60 dB SL (70 dB HL) in the good ear equal loudness was judged to be 60 dB SL (100 dB HL) in the poor ear as well. Note that Jerger allows a ±10 dB variation for recruitment and no recruitment. Hood (1969) does not advocate this leeway. However, our experience as well as that of other clinicians, would attest to the variability seen in clients administered loudness balance procedures. Thus, the 10 dB designation would seem appropriate for clinical practice.

Partial recruitment is shown if equal loudness judgments fall between those of complete and no recruitment. At the highest intensity levels (Fig. 11.2A) equal loudness was judged at 85 dB HL in the good ear and 100 dB HL for the poor. Clearly, this is not complete recruitment because these HLs are not equal. The 15 dB difference is beyond the 10 dB leeway. It is surely not absence of recruitment because the 85 and 50 dB SLs far exceed the equal levels ± 10 dB.

Decruitment has been noted less frequently than the other patterns. Decruitment is the opposite of recruitment. In this case the poor ear is less sensitive to increasing intensity than the good ear. Separation of decruitment from no recruitment is obtained when equal loudness judgments show a SL difference of 15 dB or more in the poor ear than in the good ear. In Figure 11.2B equal loudness at threshold was 5 and 40 dB HL for the good and poor ears, respectively. However, with the good ear signal at 40 dB SL (45 dB HL) an equal loudness judgment in the poor ear was not achieved until an SL of 65 dB (100 dB HL).

CLINICAL RESULTS WITH LOUDNESS BALANCE

Early Findings

Originally Fowler (1936) expected that loudness balance testing would help to differentiate those with preclinical otosclerosis from those with other hearing disorders. He found, however, that ABLB separated conductive from sensory-neural problems instead. In 1948 Dix et al. reported on the value of loudness balance procedures in separating cochlear from retrocochlear lesions. Shortly thereafter, Eby and Williams (1951) noted similar results. Those with cochlear lesions evidenced complete or partial recruitment whereas those with retrocochlear disorders showed no recruitment. Dix et al. (1948) reported decruitment in a client with an eighth nerve tumor. Similar results on several cases were later noted by Tillman (1969).

The expected result with a conductive loss is no recruitment, or equal loudness at equal SLs. For example, the ABLB pattern plotted in graphic form would be a straight line parallel to the ideal 45° function (See Fig. 11.1B). The dB difference would reflect the conductive component of the poor ear.

Loudness Balance and Differential Diagnosis

Since those early studies, ABLB and MLB have been used in test batteries to differentiate cochlear from retrocochlear disorders. In most articles attention has centered on unilateral losses and, consequently, use of ABLB. In most reports the majority of retrocochlear problems has been eighth nerve tumors.

ABLB studies consistently have shown the expected recruitment in cochlear cases a greater percentage of the time than the absence of recruitment in retrocochlear disorder. Hood (1969) reported that all 424 Ménière's patients tested evidenced recruitment. Hallpike (1965) and Tillman (1969) also noted recruitment present in 100% of cochlear ears they tested. As expected, with any diagnostic test, 100% is not always the case. Recruitment was reported in 73% of 36 Ménière's patients by Palva et al. (1978). Presence of recruitment in 85 and 84% of cochlear ears was noted by Sanders et al. (1974) and Thomsen et al. (1981), respectively. Thus, recruitment would seem very likely in ears with cochlear disorders. However, attention should be paid to "no recruitment" results, a false positive finding that could suggest a retrocochlear involvement. The previous research cited recruitment absence in as many as 15 to 27% of the cases with cochlear disorder.

"No recruitment" in a sensory-neural case suggests no cochlear pathology, which tends to support retrocochlear findings. However, the relative frequency of the expected "no recruitment" or "decruitment" in retrocochlear lesions varies considerably. Thomsen et al. (1981) noted that 90% of 44 patients with acoustic tumors showed no recruitment which can be contrasted with Hirsch et al. (1979) who reported only 33% in nine patients with acoustic neurinomas showed no recruitment. Findings of "no recruitment" by others are sprinkled throughout this range with 50% (Johnson, 1977), 57% (Clemis and Curtis, 1977), 63% (Palva et al., 1978) and 67% (Sanders et al., 1974). Thus, on the negative side, results implying cochlear disorder in confirmed acoustic neurinoma cases have ranged from 10 to 67%.

Most differential diagnostic studies have reported on acoustic tumor as the retrocochlear lesion. Two explanations commonly mentioned for the presence of recruitment in such cases are interference with cochlear blood supply (Priede and Coles, 1974; Tonndorf, 1980, 1981) and size of the tumor (Johnson, 1977). Johnson remarked that 50% of 171 patients evidenced no recruitment. Relative to tumor size the expected absence of recruitment was 72% for large tumors and 37 and 24% for medium and small tumors, respectively. In line with this, Hirsch et al. (1979) noted that in nine patients with medium to small tumors only three showed no recruitment. A third factor that often is not mentioned is the test contamination because of a coincidental high frequency cochlear loss (e.g., due to noise exposure). Under these circumstances testing is more likely to reveal appropriate results if ABLB can be carried out at 500 or 1000 Hz and not at 4000 Hz. Further discussion of the variable loudness balance test results for acoustic tumors follows discussion of the SISI test.

LOUDNESS BALANCE MODIFICATIONS

Bekesy Tracking

Miskolczy-Fodor (1964) reported on a Bekesy tracking method to assess recruitment using an ABLB format. Similar research was carried out by Carver (1970, 1978), Gelfand (1974), and Sung and Sung (1976). A Bekesy tracking of the variable tone is made by the client to match the loudness of a reference tone in the other ear. The resulting Bekesy plot is similar to the graphical form presented in Figures 11.1 and 11.2. There was more variability associated with this Bekesy form of ABLB testing than the conventional method (Gelfand, 1974; Sung and Sung, 1976).

Computer-Assisted ABLB

Fritze (1978) expressed concern about ABLB testing relative to the ear serving as the reference ear. He suggested randomization of both the reference ear and reference intensities for each equal loudness judgment. A computer in line with an audiometer was used to generate reference ear and intensity settings randomly. Loudness balance was done by the client using the method of adjustment. Test results were printed out graphically (see Figs. 11.1 and 11.2).

Results of this computerized procedure were compared to Jerger's (poor ear as reference) and Hood's (good ear as reference) methods on 26 subjects with unilateral cochlear lesions. All evidenced recruitment by the computerized format versus 23 by the Hood and 8

by the Jerger procedure. Fritze attributed the difference in results to the randomization of reference ear and HL level in the computerized procedure.

Such ABLB results would seem promising for the future relative to careful control of test conditions through computer algorithms. However, there has not been further research by Fritze relative to noncochlear disorders, such as acoustic neuroma. Although several audiometers on the market now have microprocessing capability, there have been no reports of their use relative to loudness balance measures.

SUMMARY OF LOUDNESS BALANCE PROCEDURES

Loudness balance procedures seem effective in detecting cochlear disorder but less so for retrocochlear dysfunction. As cited previously, the trend for earlier detection of acoustic tumors and lesions similarly affecting the auditory nerve may account for the high false negative rates noted by some authors. However, further research like that of Fritze (1978) in computer-assisted loudness balance testing may improve ABLB as a clinical procedure.

The Short Increment Sensitivity Index (SISI) Test

The SISI test grew out of research done in the late 1940s and the 1950s on the phenomenon of difference limen for intensity. Various authors surmised that those with cochlear lesions might show smaller difference limens for intensity (DLI) for puretones than those with normal hearing or noncochlear lesions. In most cases a reduced DLI was suggested as evidence of recruitment and that if DLI measures were not a direct measure of recruitment they were at least indirect measures of it. Lusher and Zwislocki (1949) examined DLI using the method of limits with an amplitude modulated tone presented at 40 dB SL. They reported that those with cochlear problems showed a reduced DLI relative to normals. The DLI was explored by Denes and Naunton (1950) in a different fashion; comparisons of DLI at 4 and 44 dB SL were carried out. At each level a constant intensity tone was compared to a variable intensity tone that followed it to determine the smallest intensity needed for the client to judge that there was a barely noticeable intensity difference. Other studies followed with mixed results; some found reduced DLIs in those with cochlear lesions (Lund-Iverson, 1950; Lusher, 1951; Jerger, 1952, 1953) although others reported little diagnostic value for DLI (Liden and Nillson, 1950; Hirsh, Palva and Goodman, 1954). There also was a general concensus that many clients had trouble with the DLI tasks. Problems in learning DLI tasks were discussed by Harris (1963). Thus, conventional DLI measures fell into disuse soon after they came on the diagnostic scene.

However, Jerger's (1952, 1953) early success with DLI measures led to Jerger, Shedd, and Harford's (1959) development of the SISI test. As they noted, the SISI task was much easier to administer and score than the DLI tests as the client's response was simply to report when or if a steady tone periodically increased or jumped in intensity. Jerger (1961) has noted that the SISI was not to be viewed as a direct or indirect test of recruitment but, rather, a site of lesion test. In short, results on the SISI may complement loudness balance measures but the two were not to be viewed as synonymous.

Conventional SISI Test: Procedure and Interpretation

As originally described by Jerger et al. (1959) the SISI test consisted of a steady or carrier tone presented at 20 dB SL *re:* puretone threshold with increments of intensity superimposed every 5 seconds. The client was to report whenever an increase in intensity was perceived. The test was to begin with several five-dB increment presentations, because they are easily heard by most clients. After this training period twenty 1-dB test increments were presented. Response to each of the 1-dB increments was worth 5%. Ease of perception of most of the 1-dB increments (high or positive SISI scores) was noted as the hallmark of cochlear lesions with few (low or negative SISI scores) or no increments heard for normal ears or for other auditory sites of dysfunction.

Relative to SISI results (Jerger et al., 1959), scores in the range of 0 to 20% were termed "negative" or low SISI scores, likely seen with normals, conductives, or those with VIIIth nerve problems, whereas scores of 25 to 65% were "questionable." Scores of 70 to 100% were termed "positive" or high SISI scores characteristically expected in cases of cochlear dysfunction. Scores on the SISI test may be related to test frequency. Jerger et al. (1959) and Jerger (1962, 1973) have reported SISI scores increasing with frequency from 250 to 4000 Hz. Jerger (1962) noted that results for 250 Hz were not as diagnostic as higher frequencies with clinical use focusing on the frequencies 500 to 4000 Hz. More specifically, Jerger (1973) reported that for cochlear disorders high scores of 80 to 100% are likely for 2000, 3000, and 4000 Hz with questionable scores of 40 to 60% for 1000 Hz and low scores (0 to 20%) for 250 and 500 Hz. Yantis and Decker (1964) also suggested that scores of 80 to 100% typically are seen in cochlear disorders at frequencies of 2000 Hz and above.

If the standard SISI is to be used to help detect cochlear lesions, the above information suggests giving the SISI only at frequencies 2000 Hz and above because results at 1000 Hz tend to yield equivocal ("questionable") scores and those at 250 and 500 Hz result in low (0 to 20%) scores also seen with normals and those with sites of lesion other than cochlear. Fewer frequencies tested with the SISI should be no problem because, presumably, other tests would help pinpoint the site of lesion. For example, acoustic reflex decay measures at 500 and 1000 Hz could complement high frequency results on the SISI relative to differential diagnosis because reflex decay measures above 1000 Hz typically prove to be equivocal for diagnostic purposes.

Procedural Variations on the SISI Test

Client Attention

Since the initial report on the SISI in 1959 (Jerger et al.) there has been much study aimed at improving the utility of the test. Three suggestions have been given to enhance client attention to the SISI that should improve the sensitivity of the original test and its variations (Hanley and Utting, 1965; Hughes, 1968; Owens, 1965a; Yantis and Decker, 1964). First, to orient the client at each test frequency several decreasing dB increments from five to four, etc., should be presented before reaching the 1-dB test increment. Second, during the formal test phase, some clients (presumably with cochlear lesions) will respond to the majority of the 1-dB increments. To help insure that responses are to the test increment and not false positives, resulting from a constant interincrement time interval, the clinician should randomly reduce the increment to 0 dB. Finally, if there is no or minimal response to the test increments the clinician should randomly introduce an intensity increment identifiable by the client to assure continued attention to the task.

Number of Test Increments

Owens (1965) noted that often a client either hears all the test increments or none and suggested use of 10 rather than 20 increments per frequency. Yantis and Decker remarked that SISI scores tended to be very high or very low (1964) although Griffing and Tuck (1963) reported quite high correlations between the first and second half of SISI test items in their subjects. We concur with Martin (1985) in suggesting presentation of only 10 items if, for the first 10, the client hears none or 1 (0 to 10%) or 9 or 10 (90 to 100%); otherwise all 20 should be administered. (Obviously, with only 10 items each will be worth 10 rather than 5%.)

Intensity Test Increment Size

Research has also centered on the size of the test increment with the assumption that an intensity change of less than 1 dB might prove a better divider of cochlear from noncochlear lesions or normal ears (Hanley and Utting, 1965; Sanders, 1966; Sanders and Simpson, 1966). Hanley and Utting (1965) suggested reducing the test increment to 0.75 dB. However, overall results by Sanders (1966) and Sanders and Simpson (1966) supported retention of the 1-dB level. The 1-dB increment size was the choice reported by audiologists in two polls of clinical test usage (Pennington and Martin, 1972; Martin and Forbis, 1978).

Presentation Level of the SISI and Differential Diagnosis

One modification of the SISI test that has received much attention is the presentation level of the carrier tone. In an early study Owens (1965a) reported that for mild cochlear lesions of 40 to 50 dB HL (ANSI, 1969) SISI scores often were not positive. He found that subsequent testing at a 30-dB SL presentation level would often result in positive scores. Thompson (1963) reported on two clients who later were surgically confirmed to have acoustic neuromas as showing minimal response on the SISI at the conventional 20 dB SL for either the normal or pathologic ear while at a high level (85 dB HL re: ANSI 1969) 1-dB increments could be detected by the normal but not the pathologic ear. These early findings by Owens (1965) and Thompson (1963) suggest that presentation levels higher than 20 dB SL might better separate normal and cochlear lesioned ears from those with auditory nerve dysfunction.

A few studies on presentation level have investigated normal ear performance alone. Many studies compared the results for normal versus cochlear ears although others reported on results for cochlear and retrocochlear lesions with varied presentation levels.

Owens (1965) noted that among normal subjects (thresholds 20 dB or better re: ANSI, 1969) scores of 60% or higher were not obtained until SLs of 35 to 45 dB for 500, 1000, 2000, and 4000 Hz. Cooper and Owen (1976) using 30 normal subjects, computed mean scores of slightly more than 80% at 70 dB HL at 4000 Hz and 80 dB HL at 1000 Hz; all subjects' scores were 100% at 100 dB HL. Similarly, among 231 presumed cochlear-impaired ears administered the SISI at 4000 Hz, scores usually were 80% or more at 90 dB HL (re: ANSI, 1969).

Comparing normal and cochlear lesioned ears Young and Harbert (1967) reported little difference in SISI performance at levels of 60 dB SPL or more. Among normal subjects for 500, 1000, 2000, and 4000 Hz, scores were 65% or more at 65 dB SPL (about 55 dB HL). They suggested that a high SISI score for a sensory-neural ear means that it is responding like a normal ear at the same SPL. Harbert et al. (1969) compared SISI results for normal and recruiting ears at several SPLs. At levels of 60 dB SPL or more both groups gave positive SISI scores although scores for normal and recruiting ears were the same at the same SPLs.

Swisher (1966) and Swisher et al. (1966) noted that normal subjects and those with cochlear losses performed much the same on the SISI at high HLs. For a 2000-Hz tone presented at varying HLs to 20 normal subjects and to 20 with cochlear loss, higher SISI scores were seen among the cochlear subjects relative to SL presentation but scores were quite similar for both groups as a function of HL (Swisher, 1966). Among 25 normals, 23 heard 1-dB increments with no trouble at 70 dB HL (ANSI, 1969) for a 2000 Hz tone although 24 of 25 sensorineural loss subjects heard this increment at 70 dB HL or higher (Swisher et al., 1966).

Martin and Salas (1970) investigated the relationship between loudness and SISI results at 4000 Hz for subjects with one normal ear and one cochlear-impaired ear. Four ear comparisons were obtained. One was conventional SISI (20 dB SL) for the poor versus normal ear with mean scores of 97.9 and 2.9%, respectively. Two were conventional SISI in one ear (e.g., cochlear impaired ear) and SISI at a level judged equally loud in the other (e.g., normal ear). Finally, the normal ear was evaluated at the intensity equal to the conventional 20 dB SL level in the cochlear impaired ear. For this comparison, the mean normal ear score was 98.3%, not unlike the conventional SISI mean score of 97.9% of the cochlear impaired ear. The authors concluded that SISI scores were more a product of intensity (SPL) than loudness. They suggested that high scores can be expected at 55 to 65 dB SPL (about 45 to 55 dB HL re: ANSI, 1969).

Sanders et al. (1974, 1975, 1978) have provided further information comparing the standard 20 dB SL level versus intensities well above 20 dB SL for detecting cochlear lesions. They (1974) reported that for 92 ears 76% showed high (≥70%) SISI scores at 20 dB SL although noting (1975) that for 67 cochlear ears 98% (66 ears) showed positive (≥70%) results for most at a high presentation level of 85 dB HL (a few at 80 or 90 dB HL). Finally, in a direct comparison of levels, among 26 ears with mild to moderate losses Sanders et al. (1978) found that 19% showed positive results at the standard level versus 88% at a test level of 80 dB HL.

In summary, the above evidence suggests that at high presentation levels normal ears will show high SISI scores. Cochlear loss cases also will show high scores even if some of those with mild to moderate losses did not demonstrate high scores at 20 dB SL.

The early findings for retrocochlear (mostly VIIIth nerve) problems on the SISI typically were low scores of 25% or less (Jerger et al. 1959; Jerger, 1961; Thompson, 1963; Owens, 1965). For SISI given at 20 dB SL Sanders et al. (1975) noted 83% of 24 acoustic tumor ears showed low SISI scores whereas as late as 1978 Sanders et al. reported negative SISI scores in 67 of 67 tumor ears.

Despite such promising results, many studies do not show the low scores on the standard SISI or SISI at high intensity levels typically expected in cases with retro-cochlear problems. For example, for the acoustic tumor subjects of Sanders et al. (1975, 1978) it was found that at intensities beyond 20 dB SL some SISI scores changed from negative to positive. In their 1975 study of 24 tumor cases, 48% showed positive scores at a level of 105 dB HL although in the 1978 study of 67 subjects with retrocochlear lesions 17% showed positive scores at a level of 90 dB HL. Thus, at high intensity levels some individuals with auditory nerve problems are likely to respond with high SISI scores, a false negative response suggesting a cochlear lesion site.

Furthermore, in surveys of different studies both Sanders (1982) and Olsen (1987, 1991) have reported sensitivity of the SISI to auditory nerve problems to range from 91% (Jerger, 1961) to 48% (Sanders et al., 1974) with most at 63% or less. In combining results from several studies Turner et al. (1984a, 1984b, 1984c) as well as Hall (1991) have noted that the SISI does not show the sensitivity desired for the detection of auditory nerve disorder. For example, Hall (1991) stated that among 720 acoustic tumor cases only 64% of the time did the SISI suggest such a problem.

Suggested Clinical Procedure

From the above survey it is apparent that the SISI, as was the case with loudness balance procedures, is a good test to detect cochlear problems but lacks sensitivity relative to retrocochlear lesions. Also, it would appear that to maximize separation of normal and cochlear ears from those with eighth nerve disorder, a high presentation level is suggested. To be sure, as noted above, a high level would select out most cochlear losses but also result in some high scores in some eighth nerve cases. We advocate Sanders' (1982) suggestion of a presentation level of 75 dB HL with the exception of the 20 dB SL level for those with losses of 60 dB HL or more. Furthermore, earlier research cited suggests confining testing to frequencies of 2000 Hz or above for maximum clinical utility. Relative to scoring, it would seem that the original suggestions of Jerger et al. (1959) are still adequate. High or positive scores of 70 to 100% would be expected with normal or cochlear lesioned ears. Scores of 20% or less would raise the index of suspicion of an eighth nerve problem. The high level SISI might better divide results into high or low scores with elimination of the questionable range of scores (25 to 65%) than the conventional 20 dB SL level.

CONCLUDING REMARKS

From this review of loudness balance and SISI tests it is evident that these measures are quite sensitive to coch-lear disorders but show variable results relative to retro-cochlear lesion; the latter was reported as an auditory nerve disorder in most cases. Several factors would appear to relegate these tests to a secondary role in the differential diagnostic test category. Acoustic reflex (AR) measures and auditory brainstem evoked response (ABR) (See Chapters 21 and 24) show greater sensitivity to auditory nerve disorder than either loudness balance or SISI tests. Apparently, the physiologic changes attending auditory nerve problems are more readily detected by tests of physiologic function (AR and ABR) than behavioral response tests (such as loudness balance and SISI). The loudness balance and SISI tests ask for a subjective judgment of physiologic function, at least one step removed from the more direct physiologic measures of AR and ABR. As mentioned earlier, Johnson (1977) noted a general correspondence between acoustic tumor size and classical findings with the SISI and ABLB tests; the smaller the tumor, the less likely the results of either test will point to a retrocochlear problem.

Pursuing this line of thought, this author suggests that Sanders' comments relative to the SISI and loudness balance tests seem to have merit. Sanders (1979, 1982) has suggested that the result of recruitment with loudness balance tests and high scores on the SISI test with cochlear lesioned ears at high intensities is a normal response rather than one suggesting abnormal sensitivity to intense sound. Also, the literature review for the SISI given at high intensities pointed out essentially the same results for normal and cochlear-lesioned ears. Similarly, as reported by Sanders (1979), recruitment on the ABLB is shown in normal ears when one ear is artificially given a cochlear loss with masking.

Sanders (1979, 1982) noted that negative SISI scores and no recruitment with an eighth nerve problem reflect a loudness transmission loss that is not seen in cochlear lesioned ears. However, what explanation can be offered for the variable findings reported for eighth nerve dysfunction. He suggests that results for loudness balance and SISI can range from no recruitment and negative SISI scores to recruitment and positive, high SISI scores depending on the extent of the lesion and its effect relative to loudness transmission loss. Therefore, the apparent inconsistent results on these tests in eighth nerve dysfunction is not random but related to how the lesion affects loudness transmission. However, from a clinical point of view, this author would agree with others (Hall, 1991; Jerger, 1973; Olsen, 1987, 1991; Ruth and Lambert, 1991; Sanders, 1982) that acoustic reflex and ABR measures are better for differentiating cochlear from eighth nerve dysfunction than loudness balance or SISI measures.

In certain situations these behavioral tests may be equal to or even more valuable than physiologic tests. In cochlear cases with losses of 60 dB or more acoustic reflexes are often absent (Jerger et al., 1972). Therefore, this result could suggest eighth nerve dysfunction or, simply not rule it out. Also, reflex results on moderate to severe sensorineural losses may not clearly indicate cochlear or auditory nerve site (Jerger and Jerger, 1974; Popelka, 1981; Stach and Jerger, 1991). Problems with ABR interpretation frequently arise in these cases as well, especially for high frequency sensorineural losses (Josey, 1985; Møller and Møller, 1985; Durrant and Wolf, 1991; Musiek, 1991; Schwartz and Morris, 1991). Often, the greater the loss the more likely that a tumor, if any, is quite large, thus increasing the sensitivity of both the SISI and loudness balance procedures. A similar condition exists in the case of conductive overlay in patients seen for cochlear-retrocochlear evaluation. Thus, clinically one can be faced with situations in which the physiologic tests are rendered unusable or equivocal and, therefore, more reliance must be placed on behavioral tests.

Finally, we often assume that audiologists in the United States and throughout the world have the availability of up-to-date equipment. However, we do know that in some places immittance and auditory evoked response capabilities are not readily available. In such cases the use of behavioral tests for distinguishing cochlear from retrocochlear pathology assumes much more significance.

REFERENCES

Carver WF. The reliability and precision of a modification of the ABLB test. Ann Otol Rhinol Larngol 1970;79:398–412.

Carver WF. Loudness balance procedures. In Katz J, Ed. Handbook of Clinical Audiology, 2nd ed. Baltimore: Williams & Wilkins, 1978: 168–178.

Clemis JD, and Curtis AW. Opaque cerebellopontine cisternogram. Laryngoscope 1977;87:1658–1666.

Coles RRA, and Priede VM. Factors influencing the choice of fixed-level ear in the ABLB test. Audiology 1976;15:465–479.

Cooper JC Jr, and Owen JH. In defense of SISI's. Arch Otolarygol 1976;102:396–399.

Denes P, and Naunton RF. The clinical detection of auditory recruitment. J Laryngol Otol 1950;65:375–398.

Dix MR, Hallpike CS, and Hood JD. Observations upon the loudness recruitment phenomenon, with especial reference to teh differential diagnosis of the internal ear and VIIIth nerve. Proc R Soc Med 1948;41:516–526.

Durrant JD, and Wolf KE. Auditory evoked potentials: basic aspects. pp 321-381. In Rintelmann WF, ed. Hearing Assessment, Ed. 2. Austin, TX: Pro-Ed, 1991:321–381.

Eby LG, and Williams HL. Recruitment of loudness in the differential diagnosis of end-organ and nerve fiber deafness. Laryngoscope 1951;61:400–413.

Fowler EP. Marked deafened areas in normal ears. Arch Otolaryngol 1928;8:151–155.

Fowler EP. A method for early detection of otosclerosis. Arch Otolaryngol 1936;24:731–741.

Fowler EP. The diagnosis of diseases of the neural mechanism of hearing by the aid of sounds well above threshold. Trans Am Otol Soc 1937;27:207–219.

Fritze, W. A computer controlled binaural balance test. Acta Otolaryngol (Stockh) 1978;86:89–92.

Gelfand SA. The use of an automatic-self-recording ABLB as a clilnical test of recruitment. Presented at the American Speech and Hearing Association Convention, Las Vegas, 1974.

Griffing TS, and Tuck GA. Split-half reliability of the SISI. Aud Res 1963;3:159–164.

Hall JW III. Classic site-of-lesion tests: Foundation of diagnostic audiology. In Rintelmann WF, Ed. Hearing Assessment, Ed. 2. Austin, TX: Pro-Ed, 1991:653–677.

Hallpike CS. Clinical otoneurology and its contributions in theory and practice. Proc R Soc Med 1965;58:185–196.

Hanley CN, and Utting JF. An examination of the normal hearer's response to the SISI. J Speech Hear Disord 1965;30:58–65.

Harris JD. 1963 Loudness discrimination. J Speech Hear Disord Monogr 1963;(Suppl):11.

Hirsh IJ, Palva T, and Goodman A. Difference limen and recruitment. Arch Otolaryngol 1954;60:525–540.

Hirsch A, Noren G, and Anderson H. 1979. Audiological findings after stereotaxic radiosurgery in 9 cases of acoustic neuroma. Acta Otolaryngol (Stockh) 1979;88:155–160.

Hood JD. Basic audiological requirements in neuro-otology. J Laryngol Otol 1969;83:695–711.

Hood JD. Loudness balance procedures for the measurement of recruitment. Audiology 1977;16:215–228.

Hughes RL. Atypical responses to the SISI. Ann Otolaryngol 1968; 77:332–337.

Jerger JF. Comparative evaluation of some auditory measures. J Speech Hear Res 1962b;5:3–17.

Jerger J. Diagnostic audiometry. In Jerger J, Ed. Modern Developments in Audiology, Ed. 2. New York: Academic Press, 1973:75–115.

Jerger JF. A difference limen recruitment test and its diagnostic significance. Laryngoscope 1952;62:1316–1332.

Jerger JF. DL difference test: An improved method for the clinical measurement of recruitment. Arch Otolaryngol 1953;57:490–500.

Jerger J. Hearing tests in otologic diagnosis. Asha 1962a;4:139–143.

Jerger JF. Recruitment and allied phoenomena in differential diagnosis. J Aud Res 1961;1:145–151.

Jerger J, and Jerger S. Audiological comparisonsof cochlear and eighth nerve disorders. Ann Otol Rhinol Laryngol 1974;83:1–11.

Jerger JF, Jerger S, and Mauldin L. Studies in impedance audiometry. I. Normal as sensorineural ears. Arch Otolaryngol 1972;96:513–523.

Jerger JJ, Shedd L, and Harford E. On the detection of extremely small changes in sound intensity. Arch Otolaryngol 1959;69:200–211.

Johnson EW. 1977. Auditory test results in 500 cases of acoustic neuroma. Arch Otolaryngol 1977;103:152–158.

Josey AF. Auditory brainstem response in site of lesion testing. In Katz J, Ed. Handbook of Clinical Audiology, Ed. 3. Baltimore: Williams & Wilkins, 1985;534–548.

Liden G, and Nilsson G. Differential audiometry. Acta Otolaryngol (Stockh) 1950;28:521–527.

Lund-Iverson L. An investigation on the difference limen determined by the method of Lusher and Zwislocki in normal hearing and in various forms of deafness. Acta Otolaryngol (Stockh) 1952; 42:219–224.

Lusher E. The difference limen of intensity variations of pure tones and its diagnostic significance. J Laryngol Otol 1951;65:486–510.

Lusher E, and Zwislocki J. 1949. A simple method for indirect monaural determination of the recruitment phenomenon (difference limen in intensity in different types of deafness). Acta Otolaryngol (Stockh) 1949;78(Suppl):156–168.

Martin FN. The SISI test. In Katz J, ed. Handbook of Clinical Audiology, Ed. 3. Baltimore: Williams & Wilkins, 1985:292–303.

Martin FN, and Forbis NK. The present status of audiometric practice: A follow-up study. ASHA 1978;20:531–541.

Martin FN, and Salas CR. The SISI test and subjective loudness. J Aud Res 1970;10:368–371.

Miskolczy-Fodor F. Automatically recorded loudness balance testing. Arch Otolaryngol 1964;79:355–365.

Møller MB, and Møller AR. Auditory brainstem-evoked responses (ABR) in diagnosis of eighth nerve and brainstem lesions. In Pinheiro ML, and Musiek FE, Eds. Assessment of Central Auditory Function: Foundations and Clinical Correlates. Baltimore: Williams & Wilkins, 1985:43–65.

Musiek FE. Auditory evoked responses in site-of-lesion assessment. In Rintelmann WF, Ed. Hearing Assessment, Ed. 2. Austin, TX: Pro-Ed, 1991:383–427.

Olsen WO. Differential auditory tests. In Robinette MS, and Bauch CD, Eds. Proceedings of a Symposium in Audiology. Rochester, NY: Rochester Methodist Hospital, 1987;1–29.

Olsen WO. Special auditory tests: A historical perspective. In Jacobson JT, and Northern JL, Eds. Diagnostic Audiology. Austin, TX: Pro-Ed, 1991:19–52.

Owens E. The SISI test and VIIIth nerve versus cochlear involvement. J Speech Hearing Disord 1965;30:252–262.

Palva T, Jauhiainen C, Sjoblom J, and Ylikoski J. Diagnosis and surgery of acoustic tumors. Acta Otolaryngol (Stockh) 1978;86:233–240.

Pennington CD, and Martin FN. Current trends in audiometric practices. Part II. Auditory tests for site of lesion. ASHA 1972;14:199–203.

Pohlman AG, and Kranz RW. Binaural minimum audition in a subject with ranges of deficient acuity. Proc Soc Exp Biol Med 1924; 20:335–337.

Popelka GR. The acoustic reflex in normal and pathologic ears. In Popelka GR, Ed. Hearing Assessment with the Acoustic Reflex. New York: Grune & Stratton, 1981;5–21.

Reger SN. Differences in loudness respons of normal and hard-of-hearing ears at intensity levels slightly above threshold. Ann Otol Rhinol Laryngol 1936;45:1029–1039.

Ruth RA, and Lambert PR. Evaluation and diagnosis of cochlear disorders. In Jacobson JT, and Northern JL, Eds. Diagnostic Audiology. Austin, TX: Pro-Ed, 1991:199–215.

Sanders JW. Diagnostic audiology. In Lass NJ, McReynolds LV, Northern JL, and Yoder DE, Eds. Speech, Language and Hearing: Vol. III Hearing Disorders. Philadelphia: WB Saunders Company, 1982: 944–967.

Sanders JW. 1966. The effect of increment size on the short increment sensitivity index scores. J Speech Hear Res 1966;9:297–304.

Sanders JW. Recruitment. In Rintelmann WF, Ed. Hearing Assessment, Ed 1. Baltimore: University Park Press, 1979:261–280.

Sanders JW, Josey A, and Glasscock ME III. 1974. Audiologic evaluation in cochlear and eighth nerve disorders. Arch Otolaryngol 1974; 100:283–289.

Sanders JW, Josey A, and Glasscock ME. The modified SISI in patients with VIIIth nerve tumor. Presented at the American Speech and Hearing Association Convention, Washington, D.C., 1975.

Sanders JW, Josey A, and Glasscock ME. The SISI at high intensity in normal, cochlear, and eighth nerve pathology ears. Presented at the American Speech and Hearing Association Convention, San Francisco, 1978.

Sanders JW, and Simpson ME. The effect of increment size on short increment sensitivity index scores. J Speech Hear Res 1966;9:297–304.

Schwartz DM, and Morris MD. Strategies for optimizing the detection of neuropathology from the auditory brainstem response. In Jacobson JT, and Northern JL, Eds. Diagnostic Audiology. Austin, TX: Pro-Ed, 1981:141–160.

Stach BA, and Jerger JF. Immittance measures in auditory disorders. In Jacobson JT, and Northern JL, Eds. Diagnostic Audiology. Austin, TX: Pro-Ed, 1991:113–139.

Swisher LP. Response to intensity change in cochlear pathology. Laryngoscope 1966;76:1706–1713.

Swisher LP, Doehring DG, and Rivard RC. Response to intensity change at threshold in sensory-neural hearing loss. J Aud Res 1968;8:291–298.

Sung RJ, and Sung GS. Study of the classical and modified alternate binaural loudness balance tests in normal and pathological ears. J Am Aud Soc 1976;2:49–53.

Thompson GA. Modified SISI technique for selected cases with suspected acoustic neurinoma. J Speech Hear Disord 1963;28:299–302.

Thomsen J, Nyboe J, Borum P, Tos M, and Barfoed C. 1981. Acoustic neuromas. Arch Otolaryngol 1981;107:601–607.

Tillman T. Special hearing tests in otoneurological diagnosis. Arch Otolaryngol 1969;89:25–30.

Tonndorf J. Acute cochlear disorders: the combination of hearing loss, recruitment, poor speech discrimination and tinnitus. Ann Otol Rhinol Laryngol 1980;89:353–358.

Tonndorf J. Stereociliary dysfunction, a cause of sensory hearing loss, recruitment, poor speech discrimination, and tinnitus. Acta Otolaryngol 1981;91:469–480.

Turner RG, Frazer GJ, and Shepard NT. formulating and evaluating audiologic test protocols. Ear Hearing 1984;5:321–330.

Turner RG, and Nielsen DW. Application of clinician decisioin analysis to audiological tests. Ear Hearing 1984;5:125–133.

Turner RG, Shepard NT, and Frazer GJ. Clinical performance of audiological and related diagnostic tests. Ear Hearing 1984; 5:187–194.

Yantis PA, and Decker RL. On the short increment sensitivity index (SISI test). J Speech Hear Disord 1964;29:231–246.

Young IM, and Harbert F. Significance of the SISI test. J Aud Res 1967;7:303–311.

CHAPTER 12

Tests of Retrocochlear Function

David S. Green and Lynn Huerta

Clinical audiologists use a variety of diagnostic tests for the detection of retrocochlear lesions. Behavioral tests that are currently used, although less so than in the past will be considered. Since site of lesion testing became part of the practice of clinical audiology, a significant number of new and innovative procedures for identifying retrocochlear lesions have been developed. Some of these have enjoyed limited or brief professional acceptance while others have demonstrated a greater longevity. Usually, the professional acceptance associated with a particular testing technique is dependent upon its relative availability, its cost, and its proven effectiveness in identifying a retrocochlear lesion.

We will describe a number of behavioral procedures that are available to the tester for the purpose of detecting the presence of a possible retrocochlear lesion. Several of the diagnostic tests have declined in importance because of the development of newer and more sensitive tests. However, some of the older procedures retain useful clinical functions as tests when conditions for performing the newer tests prove inappropriate. These older tests may then serve an important screening function. They might be particularly appropriate under circumstances where (*a*) newer tests are contraindicated, e.g., conductive overlay or high frequency loss, or (*b*) there is limited access to more sophisticated electrophysiological equipment.

This chapter will primarily focus on tone decay. Bekesy, high-level short increment sensitivity index (SISI), and performance intensity for phonetically balanced words (PI-PB rollover) procedures will also be discussed.

TONE DECAY

Definition

Threshold tone decay is defined as a decrease in threshold sensitivity resulting from the presence of a barely audible sound. Suprathreshold tone decay refers to a loss of audibility as a result of a stimulating tone that is delivered at a high presentation level.

History

Tone decay testing has been traced back to the late 1800s (Corradi, 1890; Rayleigh, 1882; Gradenigo, 1893), but did not come into common usage until the mid 1950s when both Bekesy (Bekesy, 1947; Reger and Kos, 1952) and conventional audiometers (Hood, 1956; Carhart, 1957) were used for tone decay measurement. As audiologists gained experience with tone decay measurements, a number of suggested modifications of the early test procedures was developed (Rosenberg, 1958; Sorensen, 1962; Green 1963; Owens, 1964; Olsen and Noffsinger 1974; Jerger and Jerger, 1975).

Auditory brainstem response (ABR) audiometry, computed axial tomography (CAT), and magnetic resonance imaging (MRI) are tests in current use that demonstrate a significantly higher degree of accuracy in identifying retrocochlear lesions than that shown by threshold tone decay tests (and other tests described in this chapter). However, while recognizing that there are more powerful diagnostic audiologic and/or medical tests, we would consider it unwise to discard tone decay tests performed with a conventional puretone audiometer. We believe that tone decay tests still serve an important diagnostic role as a *screening* procedure. This procedure continues to be clinically useful because of its availability, modest cost, and effectiveness.

When To Test for Tone Decay

Individuals who exhibit asymmetric sensory-neural hearing loss, asymmetric speech recognition abilities, sudden sensory-neural hearing loss, asymmetric tinnitus of recent origin, or vestibular symptoms such as dizziness or balance disturbance, may have retrocochlear pathology. Audiologic screening for abnormal tone decay is appropriate for subjects exhibiting these symptoms.

Instrumentation

It is well established that the presence of abnormal tone decay is a strong indicator of retrocochlear pathology (Clemis and Mastricola, 1976; Johnson, 1977; Cacace, 1981). Yet, to perform the tone decay test, minimal instrumentation is required. All that is needed is a stopwatch and a puretone audiometer. The equipment needed is readily available in audiologic settings and is relatively inexpensive. Puretone audiometers may be found not only in audiology centers, but also in schools, physicians offices, convalescent homes, homes for the elderly, and in industrial environments.

General Test Procedures

Tone decay tests can be performed at either threshold or suprathreshold levels. Both procedures appear to have good diagnostic merit and are not unduly time consuming. Because of this, it is recommended that both threshold and suprathreshold testing be done when retrocochlear lesions are suspected.

Turner et al. (1984), using techniques of clinical decision analysis, evaluated the clinical performance of audiologic tests, including the suprathreshold adaptation test (STAT) and threshold tone decay tests. This was accomplished by studying hit versus false alarm rate data garnered from a review of 15 years of clinical literature (1968 to June 1983).

From their studies, the authors concluded that the threshold and the suprathreshold tone decay tests were about equally sensitive in identifying retrocochlear pathology with a hit rate of about 70% (Turner et al., 1984).

Threshold Tone Decay Testing

Threshold tone decay measurements are usually made with conventional puretone audiometers and can be carried out at any available frequency. The quantity of tone decay in dB is usually taken as the difference between the initial threshold and the threshold at which the test is terminated. The frequencies chosen for study will depend on the patient's hearing status and tester preference. Some techniques employ a brief rest period between successive levels of stimulation. Some require a response to "tone only"; others accept a response to "any sound," tonal or not.

Comparative studies of threshold tone decay tests, with regard to their effectiveness in identifying confirmed retrocochlear pathology, suggest that the test procedure of choice should be a slight modification of the test described by Carhart (1957). The modification recommended is based on the fact that some individuals with retrocochlear pathology experience a loss of both tonality and audibility, while others experience only a loss of tonality of the test stimulus (Green, 1963). Requiring a response to the perception of tonality is thought to enhance the sensitivity of the test. The subjective change in quality of a puretone to a noise lacking tonality, which was noted by Green (1963), has been called tone perversion by Parker et al. (1968). Pestalozza and Cioce (1962), Sorensen (1962), Flottorp (1963). Harbert and Young (1964), Johnson (1966), Sung et al. (1969), and Olsen and Noffsinger (1974) have also encountered this phenomenon and take it into account when testing for tone decay.

Modified Carhart Threshold Tone Decay Test. The procedure of choice for threshold tone decay measurement is a modification of the Carhart threshold tone decay

test that requires the subject to respond to stimulus tonality. The subject is seated in an armchair and told to maintain elbow contact with the armrest while he or she is signaling. The subject is asked to raise his or her arm perpendicular to the armrest if the tonal signal is perceived, to lower it to a 45° angle if the stimulus loses tonality but remains audible and to lower his or her arm to the rest position if the sound becomes completely inaudible. The subject is cautioned against adjusting the earphones or chewing while the test is in progress, as the slightest interruption in the continuity of the signal can impair test reliability.

To facilitate the subject's judgment of "tonality," it is useful to begin the testing on the ear that is judged to be nonaffected. Since abnormal tone decay is usually confined to the ear ipsilateral to the retrocochlear lesion, the subject will be likely to hear the test stimulus as tonal in the nonaffected ear. By contrast, the listener will be better able to judge the presence or absence of tonality when the affected ear is being tested.

The modified Carhart technique entails the following steps:

1. Obtain the subject's threshold of hearing in each ear using an interrupted audiometric tone. The opposite ear should be masked when necessary.
2. Begin the tone decay test by presenting the tone stimulus continuously in the test ear at 5 dB above the established threshold.
3. As soon as the subject responds, begin timing with a stopwatch. If the test stimulus is heard with perceived tonality for a full minute, terminate the test. If the subject indicates either that the test stimulus that is heard is no longer tonal, or that it is no longer audible, before the 1-minute criterion is met, raise the intensity of the tone 5 dB *without interrupting the tone,* set the stopwatch back to zero, and begin timing for a minute again. A record may be kept of the number of seconds the tonality was perceived at each intensity level.
4. Continue raising the tone in 5-dB steps as indicated until an intensity is reached that allows the subject to perceive the tonality of the test stimulus for a full minute. When this occurs, the test at this frequency may be terminated.
5. Continue in this manner until all of the desired audiometric test frequencies have been tested.

Suprathreshold Tone Decay

Working on the hypothesis that symptoms of abnormal tone decay first appear only at the highest testable sound intensities, Jerger and Jerger (1975) proposed a simplified suprathreshold tone decay test known as the STAT (suprathreshold adaptation test). The test frequencies are 500, 1000, and 2000 Hz, and the technique incorporates the following steps:

1. The subject is instructed to signal as long as he or she hears the sound in the test ear. The nontest ear is masked with white noise at a level of 90 dB sound pressure level (SPL).
2. A continuous 500 Hz test tone at 110 dB SPL is presented until either the patient indicates that he or she no longer hears the tone, or until 60 seconds have elapsed, whichever comes first.
3. If the patient has responded for the full 60 seconds for the test frequency, the test is scored negative.
4. If the patient has failed to respond for the full 60 seconds, the test is scored positive.
5. To ensure that the patient has grasped the essential nature of the listening task, a pulsed tone is presented for 60 seconds. If the patient signals that he or she heard the pulsed but not the continuous tone for 60 seconds, it is likely that the patient is responding to the test in a proper manner.
6. The tester may then test 1000 Hz and 2000Hz, as described in steps 1 to 5.

Interpretation

Abnormal tone decay is a sign that is associated with retrocochlear lesions. Abnormal tone decay has been observed in cases of neural degeneration, inflammation and trauma, as well as by space-occupying lesions such as tumors, which press against the eighth nerve and/or the auditory brainstem. A partial list of cases in which abnormal tone decay has been observed would include: acoustic neurinoma, primary cholesteatoma (epidermoid cyst), seventh nerve neuroma, meningioma (Johnson, 1966), thermal injury to the eighth nerve (Harbert and Young, 1962), multiple sclerosis, mumps neuritis, von Recklinghausen's disease, acquired luetic deafness, Ramsay-Hunt syndrome, intracranial aneurysm, head trauma (Harbert and Young, 1968), eighth nerve atrophy, pinealoma (Kos, 1955), ninth nerve neuroma (Naunton et al., 1968), cerebellar atrophy (Miller and Daly, 1967), Arnold-Chiari malformation (Rydell and Pulec, 1971), extra-axial brainstem lesion (Jerger and Jerger, 1974a), brainstem lesions above the level of entry of the eighth nerve or lateral to the midline (Morales-Garcia and Hood, 1972) and upper and lower brainstem lesions (Katz, 1970).

Extreme tone decay can occur even when puretone thresholds are only mildly or moderately elevated. As a result, a cursory evaluation of the puretone audiogram might underestimate the potential seriousness of the condition. The tester should bear in mind that abnormal tone decay may be observed in patients with an acoustic tumor which, if untreated, could prove life threatening.

At the same time, one must be wary not to make the spurious assumption that the presence of abnormal tone decay is prima facie evidence that a life-threatening lesion exists. For both the threshold and the suprathreshold tone decay tests, positive findings warrant a medical referral and/or further audiometric testing.

For the modified Carhart method, there appears to be general agreement that a critical point in the differentiation between cochlear and retrocochlear pathology occurs as one approaches the 30-dB tone decay level. However, it would be unwise to assume that everyone with more than 30 dB of tone decay has a retrocochlear lesion or that everyone with less than that amount does not. A more productive way of looking at tone decay that approaches the 30-dB mark is that each dB of decay above 20 dB should raise the index of suspicion that a retrocochlear lesion may exist. The greater the tone decay and the number of frequencies involved, particularly the lower frequencies, the greater the possibility of serious pathology. The index of suspicion should also be raised if the rate of decay does not diminish with increasing stimulus intensity (Morales-Garcia and Hood, 1972). Patients with acoustic tumors frequently exhibit extreme, and often complete, tone decay at all frequencies. Tumor size appears related to the severity of the symptom. In support of this, Johnson (1966), reporting on 73 patients, found a positive relationship between size of tumor and tone decay results. Partial or complete tone decay was found in 63% of the patients with tumors classified as large and in only 14% of the patients in the small tumor category.

Retrocochlear lesions can coexist with any other auditory pathology (e.g., acoustic trauma, noise-induced hearing loss, middle ear pathology, presbycusis, inherited deafness, and drug ototoxicity). The audiologist is well aware that a patient whose hearing has been damaged by noise has not lessened his chances for developing an acoustic neurinoma. In addition, retrocochlear and middle ear pathologies are not mutually exclusive, and cases with both pathologies in the same person have been reported (Green, 1978).

Acoustic reflex decay testing has been cited as another relatively strong test for identifying retrocochlear pathology (Turner et al., 1984). It may be noted, however, that in the presence of conductive hearing loss, one is usually unable to measure the acoustic reflex, let alone calculate the amount of reflex decay for diagnostic purposes. The threshold tone decay test does not suffer from that limitation and can be used to screen for tone decay even in the presence of a mild to moderate conductive hearing loss.

BEKESY TESTING

Soon after Bekesy (1947) described his new automatic audiometer, Reger and Kos (1952), using Bekesy instrumentation, made the observation that an abnormally rapid temporary threshold shift occurred in an individual with an eighth cranial nerve tumor. As time passed, Bekesy audiometry proved to be a popular means of testing for retrocochlear pathology. Jerger (1960) identified a number of diagnostic configurations based on pulsed versus continuous threshold frequency sweeps (traditional Bekesy audiometry). Later refinements of Bekesy testing utilized Bekesy comfortable loudness (BCL) sweeps (Jerger and Jerger, 1974b) and also forward backward Bekesy (FBB) sweeps (Harbert and Young, 1962; Rose, 1962; Jerger et al., 1972).

Turner et al., (1984), in a study of the relevant clinical literature, calculated correct identification (hit) rates for traditional Bekesy threshold tone decay tests and tone decay tests performed on a conventional audiometer. They found that conventional audiometer tone decay tests proved to be more sensitive than traditional Bekesy audiometry in identifying retrocochlear pathology. The hit rate for traditional Bekesy audiometry was 49%, whereas the hit rate was 70% for conventional audiometer tone decay testing. However, BCL testing had a hit rate of 85% and was, on the average, more successful than either of the other two tests in identifying retrocochlear lesions.

The use of Bekesy testing is reported to have declined in recent years (Martin and Forbis, 1978; Martin and Sides, 1985). This is probably associated with reduced availability of the Bekesy test instrumentation. Where Bekesy audiometers are available, the BCL test will continue to provide useful testing for retrocochlear pathology.

PERFORMANCE-INTENSITY FUNCTION FOR PHONETI- CALLY BALANCED WORDS (PI-PB FUNCTION)

Most audiologists include some measure of word recognition abilities in their audiologic evaluation protocol as a means of assessing a patient's ability to understand speech. Word recognition abilities are often assessed at a patient's most comfortable loudness level or at some fixed sensation level above the speech reception threshold. The use of these levels of presentation, although useful in assessing a patient's ability to recognize speech, has not proven too effective in distinguishing between patients with cochlear pathology and those with retrocochlear pathology (Walsh and Goodman, 1955; Johnson, 1979; Bess, 1983).

When higher presentation levels were used for word recognition testing with patients with eighth nerve tumors, however, Jerger and Jerger (1971) noted a significant decrease in the scores of these patients at high intensity levels as compared with their patients with cochlear pathologies. This led to the development and use of the performance-intensity function for phoneti-

cally balanced words (PI-PB function) as a means of identifying patients with retrocochlear pathology (Jerger and Jerger, 1971; Dirks et al., 1977; Bess et al., 1979).

In obtaining a PI-PB function, the clinician typically presents half lists of monosyllabic words at successively higher intensities up to a maximum of 110 dB sound pressure level, or approximately 90 dB HL. The worst score (PB min) is subtracted from the best score (PB max) and this sum is then divided by the PB max score to obtain a "rollover ratio."

Rollover Ratio = (PB max − PB min) / PB max

This rollover ratio is then used to decide whether the patient is at risk for having a retrocochlear lesion. Patients with normal hearing or conductive, cochlear, or mixed hearing losses usually have a low rollover ratio, whereas those with retrocochlear pathologies often have high rollover ratios. Various rollover ratios have been used as being suggestive of retrocochlear or cochlear pathology (e.g., see Jerger and Jerger, 1971; Dirks et al., 1977; Bess et al., 1979; Meyer and Mishler, 1985).

As is true for tone decay tests, the equipment needed for PI-PB testing is readily available (audiometer equipped for speech audiometry), costs associated with the test are low, and PI-PB testing has served as a useful procedure for identifying retrocochlear pathology. However, Turner et al. (1984) reported poorer overall sensitivity for the PI-PB function test (hit rate of 74%) in the detection of retrocochlear pathology than some of the earlier studies (e.g., see Jerger and Jerger, 1971; Dirks et al., 1977; Bess et al., 1979; Meyer and Mishler, 1985).

HIGH-LEVEL SISI TEST

The short increment sensitivity index (SISI) test was introduced by Jerger et al. in 1959, as a clinical tool for differentiating cochlear from noncochlear hearing losses. Thompson (1963) suggested that, instead of using the standard 20-dB SL carrier tone, a high-level presentation could be used to identify retrocochlear pathology more effectively. In this procedure, a carrier tone is delivered at a high presentation level, usually 75–85 dB HL, and the patient is asked to identify a series of small, short-duration changes in intensity. At high presentation levels, normal-hearing subjects and those with peripheral hearing impairment are typically able to perceive and identify the small changes in intensity. Individuals with retrocochlear pathology, however, are often unable to detect these changes, perhaps because of excessive tone decay.

In the high-level SISI test procedure, as many as twenty 1-dB increments are presented at each test frequency. If a low score of correct identifications isobtained, the result is suggestive of retrocochlear pathology. Cooper and Owen (1976) and Sanders (1982) support this approach. Details about the SISI and high-level SISI tests are covered in Chapter 11.

CONCLUSIONS

Although the tests discussed in this chapter (i.e., tone decay, Bekesy audiometry, SISI, PI-PB) have declined in use in the past decade because of rapid advances in electrophysiologic techniques, these behavioral tests still retain usefulness in the differential diagnosis of retrocochlear pathology. In particular, tone decay and PI-PB are useful tools and they can be performed in a short time with readily available equipment. Bekesy audiometry and the high-level SISI can also serve a role in detecting retrocochlear pathology, especially when used as a part of a test battery approach.

REFERENCES

Bekesy GV. A new audiometer. Acta Otolaryngol 1947;35:411–422.

Bess FH. Clinical assessment of speech recognition. In Konkle DF, Rintelmann WF, Eds. Principles of speech audiometry. Baltimore: University Park Press, 1983:127–201.

Bess FH, Josey AF, and Humes LE. Performance intensity functions in cochlear and eighth nerve disorders. Am J Otol 1979;1:27–31.

Cacace A. Acoustic neuroma: an audiologic evaluation. NY State J Med 1981;81:744–748.

Carhart R. Clinical determination of abnormal auditory adaptation. Arch Otolaryngol 1957;65:32–39.

Clemis JD, and Mastricola P. Special audiometric test battery in 121 proved acoustic tumors. Arch Otolaryngol 1976;102:654–656.

Cooper JC, and Owen JH. In defense of SISI's. Arch Otolaryngol 1976;102:396–399.

Corradi C. Zur prufung der Schallperception durch die Knochen. Arch Ohrenheilk 1890;30:175–182.

Dirks DD, Kamm C, Bower D, and Bettsworth A. Use of performance-intensity functions for diagnosis. J Speech Hear Disord 1977;42:408–415.

Flottorp G. Pathological fatigue in part of the hearing nerve only. Acta Otolaryngol 1963(Suppl);188:298–307.

Gradenigo G. On the clinical signs of the affections of the auditory nerve. Arch Otol 1893;22:213–215.

Green DS. The modified tone decay test (MTDT) as a screening procedure for eighth nerve lesions. J Speech Hear Disord 1963;28:31–36.

Green DS. Tone decay. In Katz, Ed. Handbook of clinical audiology, 2nd Ed. Baltimore: Williams & Wilkins, 1978.

Harbert F, and Young IM. Threshold auditory adaptation. J Aud Res 1962;2:229–246.

Harbert F, and Young IM. Sudden deafness with complete recovery. Arch Otolaryngol 1964;79:459–471.

Harbert F, and Young IM. Clinical application of Bekesy audiometry. Laryngoscope 1968;78:487–497.

Hood JD. Fatigue and adaptation of hearing. Br Med Bull 1956;12:125–130.

Jerger J. Bekesy audiometry in analysis of auditory disorders. J Speech Hear Res 1960;3:275–287.

Jerger J, and Jerger S. Diagnostic significance of PB word functions. Arch Otolaryngol 1971;93:573–580.

Jerger J, Jerger S, and Mauldin L. The forward-backward discrepancy in Bekesy audiometry. Arch Otolaryngol 1972;72:400–406.

Jerger J, Shedd JL, and Hartford E. On the detection of extremely small changes in sound intensity. Arch Otolaryngol 1959;69:200–211.

Jerger J, and Jerger S. Auditory findings in brainstem disorders. Arch Otolaryngol 1974a;99:342–350.

Jerger J, and Jerger S. Diagnostic value of Bekesy comfortable loudness tracings. Arch Otolaryngol 1974b;99:351–360.

Jerger J, and Jerger S. A simplified tone decay test. Arch Otolaryngol 1975;101:403–407.

Johnson EW. Confirmed retrocochlear lesions. Arch Otolaryngol 1966;84:247–254.

Johnson EW. Auditory test results in 500 cases of acoustic neuroma. Arch Otolaryngol 1977;103:152–158.

Johnson EW. Results of auditory tests in acoustic tumor patients. In House WF, Luetje CM, Eds. Acoustic tumors: Vol. 1. Diagnosis. Baltimore: University Park Press, 1979:209–224.

Katz J. Audiologic diagnosis: cochlea to cortex. Menorah Med J 1970;1:25–38.

Kos CM. Auditory function as related to the complaint of dizziness. Laryngoscope 1955;65:711–721.

Martin FN, and Forbis NK. The present state of audiometric practice: a follow up study. ASHA 1978;20:531–541.

Martin FN, and Sides D. Survey of current audiometric practices. ASHA 1985;27:29–36.

Meyer D, and Mishler ET. Rollover measurements with Auditec NU-6 word lists. J Speech Hear Disord 1985;50:356–360.

Miller MH, and Daly JF. Cerebellar atrophy stimulating acoustic neurinoma. Arch Otolaryngol 1967;85:383–386.

Morales-Garcia C, and Hood JD. Tone decay test in neurotological diagnosis. Arch Otolaryngol 1972;96:231–247.

Naunton RF, Proctor L, and Elpern BS. The audiologic signs of ninth nerve neurinoma. Arch Otolaryngol 1968;87:222–227.

Olsen WO, and Noffsinger D. Comparison of one new and three old tests of auditory adaptation. Arch Otolaryngol 1974;99:94–99.

Owens E. Tone decay in eighth nerve and cochlear lesions. J Speech Hear disord 1964;29:14–22.

Parker WP, Decker RL, and Richards NG. Auditory function and lesions of the pons. Acta Otolaryngol 1968;87:228–240.

Pestalozza G, and Cioce C. Measuring auditory adaptation; the value of different clinical tests. Laryngoscope 1962;72:240–259.

Rayleigh L. Acoustical observations. IV Phil Mag 13, Series 1882;5:340–347.

Reger SN, and Kos CM. Clinical measurements and implications of recruitment. Ann Otol Rhinol Laryngol 1952;61:810–823.

Rose DW. Some effects and case histories of reversed frequency sweep in Bekesy audiometry. J Aud Res 1962;2:267–278.

Rosenberg PE. Rapid clinical measurement of tone decay. Paper presented at the American Speech and Hearing Association Convention, New York, 1958.

Rydell R, and Pulec J. Arnold-Chiari malformation. Acta Otolaryngol 1971;94:8–12.

Sanders JW. Diagnostic audiology. In Speech Language and Hearing, Vol. III; Hearing Disorders. Philadelphia: WB Saunders, 1982:944–967.

Sorensen H. Clinical application of continuous threshold recording. Acta Otolaryngol 1962;54:403–422.

Sung SS, Goetzinger CP, and Knox AW. A study of the sensitivity and reliability of three tone decay tests. Paper presented at the American Speech and Hearing Association Convention, Chicago, 1969.

Thompson G. A modified SISI technique for selected cases with suspected acoustic neurinoma. J Speech Hear Disord 1963;28:299–302.

Turner RG, Shepard NT, and Frazer GJ. Clinical performance of audiological and related diagnostic tests. Ear Hear 1984;5:187–194.

Walsh TE, and Goodman A. Speech discrimination in central auditory lesions. Laryngoscope 1955;65:1–8.

CHAPTER 13

Integrating Audiometric Results

Martin S. Robinette

DEVELOPMENT OF AUDIOLOGIC TEST BATTERIES FOR DIFFERENTIAL DIAGNOSIS

Early Years of Audiometry

As one reviews the depth and breadth of information presented in this book, one cannot help but marvel at the phenomenal growth and relevance of audiology as a professional discipline. We are but 50 years from the days when the first commercial electronic audiometer, the Western Electric 1A, was described at an American Otology Meeting by Fowler and Wegel (1922a, 1922b). They plotted hearing sensitivity on charts called "audiograms," with normal hearing as a straight line, and they received quite mixed reviews. Seashore (1899), who coined the term "audiometer," congratulated otologists "on the taking up of an entirely new point of approach to their science by introduction of measuring instruments of precision" (p. 112). Others were more skeptical of audiometry: "I have not found anything in these tests, as yet, that seems to be of any assistance" (Fowler and Wegel 1922a, p. 122); and "I plead guilty to being a mere otologist. The more I see of the audiometer the more respect I have for the tuning fork and Galton Whistle" (Fowler and Wegel 1922a, p. 118).

Despite such early skepticism, the audiometer and the puretone audiogram remain the foundation of audiologic assessment. This basic threshold evaluation affords the documentation of the degree of hearing loss, the slope of the configuration, the symmetry between ears as well as establishing a baseline for future assessments. The first audiologic test battery came into existence with the inclusion of circuitry for speech tests in an audiometer in 1924 (Jones and Knudson) and the inclusion of bone vibrators on audiometers in 1928 (Feldman, 1970).

In the early years differential diagnosis from audiologic test results was limited. The main goals were twofold: (*a*) to quantify the degree and pattern of hearing loss and (*b*) to determine if the conductive apparatus of the middle ear or the sense organ of the inner ear were at fault. At that time there were no accepted airconduction or bone-conduction calibration standards and no standard threshold testing techniques. Earphones and bone oscillators were usually handheld against the ear or mastoid area. Available masking noise

was a buzz (sawtooth noise) that provided little masking for frequencies above 1000 Hz. However, early contributions included C. C. Bunch's report of progressive high-frequency hearing loss by age group from 20 to 70 years (1929) and the audiometric configuration of noise induced hearing loss (1937). Some tuning fork tests of pseudohypocusis were modified for implementation with audiometers, such as the puretone Stenger (Guttman, 1928) and Lombard tests (Harbert, 1943). By 1937 the A.M.A. had proposed minimum standards for audiometers (Report of the Council on Physical Therapy) which encouraged the use of audiometers by otologists. Still physicians often favored tuning fork tests for the differential diagnosis of conductive versus sensory (which was referred to as perceptive) hearing loss. Puretone audiometry was accepted to quantify and monitor the degree and pattern of overall hearing loss, but bone-conduction thresholds were perceived to be uncertain with a great range of variability (Davis, 1947) despite reports to the contrary (Dean, 1930; Greenbaum, Kerridge, and Ross, 1939).

Suprathreshold audiometric tests were reported in the 1930s with limited acceptance. The tests were based on the phenomenon now known as loudness recruitment. Abnormal loudness growth was first described by Pohlman and Kranz (1924). Fowler (1928) was puzzled by a patient with a unilateral loss near 4096 Hz who perceived sound presented 5 sensation units above threshold in the affected ear to be as loud as 25 sensation units in the nonaffected ear. He suggested it may be due to some defect in Corti's organ. In concluding his report he puzzled aloud about the state of auditory testing of the day: "Is it possible that there are many normal ears like this? Is this a normal ear? Is there such a thing as a normal ear? Some day we shall find out!" (p. 155).

Fowler first described the Alternate Binaural Loudess Balance (ABLB) Test in 1936, as an early test of otosclerosis. He assumed that in the affected ear loudness would be limited or "hobbled" by the restricted excursions of the stapes. Fowler's technique required the listener match in loudness two tones, both of the same frequency presented alternately to the two ears. Reger (1936) proposed a monaural version of the test in which subjective loudness was balanced between two different frequencies in the same ear, the threshold for only one frequency being abnormally poor. In Fowler's 1937 presidential address to the American Otological Society he labeled the phenomenon "Recruitment of Loudness" (p. 207) and suggested the ABLB test for identifying sensory deafness calling it the only reliable test for neural deafness that does not require confirmation by other tests" (p. 210). Later Fowler (1938) proposed loudness balancing between air-conduction and bone-conduction to determine true bone-conduction levels from feeling vibrations at frequencies of 128 and 256 Hz.

During the 1930s and early 1940s audiometric speech testing was by no means routine and was not used for differential diagnosis. However, Fletcher and Steinberg (1929) had developed some lists of sentences that could be presented at different intensities to establish thresholds of intelligibility for speech. Hughson and Thompson (1942) used these materials for determining what they labeled "Speech Reception Threshold" (SRT).

In summary, by the mid-1940s the integration of audiometric results for differential diagnosis was in its infancy. Air-conduction audiometric configurations had been described for several pathologies. Bone-conduction thresholds and loudness balancing were being used to estimate conductive versus sensory pathology, and as a possible method of detecting pseudohypocusis; thresholds for speech reception were being advanced, but audiometry was primarily used to quantify and monitor hearing loss.

1948 Through the 1950s

The decade after World War II marked the origin of audiology as a profession and an era of dramatic progress in differential diagnosis. Four major clinical milestones occurred within a brief span of 4 years (1947—1951). These milestones included: (a) the acceptance of audiometric bone-conduction testing, (b) site of lesion tests for retrocochlear pathology, (c) clinically useful speech audiometry, and (d) the ASA standards for normal hearing thresholds.

Bone Conduction

Carhart's (1950) classical article on "Clinical Applications of Bone Conduction Audiometry" included his description of what is now known as the "Carhart notch." He described the mechanical decrease in bone conduction sensitivity of 5 dB at 500 Hz, 10 dB at 1 KHz, 15 dB at 2 KHz, and 5 dB at 4 KHz in patients with stapes fixation due to otosclerosis. To get a true measure of inner ear function preceding middle ear surgery, the above values were subtracted from the preoperative bone-conduction thresholds to estimate the "true" inner ear sensitivity. Shambaugh and Carhart (1951) also derived a

formula for predicting the results of the fenestration operation on the basis of preoperative air conduction and bone conduction thresholds. Later as stapes mobilization surgery became a significant part of otologic practice, many believed it necessary to have an audiologist in the operating room testing the patient by pure-tone air conduction audiometry at certain stages in the surgical procedure, so that the otologist might know whether the desired results were being achieved (Goodhill, 1955). This milestone established by Carhart reinforced the growing relationship between audiologist and otologist, resulting in audiograms and audiologic evaluations becoming a routine part of modern otologic practice.

Retrocochlear Pathology

The audiologist's clinical role in the differentiation of cochlear versus eighth nerve hearing loss was triggered by the classic publication of Dix et al. (1948). Using the ABLB test they found loudness recruitment present in each of 30 Ménière's disease patients, but absent in 14 of 20 eighth nerve tumor patients. The six remaining tumor patients showed partial recruitment. As noted, previous measures of loudness recruitment up to this time were seen as a replacement for bone conduction testing in determining sensory hearing loss. Distinguishing sensory from neural hearing loss demonstrated by Dix et al. (1948) ushered in the era of differential diagnostic audiology.

Bekesy's 1947 observations with his automatic audiometer led to a different approach for measuring recruitment. He suggested that excursion width on his threshold tracking procedure "is a measure of the difference limen for intensity" in noting that patients with sensory hearing loss had narrower continuous tone threshold tracings than did patients with conductive hearing loss. On this basis he stated that "This method is equivalent to the recruitment test of Fowler but permits isolated investigations of one ear" (p. 414). Unfortunately, the Bekesy automatic audiometer was not commercially available for several years. However, Luscher and Zwislocki (1948) followed up on Bekesy's observations and reported an indirect method of evaluating monaural loudness recruitment by measuring difference limens for intensity (DLI) with more readily available equipment. They initially viewed their test as an alternative to bone-conduction testing as did Fowler, but with the new diagnostic value of "recruitment" it soon became a popular site of lesion test for sensory versus neural hearing loss along with the ABLB, monaural bifrequency loudness test (MLB) (Reger, 1936) and several other DLI procedures (Denes and Naunton, 1950; Jerger, 1952, 1953). However, the enthusiasm for loudness balancing and DLI procedures waned as later studies revealed that up to 50% of patients with eighth nerve lesions also showed loudness recruitment on the ABLB test (Tillman, 1969; Sanders, et al., 1974; Johnson, 1977). Later investigators also provided evidence that the DLI tests may not be related to the loudness recruitment phenomenon (Lund-Iverson, 1952; Hirsh et al., 1954). Particularly convincing is the article by Riach et al. (1962) showing that DLI functions and loudness are not merely inverse indicies of the same auditory process since they may be controlled independently.

Speech Audiometry

Speech audiometry was established as a routine part of the audiological battery as a result of the development of speech threshold tests (Hudgins et al., 1947) and word recognition (speech discrimination) tests (Egan, 1948) at the Harvard Psychoacoustic Laboratory. Today the most common clinical methods of determining speech thresholds and speech recognition still involve the use of spondaic words and monosyllabic word lists respectively.

Using the Harvard Psychoacoustic Laboratory Phonetically Balanced word lists (PAL PB 50) recorded by Rush Hughes, speech discrimination scores helped to confirm the diagnosis of conductive hearing loss (high scores), mixed loss, and sensory loss (lower scores) (Thurlow et al., 1949). In addition, the SRT and average discrimination loss from PB 50-word lists presented at three levels (33, 48, and 63 dB SL) representing faint, average, and loud conversational speech were used together to estimate the degree of hearing handicap called the social adequacy index (SAI) (Davis, 1948). As clinical use of the CID W-1 and W-22 word lists (Hirsh et al., 1952) succeeded the Harvard PAL lists, word recognition scores became less diagnostic and the SAI fell into disuse, but the basic clinical value of speech threshold tests and word recognition has continued.

The use of the SRT to validate the accuracy of puretone thresholds became, in addition, a valuable differential diagnostic indication of pseudohypacusis as Carhart (1952) reported SRTs being obtained at much better hearing levels than puretone averages for cases of psuedohypacusis.

Normal Hearing Standards

The final milestone for the early integration of audiometric results was the establishment of a national standard of normal hearing in conjunction with standard specifications for diagnostic audiometers (ASA Z 24.5-1951). The development of these standards based on the results of a mass survey conducted by the US Public Health Service in 1935–1936, reflected advances in electronics, improvements in audiometric test environments, and audiology's growth as a scientific discipline that respected precision for clinical and research measurements. After this landmark standard, other standards quickly followed for screening audiometers (ASA Z 24.12-1952) and speech audiometers (ASA Z 24.13-1953).

Test Integration

Near the close of the 1950s Newby published his classic text "Audiology" (1958), one of the first textbooks of this growing profession. One gains insight to diagnostic audiology and test integration of the day by reviewing this text. The basic test evaluation suggested by Newby included puretone air- and bone-conduction thresholds with appropriate contralateral masking (sawtooth or white noise). Speech audiometry consisted of the SRT from CID Auditory Test W-1, most comfortable loudness (MCL) in dB above SRT, tolerance level in dB above SRT, and finally speech discrimination from CID auditory test W-22 delivered at an intensity of 40 dB greater than the SRT, or as much greater as the patient's tolerance level permitted. Contralateral masking was used if necessary for SRT and speech discrimination testing.

With the puretone audiogram, comparison of air- and bone-conduction results assisted in the diagnosis of conductive, sensory (then referred to as perceptive), or mixed-type hearing impairment. Carefully reproduced air- and bone-conduction audiometry was key in determining if a patient with otosclerosis was a good surgical candidate. Speech audiometry alone was of little diagnostic value; however, the difference in decibels between the SRT and tolerance level gave an estimate of dynamic range that, if compressed, indicated the presence of recruitment and supported a diagnosis of a loss due to an inner ear impairment. A low speech discrimination score also would be expected for a sensory rather than a conductive problem. Newby cautioned that reverse reasoning should not be applied because normal tolerance and good discrimination did not mean the lack of a cochlear problem. Newby went on to explain that retrocochlear problems were not characterized by recruitment and their speech discrimination scores depended, for the most part, on the shape of the audiogram through the speech frequencies.

Consistency of test results, particularly the puretone average loss for speech frequencies and the SRT, helped to determine the accuracy of tests and suspicion of pseudohypacusis. Special tests for detection of pseudohypacusis included the Lombard (voice reflex) test, the puretone and speech Stenger tests, the Doerfler-Stewart test (1946) for binaural functional loss (Doerfler and Epstein, 1956), the shifting voice test (Johnson et al., 1956), the delayed auditory feedback test (Lee, 1950; Black, 1951), and the psychogalvanic skin response procedure (PGSR) (Michaels and Randt, 1947; Doerfler, 1948; Bordley and Hardy, 1949).

Testing for cochlear versus retrocochlear hearing loss was based solely on tests for recruitment. Consequently a battery of several measures was not suggested; only procedures sufficient to indicate the presence or absence of recruitment were advocated. One of the recommended methods compared the most comfortable loudness (MCL) and uncomfortable loudness levels (UCL). Data for these tests were secured during standard puretone testing. If the puretone threshold, MCL, and UCL were close together for frequencies with hearing loss, the patient was judged to have recruitment suggesting a cochlear loss. If there was no air-bone gap and these levels were spread far apart, the patient did not have recruitment and an eighth nerve lesion was suspected. The interpretation of presence or degree of recruitment was based on the experienced judgment of the examiner. A corollary approach evaluated results from the SRT, MCL, and UCL with speech stimuli. Direct measures searching for presence or absence of recruitment were Fowler's ABLB test and Reger's MLB test. Indirect measures of recruitment were previously mentioned (Zwislocki, 1948; Denes and Naunton, 1950; and Jerger, 1952, 1953) and Bekesy tracings widths from a commercial Bekesy audiometer similar to one developed by Reger (1952).

A clear hierarchy of preferred tests based on clinical data was not available at this point in the development of auditory tests for differential diagnosis. However, the emphasis was clearly on the measurement of recruitment with the ABLB as the test of choice. Audiology was an established dynamic profession and its emerging role in differential diagnosis was becoming accepted by progressive otologists.

The 1960s: The Development of the Site-of-Lesion Test Battery

As audiology entered the decade of the 1960s the term "audiologic test battery" took on special meaning referring to a group of specialized audiologic tests deemed important in the differential diagnosis of retrocochlear lesions. In addition to puretone audiometry the five tests most commonly used in this battery were: speech discrimination, ABLB, SISI, Bekesy audiometry, and tone decay. The development, modification, and diagnostic criterion for these tests are discussed in greater depth in Chapters 11 and 12. Nevertheless, it is important to indicate the most popular procedures and interpretation criteria used at the time.

Speech Discrimination and ABLB

Speech discrimination testing was generally accomplished with the CID W-22 word lists (Hirsh et al., 1952) or the Northwestern University Auditory test 6 word lists (Tillman and Carhart, 1966) presented at 25 or 40 dB SL. Speech discrimination scores of 0 to 30% were considered "poor" and suggestive of eighth nerve pathology. The preferred ABLB method was suggested by Jerger (1962) using the method of adjustment with the poorer ear as the reference.

Short Increment Sensitivity Index (SISI)

The SISI test (Jerger et al. 1959) was quickly accepted as an important diagnostic test. The SISI procedure, developed as a clinical adaptation of the quantal psychophysical method (Stevens et al., 1941), was relatively quick and overcame several response variables that limited the reliability of DLI tests. Furthermore, Jerger et al. (1959) bypassed the DLI-recruitment controversy by suggesting the test did not measure either the DLI or recruitment but was a valuable site-of-lesion indicator. In the test procedure, 1-dB increments were added to a steady state 20 dB SL signal at 5-second intervals and the patient was instructed to respond to each perceived change in the loudness of the steady tone. In sensorineural cases detection of 20% or less of the 1-dB increments was considered positive, suggesting eighth nerve pathology, although scores of 70 to 100% were suggestive of cochlear involvement.

Bekesy Audiometry

Measurements of abnormal neural adaptation in eighth nerve tumor patients was reported in the 1950s (Reger and Koss, 1952; Lierle and Reger, 1955; Jerger et al., 1958), and became part of the site-of-lesion battery with Jerger's classification of Bekesy audiograms (Jerger, 1960). Tracing separate thresholds for pulsed and continuous tones provided a visual impact that became the hallmark of site-of-lesion testing for many years. In fact, the cover of the first addition of this text used Bekesy tracings as the visual (Katz, 1972). Jerger presented four basic patterns or types. The type I audiogram is characterized by an interweaving or overlapping of continuous and interrupted threshold tracings and is associated with normal hearing or conductive hearing loss. The type II tracing is characterized by the continuous tone tracing dropping mildly below the pulsed tone tracing (up to 20 dB) at high frequencies and is associated with cochlear hearing loss. The type III tracing is distinctive in that the continuous tone threshold tracing precipitously drops to levels beyond the output limits of the audiometer and is associated with eighth nerve lesions. The type IV tracing pattern was described as more closely resembling a type

II than a type III but differing in that the continuous tracing fell below the pulsed tracing at frequencies below 500 Hz. Later, Hughes et al. (1967) clarified the difference between types II and IV as being the amount of adaptation of the continuous tone. Separation of the continuous and pulsed tracing of 20 dB or less is considered a type II, tracing indicating cochlear pathology whereas a separation more than 20 dB but still within the limits of the audiometer is classified type IV and has a high probability of being associated with an eighth nerve tumor. Rose (1962) improved the measurement of neural adaptation through Bekesy tracings by introducing reversed frequency sweep (high to low frequency) tracings in addition to the traditional low frequency to high frequency direction.

Tone Decay

A different procedure for measuring neural adaptation, the tone decay test, was described by Carhart (1957) as a method that required only a conventional puretone audiometer. In Carhart's suggested procedure the patient is to indicate a response as long as a tone is audible. A continuous tone is presented below threshold and increased in 5 dB steps until the patient responds that it is audible. If the patient responds to the tone for 1 full minute, the test is concluded. If the patient does not hear the tone for 1 full minute at that level, the intensity is raised 5 dB and timing is started again. The tone is continually raised in 5 dB steps until an intensity is reached that allows the patient to perceive the tone for 1 full minute or the limit of the audiometer is reached. The amount of threshold tone decay is the difference between the hearing level of the initial response and the level at which the tone was heard for 1 minute. Several modifications of this basic procedure have been suggested to reduce the testing time (Rosenberg, 1958; Green, 1963; Owens, 1964; Olsen and Noffsinger, 1974). The amount of tone decay required for test results to be considered "positive" (suggesting the presence of a retrocochlear lesion) usually exceeds 30 dB (Rosenberg, 1969; Tillman, 1969; Olsen and Noffsinger, 1974). However, the appropriate criterion level is dependent on the psychophysical procedure used. Green (1985) suggests that each dB of decay above 15 dB "should raise the index of suspicion that a retrocochlear lesion may exist" p. 309.

Site-of-Lesion Battery Performance

Realizing no one test may be considered conclusive, audiologists generally agreed that at least three if not all five of the tests in the battery should be conducted in the attempt to provide accurate information in the differential diagnosis of retrocochlear lesions. This test battery would take as long as 1.5 to 2.5 hours. To estimate the accuracy of the test battery in correctly identifying eighth nerve tumors the results of two studies by Johnson (1965, 1977) are presented. He reported auditory test battery results on 110 surgically confirmed retrocochlear lesions in 1965, and on 500 cases in 1977 inclusive of the 1965 cases.

Column A in Table 13.1 shows the results presented in 1965. With the exception of the ABLB, all tests correctly predicted retrocochlear pathology in more than 70% of the affected patients in 1965. Test value was based primarily on the criteria of correct identification of eighth nerve lesions. Therefore by using several tests and weighing heavily any positive result as criteria for medical referral, the correct identification of retrocochlear pathology or "hit rate" was often more than 80%. Column B shows the reported data from 1977 on 500 cases. The most obvious change is the reduction in the hit rate of all tests except tone decay. For speech discrimination the hit rate dropped from 71 to 55%, for Bekesy audiometry 73 to 57%, etc. Only the tone decay test maintained a high hit rate going from 76 to 78%. Johnson attributed this general decrease in the predictive value of these tests to the increasing number of patients identified with an early diagnosis whereas the tumor was "very small" and before it involved the eighth nerve to a very large extent (Johnson, 1977). At this time Johnson reported dropping the SISI test from routine use and advocating the use of tone decay for every case of unilateral sensory-neural hearing loss.

Table 13.1.
Hearing Loss Pattern of Eighth Nerve Tumor Patients and Hit Rate (HR) of Auditory Test Battery Tests Reported by Johnson: 1965, N = 110, 1997, N = 500

	A 1965 Report % of Cases	B 1977 Report % of Cases
Unilateral/asymmetrical hearing loss	95	95
Puretone hearing loss pattern:		
High frequency loss	70	66
Flat loss	20	15
Low frequency loss	6	9
Trough-shaped loss	4	12
Auditory test battery	HR	HR
Speech discrimination ≤30%	71	55
Bekesy audiometry types III and IV	73	57
Short increment sensitivity index test 0—30%	74	55
Alternate binaural loudness balance test no recruitment	60	50
Tone decay test positive (Green 1963)	76	78

Summary

The site-of-lesion test battery of the 1960s established the clinical audiologist as a partner with the otolaryngologist. However, with the increased sensitivity of radiographic techniques and the identification of smaller lesions, the search for better diagnostic audiologic tools continued.

1970s to the Present

Several new and modified psychoacoustical tests were developed in the 1970s for use in the test battery. Space does not permit a review, but the most prominent tests included performance-intensity functions for PB words (Jerger and Jerger, 1971). Bekesy comfortable loudness test (Jerger and Jerger, 1974), and suprathreshold adaptation test (STAT) (Jerger and Jerger, 1975).

Clearly the most important advancement of the decade in site-of-lesion testing was the introduction of clinically feasible objective auditory procedures, specifically the measurement of the acoustic stapedial reflex and reflex decay (Anderson et al. 1969, 1970) and the auditory brainstem response (Selters and Brackmann, 1977). With the increased diagnostic potential of these tests, audiologists are moving from a test battery approach to a select test protocol approach for a differential diagnosis.

Acoustic Reflex

Acoustic reflex threshold testing for the purpose of measuring recruitment was reported as early as 1952 (Metz). However, routine reflex testing did not occur in the United States until electroacoustic immittance (impedance) units were commercially produced, at which time tympanometry became a popular test for middle ear disorders (Liden, 1969; Jerger, 1970). However, it was the report of Anderson et al. (1969) that focused attention to the diagnostic value of elevated/absent acoustic reflexes and abnormal reflex decay in identifying eighth nerve lesions. They noted that when stimulating 17 ears with eighth nerve lesions, the acoustic reflex was absent for 7 ears and elevated for the other 10. Furthermore, when stimulating the ears with a tone 10 dB above reflex threshold for 10 seconds, amplitude for the reflex response decreased by at least one-half within 5 seconds. Other investigators supported these findings (Jerger et al. 1974; Olsen et al. 1975; Sheehy and Inzer, 1976; Chiveralls, 1977; Hall, 1977). A definitive study of the range of the levels of acoustic reflex thresholds to be expected from patients with sensory hearing loss was presented by Silman and Gelfand (1981). Acoustic reflex thresholds higher than their 90th percentile level are considered elevated and raise the suspicion of neural pathology. Olsen et al. (1983) applied the 90th per-

centile criteria of Silman and Gelfand to a group of 30 patients with cerebellopontine angle tumors and a group of 30 patients with cochlear hearing loss configurations matched to the eighth nerve lesion group. The Silman and Gelfand criteria correctly identified 97% of the sensory hearing loss patients and 83% of the eighth nerve lesion patients. In fact, after a review of 23 studies involving 1333 ears with acoustic neuromas, Turner et al. (1984b) reported the combined use of elevated acoustic reflex thresholds and reflex decay yielded a hit rate of 84%. Not only is acoustic reflex testing more sensitive to retrocochlear lesions that the behavioral tests previously discussed, it takes less time and therefore is more economical than the other behavioral tests.

The Auditory Brainstem Response

Sohmer and Feinmesser (1967) are generally recognized as the first to report recording auditory evoked responses from the eighth nerve and brainstem using surface electrodes. Jewett and Williston's 1971 report set the basis for ABR testing by labeling the seven waves found in the first 10 millisecond of the click evoked response. They also noted that wave V had the greatest amplitude, and therefore may be the best to use for clinical comparisons. In the ensuing years ABR, using computerized signal averages, has become commonplace in the hearing clinic. The ABR is popular in assessing hearing when traditional behavioral tests are precluded or their results are equivocal. The importance of the ABR for site-of-lesion testing was initially highlighted by Selters and Brackmann (1977) when they found abnormal ABR findings for 94% of a group of eighth nerve tumor patients (43 of 46 patients). A sample of the subsequent studies supporting the hit rate of abnormal ABR results associated with eighth nerve lesions includes Selters and Brackmann (1979), Glasscock et al. (1981), Terkildsen et al. (1981), and Bauch et al. (1983). These studies presented a total of 283 eighth nerve tumor patients with ABR hit rates ranging from 96 to 98%. Although factors other than severity of hearing loss or eighth nerve lesions on occasion result in abnormal ABR findings (Bauch et al. 1982; Bauch et al., 1983) it is nevertheless clear that the ABR is the most sensitive auditory test available in identifying eighth nerve lesions.

Clinical Decision Analysis

The shift from a differential diagnostic test battery to a more streamlined test protocol approach has not been prompted by the development of objective procedures alone, but has also been due to the implementation of clinical decision analysis (CDA) to audiologic tests (Turner and Nielson, 1984; Turner, Shepard and Frazer, 1984; Turner, Frazer and Shepard, 1984; Turner,

1988). In these authoritative articles the authors explore several methods of calculating the predictive value of diagnostic tests designed to give one of two outcomes: a positive result predictive of a retrocochlear lesion or a negative result predictive of the lack of a retrocochlear lesion (retrocochlear being defined as "abnormalities of the cerebellopontine angle (CPA) including the VIIIth nerve" (Turner and Nielson, p. 125). The results of these tests ultimately fall into four categories: hit rate (HR), miss rate (MR), false alarm rate (FAR), and correct rejection rate (CRR). Hit rate (also referred to as true positive rate or *sensitivity*) is the percentage of patients with retrocochlear lesions correctly identified as positive for the lesion. Miss rate (also referred to as false negative rate) is the percentage of patients with retrocochlear lesions incorrectly identified as negative. False alarm rate (also called false positive rate) is the percentage of patients without retrocochlear lesions incorrectly identified as positive. Correct rejection rate (also called true negative rate or *specificity*) is the percentage of patients without retrocochlear lesions correctly identified as negative.

Although HR and FAR, which may be easily calculated from clinical data, are often all that is needed to determine the superior test, the use of these mutually exclusive values may become confusing. For example, if one test has an HR/FAR of 90/15% and another test has a HR/FAR of 80/15%, the first test is superior having a higher HR with the same FAR. If, however, the second test has a HR/FAR of 88/10%, the first test has a better HR but the second test has a better FAR and test superiority becomes questionable. After a thorough discussion of the relevant variables encountered in CDA, Turner and Nielson suggest that two measures, "d' and "A'" which display test performance as a single number may be useful in addition to the HR/FA, when attempting to rank order tests by performance. d' is a statistical measure of test performance; the larger the d' the better the performance. Specifically for a given test, hit rate, and false alarm rate vary significantly with diagnostic criterion. The ability of a test to distinguish patients is related to the amount of overlap of the probability distribution of the two curves for hit rate and false alarm rate. Technically defined, if the probability distribution curves are Gaussian with equal variance then d' is the difference of the means of the two curves divided by their common standard deviation. If the hit rate and false alarm rate are known, d' may be obtained by the use of published tables (Swets, 1964). A' is a nonparametric measure of test performance proposed by Pollack and Norman (1964). The measure is independent of the shape of the probability distribution curves. A' varies from 0.5 to 1.0 with a better performance being shown by a larger A'. A more complete review of d' and A'r may be found in a

chapter by Robinson and Watson (1972). Table 13.2 shows the calculations of HR, FAR, d', and A' for 11 audiologic site-of-lesion tests. The test data are combined from two tables published by Turner et al. (1984b) and are ranked ordered by HR. Turner et al. (1984b) combined results from as few as 3 studies per test to as many as 23 studies to obtain these data. The symbol "N" by HR and FAR shows the number of ears used to calculate HR and FAR, respectively.

The two objective procedures, auditory brainstem response (ABR) and acoustic reflex threshold and reflex decay tests combined (ARC), ranked first and third, respectively, for calculations of HR, d', and A'. In addition the large sample associated with these measures attests to their clinical popularity in recent years. The FAR was acceptable for all tests and was not discussed separately because it usually increases with increased HR and also because it is accounted for in calculating the d' and A'. The five traditional audiology tests reviewed in Table 13.1 (SD, BEK, SISI, ABLB, and TDT) occupy five of the last six tests ranked by HR in Table 13.2. However, they show a d' of 1.6 or less with an A' of 0.87 or less, suggesting test performance by these measures are clearly below the tests popularized in the 1970s. The performance of the modified traditional tests: SISI-M (the modified SISI test: Thompson, 1963), BCL (Bekesy comfortable loudness, Jerger and Jerger, 1974), FBB (forward backward Bekesy; Rose, 1962; Jerger et al. 1972) and PIPB (performance-intensity function for PB words (Jerger, 1971) scored higher than the traditional tests from which they were modified. Except for SISI-M, the HRs are above

Table 13.2.
Calculations of Hit Rate (HR), False Alarm Rate (FAR), d' and A' for Audiologic Tests in Rank Order by HR[a]

Rank Order HR	Test[b]	N	HR%	N	FAR%	d'	A'
1	ABR	818	95	1,289	11	2.9	0.96
2	BCL	40	85	119	8	2.5	0.94
3	ARC	1,333	84	2,719	15	2.0	0.91
4	PIPB	78	74	184	4	2.4	0.92
5	FBB	51	71	312	5	2.2	0.91
6	TDT	999	70	800	13	1.6	0.87
7	SISIM	286	69	336	10	1.8	0.88
8	SISI	490	65	410	16	1.4	0.83
9	ABLB	511	59	374	10	1.5	0.84
10	BEK	723	49	585	7	1.4	0.83
11	SD	965	45	356	18	0.8	0.73

[a]Data from review of Turner et al. (1984)
[b]Procedure key: ABR, auditory brainstem response; BCL, Bekesy comfortable loudness; ARC, acoustic reflex and reflex decay—combined; PIPB, performance intensity—phonetically balanced words; FBB, forward backward Bekesy; TDT, tone decay test; SISIM, short increment sensitivity index—Modified (Thompson 1963); SISI, short increment sensitivity index; ABLB, alternate binaural loudness balance; BEK, Bekesy audiometry; SD, speech discrimination.

70% (71 to 85), the d' above 2.0 (2.2 to 2.5), and the A' above 0.90 (0.91 to 0.94). Unfortunately the calculations for these behavioral tests are based on a relatively small number of ears, and as the authors point out, "Historically, tests seem to perform best when first developed; performance deteriorates when the test is evaluated by additional clinics. Additional data are needed to clearly demonstrate the superiority of the modified tests." (Turner et al., 1984b, p. 191).

Olsen (1987) presented a hypothetical sample of 1000 patients with sensory-neural hearing loss evaluated because of suspicion of eighth nerve tumors. Using a 5% prevalence rate 50 patients would presumably have eighth nerve lesions, and 950 patients would have sensory (cochlear) hearing losses. Hart and Davenport (1981) report 5% as the average prevalence of acoustic tumors in a clinical population suspected for retrocochlear disease. Table 13.3 shows the number of the hypothetical 1000 patients identified as true positive, false negative, true negative, and false positive by eight of the tests reviewed by Turner et al. (1984b). The test results are rank ordered by true positives. Of these patients, a positive ABR would be expected for 47 of the 50 eighth nerve tumor patients, and 104 of the cochlear hearing loss group. Abnormal acoustic reflex thresholds or reflex decay would be observed for 42 of the 50 eighth nerve lesion patients, and for 142 of the 950 with cochlear hearing loss, etc. According to Olsen's calculations for all of the diagnostic tests, more patients will have false positive identifications than true positive. This is generally true and accepted for screening tests of any type administered to raise suspicion of a pathology having a low prevalence rate.

Based on the 1984 articles, Turner and coworkers recommended that for determining retrocochlear lesions the test battery approach be abandoned in favor of a simple screening protocol that combines an audiologic screening test with a near definitive radiologic test. By definition, a definitive test has a HR/FAR of 100/0%. At present, air contrast (CT) myelography, magnetic resonance imaging (MRI), or MRI with gadolinium-DPTA are accepted as definitive tests (Kileny et al., 1991). Of course even the tests accepted as definitive have their limits. For example, MRI with gadolinium has identified acoustic tumors as small as 2 mm (Kileny et al., 1991). The proposed screening test is the ABR with its HR/FAR of 95/11%. All patients identified as positive by the screening protocol receive the definitive test that will correctly sort these patients into hits (true positive) and correct rejections (true negative). The HR of the total protocol will equal the HR of the screening test. Patients not identified in screening remain undetected because they do not receive the definitive test. The FAR of the total protocol is zero because they are correctly identified by the definitive test. Authors basically sharing this view include Schwartz (1987), Hall (1990), Musiek (personal communication), Kileny et al. (1991), and Ruth and Lambert (1991).

Regardless of the strategy used, clinicians desire to increase the HR of patients receiving the definitive test. A false alarm is preferable to a miss because the false alarm will be detected by the definitive test and the miss will be lost. Table 13.4 is designed to help review test protocol designs that use a single screening test or a battery screening to determine referral for the definitive test. Relative financial costs for each protocol are also included. Protocol evaluations assume a retrocochlear disease prevalence of 5%. The cost value assigned to most of the tests is 1.0 (ARC, ABLB, PIPB, SISI, and TDT); the ABR and the definitive test were given relative values of 5.0 and 20.0, respectively. Columns in Table 13.4 show the test protocols followed by the hit rate of the

Table 13.3.

Audiologic Test Results for Hypothetical Sample of 1000 Sensory-Neural Hearing Loss Patients of Whom 5% have Eighth Nerve Tumors, in Rank Order by True Positive Results[a]

Rank Order True Positives	Test[b]	50 Eighth Nerve Tumor		950 cochlear	
		N True Positives (Hits)	N False Negatives (Misses)	N True Negatives (Correct Rejections)	N False Positives (False Alarms)
1	ABR	47	3	846	104
2	ARC	42	8	808	142
3	PIBP	37	13	912	38
4	TDT	35	15	827	123
5	SISI-M	34	16	855	95
6	SISI	32	18	798	152
7	ABLB	29	21	855	95
8	SD	22	28	827	123

[a]Data from review of Olsen (1987).
[b]ABR, auditory brainstem response; ARC, acoustic reflex and reflex decay—combined; PIPB, performance intensity—phonetically balanced words; TDT, tone decay test; SISI-M, short increment sensitivity index—modified (Thompson 1963); SISI, short increment sensitivity index; ABLB, alternate binaural loudness balance; SD, speech discrimination.

Table 13.4.
Calculations of Predicted Performance for Selected Audiologic Protocols with Associated Hit Rates and False Alarm Rates, and Related Costs of a Hypothetical Sample of 1000 Sensory-Neural Hearing Loss Patients Having 5% Prevalence of Eighth Nerve Lesions[a]

	Protocol	$HR_{Screening}/$ $HR_{Total\ Protocol}$ (%)	$FAR_{Screening}/$ $FAR_{Total\ Protocol}$ (%)	Hypothetical 1000 SN Loss Patients		Total Cost in Units for Patients
				Hits N = 50	False Alarms N = 9501000	
1.	ABR(Pos) = Definitive (DEF)	95/95	11/0	47	104	8,020
2.	ARC(Pos) = DEF	84/84	15/0	42	142	4,680
3.	ARC(Pos) = ABR(Pos) = DEF	82/82	6/0	41	57	3,880
4.	*ABLB*ARC*PIPB*SISI[b] *TDT = DEF	92/92	31/0	46	294	11,800
5.	*ABLB*ARC*PIPB*SISI *TDT = ABR(Pos) = DEF	89/89	8/0	44	76	9,100
6.	ARC(Pos) = DEF (Neg) = ABR(Pos) = DEF	97/97	20/0	48	190	9,840
7.	DEF	100/100	0/0	50	950	20,000

[a]Modified from review of Turner et al. (1984) and Turner (1988).
[b] Between tests means tests in parallel with a loose criterion, therefore, a positive result in any test in the group signifies a positive result for the parallel group of tests.

screening protocol (HR_s) and the hit rate of the total protocol (HR_t). In all examples HR_s and HR_t are equal because any retrocochlear lesion patient missed in the screening portion is lost to the system. The next column shows false alarm rates for screening (FAR_s) and for the total protocol (FAR_t). For the total protocol the false alarms equal zero because all will be correctly identified by the definitive test. The next two columns show the number of hits and false alarms for each protocol for the hypothetical group of 1000 sensory-neural hearing loss patients suspected of having eighth nerve lesions. Note that for all protocols the numbers in these two columns (hits and false alarms) represent patients who are given the definitive test. The final column lists the relative cost of each complete protocol.

In protocol 1, recommended by Turner et al. (1984), all 1000 patients suspected of a retrocochlear lesion are screened by ABR with a HR/FAR of 95/11%. A total of 151 patients (47 hits and 104 false alarms) receive the radiologic definitive test. The relative cost is 8020 units.

In the second protocol, only the ARC is given to the 1000 suspect patients with a HR/FAR of 84/15%. A total of 184 patients (42 hits and 142 false alarms) receive the definitive test. The relative financial cost of this protocol is 4680 units which is only 58% of the total cost of protocol 1 but also misses 2.5 times as many (8 versus 3) of the true eighth nerve tumor patients in this hypothetical sample.

In the third protocol (3), the ARC is given to each suspect patient to determine which patients are tested with ABR. This procedure reduces financial cost even further but HR_t is also reduced to 82% because ARC and ABR are combined in series. In this procedure all 1000 patients are screened by ARC, in addition 184 are also

screened by ABR and finally 98 (41 hits and 57 false alarms) are given the definitive test. The relative cost of this protocol is 3880 units which is less than one-half the cost of protocol 1, but also misses three times as many of the true eighth nerve tumor patients (9 versus 3).

In protocol 4, the audiologic test battery concept is presented. Several traditional audiologic tests are combined in parallel to form the screening protocol. Using a loose referral criterion, i.e., only one of the five tests needs to be positive to refer, the approach increases HR to 92% but also increases the FAR to 31%. If a strict criterion were used (all tests must be positive to refer), the FAR would be reduced less than 4%, but the HR would be an unacceptable 59%. All other criteria for the test battery interpretation would show HR between 92 and 59%. Using the loose criterion, all 1000 patients receive all five screening tests in the battery, with a cost of 1 unit per test. A total of 340 (46 + 294) patients are referred for the radiologic test with a relative cost of 11,800 units. Assuming the protocol assumptions and the relative value scale is not far out of line, it is understandable that many clinicians would favor protocol 1 over 4 considering the increased HR and decreased cost and testing time.

Another scenario would be to combine the traditional test battery with ABR (protocol 5). Using the test battery to determine who receives ABR actually reduces the HR below ABR alone (89% versus 95%) and increases the cost to 9100 units.

Protocol 6 uses what Turner calls a "series-negative" approach within the screening portion of the protocol in that subjects that are negative on the first screening test (ARC) are still given the second screening test (ABR). In this procedure all 1000 patients are given the

ARC and patients testing positive are given the definitive test. Patients negative on the ARC are given the ABR, and subsequent positives are given the definitive test. This series-negative combination yields higher HRs (97%) and higher FARs (20%) than either ARC or ABR alone. The cost in units (9840) comes from 1000 patients being given the ARC, 816 the ABR and 238 definitive tests.

The final example, protocol 7, has the definitive test as the screening test. Consequently, all suspected patients receive the radiologic "gold standard" with its HR/FAR of 100/0% and associated high cost of 20,000 units.

Comments on CDA

This review of CDA was based primarily on a review of the work of Turner and his colleagues and is essentially an academic exercise applying several assumptions to data obtained from a literature review. Consequently, some limitations should be addressed before accepting clinical inferences. One critical assumption deals with test correlation. If two tests both identify the same patients, the tests have maximum-positive correlations. If the two tests identify different patients the tests have maximum-negative correlation. Inasmuch as actual test correlations for the tests evaluated by Turner et al. were not always available, a mid-positive correlation was assumed for all test protocols. For example, in protocol 6 of Table 13.4, the use of a mid-positive correlation assumption led to the conclusion that some patients with eighth nerve lesions will be positive for the ARC, but negative for the ABR. Although experience in our clinic shows that this will happen on occasion (Bauch et al., 1983), the actual correlation between these and other tests need to be validated by clinical studies. Another limitation of CDA as reviewed here is the requirement that test outcomes may only be (+) or (−) for the disorder being identified. This assumption, whereas appropriate for eighth nerve lesion protocols and perhaps for early identification of hearing loss (Jacobsen and Jacobsen, 1987) will not suffice for evaluations of central auditory disorder (Musiek, 1991) or the evaluation of dizzy patients. Key areas not addressed by the presentation on CDA are auditory evaluations of patients with hearing loss too severe to be adequately assessed by ABR and the evaluation of criteria that are used to categorize patients as suspect for retrocochlear lesions in the first place. Realizing that any patient with an eighth nerve tumor seen for an audiologic evaluation but not selected for a site-of-lesion protocol is lost to the system as it now functions; this caution serves to reinforce the need of continued diligence in, and evaluation of, our initial test selection, patient history, and subsequent conclusions.

The use of clinical decision analysis in audiology opens a new era for defining optimum strategies for identification and differential diagnosis of auditory disorders and a conceptual framework for clinical data analysis.

Comment on Immittance

Basic principles and clinical application of acoustic immittance are detailed in chapters 20 and 24; suffice it to say that because the seminal report of Metz (1946) and the clinical classification of tympanograms by Liden (1969) and Jerger (1970), acoustic immittance tests contribute importantly to the assessment of peripheral auditory function.

Immittance measures of tympanometry, static compliance, and the acoustic reflex are of particular value as an integrated part of the basic audiologic evaluation and should be included on the basis of history and initial audiometric results. Strong proponents have suggested immittance measurements be conducted as the initial stage of the basic evaluation and in some instances to replace puretone bone conduction testing (Hall and Ghorayeb, 1991). This author, however, views immittance measures as a strong complement to, but not a replacement for behavioral threshold measures.

Case History

The audiologist is often the first health care professional to evaluate the patient with a hearing loss complaint. This may be in a medical setting where a physician visit usually follows the audiologic evaluation, or an educational or speech and hearing facility where a medical referral is one of several potential outcomes of the evaluation. In any event a case history should be an integral part of each audiologic evaluation as the final diagnosis is based on a combination of case history and test results.

The most efficient history taking occurs as an ongoing part of the audiologic evaluation and follows the medical model. Direct, highly specific, and briefly stated questions are asked prior to the first test administered with additional questions bringing key information into focus between tests. This method provides the maximum amount of information in the minimum amount of time (Rosenberg, 1978). For example, preliminary questions designed to discover the patient's "chief complaint" may be asked as soon as the patient is seated during a brief otoscopic examination. The chief complaint should be recorded exactly as stated by the patient. The otoscopic examination quickly should establish whether the outer ears are anatomically normal, amount of cerumen, and if collapsing canals might be anticipated. By this time the audiologist should have sufficient information to decide the initial audiologic procedure, be it audiometry, immittance, speech testing, or referral for cerumen or foreign body removal.

General questions before audiologic testing may include: Reason for referral or visit? Which is the better ear? Onset of hearing loss, gradual or sudden? Associated pain? Tinnitus? One ear? Both ears? Previous diagnosis and treatment? Family history of hearing loss? Dizziness and vertigo?

Result of the initial audiologic evaluation may lead to more specific areas of inquiry such as: History of occupational and environmental noise exposure; exposure to ototoxic drugs; head injuries; childhood diseases; current medications; allergies.

For a more complete list of question strategies see Wood (1979). In addition to obtaining a history, dialogue with patients helps reveal speech and language abilities and the patient's facility in communication.

The use of long questionnaires to take medical/audiologic history generally should be avoided. A skilled interviewer can follow lines of questioning that produce relevant information and also establish rapport and confidence in the patient-clinician relationship. However, questionnaires have proven valuable with certain complaints such as dizziness where it is important to avoid suggestions that may influence the patient's response. A properly designed questionnaire forces the patient to choose from a list of symptoms those that best describe his or her experiences.

Considerations for recommending hearing aids or assistive listening devices are based in part on the patient's description of communication difficulties as well as test results. Additional questions provide information regarding: listening situations that are difficult; listening in noise versus quiet; listening in groups versus with individuals; telephone use; television listening habits; localization ability; changes in lifestyle associated with hearing problems.

Even when the initial audiologic evaluation fails to document a hearing impairment, sufficient history and discussion of the "chief complaint" should help to determine if further testing is warranted. Recall that negative definitive test results only serve to rule out the given suspect lesion or disorder. For example, central auditory processing disorders will not be ruled out with tests designed to assess dysfunction within the peripheral auditory system.

CONCLUSION

In this chapter, the evolution of audiologic evaluations and test batteries for differential diagnosis over a 70-year period have been reviewed. The puretone audiogram and basic word recognition measures remain the keystone of audiologic assessment, defining the degree and pattern of individual hearing loss and documenting au-

ditory communication difficulties. The development of test batteries is underscored by the rise and fall in popularity of several behavioral tests designed to assist in the determination of cochlear vs retrocochlear dysfunction. At present objective procedures such as immittance and auditory evoked response measures are the tests of choice to assess the site(s) of peripheral auditory lesions. The implementation of clinical decision analysis to auditory testing has led to test protocols that reduce patient time and expense while yielding increased predictive accuracy in suggesting site of lesion over test batteries of the past. As a dynamic profession, audiology has steadily advanced in its partnership with the medical community. It is essential that audiologists continue to keep pace with the expanding technology and continue to help increase our understanding of auditory disorders. Future clinical measures conducted and interpreted by audiologists may include further refinements and developments in physiologic measures of cochlear, eighth nerve, and central nervous system activity via cochlear emissions, electrical measurements of neural activity, and even measurements of blood flow and metabolic rate in response to auditory stimulation.

REFERENCES

American Standard Specifications for Audiometers for General Diagnostic Purposes. Z.24.5-1951, American Standards Association, March 21, 1951.

American Standard Specifications for Pure-Tone Audiometers for Screening Purposes. Z.24.12-1952, American Standards Association. [In Hirsh I. The Measurement of Hearing. 311–314, New York: McGraw-Hill. 1952]

American Standard Specifications for Speech Audiometers. Z.24.13-1953, American Standards Association, July 10, 1953.

Anderson H, Barr B, Wedenberg E. Intra-aural reflexes in retrocochlear lesions. In Hamberger CA and Wersall J, Eds. Nobel Symposium 10, Disorders of the Skull Base Region. Stockholm: Almquist and Wikell. 1969:48–54.

Anderson H, Barr B, and Wedenberg E. Early diagnosis of VIIIth nerve tumors by acoustic reflex tests. Acta Oto-laryngologica 1970; 263:232–237.

Bauch DC, Rose DE, and Harner SG. Auditory brainstem response results from 255 patients with suspected retrocochlear involvement. Ear Hearing 1982;3:83–86.

Bauch CD, Rose DE, and Harner SG. Auditory brainstem response and acoustic reflex test results for patients with and without tumor matched for hearing loss. Arch Otolaryngol 1983;109: 522–525.

Bekesy GV. A new audiometer. Acta Otolaryngol. (Stockh) 1947;45: 411–422.

Black J. The effect of delayed side tone upon vocal rate and intensity. J Speech Hearing Disorders 1951;16:56–60.

Bordley J, and Hardy W. A study in objective audiometry with the use of psychogalvanometric response. Ann Otol Rhinol Laryngol 1949;58:751–760.

Bunch CC. Age variations in auditory acuity. Arch Otolaryngol 1929; 9:625–636

Bunch CC. The diagnosis of occupational or traumatic deafness. A historical and audiometric study. Laryngoscope 1937;47:615.

Carhart R. Clinical application of bone conduction audiometry. Arch Otolaryngol 1950;51:798–808.

Carhart R. Speech audiometry in clinical evaluation. Acta Otolaryngol (Stockh) 1952;41:18–42.

Carhart R. Clinical determination of abnormal auditory adaptation. Arch Otolaryngol 1957;65:32–40.

Chiveralls K. A further examination of the use of the stapedius reflex in the diagnosis of acoustic neuroma. Audiology 1977; 16:331–337.

Davis H. Hearing and Deafness. Rinehart & Company, New York, 1947.

Davis H. The articulation area and the social adequacy index for hearing. Laryngoscope 1948;58:761–778.

Dean CE. Audition by bone conduction. J Acoust Soc Am 1930; 2:281–296.

Denes P, and Naunton RF. The clinical detection of auditory recruitment. J Laryngol Otol 1950;64:375–398.

Dix MR, Hallpike CS, and Hood JD. (1948). Observations upon the loudness recruitment phenomenon with especial reference to the differential diagnosis of disorders of the internal ear and VIIIth nerve. J Laryngol Otol 1948;62:671–686.

Doerfler LG. Neurophysiological clues to auditory acuity. J Speech Hearing Disorders 1948;13:227–232.

Doerfler LGT, and Epstein A. The Doerfler-Stewart (D-S) test for functional hearing loss. Monograph submitted to the Veterans Administration, 1956.

Doerfler LG, and Stewart K. Malingering and psychogenic deafness. J Speech Disorders 1946;11:181–186.

Eagan J. (1948). Articulation testing methods. Laryngoscope 1948;58:955–991.

Feldman H. A history of audiology, a comprehensive report and bibliography from the earliest beginnings to the present. In Tonndorf J, Ed. Trans for Beltone Institute for Hearing Research 1970;22:1P 1–111 [Translated by J. Tonndorf from Die Geschichtliche Entwicklung der Horprufungsmethoden, kuze Darstellung and Bibliographie von der Anfongen bis zur Gegenwart. In H. Leicher, R. Mittermaiser, Ohren-Heilkunde. Stuttgart: Georg Thieme Verlag, 1960.]

Fletcher H, and Steinberg JC. Articulation testing methods. Bell Systems Tech J 1929;7:806–854.

Fowler EP. Marked deafened areas in normal ears. Arch Otolaryngol 1928;8:151–156.

Fowler EP. A method for the early detection of otosclerosis. Arch Otolaryngol 1936;24:731–741.

Fowler EP. The diagnosis of diseases of the neural mechanisms of hearing by the aid of sounds well above threshold. Transact Am Otol Soc 1937;27:207–219.

Fowler EP. The use of threshold and louder sounds in clinical diagnosis and the prescribing of hearing aids. New methods for accurately determining the threshold for bone conduction and for measuring tinnitus and its effects on obstructive and neural deafness. Laryngoscope 1938;48:572–588.

Fowler EP, and Wegel RL. Presentation of a new instrument for determining the amount and character of auditory sensation. Transact Am Otol Soc 1922a;16:105–123.

Fowler EP, and Wegel RL. Audiometric methods and their applications. Transactions of the 28th Annual Meeting of the American Laryngological, Rhinological and Otological Society, 1922b; 98–132.

Glasscock ME, Jackson CG, and Josey AF. Brain Stem Electric Response Audiometry. New York: Grune and Stratton, 1981.

Goodhill V (1955). Surgical audiometry in stapedolysis (stapes mobilization). Arch Otolaryngol 1955;62:504–508.

Green DS. The modified tone decay test (MTDT) as a screening procedure for eighth nerve lesions. J Speech Hearing Disorders 1963; 28:31–36.

Green DS. Tone decay. In Katz J, Ed. Handbook of Clinical Audiology. Baltimore: Williams & Wilkins; 1985:304–318.

Greenbaum A, Kerridge B, and Ross E. Normal hearing by bone conduction. J Laryngol Otol 1939;59:88–92.

Guttman J. A new method of determining unilateral deafness and malingering. Laryngoscope 1928;38:686–687.

Hall CM. Stapedial reflex decay in retrocochlear and cochlear lesions. Ann Otol Rhinol Laryngol 1977;86:219–222.

Hall JW (1990) Classic site-of-lesion tests: Foundation of diagnostic audiology. In Rintelmann WF, Ed. Hearing Assessment, 2nd Ed. Austin, TX: Pro-Ed, 1990:653–677.

Hall JW, and Ghorayeb BY. Diagnosis of middle ear pathology and evaluation of conductive hearing loss, In Jacobson JT, and Northern JL, Eds. Diagnostic Audiology. Austin, TX: Pro-Ed, 1991: 161–198.

Harbert F (1943). Functional and simulated deafness. Navy Med Bull 1943;2,3:458–471, 717–728.

Hart R, and Davenport J. Diagnosis of acoustic neuroma. Neurosurgery 1981;9:450–463.

Hirsh IJ, Davis H, Silverman SR, Reynolds EG, Eldert TE, and Benson RW. Development of materials for speech audiometry. J Speech Hearing Disorders 1952;17:321–337.

Hirsh IJ, Palva T, and Goodman A. Difference limen and recruitment. Arch Otolaryngol 1954;60:525–540.

Hudgins CV, Hawkins JE, Karlin JE, and Stevens SS. The development of recorded auditory tests for measuring hearing loss for speech. Laryngoscope 1947;57:57–89.

Hughes RL, Winegar WJ, and Crabtree JA. Bekesy audiometry: Type 2 versus type 4 patterns. Arch Otolaryngol 1967;86:424–430.

Hughson W, and Thompson EA. Correlation of hearing acuity for speech with discrete frequency audiograms. Arch Otolaryngol 1942;36:526–540.

Jacobson TJ, and Jacobson CA. Principles of decision analysis in high risk infants. Semin Hearing 1987;8:133–141.

Jerger J. A difference limen recruitment test and its diagnostic significance. Laryngoscope 1952;62:1316–1332.

Jerger J. DL difference test: an improved method for the clinical measurement of recruitment. Arch Otolaryngol 1953;57:490–500.

Jerger J. Bekesy audiometry in analysis of auditory disorders. J Speech Hearing Res 1960;3:275–287.

Jerger J. Hearing tests in otologic diagnosis. ASHA 1962;4:139–145.

Jerger J. Clinical experience with impedance audiometry. Arch Otolaryngol 1970;92:311–324.

Jerger J, Carhart R, and Lassman J. Clinical observations on excessive threshold adaptation. Arch Otolaryngol 1958;68:617–623.

Jerger J, Harford E, Clemis J, and Alford B. The acoustic reflex in eighth nerve disorders. Arch Otolaryngol 1974;99:409–413.

Jerger J, and Jerger S. Critical off-time in VIIIth nerve disorders. J Speech Hearing Res 1966;9:573–580.

Jerger J, and Jerger S. Diagnostic significance of PB word functions. Arch Otolaryngol 1971;93:573–580.

Jerger J, Jerger S, and Mauldin L. The forward and backward discrepancy in Bekesy audiometry. Arch Otolaryngol 1972;96: 400–406.

Jerger J, and Jerger S. Diagnostic value of Bekesy comfortable loudness tracings. Arch Otolaryngol 1974;99:351–360.

Jerger J, and Jerger S. A simplified tone decay test. Arch Otolaryngol 1975;101:403–407.

Jerger J, Shedd J, and Harford E. On the detection of extremely small changes in sound intensity. Arch Otolaryngol 1959; 69:200–211.

Jewett DL, and Williston JS. Auditory evoked far fields averaged from the scalp of humans. Brain 1971;94:861–896.

Johnson EW. Auditory test results in 500 cases of acoustic neuroma. Arch Otolaryngol 1977;103:152–158.

Johnson EW. Auditory test results in 110 surgically confirmed retrocochlear lesions. J Speech Hearing Disorders 1965;30: 307–317.

Johnson KO, Work WP, and McCoy G. Functional deafness. Ann Otol Rhinol Laryngol 1956;65:154–170.

Jones IH, and Knudson VO. Functional tests of hearing. Transactions of the 30th Annual Meeting of the American Laryngological, Rhinological, and Otological Society. 1924;6:121--136.

Katz J, Ed. Handbook of Clinical Audiology. Baltimore: Williams & Wilkins, 1972.

Kileny PR, Telian SA, and Kemink JL. Acoustic neuroma: Diagnosis and management. In Jacobson JT, and Northern JL, Eds., Diagnostic Audiology. Austin, TX: Pro-Ed, 1991;217–233.

Lee B. Some effects of side-tone delay. J Acoust Soc Am 1950; 22:639–640.

Liden G. The scope and application of current audiometric tests. J Laryngol Otol 1969;83:507–520.

Lierle DM, and Reger SN. Experimentally induced temporary threshold shifts in ears with impaired hearing. Ann Otol Rhinol Laryngol 1955;64:263–277.

Lund-Iverson L. An investigation on the difference limen determined by the method of Luscher and Zwislocki in normal hearing and in various forms of deafness. Acta Otolaryngol (Stockh) 1952;42: 219–224.

Luscher E, and Zwislocki J. A simple method of monaural determination of the recruitment phenomenon. Pract Oto-Rhinolaryngol 1948;10:521–522.

Metz O. The acoustic impedance measured on normal and pathological ears. Acta Otolaryngol (Stockh) 1946;(Suppl):63

Metz O. Threshold of reflex contractions of muscles of middle ear and recruitment of loudness. Arch Otolaryngol 1952;55:536–543.

Michaels MW, and Randt CT. Galvanic skin response in the differential diagnosis of deafness. Arch Otolaryngol 1947;65:302–311.

Musiek FE (1990). Auditory evoked responses in site-of-lesion assessment. In Rintelmann WF, Ed. Hearing Assessment, 2nd Ed. Austin, TX: Pro-Ed, 1990:383–427.

Newby HA. Audiology. New York: Appleton-Century-Crafts Inc, 1958.

Olsen WO. Differential audiology tests. In Robinette MS, and Bauch CD, Eds. Proceedings of a Symposium in Audiology. Rochester, MN: Mayo Clinic, 1987.

Olsen WO, Bauch CD, and Harner SG. Application of Silman and Gelfand 90th percentile levels for acoustic reflex thresholds. J Speech Hearing Disorders 1983;48:330–332.

Olsen WO, and Noffsinger D. Comparison of one new and three old tests of auditory adaptation. Arch Otolaryngol 1974;99:94–99.

Olsen WO, Noffsinger D, and Kurdziel S. Acoustic reflex and reflex decay occurrence in patients with cochlear and eighth nerve lesions. Arch Otolaryngol 1975;101:622–625.

Olsen WO, Stach B, and Kurdziel S. Acoustic reflex decay in 10 seconds and in 5 seconds for Meniere's disease patients and for VIII nerve tumor patients. Ear Hearing 1981;2:180–181.

Owens E (1964). Tone decay in eighth nerve and cochlear lesions. J Speech Hearing Disorders 1964;29:14–22.

Pohlman AG, and Kranz F. Binaural minimum audition in a subject with ranges of deficient acuity. Proc Soc Exp Biol Med 1924;20: 335–337.

Pollack I, and Norman DA. A non-parametric analysis of recognition experiments. Psychonomic Sci 1964;1:125–126.

Reger SN. (1936). Differences in loudness response of the normal and hard of hearing ears at intensity levels slightly above threshold. Ann Otol Rhinol Laryngol 1936;45:1024–1039.

Reger SN. A clinical and research version of the Bekesy audiometer. Laryngoscope 1952;62:1333–1351.

Reger SN, and Kos CM. Clinical measurements and implications of recruitment. Ann Otol Rhinol Laryngol 1952;61:810–820.

Report of the Council on Physical Therapy. Tentative minimum requirements for acceptable audiometers. JAMA 1937;109:1812.

Riach W, Elliott DN, and Reed SC. Growth of loudness and its relationship to intensity discrimination under various levels of auditory fatigue. J Acoust Soc Am 1962;34:1764–1767.

Robinson DE, and Watson CS. Psychophysical methods in modern psychoacoustics. In Tobias JV Ed. Foundations of Modern Auditory Theory. New York: Academic Press, 1972:101–131.

Rose DE. Some effects and case histories of reversed frequency sweep in Bekesy audiometry. J Audiotory Res 1962;2:267–278.

Rosenberg PE. Rapid Clinical Measurement of Tone Decay. Presented at the Annual Convention of the American Speech and Hearing Association, New York, 1958.

Rosenberg PE. Tone Decay. Maico Audiol Library Series 1969;7: Report 6.

Rosenberg PE. Case history: The first test. In Katz J, Ed. Handbook of Clinical Audiology, 2nd Ed. Baltimore: Williams & Wilkins, 1978:60–66.

Ruth RA, and Lambert PR. Evaluation and diagnosis of cochlear disorders. In Jacobsen JT, and Northern JL, Eds. Diagnostic Audiol. Austin, TX: Pro-Ed, 1991:199–215.

Sanders JW, Josey AF, and Glasscock ME. Audiologic evaluation in cochlear and eighth nerve disorders. Arch Otolaryngol 1974;100: 283–293.

Schwartz DM. Neurodiagnositic audiology: Contemporary perspectives. Ear Hearing 1987;8:(Suppl).

Seashore CE. An audiometer. University of Iowa studies in Psychology, No. 2. Iowa City: University of Iowa Press, 1899.

Selters WA, Brackmann DE. Acoustic tumor detection with brainstem electric response audiometry. Arch Oolaryngol 1977;103:15–24.

Selters WA, and Brackmann DE. Brainstem electric response audiometry in acoustic tumor detection. In House WF, and Leutje CM, Eds. Acoustic Tumors: Vol. 1 Diagnosis. Baltimore: University Park Press, 1979;225–235.

Shambaugh GE, and Carhart R. Contributions of audiology to fenestration surgery, including a formula for the precise prediction of the hearing result. Arch Otolaryngol 1951;54:699–712.

Sheehy J, and Inzer B. Acoustic reflex in neuro-otologic diagnosis. Arch Otolaryngol 1976;102:647–653.

Silman S, and Gelfand SA. The relationship between magnitude of hearing loss and acoustic reflex threshold levels. J Speech Hearing Disorders 1981;46:312–316.

Sohmer H, and Feinmesser M. Cochlear action potentials recorded from the external ear in man. Ann Otol Rhinol Laryngol 1967;76:427–438.

Stevens SS, Morgan CT, and Volkmann J. Theory of the neural quantum in the discrimination of loudness and pitch. Am J Psychol 1941;54:315–345.

Swets JA. Signal Detection and Recognition by Human Observers. New York: John Wiley, 1964.

Terkildsen K, Osterhammel P, and Thomsen J. The ABR and MLR in patients with acoustic neuromas. Scand Audiol 1981; (Suppl)13:103–107.

Thompson GA. A modified SISI technique for selected cases with suspected acoustic neurinoma. J Speech Hearing Disorders 1963;28: 299–302.

Thurlow WR, Davis H, Silverman SR, and Walsh TE. Further statistical study of auditory tests in relation to the fenestration operation. Laryngoscope 1949;59:113–129.

Tillman TW. Special hearing tests in otoneurologic diagnosis. Arch Otolaryngol 1969;89:51–56.

Tillman TW, and Carhart R. An expanded test for speech discrimination utilizing CNC monosyllabic words. Brooks Air Force Base, TX: USAF School of Aerospace Medicine Technical Report, 1966.

US Public Health Service. Preliminary Report of the National Health Survey Hearing Study Series. US Public Health Service Bulletin, no. 5, 1935–1936.

Turner RG. Techniques to determine test protocol performance. Ear Hearing 1988;9:177–189.

Turner RG, Frazer GS, and Shepard NT. Formulating and evaluating audiological test protocols. Ear Hearing 1984a;5:321–330.

Turner RG, and Nielsen DW. Application of clinical decision analysis to audiological tests. Ear Hearing 1984;5:125–133.

Turner RG, Shapard FT, and Frazer CJ. Clinical performance of audiological and related diagnostic tests. Ear Hearing 1984b;5:187–194.

Wood RP. History taking in otorhinolaryngology. In Wood RR, and Northern JL, Eds. Manual of Otolaryngology: A Symptom-Oriented Text. Baltimore: Williams & Wilkins, 1979.

BEHAVIORAL EVALUATION
Central Auditory Functions

CHAPTER 14

Central Auditory Assessment : An Overview

Frank E. Musiek and Lloyd Lamb

Audiologic evaluation of the central auditory nervous system (CANS) is a relatively recent development, dating to the work of Bocca and his colleagues in the mid-1950s (Bocca et al., 1954; Bocca et al., 1955). This challenging endeavor has piqued the interest of numerous investigators but, for a number of reasons, has been slow to gain acceptance throughout the audiology community in general. One factor that has contributed to this delay is the complexity of the system under consideration. Even now the anatomy and physiology of the CANS are not completely understood, nor have its many different functions been adequately defined. The effects of CANS disorders often are quite subtle and test results may be highly variable. Moreover, there currently is a lack of standardization among clinical facilities in terms of central auditory tests and procedures, leading to a certain amount of confusion and disagreement as to what tests are most appropriate and effective.

In spite of these problems, interest in central auditory assessment seems to be increasing steadily. There is a growing body of literature showing the efficacy of both behavioral and electrophysiologic tests in identifying CANS disorders. Research with electrophysiologic techniques such as the mid-latency response (MLR) (Kraus et al., 1982; Kileny et al., 1987), the P300 event related potential (Obert and Cranford, 1990; Musiek et al., 1992), and brain electrical activity mapping (BEAM) (Duffy et al., 1981) is helping to define auditory responsive areas of the brain and further delineate normal and abnormal function. Advances in neurochemistry and neuropharmacology, particularly in the study of neurotransmitters, are contributing to our understanding of the CANS as well as the cochlea and auditory nerve (Musiek, 1989; Musiek and Hoffman, 1990). This general area of investigation should not only add to our understanding of CANS function but, theoretically, could lead to the development of pharmacological therapies for the amelioration of various auditory disorders (Musiek, 1989; Musiek and Hoffman, 1990). Further, there is evidence of increasing attention to CANS disorders by other professions, such as pediatric psychology, neuropsychology, neurology, and special education. A review of the literature of these and other professional groups revealed numerous articles dealing with issues relevant to normal and abnormal central auditory func-

tion, some of which bear directly upon topics covered in this chapter (Scherg and Von Cramon, 1986; Altman et al., 1987; Sanger et al., 1987; Corballis and Ogden, 1988; Mendez and Geehan, 1988; Secord et al., 1988; Demarco et al., 1989).

Our goal in this chapter is to present an overview of behavioral assessment of the central auditory system. First, we will consider reasons for evaluating the central auditory system as well as prerequisites for effective CANS study. Next, variables that influence central auditory assessment will be reviewed. Brief sections will address central testing of the elderly and with learning disabled children as well as applications in monitoring neurologically involved patients. The largest portion of the chapter will be devoted to specific test principles and applications in indentification and diagnosis of CANS disorders.

EVIDENCE OF NEED FOR CENTRAL AUDITORY EVALUATION

In an age of such sophisticated diagnostic tools as computed tomography (CT) scanning and magnetic resonance imaging (MRI), one might wonder about the need for neuroaudiological tests for diagnosis of CNS lesions. Keith (1983), in speculating on the future of audiology in central auditory assessment, has questioned whether the audiologist's role should lie in the prospective differential diagnosis of central nervous system (CNS) lesions or rather in describing central auditory abilities in brain-damaged adults and language-learning disabled children for purposes of remediation and education. In the authors' view it should not be an either/or situation. There is evidence that audiologists have an important contribution to make in both areas.

First, it should be remembered that the audiologist may represent the point of entry into the health care system for patients with a variety of central auditory problems. In many instances peripheral hearing will be normal, but appropriate central testing may identify higher level disorders and thus lead to medical referral. Costs, too, may be a factor in the selection of test procedures. In this regard the relative cost of central auditory testing compared with more expensive radiological or neurological procedures may make central auditory evaluation (CAE) an appropriate first choice in the diagnostic hierarchy. One should also be aware that current radiologic or magnetic imaging techniques may not be available to all patients, nor can all patients be tested with these techniques. Further, not all lesions or pathologic conditions are detectable with these techniques. Various degenerative diseases, biochemical changes, and a host of minimal neurological deficits, either acquired or congenital, may affect higher auditory processes (Dublin, 1976) but be invisible to many neurologic or radiologic studies. When these conditions occur, appropriate central auditory evaluation may provide clinical insights that cannot be obtained through other diagnostic avenues.

Further underscoring the need for central auditory evaluation is the fact that the CANS may be affected secondarily to other disorders. For example, animal research has shown that degeneration of central auditory fibers can result from auditory deprivation, cochlear ablation, and middle ear effusion (Webster and Webster, 1977), destruction of the cochlea and/or auditory nerve (Jean-Baptiste and Morest, 1975; Morest et al., 1979), noise-induced hearing loss (Theopold, 1975; Morest, 1982), and ototoxic drugs (Magee and Olszewski, 1962; Hall, 1976).

In humans, aging has been shown to result in defects of both the peripheral and central auditory systems (Hinchcliffe, 1962). Numerous examples of atrophy and degeneration of auditory areas in the brainstem and cortex have been reported in cases of presbycusis (Brody, 1955; Kirikae et al., 1964; Schuknecht, 1964; Hansen and Reske-Nielsen, 1965). For a review of auditory system defects associated with aging, the reader is directed to Gulya (1990).

There are still other disorders that may or may not affect hearing but that often result in indirect or secondary effects on the CANS. One of the most obvious is the large acoustic tumor that compresses or displaces the brainstem (Musiek, 1982). The compression could lead to hydrocephalus, which in turn could affect cortical function, or the compression could produce vascular constriction, which could compromise the brainstem or cerebrum. Other examples are head trauma and edema that might contuse, compress, or displace brain tissue far from the point of insult. Lesions such as these are capable of affecting higher auditory function in a variety of ways. In short, there are many disorders that can affect the CANS either directly or indirectly. In many instances peripheral and central auditory manifestations are so entwined that it is difficult to separate the two areas using current tests. Hence, one must always be aware of the possibility of secondary central effects.

Another area in which the CAE can provide valuable information is in monitoring the neurologic and auditory status of selected patients. Among possible monitoring applications are pre- and post-surgical testing to determine any changes in auditory function (Musiek et al., 1990b), examining central auditory abilities in patients with treatable and nontreatable CNS conditions (Musiek and Morgan, 1981), following the progress of patients with head injury (Hall et al., 1982; Harris and Hall, 1990), helping predict recovery in comatose patients (Yingling et al., 1990), and monitoring the progress of patients during rehabilitation. In addition, central testing may help document auditory function in patients with known CNS damage where an auditory problem is suspected.

While there are some commonalities among children and adults in terms of central test findings and underlying problems, the needs for CAE with children are largely different than those with adults. As with adults, some children may have medically significant neurologic conditions that could be heralded by abnormal central auditory function. Thus, CAE may result in early identification and appropriate medical referral (Musiek et al., 1985a). However, the greatest need at present seems to be in identifying and defining central auditory processing (CAP) disorders in learning-disabled (LD) children for purposes of education and remediation.

Finally, on both a practical and philosophical note, it should be emphasized that hearing, in its broadest sense, involves much more than just peripheral sensitivity and acuity. Thus, audiologists should be prepared to evaluate the function of the entire auditory system, not just the peripheral portion.

PREREQUISITES FOR STUDY OF CENTRAL AUDITORY NERVOUS SYSTEM FUNCTION

Clinical assessment of central auditory function requires broad knowledge in a number of academic areas as well as skills and insights that can be gained only through direct clinical experience. First, and perhaps foremost, those involved in CAE should be well versed in anatomy and physiology of the CANS and should understand and appreciate its subtlety and complexity. They should also be familiar with the pathologic conditions that can affect the central auditory system either directly or indirectly. Knowledge of normal anatomy and physiology and types and manifestations of CANS disorders can provide invaluable guidance in selection and interpretation of central auditory tests (see Brugge and Geisler, 1978; Keidel et al., 1983; Moller, 1983; Musiek, 1986a; 1986b; Musiek and Baran, 1986; Pickles, 1988). Discussion of CNS pathologies are also available (see Dublin, 1976; Neely, 1983; Reeves, 1985).

To understand the rationale, interpretation, and possible limitations of many central tests it is helpful if the clinician is familiar with both theories and research regarding speech perception (Spitzer, 1983). They should also be aware of the various central auditory abilities these tests purport to measure and the relevance of these abilities. Those interested in central auditory processing disorders in children will find a knowledge of learning disabilities and language development and disorders to be helpful. The clinician should be familiar with a wide variety of central tests in terms of their sensitivity and specificity, and should be comfortable in their administration and interpretation. Finally, those involved in central auditory assessment should be aware of the many variables that can influence an evaluation and their possible effects on test results.

VARIABLES INFLUENCING CENTRAL AUDITORY ASSESSMENT

In general, central auditory test variables fall into two categories: procedural variables, e.g., those having to do with instrumentation, test materials, test norms, etc., and subject, or patient, variables. If one is not mindful of these variables, test results can lead to a false impression of central auditory abilities.

Procedural Variables

When attempting to measure central auditory function in either normal or pathologic subjects, the use of a test battery is essential. The evaluation should include a case history, complete peripheral hearing assessment, as well as behavioral and electrophysiologic tests as needed to sample a variety of brainstem and cortical auditory functions (Pinheiro and Musiek, 1985).

One of the most important considerations in CAE is the availability of appropriate normative data for the various tests being used. Populations used for normative studies should reflect a wide range of ages, vocations, education, and socioeconomic levels. Linguistic factors should also be considered when establishing norms, as should the overall intelligence and medical history (specifically audiologic and neurologic aspects) of the subjects. Peripheral hearing must be carefully quantified to meet predetermined criteria. In addition, though norms may be available for a given test, it is always wise to collect one's own normative data for comparison purposes.

Properly maintained and calibrated equipment is essential to assure reliable and valid central auditory measurements (Carver, 1983; see Chapter 6). Careful attention must be given to eliminating noise or distortion that might influence test results. Tape recorded materials should be monitored for acoustical clarity and accuracy. If possible, dichotic test materials should be checked for proper temporal alignment and balance. Test tapes should be stored appropriately to preserve their quality. Finally, the test environment should be acoustically controlled to minimize the effects of environmental noise.

Patient Variables

A major factor in central auditory assessment is the effect of peripheral hearing loss on test performance. Decreased central test scores associated with peripheral loss have been reported for a variety of tests including the following: time compressed consonant-vowel-consonant monosyllables (Kurdziel et al., 1976); low pass filtered speech, rapidly alternating speech, dichotic sentences, and binaural fusion (Miltenberger et al., 1978); dichotic digits and dichotic consonant-vowels (Roeser et al., 1976). While most central auditory tests, especially those involving speech stimuli, are susceptible to contamination by peripheral loss, some tests seem to be more resistant than others. Speaks et al. (1985) studied the effects of hearing loss on four dichotic tests (digits, vowel words, consonant words, and CV syllables) and found dichotic digits to be only slightly affected by peripheral loss. From this they concluded that the dichotic digits test holds promise as a test of central auditory function even in the presence of peripheral loss. Similar claims have been made for the dichotic sentence identification (DSI) test (Fifer et al., 1983) based on findings with normal and hearing impaired subjects and patients with known or suspected lesions involving retrocochlear structures. Speaks et al. (1990) have recommended use of a monotic screening test (MST) to indicate when peripheral hearing loss is likely to produce ambiguous dichotic test results and whether a test intensity referenced to the speech reception threshold (SRT) is appropriate.

While dichotic digits and the DSI test have proven to be relatively resistant to peripheral hearing loss, there are other central tests that at times may circumvent this problem entirely. One such test is the auditory duration pattern test. In its current form, this test requires that the patient identify duration patterns (e.g., long-long-short) of tonal pulses presented at 1000 Hz. Musiek et al. (1990a) have shown duration patterns to be highly sensitive to cerebral lesions while mild to moderate cochlear hearing losses seem to have little or no effect on test results (Fig. 14.1). It is reasonable to assume that the duration pattern test could be modified to use other test frequencies for cases in which hearing loss at 1000 Hz might be sufficiently severe to preclude testing. Certain electrophysiologic tests, including the MLR (Thornton et al., 1977) and P300 (Squires and Hecox, 1983) can also be carried out using tonal stimuli of various frequencies, thus at times allowing the clinician to avoid the effects of peripheral loss by testing at the ears most sensitive or bilaterally equivalent frequencies. With the auditory brainstem response (ABR), lower frequency

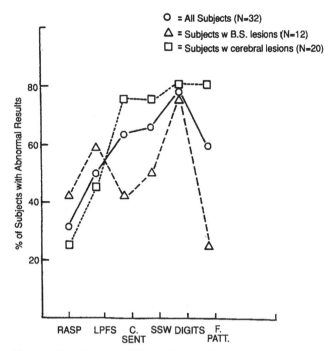

Figure 14.1. Percentage of subjects with confirmed brainstem and/or cerebral lesions that yielded abnormal results in at least one ear for the rapidly alternating speech perception (**RASP**), low pass filtered speech (**LPFS**), competing sentences (**C. SENT**) staggered spondaic words (**SSW**), dichotic digits (**DIGITS**) and frequency patterns (**F. PATT**) tests.

tone pips might be used to avoid possible effects of high frequency hearing loss (Telian and Kileny, 1989). In addition, ABR measures such as I-V, I-III, and III-V interwave latencies (IWL) and the wave V interaural latency difference (ILD) often can be obtained in spite of peripheral loss, providing valuable indices of brainstem function (Starr and Achor, 1975; Selters and Brackmann, 1977, 1979).

Age also has been shown to influence central auditory test results. Maturational effects have been noted on almost all central tests, requiring that normative data be obtained with children at each year under approximately 12—14 years (Musiek et al., 1990c). Many elderly patients, too, show reduced central test scores, presumably due to degenerative changes within the CANS (Jerger and Hayes, 1977; Stach, 1990). In light of these findings, it is critical that age-appropriate norms be used in central auditory assessment.

Among other patient characteristics of which the clinician must be aware are intellignce and linguistic background. While the effects of intelligence on central tests are not well documented, there is evidence of reduced scores on sensitized speech tests with persons of lower than normal intelligence (Bocca, 1967). Similarly, linguistic background has been shown to be a factor in reducing scores obtained with sensitized speech tests

(Davis et al., 1976; Gat and Keith, 1978) and may be an important consideration in attempting to measure central auditory abilities (Keith, 1982).

TEST FINDINGS WITH CENTRAL AUDITORY PATHOLOGY

The high level of both structural and functional redundancy in the brain serves to make the detection and localization of specific lesions a difficult task. At levels above the cochlear nucleus there is dual representation of both ears via multiple neural interconnections (Whitfield, 1967). Despite this, general trends found in central auditory test data can provide insights as to whether the brainstem, cortex, or interhemispheric areas are involved. In this section we will present an overview of test findings from some of the older as well as more recent tests as they relate to lesions in various areas of the brain. In addition, some of the more recent procedures will be described briefly. Before proceeding, however, we would like to emphasize one point. With the availability of advanced radiologic and magnetic imaging techniques, it is now possible to validate central test findings relative to a number of specific lesions. While, as suggested earlier, tests such as CT scanning and MRI may not be equally sensitive to all CNS disorders, nonetheless they should be used whenever possible to help determine the accuracy of central auditory tests. Only by relating central test findings to data on cases with known lesions can the true sensitivity and specificity of central tests be determined.

Brainstem Lesions

Because the auditory brainstem is so complex and compact a variety of central auditory effects can be found depending on the specific area and extent of involvement (Calearo and Antonelli, 1968; Parker et al., 1968; Stephens and Thornton, 1976; Lynn and Gilroy, 1977). There are a few tests such as the ABR (see Chapter 24), masking level differences (MLDs) (Olsen and Noffsinger, 1976; Lynn et al., 1981), binaural fusion (Matzker, 1959; Smith and Resnick, 1972; Willeford and Bilger, 1978), rapidly alternating speech perception (RASP) (Lynn and Gilroy, 1977), and synthetic sentence indentification with ipsilateral competing message (SSI-ICM) (Jerger and Jerger, 1975) that reportedly are sensitive to brainstem lesions but largely unaffected by cortical disorders. In our own experience there is some question as to the sensitivity of the RASP and binaural fusion tests for detection of brainstem lesions. Though these tests seem to be generally unaffected by hemispheric involvement (Musiek and Geurkink, 1982), this may be a function of their poor sensitivity. Several other tests have been shown to be of value in identifying both brainstem and cortical lesions but are unable to differentiate between the two areas. These include low pass filtered speech (LPFS) (Calearo and Antonelli, 1968; Stevens and Thornton, 1976; Musiek and Geurkink, 1982), dichotic digits (Stevens and Thornton, 1976; Musiek and Geurkink, 1982), competing sentences (Musiek and Geurkink, 1982), time compressed speech (Calearo and Antonelli, 1968), and various sound localization tests (Nordlund, 1964; Bosatra and Russolo, 1976; Stevens and Thornton, 1976; Liden and Rosenthal, 1981) to mention a few. The Staggered Spondaic Words Test (Katz, 1978), on the other hand, has been reported not only to differentiate brainstem from cortical lesions but also to yield different patterns for upper and lower brainstem lesions. Figure 14.1 illustrates results obtained using a battery of six behavioral central tests to evaluate patients with a variety of confirmed CNS lesions.

Any comprehensive approach to brainstem assessment would, of necessity, involve the use of both physiologic and psychoacoustical measures. While the ABR is probably the most sensitive and specific test for brainstem lesions in general, its contribution seems to be limited primarily to disorders that affect the pons. Thus, it is important to include other tests if one is interested in more rostral aspects of the brainstem (Musiek et al., 1988). Musiek et al. (1989a) evaluated a seven test battery with a group of patients with multiple sclerosis (MS) and found that ABR combined with MLDs or with the dichotic digits test was essentially as sensitive as the entire battery. Jerger et al. (1986), using a somewhat different test battery, reported that acoustic reflex measures (absolute threshold, absolute amplitude, relative amplitude, onset latency, and offset latency) and a combination of speech audiometry measures (intensity function, SSI-ICM, and DSI) yielded the best detection rate for MS patients. Here one should be aware that auditory effects of MS may sometimes extend beyond brainstem structures.

While interaural timing procedures have not been used routinely in clinical CANS assessment, they nonetheless seem to hold promise as tests of brainstem function (Musiek et al., 1988). Hausler and Levine (1980) studied interaural time discrimination in MS patients using a two alternative forced choice paradigm. The experimental task involved judging whether noise bursts were displaced to the left or right of a reference as stimulus lead-lag times were varied in the two ears. Eleven of 19 normal-hearing MS patients yielded abnormal results on this task. Interestingly, these same patients also had distorted ABRs with the most obvious ABR abnormalities in general being found in patients with the greatest timing disorders. Matathias et al (1985) also studied interaural timing disorders in a group of MS

patients and reported their timing task to be more sensitive than MLDs, RASP, and ABR to brainstem disorders in MS. These investigators also noted an apparent relationship among interaural timing deficiencies and ABR abnormalities. Others have also reported the use of interaural timing procedures with brainstem lesion cases (Quine et al., 1983; Russolo and Poli, 1983; Cranford et al., 1990).

Two commonly used peripheral tests, the performance-intensity function for phonetically balanced words (PI-PB) (Jerger and Jerger, 1971; Bess et al., 1979) and the acoustic reflex (Jerger and Jerger, 1977, 1981; Hall, 1985) are also valuable in detecting brainstem lesions. These tests seem to be minimally affected by cortical dysfunction (Jerger and Jerger, 1975; Gelfand and Silman, 1982).

Laterality and Brainstem Lesions

Reports of laterality, or ear, effects in patients with brainstem disorders show considerable variability for both electrophysiologic and behavioral measures. ABR abnormalities, for example, are usually found on the ear ipsilateral to the lesion (Oh et al., 1981; Musiek and Geurkink, 1982; Chiappa, 1983) although bilateral (Oh et al., 1981; Musiek and Geurkink, 1982); and, in rare instances, contralateral (Hashimoto et al., 1979; Chiappa, 1983) deficits may also occur. With behavioral tests, on the other hand, it is not uncommon to find ipsilateral, contralateral or bilateral deficits (Calearo and Antonelli; 1968; Jerger and Jerger, 1975; Lynn and Gilroy, 1977; Musiek et al., 1988). The sources of this variability, though not always clear, appear to relate primarily to the location, size, and type (intra-axial versus extra-axial) of lesion.

Jerger and Jerger (1975) suggested that extra-axial lesions mimic 8th nerve lesions and result in more ipsilateral than contralateral ear deficits. Intra-axial lesions, especially those at the low- to mid-pontine level, are likely to cause bilateral deficits through involvement of the superior olivary complex and crossing auditory fiber tracts (Musiek et al., 1988). Lesions in the rostral brainstem are often seen as contralateral ear deficits since a majority of the ascending fibers at that level reflect input from the opposite ear (Jerger and Jerger, 1974; Berlin et al., 1975a).

In the adult brain, the distance from the level of the cochlear nucleus to the nuclei of the lateral lemniscus is only about 3 cm or less. Thus, even a small to moderate size lesion could have multiple effects (Musiek et al., 1988). Large, diffuse lesions may impinge on auditory areas on both sides of the brainstem, resulting in bilateral abnormalities (Chiappa, 1983). Moreover, large space-occupying lesions might affect one side of the brainstem directly and also displace or compress the brainstem to the extent that contralateral structures or tracts are also compromised (Musiek et al., 1988).

These findings underscore the complexity of the brainstem as well as its minute dimensions. At times, laterality effects are counter to what might be expected. For instance, the typical ipsilateral ABR findings seem to be inconsistent with known neuroanatomy which shows a majority of the auditory fibers crossing to the contralateral side at the level of the superior olivary complex. One possible explanation for these seemingly contradictory findings may lie in the neural requirements for processing and transmitting different types of stimuli. For example, clicks and tone pips, being relatively simple stimuli, probably require few auditory fibers for coding and transmission. Thus, they are able to use the smaller but more rapid ipsilateral pathway. Speech, on the other hand, is much more complex and apparently needs the longer and more varied contralateral pathway (Musiek et al., 1988). These and other issues relating to brainstem function and assessment await further investigation.

Cortical and Hemispheric Lesions

A cortical lesion is one that affects only the gray matter located on the periphery of the brain. A hemispheric lesion is one that affects both the gray matter and white matter of the brain. To our knowledge none of the currently available tests are sensitive to problems in these areas to the exclusion of brainstem or peripheral lesions.

The classic central auditory findings in cortical lesions is a deficit in the ear contralateral to the side of the brain lesion (Bocca and Calearo, 1963). Dichotic speech tests, such as the SSW (Katz and Pack, 1975), competing sentences (Lynn and Gilroy, 1977), dichotic digits or words (Kimura, 1961; Speaks, 1975; Niccum et al., 1981; Musiek, 1983), dichotic consonant-vowel (CV) (Berlin et al., 1972), the synthetic sentence identification with contralateral competing message (SSI-CCM) (Jerger, 1973), and the Northwestern University Auditory Test Number 20 (NU #20) (Burke and Noffsinger, 1976), have all demonstrated primarily contralateral ear deficits in patients with documented cortical and hemispheric lesions. Monaural low redundancy speech tests and monotic speech tests, such as time-compressed speech (Kurdziel et al., 1976), LPFS (Jerger, 1960; Korsan-Bengsen, 1973), speech in noise (Morales-Garcia and Poole, 1972; Olsen et al., 1975), and interrupted speech (Korsan-Bengsen, 1973), show the same trend toward contralateral deficits. Recently, Bergman et al. (1987) described a modification of the dichotic sentence test in which competing sentences in the non-test ear are increased in intensity until they interfere with the intelligibility of "target" sentences in the test ear. The level at which the competing messages partially or totally "suppress" the target sentences is referred to as the threshold of interference. According to Bergman and his colleagues, this test is sensitive to cortical lesions (as shown by low interference, or suppression, thresholds) and for the most part yields the anticipated contralateral ear deficits.

A number of psychoacoustical procedures employing non-speech stimuli have also been used to assess cortical and hemispheric lesions. Recently, Moore et al. (1990) studied the abilities of normal subjects and a small group of subjects with various neuropathologies to track a fused auditory image (FAI) as it moved through auditory space. Movement of the FAI was achieved by systematically varying the delay between pairs of clicks presented, one each, from matched speakers placed on either side of the subject's head. The perceived location of the auditory image, which varies according to the temporal relationship of the clicks, is referred to as the precedence effect. While normal subjects were able to track the FAI accurately, those with CNS lesions had considerable difficulty with the task. Two subjects with unilateral temporal lobe lesions (one left hemisphere and one right hemisphere) exhibited auditory field deficits opposite the damaged hemispheres. Results of this investigation are consistent with earlier localization and lateralization studies that showed contralateral ear effects (Sanchez-Longo and Forester, 1958; Pinheiro and Tobin, 1969, 1971; Liden and Rosenhall, 1981). Following another line of investigation, Cranford et al. (1982) studied brief tone frequency difference limens (DLs) in a group of patients with temporal lobe lesions. While thresholds for brief tones were the same for both the experimental and control groups, the frequency DL was considerably greater in the patients with brain lesions, with the greatest difference noted in the ear contralateral to the lesion. Using a different type discrimination task, Blaettner et al. (1989) studied the abilities of normal and brain-damaged subjects to detect monaural pattern changes in dichotically presented click trains. These investigators reported that patients with telencephalic (hemispheric) lesions not only performed more poorly than normal subjects on the experimental task, but that the test also identified the involved hemisphere with a high degree of accuracy. Again, the greatest performance deficit was in the ear contralateral to the damaged hemisphere.

There seem to be two prominent exceptions to the contralateral ear effects described above. One exception is seen in the results of auditory pattern tests, such as frequency and duration patterns, and the other when auditory fibers of the corpus callosum are compromised. Both the frequency pattern and duration pattern tests are monaural tests, which require that the patient make judgments as to the pitch (frequency patterns) or duration (duration patterns) of tonal pulses presented in various patterns. In the frequency pattern test, for instance, the patient is asked to report whether the pitch of the tonal pulses is high or low. For the duration patterns the task is to report the tones as being long or short. Interestingly, both of these tests seem to yield primarily bilateral ear deficits even with cortical or hemispheric damage to only one side of the brain. This unusual finding is due to the fact that interaction between the two hemispheres is required for the patterns to be decoded (right hemisphere) and for a verbal response to occur (left hemisphere). Both the frequency pattern (Musiek and Pinheiro, 1987) and duration pattern (Musiek et al., 1990a) tests have been shown to be sensitive to cortical and hemispheric lesions, with duration patterns possibly being the more sensitive of the two (Musiek et al., 1990a). Figure 14.2 shows duration pattern test results for a group of normal subjects and for patients with either cochlear hearing loss or cerebral lesions.

At this point we should mention briefly one other area of research that bears upon the topic at hand. In a psychoacoustic experiment involving several non-linguis-

tic auditory tasks that dealt primarily with spectral or temporal processing, Divenyl and Robinson (1989) sought to answer questions relating to (*a*) hemispheric specialization of various auditory functions and (*b*) nonlinguisitic auditory capabilities of aphasics. Basically, their findings suggested bilateral representation of most of the auditory functions studied including processing of spectral information, which previously had been thought to be primarily a function of the right cerebral hemisphere. This study holds some interesting theoretical implications relative to (*a*) hemispheric specialization in auditory processing, (*b*) the relationship of nonlinguistic and linguistic auditory processing in aphasics, and (*c*) treatment strategies for aphasics and others with auditory processing disorders.

In a recent study by Thompson and Abel (1992), it was shown that patients with left temporal lobe lesions performed more poorly on frequency, duration, and consonant discrimnation tasks than did patients with right temporal lobe lesions. Generally, patients with either right or left cortical lesions performed worse than normal controls or patients with acoustic tumors. These researchers also measured response time to the various psychoacoustic tasks just mentioned. The patients with temporal lobe lesions required greater time to respond than did the control groups with the left temporal lobe lesion patients requiring the longest time (Fig. 14.3).

Interhemispheric Dysfunction

When the interhemispheric auditory fibers (corpus callosum) are damaged, even secondarily, unique patterns of results may emerge for many central tests. For example, split brain subjects show left ear deficits on dichotic tests and binaural problems on pattern tests that require verbal report (Milner et al., 1968; Sparks and Geschwind, 1968; Musiek et al., 1980; Musiek and Kibbe, 1985). Underlying these results is the fact that a large majority of the auditory fibers that project to the primary auditory cortex carry information that originates in the contralateral ear. Hence, contralateral representation is much stronger at the cortex than ipsilateral, especially in dichotic listening situations (Kimura, 1961). If a speech response is required, auditory information presented to the left ear (in a dichotic test situation) goes to the right hemisphere and must cross the corpus callosum to reach the left hemisphere so a spoken response can be mediated. Right ear stimuli are projected to the left hemisphere and therefore do not require participation of the opposite hemisphere for a speech response. According to Kimura (1961), the ipsilateral pathways are "suppressed" during dichotic testing. Given this information, one could expect left ear deficits on dichotic speech tasks if callosal fibers

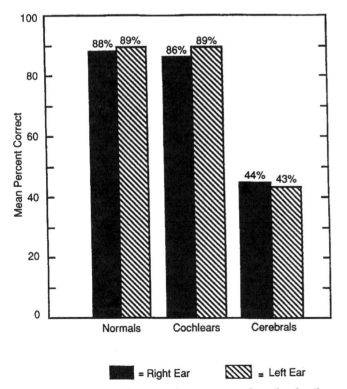

Figure 14.2. Mean performance (percent correct) on the duration pattern recognition test for normal adults (N=50), patients with cochlear hearing losses in the mild to moderate range (N=42 ears), and patients with documented lesion of the central auditory nervous system (cerebral) (N=21) (Based on data from Musiek, Baran and Pinheiro, 1990).

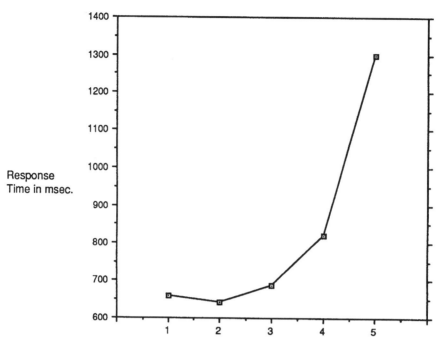

Figure 14.3. Median response times for five subject groups on a 500Hz tone duration discrimination task (Adapted from Thompson and Abel, 1992).

were compromised. Low redundancy monaural test results, however, are largely unaffected by interhemispheric dysfunction (Musiek et al., 1984).

In the case of frequency patterns, it appears that the right hemisphere must recognize the "acoustic contour" of the pattern and the left hemisphere must convert the pattern to a verbal response (e.g., "high-low-high"). Both hemispheres must interact appropriately for a correct verbal response to occur. This means that either ear tested monaurally would show a similar deficit if the auditory interhemispheric pathways were damaged (Musiek et al., 1980).

It appears that the auditory transcallosal pathways are located in the posterior half of the corpus callosum. This has been borne out by central auditory studies of patients who have undergone either partial or complete surgical section (commissurotomy) of the corpus callosum in an attempt to control intractable seizure activity (Musiek et al., 1985b; Musiek and Kibbe, 1985; Baran et al., 1986). Patients who have experienced surgical section of the posterior portion of the corpus callosum yielded expected central test results, e.g., decreased dichotic test scores on the left ear and bilaterally depressed scores on the pitch pattern test (Musiek and Kibbe, 1985; Musiek et al., 1985b). On the other hand, sectioning of the anterior portion of the corpus callosum seems to leave central auditory function relatively unchanged (Baran et al., 1986).

One interesting finding that has emerged with many split brain patients is that not only are left ear scores decreased for dichotic materials (sometimes referred to as the auditory disconnection phenomenon), but right ear scores may be considerably enhanced. This phenomenon, which has been attributed to release of the left hemisphere from central auditory competition from the right hemisphere (Berlin et al., 1975b; Musiek et al., 1985b), has been clearly demonstrated by Musiek et al. (1989b) using the dichotic rhyme task (DRT). This test, first introduced by Wexler and Halwes (1983), employs pairs of closely aligned simple rhyming words (e.g., ten-pen) which, when presented dichotically, appear to fuse into single words. Thus, instead of hearing two separate words the subject generally reports only one with slightly more than 50% of all words recognized being those presented to the right ear. Musiek et al. (1989b) showed dramatic changes in pre- and post-operative test results with the DRT with two split brain patients. Left ear scores decreased and right ear scores increased markedly, thus resulting in a large right ear-left ear (DS). The right-left asymmetry and large DSs were also found in a second group of split brain patients who were tested only post-operatively, as well as a patient with a deep left hemisphere lesion involving the transcallosal pathway. Among four dichotic tests administered to these patients, the DRT was most sensitive to interhemispheric dysfunction.

Damage to the corpus callosum, including deep brain lesions in the right hemisphere, typically produce the classic contralateral (left ear) deficits on dichotic speech tests (Musiek and Sachs, 1980). However, with lesions that affect both the left cortex and the corpus callosum, an ipsilateral (not contralateral) ear deficit may be noted (Sparks et al., 1970; Speaks, 1975; Damasio and Damasio, 1979; Musiek et al., 1989b). It is our opinion, as well as that of others (Geschwind, 1982), that callosal fibers are often affected by cortical lesions.

Monitoring Neurologically Involved Patients

Central auditory tests, when used properly, can provide a unique means of monitoring changes in CNS function over time. Both behavioral and electrophysiologic tests have provided valuable information on the neural status of patients representing a variety of disorders and monitoring needs, several of which were mentioned earlier (Musiek and Morgan, 1981; Hall et al., 1982; Musiek et al., 1983; Harris and Hall, 1990; Musiek et al., 1990b; Yingling et al., 1990).

Trauma patients who have incurred damage to the CNS may have a long and discouraging course of recovery and often it is difficult to determine whether the patient is improving. However, if the injury involves the CANS it may be possible to document changes through periodic monitoring with central auditory tests. Evidence of improvement in central auditory function may be helpful in terms of patient motivation and in planning future rehabilitation. In cases of surgery involving the CANS, pre- and post-operative measures can help in assessing changes in neurologic status as well as communication ability (Musiek et al., 1983). In one such case involving a partial temporal lobectomy in a patient with seizure disorder, Musiek et al (1990b) reported post-operative improvements in both behavioral and electrophysiologic (P300) test results that paralleled the patients overall improvement.

At times, lesions affecting the CANS are not, or cannot be, treated medically or surgically; yet it is important to track any changes in the effects of the lesions. This is often true in cases of multiple sclerosis and other degenerative neural diseases where central auditory monitoring may provide on-going information on the patient's condition and thus the progress of the disease. Similarly, clues to neural status may be obtained in cases of radiologic treatment of tumors that affect the CANS. Central testing of alcoholics also has been shown to be of value in assessing the type and degree of brain dysfunction in these patients (Squires et al., 1978; Spitzer and Ventry, 1980).

The information gained from central auditory monitoring of certain patients can serve to complement nonauditory tests. For example, audiologic monitoring might be used to help describe the functional status of the system while radiologic monitoring would yield data only on anatomic changes. Central auditory testing thus can help document overall change by its correlation with various medical tests.

Central Auditory Tests and the Elderly

In attempting to evaluate central auditory abilities in the elderly the audiologist is faced with a unique set of problems. As mentioned earlier, the pathophysiology of presbycusis encompasses both the peripheral and central auditory systems (Gulya, 1990; Stach et al., 1990). Thus, while central tests may yield abnormal results in the elderly, it may be difficult to rule out the effects of peripheral hearing loss (Marshall, 1981). Studies of time-compressed speech (Sticht and Gray, 1969; Konkle et al., 1977) and various types of speech in noise procedures (Smith and Prather, 1972; Orchik and Burgess, 1977) which have attempted to control for peripheral hearing have shown poor performance when testing elderly subjects. Deficits have also been shown on other central tests, including filtered speech (Kirikae et al., 1964; Harbert et al., 1966), interrupted speech (Bergman, 1971), the SSI-ICM (Jerger and Hayes, 1977), MLDs (Bocca and Antonelli, 1976; Olsen and Noffsinger, 1976), and the PI-PB (Gang, 1976). However, the influence of peripheral loss in these studies is difficult to differentiate from central problems. Jerger et al. (1989) studied both auditory and cognitive factors as they relate to disorders of speech understanding in elderly subjects. These investigators offered some rather compelling arguments suggesting that most of the problems of the elderly in understanding speech stem from central processing disorders rather than peripheral hearing loss. Jerger et al. (1989) and others (Martin and Cranford, 1991) have also suggested that the poor performance often seen with the elderly on dichotic speech tasks may be attributable, at least in part, to cognitive deficits. Obviously, much more study is needed before the true effects of aging on central auditory function are understood.

Apart from site of lesion information, the degree of central auditory deficits in elderly patients may be important in planning and managing rehabilitation efforts. Hayes and Jerger (1979) studied a large group of elderly subjects and found that 40% demonstrated primarily peripheral deficits while 42% showed mostly central involvement. Stach et al. (1990) found the prevalence of central auditory processing deficits (CAPD) to increase markedly with age, ranging from 17% in a group of 50-54-year-old patients to 95% in a group of patients 80 years and older. These data, and those of others (Jerger et al., 1989) that also demonstrated central involvement in a large percentage of elderly patients, appear to have important implications relative to hearing aid candidacy as well as other approaches to hearing rehabilitation with the elderly. This is borne out by research showing that patients with CAPD (*a*) do not perform as well with hearing aids as patients with only peripheral deficits, (*b*) do not appear to be as satisfied with hearing aid use, and (*c*) may not benefit as much from hearing aid use as those with a strictly peripheral loss (Hayes and Jerger, 1979; Jerger and Hayes, 1976; Stach, 1990).

Use of Central Tests with Learning Disabled Children

The current emphasis on central auditory assessment with LD children has grown out of a need to identify subtle auditory deficits that might be interfering with academic work or with social or communication skills (Baran and Musiek, 1991; see Chapter 32). There is considerable evidence indicating a relationship between learning disabilities (including dyslexia) and poor performance on various central auditory tests (Katz and Illmer, 1972; Pinheiro, 1977; Willeford and Bilger, 1978; Musiek et al., 1982; Welsh et al., 1982; Musiek et al., 1985; Jerger et al., 1987).

Development of central test procedures for children has followed two general orientations; (*a*) existing adult procedures have been adjusted for use with children, usually by modifying the expected range of normal performance, and (*b*) new central test materials and paradigms have been created that conform to children's interests and abilities (Jerger et al., 1988). Most notable among the tests developed specifically for children is the Pediatric Speech Intelligibility (PSI) test (Jerger and Jerger, 1984), which has as its basis word and sentence materials generated by normal children in the 3—6 year age range. When used with ipsilateral competing messages (PSI-ICM) and contralateral competing messages (PSI-CCM), the PSI test has demonstrated good sensitivity and specificity in identifying children with confirmed CANS lesions (Jerger, 1987; Jerger et al., 1988) and children with suspected central processing disorders (Jerger et al., 1988).

Recently, interest has developed in using central tests to screen for auditory processing disorders in LD children (Musiek et al., 1990c). Keith (1986) has published a screening battery, the SCAN test, which is composed of three subtests; competing words, auditory figure-ground, and filtered words. These tests are purported to assess auditory maturation, identify children at risk for auditory processing problems, and identify children who may benefit from rehabilitation. Hurley and Singer (1989) evaluated four central tests (dichotic digits, binaural fusion, pitch pattern, and filtered speech) within a screening context and found dichotic digits to be highly efficient in identifying central processing disorders in school children. Like Keith and his associates (1986; 1989), these investigators have advocated the use of cen-

tral auditory tests as screening tools.

Another recent development with LD children is the use of electrophysiologic tests to identify and/or confirm auditory processing disorders. In this regard, investigators have pointed to the MLR (Musiek et al., 1985a; Jerger et al., 1987; Musiek, 1989) and the late vertex response (LVR) and P300 cognitive potential (Jirsa and Clontz, 1990) as possible indices of central auditory dysfunction in children. In our view the most appropriate use of these tests, at least at present, is in concert with behavioral tests. There may be instances in which only evoked response tests or only behavioral tests will identify a central auditory disorder (Musiek et al., 1984; Musiek et al., 1985a).

One key issue with LD children has to do with the neuroauditory disorders that underlie abnormal test findings. There currently is evidence suggesting at least three general types of disorders: neurological (Musiek et al., 1985a), maturational (Musiek et al., 1984; Musiek et al., 1985a), and developmental (Galaburda and Kemper, 1979; Musiek et al., 1985a; Drake, 1968). In a neuropathologic report on a patient with dyslexia, Galabura and Kemper (1979) showed an underdeveloped (polymicrogyri) area in the left hemisphere of the brain. Dysplasia was also noted deep in the left hemisphere (insular area). Interestingly, there is a record of dichotic digit test results on this patient showing a left ear deficit. Drake (1968) reported abnormal gyri in the parietal regions of the brain and marked thinning of the corpus callosum in another patient with dyslexia. Musiek et al. (1985a) have provided evidence of central auditory problems in two LD children with suspected developmental brain disorders as well as one with apparant neuromaturational delay and two with active neurological disorders (one with a bihemispheric seizure disorder and the other with a right hemisphere subarachnoid cyst). All gave depressed central test results consistent with their known or suspected lesions. Neuropathologic data such as these are valuable from various points of view. They not only help us understand the mechanisms of auditory processing disorders in LD children, but they also demonstrate the effects of specific lesions on central test results.

Though some test results seem incisive, there is often great variability among tests and subjects, making test interpretation most difficult with LD children. Much of this variability may be related to the nature of the tests as well as the auditory problems affecting the children. Additionally, psychological (Culbertson, 1981), educational, language, (Butler, 1981) social, and maturational factors (Rees, 1981) may bear upon the validity of central tests with a given learning-disabled child. Hence, if central tests are used with LD children they should be administered and interpreted with caution with the examiner being keenly aware of their limitations. If kept in the proper perspective, central tests with learning-disabled children may help identify and define auditory processing deficits and also serve as a basis for developing habilitation/rehabilitation strategies and education programs. However, a great deal more must be known before central auditory assessment of the LD child can be approached with total confidence. Only by testing children with documented CNS lesions can the true validity of various central auditory tests be established for use with the pediatric population.

The Test Battery Approach

As suggested earlier in this chapter, assessment of a system as complex and redundant as the CANS usually requires a variety of tests. Procedures that identify problems in one area may be totally insensitive to lesions located elsewhere. Further, because of the complexity of the CANS, the effects of a given lesion may be so subtle that it will escape detection by one test but be clearly "visible" to another. Test batteries, however, do not necessarily need to be extensive because two or three appropriately selected tests often can do as well as a battery of six or seven.

The first step in any central auditory evaluation should be a comprehensive audiologic case history. Symptoms, such as tinnitus, auditory hallucinations, difficulty hearing in noisy or reverberant conditions, trouble with sound localization, difficulty following complex verbal instructions, etc., often herald central disorders and, in addition, can provide guidance in test selection. Willeford and Burleigh (1985) present an excellent discussion of auditory and behavioral symptoms and of the central auditory case history which, though directed toward children, can also be helpful when considering adult disorders.

Following the case history the patient should have a thorough peripheral hearing evaluation. This will help determine, among other things, which central tests might be performed without fear of contamination by peripheral factors, and the appropriate levels at which to administer various tests.

There may be instances when case history information or data from medical or audiologic evaluations would lead one to bias the test battery toward a given type of test or particular area of the CANS. However, it generally is recommended that a sufficient variety of tests be used to assess the entire system. The selection of appropriate tests depends on a number of factors. Tests with high levels of sensitivity and specificity generally are good choices. However, variety should not be sacrificed in an effort to include only the most powerful and efficient tests. The more central processes that are evaluated, the better the chances of identifying a problem.

At a minimum, a central auditory test battery should include the following: (*a*) several tests of brainstem auditory function, including both objective and subjective procedures; and (*b*) several tests of cortical/hemispheric and interhemispheric function, including both verbal and nonverbal materials. Possible tests of brainstem function include MLD; (Olsen and Noffsinger, 1976; Lynn et al., 1981), ABR (see Chapter 24) acoustic reflexes (Jerger and Jerger, 1977, 1981; Hall, 1985; Jerger et al., 1986), and SSI-ICM (Jerger and Jerger, 1975), all of which, as indicated earlier, have shown good sensitivity to lesions of the lower brainstem but little or no effect with higher level disorders. Dichotic speech tests, such as dichotic digits, should be included in a central battery for their sensitivity to both brainstem and cortical lesions (Stevens and Thornton, 1976; Musiek and Geurkink, 1982). To create a more linguistically challenging listening task, one might wish to consider dichotic tests, such as competing sentences (Willeford and Burleigh, 1985) or the DSI (Fifer et al., 1983). Linguistically loaded tests can be especially helpful in identifying auditory processing problems in children. Auditory sequencing tests, such as frequency patterns (Musiek and Pinheiro, 1987) and duration patterns (Musiek et al., 1990a) have shown good sensitivity to cortical and hemispheric lesions and should be strongly considered for any central test battery. For children, sequencing tasks such as that recommended by Tallal et al. (1980), might be appropriate. Sound localization tasks involving temporal processing have demonstrated promise diagnostically and might also be included in a test battery. For instance, various tests of the precedence effect have identified both brainstem (Cranford et al., 1990) and cortical (Moore et al., 1990) abnormalities. Finally, the MLR (Kraus et al., 1982; Kileny et al., 1987; Musiek et al., 1985a; Jerger et al., 1987; Musiek, 1989), the LVR (Jirsa and Clontz, 1990), and the P300 (Harris and Hall, 1990; Jirsa and Clontz, 1990; Musiek et al., 1990b; Obert and Cranford, 1990; Yingling et al., 1990) evoked responses have shown potential for identifying disorders at higher levels of the auditory system and can at times be valuable elements in a central test battery.

CONCLUSION

Auditory evaluation of the CANS has been slow to gain acceptance as a routine part of the audiologist's responsibility. This is probably due to a number of factors including the complexity of the CANS and the subtlety of many CANS disorders, as well as a lack of standardization of test procedures. Nonetheless, CANS assessment represents an interesting and vital area that demands attention if audiology as a profession is to realize its total potential.

In this chapter we have presented an overview of the central auditory evaluation, emphasizing behavioral tests. Assessment techniques have been highlighted relative to specific areas of the CANS. We have discussed several applications of central tests as well as factors which influence successful central auditory evaluation. Unique populations, such as the elderly and the LD child, have been considered as have special uses of central tests in monitoring CANS function in selected patients.

While the "cause" of central auditory assessment is being advanced there is still much work to be done. Audiologists must become better prepared if they are to understand both the normal and abnormal CANS and methods of assessing CANS function. Additional research is needed in developing and/or refining central auditory test procedures and demonstrating their clinical applicability. In the authors' view we have only seen the tip of the iceberg, so to speak, in this vital and challenging area.

REFERENCES

Altman J, Rosenblum A, and Lvova V. Lateralization of a moving auditory image in patients with focal damage of the brain hemispheres. Neuropsychologia 1987;25:435–442.

Baran J, and Musiek F. 1991. Behavioral assessment of the central auditory nervous system. In Rintelman W, Ed. Hearing Assessment, 2nd Ed. Austin, TX: Pro Ed Publishers, 1991.

Baran J, Musiek F, and Reeves A. Central auditory function following anterior sectioning of the corpus callosum. Ear Hear 1986;7: 359–362.

Bergman M, 1971. Hearing and aging. Audiology 1971;10:164–171.

Bergman M, Hirsch S, Solzi P, and Mankowitz Z. The threshold of interference test: a new test of interhemispheric suppression in brain injury. Ear Hear 1987;8:147–150.

Berlin C, Cullen J, Berlin H, Tobey E, and Mouney D. Dichotic listening in a patient with presumed lesion in the region of the medial geniculate bodies. Paper presented at the Annual Meeting of the Acoustical Society of America, San Francisco, 1975a.

Berlin C, Cullen J, Hughes L, Berlin H, Lowe-Bell S, and Thompson C. 1975b. Dichotic processing of speech: acoustic and phonetic variables. In Sullivan M, Ed. Proceedings of a Symposium on Central Auditory Processing Disorders. Omaha, NE: University of Nebraska Medical Center, 1975b.

Berlin C, Lowe-Bell S, Jannetta P, and Kline D. Central auditory deficits after temporal lobectomy. Arch Otolaryngol 1972;96:4–10.

Bess F, Josey A, and Humes L. Performance intensity functions in eighth nerve disorders. Am J Otol 1979;1:27–31.

Blaettner U, Scherg M, and Von Craman D. Diagnosis of unilateral telencephalic hearing disorders. Brain 1989;112:177–195.

Bocca E. Distorted speech tests. In Graham B, Ed. Sensorineural Hearing Processes and Disorders. Boston: Little, Brown, 1967.

Bocca E, and Antonelli A. Masking level differences: another tool for the evaluation of peripheral and cortical defects. Audiology 1976; 15:141–251.

Bocca E, and Calearo C. Central hearing processes. In Jerger J, Ed. Modern Developments in Audiology. New York: Academic Press, 1963.

Bocca E, Calearo C, and Cassinari V. A new method for testing hearing in temporal lobe tumors. Acta Otolaryngol 1954;44:219–221.

Bocca E, Calearo C, Cassinari V, and Migliavacca F. Testing cortical hearing in temporal lobe tumors. Acta Otolaryngol 1955;45:289–304.

Bosatra A. and M. Russolo M. Directional hearing, temporal order and auditory pattern in peripheral and brainstem lesions. Audiology 1976;15:141–151.

Brody H. Organization of the cerebral cortex. Study of aging in human cerebral cortex. J Comp Neurol 1955;102:511.

Brugge J. and Geisler C. Auditory mechanisms of the lower brainstem. Ann Rev Neurosci 1978;1:363–394.

Burke M, and Noffsinger D. Dichotic performance by cortical lesion patients utilizing meaningful and meaningless competition. Paper presented at the Annual Meeting of the American Speech and Hearing Association, Houston, 1976.

Butler K. Language processing disorders: factors in diagnosis and remediation. In Keith R, Ed. Central Auditory Processing and Language Disorders in Children. Houston: College-Hill Press, 1981.

Calearo C, and Antonelli A. Audiometric findings in brainstem lesions. Acta Otolaryngol 1968;66:305–319.

Carver W. Tape recordings and tape recorders: Their care and maintenance. Semin Hearing 1983;4:311–315.

Chiappa K. Evoked Potentials in Clinical Medicine. New York: Raven Press, 1983.

Corballis M, and Ogden J. Dichotic listening in commissurotomized and hemispherectomized subjects. Neuropsychologia 1988;26: 565–573.

Cranford J, Boose M, and Moore C. Tests of the precedence effect in sound localization reveal abnormalities in multiple sclerosis. Ear Hear 1990;11:282.

Cranford J, Stream R, Rye C, and Slade T. Detection v. discrimination of brief duration tones. Arch Otolaryngol 1982;108:350–356.

Culbertson J. Psychological evaluation and educational planning for children with central auditory dysfunction. In Keith R, Ed. Central Auditory and Language Disorders in Children. Houston: College-Hill Press, 1981.

Damasio H, and Damasio A. Paradoxic ear extinction in dichotic listening: possible anatomic significance. Neurology 1979;29:646–653.

Davis R, Wikastelanski, and Stephens S. Some factors influencing the results of speech tests of central auditory function. Scand Audiol 1976;5:179–186.

Demarco S, Harbour A, Hume G, and Givins G. Perception of time-altered monosyllables in a specific group of phonologically disordered children. Neuropsychologia 1989;27:753–757.

Divenyl P, and Robinson A. Nonlinguistic auditory capabilities in aphasia. Brain and Language 1989;37:290–326.

Drake W. Clinical and pathological findings in a child with developmental learning disability. J Learn Disabil 1968;1:9–25.

Dublin W. Fundamentals of Sensorineural Auditory Pathology. Springfield, IL: Charles C Thomas, 1976.

Duffy F, Bartels P, and Burchfield J. Significance of probability mapping: an aide to the topographic analysis of brain electrical activity. Electroencephalogr Clin Neurophysiol 1981;51:455–462.

Fifer R, Jerger J, Berlin C, Tobey E, and Campbell J. Development of a dichotic sentence identification test for hearing impaired adults. Ear Hear 1983;4:300–305.

Galaburda N, and Kemper T. Cytoarchetectonic abnormalities in developmental dyslexia: a case study. Ann Neurol 1979;6:94–100.

Gang R. The effects of age on the diagnostic utility of the rollover phenomenon. J Speech Hear Disord 1976;41:63–69.

Gat I, and Keith R. An effect of linguistic experience and auditory word discrimination by native and non-native speakers of English. Audiology 1978;17:339–345.

Gefland S, and Silman S. Acoustic reflex thresholds in brain damaged patients. Ear Hear 1982;3:93–95.

Geschwind N. The frequency of callosal syndromes in neurological practice. Paper presented at the Epilepsy and Corpus Callosum Conference, Hanover, New Hampshire, 1982.

Gulya J. Aging: structural and physiological changes of the auditory and vestibular mechanisms. In Cherow E, Ed. Proceedings of the Research Symposium on Communication Sciences and Disorders and Aging. ASHA Reports 1990;19:126–133.

Hall J. The cochlear nuclei in monkeys after dihydrostreptomycin or noise exposure. Arch Otolaryngol 1976;81:344–352.

Hall J. The acoustic reflex in central auditory dysfunction. In Pinheiro M, and Musiek F, Eds. Assessment of Central Auditory Dysfunction, Baltimore: Williams & Wilkins, 1985.

Hall J, Huangfu M, and Gennarelli T. Auditory function in acute head injury. Laryngoscope 1982;93:383–390.

Hansen C, and Reske-Nielsen E. Pathological studies in presbycusis. Arch Otolaryngol 1965;82:115–132.

Harbert F, Young I, and Menduke H. Audiologic findings in presbycusis. J Aud Res 1966;6:297–312.

Harris D, and Hall J. Feasibility of auditory event related potential measurement in brain injury rehabilitation. Ear Hear 1990;11:340–350.

Hashimoto I, Ishiyama Y, and Tozuka G. Bilaterally recorded brainstem auditory evoked responses: their asymmetric abnormalities and lesions of the brainstem. Arch Neurol 1979;36:161–167.

Hausler R, and Levine R. Brainstem auditory evoked potentials are related to interaural time discrimination in patients with multiple sclerosis. Brain Research 1980;191:589–594.

Hayes D, and Jerger J. Aging and the use of hearing aids. Scand Audiol 1979;8:33–40.

Hinchcliff R. The anatomical locus of presbycusis. J Speech Hear Disord. 1962;27:301–310.

Hurley R, and Singer J. The effectiveness of selected auditory processing tests as screening tests with children. Paper presented at the Annual Meeting of the American Academy of Audiology, Kiawah, SC, 1989.

Jean-Baptiste M, and Morest D. Transneuronal changes of synaptic endings and nuclear chromatin in the trapezoid body following cochlear ablation in cats. J Comp Neurol 1975;162:111–134.

Jerger J. Observations of auditory behavior in lesions of the central auditory pathways. Arch Otolaryngol 1960;73:797–806.

Jerger J. Diagnostic audiometry. In Jerger J, Ed. Modern Developments in Audiology. New York, Academic Press, 1973.

Jerger J, and Hayes D. Hearing aid evaluation: clinical experience with a new philosophy. Arch Otolaryngol 1976;102:214–225.

Jerger J, and Hayes D. Diagnostic speech audiometry. Arch Otolaryngol 1977;103:216–222.

Jerger J, and Jerger S. Diagnostic significance of PB word functions. Arch Otolaryngol 1971;93:573–580.

Jerger J, and Jerger S. Auditory findings in brainstem disorders. Arch Otolaryngol 1974;99:342–350.

Jerger J, and Jerger S. Clinical validity of central auditory tests. Scand Audiol 1975;4:147–163.

Jerger J, and Jerger S. Diagnostic value of crossed vs. uncrossed acoustic relexes in eighth nerve and brainstem disorders. Arch Otolaryngol 1977;103:445–451.

Jerger J, and Jerger S. Auditory Disorders: A Manual for Clinical Evaluation. Boston: Little, Brown, 1981.

Jerger J, Jerger S, Oliver T, and Pirozzolo F. Speech understanding in the elderly. Ear Hear 1989;10:79–89.

Jerger J, Oliver T, Chimiel R, and Rivera V. Patterns of auditory abnormality in multiple sclerosis. Audiology 1986;25:193–209.

Jerger S. Validation of the pediatric speech intelligibility test in children with central nervous system lesions. Audiology 1987;26:298–311.

Jerger S, and Jerger J. Pediatric speech intelligibility test: Manual for administration. St. Louis, MO: Auditec, 1984.

Jerger S, Martin R, and Jerger J. Specific auditory perceptual dysfunction in a learning disabled child. Ear Hear 1987;8:78–86.

Jerger S, Johnson K, and Loiselle L. Pediatric central auditory dysfunction: Comparison of children with confirmed lesions versus suspected processing disorders. Am J Otol 1988;9(Suppl):63–71.

Jirsa R, and Clontz K. Long latency auditory event-related potentials from children with auditory processing disorders. Ear Hear 1990; 11:222–232.

Katz J. Clinical use of central auditory tests. In Katz J, Ed. Handbook of Clinical Audiology. 2nd Ed. Baltimore: Williams & Wilkins, 1978.

Katz J, and Illmer R. Auditory perception in children with learning disabilities. In Katz J, Ed. Handbook of Clinical Audiology. Baltimore: Williams & Wilkins, 1972.

Katz J, and Pack G. New developments in differential diagnosis using the SSW test. In Sullivan M, Ed. Proceedings of a Symposium on Central Auditory Processing Disorders. Omaha, NE: University of Nebraska Medical Center, 1975.

Keidel W, Kallert S, and North M. The Physiological Basis of Hearing. New York: Thieme-Stratton, 1983.

Keith R. Central auditory tests. In Lass N, L. McReynolds L, Northern J, and Yoder D, Eds. Speech, Language, and Hearing. Vol. III: Hearing Disorders. Philadelphia: WB Saunders, 1982. Philadelphia.

Keith R. Comments on Spitzer, J. A central auditory evaluation protocol: a guide for training and diagnosis of lesions of the central system. Ear Hear 1983;4:229–230.

Keith R. SCAN: A screening test for auditory processing disorders: Manual. San Diego: The Psychology Corp, 1986.

Keith R, Rudy J, Donahue P, and Katbamna B. Comparison of SCAN results with auditory and language measures in a clinical population. Ear Hear 1989;10:382–386.

Kileny P, Paccioretti D, and Wilson A. Effect of cortical lesions on middle latency auditory evoked responses (MLR). Electroencephalogr Clin Neurophysiol 1987;66:108–120.

Kimura D. Some effects of temporal lobe damage on auditory perception. Can J Psychol 1961;15:157–165.

Kirikae I, Sato T, and Shitaera T. Study of hearing in advanced age. Laryngoscope 1964;74:205–221.

Konkle D, Beasley D, and Bess F. Intelligibility of time-altered speech in relation to chronological age. J Speech Hear Res 1977;20: 108–115.

Korsan-Bengsen M. Distorted speech audiometry. Acta Otolaryngol 1973;Suppl 310.

Kraus N, Ozdamar O, Hier O, and Stein L. Auditory middle latency responses (MLRs) in patients with cortical lesions. Electroencephalogr Clin Neurophysiol 1982;54:275–287.

Kurdziel S, Noffsinger D, and Olsen D. Performance by cortical lesion patients on 40 and 60% time compressed materials. J Am Audiol Soc 1976;2:3–7.

Liden G, and Rosenhall V. New developments in diagnostic auditory neurological problems. In Paparella M, and Meyerhoff W, Eds. Sensorineural Hearing Loss, Vertigo and Tinnitus. Baltimore: Williams & Wilkins, 1981.

Lynn G, and Gilroy J. Evaluation of central auditory dysfunction in patients with neurological disorders. In R. Keith, ed. Central Auditory Dysfunction. New York: Grune and Stratton, 1977.

Lynn G, Gilroy J, Taylor P, and Leiser R. Binaural masking level differences in neurological disorders. Arch Otolaryngol 1981; 107:357–362.

Magee T, and Olszewski J. Streptomycin sulfate and dihydrostreptomycin toxicity. Arch Otolaryngol 1962;75:295–311.

Marshall L. Auditory processing in aging listeners. J Speech Hear Disord. 1981;46:226–240.

Martin D, and Cranford J. Age related changes in binaural processing: II Behavioral Findings. Am J Otol 1991;12:365–369.

Matathias H, Sohmer H, and Biton V. Central auditory tests and auditory nerve–brainstem evoked responses in multiple sclerosis. Acta Otolaryngol 1985;99:369–376.

Matzger J. Two new methods for the assessment of central auditory function in cases of brain disease. Ann Otol Rhinol Laryngol 1959;68:1185–1196.

Mendez M, and Geehan G. Cortical auditory disorders: clinical and psychoacoustic features. J Neurol Neurosurg Psychiatry 1988; 51:1–9.

Milner B, Taylor S, and Sperry R. Lateralized suppression of dichotically presented digits after commissural section in man. Science 1968;161:184–185.

Miltenberger G, Dawson G, and Raica A. Central auditory testing with peripheral hearing loss. Arch Otolaryngol 1978;104:11–15.

Moller A. Auditory Physiology. New York: Academic Press, 1983.

Moore C, Cranford J, and Rahn A. Tracking of a "moving" fused auditory image under conditions that elicit the precedence effect. J Speech Hear Res 1990;33:141–148.

Morales-Garcia C, and Poole J. Masked speech audiometry in central deafness. Acta Otolaryngol 1972;74:307–316.

Morest D. Degeneration in the brain following exposure to noise. In Hamernik R, Henderson D, and Salvi R, Eds. New Perspectives on Noise Induced Hearing Loss. N York: Raven Press, 1982.

Morest D, Ard M, and Yurgelon-Todd D. Degeneration in the central auditory pathways after acoustic deprivation or overstimulation in the cat. Anat. Rec 1979;193:750.

Musiek F. ABR in eighth-nerve and brainstem disorders. Am J Otol 1982;3:242–248.

Musiek F. Assessment of central auditory dysfunction: the dichotic digits test revisited. Ear Hear 1983;4:79–83.

Musiek F. Neuroanatomy, neurophysiology and central auditory assessment. Part II: The cerebrum. Ear Hear 1986a;7:283–294.

Musiek F. Neuroanatomy, neurophysiology, and central auditory assessment. Part III: Corpus callosum and efferent pathways. Ear Hear 1986b;7:349–358.

Musiek F. Probing brain function with acoustic stimuli. ASHA 1989; 31:100–106.

Musiek F, and J. Baran. Neuroanatomy, neurophysiology, and central auditory assessment. Part I: Brainstem. Ear Hear 1986;7:207–219.

Musiek F, and Geurkink N. Auditory brainstem response and central auditory test findings for patients with brainstem lesions. Laryngoscope 1982;92:891–900.

Musiek F, and Hoffman D. An introduction to the functional neurochemistry of the auditory system. Ear Hear 1990;11:395–402.

Musiek F, and Kibbe K. An overview of audiological test results in patients with commissurotomy. In Reeves A, Ed. Epilepsy and the Corpus Callosum. New York: Plenum Press, 1985.

Musiek F, and Morgan G. The use of central auditory tests in case of vasculitis. Ear Hear 1981;2:100–102.

Musiek F, and Pinheiro M. Frequency patterns in cochlear, brainstem, and cerebral lesions. Audiology 1987;26:79–88.

Musiek F, and Sachs E. Reversible neuroaudiologic findings in a case of right frontal lobe abcess with recovery. Arch Otolaryngol. 1980; 106:280–283.

Musiek F, Baran J, and Pinheiro M. P300 results in patients with lesions of the auditory areas of the cerebrum. J Am Acad Audiol 1992;3:5–15.

Musiek F, Geurkink N, and Keitel S. Test battery assessment of auditory perceptual dysfunction in children. Laryngoscope 1982;92: 251–257.

Musiek F, Gollegly K, and Ross M. Profiles of types of central auditory processing disorders in children with learning disabilities. J Childhood Communication Disorders 1985a;9:43–63.

Musiek F, Kibbe K, and Baran J. Neuroaudiologic results from split brain patients. Semin Hear 1984;5:219–299.

Musiek F, Pinheiro M, and Wilson D. Auditory pattern perception in "split brain" patients. Arch Otolaryngol 1980;106:610–612.

Musiek F, Weider D, and Mueller R. Reversible audiologic results in a patient with an extra-axial brainstem tumor. Ear Hear 1983;4: 169–172.

Musiek F, Reeves A, and Baran J. Release from central auditory competition in the split-brain patient. Neurology 1985b;35:983–987.

Musiek F, Geurkink N, Welder D, and Donnelly K. Past, present, and future applications of auditory middle latency response. Laryngoscope 1984;94:1545–1552.

Musiek F, Gollegly K, Kibbe K, and Reeves A. Electrophysiologic and behavioral auditory findings in multiple sclerosis. Am J Otol 1989a; 10:343–350.

Musiek F, Gollegly K, Kibbe K, and Verkest S. Current concepts on the use of ABR and auditory psychophysical tests in the evaluation of brainstem lesions. Am J Otol 1988;9(Suppl):25–35.

Musiek F, Krudziel-Schwan S, Kibbe K, Gollegly K, Baran J, and Rintleman W. The dichotic rhyme test: results in split-brain patients. Ear Hear 1989b;10:33–39.

Musiek F, Baran J, and Pinheiro M. Duration pattern recognition in normal subjects and patients with cerebral and cochlear lesions. Audiology 1990a;29:304–313.

Musiek F, Bromley M, Roberts D, and Lamb L. Improvement of central auditory function after partial temporal lobectomy in a patient with seizure disorder. J Am Acad Audiol 1990b;1:146–150.

Musiek F, Gollegly K, Lamb L, and Lamb P. Selected issues in screening for central auditory processing dysfunction. Semin Hear 1990c;11:372–384.

Neely G. Disorders of the central auditory system. Seminars in Hearing 1983;4:97–107.

Niccum N, Rubens A, and Speaks C. Effects of stimulus materials on the dichotic listening performance of aphasic patients. J Speech Hear Res 1981;24:526–534.

Nordlund M. Directional audiometry. Acta Otolaryngol 1964;57:1–11.

Obert A, and Cranford J. Effects of neocortical lesions on the P300 component of the auditory evoked response. Am J Otol 1990;11: 447–453.

Oh S, Kuba T, Soyer A, Choi I, Bonikowski F, and Viter J. Lateralization of brainstem lesions by brainstem auditory evoked potentials. Neurology 1981;31:14–18.

Olsen W, and Noffsinger D. Masking level differences for cochlear and brainstem lesion. Ann Otol 1976;85:820–825.

Olsen W, Noffsinger D, and Kurdziel S. Speech discrimination in quiet and in white noise by patients with peripheral and central lesions. Acta Otolaryngol 1975;80:375–382.

Orchik D, and Burgess T. Synthetic sentences identification as a function of the age of the listener. J Am Audiol Soc 1977;3:42–46.

Parker W, Decker R, and Richards N. Auditory function and lesions of the pons. Arch Otolaryngol 1968;87:228–240.

Pickles J. An Introduction to the Physiology of Hearing. 2nd Ed. New York: Academic Press, 1988.

Pinheiro M. Tests of central auditory function in children with learning disabilities. In Keith R, Ed. Central Auditory Dysfunction. New York: Grune and Stratton, 1977.

Pinheiro M, and Musiek F. Special considerations in central auditory evaluation. In Pinheiro M, and Musiek F, Eds. Assessment of Central Auditory Dysfunction. Baltimore: Williams & Wilkins, 1985.

Pinheiro M, and Tobin H. Interaural intensity difference for intracranial lateralization. J Acoust Soc Am 1969;40:1482–1487.

Pinheiro M, and Tobin H. Interaural intensity differences as a diagnostic indicator. Acta Otolaryngol 1971;71:326–328.

Quine D, Regan D, and Murray T. Delayed auditory tone perception in multiple sclerosis. Can J Neurol Sci 1983;10:183–186.

Rees N. Saying more than we know: is auditory processing disorder a meaningful concept? In Keith R, Ed. Central Auditory Processing and Language Disorders in Children. Houston: College-Hill Press, 1981.

Reeves A. Overview of disorders of the central nervous system. In Pinheiro M, and Musiek F, Eds. Assessment of Central Auditory Function. Baltimore: Williams & Wilkins, 1985.

Roeser R, Johns D, and Price L. Dichotic listening in adults with sensorineural hearing loss. J Am Audiol Soc 1976;2:19–25.

Russolo M, and Poli P. Lateralization, impedance, auditory brainstem response, and synthetic sentence audiometry in brainstem disorders. Audiology 1983;22:50–62.

Sanchez-Longo L, and Forester F. Clinical significance of impairments in sound localizations. Neurology 1958;8:119–125.

Sanger D, Decker T, and Freed J. Early identification of children "at risk" for auditory processing problems. Education Treatment Children 1987;10:165–174.

Scherg M, and Von Cramon D. Psychoacoustic and electrophysiologic correlates of central hearing disorders in man. Eur Arch Psychiatry Neurol Sci 1986;236:56–60.

Schuknecht H. Further observations on the pathology of presbycusis. Arch Otolaryngol 1964;80:368–382.

Secord G, Erickson M, and Bush J. Neuropsychological sequelae of otitis media in children and adolescents with learning disabilities. J Pediatr Psychol 1988;13:531–542.

Selters W, and Brackmann D. Acoustic tumor detection with brainstem electric response audiometry. Arch Otolaryngol 1977;103:181–187.

Selters W, and Brackmann D. Brainstem electric response audiometry acoustic tumor detection. In House W, and Luetje C, Eds. Acoustic Tumors. Vol. 1. Baltimore: University Park Press, 1979.

Smith R, and Prather W. Phoneme discrimination in older persons under varying signal-to-noise conditions. J Speech Hear Res 1972;14:630–638.

Smith B, and Resnick D. An auditory test for assessing brainstem integrity: a preliminary report. Laryngoscope 1972;32:414–424.

Sparks R, and Geschwind N. Dichotic listening in man after section of neo-cortical commissures. Cortex 1968;4:13–16.

Sparks R, Goodglass H, and Nickel B. Ipsilateral versus contralateral extinction in dichotic listening resulting from hemispheric lesions. Cortex 1970;6:249–260.

Speaks C. Dichotic listening: a clinical or research tool? In Sullivan M, Ed. Proceedings of a Symposium on Central Auditory Processing Disorders. Omaha, NE: University of Nebraska Medical Center, 1975.

Speaks C, Niccum N, and Van Tasell D. Effects of stimulus materials on the dichotic listening performance of patients with sensorineural hearing loss. J Speech Hear Res 1985;28:16–25.

Speaks C, Olsen W, Clay J, and Niccum N. Audiometric criteria for dichotic central auditory speech tests. Paper presented at the Annual Meeting of the American Speech-Language-Hearing Association, Seattle, 1990.

Spitzer J. A central auditory evaluation protocol. Ear Hear 1983;4:221–231.

Spitzer J, and Ventry I. Central auditory dysfunction among chronic alcoholics. Arch Otolaryngol 1980;106:224–229.

Squires K, and Hecox K. Electrophysiological evaluation of higher level auditory processing. Semin in Hear 1983;4:415–432.

Squires K, Chu N, and Starr A. Auditory brainstem potentials with alcohol. Electroencephalogr Clin Neurophysiol 1978;45:577–584.

Stach B. Central auditory processing disorders and amplification applications. In Cherow E, Ed. Proceedings of the Research Symposium on Communication Sciences and Disorders and Aging. ASHA Reports 1990;19:150–156.

Stach B, Spretnjak M, and Jerger J. The prevalence of central presbycusis in clinical populations. J Am Acad Audiol 1990;1:109–115.

Starr A, and Achor J. Auditory brainstem response in neurological disease. Arch Neurol 1975;32:761–768.

Stevens S, and Thornton A. Subjective and electrophysiologic tests in brainstem lesions. Arch Otolaryngol 1976;102:608–613.

Sticht T, and Gray B. The intelligibility of time-compressed words as a function of age and hearing loss. J Speech Hear Res 1969;12:443–448.

Tallal P, Stark R, Kallman C, and Mellits D. Developmental dysphasia: relation between acoustic processing deficits and verbal processing. Neuropsychologia 1980;18:273–284.

Telian S, and Kileny P. Usefulness of 1000Hz tone burst evoked responses in the diagnosis of acoustic neuroma. Otolaryngol Head Neck Surg 1989;101:466–471.

Theopold H. Degenerative alterations in the ventral cochlear nucleus of the guinea pig after impulse noise exposure: a preliminary light and electron microscope study. Arch Otorhinolaryngol 1975;209:247–262.

Thompson M, and Abel S. Indices of hearing in patients with central auditory pathology. Scand Audiol 1992;21:(Suppl 35).

Thornton A, Mendel M, and Anderson C. Effects of stimulus frequency and intensity on the middle components of the averaged auditory electrocephalic response. J Speech Hear Res 1977;20:81–94.

Webster D, and Webster M. Neonatal sound deprivation affects brainstem auditory nuclei. Arch Otolaryngol 1977;103:392–396.

Welsh L, Welsh J, Healy M, and Cooper B. Cortical, subcortical, and brainstem dysfunction: Correlation in dyslexic children. Ann Otol Rhinol Laryngol 1982;91:310–315.

Wexler B, and Halwes T. Increasing the power of dichotic methods: the fused rhymed words test. Neuropsychologia 1983;21:59–66.

Whitfield T. The Auditory Pathway. Baltimore: Williams & Wilkins, 1967.

Willeford J, and Bilger J. Auditory perception in children with learning disabilities. In Katz J, Ed. Handbook of Clinical Audiology. 2nd Ed. Baltimore: Williams & Wilkins, 1978.

Willeford J, and Burleigh J. Handbook of Central Auditory Processing Disorders in Children. Orlando, FL: Grune and Stratton, 1985:49–86.

Yingling C, Hosobuchi Y, and Harrington M. P300 as a predictor of recovery from coma. Lancet 1990;1:873.

CHAPTER 15

Nonspeech Procedures in Central Testing

Zahrl G. Schoeny and Richard E. Talbott

This chapter will provide an overview of the various non-speech test procedures that can be used in central auditory assessment, and will suggest a reconceptualization of the role of these tests in the assessment of the auditory system. Typically the primary application of pure-tone-based procedures has been to establish threshold and for baseline information, while speech tests have served the primary role of assessing suprathreshold function. The subjectivity and variability of suprathreshold data obtained using puretone procedures has contributed to a lack of acceptance of these tests for site-of-lesion identification.

In recent years substantial development has taken place in applying evoked potential testing to the study of auditory system integrity (Davis, 1976; Ruth and Lambert, 1991). Many clinicians assume that because of the contributions of these physiologic measures to the audiologic test battery it obviates the need for behavioral tests. The opposite, however, may indeed be the case: physiologic measures may enhance the value of nonspeech behavioral tests for assessing the functional integrity of the auditory system. The objectivity and anatomical specificity of physiologic tests will enable the development and/or test procedures that specifically measure the functional attributes of central auditory processing. The contribution of audiology to the site-of-lesion evaluation is well documented and remains an integral part of the audiologists clinical services. However, the future significance of the audiology clinical contribution may rest more heavily in the ability to analyze and provide rehabilitative strategies for individuals whose auditory processing capabilities are somehow compromised. This is particularly critical where the auditory processing deficit affects educational, social, psychological, and/or vocational development and achievement. In the habilitative model of service delivery, the assessment of function is essential. To do this, it is necessary to develop tests aimed at identifying specific abilities. For this purpose puretone and other nonspeech stimuli (e.g., noises, environmental sounds, and music) provide considerable variation from which to choose. In addition, unlike speech stimuli they may be modified and measured in numerous ways without destroying the signal. Thus, nonspeech tests may be able to assess the underlying breakdowns in a manner that is not directly dependent upon language ability.

An advantage of using nonverbal materials from a clinical and research perspective is that results may be more directly related to basic behavioral studies on animals. Neff et al. (1975) and Neff (1977) provide excellent overviews of the research leading to current understanding of central auditory function. Speech based tests are well suited to identify many functional auditory capacities, but they also have limitations. Their use is not appropriate for a substantial number of subjects, e.g., those who lack adequate facility with the speech- and language-based content of the tests. Individuals who have not yet developed functional language ability, individuals with language dysfunction, and non-English speaking individuals are examples of subjects for whom the use of sensitized speech tests is of questionable validity. In addition, speech tests may not reveal important but more subtle auditory processing deficits because the listener can use linguistic or intellectual skills to compensate for the processing deficit.

Carhart (1968) outlined an approach for evaluation of the auditory system based on audiologic configurations. Once the test data were obtained it would be possible to make a sophisticated assessment; however, three assumptions were critical to the validation of this research strategy: (*a*) that there are unique properties and functions associated with various levels of the central auditory nervous system (CANS), (*b*) tests that examine such properties or functions can be devised, and (*c*) results from such tests can provide indications of the functional integrity of a particular level of the CANS.

Before any auditory signal reaches the level of conscious recognition it passes through multiple way stations containing cells that are uniquely responsive to one or more parameters of acoustic signals. It is important to keep in mind the difficulty inherent in developing noninvasive clinical tools for the assessment of such a system and the need for the selection of proper stimulus tasks to assess the range of functions involved.

ANATOMY OVERVIEW

The following simple construct of the central auditory nervous system is generally used by neurologists and anatomists, and is a valuable model for the task of conceptualizing the CANS. The system up to and including cranial nerve VIII is defined as the peripheral system, while the brainstem and the brain are defined as the central system. The low brainstem refers to the inferior portion of the brainstem, including the cochlear nuclei and the superior olivary complex. The high brainstem refers to the upper portion of the brainstem, including the inferior colliculus. The auditory reception area refers to Heschl's gyrus (the middle posterior portion of the superior temporal gyrus in each cerebral hemisphere). The nonauditory reception portion includes the entire cerebrum excluding the auditory reception areas.

For purposes of this chapter, the central auditory nervous system is considered to begin at the level of the cochlear nuclei. Peripheral lesions end at the termini of nerve VIII fibers in the cochlear nuclei. Brainstem lesions are those affecting the major decussation of CANS pathways in the brainstem and/or associated nuclei in this area. Lesions of the auditory cortex and interhemispheric networks refer primarily to those influencing the temporal lobes and adjacent tissue as well as the corpus callosum and other commissural connections between the right and left hemispheres.

The intricacy of the central projections of the auditory system is well documented (Ades, 1959; Durrant and Lovrinic, 1977). Chapter 3, 4, and 14 provide excellent information relating to the anatomy and physiology of CANS. The reader is also referred to Gelfand (1990) and Pickles (1988) for more complete coverage. Illustrations of this complexity occur before fibers of the eighth nerve enter the first major central way station, the cochlear nucleus. Notably, the work of Sando (1965) confirmed a bifurcation of the eighth nerve axons into anterior and posterior branches that were in turn distributed to the ventral and dorsal cochlear nuclei respectively.

RATIONALE FOR DEVELOPING NONSPEECH TESTS OF CENTRAL FUNCTION

The literature regarding the use of pure tones in CANS evaluation have focused primarily on the clinical utility in identifying gross lesions of the nervous system. That is, most investigations were directed toward the accuracy with which various tests using pure tone stimuli identified sites of lesion caused by tumors, demyelinating disease, cerebral vascular accident, and other disturbances to the system (Baran and Musiek, 1991). Obviously, the identification of these sites of lesion is of benefit to the neurologist and the patient; yet, as indicated before, the more significant contribution of the field of audiology in the future may lie in our ability to provide a complete assessment" of the integrity of the central auditory processing system. The effects of differences in CNS processing

of auditory stimuli are yet to be thoroughly understood, especially in terms of their impact on language development and cognition. As more becomes known about these relationships, the use of nonspeech stimuli as a significant probe may prove essential. While clicks are practical stimuli in the evaluation of the central auditory system using electrophysiologic techniques, the use of sinusoids are necessary to study frequency-related aspects of the central mechanisms (Gelfand, 1990).

It has been suggested that "it is difficult to overestimate the potential value of brainstem electric response measures" (Rintelmann, 1979 p.364); however, this emphasis on physiologic tests has led to an under utilization of behavioral procedures that may contribute to our understanding of the functional abilities of the individual. While advances in physiologic measures will continue to improve the precision with which we identify site of lesion, behavioral assessment may provide the critical information needed for developing rehabilitative strategies.

Identification of the symptomatology related to specific dysfunctions of the CANS is a difficult task. Unlike the peripheral auditory, the CANS can mask detection of even even extensive damage. For example, an entire temporal lobe may be removed and the effect on hearing is so slight that the audiologist must go to great lengths to show the system is not entirely normal (Jerger, 1963). The function of the auditory system becomes more and more differentiated as one passes upward from the periphery (Bocca and Calearo, 1963). Therefore, diagnostic tests of sufficient subtlety are essential to identification of lesions of the central auditory system. The need for the development of additional tests of central auditory function has long been apparent. The inability to specify the status of the central system has contributed greatly to the slow development in this area.

The first priority with dealing with this difficult task is to identify the critical auditory abilities that need to be assessed. Simultaneous to this process should be the development of suprathreshold tests go measure these abilities that can be applied routinely in the clinical setting. One possible scheme for selecting behaviors to study is reported by Schoeny and Hasenstab (1983) (see Chapter 32).

A rationale for the need of CANS evaluation was given by Elliott (1969, p357) more than 20 years ago and may even be more true today. "The central nervous system is only today beginning to yield its mysteries to research, so that almost yearly the practitioner finds new resources where his predecessors found only meaningless, complexities: yet so vast are the complexities of the system that the prospects of further discoveries, some dramatic, seem inexhaustible." (Elliott, 1969, p. 357.)

REVIEW AND DISCUSSION OF NONSPEECH TESTS FOR CANS ASSESSMENT

The following provides a review of the nonspeech-pure-tone–based tests that have been used for the evaluation of the central auditory mechanisms. The application of these tests to a more functionally oriented assessment will also be presented.

Masking Level Difference

Masking level difference phenomena has been studied extensively since the psychoacoustic study by Hirsh (1948). The masking level difference (MLD) is the dB difference that is necessary to maintain the listener's performance constant when changes in the interaural listening conditions are introduced Jeffress (1965) described the unexpected changes that take place under certain noise conditions, which illustrate the binaural release from masking phenomena. When (a) a noise is presented to the earphone on one ear at a comfortable listening level, and (b) a 500 Hz pulsed tone is added to it, and (c) the level of the tone is adjusted until it is just inaudible, you have obtained a standard masked threshold. When the same noise is presented to the other earphone, the listener will now find the tone in the first ear to be clearly audible. However, when the same tone is added to the noise in the second ear, the tone becomes inaudible in either ear. If the polarity of the tone to one ear is reversed, the tone is again clearly audible. Now the tone "can be reduced in level by many decibels before it again becomes inaudible." (Jeffress, 1965, p.1.)

The detectability of an auditory signal that is presented in noise has been shown to increase markedly when appropriate changes in the interaural relations between the signal and/or noise are introduced (Hirsh, 1948; Hirsh and Webster, 1949; and Schenkel, 1964). This increase in detectibility, or release from masking, is usually expressed quantitatively as a MLD. While the reference condition for computing the MLD in psychophysical has been the monaural listening condition; clinical studies have used the binaural listening condition where the signal and the noise have the same interaural phase relations because this has been found to be equivalent to the monaural condition (Jeffress et al., 1956; Blodgett et al., 1958; and Hirsh and Burgest, 1958). Thus, the MLD may be defined as the difference in dB between the monaural or the binaural in-phase condition and a particular binaural condition.

A variety of listening conditions have been used to investigate MLDs. The parameters that have been manipulated have included variations of interaural phase, interaural time delay, interaural intensity ratio, interaural noise correlation, and combinations of monaural and binaural listening. The feature common to all listening conditions is that a signal to be perceived, designated as S (signal), is combined with a masking sound, which traditionally has been a broad spectrum noise designated as M (masker). Different investigations have used N for noise in the listing of MLD conditions. However, other studies use pure tone maskers or even speech maskers, so it seems more general to use the letter M to indicate the masker condition as noise is not the only masker used in the measurement of MLDs. Subscripts are used in conjunction with these two primary symbols to designate how the combined stimuli are presented under the permutations of monaural-binaural conditions that can occur. The simplest, of course, is monaural administration of both signals, which would be coded, SmMm.

The conditions listed in Table 15.1 show the variety of combinations that can occur with variations of ear, signal, masker, and a variety of interaural conditions. This detail is given to the various conditions involved in the MLD measurement because future test development will likely tap some of these addition conditions in order to tap higher level auditory processing skills. Studies by Goldstein and Stephens (1975), Waryas and Batten (1985), and Hall, Cokely, and Grose (1988) have indicated that MLDs could be useful in the evaluation of central auditory processing ability.

A shift in the efficiency of the noise as a masker with change in listening condition is quantified in terms of

Table 15.1.
Listening Conditions and Terminology Involved in the Application of Marking Level Differences.

SmMm	The signal and the masker are in the same ear. (True monaural)
SoMo	The signal and the masker are presented binaurally and in phase at the ears. (Homophasic)
SπMπ	The signal and the masker are presented binaurally and are out of phase at one ear relative to the other. (Homophasic)
SmMo	The signal is monaural and the masker is presented in phase at the two ears.
SmMπ	The signal is monaural and the masker is presented reversed in phase at one ear relative to the other.
SπMo	The signal is reversed in phase at one ear relative to the other and the masker is presented in phase at the two ears. (Antiphasic)
SoMπ	The signal is presented in phase at the two ears and the masker is reversed in phase at one ear relative to the other. (Antiphasic)
SoMu	The signal is presented in phase at the two ears and the masker is presented at the two ears but is uncorrected (from two separate noise generators).
SπMu	The signal is reversed in phase at one ear relative to the other and the masker is uncorrelated.
SmMu	The signal is monaural and the masker is binaural but uncorrelated.

the resulting MLD. Specifically, the MLD is the difference in decibels between the signal level in the reference and out-of-phase conditions. For example, the masked threshold in dB for SoMo minus the masked threshold in dB for SπMo would yield the MLD for the SπMo condition. Typically the reference condition used to establish the magnitude of the release from masking is the condition in which masking is greatest (e.g., poorest threshold). The condition in which masking is maximal is the monaural one, SmMm.

For more detailed information on the various conditions affecting MLDs the reader is referred to the following references: Hirsh and Webster, 1949; Schenkel, 1966; Schoeny, 1968; Hall, Tyler, and Fernandes, 1984). The following is an overview of the parameters that affect a change in the character of the MLD. Many factors influence the size of MLDs. Masking level differences have seen shown to be a stable aspect of auditory behavior and can be reliably measured in the clinic (Schoeny, 1968; Schoeny and Carhart, 1971; and Stubblefield and Goldstein, 1977). The MLDs are greatest at the lower frequencies, particularly in the region of 200 to 500 Hz. The size of MLDs increase with the level of masking up to an effective masking level of about 40 to 50 dB. The MLD is greatest in the antiphasic listening condition followed by S_oM_π. At intermediate values of phase shift from 180° to 0° the function shows a gradual decrease in the size. The effect of time delay on MLD are essentially the same as those for phase shift.

The reader is referred to Green and Yost (1975) and Durlach and Colburn (1978) for comprehensive discussions regarding the underlying mechanisms supporting the ability of the binaural auditory system to utilize interaural information to improve hearing in certain binaural listening conditions. Henning (1991) and Yost (1988) have further elaborated the role of the binaural system in masking level differences in studies examining various parameters of the systems response to binaural stimulation.

Effect of Hearing Loss

Studies by a number of investigators (Schoeny and Carhart, 1971; Quaranta and Cervellera,1974; Olsen, Noffsinger, and Carhart, l976; Quaranta, Cassano, and Cervellera, 1978 and Jerger, Brown, and Smith, 1984) have shown that certain peripheral hearing losses can have a profound effect on the size of the MLD. Conductive hearing loss can reduce the MLD effect, even when the hearing has returned to normal (Pillsbury, Grose, and Hall, 1991). Cochlear hearing loss, which affects the ability of the system to preserve the temporal cues inherent in the signal, will have a marked effect on the size of the MLD (Schoeny and Carhart, 1971). It is critical to remember that peripheral changes can have a significant effect on the MLD and this must be taken into account when interpreting the results of clinical applications of MLDs.

MLDs in the Assessment of Central Auditory Function

Masking level differences can be obtained for either puretones or speech. MLDs using puretones are usually obtained at 500 Hz, although other frequencies may be used. The the masker is generally a narrow band of noise that centers around the test frequency. Typically a Bekesy type tracking method is used to obtain the thresholds. Several clinical diagnostic audiometers include the instrumentation for measuring MLDs. It is unfortunate, however, that the manufactures have not yet included the SmMo condition as that would allow for the differentiation of ear in many clinical cases. The value of this condition was reported by Schoeny and Carhart (1971). A standard clinical protocol for the measurement of MLDs can be found in the reports by Noffsinger et al. (1972) and Olsen et al. (1976). The reader is referred to Noffsinger et al. (1985) for a more complete discussion of the clinical instrumentation and procedures for the MLD test.

Brainstem lesions have been shown to reduce or eliminate the MLD (Olsen and Noffsinger, 1976; Olsen, Noffsinger, and Carhart, 1976 and Lynn et al. 1981). Cortical lesions, on the other hand, rarely affect MLDs (Cullen and Thompson, 1974; Olsen, Noffsinger, and Carhart, 1976; and Noffsinger and Kurdziel, 1979, Lynn et al., 1981). A germinal study by Noffsinger, Kurdziel, and Applebaum (1975) showed that MLDs for a 500 Hz puretone were abnormal in a patient with a focal pontine lesion. The patient was followed over time to chart the recovery course of the auditory response using several psychoacoustic tasks. The MLD in this patient remained very small long after the recovery from the focal pontine lesion. This procedure can show residual abnormality even when other tests suggest normal function and is useful in early identification of dysfunction.

While the use of MLDs to study the response of the brainstem has proven to be significant and site specific, it is important to remember that peripheral effects can alter the MLD response. Of particular interest is the study by Olsen and Noffsinger (1976) in which they compared MLDs in 12 subjects with high frequency hearing loss, 12 subjects with Ménière's disease, cause the audiologist to be cautious in interpreting the results of the MLD test without audiometric evidence of a normal peripheral system.

One specific pathology that has been studied extensively using MLDs is multiple sclerosis (MS). Noffsinger et al. (1972) first demonstrated the value of MLD in the identification of lesions in the lower brainstem associated with MS. Studies by Matathias, Sohmer, and Biton (1985); Jerger et al. (1986); and Hendler, Squires, and Emmerich (1990) have elaborated on the role of MLD testing in multiple sclerosis. Each of the above studies has showm the MLD to be a good psychoacoustic (behavioral) test for the assessment of the auditory function of lower brainstem integrity.

MLDs have been used to identify different types of presbycusis. Novak and Anderson (1982) found that older adults who were diagnosed as having "neural presbycusis" had significant reductions in the size of the MLDs. However, when the test was done without external noise (i.e., just Sπ) the neural presbycusis group had slightly larger MLDs than they demonstrated with noise. This finding seems to support the idea of increased internal noise in the subject with auditory neural involvement. Yost (1988) provided support for the internal noise hypothesis in explaining the function of the MLD.

At the other end of the continuum Nozza (1987) reported differences in the MLD as a function of maturation. In a follow-up study Hall and Grose (1990) found that the MLD for children below 5–6 years of age was smaller than that found in adults. This reduced MLD was not found to be the result of peripheral factor alone, but was attributed to developmental differences probably related to central auditory processing.

MLDs have also been used in assessing children with learning disabilities. Sweetow and Reddell (1978) found reduced MLD in children with suspected auditory perceptual problems. These authors felt that the test would be of great value especially with nonverbal children. Waryas and Battin (1985) reported the results of a study attempting to provide norms to use with a learning-disabled (LD) population. Their findings for LD cases however, were not different than those reported for normals. This led Waryas and Battin (1985) to speculate that there are probably subcategories in the learning-disabled population that require specific identification. To reinforce the preceding point Battin and Waryas (1985) reported a series of individual cases of subjects with learning disability in which the MLD results were greatly reduced. They concluded that carefully applied MLDs are very useful in the assessment of LD, but cautioned that normal MLDs did not mean the absence of auditory processing disorders.

Another application for the MLD test may in the identification of specific auditory processing abilities. A study by Hall, Cokely, and Grose (1988) suggests an added application of MLDs that might be of great value in identifying auditory functions critical to auditory processing development. Subjects with the ability to combine monaural and binaural auditory information appear to have better auditory processing skills than subjects that are unable to combine these skills. An earlier study that demonstrated the use of MLDs in measuring auditory processing capacity was done by Goldstein and Stephens (1975). These authors suggested that MLDs represent a component of auditory processing, not simply threshold detection, and should be studied further to understand the relation of MLDs to other suprathreshold auditory behaviors.

An application of the MLD test that clearly involves central function is the use of the test in evaluating subjects who stutter Kramer, Green, and Guitar, (1987) found that subjects who stutter had smaller MLDs than nonstutterers. This result was interpreted to mean that individuals who stutter have poorer auditory processing ability than nonstutter's and probably have more difficulty with temporal processing. It is clear that MLDs are of value in the assessment of central auditory function and that we have a reasonable understanding of the bases of the MLD. Data reported by Yonovitz, Thompson, and Lozar (1979) and Schaefer, Martinez, and Noffsinger (1983) demonstrate that MLDs can be assessed by using auditory evoked potentials, at the cortical level. The value of this approach combined with the behavioral assessment will provide the clinician with a powerful approach for the elaboration of auditory function.

Temporal Ordering Tests

Tests requiring subjects to make auditory discriminations on the basis of temporal ordering or sequencing have been employed for many years. Speech, noise, and tones have all been used as test signals. The variables studied have included; tonal frequency, intensity, rate of presentation, sequence of presentation, duration of components, intervals between presentations, overlapped versus nonoverlapped, and so forth. The overall goal of these studies has been to determine the behavioral limits of the auditory/neural system in making these discriminations and, secondly, to isolate the neural centers that might mediate this capability. Information regarding the selective response of certain neurons and neural centers to specific parameters of auditory input provides the basis for interpretation of the results of these studies. When specific behaviors can be associated with particular areas of the central nervous system, this has an inherent appeal both from a clincial diagnostic standpoint and from the perspective of increasing our understanding of auditory processing in general. Interpretation of the data from these studies, however, is still difficult. Results vary greatly in clinical studies using temporal ordering and sequencing depending methodology used. Musiek, et al. (1984) support the previously reported observation that interhemispheric interaction may be a critical feature in auditory pattern perception.

They studied preoperative and postoperative subjects who underwent complete commissurectomies. Results from this investigation and others (Pinheiro and Musiek, 1985) suggest that both hemispheres and their interconnections must be intact for accurate neural decoding and for verbal reporting of these patterns.

In order to evaluate central processing of auditory input, Pinheiro (1977a) developed a test to measure both pattern perception and temporal sequencing abilities called the Pitch Pattern Sequence Test (PPS). A beneficial feature of this test is that there are two separate versions, one for children and one for adults, and it has been reported to be particularly sensitive in children with LD. The adult version presents 120 test pattern sequences made up of three tone bursts, two of one frequency and one of another frequency, with a duration of 200 ms and interstimulus intervals of 150 ms. The test is administered at 50 dB above each subject's 1 kHz threshold. The response mode is varied depending on the subject's capabilities and the information desired. The listener may be asked to respond verbally, manually, or by humming the pattern. Patients with auditory cortex dysfunction, in either hemisphere, show a decrease in their ability to perform these tasks in each ear regardless of the response mode. Patients with interhemispheric dysfunction perform well in the humming condition (Pinheiro and Musiek, 1985, p. 232).

The children's version of the PPS test involves having the child respond to a three tone burst pattern that is similar to the adult version, however, the duration of both the stimulus and the interval are longer for the children. The application of this test to children with LD revealed a consistently decreased ability to perform the verbal task (Pinheiro, 1977b). In fact, all subjects with learning disabilities studied in this investigation had similar central processing profiles in that they had poor performance on the PPS-manual response and the simultaneous sentences in comparison to the eight other tests of central dysfunction used. Comparisons across the response types (verbal, manual, hummed) to the PPS test in LD children have revealed that, in contrast to normals who show little or no response differences, the learning-disabled children are able to hum the patterns but show marked difficulty in responding verbally or manually (Musiek and Geurkink, 1980; Musiek et al., 1982). The apparent ability of these children to perceive the temporal order of the patterns accurately, but inability to process the input recognition and the output sequencing, is similar to observations in split brain patients (Musiek et al., 1984).

A great deal of variability in performance across children on the PPS tasks and other tests of sequencing and ordering has been observed, as would be expected. Research combining evoked potential and/or brain mapping procedures with PPS and other psychophysical sequencing/temporal ordering measures may control for differences caused by maturational variance encountered in the past. The different insight that each measures provides can only enhance their respective contribution.

One recently developed test that shows considerable promise and overcomes some of the problems of using speech material is the Psychoacoustic Pattern Discrimination Test (PPDT) developed by Blaettner et al (1989). This test was developed to provide a measure that (a) was not confounded by perceptual deficits inherent in the use of speech materials, (b) would detect unilateral telencephalic hearing disorders, (c) would be relatively insensitive to peripheral hearing loss. The procedure uses noise bursts to assess discrimination changes in intensity and click trains to test discrimination of changes in temporal structure. The initial studies using this procedure revealed significant differences between subjects with right and left hemisphere involvement and normals. The major finding was that the most prominent abnormality consisted of greater missed discrimination on the ear opposite the telencephalic lesion. This was comparable to the contralateral ear effect previously described for dichotic tests. Patient groups not having telencephalic auditory structure lesions performed the same as normals. An interesting observation of this study was the relation between performance on the PPDT and the particular vascular involvement. Clear differences were obtained depending on which branch of the cerebral artery was involved. The small sample size upon which these site-of-lesion observations were made prohibited statistical analysis of this information, however, it is compelling with regard to further investigation.

Comparisons of the PPDT to auditory evoked potentials (AEP) results further support the use of both behavioral and electrophysiologic clinical data in the analysis of central auditory function. Blaettner et al. (1989) showed that AEPs revealed abnormal middle and/or late potentials in all cases with abnormal PPDTs without the reverse being true. This is a case in which the use of a psychophysical measure appears to have added support for the sensitivity of the AEP to structural damage preceding any functional manifestation. Scherg and von Cramon (1986) point out that this is only true when the AEP dipole activity is isolated to each hemisphere allowing interhemispheric comparisons.

As suggested earlier, behavioral assessment using puretones in conjunction with newer electrophysiological techniques may clear up some of the apparent ambiguities of the past and provide us with better clinical tools. The results of clinical studies of temporal sequencing performance in patients with cortical lesions have been varied. Results range from the need for increased stimulus intervals for discriminating stimulus differences when compared to normals (Lackner and Teuber, 1973) to loss of verbal memory code in brain-damaged patients (DeRenzi et al., 1977). The difficulty in analyzing clinical studies on human subjects with cortical lesions lies in the inability to control the specific site of lesion across patients. Almost every conceivable stimulus type and sequence has been applied in both normal and pathologic patients; however, very few clinical tests of temporal ordering or sequencing have gained widespread acceptance for site-of-lesion testing using either speech or nonspeech material.

Additional Tests That May Be Applicable To Central Evaluation

Many of the assumptions and previously accepted "truths" about the role of the various subcomponents of the central nervous system in auditory processing are being challenged. Reinterpretation of older studies in the face of new information is facilitating the evolution of a better understanding of how the system functions. As suggested at the outset of this chapter, reevaluations of the role of behavioral auditory tests is also in order in light of this new information and the development of site-specific test procedures, such as evoked response audiometry and imaging techniques. When looking at auditory tests that might be useful for the evaluation of central auditory function, it is important to keep in mind that almost all of the existing tests were initially developed for the purpose of identifying the site of lesion.

Jerger et al. (1988) raised another concern that must be factored in when considering the development of tests of central auditory function. The indicated results obtained in children using behavioral tests may not be appropriately interpreted based on the results obtained in the adult population. These generalization to children may be inappropriate as there is much less specificity of cognitive defects resulting from specific central nervous system lesions in children than in adults. In light of this need to reevaluate the application of test results to children, Jerger et al. (1988) provided a strategy that can be used for guiding future clinical application and research in pediatric central evaluations: (a) establish a database of subjects with confirmed lesions; (b) compare the results found in the database with the results of individuals with central auditory disorders; (c) establish the relation between a pattern of auditory results and functional deficit. These suggestions can just as easily be adapted to the development of tests of central auditory function in adults.

In the next section a review of selected nonspeech auditory tests is presented. While the power of some of these tests for site of lesion testing has been questioned, they are presented with the goal of stimulating consideration of their contribution for functional assessment.

ALTERNATE BINAURAL LOUDNESS BALANCE

Puretone tests using alternate binaural loudness balance (ABLB) as an indication of central dysfunction have been studied (Jerger, 1960; Davis and Goodman, 1966). It was found that in cases of lesions of the central auditory pathway, if the lesion is at a high level, then the intensity level in the contralateral ear must be much greater than in the homolateral one in order to give the same sensation of loudness. On the other hand, if the lesion is at a lower level (midbrain), then the principal disturbance will not affect the binaural assessment of loudness but will affect the localization of sound in the median plane when using a simultaneous presentation. When administering the ABLB as a test of central auditory function, the revealing finding is the demonstration of equal loudness at unequal intensity levels with the ear contralateral to the involved central site requiring the greater intensity. These results were confirmed in a novel study by Mencher, Clack, and Rupp (1973) that measured direct loudness estimations in subjects with temporal lobe lesions. Based on their results comparing the direct loudness scaling and the results using the ABLB it was suggested that the loudness imbalance in cases of temporal lobe pathology occurred due to the inability to efficiently utilize signals received through the two ears.

LOCALIZATION AND LATERALIZATION

The scholarly treatment of directional hearing in the book *Directional Hearing* by Yost and Gourevitch (1987), provides an excellent foundation for the state of the art work with localization and lateralization. Auditory localization is the ability to identify the source of a sound in space. In the lateralization task, sounds are presented through headphones. Cues for localization and lateralization include interaural time differences and interaural intensity differences.

While similar rules govern both lateralization and localization behavior, the study of lateralization might contribute more to the ability to assess the CANS. Earphone presentation of the stimuli in lateralization tasks allows for control over the stimuli and interstimulus relationships that is difficult to accomplish in the sound field. Yost (1991) provides an excellent review of the basis of auditory image perception. The material in this article gives an orientation for the development of tests and systematic investigation that will asses this critical area of central auditory behavior.

The "precedence effect" has become a central focus in studies of the auditory system (Cranford, Boose, and

Moore, 1990; Moore, Cranford, and Rahn, 1990). To elicit the precedence effect the sounds presented to the two ears must be qualitatively similar; if second sound differs significantly from the primary sound, there will be a perception of two sounds and fusion will not occur. Measurement of the gating of incoming information in the auditory system may prove to be a pivotal advancement in the near future. In everyday listening the auditory system is forced to deal with a very complex acoustical environment. The ability to focus on a specific signal of greatest informational value at the moment, may be one of the contributions of the precedence effect. The auditory system, uses temporal and intensity information not only to determine the location of the sound source, but to select the ear through which to gate the information to the CANS (Green, 1966). Age has been shown to affect lateralization and the precedence effect (Herman, Warren, and Wagener, 1977; Cranford, Boose, and Moore, 1990). Tests involving lateralization have been shown to be of value in the assessment of some patients with central auditory pathology (Shitara, Sato, and Kirikae, 1965; Groen, 1969; and Moore, Cranford, and Rahn, 1990).

Abnormal horizontal localization and lateralization have been reported in patients with eighth nerve lesions and in some with brainstem lesions (Nordlund, 1964; Stephens, 1976; Hausler, Cloburn, and Marr, 1983). The situation with regard to auditory cortical lesions is more complicated and controversial. It is probably necessary to use a complex localization task in order to identify lesions involving the cortex (Stephens, 1976). Sanchez-Longo and colleagues (Sanchez-Longo and Forster, 1958; Sanchez-Longo, Forster, and Auth, 1957) studied sound localization ability in adults with brain damage. They found the ear contralateral to the temporal lesions to show deficits in localization ability.

Studies investigating the use of simultaneous binaural median plane lateralization (SBMPL) yielded the following results. Matzker (1959) did not find errors in lateralization when he delivered tones of the same intensity and frequency to the two ears simultaneously in subjects affected with lesions of the temporal cortex. Sanchez-Longo et al. (1957) used normal subjects, subjects with extratemporal lesions and subjects with temporal lobe lesions to localize a noise source. They found that patients with temporal lobe tumors localized the noise toward the side opposite the side with the lesion. Inability to perceive the fused experience or achieving a midline image only with considerable interaural intensity difference is sometimes a product of peripheral or lower brainstem dysfunction. In a study by Noffsinger et al. (1972) several auditory tests were administered to individuals with multiple sclerosis. Of the 60 individuals in the study, 12 could not achieve a me-

dian plane image. The authors concluded that the SBMPL indicated dysfunction at a lower brainstem level rather at higher levels of the central auditory system. In another study, Noffsinger et al. (1984) used the SBMPL test on a subject with a specifically defined brainstem lesion. They found that the subject could achieve a median plane image with higher frequency stimuli (2000 Hz, for example), but could not achieve the median image with lower frequency signals. These results support the suggestions offered by Jerger and Harford (1960) that the SBMPL utilized the synchrony of the onset action potential (AP) to attain the median plane image. The superior olivary complex, in the lower brainstem, seems to be the area responsible for the attainment of a median plane image, which appears to depend on the temporal synchrony between the two ears. Noffsinger et al. (1984) confirmed the early study by Matzker (1959) showing that cortical damage does not affect performance on the SBMPL task.

SHORT INCREMENT SENSITIVITY INDEX

Jerger et al. (1969) proposed a modification of the Short Increment Sensitivity Index (SISI) procedure in which scores were plotted as a function of sensation level. In this study and one by Hodgson (1967), marked asymmetries in the bilateral SISI scores were observed in patients with temporal lobe lesions. Other investigators, however, have observed essentially normal difference limens in temporal lobectomies (Swisher, 1967; Mencher et al., 1970).

The SISI has not typically been used as a part of the CANS test battery. However, our increased understanding of the contributions of certain neurons and neural centers to the perception of intensity and duration changes may make the use of the SISI test more attractive. For a detailed review of the development and subsequent research on the SISI test the reader is referred to the thorough work of Buus, Florentine, and Redden (1982).

OTHER AUDITORY BEHAVIORS

Many other auditory procedures have been studied over the years. Among them are auditory adaptation, binaural beats, central masking, flutter fusion, gap detection, perceptual masking, temporal integration, and temporal masking (including forward and backward masking). The research reviewed in this chapter are examples of what might be easily implemented in the clinical routine. Hopefully these procedures can assist in the evaluation of central auditory function and thus speed the development of therapeutic intervention strategies and educational procedures for aiding those with auditory processing disorders.

SUMMARY

The contribution of the audiologist to the diagnostic team in the evaluation of the central auditory nervous system is an important aspect of the audiologic practice. For the most part, however, the audiologist's role in this process has been to assist in the identification of pathology that will be treated by other professionals. The scope of the audiologist's practice should include the identification and rehabilitation of the more subtle auditory processing functions of the neural system. Physiologic measures that provide specificity and insights into auditory integrity, do not reveal the functional capabilities of the individual. Nonspeech materials to assess specific auditory processing capabilities may be one of the cornerstones of our future clinical practice. The evolution of physiologic measures has opened up new potential for the behavioral evaluation and subsequent application of this knowledge.

REFERENCES

Ades H. Central auditory mechanisms. In Magoun, H.W. Eds. Handbook of Physiology: Neurophysiology. Vol I. Baltimore: William & Wilkins, 1959:585–613.

Baran JA, and Musiek FE. Behavioral assessment of the elderly. In Rintelmann WF, Ed. Hearing Assessment, 2nd ed. Austin: Pro-Ed, Inc., 1991:549–602.

Battin RR, and Waryas PA. Profiles of patients demonstrating abnormal masking level difference responses. J Child Commun Disorders 1985;8:155–164.

Blaettner U, Scherg M, and Von Cramon D. Diagnosis of unilateral telencephalic hearing disorders: evaluation of a simple psychoacoustic patten discrimination test. Brain 1989;112:177–195.

Blodgett HC, Jeffress LA, and Taylor BW. Relation of masked threshold to signal distortion for various interaural phase combinations. Am J Psychol 1958;71:283–290.

Bocca E, and Calearo C. Central hearing processes. In Jerger J, Ed. Modern Developments in Audiology. New York: Academic Press, 1963:337–370.

Buus S, Florentine M, and Redden R. The SISI test: a review. Part I and Part II. Audiology 1982;21:273–293, 365–385.

Carhart R. (1968).

Cranford JL, Boose M, and Moore CA. Effects of aging on the precedence effect in sound localization. J Speech Hearing Res 1990; 33:654–659.

Cullen JK Jr, and Thompson CL. Masking release for subjects with temporal lobe resection. Arch Otolaryngol 1974;100: 113–116.

Davis H. Principles of electric response audiometry. Ann Otol Rhinol Otolaryngol 1976;85(Suppl 28):1–96.

Davis H, and Goodman AC. Subtractive hearing loss, loudness, recruitment, and decruitment. Ann Otol Rhinol Laryngol 1966; 102:87–94.

DeRenzi E, Faglioni P, and Villa P. Sequential memory for figures in brain-damaged patients. Neuropsychologia 1977;13:43–49.

Durlach NI, and Colburn HS. Binaural phenomena. In Carterette EC, and Friedman MP, Eds. Handbook of Perception. Vol. 4. New York: Academic Press, 1978:365–466.

Durrant J and Lovrinic J. Bases of Hearing Science. Baltimore: Williams & Wilkins, 1977.

Elliott HC. Textbook of Neuroanatomy, 2nd ed. Philadelphia: JB Lippincott, 1969:375.

Gelfand, S. Hearing: An Introduction to Psychological and Physiological Acoustics. 2nd ed. New York: Marcel Dekker, 1990.

Goldstein DP, and Stephens SDG. Masking level difference: A measure of auditory processing capability. Audiology 1975;14:354–367.

Groen JJ. Diagnostic value of lateralization ability for dichotic time differences. Acta Oto-Laryngol 1969;67:326–332.

Hall JW III, and Grose JH. The masking-level difference in children. J Am Acad Audiol 1990;1:81–88.

Hall JW, Tyler RS, and Fernandes MA. Factors influencing the masking level difference in cochlear hearing-impaired and normal- hearing listeners. J Speech Hearing Res 1984;27:145–154.

Hall JW III, Cokely JA, and Grose JH. Combined monaural and binaural masking release. J Acoust Soc Am 1988;83:1839–1845.

Hausler R, Colburn S, and Marr E. Sound localization in subjects with impaired hearing: Spacial-discrimination and interaural- discrimination tests. Acta Oto-Laryngol 1983;400(suppl.):1–62.

Hendler T, Squires NK, and Emmerich DS. Psychophysical measures of central auditory dysfunction in multiple sclerosis: neurophysiological and neuroanatomical correlates. Ear Hearing 1990; 11:403–416.

Herman GE, Warren LR, and Wagener JW. Auditory lateralization: age differences in sensitivity to dichotic time and amplitude cues. J Gerontol 1977;32:187–191.

Hirsh IJ. The influence of interaural phase on interaural summation and inhibition. J Acoust Soc Am 1948;20:536–544.

Hirsh IJ, and Burgest M. Binaural effects in remote masking. J Acoust Soc Am 1958;30:827–832.

Hirsh IJ, and Webster FA. Some determinants of interaural phase effects. J Acoust Soc Am 1949;21:496–501.

Hodgson W. Audiological report of a patient with left hemispherectomy. J Speech Hear Disord 1967;32:39–45.

Jeffress, LA. Binaural signal detection: Vector theory. Defense Research Lab. Acoustical Report no. 245, University of Texas, 1965.

Jeffress LA, Blodgett HC, Sandel TT, and Wood CL. masking of tonal signals. J Acoust Soc Am 1956;28:416–426.

Jerger J. Observations on auditory behavior in lesions of the central auditory pathways. Arch Otolaryngol 1960;71:797–806.

Jerger, J. (1963)

Jerger J, and Harford E. The alternate and simultaneous balancing of pure tones. J Speech Hear Res 1960;3:17–30.

Jerger J, Weikers NJ, Sharbrough FW, and Jerger S. Bilateral lesions of the temporal lobe: a case study. Acta-Otolaryngologica 1969;258 (Suppl):1–57.

Jerger J, Brown D, and Smith S. Effect of peripheral hearing loss on masking level difference. Arch Otolaryngol 1984;110:290–296.

Jerger J, Oliver TA, Chmiel R, and Rivera V. Patterns of auditory abnormality in multiple sclerosis. Audiology 1986;25:193–209.

Jerger S, Johnson K, and Loiselle L. Pediatric central auditory dysfunction. Am J Otolaryngol 1988;9(suppl.):63–70.

Kramer MB, Green D, and Guitar B. A comparison of stutterers and nonstutterers on masking level differences and synthetic sentence identification tasks. J Commun Disord 1987;20:379–390.

Lackner J, and Teuber HL. Alterations in auditory fusion thresholds after cerebral injury in man. Neuropsychologia 1973;11:409–415.

Lynn GE, Gilroy J, Taylor, PC, and Leiser RP. Binaural masking-level differences in neurological disorders. Arch Otolaryngol 1981;107: 357–362.

Matthias D, Sohmer H, and Biton V. Central auditory tests and auditory nerve-brainstem evoked responses in multiple sclerosis. Acta Otolaryngol 1985;99:369–376.

Matzker J. Two methods for the assessment of central auditory functions in cases of brain disease. Ann Otol Rhinol Laryngol 1959;68: 1155–1197.

Mencher G, Clack D, and Rupp R. The different limen for intensity and central auditory pathology. J Aud Res 1970;10:372–377.

Mencher G, Clack D, and Rupp R. Decruitment and the growth of loudness in the ears of brain-damaged adults. Cortex 1973; 9:335–345.

Moore CA, Cranford JL, and Rhan AE. Tracking of a "moving" fused auditory image under conditions that elicit the precedence effect. Speech Hear Res 1990;90:141–148.

Musiek FE, and Geurkink NA. Auditory perceptual problems in children: Considerations for the otolaryngologist and audiologist. Laryngoscope 1980;90:962–971.

Musiek FE, Geurkink NA, and Keitel S. Test battery assessment of auditory perceptual dysfunction in children. Laryngoscope 1982;92: 251–257.

Musiek FE, Kibbe K, and Baran JA. Neuroaudiological results from split-brain patients. Semin Hear 1984;5:219–229.

Neff WD. The brain and hearing: auditory discrimination affected by brain lesions. Ann Otol 1977;86:500–506.

Neff WD, Diamond IT, and Cassedy TH. Behavioral studies of auditory discrimination: central nervous system. In Keidel WD, and Neff WD, Eds. Auditory System, 1975.

Noffsinger D, and Kurdziel. Assessment of central auditory lesions. In Rintelman W, Ed. Hearing Assessment. Baltimore: University Park Press, 1979.

Noffsinger D, Olsen WO, Carhart R, Hart, CW, and Sahgal V. Auditory and vestibular aberrations in multiple sclerosis. Acta Oto-Laryngologica 1972;303(Suppl):1–63.

Noffsinger D, Kurdziel S, and Applebaum EL. Value ofspecial auditory tests in the latero-medial inferior pontine syndrome. Ann Otol Rhinol Laryngol 1975;84:384–390.

Noffsinger D, Schaefer AB, and Martinez CD. Behavioral and objective estimates of auditory brainstem integrity. Semin Hear 1984;5: 337–349.

Noffsinger D, Schaefer AB, and Martinez CD. Puretone techniques in evaluations of central auditory function. In Katz J, Ed. Handbook of Clinical Audiology, 3rd ed. Baltimore: Williams & Wilkins, 1985: 337–354.

Norland B. Directional audiometry. Acta Oto-Laryngol 1964;57:1–18.

Novak RE, and Anderson CV. Differentiation of types of presbycusis using the masking-level difference. J Speech Hear Res 1982; 25:504–508.

Nozza RJ. The binaural masking level difference in infants and adults: Development change in binaural hearing. Infant Behav Dev 1987; 10:105–110.

Olsen WO, and Noffsinger D. Masking level differencesfor cochlear and brain stem lesions. Ann Otol Rhinol Laryngol 1976;86:820–825.

Olsen WO, Noffsinger D, and Carhart R. Masking level differences encountered in clinical populations. Audiology 1976;15:287–301.

Pickles JO. An Introduction to the Physiology of Hearing. 2nd Ed. New York: Academic Press, 1988.

Pillsbury HC, Grose JH, and Hall JW. Otitis-media with effusion in children—binaural hearing before and after corrective surgery. Arch Otolaryngol Head Neck Surg 1991;17:718–723.

Pinheiro ML. Auditory patten reversal in auditory perception in patents with left and right hemisphere lesions. Ohio J Speech Hear 1977a;12:9–20.

Pinheiro ML. Tests of central auditory function in children with learning disabilities. In Keith RW, Ed. Central Auditory Dysfunction. New York: Grune and Stratton, 1977b:223–256.

Pinheiro ML, and Musiek FE. Sequencing and temporal ordering in the auditory system. In Pinheiro ML, and Musiek FE, Eds. Assessment of Central Auditory Dysfunction: Foundations and Clinical Correlates. Baltimore: Williams & Wilkins, 1985:219–238.

Quaranta A, Cassano P, and Cervellera G. Clinicalvalue of the tonal masking level difference. Audiology 1978;17:232–238.

Quaranta A, and Cervellera G. Masking level difference in normal and pathological ears. Audiology 1974;13:428–431.

Rintlemann, WF, Ed. Hearing Assessment. Baltimore: University Park Press, 1979:364.

Ruth R and Lambert P. Auditory Evoked Potentials. Otolaryngol Clin North Am. Philadelphia: WB Saunders, 1991;24:349–370.

Sanchez-Longo LP, Forster FM, and Auth TL. A clinical test for sound localization and its applications. Neurology 1957;7:653–655.

Sanchez-Longo LP, and Forster FM. Clinical significance of impairment of sound localization. Neurology 1958;8:119–125.

Sando I. The anatomical interrelationships of the cochlear nerve fibers. Acta Otolaryngol 1965;59:417–436.

Schaefer AB, Martiniez CD, and Noffsinger D. The effects of signal-masker phase conditions on the late cortical responses. San Diego: The Acoustical Society of America, 1983.

von Schenkel KD. Uber die abhangigheit der mithorschwellen von der interauralen phasenlage des testschalls. Acustica 1964;14:337–346.

Schenkel KD. Accumulation theory of binaural-masked thresholds. The J Acoust Soc Am 1966;41:20–31.

Scherg M, and von Cramon D. Psychoacoustic and electrophysiologic correlates of central hearing disorder in man. Eur Arch Psychiatry Neurol Sci 1986;236:56–60.

Shitara T, Sato T, and Kirikae I. Clinical application of directional hearing test. Internat Audiol 1965;4:35–36.

Schoeny ZG. Comparisons of Masking Level Differences for Normal Hearing Subjects and Subjects with Unilateral Ménière's Disease. Northwestern University. University Microfilms, 1968.

Schoeny ZG, and Carhart R. Effects of unilateral Ménière's disease on masking level differences. J Acoust Soc Am 1971;50:1143–1150.

Schoeny ZG, and Hasenstab MS. "Auditory Processing" Short Course. Virginia Speech and Hearing Association Convention, Charlottesville, VA, April, 1983.

Stephens SDG. Auditory temporal summation in patients with central nervous system lesions. In Stephens SDG, Ed. Disorders of Auditory Function. London: Academic Press, 1976:243–252.

Stubblefield JH, and Goldstein DP. A test-retest reliability study on clinical measurement of masking level difference. Audiology 1977; 16:419–431.

Sweetow RW, and Reddell RC. The use of masking level differences in the identification of children with perceptual problems. J Am Aud Soc 1978;4:52–56.

Swisher L. Auditory intensity discrimination in patients with temporal lobe damager. Cortex 1967;3:179–193.

Waryas PA, and Batten RR. Masking level difference response norms from learning disabled individuals. J Child Commun Dis 1985; 8:147–153.

Webster FA. The influence of interaural phase on masked thresholds. I: The role of interaural time-deviation. J Acoust Soc Am 1951;23: 452–462.

Yonovitz A, Thompson CL, and Lozar J. Masking level differences; Auditory evoked responses with homophasic and antiphasic signal and noise. J Speech Hear Res 1979;22:403–411.

Yost WA. The masking-level difference and overall masker level: Restating the internal noise hypothesis. J Acoust Soc Am 1988;83: 1517–1521.

Yost WA, and Gourevitch G, Eds. Directional Hearing. New York: Springer-Verlag, 1987.

Yost WA. Auditory image perception and analysis: the basis of hearing. Hearing Res 1991;56:8–18.

CHAPTER 16

Monosyllabic Procedures
In Central Testing

H. Gustav Mueller and Kathryn E. Bright

In 1963, in their now classic chapter in Jerger's *Modern Developments in Audiology*, the Italian researchers Bocca and Calearo described the basic considerations of central hearing processes and summarized much of their own work in this area. These authors explained and illustrated such important concepts as the redundancy principle, the contralateral ear effect, the "rollover" phenomenon (although not labeled as such), and the neuroanatomical correlates related to these observations.

Jerger (1964) summarized his early research in the area of central auditory testing, with clinical conclusions in agreement with the work of the Italian researchers. In a third germinal book chapter, published in the first edition of *Handbook of Clinical Audiology*, Berlin and Lowe (1972) discussed the interaction of temporal factors with frequency and intensity, and the effects of temporal lobe lesions on speech audiometry; they also summarized the research from their laboratory relating to dichotic speech testing. The basic principles and test strategies outlined in these early writings have remained timely and relevant and are reflected in much of the current clinical work.

This chapter will focus on only one category of central auditory nervous system (CANS) speech tests: those tests employing monosyllables as the stimulus. As discussed by Musiek and Lamb in Chapter 14, it is common to use a test battery approach for the detection of a central auditory pathology. Because of the complexities and subtleties of the central auditory nervous system, it is generally believed that no single speech test is sensitive to all pathologies or dysfunctions of the CANS. When a test battery is selected, therefore, for a given patient three factors usually are considered: (*a*) the neuroanatomical site for which the test is the most sensitive (e.g., low brainstem versus auditory cortex), (*b*) whether the test is monaural, binaural or dichotic, and (*c*) the difficulty of the test (relatively easy CANS tests may not be sensitive to subtle CANS pathologies). Note that the character of speech material, whether monosyllabic, bisyllabic, or sentence length, is not a critical clinical consideration. Hence, the beginning student of audiology should not view this chapter in isolation, but rather as it relates to the other four chapters within this section.

This chapter will review contemporary CANS speech tests that utilize monosyllables and provide a brief description of each test. Several monosyllabic tests have been designed especially for use with children, and these tests will be reviewed separately. The interpretation of CANS test results cannot be conducted without considering such factors as peripheral hearing status, age of the patient, and the reliability, sensitivity and specificity of the test employed. These factors will be addressed as they apply to the various monosyllabic tests.

UNDERLYING PRINCIPLES

There are three primary concepts that must be kept in mind when monosyllabic CANS speech tests are reviewed and selected for clinical use, and when the results of these tests are interpreted. The first of these concepts is the redundancy principle. As described by Bocca and Calearo (1963), the ease with which one is able to perceive speech is due in part to the extrinsic redundancy within the speech signal and the intrinsic redundancy within the auditory system. Extrinsic redundancy refers to the numerous overlapping cues within speech itself; intrinsic redundancy refers to the multiple CANS pathways and sources of information that the human system possesses for processing speech. Individuals usually will perform at or near normal for a speech-processing task if only one of these two types of redundancy has been reduced (e.g., clear speech with a CANS disorder, or mildly distorted speech with a normal CANS). If both extrinsic and intrinsic redundancy have been reduced, however, then abnormal performance often is observed. Clearly, this interaction is the basis for using speech audiometry for the detection of CANS dysfunction. The sensitivity and specificity of a selected speech test depends heavily on the degree to which each type of redundancy is reduced for a given patient/test combination.

The second important concept concerns the relationship between the neuroanatomical location of the pathology or dysfunction and the ear that is expected to demonstrate the reduced performance. The contralateral ear effect, observed because of the dominant crossing auditory fiber tract, was described in early research by Bocca and his colleagues (Bocca et al., 1954, 1955), Goldstein et al. (1956), and Jerger (1960 a, b). Today, this diagnostic pattern continues to be the expected finding for most disorders of the auditory cortex. This pattern sometimes is altered, however, when a deep posterior left temporal lobe lesion is present. A pathology in this region may cause abnormal test results bilaterally, or only in the ipsilateral ear. For adults or children with generalized auditory processing deficits, the contralateral ear concept is less straightforward, as typically there is no specific site of lesion or dysfunction. Disorders of the interhemispheric connections (corpus callosum) also can produce abnormal CANS test results, especially for dichotic stimuli. This type of pathology typically causes a reduced score for the left ear (see Baran and Musiek, 1991, for review).

When speech tests are used to detect brainstem rather than cortical pathology, abnormal findings may be observed for either the ipsilateral or contralateral ear. Jerger and Jerger (1975a) reported that the ear effect for brainstem disorders is related to whether the pathology is extra-axial or intra-axial. Intra-axial pathologies often show a subtle effect for one or both ears, whereas extra-axial pathologies more commonly show an ipsilateral effect due to the frequent involvement of the cochlear nuclei and the fibers of cranial nerve VIII.

The third principle concerning the clinical use of CANS tests relates to the task presented to the patient. Speech tests can be used to create different types of listening tasks, the combination of which can enhance the sensitivity of the CANS test battery. For example, monosyllables can be mixed with noise to create a *figure/ground* task. Or, different frequency bands of the same monosyllable can be presented to each ear simultaneously to create a *fusion* task. Or finally, different monosyllables can be presented to each ear dichotically to create a *separation* task. Monosyllables can also be distorted by time compression or by altering their spectral content with filters.

The three principles described here are critical to the interpretation of CANS tests and the selection of a test battery for a given patient. By relating the intrinsic and extrinsic redundancy to the expected ear effect for a degraded speech, fusion, or separation task, monosyllables can be used effectively in the clinical evaluation of CANS disorders.

CLINICAL APPLICATIONS OF CANS TESTS

In a text on *clinical* audiology, it is important to discuss how these procedures can be implemented into the day-to-day test protocol of the clinical audiologist. Given that there are CANS tests that can be administered and

scored in as little as ten minutes, one might suggest that at least one CANS screening test should be given to the majority of patients evaluated. As previously discussed, it is common for individuals with central auditory disorders to perform normally on the peripheral battery, and hence, even a CANS screening test can add useful information for forming a diagnostic impression.

While there would seem to be some merit in routinely conducting a CANS screening test, there are few audiology clinics that follow this practice. In a 1988 survey by Mueller of 24 audiology clinics, not one facility reported frequent use of a CANS speech test (Hood and Mueller, 1988). Most clinics reported that CANS speech tests either were not used at all, or that they were only used when a CANS disorder was suspected. The most common reasons given for not using CANS tests were: (*a*) the tests are not diagnostically efficient (poor sensitivity/specificity), (*b*) the treatment/disposition plan for a positive finding is poorly defined, (*c*) the tests take too long to administer and score, and (*d*) "our clinic rarely sees patients with CANS disorders." Mueller reported, however, that in many cases the audiologist's reluctance to use CANS tests was not based on empirical findings, but rather on a general belief that had been passed along from instructors and co-workers.

If one considers adding CANS testing to the clinic protocol, it is useful to categorize the different reasons for conducting this testing. In general, the clinical application of CANS testing falls within one of four different areas: (*a*) to detect space–occupying lesions (Musiek, 1983b, Jerger and Jerger, 1981), (*b*) to detect generalized CANS processing deficits (Stach et al., 1990a, b; Grimes et al., 1985), (*c*) to monitor the change in a CANS disorder (Grimes, 1985; Stach et al., 1985; Grimes, 1990), and (*d*) to provide a framework for counseling patients fitted with hearing aids (Davies and Mueller, 1987; Mueller and Calkins, 1988; Stach, 1990a, b). As the following tests are described, it is important to consider how each test can be used in one or more of these areas.

MONAURAL CANS TESTS

Monosyllabic words are commonly used for CANS testing. Historically, standard monaural phonetically balanced word recognition procedures led to the development of CANS tests using degraded speech to make the listening task more difficult. Because monosyllables represent the linguistic unit with the least extrinsic redundancy, distorting the stimulus by filtering, time compression, or introducing background noise can easily affect patient performance. For dichotic tests, monosyllables are frequently chosen frequently because of the relative ease of obtaining precise temporal alignment of the stimuli presented to each ear. As a result, a dichotic CANS test using monosyllables presents a more difficult task than when bisyllables or sentences are employed for dichotic testing.

In general, presentation of conventional monosyllabic, phonetically balanced (PB) word lists (e.g., NU 6 or W-22) does not constitute a CANS test because these lists do not present a difficult enough task to cause a breakdown in performance when central pathology exists (Katz and Pack, 1975; Lynn and Gilroy, 1977). In some studies, however, PB-max performance has been reported as abnormal when individuals have pathology or space-occupying lesions of the brainstem (e.g., Jerger and Jerger, 1975 a,b; Stach et al., 1990a). Performance–intensity-PB (PI-PB) rollover has been found to be more sensitive to CANS pathology than PB-max measures, but again, normal results are often present (Rintelmann, 1985; Mueller, 1987; Chandler and Sedge, 1987). It is apparent, therefore, that when monosyllables are presented monaurally, this speech material must be degraded in some manner in order for the test to serve as an effective measure of CANS dysfunction. This section will review three commonly used monaural degraded monosyllabic procedures: filtered speech, speech-in-noise, and time-compressed speech.

Filtered Speech

Low-pass filtered speech was one of the first methods used to construct a low redundancy CANS speech test. As early as 1954, Bocca et al. reported reduced performance (contralateral ear effect) on this task for a patient with a temporal lobe tumor. Subsequent research by Bocca and colleagues (1955) and Jerger (1960 a, b; 1964) revealed that low-pass filtered speech was a relatively sensitive test for tumors affecting the temporal cortex.

In the 1970s, Lynn and Gilroy presented extensive data related to filtered speech testing in a series of studies of tumors of the frontal, parietal, and temporal lobes (Lynn and Gilroy, 1972, 1977). In one study, Lynn and Gilroy (1977) reported a 74% sensitivity rating for the low-pass filtered speech test (NU 6 word lists) for detecting temporal lobe lesions. Numerous other studies have examined the effectiveness of low-pass filtered speech in detecting CANS dysfunction. A review of these studies can be found elsewhere (Mueller, 1985; Rintelmann, 1985).

While low-pass filtered speech has been one of the most commonly used monosyllabic CANS tests, there is little standardization of these test materials. Different word lists, cut-off frequencies, and filter rejection rates have been used, often with little published normative data. In the late 1970s and early 1980s the low-pass filtered test of Ivey (1969) was perhaps the most widely used, as it was part of the CANS speech test battery rec-

ommended by Willeford (1976). The Ivey filtered speech test (500 Hz cut-off, 18 dB/octave filter) consists of two 50-word lists of the Michigan consonant-nucleus-consonant (CNC) material. The words were especially selected to be intelligible to normal adults even when filtered, as reflected in their mean score of 88% and a range of 74–98% (Ivey, 1969).

When peripheral hearing loss is present, it is helpful to make a direct comparison between the patient's performance on low-pass filtered material and a non-distorted version of the same test. The difference score then becomes the value used for predicting the integrity of the CANS. For this purpose, it is convenient to use a filtered version of a commonly used monosyllabic word list, such as the NU 6 (see Chapter 10). Low-pass filtered versions of the NU 6 lists, at three different cut-off frequencies (500, 750 and 1000 Hz), are available commercially from Auditec of St Louis. Wilson and Mueller (1984) reported on the normative results for the Auditec filtered speech tapes and their findings are summarized in Table 16.1. Observe that the list equivalency of the NU 6 material is maintained, except for the 500-Hz filter recording. The poor performance obtained for normals for the 500 Hz filter cut-off also suggests that this recording probably would not be appropriate for differentiation of CANS pathology.

Speech-in-Noise

A second method of reducing the redundancy of monosyllabic speech material is to present an ipsilateral competing noise. Most commonly, white noise is used in conjunction with a standardized PB list, such as the NU 6, although speech spectrum noise is also used. The signal-to-noise ratio (S/N) that is selected is criti-

Table 16.1.
Normative Data for Adult Subjects on the Auditec NU 6 Filtered-Speech Tests.[a]

Test		List 1	List 2	List 3	List 4
500 Hz	Mean	46.1	49.9	40.6	43.9
(Form A)	S.D.[b]	13.3	12.0	12.1	10.5
	Range	26–76	20–66	8–64	8–64
750 Hz	Mean	78.4	75.2	74.0	79.3
(Form B)	S.D.	10.2	12.0	13.2	11.9
	Range	64–100	50–94	48–94	52–94
1000 Hz	Mean	89.3	91.5	93.3	91.0
(Form C)	S.D.	7.1	5.8	5.0	6.4
	Range	68–100	76–100	80–100	76–100

[a]From Wilson and Mueller, 1984.
[b]S.D., standard deviation.

cal; usually a value somewhere between 0 and +10 dB is employed.

As part of an extensive survey of clinical trends in audiology, Martin and Morris (1989) reported on the popularity of various CANS tests. Observe in Table 16.2 that speech-in-noise was found to be one of the most popular CANS tests, as 53% of the audiologists surveyed reported using this procedure. A plausible explanation for the popularity of this procedure is that the speech-in-noise test is easily used. Only a conventional audiometer and standardized recorded monosyllabic word lists are required for administration of the test. (While not recommended, a more cavalier clinician might even substitute monitored live voice for the recorded speech material.) It is this ease of administration that has caused speech-in-noise testing to be not only among the most used, but probably the most *misused* test of CANS function.

Before conducting speech-in-noise testing it is important to obtain normative data for the material used, and to assure that the signal-to-noise ratio reported is indeed the signal-to-noise ratio delivered to the ear. (It is necessary to measure earphone output for the speech and noise signals, as equal audiometric dial settings do not necessarily guarantee a 0 dB signal-to-noise ratio at the ear). One way to assure appropriate and consistent signal-to-noise ratios is to record the monosyllables and the noise at the desired signal-to-noise ratio on the same tape track.

Conflicting reports concerning the clinical application of speech-in-noise testing also have led to poor understanding of normal performance. Consider, for example, that one study reported that nine-year-old children with PBK-in-noise scores (S/N = 0 dB) at or near 60% have auditory perceptual deficits (Cohen, 1980). In contrast, Rupp (1983) reported that the mean PBK-in-noise score (S/N = 0 dB) for *normal* nine-year-old children was 39%.

As discussed by Bess (1983) the reliability of speech-in-noise testing also is a concern. Observe, for example, the variability of mean scores, and the dispersion measurements shown in Table 16.3. These results were obtained from normal adults using white noise at a 0 dB S/N ration. Clearly, when one finds small differences of 6–10% between ears, these could easily be a function of the test variability, and hence, should not be interpreted as clinically significant.

With the above issues in mind, it is relevant to review some of the research that has used speech-in-noise testing for the detection of CANS pathology. In 1959, Sinha reported reduced performance on a speech-in-noise task for the contralateral ears of individuals with cortical lesions. Subsequent studies have shown abnormal scores associated with cranial nerve VIII lesions (Dayal et al., 1966; Katinsky et al., 1972; Olsen et al., 1975), extra-axial (Dayal et al., 1966) and intra-axial brainstem lesions (Morales-Garcia and Poole, 1972; Noffsinger et al., 1972), temporal lobe pathology (Heilman et al., 1973; Morales-Garcia and Poole, 1972; Olsen et al., 1975), as well as in split-brain patients (Musiek et al., 1979), patients with multiple sclerosis (Dayal et al., 1966; Fowler and Noffsinger, 1984; Noffsinger at al, 1972; Olsen et al., 1975), and learning-disabled adults (Chermak et al., 1989).

Olsen et al. (1975) collected normative data for a large group of normal listeners using the NU 6 monosyllabic lists in white noise with a signal-to-noise ratio of 0 dB. They also tested groups of patients with cochlear, cranial nerve VIII, and temporal lobe pathology, as well

Table 16.2.

Reported Use of Speech Tests for the Diagnosis of Central Auditory Lesions (N = 325 Audiologists).[a]

Test	Number	Percentage
Monaural filtered speech	48	14.8
Binaural filtered speech	22	6.8
Staggered Spondaic Words (SSW)	172	52.9
Speech in noise	173	53.2
Synthetic Sentence Identification test with ipsilateral competing message (SSI-ICM)	112	34.5
Synthetic Sentence Identification test with contralateral competing message (SSI-CCM)	101	31.1
Performance intensity function for PB words	235	72.3
Competing-sentences test	67	20.6
Willeford Battery	75	23.0
Other	78	23.9
Do not test	129	28.4

[a]From Martin and Morris, 1989.

Table 16.3.

Mean Word Recognition Scores and Dispersion Measurements in Normal Hearing Subjects Obtained in the Presence of a Broadband Noise (Signal-to-Noise Ratio = 0 dB) for Several Representative Studies.[a]

Investigator(s)	Material	Mean word recognition (%)	SD	Range
Rupp and Phillips (1969)	CID W-22	72	—	36–92
Keith and Talis (1972)	CID W-22	82	—	10
Sever (1973)	NU #6	48	11	30–66
Olsen, Noffsinger, and Kurdziel (1975)	NU #6	74	—	56–94
Schwartz, Bess, and Larson (1977)	NU #6	63	21	—
Humes, Bess, and Schwartz (1978)	NU #6	68	21	—

[a]From Bass, 1983.

as patients diagnosed as having multiple sclerosis. They reported significant reduction in speech recognition for patients in all of the disordered groups. Difference scores for each group were calculated by comparing scores obtained in quiet with scores obtained in noise and are reported in Table 16.4. A difference of 40% or more between the two conditions was considered significant. Olsen et al. concluded that speech-in-noise testing may be useful for suggesting abnormal auditory function but not for identifying a specific site.

Little research has been published in recent years regarding the use of speech-in-noise as a test of central auditory dysfunction in adults. It should be noted that speech-in-noise tests are particularly affected by peripheral hearing loss. It is well known that individuals with even mild hearing losses have difficulty understanding speech in the presence of background noise. In addition, speech recognition in noise has been shown to deteriorate with advancing age (Dubno et al., 1984; Plomp and Mimpen, 1979).

Time-Compressed Speech

Another way to reduce the redundancy of a speech signal is to alter the temporal characteristics of the signal. Speech can be temporally altered in a variety of ways. The speaker can simply talk faster, or recorded material can be played back at a higher speed. The result of these techniques is termed accelerated speech. Bocca (1958) and Calearo and Lazzaroni (1957) were the first to use recorded accelerated speech to evaluate patients with lesions of the auditory cortex. Currently, electronic time compression is used to reduce the duration of a tape-recorded speech signal without altering its frequency characteristics (Fairbanks et al., 1954; Lee, 1972). Time-compressed speech is generally described in terms of the percentage of temporal reduction, that is, 30% time-compressed speech is speech in which 30% of the signal has been removed in small units.

Beasley et al. (1972 a, b) found that recognition of monosyllables decreased gradually for normal listeners as time compression increased from 30% to 60% and that recognition was drastically reduced for 70% compression. When sensation level was also varied, recognition of compressed speech increased to a 32 dB sensation level and then remained relatively unchanged. There is evidence, however, that the time-compressed NU 6 lists, commercially available from Auditec since 1978, are significantly more difficult for normal listeners than the recordings used by Beasley and colleagues (deChicchis et al., 1981; Grimes et al., 1984). In addition, results differ for time-compressed NU 6 lists versus CID W-22 lists (deChicchis et al., 1981), and there is an apparent lack of equivalency among lists in the commercial 60% time compression version of the NU 6 material (Grimes et al., 1984). It is highly recommended that normative data be obtained for specific time-compressed test materials before applying the tests to clinical populations.

Time-compressed speech has typically been used to assess patients with cortical lesions. Kurdziel et al. (1976) reported reduced performance for the contralateral ears of patients with diffuse temporal lobe lesions primarily due to cerebrovascular accidents, especially for the 60% compression condition (see Figure 16.1). Patients with discrete lesions, however, showed normal overall performance bilaterally. Others have reported similar results (Rintelmann et al., 1974; Baran et al., 1985; Mueller et al., 1987).

As with most CANS monosyllabic tests, peripheral hearing loss, even mild high frequency deficit, can have a significant impact on the test outcome for compressed speech. Grimes et al. (1984) obtained depressed scores from subjects with high frequency hearing loss on 60% time-compressed speech (Auditec). The subjects with hearing loss had a mean score of 34% compared to mean scores for the normal-hearing subjects of 71%. The reduction in performance for those with peripheral hearing loss is greater than that reported by Kurdziel et

Table 16.4.
Incidence (in Percent) of Differences in Speech Discrimination Scores for Normals and Five Pathology Groups.[a]

Group	Difference Scores (Quiet Minus White Noise Scores)								
	0–8	10–18	20–28	30–38	40–48	50–58	60–68	70–78	80–88	90–98
Normal	0.7	16.0	60.6	22.0	0.7				
Noise Trauma	2.0	10.0	40.0	40.0	8.0				
Ménière's disease		8.0	20.0	24.0	16.0	24.0		4.0	4.0
Eighth nerve tumor			23.8	14.3	14.3	23.8	14.3	4.8		4.8
Multiple sclerosis	4.0	16.0	44.0	22.0	6.0	8.0			
Temporal lobe lesion			22.8	35.0	19.2	7.7	3.8	7.7	3.8

[a]From Olsen et al., 1975.

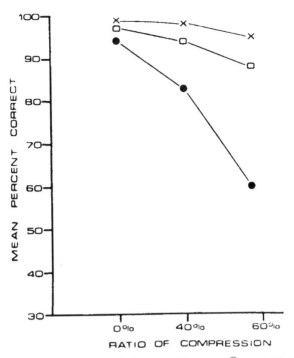

Figure 16.1. Performance for X, normal listeners; ○, ear ipsilateral to absent or damaged temporal lobe; and ●, ear contralateral to absent or damaged temporal lobe. (From Kurdziel et al., 1976.)

al. and others for subjects with temporal lobe pathology (see Figure 16.1). In addition, given the low scores obtained by the individuals with hearing loss, it would be extremely difficult to identify a concomitant central auditory dysfunction.

BINAURAL INTEGRATION TESTS

Monosyllables are also used in binaural integration techniques. These tests do not identify disorders by ear or side, but rather reflect fusion (resynthesis) or integration capabilities believed to be centered primarily in the low brainstem. The binaural integration tasks should not be confused with the dichotic separation tasks, which will be discussed in the following section.

Perhaps the best-known binaural fusion technique for assessing central auditory function was developed by Matzker (1959). A low frequency bandpass version of the stimulus is presented to one ear while a high frequency bandpass version is presented simultaneously to the other ear. When either bandpass segment is presented monaurally, word recognition ability is very poor. When both segments of the signal are presented simultaneously to opposite ears, it is perceived as a single word and high recognition scores are obtained for normal listeners.

Much of the research in binaural fusion has involved the use of bisyllabic speech stimuli; however, Smith and

Resnick (1972) believed that monosyllables would further reduce the redundancy of the speech signal and make the test more sensitive. They used CNC monosyllables filtered to obtain a low band from 360 to 890 Hz and a high band from 1750 to 2220 Hz. Using a presentation procedure similar to that of Matzker (1959), Smith and Resnick studied four groups of adult patients: normal, bilateral hearing loss (presumably cochlear), temporal lobe lesion, and brainstem pathology. Scores for the dichotic task (one band to each ear) were compared to scores obtained when both bands were presented to both ears (diotic task). Diotic scores were not significantly higher than dichotic scores for the normal, peripheral hearing loss, and temporal lobe groups, indicating the presence of normal central resynthesis. Significant differences, however, were observed for all four brainstem cases with results showing from 18 to 24% enhancement for the diotic task.

Noffsinger et al. (1972) used filtered NU 6 lists in bands from 250 to 750 Hz and 1250 to 1750 Hz with multiple sclerosis patients. Abnormal scores were reported for 8 of the 36 subjects. In contrast to the results of Smith and Resnick (1972), Noffsinger et al. found that abnormal performance usually occurred in the diotic rather than the dichotic condition and was much more common in persons whose lesions were inferred to be above the binaural integrative mechanisms of the brainstem.

For the past several years an NU 6 binaural fusion test has been available commercially; however, little research has been conducted using these tapes with individuals having CANS pathology. Wilson and Mueller (1984) reported data for the Auditec version of this test, and these findings are displayed in Table 16.5. These normative data are helpful for interpreting results when using the NU 6 binaural fusion test.

Because of the inconclusive nature of the work on binaural fusion with disordered populations, binaural fusion tests should be used cautiously. Further discussion of binaural fusion with bisyllables can be found in Chapter 17.

Table 16.5.
Normative Data for Adult Subjects on the Auditec NU 6 Binaural Fusion Speech Test.[a]

Test		Left Ear— Low Freq Right Ear— High Freq	Right Ear— Low Freq Left Ear— High Freq	Left Ear Both Bands	Right Ear Both Bands
Form A	Mean	81.5	83.2	77.8	76.9
	S.D.[b]	8.9	7.5	9.8	9.9
	Range	66–92	66–94	58–92	48–88

[a]From Wilson and Mueller, 1984.
[b]S.D., standard deviation.

Other binaural monosyllabic interaction techniques that have not received a great deal of attention are faint filtered speech (Bocca, 1955; Calearo, 1957; Jerger, 1960 a, b) and the masking level difference (MLD) with monosyllables (Cullen and Thompson, 1974). Limited clinical use may be due in part to a lack of commercially available test materials.

DICHOTIC TESTS

The term dichotic refers to the simultaneous competing presentation of two different speech signals to opposite ears. Subjects are asked to repeat back what is heard in one or both ears a separation task. Generally, when speech is presented dichotically to normal listeners, higher scores are obtained from the material to the right ear than to the left. This has been referred to as the right ear advantage and is believed to reflect the dominance of the left hemisphere for speech and language perception (Studdert-Kennedy and Shankweiler, 1970). Figure 16.2, which is based on the work of Kimura (1961a, b) and Sparks et al. (1970), illustrates the pathways of dichotic speech. According to this model, when the left hemisphere is dominant for lan-

guage, the right hemisphere acts as a relay station for information from the left ear which is transferred across the corpus callosum to the left hemisphere. As with most other speech tests designed to detect CANS pathology, when dichotic speech is presented to individuals with temporal lobe lesions, reduced performance is expected for the ear contralateral to the disorder because of the dominant crossed auditory fiber tracts.

There are a number of procedural details that must be addressed when administering dichotic tests, including quality of recordings, onset and offset alignment of stimuli, and intensity of presentation. For a discussion of these issues, see Musiek and Pinheiro (1985).

Dichotic Digits

Kimura (1961a, b) is credited with being first to use dichotic digits to test subjects with brain damage. She used three digits presented to each ear of subjects who had temporal lobectomies for treatment of epileptic seizures. Kimura reported a decrease in scores for the ear contralateral to the lesion, but when the left temporal lobe was affected, bilaterally decreased scores were seen.

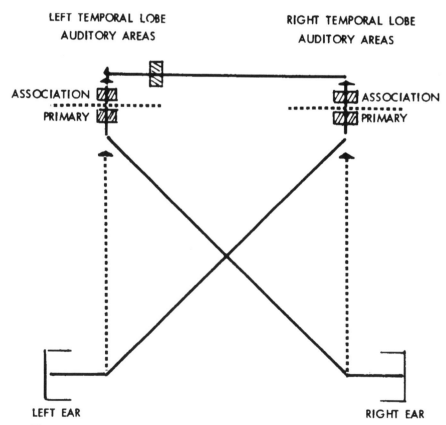

Figure 16.2. Ipsilateral and decussating auditory pathways to the temporal lobe and across the corpus callosum. (Adapted from Sparks et al., 1970.)

In a version of the dichotic digits test recommended by Musiek (1983a), two digits are presented to each ear simultaneously. For example, the digits 2,5 may be presented to the right ear and 3,8 to the left ear. The subject is asked to repeat all four digits in any order. Only the digits one through ten (except seven) are used, and the recommended presentation level is 50 dB sensation level (re: SRT or puretone average).

Musiek (1983a, b) has reported that the dichotic digits test is highly sensitive for detecting both brainstem and hemispheric pathology. In a study of nine subjects with brainstem pathology and 12 subjects with hemispheric lesions, Musiek (1983b) reported that 18 showed abnormal results in at least one ear. Because of the test's apparent sensitivity, as well as the fact that it is relatively unaffected by peripheral hearing loss, the dichotic digits test has been recommended by Musiek and his colleagues as a quick and easy screening test for CANS dysfunction (Musiek, 1983a; Musiek et al., 1991). Subjects with normal hearing typically score above 90% and subjects with peripheral hearing loss obtain scores of 80% or higher. Scores below 80% suggest that further CANS testing is indicated.

As part of a study of head-injured Vietnam veterans Mueller et al. (1987) used a dichotic digits task in which three digits were presented to each ear. The authors note that reduced scores for some of the patients may have reflected an inability to remember six digits and repeat them back rather than CANS dysfunction. Results for patients with temporal lobe injuries were similar to those reported by other investigators (Kimura, 1961b; Oxbury and Oxbury, 1969; Sparks et al., 1970). When the left temporal lobe was injured, both right and left ear scores were reduced, whereas right temporal lobe damage affected only the scores for the left ear. Individuals with injury in other brain areas performed normally.

In an attempt to explain the ipsilateral ear effect often reported for left temporal lobe lesions but not for right (Kimura, 1961b; Oxbury and Oxbury, 1969; Sparks et al., 1970; Mueller et al., 1987), Sparks et al. (1970) proposed a model for the pathways of dichotic speech suggesting areas where lesions could cause a reduction in either right or left ear performance (see Figure 16.2). According to the model, deep lesions affecting the callosal fiber tracts from the right hemisphere would be responsible for test results similar to those of a right hemisphere lesion, that is, decreased scores for the left ear but not for the right ear. The absence of an ipsilateral effect for the right hemisphere added support to the notion that a dominant path exists to the left hemisphere for dichotic speech. This model would also appear to explain dichotic digit results for patients with lesions of the interhemispheric connections where

marked reduction is normally found for the left ear while the right ear performs at or above normal (Milner et al., 1968; Sparks and Geschwind, 1968; Musiek and Wilson, 1979; Musiek et al., 1979).

It is clear dichotic testing can yield important diagnostic information that could be missed by monaural measures. While the dichotic digits test is relatively unaffected by peripheral hearing loss, Rodriguez et al. (1990) have reported a decrease in performance with advancing age in elderly adults. In general, however, the dichotic digits test is relatively easy to administer and score, can be used when mild hearing loss is present, and, given the closed set response, is applicable for a wide range of patients.

Dichotic Consonant-Vowels

The dichotic consonant-vowel (CV) test (developed by Berlin and available from Auditec) is considered a more difficult task than dichotic digits (Niccum et al., 1981). The material consists of six stop consonant-vowel syllables (pa, ta, ka, ba, da, ga). Dichotically presented CVs have an apparent advantage over digits in that alignment of acoustic energy is relatively simple because of the high degree of similarity among the syllables. This allows for a more simultaneous presentation than is possible for digits, which reduces the linguistic value of the CV task and maximizes the acoustic and phonetic competition (Berlin and McNeil, 1976). The CV dichotic task also relies less heavily on short term memory than the digit test in which as many as six digits must be remembered. It is likely that these two dichotic tests measure slightly different perceptual processes.

Dichotic CVs are often presented so that the onset of the CV to one ear lags behind the onset of the CV to the other ear by 15, 30, 60, or 90 msec. Berlin et al. (1975) and Olsen (1983) have reported that normal subjects show an improvement in scores with lag times of 30 to 90 msec when compared with scores obtained for simultaneous presentation. Similar improvements in scores have not been seen, however, with patients with temporal lobectomies. Table 16.6 shows scores for normal listeners obtained by Olsen (1983) for various lag times.

Much of the background research and current understanding surrounding the dichotic CV procedure has been contributed by Berlin and his colleagues and summarized by Berlin and McNeil (1976). Research findings with CVs have generally paralleled the studies with dichotic digits. Berlin et al. (1975) evaluated three temporal lobectomy patients and four hemispherectomy patients using dichotic CVs. As expected, the ear contralateral to the affected side showed reduced scores for the patients with temporal lobectomies. The hemispherectomy

Table 16.6.
Mean Scores and Ranges of Scores (in Percent) for Dichotic CV Test Materials for 50 Normal Subjects.[a]

	Test Condition							
	Left ear lag: 90 msec		0 msec		Right ear lag: 90 msec		Average	
	R	L	R	L	R	L	R	L
Mean	86.3	79.3	69.3	59.2	87.7	79.2	81.1	72.5
Range	63–100	56–100	47–93	43–77	69–100	50–100	66–95	60–89

[a]From Olsen, 1983.

patients also had reduced scores for contralateral ears, but when the CVs were presented monaurally to the same ear, scores were better than those expected from normal listeners. To explain these findings, Cullen et al. (1975) suggested that the right ear advantage observed in normals for dichotic CVs is the result of noise associated with transcallosal relay of information from the right to the left hemisphere. During monaural listening or when the right ear receives the information during dichotic listening, transcallosal noise would not be an issue and scores would therefore be enhanced.

Subsequent studies have demonstrated that results from brain-damaged patients on tasks using dichotic CVs are not always easy to interpret. Olsen (1983) administered dichotic CVs to 50 normal listeners and 67 patients with the anterior portion of either the left or right temporal lobe removed. He reported a wide range of performance for normal listeners, and over 40% of the temporal lobe patients obtained scores that fell within normal limits. Ipsilateral ear effects were also observed by Olsen, and he concluded that determination of the side of a cortical lesion cannot be accomplished using dichotic listening tests. Speaks (1975) reported similar results and drew the same conclusion. This criticism may apply to other CANS tests as well.

Dichotic CV testing was performed as part of the study of head-injured Vietnam veterans mentioned previously (Mueller et al., 1987). For their subjects with posterior temporal lobe injuries, Mueller et al. (1987) reported contralateral ear effects as well as an ipsilateral ear effect when the left temporal lobe was injured. In addition to obtaining percent correct scores for each ear, Mueller et al. calculated the double-correct score (when both CVs were correctly identified) for a paired presentation. Dichotic CVs are typically fused and heard as a single unit, making double-correct scores relatively low. Normal listeners achieve only about 40 to 45% double-correct responses. Double-correct scores for subjects with temporal lobe injury were significantly lower than those obtained from normal listeners (Figure 16.3). They concluded that double-correct scores may be a useful indicator of posterior temporal lobe dysfunction, although they are not likely to be useful in determining which hemisphere is involved.

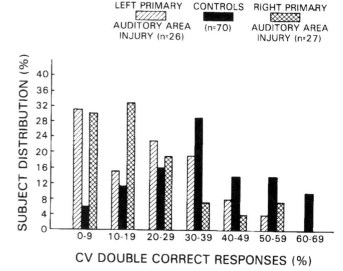

Figure 16.3. Distribution of CV double-correct responses for individuals with injury to the right or left primary auditory processing region. (From Mueller et al., 1987.)

Because it is a difficult test, dichotic CVs may be inappropriate for some patients, and an easier test (e.g., Dichotic Sentence Identification, digits, Staggered Spodaic Words [SSW]) may need to be substituted. In general, however, dichotic CV tests can be given to a wide range of patients with relative ease.

Dichotic Rhyme Test

The dichotic rhyme task was introduced by Wexler and Halwes (1983) and modified by Musiek et al. (1989). It is composed of rhyming pairs of consonant-vowel-consonant words that begin with one of the stop consonants (p,t,k,b,d,g). Each pair of words differs by the initial consonant (e.g., bill, pill; ten, pen).

The dichotic rhyme test consists of digitized words that have been cross-spliced so that the final portions of the words are identical. This results in good temporal alignment and the words are often fused and perceived as a single word.

Musiek et al. (1989) have collected normative data for the dichotic rhyme test as well as preliminary data for split-brain patients. For 115 normal listeners, scores were near 50%, suggesting that only one word of the two was identified. Dichotic rhyme scores for six split-brain patients fell outside the range of scores for normals (Figure 16.4). Left ear scores were significantly lower than normal, and right ear scores were enhanced. The authors suggest that the relatively large enhancement in right ear scores is due to a release from central auditory competition in the left hemisphere, that is, the left hemisphere no longer receives information from the right hemisphere and need only process information from the right ear.

Although other researchers have also observed enhancements in right ear scores on dichotic tasks for split brain patients or for ears ipsilateral to hemispherectomy (Berlin et al., 1975; Springer and Gazzaniga, 1975; Musiek et al., 1985), Musiek et al. (1989) suggest that the dichotic rhyme test may be uniquely suited to assess such enhancements because of the relatively low scores obtained by normal listeners (near 50%). For many dichotic tasks, normal listeners perform near 100% and there is not sufficient room for enhanced scores to be evaluated. With further study, the dichotic rhyme test promises to become a valuable addition to the central auditory test battery for the identification of interhemispheric or transcallosal pathology.

COMPARISON OF THE EFFICIENCY OF MONOSYLLABIC TASKS

An interesting case from the study of head-injured veterans (Mueller et al. 1987) will serve to illustrate the some of the differences among three dichotic tests—the SSW, dichotic digits, and dichotic CVs. The patient received a high-velocity gunshot wound to the left frontal-parietal region. The left temporal lobe is missing anteriorly with significant damage extending posteriorly. Large portions of the left frontal and parietal lobes are also missing.

As shown in Table 16.7, performance for the right ear of this patient is extremely poor on all three tests. Of interest is the fact that right ear performance is as good for the more difficult CV material as it is for the meaningful words of the SSW or the dichotic digits. This may be due to greater control of the stimulus onset time for the CVs, providing a consistent advantage for the left ear CV in the right hemisphere. In essence, the task is no longer a truly dichotic one for this patient. When a 90 msec right-ear lead was introduced for the CV material, the left ear score was reduced to 43% and no double-correct scores were obtained. With a 90 msec left-ear lead, however, the score for the left ear was 63% and 7% double correct scores were present.

In general, dichotic speech tests are uniquely suited to the study of temporal lobe dysfunction. While ipsilateral ear effects are sometimes present, significant findings are normally only observed for the contralateral ear, especially if the lesion or pathology is discrete. This relationship was illustrated by Mueller et al. (1987) and is displayed in Table 16.8. These authors studied 78 individuals with injury to either the right or left temporal lobe and categorized the extent of injury according to the 13 anatomical areas shown in Table 16.8. All subjects were given three dichotic tests: the monosyllabic digits, CVs, and the bisyllabic SSW. Observe that none of the

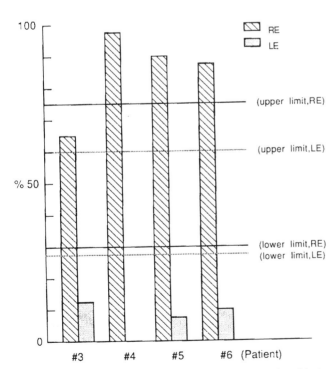

Figure 16.4. Dichotic rhyme test results for four split-brain subjects. The solid lines encompass the 95% confidence limits for the right ear; the dotted lines, the 95% confidence intervals for the left ear. (From Musiek et al., 1989.)

Table 16.7.
Dichotic Test Results for a Patient with Left Temporal Lobe Injury. Control Group Data Shown for Comparison. (Scores shown in percent correct)

	SSW		Dichotic Digits		Dichotic CVs		
	Right	Left	Right	Left	Right	Left	Double Correct
Temporal Lobe Injury Patient	2	78	10	69	7	73	0
Control group[b]							
Mean	98	94	93	91	76	52	36
S.D.	4	6	7	8	14	19	18
90th percentile cutoff	93	89	84	73	60	31	10

[a]From Mueller et al., 1987.
[b]Control group data shown for comparison.

Table 16.8.
Summary of Significant Associations between Dichotic Speech Test Results and Injury to Specific Temporal Lobe Regions.[a]

	Significant Associations	
	Right Ear Score	Left Ear Score
Right injury		
SSW		I, K, L
Dichotic digits		
Dichotic CVs		E, F, H, I, K, M
Left injury		
SSW	B, G, L, M	
Dichotic digits	I, J, H. L	L
Dichotic CVs	I, J, K, L	
Temporal lobe areas		
A.- Mesial temporal pole		
B.- Lateral temporal pole		
C.- Uncus (including amygdala)		
D.- Rostral hippocampus		
E.- Anterior mesial superior temporal gyrus		
F.- Anterior middle and inferior temporal gyrus		
G.- Posterior middle and inferior temporal gyrus		
H.- Middle superior temporal gyrus		
I.- Rostral posterior superior temporal gyrus		
J.- Posterior middle temporal gyrus		
K.- Posterior superior temporal gyrus		
L.- Anterior temporal white matter		
M.- Posterior temporal white matter		

[a]From Mueller et al., 1987.

dichotic right ear scores were significantly associated ($p > 0.01$) with right temporal lobe injury and only one left ear score (dichotic digits) was related to left temporal lobe injury (anterior temporal white matter). As expected, few significant associations occurred for anterior temporal lobe injury. In summary, these findings illustrate the notion that the various dichotic tasks may actually assess different processes.

Few studies have examined and compared both monaural and dichotic CANS tests, however, Grady et al. (1989); obtained results for both dichotic (SSW) and monotic (time compression and low-pass filtered speech) tasks for a group of Alzheimer patients. They found that the SSW was more sensitive than either monotic task although performance for both time-compressed speech and filtered speech was abnormal (see Figure 16.5). Grady et al. concluded that performance on dichotic tasks depends on the integrity of the temporal lobe, whereas decreased performance on degraded monotic tasks reflects a more general deficit for Alzheimer patients.

Musiek (1983b) compared results on the dichotic digits test, the SSW, and the competing sentences subtest of the Willeford battery for normally hearing subjects with brainstem and hemispheric lesions. Tables 16.9 and 16.10 provide a summary of the results for

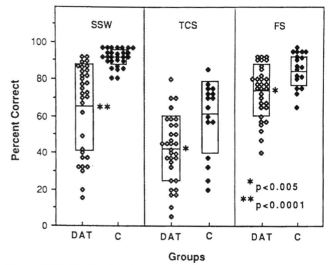

Figure 16.5. Scatterplot of scores on three central auditory speech tests for Dementia of Alzheimer Type (DAT) patients and controls (C). Boxes represent mean ± standard deviation. (SSW = staggered spondaic word; TCS = time compressed speech; FS = filtered speech.) (From Grady et al., 1989.)

Table 16.9.
Ipsilateral versus Contralateral Scores on Three Speech Tests for Subjects with Unilateral Hemispheric Lesions (N = 15).[a]

	Competing Sentences: Ipsilateral/ Contralateral	SSW: Ipsilateral/ Contralateral	Dichotic Digits: Ipsilateral/ Contralateral
Mean (%)	91.4/68.2	90.2/64.5	85.1/54.2
S.D. (%)	18.5/33.4	9.1/29.9	14.5/30.8
Range (%)	32–100/0–100	62–100/8–100	55–100/0–93

[a]From Musiek, 1983b.

Table 16.10.
Ipsilateral (versus) Contralateral Scores on Three Speech Tests for Subjects with Unilateral Brainstem Lesions (N = 7).[a]

	Competing Sentences: Ipsilateral/ Contralateral	SSW: Ipsilateral/ Contralateral	Dichotic Words: Ipsilateral/ Contralateral
Mean (%)	52.4/92.1	66.0/90.0	68.0/88.1
S.D. (%)	41.2/15.2	27.2/6.0	21.0/9.1
Range (%)	0–100/60–100	30–100/80–98	30–95/78–100

[a]From Musiek, 1983b.

both groups. The dichotic digits test was most sensitive to the presence of central pathology followed by the SSW and then the competing sentences, although there was no significant statistical difference among the tests. All three tests resulted in expected ear effects: subjects with brainstem lesions obtained the poorest scores for the ear ipsilateral to the lesion and subjects with hemispheric lesions typically obtained the poorest scores for the contralateral ear.

The findings of Musiek (1983b) suggest that CANS tests provide an efficient method of detecting space-occupying lesions. What must be remembered, however, is that the data presented in many studies were collected from patients referred to the audiology clinic *because it was already known that the patient had a space-occupying lesion*. In routine clinical practice, it is usually not known if a pathology exists, or what is the cause of the abnormal test results. If CANS tests are to be part of a clinical protocol for site-of-lesion testing, it is critical to understand the operating characteristics of these tests, and to conduct a cost-benefit analysis (see Turner, 1991; Hyde et al., 1991).

A final clinical issue related to the efficiency of monosyllabic speech tests for detection of CANS disorders is the cost-to-benefit ratio. The cost-to-benefit analysis is related not only to the monetary costs of conducting the tests, but also the costs to the patient if a lesion or pathology goes undetected. For example, if a clinic implements an aggressive CANS testing program, a decision must be made regarding the disposition of those individuals that perform abnormally. One possible outcome is that these patients all receive a magnetic resonance imaging (MRI) scan, the test considered to be the definitive measure for space-occupying lesions. Given the low prevalence of CANS lesions in the average audiology clinic caseload, and the false alarm rate of CANS tests, it is probable that nearly all individuals receiving the MRI test will not have a lesion. While this protocol will result in considerable unnecessary expense, it is possible that a CANS lesion will be detected that otherwise would have been missed. Does this benefit justify the cost?

MONOSYLLABIC TESTS FOR CHILDREN

Although CANS tests for adults and children are similar, the reason for conducting the test is usually different. CANS testing with adults is usually lesion oriented, with tests designed to detect the specific anatomic regions of a disorder. Although tumors and other central lesions also exist in children, most of the testing with this population is conducted because of suspected auditory processing problems or learning disabilities. In these cases, there probably is not a specific central auditory site of involvement. It has been suggested that CANS dysfunction in children is related to delays in neuromaturational development of the auditory system (Musiek et al., 1984) or to diffuse neurological involvement (Musiek et al., 1985). Test results, therefore, might not be directly related to a specific neuroanatomical region of the CANS.

In the 1970s, methods for assessing the central auditory function of children began to receive an increasing amount of attention. Children with a variety of problems including auditory attention deficits, academic deficiencies, behavior problems, learning difficulties, and language disorders began to be referred for CANS testing with the belief that the test results might provide some insight relative to effective management of these children.

In an attempt to develop adequate testing techniques, many of the CANS tests for assessing adults were adapted for use with children. Table 16.11 is a summary of some studies in which adult testing techniques were used with children. Since the mid-1980s, new tests tended not to be modifications, but rather specifically developed for use with children, and physiologic methods.

When using CANS tests that have been modified for children, it is critical that appropriate age-related norms be used and that an adequate normative data

Table 16.11.
Studies Using Monosyllabic Tests Modified for Children

Low-pass filtered speech	Willeford (1976)
	Martin and Clark (1977)
	Farrer and Keith (1981)
Filtered speech (binaural fusion)	Palva and Jokinen (1975)
	Martin and Clark (1977)
	Davis and McCroskey (1980)
	Plakke et al. (1981)
	Roush and Tait (1984)
Speech-in-noise (figure-ground)	Cohen (1980)
	Rupp (1983)
	Papso and Blood (1989)
Time compressed speech	Beasley et al. (1976)
	Manning et al. (1977)
	Orchik and Oelschlager (1977)
Dichotic CVs	Berlin et al. (1973)
	Hynd and Obrzut (1977)
	Mirabile et al. (1978)
	Tobey et al. (1979)
	Koomar and Cermak (1981)
	Dermody et al. (1983)
	Harris et al. (1983)
	Hynd et al. (1983)
	Roeser et al. (1983)
Dichotic digits	Sommers and Taylor (1972)
	Witelson and Rabinovitch (1972)
	Bakker et al. (1979)
	Pettit and Helms (1979)
	Hiscock and Kinsbourne (1980)
	Musiek and Geurkink (1980)
	Koomar and Cermak (1981)
	Newell and Rugel (1981)
	Musiek et al. (1982)
	Kraft (1984)
	Musiek et al. (1984)

base be available for interpretation of the results. For all of the techniques listed in Table 16.11, maturational effects have been reported, that is, performance improves with age. In addition, at each age level, there is high variability among normal subjects, and scores from normal and disordered subjects often overlap. Based on these observations, it is necessary to use a battery approach to CANS testing. Abnormal performance on a single test may simply reflect the variability inherent in the test results obtained from children, whereas abnormal performance on a variety of tests is more compelling evidence that CANS dysfunction exists. In addition, variables such as stimulus presentation levels, test instructions, scoring methods, types of speech material (PBK, WIPI, CVs, digits), and methods of response (picture pointing versus verbal) must be considered when attempting to compare test results to normative data or to results collected by other clinicians. Clearly, every attempt must be made to control as many variables as possible, and test results must be interpreted cautiously when adult procedures are adapted for testing children.

Two tests that use monosyllabic stimuli have been developed specifically for children: the Pediatric Speech Intelligibility (PSI) test (Jerger and Jerger, 1984) and the SCAN (Keith, 1986). The PSI consists of both monosyllabic word and sentence stimuli with either ipsilateral or contralateral competing messages. According to the authors, it was developed in an attempt to provide a test that is insensitive to developmental differences in cognitive skills and that is difficult enough to be sensitive to the presence of central auditory deficits. It was designed for use with children as young as 3 years of age.

Preliminary reports of results for children with confirmed or suspected central lesions suggest that the PSI is able to distinguish between children with central auditory lesions and those with nonauditory central lesions (Jerger, 1987; Jerger et al., 1988; Jerger and Zeller, 1989).

The SCAN is a screening test of CANS dysfunction for children ages 3 to 11. The purposes of the SCAN are to provide preliminary information about a child's maturation and auditory processing abilities; to identify children at risk for auditory processing problems; and to identify children who might benefit from intervention to improve auditory learning abilities (Keith, 1986). It was specifically designed for use in the schools where time and equipment are limited. The SCAN is a taped test that can be administered in 20 minutes and requires only a stereo tape cassette with headphones and a quiet room.

The SCAN consists of three subtests: low-pass filtered words, auditory figure-ground, and competing words.

Both the filtered word and figure-ground subtests were included to identify problems that might occur due to poor listening environments. The competing words subtest was included in the battery to provide information about the maturation of a child's auditory system by comparing right- and left-ear advantages to those for a normative group. If a child's ear advantage scores are abnormal, it might suggest delayed maturation of the auditory system or an abnormality of the central auditory nervous system (Keith, 1984).

Normative data for 1034 children are provided in the manual accompanying the SCAN. The author suggests, however, that the data for the 3- and 4-year-olds be considered experimental because of the small sample size and difficulty administering the test to this age group. Data are also provided for children of varying ethnic backgrounds.

One advantage of the SCAN is that it considers the high degree of variability inherent at each age level when testing children. Confidence intervals may be established around a child's score that reflect the measurement error associated with the test. For example, if a 7-year-old child obtained a composite standardized score of 75 on one occasion and a score of 70 on retest, it is helpful to know the likelihood that the difference is due to test-retest variability and not to a true deterioration in performance. By using the norms and tables provided in the SCAN test manual, it can be determined that, for the above example, there is an 80% likelihood that the second score is not significantly different from the first.

In a study comparing the SCAN to several other CANS and language tests, results for the competing words subtest of the SCAN correlated highly with the SSW and the competing sentences subtest of the Willeford battery (Keith et al., 1989). The SCAN battery, as a whole, was more sensitive than either the Willeford competing sentences or the SSW in identifying children with histories of attention deficit disorder (ADD). Further research is warranted to determine the sensitivity and specificity of the SCAN in identifying the presence of CANS disorders; however, the SCAN appears to be a well-designed screening test for central auditory function. Adequate normative data have been obtained for the SCAN, and a minimal amount of time and equipment are needed to administer the test. While the SCAN is referred to as a *screening* test, so too are all the other tests discussed in this chapter, although not always labeled as such.

Some audiology clinics conduct several CANS tests and consider a positive finding on any one of them to identify a "hit" (see figure 16.6). While this approach will enhance the sensitivity of the test battery, it also will substantially increase the false alarm rate. In the

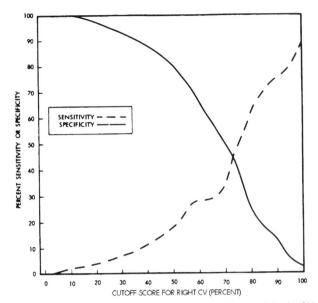

Figure 16.6. Plots of sensitivity and specificity for the dichotic *CVs* as a function of cut off value.

case of an adult suspected of having a space-occupying lesion, the "cost" of making a diagnostic mistake is financial (i.e., unnecessary imaging studies); with children, the cost of misdiagnosis may be to delay or prevent further evaluation and remediation of the problem. When a test battery is selected, therefore, the tests should be chosen because they assess different processes, not simply because "more is better." Hurley (1989) provides a review of commonly used CANS tests for children and reports on their sensitivity and specificity.

In summary, there are a variety of available CANS tests that use monosyllabic stimuli for the evaluation of children. In general, they can be helpful in describing the maturation level of the central auditory system, ruling out auditory abnormalities that could contribute to a language or learning problem (Keith, 1981), or in identifying children who have difficulty learning via auditory channels.

REFERENCES

Bakker DJ, Hoefkens M, and Van der Vlugt H. Hemispheric specialization in children as reflected in the longitudinal development of ear asymmetry. Cortex 1979;15:619–625.

Baran JA, and Musiek FE. Behavioral assessment of the central auditory nervous system. In Rintelmann WF, Ed. Hearing Assessment. Austin, TX: Pro-Ed, 1991.

Baran JA, Verkest S. Gollegly K, Kibbe-Michal K, Rintelmann WF, and Musiek FE. Use of compressed speech in the assessment of central nervous system disorder. J Acoust Soc Am 1985; 78(suppl 1):S41.

Beasley DS, Forman B, and Rintelmann WF. Intelligibility of time-compressed CNC monosyllables by normal listeners. J Aud Res 1972a;12:71–75.

Beasley DS, Maki J, and Orchik D. Children's perception of time-compressed speech using two measures of speech discrimination. J Speech Hear Dis 1976;41:216–225.

Beasley DS, Schwimmer S, and Rintelmann WF. Intelligibility of time-compressed monosyllables. J Speech Hear Res 1972b;15: 340–350.

Berlin CI, and Lowe SS. Temporal and dichotic factors in central auditory testing. In Katz J, Ed. Handbook of Clinical Audiology. Baltimore: Williams & Wilkins, 1972.

Berlin C, and McNeil M. Dichotic listening. In Lass N, Ed. Contemporary Issues in Experimental Phonetics. New York: Academic Press, 1976.

Berlin CI, Cullen JK, Hughes LF, Berlin JL, Lowe-Bell SS, and Thompson CL. Dichotic processing of speech: acoustic and phonetic variables. In Sullivan MD, Ed. Central Auditory Processing Disorders. Proceedings of a conference at the University of Nebraska Medical Center, Omaha, 1975.

Berlin CI, Hughes LF, Lowe-Bell SS, and Berlin HL. Dichotic right ear advantage in children 5 to 13. Cortex 1973;9:394–402.

Bess FH. Clinical assessment of speech recognition. In Konkle DF, and Rintelmann WF, Eds. Principles of Speech Audiometry. Baltimore: University Park Press, 1983.

Bocca E. Binaural hearing: another approach. Laryngoscope 1955;65:1164–1171.

Bocca E. Clinical aspects of cortical deafness. Laryngoscope 1958;68:301–311.

Bocca E, and Calearo C. Central hearing processes. In Jerger J, Ed. Modern Developments in Audiology. New York: Academic Press, 1963.

Bocca E, Calearo C, and Cassinari V. A new method for testing hearing in temporal lobe tumors. Acta Otolaryngol (Stockh) 1954;44:219–221.

Bocca E, Calearo C, Cassinari V, and Migliavacca F. Testing "cortical" hearing in temporal lobe tumors. Acta Otolaryngol (Stockh) 1955;45:289–304.

Calearo C. Binaural summation in lesions of the temporal lobe. Acta Otolaryngol (Stockh) 1957;47:392–397.

Calearo C, and Lazzaroni A. Speech intelligibility in relation to the speed of the message. Laryngoscope 1957;67:410–419.

Chandler D, and Sedge RK. Pure-tone sensitivity and speech recognition findings following head injury. Semin Hear 1987: 8;241–251.

Chermak GD, Vonhof MR, and Bendel RB. Word identification performance in the presence of competing speech and noise in learning disabled adults. Ear Hear 1989;10:90–93.

Cohen RL. Auditory skills and the communicative process. Semin Speech Lang Hear 1980;1:107–116.

Cullen J, Berlin C, Hughes L, Thompson C, and Samson D. Speech information follow: A model. In Sullivan MD, Ed. Central Auditory Processing Disorders. Proceedings of a conference at the University of Nebraska Medical Center, Omaha, 1975.

Cullen JK, and Thompson CL. Masking release for subjects with temporal lobe resections. Arch Otolaryngol 1974;100:113–116.

Davies J, and Mueller HG. Hearing aid selection. In Mueller HG, and Geoffrey V, Eds. Communication Disorders in Aging. Washington DC: Gallaudet Press, 1987.

Davis S, and McCroskey RL. Auditory fusion in children. Child Dev 1980;51:75–80.

Dayal VS, Tarantino L, and Swisher LP. Neuro-otologic studies in multiple sclerosis. Laryngoscope 1966;76:1798–1809.

deChicchis A, Orchik DJ, and Tecca J. The effect of word list and talker variation on word recognition scores using time-altered speech. J Speech Hear Disord 1981;46:213–216.

Dermody P, Katsch R, and Mackie K. Auditory processing limitations in low verbal children: evidence from a two-response dichotic listening task. Ear Hear 1983;4:272–277.

Dubno JR, Dirks DD, and Morgan DE. Effects of age and mild hearing loss on speech recognition in noise. J Acoust Soc Am 1984;76:87–96.

Fairbanks G, Everitt W, and Jaeger R. Methods for time or frequency compression-expansion of speech Trans IRE-PGA AU-2, 1954: 7–12.

Farrer SM, and Keith RW. Filtered word testing in the assessment of children's central auditory abilities. Ear Hear 1981; 2:267–269.

Fowler CG, and Noffsinger PD. Effects of stimulus rate and frequency on the auditory brainstem response in normal, cochlear-impaired and VIII nerve/brainstem-impaired subjects. J Speech Hear Res 1984;26:560–567.

Goldstein R, Goodman AC, and King RB. Hearing and speech in infantile hemiplegia before and after left hemispherectomy. Neurology 1956;56:295–306.

Grady CL, Grimes AM, Patronas N, Sunderland T, Foster NL, and Rapoport SI. Divided attention, as measured by dichotic speech performance, in dementia of the Alzheimer type. Arch Neurol 1989;46:317.

Grimes AM. Auditory changes. In Lubinski R, Ed. Dementia and Communication. Philadelphia: BC Decker, 1991:175–197.

Grimes AM, Grady CL, Foster NL, Sunderland T, and Patronas NJ. Central auditory function in Alzheimer's disease. Neurology 1985;35:352–358.

Grimes AM, Mueller HG, and Williams DL. Clinical considerations in the use of time-compressed speech. Ear Hear 1984;5:114–117.

Harris VL, Keith RW, and Novak KK. Relationship between two dichotic listening tests and the token test for children. Ear Hear 1983;4:278–282.

Heilman KM, Hammer LC, and Wilder BJ. An audiometric defect in temporal lobe dysfunction. Neurology (NY) 1973;23:384–386.

Hiscock M, and Kinsbourne M. Asymmetries of selective listening and attention switching in children. Developmental Psych 1980;16:70–82.

Hood LJ, and Mueller HG. Central auditory testing—What does it tell us? ASHA 1988;31:47[Abstract].

Hurley RM. Decision matrix analysis of selected children's central processing tests. Paper presented at the annual meeting of the American Academy of Audiology. Kiawah Island, SC, April, 1989.

Hyde ML, Davidson MJ, and Alberti PW. Auditory test strategy. In Jacobson JT, and Northern JL, Eds. Diagnostic Audiology. Austin: Pro-Ed, 1991:295–322.

Hynd GW, and Obrzut JE. Effects of grade level and sex on the magnitude of the dichotic ear advantage. Neuropsychologia 1977;15:669–692.

Hynd GW, Cohen M, and Obrzut JE. Dichotic consonant–vowel (CV) testing in the diagnosis of learning disabilities in children. Ear Hear 1983;4:283–286.

Ivey R. Tests of CNS auditory function. [Thesis] Fort Collins, CO: Colorado State University, 1969.

Jerger JF. Observations on auditory behavior in lesions of the central auditory pathways. Arch Otolaryngol 1960b;71:797–806.

Jerger JF. Audiological manifestations of lesions in the auditory nervous system. Laryngoscope 1960b;70:417–425.

Jerger JF. Auditory tests for disorders of the central auditory mechanisms. In Fields W, and Alford B, Eds. Neurological Aspects of Auditory and Vestibular Disorders. Springfield, IL: Charles C Thomas, 1964.

Jerger JF, and Jerger SW. Extra- and intra-axial brain stem auditory disorders. Audiology 1975a;14:93–117.

Jerger JF, and Jerger SW. Clinical validity of central auditory tests. Scand Audiol 1975b;4:147–163.

Jerger JF, and Jordan C. Normal audiometric findings. Am J Otol 1980;1:157–159.

Jerger S. Validation of the Pediatric Speech Intelligibility Test in children with central nervous system lesions. Audiology 1987;26:298–311.

Jerger SW, and Jerger JF. Auditory Disorders. Boston: Little, Brown, 1981.

Jerger SW, and Jerger JF. Pediatric speech intelligibility test: Manual for administration. St Louis: Auditec, 1984.

Jerger S, Johnson K, and Loiselle L. Pediatric central auditory dysfunction: comparison of children with confirmed lesions versus suspected processing disorders. Am J Otol 1988;9:63–71.

Jerger S, and Zeller RS. Dichotic listening in a child with a cerebral lesion: The "paradoxical" ipsilateral ear deficit. Ear Hear 1989;10:167–172.

Katinsky S, Lovrinic J, Buchheit W. Cochlear findings in VIIIth nerve tumors. Audiology 1972;11:213–217.

Katz J, and Pack G. New developments in differential diagnosis using the SSW test. In Sullivan M, Ed. Central Auditory Processing Disorders. Omaha: University of Nebraska Press, 1975.

Keith RW. Audiological and auditory language tests of central auditory function. In Keith RW, Ed. Central Auditory and Language Disorders in Children. Houston: College-Hill Press, 1981.

Keith RW. Dichotic listening in children. In Beasley D, Ed. Audition in Childhood: Methods of Study. San Diego: College Hill Press, 1984.

Keith RW. SCAN, a screening test for auditory processing disorders. San Antonio, TX: The Psychology Corporation, 1986.

Keith RW, Rudy J, Dona PA, and Katbamna B. Comparison of SCAN results with other auditory and language measures in a clinical population. Ear Hear 1989;10:382–386.

Kimura D. Cerebral dominance and the perception of verbal stimuli. Can J Psychol 1961a;15:166–171.

Kimura D. Some effects of temporal lobe damage on auditory perception. Can J Psychol 1961b;15:157–165.

Koomar JA, and Cermak SA. Reliability of dichotic listening using two stimulus formats with normal and learning-disabled children. Am J Occup Ther 1981;35:456–463.

Kraft RH. Lateral specialization and verbal/spatial ability in preschool children: age, sex and familial handedness differences. Neuropsychologia 1984;22:319–335.

Kurdziel SA, Noffsinger PD, and Olsen W. Performance by cortical lesion patients on 40 and 60 percent time-compressed materials. J Am Audiol Soc 1976;2:3–7.

Lee F. Time compression and expansion of speech by the sampling method. J Audio Eng Soc 1972;20:738–742.

Lynn GE, and Gilroy J. Neuro-audiological abnormalities in patients with temporal lobe tumors. J Neurol Sci 1972;17:167–184.

Lynn GE, and Gilroy J. Evaluation of central auditory dysfunction in patients with neurological disorders. In Keith RW, Ed. Central Auditory Dysfunction. New York: Grune & Stratton, 1977.

Manning WH, Johnston KL, and Beasley DS. The performance of children with auditory perceptual disorders on a time-compressed speech discrimination measure. J Speech Hear Disord 1977;42: 77–84.

Martin F, and Clark J. Audiologic detection of auditory processing disorders in children. J Am Audiol Soc 1977;3:140–146.

Martin FN, and Morris LJ. Current audiologic practices in the United States. Hear J 1989;42:25–44.

Matzker J. Two new methods for the assessment of central auditory functions in cases of brain disease. Ann Oto Rhino Laryngol 1959;68:1155–1197.

Milner B, Taylor S, and Sperry R. Lateralized suppression of dichotically presented digits after commissural section in man. Science 1968;161:184–185.

Mirabile PJ, Porter RJ, Hughes LF, and Berlin CI. Dichotic lag effect in children 7 to 15. Dev Psychobiol 1978;14:277–285.

Morales-Garcia C, and Poole JO. Masked speech audiometry in central deafness. Acta Otolaryngol (Stockh) 1972;74:307–316.

Mueller HG. Monosyllabic procedures In Katz J, Ed. Handbook of Clinical Audiology. 3rd Ed. Baltimore: Williams & Wilkins, 1985.

Mueller HG. An auditory test protocol for evaluation of neural trauma. Semin Hear 1987;8:223–239.

Mueller HG, and Calkins AM. Dichotic speech measures for predicting hearing aid benefit. [Abstract]. ASHA 1988;30:104.

Mueller HG, Beck WG, and Sedge RK. Comparison of the efficiency of cortical level speech tests. Semin Hear 1987;8:279–298.

Musiek FE. Assessment of central auditory dysfunction: the dichotic digit test revisited. Ear Hear 1983a;4:79–83.

Musiek FE. Assessment of three dichotic speech tests on subjects with intracranial lesions. Ear Hear 1983b;4:318–323.

Musiek FE, and Geurkink NA. Auditory perceptual problems in children: considerations for the otolaryngologist and audiologist. Laryngoscope 1980;90:962–971.

Musiek FE, and Pinheiro ML. Dichotic speech tests in the detection of central auditory dysfunction. In Pinheiro ML, and Musiek FE. Assessment of Central Auditory Dysfunction: Foundations and Clinical Correlates. Baltimore: Williams & Wilkins, 1985.

Musiek FE, and Wilson DH. SSW and dichotic digit results pre- and postcommissurotomy: A case report. J Speech Hear Disord 1979;44:528–533.

Musiek FE, Geurkink NA, and Keitel S. Test battery assessment of auditory perceptual dysfunction in children. Laryngoscope 1982;92:251–257.

Musiek FE, Gollegly KM, and Baran JA. Myelination of the corpus callosum in learning disabled children: Theoretical and clinical correlates. Semin Hear 1984;5:219–229.

Musiek FE, Gollegly KM, Kibbe KS, and Verkest-Lenz SB. Proposed screening test for central auditory disorders: Follow–up on the dichotic digits test. Am J Otol 1991;12:109–113.

Musiek FE, Gollegly KM, and Ross MK. Profiles of types of central auditory processing disorders in children with learning disabilities. J Childhood Comm Dis 1985;9:43–61.

Musiek FE, Kurdziel-Schwan S, Kibbe KS, Gollegly KM, Baran JA, and Rintelmann WF. The dichotic rhyme task: results in split–brain patients. Ear Hear 1989;10:33–39.

Musiek FE, Reeves A, and Baran J. Release from central auditory competition in the split-brain patient. Neurology 1985;35: 983–987.

Musiek FE, Wilson DH, and Pinheiro ML. Audiological manifestations in "split–brain" patients. J Am Audiol Soc 1979;5:25–29.

Newell D, and Rugel RP. Hemispheric specialization in normal and disabled readers. J Learn Disabil 1981;14:296–297.

Niccum N, Rubens A, and Speaks C. Effects of stimulus material on the dichotic listening performance of aphasic patients. J Speech Hear Res 1981;24:526–534.

Noffsinger PD, Olsen WO, Carhart R, Hart CW, and Sahgal V. Auditory and vestibular aberrations in multiple sclerosis. Acta Otolaryngol (Stockh) 1972;303(Suppl 1):1–63.

Olsen WO. Dichotic test results for normal subjects and for temporal lobectomy patients. Ear Hear 1983;4:324–330.

Olsen WO, Noffsinger PD, and Kurdziel SA. Speech discrimination in quiet and in white noise by patients with peripheral and central lesions. Acta Otolaryngol (Stockh) 1975;80:375–382.

Orchik DJ, and Oelschlaeger ML. Time-compressed speech discrimination in children and its relationship to articulation. J Am Audiol Soc 1977;3:37–41.

Oxbury J, and Oxbury S. Effect of temporal lobectomy on the report of dichotically presented digits. Cortex 1969;5:3–14.

Palva A, and Jokinen K. Undistorted and filtered speech audiometry in children with normal hearing. Acta Otolaryngol 1975;80: 383–388.

Papso CF, and Blood IM. Word recognition skills of children and adults in background noise. Ear Hear 1989;10:235–236.

Pettit JM, and Helms S. Hemispheric language dominance of language-disordered, articulation-disordered, and normal children. J Learn Disabil 1979;12:12–17.

Plakke BL, Orchik DJ, and Beasley DS. Children's performance on a binaural fusion task. J Speech Hear Res 1981;24:520–525.

Plomp R, and Mimpen AM. Speech-reception threshold for sentences as a function of age and noise level. J Acoust Soc Am 1979;66:1333–1342.

Rintelmann WF. Monaural speech tests in the detection of central auditory disorders. In Pinheiro ML and Musiek FE, eds. Assessment of Central Auditory Dysfunction: Foundations and Clinical Correlates. Baltimore: Williams & Wilkins, 1985.

Rintelmann WF, Beasley D, and Lynn G. Time-compressed CNC monosyllables: case findings in central auditory disorders. Paper presented at the meeting of the Michigan Speech and Hearing Association, Detroit, 1974.

Roeser RJ, Millay KK, and Morrow JM. Dichotic consonant-vowel (CV) perception in normal and learning-impaired children. Ear Hear 1983;4:293–299.

Roush J, and Tait CA. Binaural fusion, masking level differences, and auditory brain stem responses in children with language-learning disabilities. Ear Hear 1984;5:37–41.

Rodriguez GP, DiSarno NJ, and Hardiman CJ. Central auditory processing in normal–hearing elderly adults. Audiology 1990; 29:85–92.

Rupp RR. Establishing norms for speech-in-noise skills in children. Hear J 1983;36:16–19.

Sinha SO. The role of the temporal lobe in hearing. [Thesis] Montreal, Canada: McGill University, 1959.

Smith BB, and Resnick DM. An auditory test for assessing brain stem integrity: preliminary report. Laryngoscope 1972;84: 414–424.

Sommers RK, and Taylor ML. Cerebral speech dominance in language-disordered and normal children. Cortex 1972;8:224–232.

Sparks R, and Geschwind N. Dichotic listening in man after section of neocortical commissures. Cortex 1968;4:3–16.

Sparks R, Goodglass H, and Nickel B. Ipsilateral versus contralateral extinction in dichotic listening resulting from hemisphere lesions. Cortex 1970;6:249–260.

Speaks C. Dichotic listening: a clinical or research tool? In Sullivan MD, Ed. Central Auditory Processing Disorders. Proceedings of a conference at the University of Nebraska Medical Center, Omaha, NE, 1975.

Springer S, and Gazzaniga M. Dichotic testing of partial and complete split brain patients. Neuropsychologia 1975;3:341–346.

Stach BA. Central auditory processing disorders and amplification applications. In Cherow E, Ed. Proceedings of the Research Symposium on Communication Sciences and Disorders and Aging. ASHA Reports 1990a;19:150–156.

Stach BA. Hearing aid amplification and central processing disorders. In Sandlin R, Ed. Handbook of Hearing Aid Amplification. Vol. 2. Boston: College-Hill Press, 1990b.

Stach BA, Jerger JF, and Fleming KA. Central presbyacusis: A longitudinal case study. Ear Hear 1985;6:304–306.

Stach BA, Degado-Vilches G, and Smith-Farach S. Hearing loss in multiple sclerosis. Semin Hear 1990a;11:221–230.

Stach BA, Spretnjak ML, and Jerger JF. The prevalence of central presbyacusis in a clinical population. J Am Acad Audiol 1990b; 1:109–115.

Studdert-Kennedy M, and Shankweiler D. Hemispheric specialization for speech perception. J Acoust Soc Am 1970;48:579–594.

Tobey EA, Cullen JK, and Rampp DL. Effects of stimulus-onset asynchrony on the dichotic performance of children with auditory-processing disorders. J Speech Hear Res 1979;22: 197–211.

Turner RT. Making clinical decisions. In Rintelmann WF, Ed. Hearing Assessment. 2nd ed. Austin, TX: Pro-Ed, 1991:679–738.

Wexler B, and Halwes T. Increasing the power of dichotic methods: the fused rhymed words test. Neuropsychologia 1983;21:59–66.

Willeford JA. Central auditory function in children with learning disabilities. Audiol Hear Educ 1976;2:12–20.

Wilson L, and Mueller HG. Performance of normal hearing individuals on Auditec filtered speech tests. [Abstract] ASHA 1984; 27:189.

Witelson DR, and Rabinovitch MS. Hemispheric speech lateralization in children with auditory-linguistic deficits. Cortex 1972;8:412–424.

CHAPTER 17

Spondaic Procedures in Central Testing

Jack Katz and Robert G. Ivey

This chapter focuses on two well-known audiological tests of central function that make use of spondaic words. The chapter is arranged in a "bottom-up" fashion, starting with the binaural fusion (BF) procedure that challenges functions at the brainstem level, and then the staggered spondaic word (SSW) test that is best known for its challenge at the cortical level. The masking level difference (MLD) test for spondaic words, another central test, is covered in Chapter 15 along with the puretone MLD.

Spondees are two-syllable words with equal stress on each syllable (e.g., baseball, cowboy). The properties of spondaic words lend themselves to the assessment of the threshold of intelligibility (see Chapter 10) as well as to a number of central auditory tests.

Spondees rise rapidly in intelligibility with small increases in intensity. Therefore, they are ideal for the measurement of speech thresholds. Beyond 10 dBSL the percentage of words that are correctly identified remains fairly constant. The stability in measurement of spondaic words is most likely related to the high level of redundancy of these compound words. Thus, even at 5dB above threshold spondees are easily recognized by the listener.

There are relatively few spondaic words in English. When one hears the spondaic meter and a portion of the phonemic elements (e.g., one syllable or the vowels), there is a high probability of identifying the entire compound word. If the word "base" is recognized as the first syllable there are very few alternatives other than "ball" to complete the spondee. If, however, "ball" was identified one could choose from "base, foot, white, fast", but the vowel, which is generally easy to recognize, would encourage the correct selection of the first syllable.

In the BF test two small frequency bands of energy are delivered to the listener. This small portion of the spondaic word is sufficient for easy recognition by normal listeners. The two-syllable nature of the spondee is expected in the staggered spondaic word test. In this procedure one of the spondees is presented one-syllable earlier than the word to the other ear. This temporal-linguistic offset provides a number of subscales for analyzing central dysfunction.

BINAURAL FUSION TEST

The BF test is modeled after a dichotic procedure that was developed by Matzker (1959). The listener was required to combine the high frequency band portion of a message that was presented to one ear with the low frequency band portion that was directed to the other ear. Matzker indicated that his BF test evaluated the brainstem fusion mechanism.

The BF test appears to be more a test of binaural resynthesis than fusion. That is, we now consider fusion the joining of equal signals in each ear into one midline image. Resynthesis would be a better term to describe the combination of simultaneous complementary signals from the two ears into one composite item. The perception of each filtered segment is at each ear. There is no perception of a whole word in the midline, as would be the case in true binaural fusion.

The BF test (Ivey, 1969) was developed for inclusion in the Colorado State University Central Auditory Test battery to provide a procedure that would be sensitive to dysfunction at the brainstem level. Like the other tests in the battery, it was intended for use with adults who had auditory complaints despite the finding of normal puretone hearing (Ivey and Willeford, 1988). The test is available through Robert Ivey, Suite 205, 215 Piccadilly St., London, Ontario N6A 1S2 (Canada) or Jack Willeford, 555 North Pantano Rd., Tucson, AZ 85710.

Procedure

The BF test was constructed using 40 spondees in two lists. The words were filtered using 500 to 700 Hz and 1900 to 2100 band-pass filters with a 36 dB/octave rejection rate. Items were initially presented at 25 dBSL re: puretone thresholds at 500 Hz and 2000 Hz for the low band-pass (LBP) and high band-pass (HBP) conditions respectively. Words selected to be included in the test were required to demonstrate low intelligibility for each band-pass condition alone, but high intelligibility when presented in the dichotic condition. A pilot project using normal young adults showed the intelligibility of the LBP segment to be 18% while the HBP segment was 29% (Ivey and Willeford, 1988). In the dichotic condition intelligibility was 94%. Two lists were constructed for approximately equal intelligibility based on the pilot study. Each list contains 20 words, which are scored with a value of 5% per word. The band-pass presentations to the two ears on the first list are reversed for the second list in order to avoid a specific ear-frequency effect. The score is arbitrarily assigned to the ear receiving the LBP segment.

The BF test is easy to administer. It requires a two-channel audiometer with a stereo tape deck. Responses consist of repeating the words, a familiar task following the speech reception thresholds and word discrimination testing. These instructions work well with children and adults: "The man says 'ready . . . cowboy' or 'ready . . . hotdog' or 'ready . . . sailboat.' He says the same word to both ears at the same time, but they sound different. So listen to both ears and tell me the word you think he says. If you are not sure, take a guess. He says 'ready' every time, so you don't need to tell me that. Just tell me the word each time." If the patient persists in repeating "ready" it may be eliminated by pressing the interrupter switch on the audiometer.

Normative Studies

In the normative study (Ivey, 1969) the BF test was presented at 25 dBSL in the dichotic condition. Twenty young adults showed an average intelligibility of 90% (List 1 x = 94%, SD = 7; List 2 x = 86%, SD = 8). The difference between the scores on Lists 1 and 2 (8%) was found to be statistically significant. It was suggested that because the difference is known, it can be accommodated. The difference is due to more words in List 2 being less familiar and therefore less intelligible. There was no significant difference found between ears (Right ear x = 89%, SD = 8, Left ear x = 90%, SD = 8).

The test battery including BF was normed for use with children (Willeford, 1977a). Revised norms were published by Willeford and Burleigh in 1985 (see Table 17.1). These norms were obtained at presentation levels of 30 dBSL. The recommended level for presentation to children is 30 dBSL, because the child norms were col-

lected with tapes on which the calibration tone was recorded 5 dB above the level on the master tape. Therefore the presentation SL was increased by 5 dB in order to maintain the speech at the same level as before (Ivey and Willeford, 1988). Subsequent tapes were copied in this manner. Willeford suggested that if poor scores are obtained, a higher sensation level (e.g., 40 dBSL) could be used. If the listener's scores remain low it suggests a brainstem level deficit (Willeford, 1977b).

White (1977), in a normative study of 49 children (age range 6 to 10 years), found an overall difference of 13% between List 1 (71%) and List 2 (58%). She suggests that children should be familiarized with the words prior to testing in order to accommodate for the more difficult vocabulary of List 2. Willeford and Burleigh (1985) suggested another approach. Ten percent may be added to the score for List 2 in order to compensate for the difference.

Windham et al. (1986) evaluated 40 urban black children (age range 7.4 to 11.4 years) with a battery of central auditory tests including BF. These children were selected as "intellectually, functionally, and behaviorally normal." All subjects had normal hearing. The test was presented at 30 dBSL. They found the performance of their children was ". . . not qualitatively nor quantitatively different from the performance of 'normal' white children" (p. 13).

Figure 17.1 represents the results of a study (Ivey et al., 1982) intended to explore intelligibility of the two lists across intensity. Each of the two band pass segments was evaluated separately, as was the dichotic binaural condition. Each of these conditions was evaluated on a separate group of 11 young adults.

The results of this study showed a relatively rapid rise of intelligibility (approximately 24% per 5 dB step) for the HBP segment as intensity increased. The LBP segment showed a shallower slope (approximately 5% per 5 dB step) that does not reach 50% by 40 dBHL. When the materials were presented dichotically, intelligibility was relatively high at all levels with a slope of approximately 10% per 5 dB step. It appears that presentation levels of 25 or 30 dBSL are most appropriate for maintaining low intelligibility for the band-pass segments while obtaining high intelligibility for the dichotic condition. The difference between lists is evident in the individual band-pass data but less obvious for the dichotic condition. (An average of 1.3% difference over the six presentation levels.)

Miltenberger et al. (1978) evaluated central audition in 70 patients with a variety of sensory-neural hearing losses. Twenty-four percent of the group performed below normal on BF. They suggested that because most of the patients had sloping hearing losses and required elevated presentation levels, there may have been a

Table 17.1.
Binaural Fusion Child Norms Collected at 30 dBSL[a]

Age	N	Mean (%)		Range (%)	
		right	left	right	left
6	40	74.1	75.0	55–95	55–100
7	40	76.0	75.5	55–100	55–100
8	40	76.8	76.8	65–100	60–100
9	40	79.9	78.8	55–100	55–100
10	40	89.2	87.6	80–95	75–95
Adult	20	89.3	90.5	75–100	75–100

[a]A 10% correction factor is added to List 2 scores for the child norms. From Willeford and Burleigh (1985). Adult norms from Ivey (1969) and Ivey and Willeford (1988).

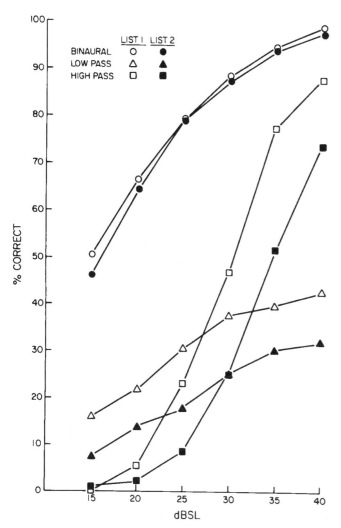

Figure 17.1. Performance-intensity function on Lists 1 and 2 of the Binaural Fusion/Resynthesis test for normal adult subjects. Separate information is shown for the high frequency and low frequency bands in each ear, as well as for the binaural condition (Ivey et al., 1982).

band-pass spread to adjacent areas that had better hearing sensitivity. They concluded however that central auditory tests including binaural fusion could be administered to persons with sensory-neural hearing losses as long as the audiometric results were considered and that the test results were interpreted with caution.

Grady et al. (1984) studied a group of 36 normal males (age range 21–83) in order to determine if aging affects the ability to process speech stimuli. They found that although word discrimination and low-pass filtered speech scores were negatively correlated (p < 0.05) with increasing age, BF scores were not significantly correlated with age.

Wilimas et al. (1988) studied a group of 22 patients with sickle cell anemia and a control group of 19 individuals. Of the patient group, 13 were chronically transfused and 9 were untransfused. There was no significant difference found for the three groups of subjects for BF or competing sentences. They concluded that central auditory dysfunction is not a common finding in patients with sickle cell anemia.

Pathologic Findings

Early researchers, such as Matzker (1959), Linden (1964), Hayashi (1966) and Ohta et al. (1967), showed in their work with patients that binaural fusion or resynthesis is a function of the brainstem. Further studies with adults having central nervous system lesions showed the test to be sensitive to lesions that compromise the brainstem through compression (Lynn et al., 1972), trauma (Pinheiro et al., 1982), and due to decompression sickness (Miltenberger et al., 1979). However, poor scores on binaural resynthesis tests have been found in cases with normal auditory brainstem responses (Smith and Resnick, 1972; Welsh et al., 1982; Musiek and Geurkink, 1982). There is no reason to believe that the on-effect type of processing reflected in the ABR is the only transmission device in the brainstem. Complex stimuli that exist over time also depend on temporal integration. Binaural mechanisms depend on input from the two ears. The first level of interaction is at the superior olivary complex allowing the fusion of similar inputs from the two ears into a single auditory image. In addition, binaural resynthesis depends on a mechanism in the brainstem above the superior olivary complex that allows for the resynthesis of different but complementary information (Ivey and Willeford, 1988).

Children Having Difficulty in School

Willeford (1977a) was the first to apply the BF test to children having difficulty in school. He used a test battery including competing sentences, low-pass filtered speech, binaural fusion, and rapidly alternating speech. He found in a study of 150 learning-disabled (LD) children that the BF test was the one most frequently failed (64%). Other studies (Willeford, 1977b; Welsh et al., 1980; Welsh et al., 1982) have found high failure rates in LD children. Welsh et al. (1980) found that of 20 dyslexics 85% fell below the range of normal on the BF test. Welsh et al. (1982) studied 77 dyslexics (age range 7 to 18 years) and found that 79% failed the BF test in one or both ears. Although there was a general improvement in test scores with increasing age, the older students' results remained below the 7 year old norm. In a study of 103 children referred for central auditory evaluation because of difficulty in school, Ivey (1986) found that 49% failed BF in one or both ears.

Eighty children who were referred for central auditory evaluation took part in a study to explore list and ear differences. List 1 was presented first and then List 2.

For 40 children the words were presented LBP-RE, HBP-LE first, while the other 40 children received HBP-RE, LBP-LE first. The band-pass-ear condition was reversed after each set of 10 words. The test was presented at 30 dBSL (re: puretone thresholds at 500 and 2000 Hz). Table 17.2 shows the error rates for each item in each list in the order of difficulty, the total errors for each list and the total errors for each ear. There were a total of 3200 responses collected (1600 per ear or list). Eighty responses were collected per word across ears and lists. The errors represented an average score (correct responses) of 67% for List 1 and 57% for List 2. This finding supports the recommendation made by Willeford to add 10% to the score for List 2 in order to compensate for the list difference. The score for the right ear was 63% and for the left ear 61%. No systematic ear difference was found for either band-pass-ear condition.

Poor scores may be due to a failure of the binaural resynthesis mechanism of the brainstem or to difficulty discriminating words having reduced redundancy which may be due to a left hemisphere deficit (Dempsey, 1977). This question may be resolved by a retest with both frequency bands to both ears (Matzker, 1959; Lynn et al., 1972; Smith and Resnick, 1972). If the diotic score improves to a normal level, then there is a binaural resynthesis deficit.

There is evidence of visual involvement in children with binaural resynthesis deficits. Willeford and Bilger (1978) observed that ". . . children who perform poorly on tests of brainstem integrity may have their auditory attention diverted by visual distractions as well as by ambient auditory events" (p. 419). They speculated that this may be due to a breakdown in coordinated access to multisensory processors of the brainstem reticular formation, the thalamus or other limbic-system mechanisms. Welsh et al. (1980) and Welsh et al. (1982) studied groups of dyslexic children and found various central auditory deficits including a high rate of binaural resynthesis deficits. Reading is a highly auditory behavior dependent on visual-auditory interaction at various levels. Poor scores in BF in dyslexics may implicate a dysfunction at the earliest level of visual-auditory (multisensory) interaction in the brainstem.

These observations are not surprising given the proximity of the superior colliculi (visual nuclei) to the inferior colliculi (auditory nuclei) in the brainstem. There may be a relationship between poor BF test scores and failure to learn to read by a "phonics" approach. Difficulty with both sound-symbol association and visual distractibility would be consistent with a failure to adequately relate visual to auditory stimuli that are different but complementary. An analogous condition may occur when the sound track of a movie is not synchronous with the picture, so that the illusion of sound coming from the screen is lost. In other words, an automatic association of the two stimuli is not made at the brainstem level (Ivey, 1986).

THE STAGGERED SPONDAIC WORD TEST

The Staggered Spondaic Word test, one of the early central procedures employed by audiologists in the United States, has been used extensively over the past 30 years. It continues to be one of the most frequently administered tests of central auditory function (Oliver, 1987; Martin and Morris, 1989).

The original application of the SSW was for localizing the site-of-dysfunction in cases with suspected brain or brainstem lesions (Katz, 1962). When professional attention turned to the study of auditory processing problems, as seen in learning-disabled children, the data that were obtained from brain lesion patients formed the basis for understanding processing difficulties.

The features that make the SSW test especially useful, include (a) its resistance to the influence of peripheral hearing distortion (Katz, 1968; Cafarelli et al., 1977; Arnst, 1980), (b) its simplicity, which makes it applicable to a wide variety of ages (Brunt, 1965; Ammerman and Parnell, 1980) and disordered populations, such as the mentally retarded (Hadaway, 1969), autistic (Miller et al., 1981), Alzheimer's disease patients (Grimes et al., 1985), and others (Winn, 1965; Hall and Jerger, 1978; Air, 1979), (c) coherent normative data to evaluate individuals 5 to 70 years of age, (d) evidence of strong reliability and validity (Katz and Arndt, 1982; Katz et al.,

Table 17.2.
Error Rate for Each Word for 80 Children

List 1		List 2	
RAINBOW	2	WILDCAT	8
BASEBALL	4	HORSESHOE	11
EYEBROW	4	SCARECROW	16
CHURCHBELL	7	FOOTSTOOL	21
BEDROOM	12	YARDSTICK	22
BLUEJAY	12	WATCHWORD	23
BAGPIPE	13	BOBWHITE	25
WOODCHUCK	14	WORKSHOP	29
DAYLIGHT	18	WIGWAM	30
SHOELACE	20	PLATFORM	31
NORTHWEST	22	THEREFORE	33
BIRDNEST	27	HOUSEWORK	35
MEATBALL	32	DOORMAT	36
DRUGSTORE	35	STAIRWAY	38
BUCKWHEAT	41	LIFEBOAT	40
ALTHOUGH	41	DOLLHOUSE	49
BONBON	45	NUTMEG	53
PADLOCK	49	WHIZBANG	60
BLOODHOUND	51	MISHAP	66
DOVETAIL	75	SOYBEAN	67

LIST ERRORS	524		693
EAR ERRORS ACROSS LISTS:		RIGHT EAR	597
		LEFT EAR	620

1980; Katz et al., 1985; Hurley, 1990), and (*e*) brevity, making the procedure cost effective.

The Competing Environmental Sound (CES) test is a companion procedure to the SSW (Katz et al., 1975; Johnson and Sherman, 1980). Its main purpose is to help identify commissural pathway dysfunction (e.g., corpus callosum). This test will be mentioned briefly to show how it helps to reduce the ambiguity that may occur when there is poor performance in the left ear on the SSW.

Administration of the SSW Test

The SSW test is delivered via a two-channel tape player and audiometer. The standard presentation is 50 dB SL (± 5 dB); however, if the listener is intolerant of this intensity, it can be reduced to as low as 25 dB SL, if necessary. In case of significant conductive loss (20 dB or greater), the presentation to that ear should be lowered to 30 dB SL.

The test tape (available from Precision Acoustics, 411 NE 87th Avenue, Suite B, Vancouver, WA 98664) takes about 10 minutes to administer. Each SSW item is made up of two spondaic or compound words as shown in Figure 17.2. The first item generally begins in the right ear with the word "up", a right noncompeting (RNC) condition. The words "stairs" and "down", which are presented simultaneously to opposite ears, are designated as the right competing (RC) and left competing (LC) conditions, respectively. The last word "town" is the left noncompeting (LNC) condition. Test items, which follow this pattern, are designated as right-ear-first (REF) items. The second item, which is left-ear-first (LEF), is "outside, inlaw". It follows the opposite sequence from LNC to RNC. The 40 items of the standard EC list alternate between REF and LEF. It is critical that the routing of the tape (i.e., REF or LEF) be designated on the first page of the scoring form, and

	Sequence		
	First	Second	Third
Item 1 (REF)	**RNC**	**RC**	
	up	stairs	
		down	town
		LC	**LNC**
Item 2 (LEF)	**LNC**	**LC**	
	out	side	
		in	law
		RC	**RNC**

Figure 17.2. The first two items of the SSW test. The first item is given right-ear-first (REF) and the second one left-ear-first (LEF). Each of the four component words of an item represent different conditions. The four conditions are right noncompeting (RNC), right competing (RC), left competing (LC), and left noncompeting (LNC).

preferably on the succeeding pages. Figure 17.3 shows the last 10 items of the test.

The instructions state that words will be presented to one or both ears and that the listener should repeat them. It is appropriate to add that the phrase, "Are you ready?" precedes each item and that this is simply to prepare the listener that the item will be coming. The listener is not to repeat or respond to that phrase.

Scoring of the SSW Test

The SSW test should be scored both quantitatively and qualitatively. Each of the approaches can provide support or complementary information to indicate the scope of the auditory dysfunction. The quantitative components include the raw (R-SSW), corrected (C-SSW) and adjusted SSW (A-SSW) scores. The qualitative procedures include: (*a*) response bias, which refers to defined patterns of response such as reversals and order effects, and (*b*) qualifiers, which refer to test-taking behaviors, such as quick responses and delays.

Scoring Words and Items

Responses to each of the 160 test words must be considered individually, as either right or wrong. If a word is wrong (omitted or substituted) ignoring the sequence, then a horizontal line is drawn through the word on the scoring form, and the error is shown above it. An omitted word is designated by a dash (see Figure 17.3, items 31, 34, and 37). If the error entails the substitution of another word, or a nonsense word, then it is written in (see items 32, 36, and 39). The number of errors on each item is shown in the column labeled "Wrong". If all four words are correct, regardless of the order in which they are repeated, a dot (•) is entered in the "Wrong" column (see items 33 and 40).

The sequence of the words in the response does not enter into the scoring of errors. However, the incorrect order is specified by numbers shown below the words (see items 34, 38, and 39). An item out of sequence with no more than one error is considered a reversal (see items 38, 39, and 40). Reversals are designated by circling the "R" in the "Rev" column.

Figure 17.3 shows the eight columns on the scoring form, four for REF words (columns A–D) and four for LEF words (columns E–H). The total errors for each column provide the most important information. These totals, which are referred to as the "eight cardinal numbers", are used in various ways to study the person's performance.

Quantitative Scoring

The R-SSW Score. This score provides the percentage of error for each of the four conditions, the average

	(A)	(B)	(C)	(D)	Rev	WRONG
31.	bird	~~cage~~	crow's	nest	R	1
33.	book	shelf	drug	store	R	•
35.	hand	**fall** ~~ball~~	milk	shake	R	1
37.	for	— ~~give~~	**masked** ~~milk~~	man	R	2
39.	race 1	horse 4	**straight** ~~street~~ 3	car 2	Ⓡ	•
SUM Page 3	O	4	3	1		
SUM Page 2	O	3	3	2		
TOTAL	O	7	6	3		16
		(CARDINAL NUMBERS)				
~~Left~~ First	~~L-NC~~ (A) R-NC	~~L-C~~ (B) R-C	~~R-C~~ (C) L-C	~~R-NC~~ (D) L-NC		
Right First						

	(E)	(F)	(G)	(H)	Rev	WRONG
32.	week	**day** ~~end~~	work	day	R	1
34.	wood 2	work 1	— ~~beach~~	— ~~craft~~	R	2
36.	fish	net	/ʃæ/ ~~sky~~	line	R	1
38.	sheep 3	— ~~skin~~	bull 1	dog 2	Ⓡ	1
40.	green 3	house 4	string 1	bean 2	Ⓡ	•
SUM Page 3	O	3	4	2		
SUM Page 2	1	2	4	O		
TOTAL	1	5	8	2		16
		(CARDINAL NUMBERS)				
~~R-NC~~ ~~R-C~~ ~~L-C~~ ~~L-NC~~	(E) L-NC	(F) L-C	(G) R-C	(H) R-NC		

EAR EFFECT		
Total Errors	REF	LEF
☐ Sig. ☒ N. Sig.	16	16

REVERSALS	
TOTAL =	8

ORDER EFFECT			
1	2	3	4
(A+E)	(B+F)	(C+G)	(D+H)
1	12	14	5
TOTAL 13 1st SPONDEE		TOTAL 19 2nd SPONDEE	
☒ Sig		☐ N. Sig	

COMBINED TOTALS				
	RNC	RC	LC	LNC
(A) - (D) or (E) - (H)	0	7	6	3
(H) - (E) or (D) - (A)	2	8	5	1
GRAND TOTALS	2	15	11	4

Enter these figures on Page 1

Figure 17.3. The last 10 items of the test and the calculations on the bottom of the third page of the scoring form.

error for each ear, and the average error for the entire test (total). This is accomplished by combining the eight cardinal numbers to obtain the four condition scores. The calculations are made on the bottom of the third page of the scoring form (see Figure 17.3). If the test is given REF, then the number of errors for columns A through D are entered in alphabetical order. LEF entries must be reversed (H through E) to combine the RNC errors from the first half of the test with the RNC errors from the second half, and so on. The grand totals

for the four conditions are then carried over to the upper right-hand side of the first page (see Figure 17.4). The maximum number of errors for any condition is 40, therefore, to convert the numbers to percent, each error must be multiplied by 2.5. It is customary to round 0.5's to the nearest *even* number. The condition scores (in percent) are averaged to obtain a right-ear (RNC + RC ÷ 2) and left-ear (LC + LNC ÷ 2) scores. Finally, these two scores are averaged (RE + LE ÷ 2) to obtain the total R-SSW score.

STANDARD SSW TEST-LIST EC

Name __Anna Morris__ Date __Nov. 15, 1993__ (REF) LEF

AGE __47__ Sex: M (F) Handed: (R) L A Tester __M. M.__

1. R-SSW
Enter totals from page 3

CONDITION	RNC	RC	LC	LNC
Total Errors	2	15	11	4
Multiplier	x 2.5	x	x	x
R-SSW %Error	5	38	28	10

EAR	RE		LE	
R-SSW %Error	22		19	

TOTAL		T		
R-SSW % Error		20		

2. C-SSW
Enter R-SSW % error

CONDITION	RNC	RC	LC	LNC
R-SSW % Error	5	38	28	10
-WDS % Error	-4	-4	-0	-0
C-SSW % Error	1	34	28	10

EAR	RE		LE	
C-SSW % Error	18		19	

TOTAL		T		
C-SSW % Error		18		

3. A - SSW
Enter least biased errors from page 3

CONDITION	RNC	RC	LC	LNC
Least Biased Errors				
Multiplier	x	x	x	x
Least Biased % Errors				
-WDS % Error	−	−	−	−
A-SSW % Error				

EAR	RE		LE	
A-SSW % Error				

TOTAL		T		
A-SSW % Error				

Graph (PERCENT ERROR, 100–0 to (-25)):
RIGHT NC C — LEFT C NC
X=R-SSW
O=C-SSW
A=A-SSW

SSW SUMMARY
Score

Response Bias

Reversals __8__ (SIG) NS
Sig-Order __13__ / __19__ H/L (L/H)
Sig-Ear ____ / ____ L/H H/L
Type A LC RC
Other: _____

COMMENTS: _____

AUDIOMETRIC SUMMARY

	3-FREQ SP AVG	SRT	WDS	SSW HL
RE	15		96	65
LE	8		100	60

PRECISION ACOUSTICS
411 N.E. 87th. Avenue, Suite B
Vancouver. WA. 98664
(206) 892-9367

Multipliers

#ITEMS	R-SSW	A-SSW
20	5	10
25	4	8
30	3.3	6.7
(40)	2.5	5

If other: _____
( ) _____

TEC ANALYSIS

	C-SSW			A-SSW		
	Total	Ear	Cond.	Total	Ear	Cond.
#	18	19	34			
CAT	MO	MI	MO			

Combined TEC	MO	Combined TEC	

©Jack Katz, 1965, 1970, 1977, 1986

Figure 17.4. The first page of scoring form where calculations for the R-SSW, C-SSW, and A-SSW (not shown) are made. In addition, there is room to show response bias and other information.

The C-SSW Scores. These scores are generally used for interpreting the test results. To obtain the C-SSWs, the R-SSW scores are corrected by subtracting the percentage of word recognition error from the respective condition scores. The standard procedure is to use the Hirsh W-22 recording (Technisonic Corporation), because it tends to offset the error associated with cochlear distortion (Katz, 1977). Figure 17.4, on the upper right, shows the corrections based on discrimination scores of 96% and 100% for the right and left ears, respectively. These C-SSW scores are then averaged in the same way as for the R-SSW, to provide ear and total scores. Both the R-SSW and C-SSW scores for the four conditions are graphed on the first page of the scoring form. The figure is referred to as the SSW-Gram.

Although a correction factor could add an element of error to a score, the SSW correction is considered justified because it provides two important advantages over the raw scores. First, it permits one to evaluate a patient with as much as a 40 dB HL threshold in the speech frequencies, without major concern for contamination (Arnst, 1980a and b).

The second advantage of the C-SSW score is that although there is a close relationship between the R-SSW and word recognition scores for cochlear cases, a large overcorrection generally occurs in retrocochlear cases when the disorder is sufficient to affect discrimination. Thus, a significantly negative C-SSW score is likely to result, helping to differentiate the site of lesion in certain cases with sensory-neural hearing losses.

Figure 17.5 shows the remarkable similarity between the R-SSW and the Hirsh W-22 scores for 100 ears with cochlear pathology. Various studies have shown correlations of about 0.85 for each ear when comparing the W-22s and R-SSW scores (Katz and Pack, 1975; Arnst, 1980a). Although, some investigators have expressed reluctance, on theoretical grounds, to subtract a monosyllabic score from a spondaic score (Lynn and Gilroy, 1975), there is ample evidence that the correction does work, especially when the loss does not exceed 40 dB (Cafarelli et al., 1979; Arnst, 1982a and b).

Quantitative Analysis for Site-of-Dysfunction

Unless stated otherwise, the data in this section come from Katz (1976). As previously noted, in cases of cochlear hearing impairment, C-SSW scores generally are neither extremely positive nor extremely negative, when there is no more than a moderate hearing loss in the speech frequencies. Mean C-SSW scores for groups of cochlear cases are usually very close to zero. However, eighth nerve cases often have such poor discrimination for monosyllabic words that the correction is extensive. The percent of SSW error is generally far less than on monosyllabic word discrimination test. This results in a significantly large overcorrected score in the affected ear. For example, in eighth nerve cases, the mean C-SSW score for the affected ear was a dramatic −27. The specific criteria for overcorrected scores are shown in Table 17.3 and discussed in the section on total, ear, and condition analysis.

Patients with low auditory brainstem tumors had an average C-SSW score of −13 in the affected ear. The affected ear was almost always *ipsilateral* to the lesion, whether the tumor was intra- or extra-axial (Katz, 1971, 1976). Other behavioral tests as well as acoustic reflex and auditory brainstem response findings tend to show ipsilateral abnormalities, which is not consistent with the traditional notion but is supported by other researchers (Marsh et al., 1974; Musiek et al., 1988). Rather, the pathophysiology seems to suggest that the cumulative decussation necessary to produce a contralateral effect on the SSW is higher than the superior olivary complex.

Even upper brainstem cases generally show an ipsilateral effect on the SSW. In these cases a similar puretone pattern may be noted bilaterally, but the extent of loss is greater ipsilaterally. Upper brainstem tumor cases had a mean C-SSW score of +53 in the ear ipsilateral to the lesion.

In contrast to the previously mentioned sites, lesions of the auditory reception (AR) center, located in Heschl's gyrus in each hemisphere, display a *contralateral* effect. AR cases had a mean C-SSW score of +52 in the ear contralateral to the damaged side. These findings suggest that somewhere between the upper brainstem and the AR center, the affected ear on the SSW shifts from ipsilateral to contralateral.

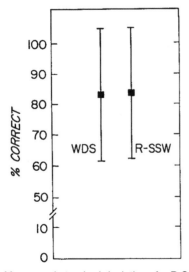

Figure 17.5. Means and standard deviations for R-SSW and word discrimination scores (WDS) based on 100 ears with cochlear pathology (Katz, 1977:111).

Table 17.3.
C-SSW/A-SSW Category Table: Adult Site-of-Dysfunction Information[a]

Score	Category				
	Over Corrected	Normal	Mildly Abnormal	Moderately Abnormal	Severely Abnormal
TOTAL	— to –5	–4 to 5	6 to 15	16 to 35	36 to 100
EAR	— to –7	–6 to 10	11 to 20	21 to 40	41 to 100
CONDITION	— to –10	–9 to 15	16 to 25	26 to 45	46 to 100

[a]This information was set up to differentiate the loci of auditory disorders such as auditory reception problems versus cerebral disorders outside of the auditory reception region. These criteria may also be used to distinguish upper from lower auditory brainstem dysfunction, etc.

The last pathological group is referred to as non-auditory reception (NAR). These individuals have cerebral lesions which do not effect the AR centers. NAR lesions include cases as diverse as a lobectomy of the anterior temporal lobe which does not impinge on Heschl's gyrus, a frontal lobe tumor and an occipital lobe stroke. NAR cases generally have pretty good or even normal SSW scores. Their mean C-SSW score was +8 in the ear opposite the lesion, as compared to the moderate or severe scores of AR cases.

In most instances, NAR patients are easily distinguished from AR cases; however, this may not be true for those with corpus callosum lesions. Corpus callosum patients are considered NAR if Heschl's gyrus is spared. Damage to the middle and posterior portions of the corpus callosum was found to have a significant effect on SSW performance in the *(LC)* condition, regardless of the involved hemisphere (Katz et al., 1980). Commissural pathway lesions seem to be unique in that they show left ear disability on dichotic tests in those with left-hemisphere dominance for language (Lynn, 1975; Musiek and Wilson, 1979). Involvement of the anterior portion of the corpus callosum does not seem to produce a major deficit except in elderly cases (Katz et al., 1980). Findings suggest that elderly individuals with anterior corpus callosum tumors have SSW patterns similar to those with posterior corpus callosum lesions.

Not all portions of the central nervous system can be identified by the SSW. Regions that are not generally identifiable by a test are referred to as *silent areas.* Certain areas of the brain are known to be silent on the SSW. These areas include the visual cortex (occipital lobe) and the posterosuperior parietal region. Thus, we cannot expect to find quantitative or even qualitative signs when a lesion is confined to silent areas.

Obtaining a Total-Ear-Condition Analysis

The TEC analysis refers to a total (T), ear (E) and condition (C) analysis for C-SSW scores. It is used in site-of-dysfunction studies with adults. The TEC analysis is *not* appropriate for evaluating children who are being tested for auditory processing (AP) disorders.

The first step in the TEC analysis is to narrow down the significant C-SSW options. There is no problem in selecting the appropriate T score because there is only one from which to choose. This information is entered on the lower right-hand side of page one (see Figure 17.4). The corresponding category is obtained from Table 17.3. For example, for a total score of +3 would be normal (N) while +40 would be severe (S). For the illustration shown in the figure the total is 18 and the category MO.

Next, we choose the more extreme of the two E scores. For example, 20 is more extreme than 10, and –20 is more extreme than –10. If both choices are positive (or negative), then the task is simplified. However, if there is a positive and negative value they must be considered separately. If we have –20 for one ear and +20 for the other, the corresponding categories for E are overcorrected (O) and mild (MI), respectively. Such a case would require a double entry. In the figure the ear score was 19 and the category MI.

The same procedures are now followed to obtain a single condition score and its corresponding category. If there are significant positive and negative scores, then the most extreme for each is used. Consider the following TEC example: RNC = –30, RC = –10, LC = +40, LNC = +30. The –30 represents the most extreme negative score and +40 the most extreme positive. The TEC category table shows that a –30 condition is O, while +40 is moderate (MO). Because both scores are significant (not N), we must deal with *both* categories. In this illustration, the two E scores would be –20 and +35, with corresponding categories of O and MO, respectively. Because one is significant in the negative direction and the other significant in the positive direction, we must utilize both categories. The total score in this case would be 7.5, which, when rounded to the nearest even number, is 8, a MI score.

Figure 17.4 shows a more typical case than the complex one above. In any event, once the extreme scores are selected for T, E, and C and the respective categories are derived from Table 17.3, one can complete the TEC analysis.

Combining T, E, and C Scores

The rules for combining T, E, and C into one representative category are logical:

1. Significant positive and significant negative scores must be considered separately. For example, a positive score that is associated with a high brainstem lesion may be found in one ear and a negative score due to a severe cochlear problem could be identified in the other. Each is significant and should be identified audiometrically. If both positive and negative scores are significant then the combined TEC will be a dual category, that is, part of the result will be O and the other part MI, MO, or S.

2. The N category is of importance only when there is no abnormal finding to supersede it. For example, if a person has three normal conditions, but the fourth is abnormal, then we ignore the normal portions to find out about the problem.

3. To combine the T, E and C, we consider each of the three indicators. The most common category, rather than the best or poorest, is taken as the combined category. Often, the T, E, and C categories are the same. For example, if T, E, and C are MI, MI, MI, it is easy to see that the combined category is also MI. However, if they are MO, MI, MO, then the common category (MO) is taken as the combined category. Of course, considering point number 2, if the categories are N, N, MI, we must ignore the N findings and take the MI as the combined category. If there is no common category then the median is used. For example, MI, MO, S would be combined to MO.

4. These three rules will enable the user to arrive at the combined TEC quickly and reliably. The major complication is when there are one or two dual categories. While O, O, O would be simple to combine (O), the following may prove more difficult: MI, O-MO, O-S. In this case there are both overcorrected and some strongly positive scores. The rule to solve this problem is that when there is a dual category, simply remove the O (or Os), and use it as half of the combined category. Then combine the T, E and C in this simplified form. The MI, MO, and S yields MO as the median which is used as the other half of the combined category (O-MO).

The next section will discuss how the combined TEC helps in interpreting the SSW. It is based on information in the SSW Workshop Manual (Katz, 1987).

Selecting Site-of-Dysfunction Based on Quantitative Results

The TEC information can now be used to determine the presumed site-of-dysfunction.

Normal TEC. Essentially all cases with normal peripheral and central auditory systems (exclusive of special groups such as foreign born listeners) should fall into this category. The same is true for those with conductive hearing losses, when a presentation level of 30 dB SL is used. In addition, about half of the cochlear cases demonstrate normal TECs, as expected because of the correction factor. It is important to note that about half of the NAR cases also demonstrate normal TECs. This is in part because some areas of the brain are silent on the SSW.

Overcorrected TEC. In order to have an O TEC, it is necessary to have a significantly reduced word recognition score relative to the R-SSW score. Thus, regardless of the etiology, if there is no influence on discrimination, we cannot expect to see an O. Almost all of the eighth nerve and low brainstem cases tested had O TECs in the ear ipsilateral to the lesion. In addition, about half of the cochlear cases, especially those with unilateral losses, fell into this category.

Mild TEC. About half of the NAR cases had MI combined TEC categories. About 20% of cochlear cases, especially those with unilateral losses, fell into the MI category, as well as fewer than 10% of the conductives. Diagnostic confusion arose in less than 10% of the AR cases who had MI TECs.

Moderate/Severe TEC. Almost all of the high brainstem cases had MO or S scores when the lesion involved the auditory pathways (Katz, 1976). In addition, over 90% of the ARs were so classified. A MO score is considered a false positive finding in NAR cases. This was noted in about 5% of the NARs and 5% of the unilateral cochlear cases. Figure 17.6 shows the mean condition scores and SDs for right and left hemisphere AR cases. Site of lesion was determined by physicians independent of SSW results.

Other Pathways. Two commissural pathways, the corpus callosum and anterior commissure, are dealt with separately here. These are more difficult to specify because we have fewer verified cases to generalize from and because location, age, and gender seem to complicate the picture. For patients with tumors involving the anterior commissure and/or the middle or posterior portions of the corpus callosum, MO or S TECs have been found in about 80% of the cases. Anterior corpus callosum cases have demonstrated MI scores, except for those individuals over 60 years of age. The elderly cases had MO TECs with the primary abnormality in the left ear, especially the LC condition. Means and standard deviations for 24 cases with adventitious tumors of the corpus callosum are shown in Figure 17.7.

To simplify the diagnostic task, the audiologist can employ Table 17.4, which is divided into three parts. The top section provides typical TEC categories, the

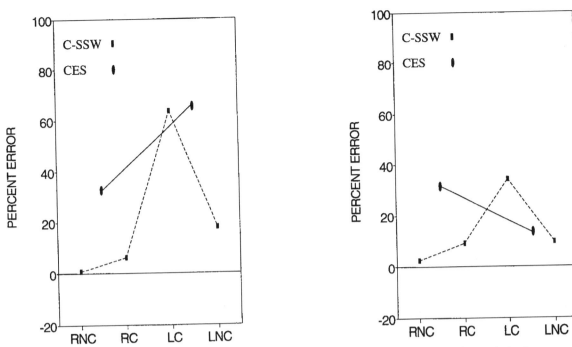

Figure 17.6. C-SSW scores and CES results for 12 right AR and 30 left AR cases. This demonstrates the contralateral effect in AR cases. The SSW and CES tests peak on the same side.

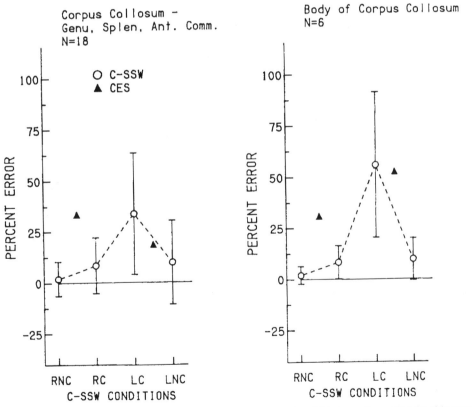

Figure 17.7. C-SSW and CES results for corpus callosum and/or anterior commissure tumor cases. The figure on the left shows the results for 18 cases in which lesions involved the posterior or anterior portion of the corpus callosum and/or the anterior commissure. The figure on the right shows the results for six cases in which lesions involve the body of the corpus callosum (Katz et al., 1980). The CES test peaks in opposite ears (Katz and Smith, 1991:244).

Table 17.4.
Selecting Site-of-Dysfunction Based on Quantitative Results[a]

Combined TEC Categories	Overcorrected				Normal	Mild				Moderate/Severe		
Most typical patterns Total	O	N	O	O	N	MI	MI	MI	N	MO	MO	S
Ear	O	N	O	N	N	MI	N	MI	N	MO	MO	S
Cond	O	O	N	N	N	MI	N	MO	MI	MO	S	S

Diagnostic considerations			
1. Cochlear 2. Eighth nerve 3. Low brainstem	1. Normal 2. NAR 3. Cochlear	1. NAR if no hearing loss 2. Cochlear 3. NAR and cochlear 4. Mid brainstem if MI-O and retrocochlear signs	1. AR 2. Corpus callosum/ anterior commissure 3. High brainstem

Additional audiometric tests to narrow diagnosis			
1–3. Cochlear and retrocochlear tests	1&2. Use response bias and other central tests 3. Threshold and cochlear tests	1. Response bias and other central tests 2&3. In some cases these cannot be differentiated 4. ABR, reflex decay and central tests	1&2. CES and other central tests 3. Tone and reflex decay, ABR and other cochlear and retrocochlear tests

[a]This table provides reasonable alternatives to consider when evaluating adults, up to 60 years of age, for site-of-dysfunction. Select the appropriate TEC category or find the T (total), E (ear), and C (condition) that correspond to the typical patterns. Consider the diagnostic levels shown and then, if further differentiation is needed, see which additional tests would be most helpful. The regions listed are not exhaustive and multiple sites of lesion are also possible. This table is a modification of Table 14.2 in Kaplan, Gladstone, and Katz, 1984:300.

middle portion shows the major diagnostic considerations for each and the bottom offers additional tests helpful in differentiating among the primary diagnostic considerations.

Comparing SSW and CES Test Results

A comparison of the depressed ear scores on the SSW and CES tests can provide evidence to help distinguish between right AR center and certain commissural pathway lesions. It should be noted that involvement of the right AR center, the corpus callosum and/or the anterior commissure all produce an error peak in the left ear on the SSW-Gram. Thus, one cannot simply assume that a left ear peak is the result of a right hemisphere involvement (Lynn, 1975). The CES test may be administered to reduce the ambiguity of a left ear peak.

Although the patterns are similar on the SSW, the CES peak of errors is in the opposite ear. This "crossed pattern" between SSW and CES results suggests a commissural disconnection (Figure 17.7). When the results for both tests peak in the left ear, this indicates a right AR disorder. The apparent exception to this rule is when the middle portion of the corpus callosum is dam-

aged. In this case, like the right AR cases, the peak for both tests is generally in the left ear.

When both tests show significant errors in the left ear, one might distinguish a right AR disorder from a mid corpus callosum problem by use of the Pinheiro Pitch Pattern Sequence test (see Chapter 15) or filtered speech tests (Lynn and Gilroy, 1977). Another approach is to consider the word recognition scores, which are assumed to be normal relative to puretone thresholds when the commissural pathways are damaged (Katz et al., 1980).

Response Bias

One unique feature of the SSW test is a group of qualitative indicators known as response bias (RB). RB refers to peculiarities in a person's responses. The major RBs are reversals, order effects, ear effects, and type A patterns. A reversal refers to an item in which the words are repeated out of order, *as long as there is no more than one error on the item* (see Figure 17.3, items 38–40). Note that item 34 is not a reversal, because there are two errors. Two or more reversals on the test is significant for an adult.

Another RB, order effect, refers to significantly fewer errors on the first halves of items (i.e., the first two words) compared to the second halves or vice versa. Ear effects indicate significant differences between the number of errors made on REF versus LEF items. A significant difference for adults for ear or order effects is five errors. Figure 17.4 (lower portion) shows the significant order effect (13/19) but not the non-significant ear effect (16/16).

Order and ear effects are classified as either *high-low* or *low-high*. High refers to the larger number of errors. An order effect with significantly more errors on the first spondee is called an order high-low. When there are more errors on the second spondee it is low-high. Ear effects are similarly labeled. When more errors are found on REF words, it is high-low, but if the LEF errors are significantly greater it is referred to as an ear effect low-high. Table 17.5 shows the regions associated with these RBs. Because an order effect low-high is exactly the opposite of an order high-low, in cases of widespread difficulties these signs may be cancelled. A rule of thumb is that when there are many errors signifying poor CANS functioning (at a cerebral level), but there are no significant ear or order effects indicating which processing center is affected, one can assume that both the anterior cerebral and the posterior temporal regions have been compromised. In fact, when the results of a stroke begin to resolve, ear or order effects may show up as the global effects disappear. The same cancellation effect is seen in children who are evaluated for AP problems.

A third major RB is the type A pattern. The error pattern in type A cases is a highly asymmetrical when looking at the eight cardinal numbers. An illustration of this is:

$$
\begin{array}{cccc cccc}
A & B & C & D & E & F & G & H \\
0 & 1 & 0 & 0 & 1 & 7 & 1 & 0
\end{array}
$$

Table 17.5.
Site-of-Dysfunction as Suggested by SSW[a]

Significant Response bias		Suggested Locus of Involvement (Site-of-Dysfunction Adult Cases Only)
Order effect	low-high	Posterior temporal, auditory cortex
	high-low	Anterior half of brain
Ear effect	high-low	Posterior temporal, auditory cortex
	low-high	Fronto-temporal
Reversals		Anterior temporal, sensory-motor strip and adjacent frontal region
Type A		Not very effective for locating lesions, but is seen in one third of corpus callosum cases and in a high percentage of thalamic cases

[a]The response biases often noted on the SSW test and the loci of dysfunction that are suggested by each. Extreme caution is required in cases with hearing loss as this alone can produce response bias.

It can be seen that a large number of the errors are in just one column. The three criteria for a Type A are met when (*a*) the column with the major errors has at least twice as many errors as the next highest column, (*b*) there must be a difference between these two columns of at least 3 points, and (*c*) the column having the largest number of errors must be F or B (usually column F).

The following example illustrates how RB can be used to locate the site of the cerebral dysfunction. A patient has a MI combined TEC suggesting a NAR disorder. While this information is of value, it does not indicate where in the vast NAR region the disorder may be found. RB can be effective in suggesting the compromised region. It should be noted, however, that RB does not indicate which hemisphere is involved and can be offset by hearing loss.

Qualifiers

The use of qualifiers is the second form of qualitative analysis. Qualifiers are based on observable test behaviors which may provide clues regarding the underlying problem. A few examples will be discussed here.

Individuals tend to respond in a certain cadence to SSW items. Therefore, when a response is too quick or two slow this is obvious to the experienced tester. For many years it has been noted that some individuals respond in a slow fashion (e.g., with a 3 second delay) to various items, while other listeners may begin to respond very quickly (e.g., in < 0.5 seconds) on some items. Occasionally, they begin to respond even before an item presentation has been completed. A third pattern related to the temporal response pattern is the extreme delay. In this case the delay may be many seconds, but surprisingly the response is generally correct. These extreme delays are labeled by two Xs circled at the point of infraction. The more typical delayed responses, which are associated with slow phonemic decoding, are designated by a circled X. Quick responses, which are generally found in those with a rapidly fading memory, are designated by a circled Q in the box with the item number.

Evaluation of Auditory Processing Problems

The SSW may be used to determine if an auditory processing problem is present, and if so, its characteristics. The SSW test is particularly useful as a test of AP function when there is a concern for the management of an AP disorder in a child or an adult with a learning or speech-language problem. The multidimensional scoring of the SSW, the many diagnostic indicators that it has, and the considerable knowledge that we have gained from the evaluation patients with CNS and AP disorders, provides

Table 17.6.
C-SSW Data: Combined National Sample, 1985 and National Sample for Elderly, 1990[a]

	Age Group	RNC			RC			LC			LNC		
		M	SD	NL	M	SD	NL	M	SD	NL	M	SD	NL
	5	5	8	13	36	15	51	40	19	59	7	13	20
	6	3	7	10	17	13	30	30	17	47	2	8	10
	7	1	5	6	8	7	15	18	11	29	1	5	6
	8	1	4	5	6	7	13	10	8	18	0[b]	4	4
	9	1	3	4	4	5	9	8	8	16	0[b]	3	3
	10	−1	4	3	3	5[c]	8	7	7	14	0	3	3
	11	−1	3	2	1	3	4	5	6	11	−1	4	3
(1 SD)	12–59	−1	2[c]	1	1	2	3	1	4	5	−1	2	1
(2 SD)	12–59	−1	2[c]	3	1	2	4	1	4	9	−1	2	3
	60–69	−2[c]	5	3	1	7	9	49	9	14	−3	6	3

[a]Means (M), standard deviation (SD) and normal limits (NL) for normal control subjects, ages 5 through 69 years. C-SSW scores for each of the four conditions is shown. The limits of normal were set at one SD above the mean for children and 60- to 69-year-olds. For young adults, both 1 and 2 SD limits are shown. In three cases small changes were made to retain coherent limits. The data for 5-year-olds are based on the first 20 items of the EC list.
[b]Rounded *up* instead of down.
[c]Rounded *down* instead of up.

us with information that may be useful in guiding the management of those who have AP disorders.

SSW administration for AP cases is essentially the same as that used for locating the site of dysfunction. The one exception is that 5-year-olds, who are tested for AP difficulty, should receive only the first 20 items of the EC list instead of all 40 items. For these children as well as 6-year-olds, live voice and/or the use of kindergarten phonemically balanced (PBK) words (Haskins, 1949) is preferred. The major difference between AP and site-of-dysfunction evaluations is the interpretive criteria.

Criteria for AP Evaluations

In site-of-dysfunction cases the major consideration is *where* the problem may be found; however, in those seen for AP testing, the focus is generally on whether there is a problem and *what* the problem is. Often there is also the question of rehabilitation for the person with AP difficulties.

The SSW statistical norms incorporate data from more than 60 audiologists (who attended at least one SSW workshop), from across the U.S. and Canada, who contributed up to 5 normal control cases for a total of 287 individuals, 5 to 60 years of age (Katz, 1986). Table 17.5 shows the means, standard deviations (SD), and normal limits (NL) for the four C-SSW conditions for the various age groups. The +1 SD point was used as the NL except for the 12 to 60 year group for which the +2 SD values are also given. Table 17.7 shows the normal limits for response bias information. It should be noted that the apparent discrepancy for 5-year-olds is due to the use of only half of the items for these children.

Table 17.7.
Response Bias Criteria—Limits of Normal[a]

Age Group (years)	Reversals (number)	Order[b] H/L	L/H	Ear[b] L/H	H/L	Type A Differences[c]
5	3	7	7	4	4	4
6	6	7	7	7	5	5
7	5	7	7	7	5	5
8	4	6	6	7	5	5
9	3	6	4	7	5	4
10	3	4	4	5	5	4
11	3	4	4	5	5	2
12–59	1	4	4	4	4	2
60–69	4	6	6	6	6	2

[a]Response bias information from the national samples is shown for reversals, order effects, ear effects and type A patterns. The figures shown represent the permissible limits. Data for 5-year-olds are based on the first 20 items. These data are to be used to determine how a person compares to a normal population, for purpose of AP evaluations.
[b]Refers to *differences* for order and ear effects.
[c]Only for columns B or F when it is 2 times each of the other seven columns.

Learning Disabled versus Controls

Audiologists are typically asked to provide information about AP abilities for individuals having academic difficulties. Therefore, this population generally serves as the criterion group for deciding the sensitivity of various central tests. Many studies have shown the effectiveness of the SSW in identifying AP problems in learning disabled and other groups (Stubblefield and Young, 1975; Lukas and Eschenheimer, 1978; Lucker, 1980; Stecker, 1983; Hurley, 1990). Data for 287 controls (Katz, 1985a) were compared with the results for 171 clients who were seen by audiologists in the U.S. and Canada because of suspected AP problems associated with LD (Katz, 1985b). Table 17.8 shows the hit-miss relationship of younger (5 to 10 years of age) and

Table 17.8.
SSW Test Results for Learning Disabled and Control Subjects

Group	All Normal	Significant Findings		
	%	Conditions only (%)	RB only (%)	Conditions and RB (%)
Younger Control	70	12	10	8
Younger LD	6	35	4	55
Older Control	87	4	5	3
Older LD	15	15	10	59

[a]Hit-miss information for a large sample of learning disabled and control subjects that were obtained in two national samples. The younger group was 5 through 10 years of age and the older group over 10 years. For consistency the 1 SD cutoff point was used for condition scores regardless of age.

older (over 10 years of age) control and experimental subjects. Overall, 92% of the experimental subjects failed one or more aspects of the SSW versus 23% of the controls. Although the hit ratio was slightly higher than expected, Stecker (1983), using the same criteria, found a similar percentage in her study.

Interpretations of Auditory Processing Evaluations

Recently, four major categories of AP dysfunction have been suggested (Katz and Smith, 1991, Katz, 1992). The categories are not mutually exclusive and their characteristics may range from borderline to severe. By use of the SSW and other central tests, characteristics of these categories may be noted and thus contribute to the understanding of the problem and how to manage it (see Chapter 32).

Decoding Type. Abnormal performance in the RC and LNC conditions as well as order effect low/high and ear effect high/low RBs are associated with poor *phonemic* decoding skills. Those who demonstrate these SSW signs are likely to have some or all of the following: poor phonic skills (affecting reading and spelling), as well as receptive language and articulation difficulties in their early years.

Tolerance-Fading Memory Type. In tolerance-fading memory (TFM) types, the order high/low and ear low/high are signs of one or both of the following: (*a*) difficulty in blocking out background sounds, and (*b*) short term memory problem. In LD cases, it is generally a safe guess that both problems exist when the order high/low or ear low/high are found. These children are not as educationally handicapped as the poor decoders, but their classroom behavior is generally more noticeable. For example, they are typically inattentive and may be hyperactive as well. The educational concomitants are generally reading comprehension problems and ex-

pressive difficulties in speaking or writing. Poor, but not impossible, handwriting is often seen in these individuals. On the SSW test the TFM is one of the two categories that is primarily associated with poor performance in the LC condition.

Integration Type. The type A pattern is associated with auditory-visual or other integration problems. The SSW-Gram often shows a sharp LC peak of errors in these cases, even when the type A criteria are not satisfied. Another characteristic of this group is that they may show very long delays in responding on the SSW or, even more likely, on the CES test or simply when questioned. There appears to be two major subtypes of integration problems. One of the subtypes has severe auditory-visual integration difficulties and severe reading and spelling dysfunction. This is the group that is likely to be extremely poor in phonics and may by labeled "dyslexic".

The second group is less severe in its learning problems, performing much like the TFM subjects. These individuals sometimes demonstrate peculiar behaviors. For example, they may be poor responders on puretone tests and may be considered "nonorganic" or "willful" because they fail follow directions in a consistent manner.

Organization type. A significant number of reversals on the SSW test is often indicative of an organizational problem. It may manifest itself in sloppiness, poor spelling, and difficulty in keeping things in order. Visual reversals (e.g., b/d) has also been noted in this group of children. Organizational difficulty is associated mostly with the TFM group, but the most reversals are generally seen in cases with both TFM and phonemic decoding deficits.

Management Approaches

Different strategies may be used to manage AP problems based on the affected categories and their severity as revealed by the central test battery. Classroom controls that reduce the noise and improve the signal-to-noise ratio will benefit all of the children, but will be especially important for the TFM group. Direct therapeutic intervention has been extremely effective in dealing with the poor phonemic decoders (Katz, 1983). A computer program, SSW CIR (Katz et al., 1988), has been devised to calculate, interpret and recommend from the SSW test results (available from JIMM Co., 113 Kaymar Dr., Amherst, NY 14228). Chapter 31 contains further information on management.

REFERENCES

Air DH. A study of central auditory functioning in aphasics. [Ph.D. Dissertation] Cincinnati, OH: University of Cincinnati, 1980.
Amerman JD, and Parnell MM. The staggered spondaic word test: a normative investigation of older adults. Ear Hear 1980;1:42–45.

Arnst D, and Katz J, Eds. The SSW Test: Development and Clinical Use. San Diego, CA: College-Hill Press, 1982.

Arnst DJ. SSW test results with peripheral hearing loss. In Arnst D, and Katz J, Eds. The SSW Test: Development and Clinical Use. San Diego, CA: College-Hill Press, 1982a:287–293.

Arnst DJ. Performance of older adults on the SSW test. In Arnst D, and Katz J, Eds. The SSW Test: Development and Clinical Use. San Diego, CA: College-Hill Press, 1982b:449–456.

Berrick JM, Shubow GF, Schultz MC, Freed H, Fournier SR, and Hughes JP. Auditory processing results for children: Normative and clinical results on the SSW test. J Speech Hear Dis 1984;49:318–325.

Bruder GE. Cerebral laterality and psychopathology: Dichotic listening studies in schizophrenia and affective disorders. Schizo Bull 1983;9:134–151.

Brunt MA. Performance on three auditory tests by children with functional articulation disorders. [Thesis] Pittsburgh, PA: University of Pittsburgh, 1965.

Cafarelli DL, Nodar RH, Collard M, and Larkins DA. 1979. SSW test results on patients with Ménière's disease. Paper presented at American Speech-Language-Hearing Association convention, Atlanta, GA, 1979.

Dempsey C. Some thoughts concerning alternate explanations of central auditory test results. In Keith RW, Ed. Central Auditory Dysfunction. New York: Grune & Stratton, 1977:293–317.

Grady CL, Grimes AM, Pinkus A, Schwartz M, Rapoport SI, and Cutler NR. Alterations in auditory processing of speech stimuli during aging in healthy subjects. Cortex 1984;20:101–110.

Grimes AM, Grady CL, Foster NL, Sunderland T, and Patronas NJ. Central auditory function in Alzheimer's disease. Neurology 1985;35:352–358.

Hadaway S. An investigation of the relationship between measured intelligence and performance on the Staggered Spondaic Word test. [Thesis] Stillwater, OK: Oklahoma State University, 1964.

Hall JW, and Jerger J. Central auditory function in stutterers. J Speech Hear Res 1978;21:324–337.

Haskins HA. A phonetically balanced test of speech discrimination for children. [Thesis] Evanston, IL: Northwestern University, 1949.

Hayashi R. Binaural fusion test: A diagnostic approach to central auditory disorders. DSH Abstracts 1966; 6.

Hurley RM. Decision matrix analysis of selected children's central auditory processing tests. J Am Acad Audiol 1990;1:50.

Ivey RG. 1969. Tests of CNS auditory function. [Thesis] Fort Collins, CO: Colorado State University, 1969.

Ivey RG. A survey of school age children referred for central auditory assessment. Hum Commun Can/Commun Hum Can 1986; 10:5–10.

Ivey RG, Field B, Gibson N, Maschas S, Wickham K, and Zoller K. Performance-intensity curves for binaural fusion. [Unpublished graduate project] London, Ontario: University of Western Ontario, 1982.

Ivey RG, and Willeford JA. Three tests of CNS auditory function. Hum Commun Can/Commun Hum Can 1988;12:35–43.

Jerger J, and Jerger S. Clinical validity of central auditory tests. Scand Audiol 1975;4:147–163.

Johnson DW, and Sherman RE. The new SSW test (list EE) and the CES test: Preliminary analysis of central auditory function in children ages 6–12 years. Audiol Hear Educ 1979;6:5–8.

Kaplan H, Gladstone VS, and Katz J. Basic Interpretation: Staggered Spondaic Word Test. Site of Lesion Testing. Baltimore: University Park Press, 1984:287–326.

Katz J. The use of staggered spondaic words for assessing the integrity of the central auditory nervous system. J Aud Res 1962;2:327–337.

Katz J. The SSW test: An interim report. J Speech Hear Dis 1968;33:132–146.

Katz, J. Differential diagnosis of auditory impairments. In Fulton R,

and Lloyd LL, Eds. Auditory Assessment of the Difficult-to-Test. Baltimore: Williams & Wilkins, 1969:120–153.

Katz J. Audiologic diagnosis: Cochlea to cortex. Menorah Med J 1971;1:25–38.

Katz J. The staggered spondaic word test. In Keith RW, Ed. Central Auditory Dysfunction. New York: Grune & Stratton, 1977:103–121.

Katz, J. SSW Workshop Manual. Buffalo, NY: Allentown Industries, 1978.

Katz J. Phonemic synthesis. In Lasky E, and Katz J, Eds. Central Auditory Processing Disorders: Problems of Speech, Language and Learning. Baltimore: University Park Press (Pro Ed), 1983a.

Katz J. C-SSW norms: The learning disabled 12–60 years of age. SSW Reports 1983b;5:21–24.

Katz J. SSW Test User's Manual. Vancouver, WA: Precision Acoustics, 1986.

Katz, J. Older vs. younger subjects. SSW Reports 1987;9:11–12.

Katz, J. Tentative criteria for individuals 60 through 79 years of age. SSW Reports 1990;12:1–6.

Katz, J. Classification of auditory processing disorders. In Katz J, Stecker NA, and Henderson D, Eds. Central Auditory Processing: A Transdisciplinary View. Boston: CV Mosby, 1992.

Katz J, et al. Combined National Sample norms: ages 5–60 years. SSW Reports 1985;7:1–4.

Katz J, and Arndt WB. A split-half evaluation of the SSW test. In Arnst D, and Katz J, Eds. The SSW Test: Development and Clinical Use. San Diego, CA: College-Hill Press, 1979:179–181.

Katz J, and Cummings D. Split-half reliability of the SSW test with learning disabled children. Unpublished study, 1974.

Katz J, and Illmer R. Auditory perception in children with learning disabilities. In Katz J, Ed. Handbook of Clinical Audiology. Baltimore: Williams & Wilkins, 1972:540–563.

Katz J, and Lawrence-Dederich S. Central nervous system, cerebral dominance, and dyslexia. Proceedings Second Annual Conference on Dyslexia: Psychologic and neurologic. Aalborg, Denmark, 1986.

Katz J, and Pack G. New developments in differential diagnosis using the SSW test. In Sullivan M, Ed. Central Auditory Processing Disorders. Omaha, NE: University of Nebraska Press, 1975:84–107.

Katz J, and Smith P. 1991. The SSW test: A ten minute look at the CNS through the ears. In Zappulla RA, et al., Eds. Windows on the brain. Ann N Y Acad Sci 1991;620:233–252.

Katz J, and Wilde L. Auditory perceptual disorders in children. In Katz J, Ed. Handbook of Clinical Audiology. 3rd ed. Baltimore: Williams & Wilkins, 1985:664–688.

Katz J, Avellanosa AA, and Aguilar-Markulis NV. Evaluation of corpus callosum tumors using SSW, CES and PICA. Paper presented at American Speech-Language Hearing Association convention, Detroit, MI, 1980.

Katz J, Basil RA, and Smith JM. A staggered spondaic word test for detecting central auditory lesions. Ann Otol Rhinol Laryngol 1963;72:908–918.

Katz J, McCarthy D, Jacobs L, and Wilson L. Cross validation of the SSW test using CT scan verification. [Unpublished study] 1985.

Katz J, Singer S, Fanning J, and Harrison SS. Unusual central auditory processing functions in incarcerated youths. Presented at New York State Speech-Language-Hearing Association convention, Buffalo, NY, 1988.

Katz J, Yeung E, and Medwetsky L. SSW CIR: Calculations, Interpretations and Recommendations. Amherst, NY: JIMM Co, 1988.

Linden A. Distorted speech and binaural speech resynthesis tests. Acta Oto-laryngologica 1964;58:32–48.

Lynn GE, Benitez JT, Eisenbray AB, Gilroy J, and Wilner HI. Neuro-audiological correlates in cerebral hemisphere lesions. Audiology 1972;11:115–134.

Lynn GE. Dichotic speech discrimination in patients with deep cerebral hemisphere lesions. Presented at the Ninth Colorado Medical Audiology Workshop, Vail, CO, 1975.

Lynn GE, and Gilroy J. Effects of brain lesions on the perception of monotic and dichotic speech stimuli. In Sullivan M, Ed. Central Auditory Processing Disorders, Omaha, NE: University of Nebraska Press, 1975.

Marsh T, Brown WS, and Smith JC. Differential brainstem pathways for the conduction of auditory frequency-following responses. Electroencephalogr Clin Neurophysiol 1974;36:415–424.

Martin FN, and Morris LJ. Current audiologic practices in the United States. Hear J 1989; (April):25–44.

Matzker J. Two new methods for the assessment of central auditory functions in cases of brain disease. Ann Otol Rhinol Laryngol 1959;68:1185–1197.

Miltenberger GE, Caruso VG, Correia MJ, Love JT, and Winkelmann P. Utilization of a central auditory processing test battery in evaluating residual effects of decompression sickness. J Speech Hear Dis 1979;44:111–120.

Miltenberger GE, Dawson GJ, and Raica AN. Central auditory testing with peripheral hearing loss. Arch Otolaryngol 1978;104:11–15.

Musiek FE, and Geurkink NA. Auditory brain stem response and central auditory test findings for patients with brain stem lesions: A preliminary report. Laryngoscope 1982;92:891–900.

Musiek FE, Gollegly KM, Kibbe KS, and Verkest SB. Current concepts on the use of ABR and auditory psychophysical tests in the evaluation of brain stem lesions. Am J Otol 1988;9 Suppl:25–35.

Ohta F, Hayashi R, and Morimoto M. Differential diagnosis of retrocochlear deafness: Binaural fusion test and binaural separation test. J Int Audiol 1967;6:58–62.

Oliver SK. Current trends in central auditory processing testing. Paper presented at the California Speech-Language-Hearing Association, San Francisco, 1987.

Pinheiro ML, Jacobson GP, and Boller F. Auditory dysfunction following a gunshot wound of the pons. J Speech Hear Dis 1982;47:296–300.

Smith BB, and Resnick DM. An auditory test for assessing brain-stem integrity: Preliminary report. Laryngoscope 1972;82:414–424.

Stecker NA. A comparison of efferent auditory system functioning in three groups of children. [Ph.D. dissertation] Buffalo, NY: State University of New York at Buffalo, 1983.

Welsh LW, Welsh JJ, Healy M. Central auditory testing and dyslexia. Laryngoscope 1980;90:972–984.

Welsh LW, Welsh JJ, Healy M, and Cooper B. Cortical, subcortical, and brainstem dysfunction: a correlation in dyslexic children. Ann Otol Rhinol Laryngol 1982;91:310–315.

White EJ. Children's performance on the SSW test and Willeford battery: Interim clinical data. In Keith RW, Ed. Central Auditory Dysfunction. New York: Grune & Stratton, 1977:319–340.

Wilimas JA, McHaney VA, Presbury G, Dahl J, and Wang W. Auditory function in sickle cell anemia. Am J Pediatr Hematol/Oncol 1988;10:214–216.

Willeford JA. Assessing central auditory behavior in children: A test battery approach. In Keith RW, Ed. Central Auditory Dysfunction. New York: Grune & Stratton, 1977a:43–68.

Willeford JA. Differential diagnosis of central auditory dysfunction. Audiology: An Audio Journal for Continuing Education, Grune & Stratton, New York, 1977b.

Willeford JA, and Bilger JM. Auditory perception in children with learning disabilities. In Katz J, Ed. Handbook of Clinical Audiology, 2nd ed. Baltimore: Williams & Wilkins, 1978:410–425.

Willeford JA, and Burleigh JM. Handbook of Central Auditory Processing Disorders in Children. New York: Grune & Stratton, 1985.

Windham R, Parks M, and Mitchener-Colston, W. Central auditory processing in urban black children: a normative study. Dev Behav Pediatr 1986;7:8–13.

CHAPTER 18

Sentence Procedures in Central Testing

Jack A. Willeford and Joan M. Burleigh

Sentence-type materials have been used clinically for the purpose of identifying site-of-lesion in adult patients who have sustained damage to the brain. Sentence tests have also been used to confirm the presence and determine the nature of central auditory processing difficulties, primarily involving children. It is the purpose of this chapter to review the major types of sentence tests, their applications to adults and children, and their relationships to other types of central auditory measures.

SYNTHETIC SENTENCE IDENTIFICATION TEST

Sentences that are systematically altered from the standard rules of grammar and syntax were developed into a test to serve as an adjunct to standard speech audiometry (Speaks and Jerger, 1965). When they were found to be too easy, the same synthetic sentences were used in a competing message paradigm for measuring functions of the central nervous system (Jerger and Jerger, 1974; Speaks, 1975; Jerger and Jerger, 1975). The rationale for using this technique was to benefit from the sentence structure, a rapidly changing acoustical pattern with time, and avoiding the use of monosyllabic words. Both the limited meaningfulness of the sentences and the use of a closed message set response mode reduced the dependence on linguistic and memory skills. Thus, in this procedure, one would need only identify (by number) which of the 10 sentences was presented (Speaks and Jerger, 1965; Jerger, Speaks and Trammell, 1968).

A group of synthetic sentences was selected from among the various word-orders and sentence lengths for two major studies (Jerger and Jerger, 1974, 1975). Several lists of randomly ordered seven-word sentences were produced. The sentences are shown in Table 18.1.

The synthetic sentence identification (SSI) procedure uses synthetic sentences by a male speaker with competition (a narrative by the same speaker about the life of Davy Crockett) in the same ear or in opposite ears. When the sentences and the competition were directed to opposite ears it was referred to as contralateral competing message (CCM) and when both the sentences and the competition were presented to the same ear it was termed ipsilateral competing message (ICM). For the ICM each ear is tested separately. In both the CCM and ICM conditions various message-to-competition ratios (MCR) were

used. Sentences were presented at levels that yielded 100% performance (generally about 50 dB SL) and then MCR for the CCM procedure were varied in 20-dB steps 0 to −40 dB (from equal SPL to competition 40 dB above the primary message). In the more challenging ICM condition the competition was varied in 10-dB steps for MCR of +10 to −20dB. For the SSI-CCM normal performance was 100% correct for all MCR. For the ICM the scores ranged from 100% to about 20% with increasing competition. Figure 18.1 shows the means for the SSI-ICM condition from +10 to −30dB MCR.

Jerger and Jerger (1974) used the SSI test with patients who were carefully defined as intra-axial brainstem cases, with lesions above the level of the cochlear nuclei. Their performance on the CCM and ICM versions were strikingly dissimilar. All 11 subjects performed poorly on the ICM condition, 6 failing in each ear and 5 failing just in the contralateral ear (CE). None of the patients performed poorly on the ipsilateral ear (IE) only. When performance was averaged across the MCR 0 to −20 dB for the IE and CE, the brainstem cases had a score of 36% correct compared to the normal group with 76%.

In contrast to the poor performance on the ICM procedure, on the CCM the brainstem patients had relatively little difficulty. Eight of them had normal performance in both ears and only three failed in one ear.

Figure 18.2 shows SSI results for a typical brainstem case. The data are for a 17-year-old girl with a left-sided pontine glioma. This patient, who had normal puretone

Table 18.1.
Synthetic Sentence Identification (SSI)[a]

1. Small boat with a picture has become
2. Built the government with the force almost
3. Go change your car color is red
4. Forward march said the boy had a
5. March around without a care in your
6. That neighbor who said business is better
7. Battle cry and be better than ever
8. Down by the time is real enough
9. Agree with him only to find out
10. Women view men with green paper should

[a]Supplied by Jerger J, personal communication; and Jerger J, Speaks C, and Trammell J. J Speech Hear Disord 1968;33:318–328.

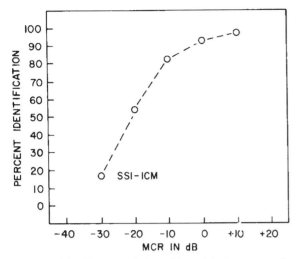

Figure 18.1. SSI-ICM norms (adapted from data in a personal communication from Jerger, 1975).

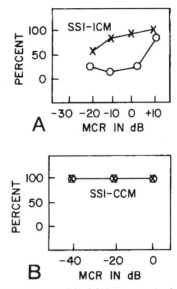

Figure 18.2. SSI-ICM and SSI-CCM test results for a 17-year-old girl with an intra-axial brainstem lesion on the left side (adapted from Jerger and Jerger, 1974).

sensitivity, had a deficit on the ICM procedure in the CE, with normal scores in the IE and in the CCM conditions. The major finding in this study was that brainstem cases were consistently poorer on the ICM condition than on the CCM. Although there was some variability in the findings across subjects, this study showed SSI-ICM to be very sensitive to the presence of brainstem dysfunction.

The second investigation (Jerger and Jerger, 1975) compared the results of the SSI with the staggered spondaic word (SSW) test (Katz, 1962) (see Chapter 17) in two groups of patients with medically diagnosed disorders of the central auditory system. One group consisted of 10 patients with intra-axial brainstem lesions and the other group was composed of 10 individuals with temporal lobe lesions.

The results for the brainstem group were in general agreement with their earlier findings. In this study performance for the ICM condition the CE was depressed by 40% for the brainstem group. Failure for the temporal lobe group showed up in both the ICM and CCM conditions. For ICM the temporal lobe group had a mean score that was depressed about 40% in the CE and 30% in the IE. On the CCM the brainstem group had normal results in each ear, whereas the temporal lobe group had normal IE performance and a deficit of 20% in the CE.

The Jergers indicated from their research that on the SSI-ICM, brainstem cases showed poor performance only in the CE. On the SSI-CCM these patients had relatively good performance, within normal limits in each ear. However, in temporal lobe cases both ICM and CCM were affected. The ICM deficits were shown in both ears and on the CCM the failure was shown only in the ear contralateral to the damaged hemisphere.

A few differences may be noted between the results of the two studies above. The authors account for these dif-

ferences by acknowledging that exceptional findings had occurred in the later study. In general, brainstem cases have "relatively more" difficulty on the ICM task than on the CCM, whereas the opposite is true for the temporal lobe cases.

The Jergers' comparison of the SSI and SSW tests is of interest, especially because the SSW test results are compared with other sentence procedures in a later section. They indicate that the SSW scores were consistently reduced in temporal lobe cases, but that variable results were found in the brainstem group. These findings led Jerger and Jerger to conclude, ". . . the overriding principle that characterized the combination of the two procedures was that the brainstem patients consistently showed SSI-ICM deficits whereas the temporal lobe patients consistently showed SSW deficits (p. 20)".

A possible limitation of the SSI test, using the technique of Jerger and Jerger, is that it involves visual as well as auditory tasks. This might penalize adults who have reading impairments or those with visual handicaps and have limited application. Its use would also be precluded for younger children with undeveloped reading skills, or those in whom central visual and auditory processes are not mutually facilitating. The latter appears to be the case, in the writers' experience, for certain children with learning disabilities. This may be circumvented by simply having the subject repeat the stimulus as Speaks (1975) suggested as an optional response method. However, this procedure makes scoring much more difficult and the SSI has not been normed for this response mode.

Martin and Mussell (1979) proposed a modification of the SSI. They observed that the Davy Crockett story

Table 18.2.
Selected Examples of Willeford's Competing Sentences

(Weather)	a.	I think we'll have rain today.
	b.	There was frost on the ground.
(Time)	a.	This watch keeps good time.
	b.	I was late to work today.
(Family)	a.	My mother is a good cook.
	b.	Your brother is a tall boy.
(Food)	a.	Please pass the salt and pepper.
	b.	The roast beef is very good.
(Safety)	a.	Fasten your seat belt.
	b.	Get read for take-off.

that serves as competition for the synthetic sentences contains pauses that enable sentence identification because of an unopposed word(s). They used a speech spectrum noise with the Davy Crockett competition (6 dB below the connected speech) to fill in the pauses. They found that the noise was sufficient to increase the difficulty level of the SSI task. Another modification of the SSI was reported by Beattie and Clark (1982). They replaced the Davy Crockett story with four-talker babble (FT) to eliminate the acoustic windows in the SSI task. In this version, the SSI-FT, the synthetic sentences were recorded on one channel and the multitalker competition was recorded on the other. Whether these two modifications are more useful than the original SSI procedure remains to be determined.

As in the case of most central auditory tests, the SSI appears to be sensitive to maturational effects (Orchik and Burgess, 1977; Decker and Nelson, 1981). Decker and Nelson tested six groups of six subjects each (8–25 years) with the SSI-ICM. Test scores improved in successive age groups. Therefore, they recommended that normative data be established to make the SSI-ICM a useful test for children.

COMPETING SENTENCE TEST

Willeford (1968) developed the competing sentence test (CST) to evaluate central auditory function. The test was first described by Ivey (1969). Unlike the SSI, the CST is composed of simple, natural English sentences. Inspiration for the test evolved, in part, from consideration of some early tests designed by Jerger (1964) and a test that Frager (1968) used in a study under Willeford's direction. In each of the studies sentences were used in a variety of ways.

Design of the CST

As in the case of the SSI, the CST was developed to avoid dependence on the identification of highly transient sin-

gle words, particularly monosyllabic words. Brief utterances place a premium on concentration and attention. Another reason for using sentences was to simulate language constructions that might occur in everyday life. It was hoped that the test might provide insight into a subject's ability to process standard forms of spoken language. Thus, temporal patterns, acoustic spectra, linguistic features, and syntactical characteristics were considered important attributes of the signal.

In contrast to the SSI, the CST was designed to provide a broader message perception and to minimize perception by key words alone. CST sentences are used in an open-set paradigm that brings some language performance and skill to bear on the success of the listener in decoding the message. However, an effort was made to select a level of language that did not penalize children, persons with low intelligence, or patients whose reduced physical well-being might compromise their maximum test performance.

Although one major consideration in test construction dealt with the test stimuli, an equally important factor was the nature of the competing message. In many dichotic tests (e.g., the SSW, dichotic digits, and dichotic CV are notable exceptions), and most tests in which the primary messages are sentences, the competition is of another form. For example, continuous discourse by a single speaker, a babble of several voices, environmental noise, white noise, accelerated speech, and backward speech have been used as the competing signals. The point at issue is that the competition "differs" from the test stimulus. Influenced by the work of Treisman (1964), competing signals were sought for the CST that were similar in character to the test items. She showed that attention to a target message in a dichotic sentence task was influenced by contextual cues or the expectancy of a relationship between words. Irrelevant (competing) words tended to be discarded during the identification phase of processing. She found that an irrelevant message by the same talker and involving similar content, was a more difficult task than that presented by two different talkers, different languages or by reversed speech. Others have shown similar results (Speaks, 1975; Berlin and McNeil, 1976). The latter reference and Segalowitz and Gruber (1977) present comprehensive information regarding dichotic listening and dichotic test construction.

A sample of CST items are shown in Table 18.2. It may be observed that the content of the paired sentences concerns time, weather, or other common themes. The two sentences are presented simultaneously, one to each ear. Although the sentences are of similar lengths, no attempt was made to time-match the onsets of the paired stimuli precisely. Berlin et al. (1973a) have shown that matching of onsets is critical when subjects are asked to respond to dichotic CV (brief consonant-vowel combinations) in which the two signals differ by only a single consonant. However, the two sentences on the CST begin and end very nearly at the same time. Precise time matching was not considered essential because it was believed that correct responses would be dependent on a combination of the several ongoing factors mentioned earlier. In this sense CST resembles normal communication in which the acoustic competition is more or less random.

Wingfield (1975) has suggested that the perceptual act of listening to sentences is not a passive handling of the speech on a word-by-word basis. He maintains that as long as there is minimal intelligibility, a person actively reconstructs the fragments that are heard so as to produce responses that are meaningful, fully grammatical, and that match the syntactic form of the heard speech when it can be detected. He concluded that speech perception on the sentence level is based on the analysis of components larger than individual words that probably correspond to higher syntactic constituents. Thus, the CST would seem to challenge a subject's ability for a task that occurs continuously in everyday living.

Recording and Standardization of the CST

Both sentences of the competing pair are recorded on magnetic stereo tape by the same male talker with a general American dialect. An attempt was made to avoid emphasizing important words, pauses, and intonation patterns that might aid the perception process.

Three lists were recorded with 25 sentence pairs each. To date only one of the lists has had major use. Thus, discussion will be restricted to that list. On the basis of pilot experiments, 35 dB SL (re puretone average for 500, 1000, and 2000 Hz) was established as the test level for the primary message. The level of the competition sentence was set at of 50dB SL (re PTA). Thus, a signal-to-competition ratio (SCR) of −15 dB was adopted.

Ivey (1969) standardized 25 pairs of CST sentences using 20 normal hearing adult subjects, 19 and 33 years old, who had negative otological and neurologic histories. The instructions to the subjects was to listen to and repeat the "signal" message (35 dB SL) and ignore the "competing" message (50 dB SL) in the other ear. This procedure was based on Kimura's (1963) statement that hemispheric dominance must be controlled in the dichotic mode by having the subjects listen to the material in one ear and ignoring the material in the other.

To control for any ear or sentence list differences, half of the subjects received the "A" sentences in the right ear and "B" sentences in the left, whereas the other half of the subjects had the reversed order (results are shown in Table 18.3). For normal adults: (a) lists A and

B were approximately equal in difficulty; (b) differences between the ears slightly favored the right ear (by a difference of 14 errors of 1000 items), and (c) for these subjects the CST was a very easy task.

The original test was subsequently shortened to two lists of 10 competing sentence pairs. This decision was based on the findings with clinical patients that only 10 items were needed to identify adult patients with confirmed cortical lesions. Thus, the 25 items provided enough stimuli to test both ears (10 to each ear). The remaining five may be used to assess the patient's ability for repeating both messages (in a simultaneous or bilateral-response mode). In the later case both sentences are delivered at 50 dB SL, or at an SCR of 0 dB. Performance on the shortened version of the test has become the standard for clinical use. This procedure has been found to be an easy task for young normal adults. Lynn and Gilroy (1977) found that they scored 100% in each ear which agrees with Willeford's informal observation of a large college-age population over several years.

Children's norms that were generated from 1976 to 1978 reflect quite a different pattern of results (Table 18.4). Subjects 5–10 years old age generally score 100% in one ear (the right ear in 212 of 225 subjects). The other ear may score anywhere from 0 to 100%. Thus, normal children commonly show a strong ear and a weak ear. In fact, 0% scores are frequently observed for the weak ear for children 5 and 6 years old. However, scores in the weak ear improve progressively with increasing age until 8 to 10 years, at which time performance in the right and left ears are equal. Thus, adult performance is achieved by about age 10. When parity between the ears is not achieved by that age or when the strong-ear score is less than 90%, the results are considered clinically significant. The latter case is abnormal because the child does not have a truly strong ear, even if the weak ear score is within the appropriate range. The SD and ranges of scores reflect considerable variability in children less than age 10, with greater variability for younger age groups. The progressive increase in performance and decrease in variability with increasing age in children is most likely due to maturation. This result is in general correspondence with other dichotic tests.

Table 18.3.

Response Performance for 20 Normal Adult Subjects on Dichotic Competing Sentence Test (adapted from Ivey, 1969)

Ear	Number of Sentences Presented	Test List A		Test List B		Total	
		Correct	Incorrect	Correct	Incorrect	Correct	Incorrect
Right	500	497	3	497	3	994	6
Left	500	494	6	486	14	980	20
Total	1000	991	9	983	17	1974	26

Table 18.4.
Willeford Competing Sentence Test Norms (in %) for Children

Age	n	Expected Results		Mean		SD		Range	
		Weak Ear	Strong Ear[a]	Weak Ear	Strong Ear[a]	Weak Ear	Strong Ear[a]	Weak Ear	Strong Ear[a]
5	25	20	90/100	24.8	94.0	35.9	4.4	0/80	90/100
6	40	60	90/100	59.5	96.5	33.2	4.0	0/100	90/100
7	40	70	100	67.8	97.5	31.2	3.6	0/100	90/100
8	40	80	100	83.0	98.0	22.2	3.2	10/100	90/100
9	40	90	100	93.0	98.8	9.8	2.6	70/100	90/100
10	40	100	100	98.4	99.2	3.6	2.6	90/100	90/100

[a]Strong ears were predominantly right ears. Left ears were the strong ears in only 13 of the 225 subjects.

An interesting observation in youngsters 11 years old or more, is that once the bilateral skill is achieved, the primary message in either ear can be reduced from 35 to 10 dB SL before performance deteriorates. Stated differently, selective attention to the primary sentence remains undiverted by the 50-dB competing sentence even when the primary message is very faint. However, it is reasonable to assume that children whose dichotic listening skills are not yet fully developed may be as functionally handicapped in central auditory skills as a mature person who fails the test as a result of a cortical lesion.

This test may be used in a bilateral response mode (CST-BR) in which sentences to each ear are repeated. Encouraged by comments and experiences of colleagues (M. Pinheiro and N. Matkin) about the sensitivity of the CST-BR, norms were established in 1979 (see Table 18.5). For the CST-BR two lists of 10 paired sentences were presented in which the subjects were scored 0 to 100% for each. The sentence in each ear had a value of 5% and therefore 10% was assigned if both were correct. The five remaining sentences were given initially for practice. As expected, the mean score correct increased with age. It was observed that younger children tended to report the right ear sentence before the left ear; however, this pattern dissipated in the older children. It is difficult to interpret this finding because some children who had dramatic ear-order response had remarkably similar test-retest scores. Therefore, the response order may simply be a strategy used by the listener. No differences were found in the performance of males and females and lists 1 and 2 were equivalent to one another. It is recommended that CST-BR be used for clinical testing. Readers interested in further details are invited to write to Willeford.

Clinical Use of the CST with Adults

The CST has been widely used with adults who had carefully defined neurologic lesions. Lynn and colleagues have reported results showing that the CST, as one of a battery of central auditory measures, is valuable in de-

Table 18.5.
Test Norms for Willeford Competing Sentences-Bilateral-Response Test (in % for SL = 50 in each Ear)

n	Age (Year)	Mean Score[a]	S.D.	Range	Mean Ear Response Order[b]		
					L	R	
20	6	46.0	16.3	20/70	3.6	6.5	(of 10)
0	7[c]	54.5		30/80	3.5	6.5	(of 10)
20	8	62.8	13.6	45/100	3.6	6.4	(of 10)
20	9	73.0	11.8	45/90	3.7	6.3	(of 10)
20	10	80.5	10.4	50/100	4.3	6.7	(of 10)
20	11	83.5	10.0	65/10	5.1	4.9	(of 10)
20	12	85.3	9.9	65/100	4.8	5.2	(of 10)

[a]Single-correct responses = 5%. Double-correct responses = 10%.
[b]Ear stimulus to which subject responded first.
[c]7-year-old data are interpolated.

tecting the presence of structural lesions in the brain (Lynn and Gilroy, 1972, 1975; Lynn et al., 1972; Lynn 1973; Gilroy and Lynn, 1974). In addition they found it useful for monitoring changes in the neurologic status of patients or as a result of treatment or surgery.

Temporal Lobe Tumors

Table 18.6 presents the mean scores for a series of tests for 10 patients with tumors in the posterior region of the temporal lobe (Lynn and Gilroy, 1975). The patients ranged in age from 23 to 66 years. Five patients had lesions in the left hemisphere and five in the right. The mean undistorted speech discrimination (UD PB) score was slightly poorer in the ear contralateral to the brain lesion, but was thought to be influenced by significant sensory-neural hearing loss and inner ear distortion that was combined with the effect of the temporal lobe tumor. Low-pass filtered speech (LPFS) and each of the other tests show unilateral asymmetries with poor scores in the CE. The alternate binaural and simultaneous binaural scores refer to Lynn and Gilroy's analysis of Katz' SSW procedure. The simultaneous binaural condition represents the overlapping (ipsilateral competing or

Table 18.6.
Subjects with Tumors in Posterior Region of Temporal Lobe[a]

Test	Ear	Mean	Range
UD PB	IE	95.8	88–100
	CE	84.0	48–100
LPFS	IE	45.1	2–92
	CE	35.5	0–68
Alt Bin	IE	93.7	82–100
	CE	70.5	25–95
Sim Bin	IE	77.4	38–100
	CE	42.9	0–88
Comp Sent	IE	84.0	0–100
	CE	33.0	0–100

[a]Mean scores in percentage correct; n = 10. UD PB, undistorted speech discrimination; LPFS, low-pass filtered speech; Alt Bin, alternating speech, binaural; Sim Bin, simultaneous speech, binaural; Comp Sent, competing sentence; IE, ipsilateral ear; CE, contralateral ear (after Lynn and Gilroy, 1975).

Table 18.7.
Auditory Findings (in %) in a Patient (Male, Age 66) with Left Temporal Lobe Ostrocytoma and Evidence of Upper Brainstem Involvement[a]

Ear	UD PB	LPFS	Alt Bin	Sim Bin	Comp Sent	Binaural Fusion
Right	100	32	70	0	0	10
Left	100	46	100	98	100	0
Binaural						10

[a]Abbreviations as in Table 18.6 (after Lynn and Gilroy, 1975).

Table 18.8.
Auditory Findings (in %) in a Patient (Female, Age 23) with Left Temporal Lobe Astrocytoma Inferior Region[a]

Ear	UD PB	LPFS	Alt Bin	Sim Bin	Comp Sent
Right	100	32	100	98	100
Left	100	56	100	98	100

[a]Abbreviations as in Table 18.6 (after Lynn and Gilroy, 1975).

Table 18.9.
Subjects with Temporal Lobe Tumors in Anterior-Inferior Regions[a]

Test	Ear	Mean	Range
UD PB	IE	98.0	96–100
	CE	99.0	96–100
LPFS	IE	47.7	28–72
	CE	32.7	20–56
Alt Bin	IE	95.8	85–100
	CE	91.8	73–100
Sim Bin	IE	90.8	73–98
	CE	75.8	28–98
Comp Sent	IE	100.0	100–100
	CE	96.7	90–100

[a]Mean scores in percentage correct; n = 6.
Abbreviations as in Table 18.6 (from Lynn and Gilroy, 1975).

contralateral competing) portions of the SSW, while the alternate binaural represents the nonoverlapping (noncompeting) portions. This permitted a comparison of the CST and SSW, both dichotic tests.

The data presented in Table 18.6 show the expected contralateral effect for both dichotically competing speech and monotically degraded-speech procedures. It may be observed that the pattern of scores for the SSW and the CST correspond with one another. Group data may be misleading because of exceptions of the contralateral ear effect in some patients. Moreover, the ear-difference scores may range from slight in some patients to 100% in others. It seems that variation in performance is dependent on factors such as size and location of lesion. For example, for most patients with temporal lobe lesions there is a dramatic CE effect for the CST. Table 18.7 provides data for such a case in which the dichotic tests identify the left hemisphere involvement. For both the CST and the SSW the difference scores are also extreme. However, Table 18.8 shows another case in which the CST and the SSW are normal bilaterally and only the monotic distorted speech provided a clue to the abnormality by the score in the CE. It is of interest that the lesion in this patient was in the inferior portion of the temporal lobe. Lynn and colleagues have noted a trend that suggests that both the CST and the SSW are highly sensitive to lesions in the posterior regions of the temporal lobe and the SSW to posterior and slightly anterior regions of the lobe, whereas monotic distorted speech is sensitive to lower and more anterior aspects of the temporal lobe. These factors are evident in the data in Tables 18.8 and 18.9.

Such results lead one to wonder whether the differences noted in these tests are a matter of relative sensitivity of the various procedures for identifying deficiencies in the higher auditory system or whether each is looking at the critical neural processing areas associated with its specific auditory tasks. Some investigators have suggested that certain types of central tests have greater sensitivity in exposing a processing breakdown (Speaks, 1975; Bellaire and Noffsinger, 1978; Olsen and Kurdziel, 1978). Although that may be true, it also seems likely that different types of tests challenge the integrity of the central processors in different ways. Thus, different tests appear to have relative strengths and weaknesses in challenging various regions or for specific purposes. Porter and Berlin (1975), who support this view, present a theoretical discussion relating certain dichotic tests to language processing and age.

Parietal Lobe Tumors

Lynn and Gilroy (1975, 1976) reported on the use of the CST with extratemporal tumors. When parietal lobe tumors were deeply situated (and involved the corpus callosum), no difference between ears was noted on monotic distorted-speech tests. However, for dichotic tests (including sentences) average performance was poorer in the LE regardless of which hemisphere was damaged. They attribute this result to the poor access that the LE has to the language-dominant left hemisphere. Similar results have been reported by other authors using dichotic tests (Sparks et al., 1970; Speaks, 1975; Olsen, 1983; Musiek et al., 1984). Lynn and Gilroy (1975) also described two left-handed patients that had poorer performance in their right ears although one patient had a tumor in the right hemisphere and the other patient had one in the left. Lynn and Gilroy (1975, 1976) have also described patients who had superficial tumors of the parietal lobe who performed normally on the central tests. It seems apparent from these reports that we still have a great deal to learn about relating auditory test results to specific sites of damage in the CNS.

Frontal Lobe Tumors

The presence of frontal lobe tumors in 11 patients produced widely varying results on their battery of central auditory tests (Lynn and Gilroy, 1975, 1976). Although five subjects had normal results on all of the tests, four of the frontal lobe cases had abnormal results on the CST and SSW tests for the IE. They believed that such results depend on the size and location of the lesion as well as on the secondary effects of pressure and infiltration.

Other Brain Applications

Lynn and Gilroy (1975, 1976) reported on additional cases that had intracranial damage other than tumors. These involved vascular and degenerative-type lesions. In each instance the results of the CST were highly significant.

Bergman et al. (1987a) have also found sentence tests effective in providing insight into central auditory function. They used the Willeford (1978) CST technique as a model to test two groups of brain-damaged adults. One group of patients had suffered diffuse cerebrocranial injuries (CCI) and the other cerebrovascular accidents

(CVA) that did not involve the temporal lobes. They were particularly interested in the Willeford technique because it is a dichotic task that requires attention and responses from only one ear at a time. Thus, it permits exploration of each ear separately without requiring the auditory system to hold the other ear's material in memory. This study was conducted in Israel, thus the sentences were recorded in Hebrew by a male talker and the scoring procedure slightly modified.

Findings showed a high incidence of central auditory dysfunction in both the CCI and CVA study populations. Specifically, ". . . an astonishing 43% . . . " of 142 serially admitted CCI patients gave abnormal responses. Among those 61 patients, 79% had abnormal left ear scores although only 15% had abnormal scores in the right ear. Four of their subjects were deficient bilaterally. The authors considered this a compelling clinical finding because the head injuries were of a diffuse nature (unclearly defined site-of-lesion), and because the patients with abnormal performances on competing sentences had no difficulty with the test material when it was presented without competition. The dichotic test results were in striking contrast to their normal/control subjects who scored at or near 100% in each ear.

In their other experimental study group of 34 patients with CVA, all had normal hearing, and their symptoms of aphasia were either mild or absent. This group also demonstrated considerable difficulty on the dichotic sentence test. In those patients with right hemisphere damage, scores were markedly poorer in the left/contralateral ear. In fact, more than half of them exhibited complete inability to repeat the test sentences correctly. However, they did well in the right/ipsilateral ear. Conversely, patients with lesions in the left hemisphere tended to score either equally poorly between ears or more poorly in the left/ipsilateral ear.

Competing Sentences in Soundfield

Because they were interested in rehabilitation aspects of brain-damaged adults, Bergman et al. (1987a) also designed a procedure for testing patients with a soundfield version of competing sentences. They wanted to determine whether there was a more real-life auditory disturbance under nonearphone conditions. In their soundfield test protocol, they used three loudspeakers, of which only two were activated at one time. The test sentence was presented through the facing loudspeaker although the competing sentence is presented at a distance of 1 meter from either the subject's left or right ear in a given test sequence. The signal-to-competition ratio was −10 dB. Ten competing sentences of three words each were used for this procedure. The subject populations were similar to those discussed above.

The overall performance on the soundfield competing-sentence test was 2 to 3 SD poorer for both CCI and CVA patients (especially for the CVA) than they were for a control group of normals. However, all three groups showed superior performances when the competing message was at the left side of the head than when the competition was at the right side.

From this series of studies, the Israeli group demonstrated that in patients with normal findings on routine audiologic tests and negative examination results for aphasia, dysfunctions of central auditory processing may be revealed through dichotic sentence tests and other variations of diagnostic competing sentence material. They concluded from their studies that central auditory processing dysfunctions can be identified even in subjects with normal hearing and no evidence of aphasia.

Threshold-of-Interference Test Using Sentences

In another interesting technique using competing sentences, Bergman et al. (1987b) normed a measure for establishing a criterion level of interference from a competing sentence on the intelligibility of a prime sentence at the test ear. As in one of the dichotic-mode experiments described earlier, three-word Hebrew sentences were used because they can be used to express complete thoughts, thus minimizing the memory load for the listener. When the SL of the test ear was set at 20 dB, a mean competing-ear SL of 75 dB was necessary in the average normal subject before it met the interference-level criterion. They also described a variation of that technique that could be applied to some normals if such interference did not occur with that test protocol. They then applied this test technique to a series of nine CVA patients. Seven of the nine patients with parietal-lobe involvement suffered left-ear suppression/right-ear advantage when the competition was near or only slightly above threshold.

In a subsequent report of 18 additional cases, findings were mixed in terms of their application to the assorted neurologic sites-of-lesion and less conclusive in terms of the results. For example, some patients showed complete suppression in one ear, predominantly the left one, although other patients scored within normal limits in both ears. However, the nature of their neurologic damage varied considerably. In summary, the authors found it interesting that the threshold-of-interference test confirmed the right-ear advantage that has been often reported for the classical dichotic listening task. They recommend the interference procedure as a rapid and efficient method to expose strong hemisphere suppression, particularly in patients with right-hemisphere damage.

CLINICAL USE OF COMPETING SENTENCE TESTS IN CHILDREN WITH LEARNING DISABILITIES

We have been using the CST since 1973 as part of a battery of tests with children. All of the children seen to date were referred because they were known to have, or else were suspected of having, some kind of "auditory problem."

The test battery consisted of the CST, a monotic test of low-pass filtered speech (FS) that used "selected" CNC words as stimuli, a binaural-fusion (BF) task that Ivey adapted from the technique by Matzker (1959, 1962), and an alternating-speech (AS) test similar to one described by Lynn and Gilroy (1975). The Ipsilateral/Contralateral Competing Sentence Test (Willeford, 1985; Willeford and Burleigh, 1985) and other selected measures have also been used. The CS and BF tests were used by Lynn et al., together with different versions of the FS and AS tasks. This fact has permitted continuing comparisons between the data on adults with well-documented lesions and those of children with irregular auditory, academic, and social histories. In the case of children, the tests are used to help identify subtle dysfunctions in auditory behavior and to follow changes in performance with maturation, training, counseling, and environmental controls.

Scoring the CST for young children should and can be more liberal. In the single-ear response task their responses are counted as correct, even if they (a) paraphrase the sentence to a lower language level as long as they do not alter the essential content or meaning of the sentence, and (b) do not interchange the language of the two competing sentences. For the bilateral response (the two-ear task), the same rules apply except that the subject is permitted some word intrusions from one ear to the other as long as the basic meaning of each sentence is preserved. Scoring for adults should be more strict, requiring essentially verbatim responses and permitting no intrusion of words from the competing sentence in either the one- or two-ear response modes. The scoring tasks require the examiner to make only simple judgments. The job is frequently made easier by the fact that there are often all-or-none-type responses. The child responds easily and correctly, or is unable to respond at all. Reasons for failing to respond include such statements as, "There was no sound in this [pointing] ear," "I couldn't hear it," "I don't know," "I couldn't understand," or "This ear [pointing] won't let the other ear listen." An example of acceptable language level transitions are as follows:

Test Pair

Primary message (35 dB SL)

The roast beef is very good.

Competition message (50 dB SL)
Please pass the salt and pepper.

Correct Response
I like the roast.
The meat is good.
The roast is good to eat.
Roast beef is good.

Incorrect Response
I don't know.
Put salt on the beef.
The salt and pepper are very good.
The roast has too much pepper.

Referring to young children, Menyuk (1969, p. 32) indicated, "We can definitely state that the child does not simply repeat what he hears, although there are instances in which he will. . . . The child is using the items in his lexicon generatively to create new utterances." Moreover, Dennis (1980, p. 163) stated that, "The interpretation of a sentence is more than the sum of its individual words. Sentences exhibit a variety of semantic properties now shown by words, for example, questioning, promising, pre-supposing."

Table 18.10 presents the clinical results obtained for a group of selected 5- to 7-year-olds. Each child had normal intelligence and normal hearing by traditional audiometric standards and all but one was right handed. Each had also been labeled as a LD child despite the fact that a multitude of tests by public-school diagnostic teams failed to identify abnormal behaviors on diagnostic tests. All were referred because their academic performances were less than the levels expected of them and their auditory perception ability appeared to be impaired. The highlight of these results is the tremendous variability in both scores and ear advantage among these youngsters on the CST. The same was also true on a number of additional measures. These results can best be described as astonishingly diverse. And, although these cases were chosen to show the extremes of test performance that we have observed, they are unique only in terms of the magnitude of score differences. Results in many children are readily judged as abnormal, but most are not this dramatic. However, in view of the wide variability among normals, we do not judge a child's performance as abnormal unless he falls below the *range* of normal responses. Some people consider abnormality to

be any score below 1 SD from the mean. However, because of the wide spread in scores for the weak ear with the CST for normals, we believe that using the range is more appropriate. Identification of unique auditory behavior in these children together with counseling has, in most cases, remarkably altered the child's self-image as well as the opinion in which the child is held by parents and teachers.

Table 18.11 illustrates similar results in a group of older children, all of whom are right-handed, have normal IQs, and normal peripheral hearing. It is almost superfluous to add that these youngsters lack self-confidence, avoid social events, are noted for misunderstanding instructions at home and assignments at school. Typically such children and their perplexed parents have spent many hours with school teachers, counselors, in mental health centers, juvenile courts, etc. Thus, evaluation of central auditory functions in children have proved to be of value for literally legions of public school children, and dichotic sentences have been found capable of contributing to this evaluation process.

Table 18.10.
Competing Sentence Test Results (in %) on Selected 5- to 7-year- olds with Hearing Disabilities

| Subject | Sex | Age | CST | |
			L	R
JO	M	5.8	100	60
SR	F	6.4	70	30
TM[a]	F	6.5	70	0
AM	M	6.5	0	0
CI	M	6.5	0	100
SP	M	6.6	100	100
TW	M	6.7	30	60
GB	F	7.2	20	70
LH	F	7.6	50	100

[a]Only left-handed subject.

Table 18.11.
Sentence Test Results (in %) on Selected Older Children with Learning Disabilities[a]

| Subject | Sex | Age | CST | |
			L	R
JL	M	9	0	30
GC	M	10	70	80
FC	M	11	60	100
MP	M	11	100	40
RW	M	13	100	100
LH	F	13	80	10
MB	M	14	90	100
BZ	M	15	90	70

Other Sentence Applications

Sentences have also been used in many ways for central auditory evaluation (Bocca and Calearo, 1963; Jerger, 1964; Calearo and Antonelli, 1968; Frager, 1968; Haggard and Parkinson, 1971; Marston and Goetzinger, 1972; Beasley and Shriner, 1973; Lynn and Gilroy, 1975; Masterson, 1975; Beasley and Flaherty-Rintleman, 1976; McNutt and Chia-Yen Li, 1980; Elliott, 1982. The reader is referred to these references for details or to a 1976 review by Berlin and McNeil. These studies used sentence stimuli in a variety of ways that included time-compressed sentence materials that were presented against a background of noise, asked simple questions that required yes-no answers against continuous discourse competition as well as a variety of other tasks to assess central auditory integrity.

A procedure that has received less attention is one in which sentence material is switched at periodic intervals between the two ears, each ear receiving alternate bursts of unintelligible spoken messages in a sequential manner. In normal listeners the rapid shifting of the message from one ear to the other provides a message that can be easily understood. Bocca and Calearo (1963), Calearo and Antonelli (1968), and Lynn and Gilroy (1976) stated that this binaural integrative function is mediated in the lower pons region of the brainstem, but may also be sensitive to diffuse cortical damage. Lynn and Gilroy (1977), using sentences at a switching rate of 300 ms, confirmed their belief by reporting low scores on five patients with low pons lesions, whereas patients with lesions in the eighth nerve, upper brainstem, and in unilateral cerebral areas had little difficulty with the test.

Willeford and Billger (1978) also reported on the use of an alternating speech test that used a 300 ms switching rate with sentences. They found it to be a very simple task, even for typical 5-year-olds, who achieved nearly perfect scores. They have also found that few children with central auditory problems have difficulty with the test, even at a presentation level of 30 dB SL. Interestingly, this same alternating speech test produced dramatically poor performance in certain deep-sea divers suffering from decompression (the "bends") sickness (Winkleman et al., 1977; Miltenberger et al., 1979).

Some current developments in sentence tasks also appear to have implications for evaluation of central auditory function. Jerger (1980) and Jerger et al. (1983) have described the development of the Pediatric Speech Intelligibility (PSI) test. It was designed to fill the present void for testing *young* children (3–6 years of age) with central auditory disorders. Both the words and sentences used in the PSI were generated by showing stimulus picture cards to normal children between 3 and 6

years of age, who were asked to name the noun words pictured and to describe (sentences) the action (verb) that the pictures suggested. After analyzing the children's responses, a series of 10 sentence constructions were chosen that were divided into two different formats. The formats were labeled I and II to correspond with performance differences related to chronologic age (between 3 and 6) and receptive language ability. Thus, the test format can be selected to be appropriate for a given child's receptive language level. They subsequently found the test had high reliability, and that it appeared to be a valid measure of central auditory dysfunction. If this test continues to prove to be feasible for practical clinical application with children between 3 and 6 years of age, it will fill an important need among current diagnostic tools for identifying central auditory disorders. It appears to be a positive step in clarifying the uncertainties about the relationship between auditory processing ability and linguistic competence.

Flowers et al. (1973) designed the test of central auditory abilities (CAA) that is a test battery for identifying young children who have difficulty listening when an auditory stimulus is distorted or when competing messages are presented. It is divided into two subtests, the intent of which are to assess selective or attentional listening. The first portion of the test consists of passing 24 sentences through a low-pass filter. The child is asked to identify each of these distorted sentences by pointing to a picture representing the word that would complete the sentence. The second subtest is also composed of 24 sentences that have been recorded against a competing background, a children's story. These competing stimuli are mixed in one channel and presented to both ears simultaneously through earphones. The relative strengths of the two ears are, therefore, not defined in this procedure. It does appear to assess, to some degree, the presence of perceptual factors when the child is experiencing difficulty in unfavorable listening environments. Therefore, use of the CAA may be justifiably used as a screening measure.

An alternative use of sentences developed by Willeford and Burleigh (Willeford, 1985; Willeford and Burleigh, 1985) is termed the ipsilateral-contralateral competing sentence (IC-CS) test. This is also a meaningful, or *natural*, sentence test that offers a multiple-task paradigm, pitting a male versus a female speaker. The IC-CS was designed to offer three test protocols in which the listener must respond to either the male speaker, the female speaker, or both. The test was inspired by certain features of the SSI except that it does not require the subject to read, and is an open-set procedure. It consists of five different lists (tests) of competing sentences, each list composed of ten sentence pairs that are administered as follows:

Dichotic (Contralateral) Competition

List 1:   A male voice to one ear and a female voice to the other ear. The response must be made to the *female voice* which is presented at 35 dB SL (re PTA) to the test ear, whereas the dichotic competition, the male voice, is presented at 50 dB SL to the nontest ear.

List 2:   The female voice provides the target sentence, as above, however the test ear is reversed. The same MCR of −15 is used.

List 3:   The male and female voices are presented to opposite ears at equal SLs (50 dB SL in each ear, SCR = 0). Subject repeats the sentences in each ear.

Nondichotic (Ipsilateral) Competition

List 4:   Both sentences (for the male and female speaker) are presented to one ear. The response is to the *female voice* only, as in lists 1 and 2. The SCR, for subjects 12 years and older, is −5 for this procedure with the female voice at 45 dB SL (re PTA) and the male voice at 50 dB SL. For subjects under age 12, the presentation level is 50 dB SL in each ear (SCR = 0).

List 5:   This is the same procedure as for list 4 but the test ear with the female voice is reversed.

As in the CST, the sentences are six to eight words in length, and each competing sentence has a common word near the middle of the sentence that is offset from its counterpart by one syllable. That is, the common words do not overlap. The purpose of the common word was to make the task more semantically competitive by allowing both ears to hear the same word. The norms for each of these conditions are shown in Table 18.12.

Scoring of the IC-CS is based on the degree to which language and meaning of each target sentence is pre-served despite the competition. Two errors per test sentence of any of the following combinations constitute an incorrect response: (*a*) borrowing from the competing sentence; (*b*) omitting a word; (*c*) adding a word; (*d*) substituting a word not found in either sentence; or (*e*) any single word error that alters the meaning or intent of the sentence.

As discussed earlier, the contralateral (dichotic) test conditions (*a, b,* and *c*) primarily assess the integrity of the temporal lobes, based on information from studies of adults with CNS lesions. However, the ipsilateral conditions (*d* and *e*), no doubt challenge the proficiency of the brainstem, as shown by Jerger and Jerger (1974). Although the precise nature and implications of below par performance on these tests with children remain vague, similar measures have been shown to be useful methods for identifying inferior auditory ability in children.

Some interesting aspects of the IC-CS are: (*a*) no ear-advantage was shown in the dichotic mode (as this is often shown on central tests in children), and (*b*) although scores did improve with age and the range of scores decreased, both varied less than these same factors on the CST. The reason why an ear advantage was not observed on the IC-CS is not known at this point, but it may be that the acoustic characteristics of the male voice are sufficiently different from those of the female voice that the degree of competition is less than that produced by the same voice uttering different sentences. Perhaps psychologic factors also play a role.

Examples of IC-CS results are shown in Table 18.13. The first subject, a 9-year-old boy, scored poorly on nearly every central auditory test. However, he had developed enough compensatory skills to survive quite well except in classes in which group discussion was required and in complex social environments. The two college students who are listed in the table have difficulty in most lecture classes and require note takers.

Table 18.12.
IC-CS Norms (in %)

Age		Test List				
		1	2	3	4	5
6 and 7	Mean	81.5	89.6	44.8	82.6	87.0
(*n* = 27)	SD	13.2	9.8	11.3	12.6	9.9
	Range	50/100	70/100	30/75	60/100	70/100
8 and 9	Mean	89.6	90.4	61.9	85.5	92.6
(*n* = 27)	SD	10.6	12.9	12.7	10.9	9.8
	Range	70/100	60/100	40/85	60/100	70/100
10 and 11	Mean	93.0	94.1	70.0	96.7	97.0
(*n* = 27)	SD	7.8	8.9	11.2	4.8	5.4
	Range	80/100	70/100	50/85	90/100	80/100
12 through	Mean	98.2	99.3	83.7	96.9	96.3
adult	SD	4.0	2.7	9.1	6.9	6.3
(*n* = 27)	Range	90/100	90/100	65/100	80/100	80/100

Table 18.13.
IC-CS Test Results (in %) for Three Patients with Learning Disabilities[a]

Subject/Age	Ear	Contralateral Single-Ear	Contralateral Both Ears	Ipsilateral	Other Tests Failed
DS/9	L	20[b]	45	60[b]	6
	R	100		30[b]	
JI/19	L	10[b]	10[b]	0[b]	5
	R	40[b]		30[b]	
KP/23	L	60[b]	40[b]	30[b]	4
	R	60[b]		40[b]	

[a] One is an elementary school child, and the other two are college students who require note takers for class lectures.
[b] Abnormal response—below the range of normal responses.

SUMMARY

This chapter presented a review of sentence tests of central auditory function. Some of these tests have been in clinical use for a number of years, whereas others are relatively recent developments. Sentence stimuli lend themselves to a wide variety of protocols and probably challenge central auditory processes in ways that words and phonemic elements do not. Their complex acoustic natures and their linguistic elements make scoring and interpretation more difficult than for tests using shorter auditory signals. However, sentences are particularly attractive as test stimuli because they more closely approximate the acoustic variables found in conversational speech. For this reason they play a unique role in the clinical evaluation of central auditory disorders.

REFERENCES

Beasley DS, and Shriner TH. Auditory analysis of temporally distorted sentential approximations. Audiology 1973;12:262–271.

Beasley DS, and Flaherty-Rintleman AK. Children's perception of temporally distorted sentential approximations of varying length. Audiology 1976;14:315–325.

Beattie RC, and Clark N. Practice effects of a four-talker babble on the synthetic sentence identification test. Ear Hear 1982;3:202–206.

Bellaire DR, and Noffsinger PD. 1978. Interpreting dichotic test results. Presented at the American Speech and Hearing Association Convention, San Francisco.

Bergman M, Hirsch S, and Solzi P. Interhemispheric suppression: A test of central auditory function. Ear Hear 1987a;8:87–91.

Bergman M, Hirsch S, Solzi P, and Mankowitz Z. The threshold-of-interference test: A new test of interhemispheric suppression in brain injury. Ear Hear 1987b;8:147–150.

Berlin CI, Hughes LF, Lowe-Bell SS, and Berlin HL. Dichotic right-ear advantage in children 5 to 13. Cortex 1973b;9:394–402.

Berlin CI, Lowe-Bell SS, Cullen JK, Thompson CL, and Loovis CF. Dichotic speech perception: An interpretation of right-ear advantage and temporal offset effects. J Acoust Soc Am 1973a;53:699–709.

Berlin CI, and McNeil MR. Dichotic listening. In Lass NJ, Ed. Contemporary Issues in Experimental Phonetics. New York: Academic Press, 1976:327–386.

Bocca E, and Calearo C. Central hearing processes. In Jerger J, Ed. Modern Developments in Audiology. New York: Academic Press, 1963:337–370.

Butler KE, Hedrick DL, and Manning CC. 1973. In Witkin R, Ed. Composite Auditory Perceptual Test. Hayward, CA: Alameda County Social Department.

Calearo C, and Antonelli AR. Audiometric findings in brainstem lesions. Acta Otolaryngol 1968;66:305–315.

Decker TN, and Nelson PW. Maturation effects on the synthetic sentence identification-ipsilateral competing message. Ear Hear 1981;2:165–169.

Dennis M. Language acquisition in a single hemisphere. In Caplan D, Ed. Biological Studies of Mental Processes. Cambridge: MIT Press, 1980:159–185.

Elliott LL. Effects of noise on perception of speech by children and certain handicapped individuals. Sound Vib 1982;(December):10–14.

Flowers A, Costello MR, and Small V. Flowers-Costello Tests of Central Auditory Abilities. Dearborn, MI: Perceptual Learning Systems, 1973.

Frager CR. Auditory integration in geriatrics [Thesis]. Fort Collins, CO: Colorado State University, 1968.

Gilroy J, and Lynn GE. Reversibility of abnormal auditory findings in cerebral hemisphere lesions. J Neurol Sci 1974;21:117–131.

Haggard MP, and Parkinson AM. Stimulus and task factors as determinants of ear advantages. Q J Exp Psychol 1971;23:168–177.

Ivey RG. Tests of CNS auditory function. [Thesis]. Fort Collins, CO: Colorado State University, 1969.

Jerger, JF. Auditory tests for disorders of the central auditory mechanism. In Fields WW, and Alford BR, Eds. Neurological Aspects of Auditory and Vestibular Disorders. Springfield, IL: Charles C Thomas, 1964:77–93.

Jerger JF, and Jerger SW. Auditory findings in brainstem disorders. Arch Otolaryngol 1974;99:342–349.

Jerger JF, and Jerger SW. Clinical validity of central auditory tests. Scand Audiol 1975;4:147–163.

Jerger JF, Speaks C, and Trammell JA. A new approach to speech audiometry. J Speech Hear Disord 1968;33:318–328.

Jerger SW. Evaluation of central auditory function in children. In Keith RW, Ed. Central Auditory and Language Disorders in Children. Houston: College-Hill Press, 1980:30–60.

Jerger SW, Jerger JF, and Abrams S. Speech audiometry in young children. Ear Hear 1983;4:56–66.

Katz J. The use of staggered spondaic words for assessing the integrity of the central auditory nervous system. J Aud Res 1962;2:327–337.

Kimura D. A note on cerebral dominance in hearing. Acta Otolaryngol 1963;56:617–618.

Lynn GE. Auditory correlates of neurological insult. Address delivered as part of "Guest Lectures in Science" series. Fort Collins, CO: Colorado State University, 1973.

Lynn JE, Benitz JT, Eisenbrey AB, Gilroy J, and Wilner HI. Neuro-audiological correlates in cerebral hemisphere lesions: temporal and parietal lobe tumors. Audiology 1972;11:115–134.

Lynn GE, and Gilroy J. Neuro-audiological abnormalities in patients with temporal lobe tumors. J Neurol Sci 1972;17:167–184.

Lynn GE, and Gilroy J. Effects of brain lesions on the perception of monotic and dichotic speech stimuli. Proceedings of a symposium on central auditory processing disorders. Omaha: University of Nebraska Medical Center, 1975:47–83.

Lynn GE, and Gilroy J. Central aspects of audition. In Northern JL, Ed. Hearing Disorders. Boston: Little, Brown & Co., 1976:102–118.

Lynn GE, and Gilroy J. Evaluation of central auditory dysfunction in patients with neurological disorders. In Keith RW, Ed. Central Auditory Dysfunction. New York: Grune & Stratton, 1977:177–222.

Marston LE, and Goetzinger CP. A comparison of sensitized words and sentences for distinguishing nonperipheral auditory changes as a function of aging. Cortex 1972;8:213–223.

Martin FN, and Mussell SA. The influence of pauses in the competing signal on synthetic sentence identification score. J Speech Hear Disord 1979;44:282–292.

Masterson P. Psychoacoustic processing of dichotic sentences by preschool children. J Aud Res 1975;15:130–139.

Matzker J. Two new methods for the assessment of central auditory functioning in cases of brain disease. Ann Otol 1959;68:1185–1197.

Matzker J. The binaural test. J Int Audiol 1962;1:209–211.

McNutt CJ, and Chia-Yen Li J. Repetition of time-altered sentences by normal and learning disabled children. J Learn Disabil 1980;13:25–34.

Menyuk P. Sentences children use. Cambridge, MA: MIT Research Monograph no. 52, 1969.

Miltenberger GE, Caruso VG, Correia MJ, Love T, and Winkleman P. Utilization of a central auditory processing test battery in diagnosing decompression sickness. J Speech Hear Disord 1979;44:110–120.

Musiek FE, Kibbe K, and Baran J. Neurological results from split-brain patients. Semin Hear 1984;5:219–229.

Olsen WO. Dichotic test results for normal subjects and for temporal lobectomy patients. Ear Hear 1983;4:324–330.

Olsen WO, and Kurdziel SA. Dichotic and SSW Test for temporal lobe lesion patients. Presented at American Speech and Hearing Association Convention, San Francisco, 1978.

Orchik D, and Burgess J. Synthetic sentence identification as a function of the age of the listener. J Am Aud Soc 1977;3:42–46.

Porter RJ, and Berlin CI. On interpreting developmental changes in the dichotic right-ear advantage. Brain Lang 1975;2:186–200.

Segalowitz SJ, and Gruber FA, Eds. Language development and neurological theory. New York: Academic Press, 1977.

Sparks R, Goodglass H, and Nickel B. Ipsilateral vs. contralateral extinction in dichotic listening resulting from hemisphere lesions. Cortex 1970;6:249–260.

Speaks C. Dichotic listening: a clinical or research tool? Proceedings of the symposium on central auditory processing disorders. Omaha: University of Nebraska Medical Center, 1975.

Speaks C, and Jerger J. Method for measurement of speech identification. J Speech Hear Res 1965;8:185–194.

Triesman AM. The effect of irrelevant material on the efficiency of selective listening. Am J Psychol 1964;77:533–546.

Willeford JA. Sentence tests of central auditory dysfunction. In Katz J, Ed. Handbook of Clinical Audiology, 2nd ed. Baltimore: Williams & Wilkins, 1978:252–261.

Willeford J. Sentence tests of central auditory dysfunction. In Katz J, Ed. Handbook of Clinical Audiology, 3rd ed. Baltimore: Williams & Wilkins, 1985:404–420.

Willeford JA, and Billger JM. Auditory perception in children with learning disabilities. In Katz J, Ed. Handbook of Clinical Audiology, 2nd ed. Baltimore: Williams & Wilkins, 1978:410–425.

Willeford J, and Burleigh J. Handbook of Central Auditory Processing Disorders in Children. Orlando, FL: Grune and Stratton, 1985.

Wingfield A. Acoustic redundancy and the perception of time-compressed speech. J Speech Hear Res 1975;18:96–104.

Winkleman P, Caruso VG, Correia MJ, Love T, and Miltenberger GE. Otoneurologic findings in injured commercial and sport divers. Laryngoscope 1977;87:508–521.

Sentence Test Sources

SSI and PSI: Auditec of St. Louis, 330 Selma Avenue, St. Louis, MO 63113.

CST and IC-CS: Jack A. Willeford, Ph.D., 2121 South Pantano Road, #326, Tucson, AZ 85710.

PHYSIOLOGICAL EVALUATION
Auditory System

CHAPTER 19

Overview and Basic Principles of Acoustic Immittance

Michael G. Block and Terry L. Wiley

The term *acoustic immittance* refers to acoustic impedance, to acoustic admittance, or to both quantities (ANSI, 1987). *Acoustic admittance* is a general term expressing the ease with which sound energy flows through a system and *acoustic impedance* represents the total opposition to the flow of sound energy. Acoustic admittance and acoustic impedance are reciprocal quantities. A system that offers high acoustic impedance (opposition) to sound energy transfer, for example, presents a low acoustic admittance. For a full discussion of tympanometric terms and procedures the reader is referred to Shanks et al. 1988.

HISTORICAL NOTE

The history of clinical acoustic immittance measures is well over 100 years old. According to Feldmann (1970), the first attempts at objective assessment of middle ear function using acoustic impedance measures were performed by Lucae in 1867. Lucae used an instrument that was a distant forerunner of the Schuster (1934) and Zwislocki (1963) mechanical acoustic impedance bridges. He obtained measures of acoustic impedance on models of the middle ear for which the tension of the tympanic membrane could be systematically varied. Lucae also performed such measurements in human subjects. There is a substantial literature on the measurement of acoustic immittance characteristics of human ears dating back to the early 1900s (see Wiley, 1991, for a complete list of references). The clinical popularity of acoustic immittance measures in the United States, however, did not grow dramatically until the 1950s and 1960s when electroacoustic impedance instruments became commercially available. Over the past 30 to 35 years, acoustic immittance techniques, procedures, and instruments have progressed from an experimental procedure used in a few isolated clinics and laboratories to a routine clinical tool used in most audiologic and otologic facilities and screening programs. The clinical and experimental literature on the topic has had a similar dramatic growth. The 1967 program for the annual meeting of the American Speech-Language-Hearing Association, for example, included only one technical paper devoted to the topic. Fifteen years later the program included more than 30 papers concerned with acoustic immittance measures in human ears. Today

computer-assisted, multiple probe frequency acoustic immittance instruments are commercially available for diagnostic applications.

Historically, early clinical acoustic immittance measures were restricted to measures of the resting state (static) acoustic impedance at the eardrum. The term static was used to refer to the case in which the ear canal pressure was at an ambient or atmospheric level and the middle ear muscles were relaxed (not contracted). These measures were used in the diagnostic categorization of middle ear disorders. As the literature has grown, the clinical application of acoustic immittance techniques has expanded into many areas encompassing almost all aspects of diagnostic audiology. Acoustic immittance measures, for example, have been applied to screening as well as diagnostic tests, to the diagnosis of peripheral and central disorders of the auditory system, and to the estimation of auditory sensitivity in patients for whom behavioral audiometry is equivocal. Acoustic immittance instruments and procedures are now commonplace not only in audiology clinics, but in ear-nose-throat clinics, public school screening programs, and other diagnostic facilities. The American Speech-Language-Hearing Association, for example, recommends the use of acoustic immittance techniques in screening for middle ear disease (Asha, 1990).

In the chapters that follow, the reader will encounter presentations dealing with the clinical applications of acoustic immittance measures. Separate chapters on tympanometry and acoustic reflex procedures will provide important background on basic clinical techniques. The application of acoustic immittance measures in screening is treated in a separate chapter, and still other chapters will include discussions of acoustic immittance techniques applied to the diagnosis of specific auditory pathologies and to particular clinical populations (such as the difficult-to-test). Our purpose is to prepare the reader for these discussions. Specifically, we will introduce the basic concepts, terminology, and measures that form the bases of clinical acoustic immittance procedures.

BASIC CONCEPTS AND TERMINOLOGY

To use acoustic immittance measures effectively in clinical diagnosis, one must first understand the underlying principles involved in these measures. One must also become familiar with the associated terminology, units of measurement, and instrumentation. The reader will be introduced to the concept of acoustic immittance, to underlying mathematical and physical concepts, and to the basic types of instrumentation in clinical use.

Throughout our discussions, we have attempted to maintain consistency with American National Standards Institute (ANSI) specifications regarding terminology, instrumentation, and variables and units of measure. The reader is referred to ANSI Standard S3.39–1987 for full detail on these specifications. Traditional units of measure cited in the standard are used throughout this chapter.

Acoustic Immittance

Acoustic immittance is a general term that describes the ease of, or opposition to sound flow through a system. Energy is transferred when sound waves reach the ear canal and sound pressure is applied to the eardrum. When sufficient sound pressure is applied, the eardrum and the entire middle ear and inner ear systems are set into motion and energy begins to flow. The transfer of energy from the pressure alterations of air particles in the ear canal to the electromechanical activity initiated within the cochlea can be described, in part, by measuring the energy flow taking place at the lateral surface of the eardrum. The middle ear system is not a perfect transducer of energy; not all of the energy that impinges on the tympanic membrane actually flows through the middle ear transmission system. The middle ear system opposes the transfer of energy to some extent. This opposition to the transfer of acoustic energy is termed acoustic impedance (Z_a). The reciprocal of this opposition, or the ease of energy flow or transfer of air pressure changes at the eardrum into movements of the ossicular chain and within the cochlear fluids, is termed acoustic admittance (Y_a). Inasmuch as either measurement approach can be used, the term acoustic immittance refers to acoustic impedance *or* acoustic admittance.

Plane of Measurement

Regardless of whether acoustic immittance measures are expressed in terms of acoustic admittance (ease of sound flow) or acoustic impedance (opposition to sound flow), the basic method of measurement is the same. The measurement of acoustic immittance is performed by presenting an acoustic signal to the ear and measuring the resulting sound energy. Specifically, a probe signal (tone) is presented in the ear canal and the sound pressure level (SPL) of that probe signal serves as an indirect index of acoustic immittance. The SPL of the probe signal measured at the probe tip is proportional to the

acoustic immittance. The greater the measured SPL, for example, the lower the equivalent acoustic admittance. A block diagram of such a system is shown in Figure 19.1. Three separate subsystems are coupled to provide a sound pressure source (e.g., a probe tone), an analysis of the sound pressure, and control over pressure in the ear canal. The coupling is by means of an hermetic seal in the ear canal. The tip of the coupling probe is the point at which the measuring system receives input. Thus, the plane of measurement of the input acoustic immittance of the auditory system is at the probe tip. This plane of measurement is remote from the tympanic membrane (eardrum), the desired point of measurement. To define the input acoustic immittance of the middle ear system at the tympanic membrane, we must first eliminate or subtract the contributions of the ear canal.

The measurement of total acoustic immittance at the probe tip made at ambient or atmospheric pressure includes contributions of the ear canal, the tympanic membrane, and the entire middle ear system. To correct or reference measurements to the plane of the tympanic membrane, the contribution of the ear canal must be subtracted from the total acoustic immittance. The contribution of the ear canal is determined by taking acoustic immittance measures with substantial air pressure in the ear canal. If the ear canal pressure is changed appreciably from ambient, the acoustic impedance at the probe tip increases. The introduction of air pressure change in the ear canal effectively stiffens the tympanic membrane and middle ear transmission system (Shanks and Lilly, 1981). When sufficient pressure is applied, the acoustic admittance declines to a minimal value (whereas acoustic impedance is maximal). At this point, the acoustic immittance at the probe tip represents that portion of the total acoustic immittance contributed by the volume of air within the ear canal. Once the acoustic immittance of the ear canal is known it can serve as a baseline and be subtracted from the total acoustic immittance measured at the probe tip. The remaining quantity (after subtraction) represents the input acoustic immittance of the middle ear system at the plane of the tympanic membrane. By removing the contribution of the ear canal to the total acoustic immittance, we establish a standard of measurement that is independent of the size of the ear canal and the depth to which the probe tip is inserted into the ear canal. These measures are referred to as *compensated* static acoustic immittance measures. Values taken at the probe tip are termed *measurement plane* measures.

Transmission of Energy

The concept of acoustic immittance is used to relate the movements of the mechanical structures of the middle ear and the transfer of energy within the middle ear sys-

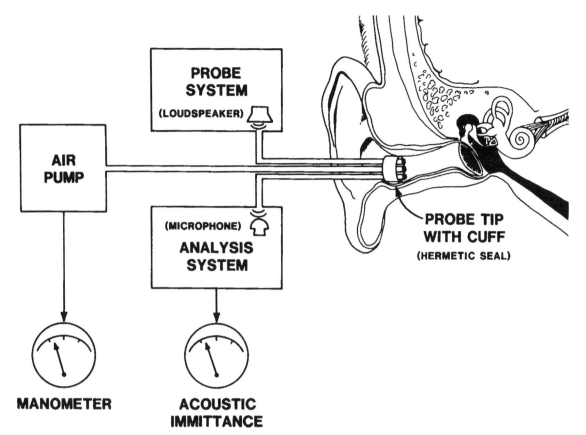

Figure 19.1. Simplified block diagram of an electroacoustic immittance instrument and its coupling to the human ear. The instrument is coupled to the ear by means of a probe tip that is hermetically sealed in the ear canal by means of a soft rubber cuff. The probe tip contains openings connected to the three basic subsystems of the instrument. One opening is directed from an air pump system used to introduce air pressure changes in the ear canal during tympanometry. Another probe tip opening connects the loudspeaker of a probe system to the ear canal for the introduction of probe tones and/or reflex-activating signals. The probe tip also connects the microphone of an analysis system to the ear canal to monitor sound pressure levels. The probe and analysis systems indirectly estimate the acoustic immittance of the ear by monitoring sound pressure levels in the ear canal (at the probe tip). The acoustic immittance at the tympanic membrane is proportional to the sound pressure level of the probe tone developed in the ear canal.

tem to the driving sinusoidal forces introduced by a probe signal. Additional and in-depth information on this topic is available (Beranek, 1949, 1954; Firestone, 1956; Lilly, 1972; Margolis, 1981; and Van Camp et al. 1986). Energy transfer occurs when the tympanic membrane and middle ear structures are set in motion. A key factor in our understanding of energy transfer in the middle ear system is that the energy transfer does not occur instantaneously with the applied force. The middle ear system is composed of different mechanical structures that react to force in a variety of ways. Acoustic immittance is a complex ratio of a force (pressure) and a velocity (movement of structures). By complex, we refer to the mathematical concept applied when two quantities or forces are varying together in different directions or at different relative times. When two mechanical forces act or react in different directions the resultant force is the vector sum of the two. The vector sum is the net magnitude plus a direction that results when the two divergent forces are com-

bined. The total opposition to the transfer of acoustic energy created by the divergent actions of these forces is termed acoustic impedance (Z_a). Specifically, the complex ratio of a sound pressure to a volume velocity at a given surface defines the acoustic impedance. The inverse ratio, or volume velocity to sound pressure, is termed acoustic admittance (Y_a). The opposition to acoustic energy transfer or Z_a is measured in *acoustic ohms*. From an instrumentation and computation point of view, it is often easier to measure acoustic admittance (Y_a) or ease of energy flow. Acoustic admittance (Y_a) is the reciprocal of Z_a, that is $Y_a = 1/Z_a$. We express acoustic admittance in measurement units of *acoustic mhos* (ohm spelled backward).

When two forces act at different times rather than in divergent directions, a similar complex ratio may be used to describe the result. We use time differences between forces primarily when we are using sinusoids. Sinusoids are forces that vary from a maximum energy flow to a minimum energy flow in a regular time pattern. When two sinusoids start at different times relative to each other they are said to be out of phase. The resultant energy contained in the combination of these sinusoidal forces is described by the phasor or vector sum of the two. A phasor is a specific vector that always arises from the origin or zero. The phasor sum, like the vector sum, is the net magnitude and the time difference that results when the two forces are combined. The time difference is expressed in degrees where 360° equals a complete cycle for a sinusoid.

Thus, complex forces are described by vectors or phasors which represent a magnitude and a direction (or phase) of force. Acoustic immittance is the complex ratio of force magnitudes occurring out of phase and is described by the contributions of the mechanical structures of the middle ear system. Acoustic immittance at the tympanic membrane is controlled by the mass of the three middle ear ossicles, by the stiffness of the ossicular ligaments and muscles, by the stiffness of the tympanic membrane and round window membrane, by the stiffness of the air contained in the tympanum, by the mass and friction that result from air movement within the tympanum and, finally, by the total immittance offered by the cochlea at the oval window (Zwislocki, 1976). The input acoustic immittance of the middle ear system, then, is controlled by a variety of masses, stiffnesses, and frictions. Basically, however, there are two main components to consider when measuring the transfer of acoustic energy: the in-phase component (i.e., that occurs simultaneously with the applied force) and the out-of-phase components (i.e., those that occur after the applied force.)

In-Phase Component

In mechanical systems, two structures may come in contact and the resultant friction transduces the motion into heat. In other words the energy is dissipated in the form of heat. This effect occurs in direct proportion to the force and in phase with the applied force. *Acoustic resistance* (R_a) (Fig. 19.2) is the dissipation of sound pressure or acoustic energy. *Acoustic conductance* (G_a) (Fig. 19.2), an admittance term, is the reciprocal of acoustic resistance. As acoustic resistance increases, acoustic conductance decreases. A physical example of an acoustic resistance is a fine mesh screen (Fig. 19.3, **top panel**). The size of the apertures (openings) is inversely proportional to the acoustic resistance offered by the screen or the resultant energy flow through the screen. Over the frequency range common in clinical acoustic immittance measures, acoustic resistance is independent of frequency. That is, acoustic resistance remains relatively constant as a function of probe frequency.

Out-of-Phase Components

The out-of-phase component affecting the transfer of acoustic energy is **acoustic reactance** (X_a) or *acoustic susceptance* (B_a) (Fig. 19.2). Acoustic reactance and acoustic susceptance are out of phase with the applied force. Recall that (Y_a) or (Z_a) are determined by the ratio of force (sound pressure) and volume velocity (sound flow). Specifically, the acoustic impedance is directly proportional to the measured sound pressure at the probe tip and acoustic admittance is directly proportional to the volume velocity at the probe tip. Accordingly, for a given acoustic system, the higher the measured sound pressure, the greater the equivalent acoustic impedance and the lower the acoustic admittance. Conversely, increases in volume velocity are associated with higher acoustic admittances and lower acoustic impedances. Out-of-phase components oppose energy flow by storing the energy in a stiffness or mass

Acoustic Immittance		
Acoustic Impedance (X_a)	<--Reciprocals-->	**Acoustic Admittance (Y_a)**
Opposition to Energy Flow (Storage) Compliant Acoustic Reactance ($-jX_a$) Mass Acoustic Reactance (jX_a)	<--Reciprocals--> <--Reciprocals-->	**Ease of Energy Flow (Storage)** Compliant Acoustic Susceptance (jB_a) Mass Acoustic Susceptance ($-jB_a$)
Opposition to Energy Flow (Dissipative) Acoustic Resistance (R_a)	<--Reciprocals-->	**Ease of Energy Flow (Dissipative)** Acoustic Conductance (G_a)

Figure 19.2. Acoustic impedance and acoustic admittance terms and their reciprocal relations.

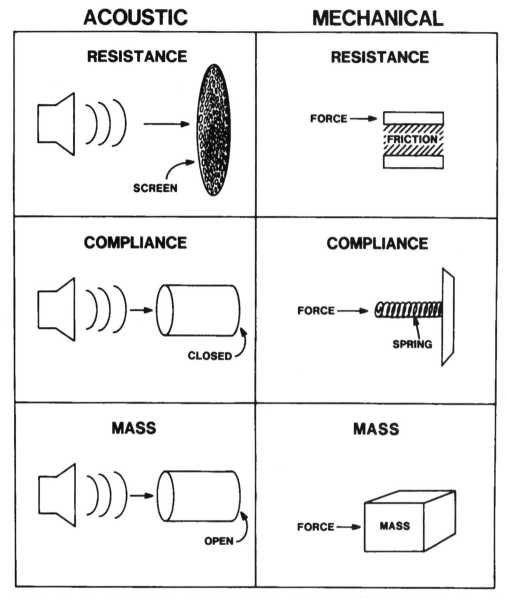

Figure 19.3. A schematic representation of the resistive and reactive components of acoustic and mechanical impedance. Further description is provided in the text.

before producing a velocity. In other words, movement of structures is delayed relative to the applied force. In mechanical systems, stiffness (compliance) is a characteristic of a spring (Fig. 19.3, **middle panel**). The stiffer a spring the greater the opposition to compression and the more energy it reflects. In acoustic systems, the stiffness characteristic may be modelled as a column of air in a tube closed at one end (Fig. 19.3, **middle panel**). The acoustic force (sound pressure) compresses the air in the tube, because one end is closed. The opposition to compression offered by the closed tube is described as *compliant acoustic reactance* or $-jX_a$ (Fig. 19.2). The tubal volume is inversely related to $-jX_a$. The admittance reciprocal of compliant acoustic reactance is *compliant acoustic susceptance* or jB_a (Fig. 19.2). The use of the j operator will be discussed later. Unlike acoustic resistance and acoustic conductance, compliant acoustic reactance and susceptance vary with probe frequency. Compliant acoustic reactances, for example, are greatest at low probe frequencies and least at higher probe frequencies.

The second form of energy storage is analogous to the inertia that exists within a mechanical or acoustic mass (Fig. 19.3, **bottom panel**). The mass tends to remain in its present state until sufficient energy is absorbed to change that state. In acoustic systems an acoustic mass may be represented as a column of air in an open tube (Fig. 19.3, **bottom panel**). Because the tube is open an acoustic force (sound pressure) will move the column without compressing the air. The opposition to displacement offered by the slug of air is described as *mass acoustic reactance* (jX$_a$) (Fig. 19.2). The admittance reciprocal of mass acoustic reactance is *mass acoustic susceptance* (–jB$_a$) (Fig. 19.2). Mass components are the complex reciprocals of compliant components. Mass components are greatest at high probe frequencies and least at lower probe frequencies.

The total acoustic reactance or susceptance is the sum of mass components and compliant components. The total acoustic reactance or susceptance will either be controlled by an acoustic mass or by an acoustic stiffness. The term control simply indicates which element is larger. If jX$_a$ and –jX$_a$ are equal or if –rjB$_a$ and jB$_a$ are equal, the system is said to be at resonance. Acoustic reactances have units of acoustic ohms; acoustic susceptances are expressed in acoustic millimhos (mmho).

Complex Numbers

As noted earlier, when a force acts on a mechanical system there is a time delay between the applied force and movements within the system. If the force is sinusoidal, such as in the case of a probe tone, then the time delay between the application of the force and resultant energy transfer is one-fourth of a cycle. That is, the response of the system to the applied force is 90° out of phase. The only effect that occurs at the instant of the force is the frictional effect; thus resistive or conductive effects are in phase with the force and reactive effects are out of phase. The extent to which each quantity contributes to the total effect is determined by their magnitude and by their phase relation (in degrees).

The phase relations between conductive-resistive elements and susceptance-reactance elements are described by their relative direction to each other on the perpendicular axes shown in Figure 19.4. The resistive-conductive elements are represented on the horizontal plane. Numbers on the horizontal plane are called real numbers. Real numbers have two directions: 0° and 180°. We omit the 0° operator for numbers in that direction and instead refer to them as positive (+). Similarly, numbers in the 180° direction are called negative (–). The factors + and – are used to represent 0° and 180°, respectively. Thus, 3 units with a 0° operator is written 3 or +3. Conversely, 3 units with a 180° operator is –3.

Reactance and susceptance are represented on the vertical plane. Numbers on the vertical plane are called imaginary numbers. Imaginary numbers, like real numbers, have two directions: 90° and –90° (or 270°). By convention, 90° is given the factor j or +j and –90° is given the factor –j. (the j factor is equal to $\sqrt{-1}$.) Thus, 4 units with a 90° operator is written j4, and 4 units with a –90° operator is written –j4. The factor j represents 90°

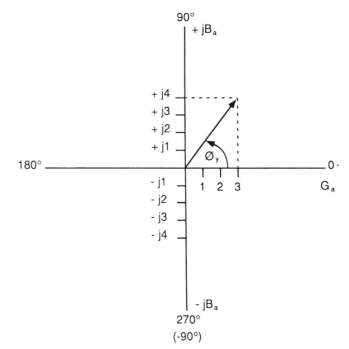

Figure 19.4. The rectangular coordinate system used for representing the complex conductance and susceptance components of acoustic admittance. The horizontal or real axis is used to represent the in-phase component: acoustic conductance (G$_a$). The in-phase component is plotted from the origin in the positive (0°) direction. The vertical or imaginary axis is used to represent the out-of-phase component: acoustic susceptance (B$_a$). By convention, mass acoustic susceptance (–jB$_a$) is plotted from the origin in the negative (270° or –90°) direction; compliant acoustic susceptance (jB$_a$) is plotted from the origin in the positive (+90°) direction. In the example shown, the complex acoustic admittance (Y$_a$) is 3+j4, indicating a stiffness-dominant system. The angle of the acoustic admittance phasor is represented by Ø$_y$. Further details are provided in the text.

and the factor –j represents –90°. A complex number contains both real and imaginary parts. For example, the complex number 3+j4 means 3 real units with a 0° operator and 4 j units with a 90° operator.

Rectangular Notation

When complex numbers are used to represent acoustic immittance quantities, we refer to this as rectangular notation. Rectangular notation means that both the in-phase (real) and out-of-phase (imaginary) quantities are explicitly expressed, such as in our example, 3+j4. In terms of our coordinate system, the real, or in-phase, element is represented on the horizontal axis. The imaginary, or out-of-phase, element is represented on the vertical or j axis, or 90° with respect to the real axis. Values plotted on the j axis indicate that they are 90° out of phase with the real values (Fig. 19.4). Out-of-phase components are reactances (X) or susceptances (B) and in-phase components are resistances (R) or conductances (G). Acoustic susceptance, for example, is the linear sum (i.e., along the same axis) of two opposing forces: the susceptance offered by an acoustic mass and the susceptance offered by an acoustic compliance or stiffness. In a mechanical system, such as the middle ear, the linear sum of the out-of-phase components determines whether the system is stiffness dominant ($-jX_a$ or jB_a) or mass dominant (jX_a or $-jB_a$). Specifically, the larger of the two reactive elements determines whether the system is stiffness or mass dominant. Mechanical systems are frequency dependent and, therefore, the frequency of oscillation of the applied force must be considered when discussing impedance or admittance. In normal systems, mass effects dominate at high frequencies and stiffness effects dominate at low frequencies. The total opposition to sound flow of a system is the result of resistive and reactive actions, each 90° out-of-phase with the other. As a result, the simple linear sum of the two components will not account for the time difference (or resultant phase) between them. Because the components are 90° apart, their vector (or phasor) sum can be derived by finding the square root of their summed squares (Pythagorean theorem). We use the fact that jX_a and R_a form the sides of a right triangle. The vector sum is the hypotenuse. Thus:

$$/Z_a/ = \sqrt{R^2 + [jX_a + (-jX_a)]^2}$$

$$\text{and } /Y_a/ = \sqrt{G^2 + [jB_a + (-jB_a)]^2}.$$

From these formulae we can see that acoustic impedance and admittance are actually quantities composed of two related effects. An easy way to describe the net result of these effects is to plot them (Fig. 19.4). We use the Cartesian coordinate system mentioned above to illustrate graphically this combination of forces in *rectangular notation*.

As was noted earlier, the horizontal axis is used to express the real or in-phase effect. Here, we plot the resistive or conductive quantity. The vertical axis (also called the j axis) is used to express the imaginary or out-of-phase effect. The reactive quantity (X or B) is plotted along this dimension. By convention, the portion above the real axis is the positive direction (j) and the portion below the real axis is the negative direction (–j). As shown in Figure 19.4 the in-phase component is represented by plotting its value along the real axis from the intersection or zero point. The total out-of-phase component is the linear sum of the mass effects and compliant effects along the j axis. The net admittance or impedance is either in the positive direction or in the negative direction.

Polar Notation

In rectangular notation, both the in-phase and out-of-phase components are expressed by using a complex number. For example, 3+j4 simply means that there are 3 in-phase units and 4 positively directed out-of-phase units. The total effect, $/Z_a/$ or $/Y_a/$, is the phasor sum of these effects. However, the force magnitude alone does not describe the phase relation among the divergent forces. The phase relation is described by the angle the vector sum makes with the real axis. This angle, Ø, is one whose tangent is the ratio of the real (in-phase) and imaginary (out-of-phase) components. We compute Ø for impedance (Ø$_Z$) and admittance (Ø$_Y$) as:

$$\text{Ø}_Z = \tan^{-1} \pm jX_a/R_a \text{ and } \text{Ø}_Y = \tan^{-1} \pm jB_a/G_a.$$

Thus, a complete polar description of Z_a or Y_a must include the phase or direction as well as the magnitude. When the magnitude and phase angle are provided we refer to this as *polar notation*. In this way, once we know the magnitude of Z_a and its phase we can compute the resistive element ($R_a = Z_a \cos Ø_Z$) and the reactive element ($\pm jX_a = Z_a \sin Ø_Z$). Also, once we know Y_a and its phase we can compute the conductive element ($G_a = Y_a \cos Ø_Y$) and the susceptive element ($\pm B_a = Y_a \sin Ø_Y$). It should be apparent, then, that if we consider the absolute magnitude of the force, or reciprocal energy transfer without considering the phase relations, we do not know to what extent friction (resistance or conductance), mass or stiffness affect the energy transfer. In the example used earlier, 3+j4 is actually a resultant magnitude of 5 with a net direction (or phase) of 53° (5/*53°*] acoustic ohms).

Acoustic Admittance

Most clinical instruments used for the measurement of acoustic immittance provide such measures in terms of acoustic admittance. The phase relation between acoustic admittance components remains the same as that for acoustic impedance components except the direction is reversed for the out-of-phase components. By convention, the real component of acoustic admittance is plotted on the same axis and direction as the real component of acoustic impedance. The real or in-phase component of acoustic admittance is acoustic conductance (G_a). Acoustic conductance is the complex reciprocal of acoustic resistance. The acoustic admittance corollary of acoustic reactance is acoustic susceptance (B_a). In a manner similar to that for acoustic impedance, the reactive elements of admittance are plotted on the imaginary (j) axis but in a reverse manner. For example, a compliant acoustic susceptance is plotted in the same direction as a mass acoustic reactance. Thus, negative-directed reactance ($-jXa$) is positive-directed susceptance (jB_a); similarly, positive-directed reactance (jX_a) is negative-directed susceptance ($-jB_a$). Conversion equations for acoustic admittance and acoustic impedance can be found in Wiley and Block (1979).

Compliance and Compliant Reactance

When considering the relation between Z_a and Y_a recall that stiffness-dominant systems are represented by $-jX_a$ and jB_a whereas mass-dominant systems are represented by jX_a and $-jB_a$. Theoretically, it is possible to have a system that offers a pure acoustic susceptance, in which case acoustic conductance is zero. This would indicate that only mass ($-jB_a$) and/or stiffness (jB_a) exists. In the human ear, however, there is always an acoustic conductance (resistive element). As mentioned earlier, at low frequencies (e.g., 226 Hz) the normal human ear is stiffness dominant. The mass or inertia of the ossicles, tympanic membrane and ligaments plays a negligible role in the control of sound flow for a 226-Hz probe tone. Acoustic conductances persist especially where joints are concerned (e.g., ossicular joints and coupling between the stapes and the vestibule). When significant ear canal pressure is applied, as in tympanometry, the tympanic membrane and ossicular chain become so stiff that the admittance approximates pure stiffness. In other words, where

$$Y_a = \sqrt{G_a^2 + jB_a^2}$$

and where G_a^2 is a very small quantity, then $Y_a \approx jB_a$. Under these circumstances Y_a has been described as a compliance. That is, the acoustic admittance may be approximated by the stiffness or compliance offered by an air column in a hard-walled right cylinder. This means that Y_a can be represented by an *equivalent volume* of air in cubic centimeters (cc). For example, if the acoustic admittance of the ear at -400 daPa ear canal pressure was the same as the acoustic admittance offered by a hard-walled cylinder of 1-cc volume, one might express the admittance as an equivalent volume of 1 cc. Indeed, some clinicians report their acoustic immittance measures as compliance values in cc. The compliance value in cc represents a hard-walled walled right cylinder of the designated volume (in cc or ml) that offers the equivalent acoustic immittance. It is important to understand that the volume measure *does not represent a real physical volume measure* of the ear canal or middle ear, but, rather, represents a volume that offers an acoustic immittance equivalent to that offered by the ear under test. Further, this representation is often associated with the assumption that the acoustic immittance measure can be modeled as a pure acoustic stiffness or acoustic compliance. This situation does not truly exist for human ears, however, because acoustic conductances (resistive elements) are always finite. Accordingly, equivalent volume measures based on such an assumption present some degree of error.

INSTRUMENTATION

To measure acoustic immittance as a function of ear canal pressure, as in tympanometry, it is necessary to maintain the probe tone at a standard or constant sound pressure level. As the acoustic immittance changes with ear canal pressure, the sound flow changes. This is reflected in a change in the probe tone sound pressure level measured at the probe tip. The acoustic immittance measuring instrument detects this change as an increase or decrease in voltage at the microphone. This voltage change is proportional to the acoustic immittance of the middle ear system at the plane of the probe tip. If the voltage compensation system operates continuously as ear canal pressure changes then the instrument can be calibrated to display the acoustic immittance of the ear in basic physical units. In contrast, instruments without a voltage compensation system usually are not calibrated in basic physical units because changes in sound flow with changes in ear canal pressure is related to an arbitrary starting point rather than to a standard voltage.

Sound energy measurements made without a voltage compensation system often are expressed in arbitrary units; they are termed arbitrary because they are idiosyncratic to the specific middle ear system and measurement device. The pressure-immittance function generated in this manner usually relates ear canal pressure only to empirically derived arbitrary units. These are used as a local, specific reference for comparison among functions. When the sound energy in the ear canal is maintained at a constant level, deviations from this constant are proportional to the acoustic immittance of the middle ear system and, thus, can be easily expressed in physical units common to all devices. In the case of acoustic admittance, for example, we can express our measures in units of acoustic mhos (actually we use mmho, because the units associated with measures in human ears are so small). When the measurement is subjected to a phase-shifting circuit, the phase relations between susceptance (jB_a or $-jB_a$) and conductance (G_a) are known and the contributions of resistive and reactive elements can be expressed. Thus, by designing an instrument with a feedback (voltage compensation) circuit and a phase-shifting circuit we are able to express the immittance characteristics of the ear in basic physical units for both resistive and reactive elements. The major advantage of this system is that it permits comparable measurements to be obtained at different facilities. The measurements themselves do not require the use of one particular instrument to be valid and comparable from clinic to clinic.

Bridges and Meters

Both types of measurement systems described are in clinical use today. One type is the electroacoustic impedance bridge which compares the sound pressure level in the ear canal (represented in volts) to a preset standard (also in volts). Once the SPL associated with the acoustic admittance of the ear canal is compensated or balanced with the standard, changes in acoustic admittance caused by changes in ear canal pressure or by contraction of middle-ear muscles can be measured by rebalancing the ear canal SPL with the standard. The amount of sound pressure needed to rebalance the bridge is inversely proportional to the change in acoustic admittance associated with the ear canal pressure change or the acoustic reflex. However, in its dynamic mode with ear canal pressure sweeping across its measurement range, often no balancing is done so the result is an arbitrary unit function.

The other type of instrument is called an electroacoustic admittance meter. This device has a feedback circuit to maintain a constant SPL in the ear canal regardless of changes in acoustic admittance. Each instantaneous change in ear canal pressure is associated with an acoustic admittance value. In some cases Y_a is assumed to be purely acoustic compliance and is expressed in cc (or ml) of equivalent volume. Other acoustic admittance meters actually measure the flow and, by phase shifting, also extract the effects of acoustic conductance and acoustic susceptance. These systems enable the clinician to evaluate both the resistance (or conductance) and reactance (or susceptance) components that contribute to the total measure. In certain middle ear pathologies, this component analysis provides important clinical information for differential diagnosis. Component information is useful, for example, in cases of ossicular discontinuity. The natural stiffness of the middle ear system is almost eliminated and the mass of the system is the dominant reactance. This mass control is manifested in undulating, notched acoustic susceptance tympanograms for cases of ossicular discontinuity (see Chapter 20).

Measurement Requirements

The measurement of acoustic energy transfer within the auditory mechanism has certain basic requirements regardless of the system used to acquire such measures. They all need a means to: (a) ensure a hermetic seal of the probe unit in the ear canal; (b) vary and monitor air pressure in the ear canal; (c) introduce a probe tone into the ear canal; (d) monitor ear canal sound pressure level; and (e) display the results calibrated in acoustic immittance terms. These basic system components are shown graphically in Figure 19.1.

Calibration

The ANSI standard, S3.39-1987, (ANSI, 1987) on acoustic immittance instruments provides necessary tolerances and required calibrations for various types of devices. The standard includes capabilities and tolerance requirements for instruments ranging in complexity from screening devices to full-range measurement systems. The clinician should be aware of all required tolerances and calibrations for their particular instrument. We review selected calibrations common to most clinical systems.

Probe Signal

Regardless of the specific probe signal frequency, the user should determine that the probe signal is accurate in frequency, at the specified level and free of unwanted distortion and noise. Measurement of these probe signal characteristics can be conducted by coupling the probe unit with a standard coupler. The SPL developed in the coupler can be measured with a standard microphone and sound level meter. The output levels, frequency accuracy, and harmonic distortion (and noise) should be evaluated and documented in the manner stipulated in the ANSI standard.

Manometer System

The pneumatic (air pressure) system should be evaluated to determine the rate of air pressure changes and the accuracy of the graduated steps on the air pressure indicator (manometer). Manometer accuracy should be within the tolerance specified by ANSI and can be determined with a U-tube manometer graduated in calibrated units. If an X-Y plotter is used to record the output as a function of air pressure changes (e.g., in tympanometry), the correspondence between the manometer readings and the pressure readings on the recorder chart must be determined.

Acoustic Immittance Monitor System

Regardless of the variables and units of measurement, the acoustic admittance or acoustic impedance value indicated by the instrument must correspond to known values for fixed cavity volumes over the range of interest. The exact test cavities and tolerances should conform to those required in the ANSI standard. Care should be taken to account for the atmospheric conditions (altitude, barometric pressure, etc.) common to the specific location (Lilly and Shanks, 1981). Also, if an external recording device is used (e.g., X-Y plotter), the meter calibration must be consistent with the recording device. That is, the value indicated on the acoustic immittance meter must correspond with the appropriate value marking on the chart paper for a set calibration cavity.

In addition to acoustic immittance values, the response times of the instrument must be specified. If a recording device is used, the response time of the recorder also must be included in the specification. These time constants are particularly important if the unit is used to measure the temporal characteristics of acoustic immittance changes. The ANSI standard provides recommended methods for these measures.

Acoustic Reflex Activator System

The specification and calibration of acoustic reflex-activating signals also must be completed according to ANSI specifications. (Acoustic reflex measures are discussed in a later section of this chapter.) The required measures include frequency accuracy, output levels, attenuator linearity, and harmonic distortion for both contralateral and ipsilateral acoustic reflex signals.

BASIC MEASURES

A variety of acoustic immittance measures are used in present audiology/otology clinics. A major clinical application of such measures is the identification and classification of middle ear disorders (see Chapters 2, 20, and 21). A significant number of patients with middle ear disease do not present significant hearing losses (Eagles et al., 1967; Eagles, 1972). This limits the clinical efficacy of audiometry in the detection of middle ear disorders. Acoustic immittance measures, in contrast, are quite effective in the early identification of middle ear abnormalities (Brooks, 1973, 1978; ASHA, 1990). Indeed, there are several reports documenting the superiority of acoustic immittance measures compared to audiometry in the detection of middle ear disorders (Brooks, 1973; Paradise et al., 1976; Liden and Renvall, 1980).

In addition to middle ear status, acoustic immittance measures are potentially useful in revealing information on specific disorders of the auditory brainstem and peripheral auditory nervous system. Abnormalities of the auditory periphery and brainstem often manifest abnormalities in acoustic reflex characteristics. Accordingly, reflex measures, which form a part of a complete acoustic immittance test procedure, are useful in determining diagnostic profiles typical of specific lesions to the peripheral and central auditory systems (Wiley and Block, 1984) (these measures are detailed in Chapter 21). We wish to emphasize that the clinical application of acoustic immittance measures is not limited to disorders of the middle ear, but may encompass audiologic diagnosis of disorders throughout major portions of the auditory system.

Finally, a major clinical advantage of acoustic immittance procedures is that no overt behavioral response is required on the part of the patient. In contrast to most audiometric techniques, acoustic immittance measures are quite valuable in the audiologic evaluation of infants, young children, and other populations for which behavioral audiometry is not always a feasible alternative.

In the chapters that follow, the clinical applications of acoustic immittance measures will be detailed along with typical findings for various pathologic conditions. In preparation for these discussions, we present basic descriptions and concepts that underlie the measures typically incorporated in clinical acoustic immittance protocols. We have organized our discussion into two major measurement sections: tympanometry and stapedial-reflex measures.

Tympanometry

Tympanometry is the measurement of acoustic immittance at the probe tip (measurement plane) or at the eardrum (compensated) as a function of air pressure variations. Air pressure (in units deca Pascals or daPa) is varied positive and negative relative to ambient or atmospheric pressure and the dynamic effects of air pressure changes on the acoustic immittance properties of the middle ear transmission system are measured. The graphic representation of acoustic immittance as a function of ear canal pressure is called a tympanogram. A representative acoustic admittance tympanogram (measurement plane) for subjects with normal middle ear systems is shown in Figure 19.5. Note that the acoustic admittance is maximal near ambient pressure and decreases as the ear canal pressure is increased or decreased relative to atmospheric pressure. The air pressure changes have the effect of stiffening the tympanic membrane and ossicular chain, resulting in a decrease in acoustic admittance at the probe tip. The normal amplitude, gradient (slope), and width characteristics of tympanograms are altered in patients with middle ear disorders. In cases of serous otitis media, for example,

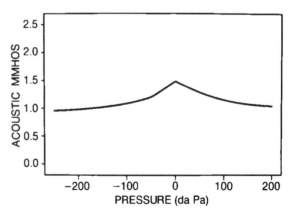

Figure 19.5. Representative acoustic admittance tympanogram (measurement plane) for individuals with normal middle ear systems. The tympanogram shown is the average (mean) of 106 normal adult ears. The probe frequency is 220 Hz.

there will be little change in acoustic immittance at the tympanic membrane with changes in ear-canal pressure. The liquid (effusion) in the middle ear, characteristic of serous otitis media, reduces the normal mobility of the tympanic membrane and ossicular chain. This results in a flat tympanometric configuration; ear canal pressure changes produce little or no effect on the acoustic immittance measured at the tympanic membrane.

Eustachian Tube Function

An assumption that underlies tympanometry is that the acoustic admittance measured at the probe tip is maximal when the air pressure on both sides of the tympanic membrane is equal. Accordingly, the air pressure at the tympanogram peak is used as an approximation of the middle ear resting pressure. This, in turn, provides a means of evaluating the ventilatory function of the Eustachian tube. In the case of a normal middle ear and Eustachian tube, the tympanogram peak will occur near ambient pressure. The normal opening and closing of the Eustachian tube maintains equilibrium between ambient or atmospheric pressure and the pressure in the middle ear space. In cases of Eustachian tube obstruction, however, the tympanogram peak typically will show a significantly negative resting pressure in the middle ear. This is diagnostically significant because Eustachian tube obstruction is often a precursor of middle ear disease, such as otitis media. The normal function of the Eustachian tube also can be tested by observation of shifts in the tympanogram peaks as the patient performs tasks such as swallowing or holding the mouth and nose shut and blowing. These tasks normally alter the middle ear resting pressure if the Eustachian tube is functioning normally.

Compensated Static Acoustic Immittance Measures

The tympanogram also can be used to estimate the resting acoustic immittance at the lateral surface of the tympanic membrane (Lilly, 1973). This is termed compensated static acoustic immittance and can be expressed in acoustic admittance or acoustic impedance notation (see ANSI, 1987). Compensated measures are those taken at the lateral surface of the tympanic membrane when the middle ear muscles are relaxed (not contracted) and when the pressure in the ear canal is at atmospheric (*ambient*) level or at the pressure corresponding to the tympanogram peak (*peak*). Compensated measures are useful in differentiating pathologies of the middle ear. Certain lesions, such as middle ear effusion and otosclerosis, will present compensated static acoustic admittance values that are substantially lower than normal. Cases of ossicular discontinuity, in contrast, are exemplified by compensated static acoustic admittance values that are much higher than normal.

Stapedial Reflex Measures

In a normal individual, a stapedius muscle contraction changes the acoustic immittance of the middle ear. The stapedius muscle will contract in response to an acoustic signal of sufficient intensity and duration. This is termed an *acoustic reflex*. The acoustic reflex in normal subjects is bilateral; if the stapedius on the right side contracts in response to sound, the stapedius on the left side also contracts. Because the stapedial reflex is bilateral, stapedius muscle activity can be elicited by presentation of an acoustic signal to either ear. An *ipsilateral* acoustic reflex is the case in which an acoustic signal (activator) is presented in the same ear housing the acoustic immittance probe unit. That is, acoustic immittance changes are measured in the same ear receiving the acoustic activating signal. A *contralateral* acoustic reflex is the case in which an activating signal (sound) is delivered to one ear and stapedius contractions (acoustic immittance changes) are monitored in the opposite ear.

Acoustic reflexes are measured clinically by recording acoustic immittance changes at the probe tip of an acoustic immittance measurement system. The tendon of the stapedius muscle attaches to the head of the stapes and when the stapedius contracts, the stapes is pulled down and out relative to the oval window. This alters the energy transfer characteristics of the middle ear system that, in turn, is manifested as a decrease in acoustic admittance at the tympanic membrane. Thus, by monitoring acoustic immittance changes we can indirectly evaluate stapedial reflex dynamics.

Because our measurements of acoustic reflex activity are based on indirect estimates of acoustic immittance changes, the integrity of our measures is dependent on an intact (normal) middle ear system and intact (normal) afferent (sensory) and efferent (motor) neuronal systems associated with the stapedius reflex arc. Abnormalities in any of these systems may be associated with abnormal stapedial reflex characteristics (Wiley and Block, 1984). Specific profiles or patterns of acoustic reflex measures often are associated with specific lesions to the peripheral and central auditory system.

Future Applications

As microprocessor technology becomes more widespread it is likely that acoustic immittance instruments will also undergo associated technologic changes. One may expect the next generation of clinical instruments to be digital rather than analog. The data displays will be stored in computer memory rather than simply being copied to a preprinted chart. Once the data are in digital form a vast array of mathematical transformations can be performed. The data can be associated with information retrieval systems for enhancement of analysis and interpretation. The data can be readily stored in such systems for easy access and cross-correlation in diagnostic decision making and in the maintenance of patient and experimental records. The acoustic-immittance system, an audiometric system and even a hearing aid analysis system may all be part of a microprocessor-based audiologic data collection system set up as a work station within a network of other computer systems. In this manner, acoustic immittance measures and data collected during an audiologic evaluation could be compared with a large interclinic data base.

An additional development of the digital era will be the routine use of multiple probe frequencies and different ways of viewing and interpreting tympanometric data. The use of multiple probe frequencies will enable clinicians to observe the resonance characteristic of the middle ear system. We may discover that shifting patterns of resonance will enhance differential diagnosis of middle ear abnormalities compared to a single frequency pressure-immittance function. Furthermore, the separation of the components of complex acoustic immittance coupled with the use of multiple probe frequencies may enhance the detection of subtle changes in middle ear function underlying specific pathologies (see Lilly, 1984; Shanks, 1984, for additional material on multifrequency applications).

REFERENCES

ANSI, American National Standards Institute. American national standard specifications for instruments to measure aural acoustic impedance and admittance (aural acoustic immittance). New York: American National Standards Institute, ANSI S3.39-1987, 1987.

ASHA, American Speech-Language-Hearing Association. Guidelines for screening for hearing impairment and middle ear disorders. Asha 1990;32(Suppl. 2):17–24.

Beranek LL. Acoustic Measurements. New York: John Wiley & Sons, 1949.

Beranek LL. Acoustics. New York: McGraw-Hill, 1954.

Brooks D. Hearing screening: A comparative study of an impedance method and pure tone screening. Scand Audiol 1973;2:67–76.

Brooks D. Acoustic impedance testing for screening auditory function in school children. Maico Aud Lib Ser 1978;15:8–9.

Eagles EL. Selected findings from the Pittsburgh study. Trans Am Acad Ophthalmol Otol 1972;76:343–348.

Eagles EL, Wishik SM, and Doerfler LG. Hearing sensitivity and ear disease in children: A prospective study. Laryngoscope 1967;(Monograph Suppl.):1–274

Feldmann H. A history of audiology. Transl Beltone Inst Hear Res 1970;22.

Firestone FA. Twixt earth and sky with rod and tube; the mobility and classical impedance analogies. J Acoust Soc Am 1956;28:1117–1153.

Liden G, and Renvall U. Impedance and tone screening of school children. Scand Audiol 1980;9:121–126.

Lilly DJ. 1972. Acoustic impedance at the tympanic membrane. In Katz J, Ed. Handbook of Clinical Audiology. Baltimore: Williams & Wilkins, 1972:434–469.

Lilly DJ. 1973. Measurement of acoustic impedance at the tympanic membrane. In Jerger J, Ed. Modern Developments in Audiology, 2nd ed. New York: Academic Press, 1973:345–406.

Lilly DJ. Multiple frequency, multiple component tympanometry: New approaches to an old diagnostic problem. Ear Hear 1984;5:300–308.

Lilly DJ, and Shanks JE. Acoustic immittance of an enclosed volume of air. In Popelka GR, Ed. Hearing Assessment with the Acoustic Reflex. New York: Grune & Stratton, 1981:145–160.

Margolis RH. Fundamentals of acoustic immittance. In Popelka GR, Ed. Hearing Assessment with the Acoustic Reflex. New York: Grune & Stratton, 1981:117–143.

Paradise J, Smith C, and Bluestone C. Tympanometric detection of middle ear effusion in infants and young children. Pediatrics 1976;58:198–210.

Schuster K. Eine methode zum vergleich akusticher impedanzen. Psysikalische Z 1934;35:408–409.

Shanks JE. Tympanometry. Ear Hear 1984;5:268–280.

Shanks JE, and Lilly DJ. An evaluation of tympanometric estimates of ear canal volume. J Speech Hear Res 1981;24:557–566.

Shanks JE, Lilly DJ, Margolis RH, Wiley TL, and Wilson RH. Tympanometry. J Speech Hear Disord 1988;53:354–377.

Van Camp KJ, Margolis RH, Wilson RH, Creten WL, and Shanks JE. Principles of Tympanometry. ASHA Monograph, 1986:24.

Wiley TL. Acoustic immittance measures: A bibliography. ASHA 1991;33(Suppl 4)3.

Wiley TL, and Block MG. Static acoustic-immittance measurements. J Speech Hear Res 1979;22:677–696.

Wiley TL, and Block MG. 1984. Acoustic and nonacoustic reflex patterns in audiologic diagnosis. In Silman S, Ed. The Acoustic Reflex: Basic Principles and Clinical Applications. New York: Academic Press, 1984:387–411.

Zwislocki J. An acoustic method for clinical examination of the ear. J Speech Hear Res 1963;6:303–314.

Zwislocki J. The acoustic middle ear function. In Feldman A, and Wilbur L, Eds. Acoustic Impedance and Admittance—The Measurement of Middle Ear Function. Baltimore: Williams & Wilkins, 1976.

CHAPTER 20

Tympanometry in Clinical Audiology

James W. Hall III and David Chandler

In 1946, Otto Metz systematically evaluated the acoustic *immittance* of normal and abnormal ears. Metz described distinct changes in acoustic immittance associated with different middle ear disorders. Over the next 25 years, his findings were sporadically confirmed (e.g., Feldman, 1963). Then, beginning in 1970 (Jerger, 1970), immittance measurements began to be incorporated into the routine audiometric test battery (Fig. 20.1). We review established principles and current clinical applications of tympanometry. Important terminology (indicated in italics) is defined in a glossary at the end of the chapter. This chapter emphasizes clinical measurement and applications of tympanometry. Readers who do not have an understanding of the physics of sound or the physical concepts underlying aural immittance, such as vector and rectangular notation, are encouraged to read Chapter 19, basic texts on acoustical physics or technical accounts of tympanometry (e.g., Van Camp et al., 1986).

Tympanometry reflects change in the physical properties of the middle ear system and tympanic membrane (TM) as air pressure in the external ear canal is varied. Tympanometry requires an airtight or *hermetic* seal between the immittance probe cuff and external ear canal walls. Tympanometry begins with the introduction of relatively high (e.g., +200 daPa) or low (e.g., –400 daPa) pressure into the external ear canal. At these pressures, *impedance* (Z) of the middle ear and TM, for practical purposes, is infinitely high and *admittance* (Y) is virtually zero. Therefore, immittance is measured only for the volume of air enclosed within the ear canal between the probe tip and TM. Actually, the volume is measured most accurately by tympanometry at –400 daPa, whereas estimations at +200 daPa may generate a relatively large error (Shanks and Lilly, 1986). In other words, the negative pressure "tail" of the admittance tympanogram is generally lower (closer to zero) than the positive pressure tail.

EAR CANAL VOLUME

Ear canal volume (admittance) is conventionally subtracted from measures of total aural admittance to yield an estimate of middle ear admittance. This is referred to as *compensated* admittance. Ear volume estimation is a routine component of tympanometry with commercially available instruments (Fig. 20.4). Ear canal volumes vary widely as a function of age. For neonates, ear canal volumes are less than 0.50 cm^3 and tympanograms are usually uninterpretable (Geddes, 1987). In one recent investigation, Holte et al. (1991) reported that external auditory canal wall and middle ear mobility, as well as tympanometric characteristics, change over the first 4 months of life. Results of this study demonstrate that resting ear canal diameter changes in response to pneumatic stimulation, and that this change steadily decreases with age until about 56 days of age. One implication of this research is that by 2 months of age, tympanograms in neonates are not affected by external auditory canal movement and hence, may be clinically useful. The topic of tympanometry in newborn infants is discussed in greater detail later in the chapter. Ear canal volumes are in the range of 0.30

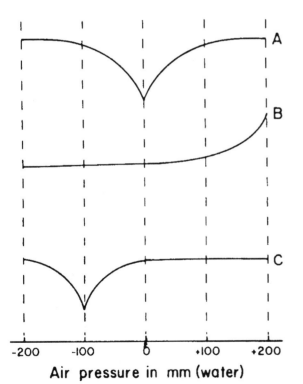

Figure 20.1. Three tympanogram types reproduced from the original article by Jerger (1970) entitled "Clinical Experience with Impedance Audiometry" which introduced the popular classification system. Note that an increase in compliance is plotted downward. See Table 20.1 for methodology of the study and Jerger's definitions of each type.

to 1.00 cm³ in children and 0.65 to 1.75 cm³ in adults (Hall, 1979; Shanks, 1985; Margolis and Heller, 1987; Holte et al., 1991). Volumes are typically somewhat smaller in females than males (Hall, 1979; Margolis and Heller, 1987).

Tympanometry

Single-Component or Single-Frequency Tympanometry

The vast majority of early clinical immittance studies was conducted with single-component or single-frequency tympanometry. With single-component tympanometry, admittance (Y) of the middle ear system increases (Fig. 20.1), and impedance (Z) decreases, as ear canal pressure approaches approximately 0 daPa. At 0 daPa, or often at a slightly negative pressure, such as from 0 to −25 daPa, admittance is maximal (impedance is minimal). Then, with further variation in air pressure (e.g., toward −200 or +200 daPa) the magnitude of these middle ear physical quantities approach their respective baseline values. Immittance values may differ for the positive versus negative pressure extremes, a point that is supported with clinical data in a subsequent section of the chapter. Immittance pressure functions may be recorded continuously on a strip-chart recorder or X-Y plotter, or immittance values at different pressure readings may be plotted manually. With modern computer-based immittance instruments, multiple sequential tympanograms can be averaged to produce a more stable immittance pressure function.

Tympanogram Classification

Over the years, various classification systems for single-component (admittance or impedance), low probe-tone frequency (226 Hz) tympanograms have been reported (Jerger, 1970; Bluestone et al., 1973; Feldman, 1976; Cooper et al., 1982). Jerger's (1970) system is simple and clinically popular. With this system, tympanograms are classified as type A, B, or C (Fig. 20.1), and defined as summarized in Table 20.1. Briefly, the type A, or normal tympanogram, has a peak (point of maximum admittance) at or near normal atmospheric pressure, within the range of 0 to −100 daPa. The peak may actually be slightly positive (e.g., +25 daPa). The type B tympanogram has no distinct point of maximum admittance. As pressure in the ear canal is varied, there is relatively little change in admittance. In some cases, the type B tympanogram is virtually flat. However, the type B tympanogram may more closely resemble a "rounded" type A. In another variation of the type B tympanogram, there is a gradual increase in admittance with pressure change throughout the range of +200 to −400 daPa without a peak. The most common clinical correlate of type B is fluid in the middle ear space. Tympanogram type C

Table 20.1.
Test Protocol and Tympanogram Type Criteria as Reported by Jerger in 1970; Typanometric Data were Reported for 554 Ears of 316 Subjects with Varied Types of Hearing Impairment (Normal Hearing, Conductive Impairment, Sensory-Neural Impairment); Original illustration of Tympanogram Types Is Reproduced in Figure 20.2[a]

Measurement parameters
Instrument: Madsen (type ZO-70) **Probe tone frequency:** 220 Hz **Air pressure range/direction:** +200 to -200 or -400 daPa **Rate of pressure change:** not specified

[a] *Tympanogram type definitions* (Jerger, 1970, p. 312).
Type A: The type A function is characterized by a relatively sharp maximum at or near 0 mm. Type A functions are found in normal and otosclerotic ears.
Type B: The type B functions shows little or no maximum. Compliance remains essentially unchanged over a large range of pressure variation. Type B functions are found in ears with serous or adhesive otitis media.
Type C: In the type C function the maximum is shifted to the left of zero by negative pressure in the middle ear. Slight negative pressure is quite common in many otherwise normal ears, but when the maximum equals or exceeds approximately 100 daPa significant negative pressure in the middle ear may be presumed.

has a distinct point of maximum admittance. The peak, however, occurs when air pressure in the ear canal exceeds −100 daPa relative to normal atmospheric pressure. This tympanogram type usually reflects eustachian tube dysfunction and may be a precursor of serous otitis media. The type C tympanogram may also eventually evolve into a type B.

The three single-component tympanogram types described in Jerger's (1970) classification system (Fig. 20.1 and Table 20.1) adequately differentiate many middle ear pathologic entities. Variations of these types, however, have been described (Fig. 20.2). Reduced mobility of the ossicular chain, as in patients with ossicular or stapes fixation, often produces an A-shallow (A_s) tympanogram. The type A tympanogram may be excessively deep (A_d), reflecting a highly compliant middle ear system (e.g., ossicular chain disruption) or a scarred or flaccid TM (Jerger, 1970). Early investigators noted that a higher probe-tone frequency (such as 600 or 800 Hz) may yield a W-shaped tympanogram or an undulating tympanogram, even in persons with unequivocally normal hearing (Feldman, 1963). Such tympanogram variations are sometimes classified as types D and E (Jerger, 1970).

Static Immittance

Static immittance is acoustic immittance of the middle ear at rest, i.e., under normal atmospheric pressure. Although often calculated during tympanometry, static immittance is in contrast to the immittance-pressure function (tympanogram), which is a dynamic measure

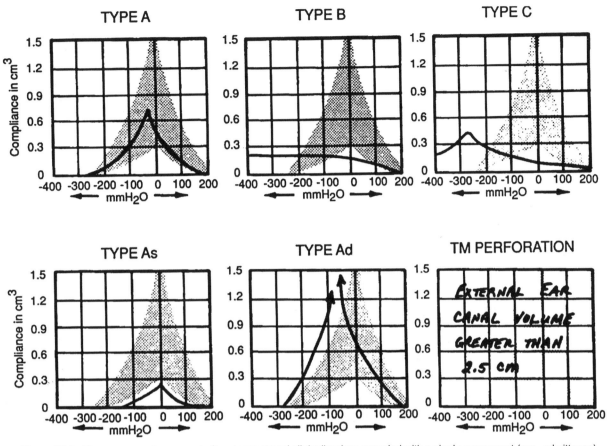

Figure 20.2. Tympanogram types most often encountered clinically when recorded with a single component (e.g., admittance) and a common relatively low (e.g., 226 Hz) probe tone frequency.

of middle ear physical properties. Static immittance is best measured at 226 Hz, for practical and scientific reasons (Van Camp et al., 1986). Clinically, static immittance is determined by first estimating physical volume of air in the external ear canal. This measurement is made at an extreme air pressure that produces minimal compliance. This serves as a baseline with minimal admittance (maximal impedance), as already noted. Then, static immittance of the middle ear system is calculated by subtracting estimated ear canal volume from the peak immittance value from tympanometry. Such calculations, either manual or automatic, may be subject to quantitative error if only vector magnitude information is used (e.g., admittance in single-component instruments), without regard to quantity phase angle (Shanks, 1984). However, calculations based on a 226 Hz probe tone in normal ears probably produce clinically negligible errors.

Normal static immittance values, when measured at 226 Hz and described as compliance of an equivalent volume of air, range from about 0.30 to 1.60 cm^3 (Jerger et al., 1972; Hall, 1979). There are no interaural differences in static compliance (Osterhammel and Osterhammel, 1979). That is, in a group of normal subjects

right and left ear performance is indistinguishable. However, static immittance is influenced to some extent by the age and sex of the patient. Static compliance tends to increase with chronologic age from 1 to 35 years (Jerger et al., 1972; Hall, 1979). The increase during this age range is greater for males than for females. Above age 35 years, static compliance gradually decreases with age. The average values above age 70 years approach the lower limit of the normal range (0.30 cm^3). In general, static compliance is greater in males than in females. However, both the age and sex effects are small with respect to the considerable variability inherent in static compliance measurements and not statistically significant (Osterhammel and Osterhammel, 1979). There are, as Van Camp et al. (1986) point out, little unified normative data on static immittance in physical units, such as admittance in *acoustic mmhos*, collected according to well-defined and clinically applicable methodology.

Early clinical tympanometry research confirmed the usefulness of static immittance in the identification and differentiation of middle ear disorders (e.g., Jerger et al., 1974). Static immittance is characteristically altered by most common middle ear disorders, such as fixation of the ossicular chain, middle ear fluid, and discontinuity of the ossicular chain. Fixation, the mechanical effect on the ossicular chain that usually results from otosclerosis, reduces mobility of the middle ear system. On the average, static compliance values in this disorder are lower, 0.35 cm³, than in the normal population, 0.67 cm³ (Jerger et al., 1974). However, the range of static compliance values for normal ears versus fixed ears overlap to some extent. It is likely that few otosclerotic ears will be identified by static compliance alone. In fact, increased ossicular chain stiffness (the mechanical effect of otosclerosis on middle ear function) is not invariably associated with otosclerosis. Other clinical entities, for example adhesive otitis media, may similarly restrict ossicular chain mobility.

Clearly, when evaluated in isolation static immittance is of little value in the identification and differentiation of middle ear disorders. This is due to the lack of normative data in physical units, the considerable overlap of normal and clinical expectations, and the methodologic factors affecting measurement. However, interpreted in conjunction with other audiometric tests, static immittance can be an important clinical measure of middle ear status. One must always keep in mind, in the clinical interpretation of static immittance values, a fundamental, but often unappreciated, principle of immittance measurements: Although immittance findings reflect the function of the middle ear system, they do not define or diagnose middle ear disease.

Tympanogram Gradient

Finally, *gradient* has received renewed interest as a clinically useful tympanometric parameter (Cooper et al.,

1982; de Jonge, 1986; Koebsell and Margolis, 1986; Tompkins and Hall, 1990). It can be used to supplement measurement of ear canal volume, pressure for peak admittance, and static admittance. An example of one measure of gradient, a computation of tympanogram admittance relative to a pressure range, is illustrated in Figure 20.3. Briefly, a half-amplitude admittance (Y) point is determined on each side (positive and negative pressure directions) by dividing the total amplitude on each side by 2 (Yx-Yc pos/2=Yb, Yx-Yc neg/2=Ya), as in Figure 20.3. The difference in air pressure between each of these points on the slope of the tympanogram (pressure for Ya, Pa; pressure for Yb, Pb) is referred to as delta (difference) pressure (dP) and is stated in daPa.

Each of the tympanograms shown in Figure 20.3 is from a subject with normal hearing sensitivity, including absence of an airbone gap. Subject JH, however, reported that as a child he had numerous ear infections, with frequent spontaneous TM ruptures and myringotomies. Otoscopic examination indicated marked TM scarring. The gradient pressure difference (GdP) for a patient is interpreted in the context of normative data that are either available from the literature or generated for the specific immittance test protocol used in the audiology facility. Normative data reported by deJonge (1986) and Koebsell and Margolis (1986) are summarized in Table 20.2. Referring back to Figure 20.3, the tympanogram Gdp for subject DC is well within the normal region, whereas JH has an abnormally small pressure difference.

The GdP index is quite easy to calculate, which is a clinical asset and, based on the findings of deJonge (1986) and Koebsell and Margolis (1986), contributes information not available from the simple static admit-

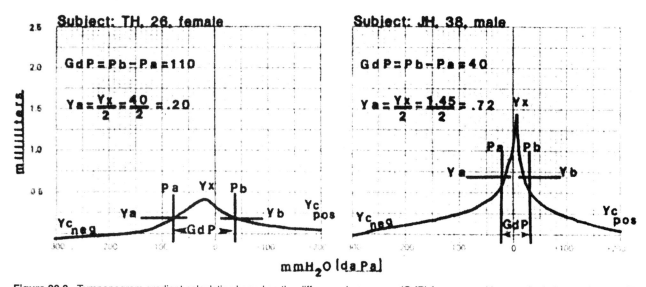

Figure 20.3. Tympanogram gradient calculation based on the difference in pressure (**GdP**) for an ear with normal admittance (subject TH) and an ear with high admittance (JH). Both subjects had normal hearing sensitivity.

Table 20.2.
Normative Data for Children and Adults for Tympanometric Gradient (GdP) Based on the Difference in Pressure between Half-Amplitude Points on the Admittance Tympanogram; Data Were Collected for a 226-Hz Probe Tone Frequency at a Standard Air Pump Speed of 50 daPa/sec; Calculation of GdP Is Described in the Text

Population	Index	GdP (da Pa)
Children[a]	Mean	133
	10th percentile	80
	90th percentile	200
Adults[b]	50th percentile	110
	5th percentile	63
	90th percentile	162

[a]Data for 88 ears of 46 children between the ages of 3.7 and 5.8 years, as reported by Koebsell and Margolis (1986).
[b]Data for right ears of 83 college students with an average age of 22 years, as reported by de Jonge (1986).

tance measures. These investigators speculate that the Gdp may have more desirable sensitivity and specificity characteristics for detection of high impedance (low admittance) middle ear disease. Although this theory is clinically attractive, documentation in patient populations is not yet available. To the contrary, in a study of 80 subjects with otologically confirmed normal middle ear function and 80 subjects with otologically diagnosed otitis media, Tompkins and Hall (1990) found only a few in the otitis media group who would have been classified as normal by conventional tympanometric analysis (i.e., using type A, B, or C). These authors calculated tympanogram gradient both according to ASHA Guidelines for Screening for Middle Ear Disease and Hearing Loss and with the method incorporated into the Grason-Stadler 33 Middle Ear Analyzer. Mean gradient values for the GS 33 were 0.53 for normal ears and abnormally lower (0.20) for otitis media ears. One major clinical limitation for routine use of gradient emerged from this study. The GS 33 did not produce a gradient calculation for lack of a tympanogram peak in approximately one-third of subjects with otitis media. Exact gradient values were lacking for an additional 20 tympanograms with the ASHA method. Thus, it should be recognized that gradient is not applicable to a significant proportion of individuals with otitis media. Further studies of the gradient measure, carried out with real physical units of immittance (such as acoustic ohms or mmho), are required to verify its actual clinical value.

Multiple-Frequency or Multiple-Component Tympanometry

Since the introduction of clinical acoustic immittance, most often measurements have been made using single component, usually compliant reactance, with a single-probe frequency (approximately 226 Hz). There are three likely explanations for this trend. First, until recently, only one manufacturer (Grason-Stadler) marketed an instrument with the capacity for more sophisticated measurements. There are now several different brands available commercially. Second, the most commonly encountered otologic diseases, such as otitis media, eustachian tube dysfunction with TM retraction, or otosclerosis, increase middle ear impedance or stiffness. In many cases, these diseases can be detected and adequately described with a low-frequency probe tone and acoustic compliance (the reciprocal of stiffness). Finally, tympanograms generated for multiple components with higher frequencies tend to be more complex, and not as straightforward to categorize and interpret clinically, as single frequency/single component tympanograms. Van Camp et al. (1986) present three arguments for adding high-frequency two-component tympanometry to the routine immittance test battery. They recommend either 660 or preferably 678 Hz, an integral multiple of 226 Hz. The three arguments for using the higher frequency probe tone are: (a) low-impedance abnormalities produce unique tympanogram shapes only for high-probe frequencies; (b) contralateral acoustic-reflex measurement in both adult and neonatal populations is possible with a higher frequency probe tone. The 226 Hz probe tone is only appropriate for adults, but unsuitable for neonates (Bennett and Weatherby, 1982), as described in more detail later in the chapter, and (c) ipsilateral acoustic reflexes, which are very useful clinically, are contaminated by artifacts at 226 Hz, but not at 660 Hz (Green and Margolis, 1983).

The literature contains comprehensive descriptions of multi-frequency/multi-component tympanometric patterns and the rules used in their clinical application (e.g., Bluestone et al., 1973; Holte et al., 1991; Margolis and Heller, 1987; Margolis and Shanks, 1991; Van Camp et al., 1986). The following is a review of some of the important factors in multi-frequency/multi-component immittance measurement and an outline of the terminology used in the categorization of *susceptance, conductance,* and admittance tympanograms with commercially available equipment (also see Glossary). Additional information found in the references will be invaluable for clinicians preparing to apply these techniques clinically.

Skill in tympanogram pattern recognition and an understanding of one of the existing classification systems are important for the interpretation of multi-component/multi-frequency tympanometry. At this point, clinical conclusions are based primarily on qualitative rather than quantitative analysis. Complexity of tympanograms varies, depending on the number of peaks and troughs (i.e., extrema), for each component at each frequency (Fig.

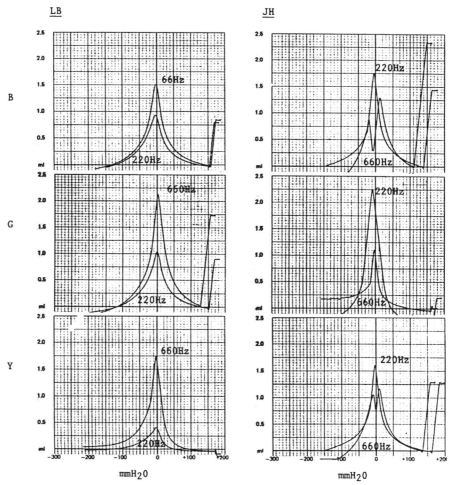

Figure 20.4. Multi-probe frequency, multi-component admittance tympanograms for an ear with scarred tympanic membrane but normal hearing (subject JH from Fig. 3) and a subject with normal tympanometry and normal hearing (subject LB). Pa and Pb refer to the negative and positive pressure values, respectively, of the maximum admittance peaks. Components are as follows: **Y** = admittance; **B** = susceptance; **G** = conductance. Classification of multi-component tympanograms is according to the number of positive and negative peaks (or extrema) that occur for each component (**B, G,** and **Y**). Normal variations are listed in Table 20.3.

20.4). An extrema may be referred to a maximum (increased admittance) or minimum (decreased admittance). The simplest normal pattern has one peak for susceptance (B), one for conductance (G), and one for admittance (Y), or a 1B1G1Y tympanogram. The admittance component is not always included in such classifications. A bell-shaped tympanogram for each component is found for the majority of normal ears, but there are other normal patterns, as displayed in Table 20.3 and illustrated by the curves in Figure 20.4. A pattern occurring in 4.5% of the normal population studied by Creten et al. (1983) is a 3B3G3Y tympanogram. This middle ear is mass controlled at ambient ear canal pressure (0 daPa) and both susceptance and conductance tympanograms have a minimum peak in the center and a maximum on either side. This tympanogram pattern met two criteria to be classified as normal. First, the pressure interval between the two maximum peaks was greater for the suscep-

Table 20.3.
Proportion of Different Types of Normal Multi-component Tympanograms (Adapted from Creten et al., 1985)

Tympanogram Type	Percentage of Subjects
1B 1G 1Y 10°[a]	56.8
3B 1G 1Y 10°	25.8
3B 1G 3Y 10°	2.3
3B 3G 3Y 10°	4.5
3B 3G 3Y 30°	1.5
5B 3G 3Y 30°	9.1

[a]Phase in degrees.

tance than conductance curve. Also, in accordance with data of Van de Heyning et al. (1982) for this 3B3G3Y tympanogram type (at 660 Hz), the two susceptance maxima were within a pressure range of no more than 75 daPa.

This pattern schema includes an admittance phase angle quantity, YФ, because phase was reported in some of the basic studies of multi-frequency, multi-component tympanometry (Creten et al. 1985; Creten et al., 1981; Van Camp et al., 1983). Phase angle measurement is now commercially available on immittance instruments. Another feature of selected modern immittance systems is the sweep-frequency probe tone, as described by Funasaka and Kumakawa (1988), Wada et al., (1989), and Holte et al., 1991) that sweeps several frequencies (e.g., 200–2000 Hz) in a brief period (4 seconds). The reason for this was to develop a stimulus that approximated the frequency response of the middle ear (i.e., 1500 Hz) and better assessed the dynamic characteristics of the middle ear. Advocates of this system report that the sweep-frequency probe is more accurate than conventional tympanometry (which uses a fixed low frequency probe tone) in its assessment of ossicular chain disorders such as discontinuity or fixation. The sweep-frequency probe, although holding promise, has not yet been extensively investigated clinically.

Test Variables in Tympanometry

Introduction. Successful clinical application of tympanometry depends on an appreciation of the influences of test variables including, in addition to probe frequency and the admittance component measured, the direction (positive-to-negative versus negative-to-positive) and rate (e.g., 25, 50, or 100 daPa/second) of pressure change and the number of successive tympanometry trials for a patient while the ear canal remains sealed (Wilson et al., 1984). An excellent summary of research on the effects of direction, and rate, of pressure change is provided by Wilson et al. (1984) and Shanks and Wilson (1986).

Direction of air pressure change in the external ear canal. Direction of pressure change affects tympanometric shape producing a higher incidence of notching, and/or deeper notch, for changes in an ascending (negative to positive) direction. Peak static admittance is also affected by direction. Also, phase angle typically decreases with ascending pressure changes. Finally, tympanometric peak pressure shifts with changes in direction.

At this juncture, it is reasonable to ask whether pressure direction could actually alter clinical interpretation of tympanograms with, e.g., the Jerger classification system. To answer this question, we analyzed tympanometric data for a series of 182 patients undergoing routine tympanometry as part of comprehensive audiologic assessment at the Vanderbilt University Hospital audiology clinic. Admittance tympanograms were recorded with a Grason-Stadler Middle Ear Analyzer. The probe tone was 226 Hz and air pressure within the ear canal was changed at a rate of 50 daPa/second. Tympanograms

for all patients were recorded separately for a positive-to-negative (descending) pressure direction beginning at +200 daPa and also a negative-to-positive (ascending) pressure direction beginning at –300 or –400 daPa. Examples of descending and ascending pressure tympanograms are shown in Figure 20.5.

Clearly, pressure direction can influence the pressure at which the tympanogram peak occurs as well as tympanogram amplitude. Tympanogram pressure peak differences between descending versus ascending ranged from –110 daPa (pressure peak more negative with descending) to +170 daPa (pressure peak more negative with ascending). The average pressure peak difference between the two directions was 31.2 daPa. Overall, most (97%) of the ears showed more negative pressure peaks in the descending direction, whereas only 2% were more negative with ascending and for a mere 1% was there no difference at all. When the peak compliance was greater for the ascending direction, it was as much as 1.15 ml above the descending tympanogram; however, when the descending tympanogram was greater it was only as much as 0.5 ml above the ascending peak. Average amplitude change with direction, however, was minimal (0.1 ml). The majority of ears (62%) had lower amplitude for the descending than the ascending (21%) pressure change. There was no amplitude difference as a function of pressure direction change for 16% of the ears.

We found that the direction of pressure change altered the Jerger classification typing for 23 ears (13% of the total), as summarized in Table 20.4. Two of these ears had confirmed pathologies (otosclerosis and cholesteatoma) that would not have been viewed as abnormal if only the ascending pressure direction were used. The implications of this simple study are evident. In the original tympanometric reports by Jerger in which the now familiar classification system was initially introduced and then documented clinically (Jerger, 1970; Jerger et al., 1972; Jerger et al., 1974), pressure in the external ear canal was varied from positive to negative (usually +200 daPa down to –200, 300, or 400 daPa). This convention should be maintained for valid tympanometric interpretation with the Jerger classification system. Of course, with commercially available immittance instruments pressure can be changed in either direction, usually under manual or automatic control. At least one study has investigated the effect of direction of pressure change on obtaining an airtight seal during tympanometry (Rubenstein et al., 1989). This study suggests that when tympanometry is initiated with an ascending direction of pressure change, there is greater likelihood of maintaining an air-tight seal. This observation, made independently by clinicians, may account for the apparent popularity of routinely using an as-

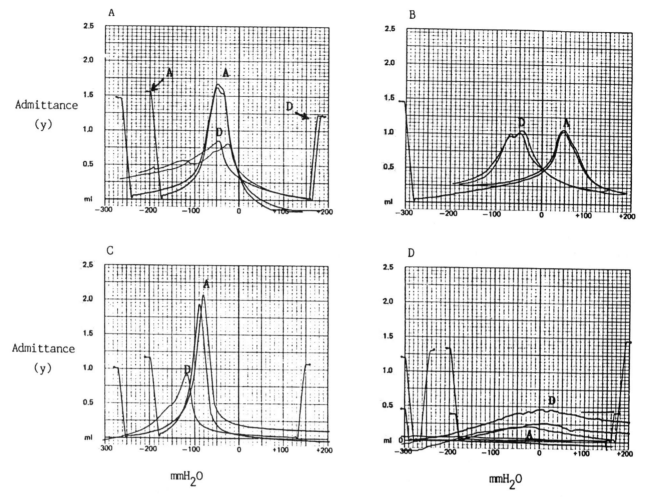

Figure 20.5. Tympanograms recorded from four different patients with positive-to-negative (descending or **D**) and negative-to-positive (ascending or **A**) pressure change. Note the differences in the pres-

sure peak (in mm H_2O) and amplitude (in ml) for tympanograms recorded in each pressure direction. Data on the effect of pressure direction on tympanometry are summarized in Table 20.4.

Table 20.4.
Tympanogram Type (Jerger, 1970) as a Function of Direction of Pressure Change in 186 Ears; Type Descending Refers to the Tympanometric Type that Was Obtained when Recording from Positive to Negative Pressure; Type Ascending Refers to the Classification of the Tympanogram when the Recording Was Made in the Opposite Direction

Type Descending (+ to - Pressure)	Type Ascending (- to + Pressure)					
	A	As	Ad	B	C	Cpos
A	123	0	4	0	7	0
As	7	4	0	0	0	0
Ad	1	0	4	0	0	0
B	0	0	0	2	0	0
C	4	0	0	0	17	0
Cpos	0	0	0	0	0	6

cending pressure technique. Published reports on the effect of pressure change are mixed. Margolis and Shanks (1991) state that "because the effect of direc-

tion of pressure change is small at 226 Hz, it is probably reasonable to use the same norms for both pressure directions" (p. 207). However, our original data confirm the clinical importance of pressure change in tympanometry. A prudent recommendation to clinicians who notice shifts in peak pressure with changes in direction is to average peak pressures recorded with forward and backward tracings, rather than depending on a unidirectional tracing.

Rate of pressure change. In addition to direction of pressure change, rate of pressure change can affect tympanometry. The primary effect of rate is on peak static admittance; i.e., peak static admittance decreases as rate of pressure change increases (Shanks and Wilson, 1986). Conflicting data have been reported on the effect of rate on tympanometric peak pressure. Although some investigators reported no effect of rate of ear canal pressure change on tympanometric peak pressure (Elner et al., 1971; Williams, 1976; Decraemer, 1984), other studies have shown that peak pressure changes as a function of rate (Woodford et al., 1975; Ivarsson et al., 1983; Feldman et al., 1984; Shanks and Wilson, 1986). At least one study has investigated the effects of rapid change in immittance on the temporal response characteristics of different commercially available immittance instruments (Thompson and Robinette, 1988). These investigators reported that temporal characteristics of these devices varied greatly, and that digital systems tended to be faster than analog devices. The temporal response of the immittance unit can confound measures of temporal characteristics (e.g., acoustic reflex response), or affect the tympanometric measures previously discussed.

Developmental changes in tympanometry. Attempts to apply immittance measures, including tympanometry and acoustic reflexes in pediatric populations were a logical step in the search for clinically feasible techniques for objective auditory assessment in children, particularly those who were very young or difficult-to-test with behavioral audiometry (Table 20.5). As a result, published clinical experiences with immittance measures in children are numerous and date back over 20 years (e.g., Feldman, 1963; Bluestone et al., 1973; Jerger et al., 1974; Keith, 1975; Margolis and Popelka, 1975). With the recent introduction of several sophisticated clinical devices

Table 20.5.
Hearing and Tympanometric Criteria for Audiologic and/or Medical Referral (Adapted from American Speech-Language-Hearing Association, 1990)

I. History
    A. Otalgia
    B. Otorrhea
II. Visual Inspection of the Ear
    A. Structural defect of the ear, head, or neck
    B. Ear canal abnormalities
        1. blood or effusion
        2. occlusion
        3. inflammation
        4. excessive cerumen, tumor, foreign material
    C. Eardrum abnormalities
        1. abnormal color
        2. bulging ear drum
        3. fluid line or bubbles
        4. perforation
        5. retraction
III. Identification Audiometry
    Fail air conduction screening at 20 dB HL at 1000, 2000, or 4000 Hz in either ear (see ASHA, 1985 for further definition). These criteria may require alteration for various clinical settings and populations.
IV. Tympanometry
    A. Flat tympanogram and equivalent ear canal volume (V$_{ec}$) outside normal range.
    B. Low static admittance (peak Y) on two successive occurrences in a 4- to 6-week interval.
    C. Abnormally wide tympanometric width (TW) on two successive occurrences in a 4- to 6-week interval.

for multi-component, multi-frequency immittance measurements, there has been a resurgence in research of tympanometry in children in general, and newborn infants in particular (Gates et al., 1986; Geddes, 1987; Marchant et al., 1986).

Holte et al. (1991) reported the most comprehensive investigation of tympanometric maturation. Differences between the middle ear properties of neonates versus older children and adults, as assessed by tympanometry, have long been appreciated (Keith, 1975; Bennett, 1975; Himmelfarb et al., 1979; Margolis and Popelka, 1975). Among the characteristic features of neonatal tympanograms are double peaks, even at low probe tone frequencies (e.g., 226 Hz). This indicates that the neonatal middle ear system is dominated more by mass and resistance than the adult middle ear system, which is mostly controlled by compliance. It is also commonly assumed that hypermobility of the ear canal wall confounds tympanometry in infants, although there is no published experimental confirmation of this popular assumption.

Holte et al. (1991) studied ear canal mobility and acoustic (tympanic membrane and middle ear) susceptance, conductance, and admittance over the age range of 1 day to 4 months in 23 healthy, full-term newborn infants using commercially available instrumentation (Virtual 310). Examples of their findings are illustrated in Figures 20.6 and 20.7. First, on the basis of video recordings of ear canal wall movement, these authors dispel the belief that ear canal mobility is the sole factor producing atypical tympanogram shapes in neonates. Tympanometric changes as a function of age in infants are clear from the data displayed in Figures 20.6 and 20.7. The age-related changes can be summarized as follows: (*a*) the mass and resistive components of tympanic membrane/middle ear function are indeed more pronounced for neonates than for older children and adults; (*b*) related to this finding, phase angle increases with age reflecting a greater role of middle ear compliance; (*c*) resonant frequency of the middle ear increases as a function of age; (*d*) admittance amplitude (magnitude) increases with age; (*e*) the direction of air pressure change was an important factor in neonatal tympanometry; (*f*) less than 1 month old, a positive-to-negative pressure change is definitely preferable because ear canal collapse was often caused with a negative-to-positive (ascending) pressure; (*g*) there was considerable, unexplained intersubject variability in admittance in these healthy neonates, arguing against the usefulness of normative data for probe frequencies of 450 Hz and higher in this population (Table 20.6); and (*h*) less than 4 months old, multi-component tympanograms at only 226 Hz are recommended since higher frequencies produce highly variable tympanograms that are difficult to

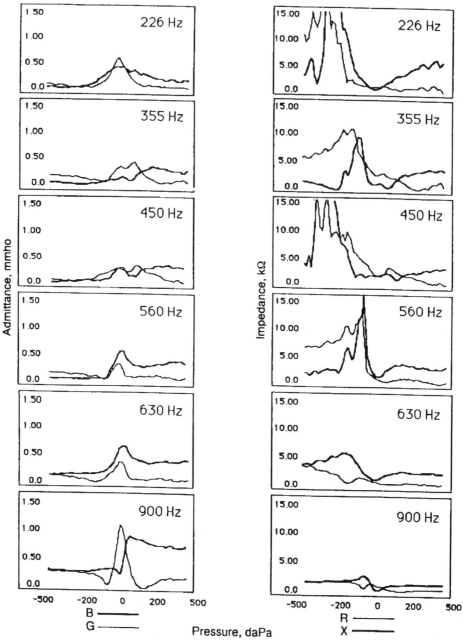

Figure 20.6. Multi-component tympanograms recorded from one ear of a neonate at 2 days of age. Pressure change was from positive-to-negative (descending). Components are as follows: **B** = susceptance; **G** = conductance; **R** = resistance; **X** = absolute value of reactance (From Holte et al., 1991).

interpret (using the model described earlier in this chapter and displayed in Table 20.3).

It is likely that the current excitement about otoacoustic emissions as a tool for pediatric auditory assessment (Norton and Widen, 1990; Stevens et al., 1990) will fuel further interest in infant tympanometry. Otoacoustic emissions are not recorded from patients with abnormal middle ear function. Tympanometry in neonates might contribute to the screening and diagnostic

value of otoacoustic emissions by differentiation of middle ear versus cochlear dysfunction.

The Role of Tympanometry

The effect of different variables encourages restraint and caution in clinical application of tympanometry. As noted above, diagnosis of middle ear disease can rarely be made on the basis of tympanometry alone (Gates et al., 1986; Shanks, 1984; Van Camp et al.,

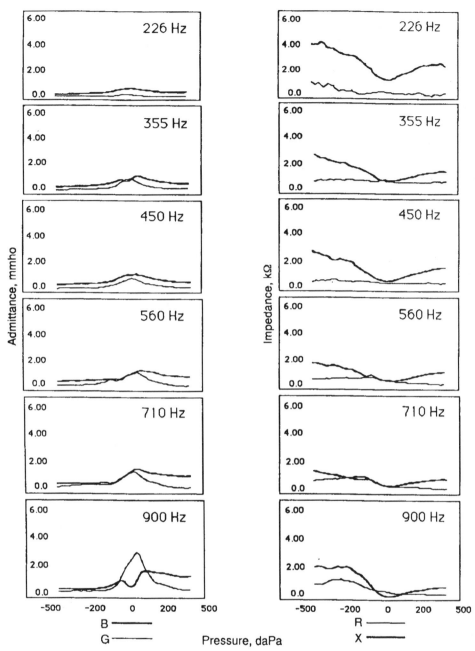

Figure 20.7. Multi-component tympanograms recorded from one ear of a neonate at 62 days of age. Tympanometric data from this infant at 2 days of age are shown in Figure 20.6. Pressure change was from positive-to-negative (descending) at a rate of 250 daPa/sec. Components are as follows: **B** = susceptance; **G** + conductance; **R** = resistance; **X** + absolute value of reactance. (From Holte et al., 1991).

1986), whereas routine otoscopic examination is sufficiently sensitive for differential diagnosis of certain diseases (Hall and Ghorayeb, 1991). Furthermore, as Van Camp et al. (1986) point out, the sensitivity of tympanometry exceeds specificity. In other words, middle ear disease will generally be detected by an abnormal tympanometric pattern (high sensitivity), but it is not uncommon to record abnormal patterns in normal ears as well. However, the converse relation may also occur. For example, Muchnik et al. (1989)

studied the clinical validity of static admittance measures in 42 confirmed otosclerotic ears using 220 and 660 Hz probe tones. They found no significant differences between otosclerotic and normal ears as a function of probe tone frequency. It is of interest that normal or above-normal compliance was found in 67% of the otosclerotic ears. Furthermore, one disease may produce distinctly different tympanograms in different patients. These clinical problems are certainly not unique to tympanometry. Confirmation, or

Table 20.6.
Interim Normative Data for Static Admittance (Peak Y), Equivalent Ear Canal Volume (V$_{cc}$), and Typanometric Width (TW) Suggested in Guidelines for Screening Hearing Impairment and Middle-Ear Disorders (adapted from American Speech-Language-Hearing Association, 1990)[a]

Group	Admittance Measure		
	Peak Y (mmho or cc)	Vec (cc)	TW (daPa)
Children (age 3–5 years)			
Mean	0.5	0.7	100
(90% range)	(0.2–0.9)	(0.4–1.0)	(60–100)
Adults			
mean	0.8	1.1	80
(90% range)	(0.3–1.4)	(0.6–1.5)	(50–100)

[a]Data are from Margolis and Heller (1987) and were collected with an acoustic immittance instrument with a 226 Hz probe tone, a pump speed of 200 daPa/sec, and automatically compensated era canal volume.

cross-check of the results of a single test procedure, such as tympanometry, with independent measures of auditory function, such as puretone audiometry, is a proper clinical practice (Jerger and Hayes, 1976). We find the form illustrated in Figure 20.8 quite useful for rapid detection of the pattern of clinical audiometric findings, including tympanometry. By plotting puretone, speech, and immittance data on the same sheet, separately for each ear, it is possible to correlate at a glance tympanometry with independent auditory measures. This point was emphasized in a recent review of middle ear pathology and conductive hearing loss (Hall and Ghorayeb, 1991).

Attitudes Toward Tympanometry by Physicians

The clinical effectiveness of tympanometry has been restricted, in part, due to its limited acceptance in the medical profession. Apart from audiology and otolaryngology, few other health care disciplines have realized the potential use of tympanometry. This is particularly important for the pediatrician, family practice physician, health nurse, and other health care providers who may encounter patients with middle ear disorders. Teele (1983) reported that otitis media accounts for more than one-third of all office visits to the pediatrician. Our experience suggests that the pediatrician treats otitis media more often than the otolaryngologist, who typically sees only the chronic cases. If tympanometry is clinically valuable, why then is it not widely used within the medical community?

The predictive value of tympanometry in middle ear effusion has been well established by otolaryngology (e.g., Gates et al., 1986). Despite this experimental evi-

dence, there continues to be debate even among otolaryngologists as to the benefit of tympanometry. Stoney and Rogers (1989) surveyed more than 300 otolaryngologists throughout the United Kingdom about their reliance upon immittance audiometry in managing middle ear disorders. These authors reported that only 17% of the physicians surveyed responded that they used immittance routinely for every otologic patient. Of those who used the technique, only about one-half reported that it was a "very useful" aid in making their clinical diagnosis. These authors further criticize the attitude of the profession of audiology toward tympanometry as "simplistic." They called for a more critical attitude toward tympanometry, contending that it is not the panacea diagnostic measure that the audiology world would make it out to be.

The validity of the questionnaire survey by Stoney and Rogers was questioned by Haggard and Lutman (1990). Haggard and Lutman (1990) further cited four advantages of tympanometry that were overlooked by Stoney and Rogers. First, tympanometry is easy to perform. This advantage is particularly enhanced with recently introduced hand-held tympanometric devices, such as the "MicroTymp" (illustrated in Fig. 20.9). Second, comparison of data from different clinicians or different test sites is straightforward for tympanometry, but not for conventional otoscopy. Three, immittance measures provide a cross-check advantage when they are included as part of a clinical battery. Finally, immittance audiometry documents the persistence of otitis media with effusion and the results of treatment. It is possible that this type of disagreement regarding the benefit of tympanometry has contributed to the evolution of clinical alternatives to tympanometry, such as the pneumatic otoscope and the acoustic otoscope.

PNEUMATIC OTOSCOPY AND ACOUSTIC REFLECTIVITY

The pneumatic otoscope has a rubber bulb joined by rubber tubing to the head of the otoscope. This device permits routine otoscopy while introducing air pressure so that movement of the tympanic membrane can be visualized. Pneumatic otoscopy is simple, expedient, and can be reliable in the hands of an experienced clinician. Pneumatic otoscopy preceded tympanometry. However, in recent years its clinical usefulness has been seriously questioned by those most likely to use it—the otolaryngologist and the pediatrician.

Studies that have compared the efficiency of pneumatic otoscopy and tympanometry in detecting middle ear effusion have provided mixed results. One recent investigation compared the predictive accuracy of both procedures independently, and in conjunction with one another (Toner and Mains, 1990). For 222 ears preoperatively examined with middle ear effusion, there was essentially no difference in sensitivity between tympanometry (89%) and pneumatic otoscopy (88%). Furthermore, there was no significant increase in their predictive accuracy when used in conjunction. Conversely, after reviewing investigations of this controversy, Barr (1990) concluded that the best results will be ascertained from a combination of pneumatic otoscopy and tympanometry. In another study, Cavanaugh (1989) reported that a significant disadvantage of pneumatic otoscopy is its subjectivity due to lack of standardization, and wide variations in its delivered pressure (ranging from 338 to 1134 daPa). From this review it is evident that debate on the validity of pneumatic otoscopy versus tympanometry continues.

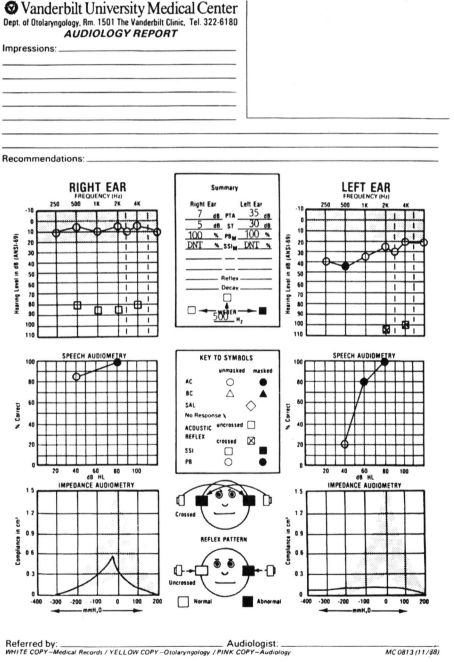

Figure 20.8. Auditory findings for a young child with unilateral (left ear) otitis media with effusion. Audiometric pattern, including pure tone, speech, and immittance (tympanograms and acoustic reflexes) is consistent with the diagnosis of otitis media with effusion, and defines the type and degree of hearing loss. Tympanograms interpreted in isolation do not adequately describe auditory status.

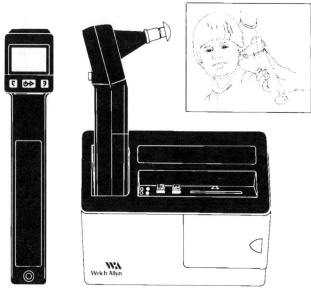

Figure 20.9. The Micro Tymp analyzer, a hand-held (10 ounce) tympanometer. Tympanogram is displayed with a liquid crystal diode (LCD) readout and can be printed on a miniature strip chart that includes guidelines for interpretation (Courtesy of Welch Allyn, Skaneateles Falls, NY).

The advent of the acoustic reflectivity otoscope has attempted to reconcile some of the aforementioned differences by combining tympanometry with the pneumatic otoscope in one instrument. This is a hand-held device (Fig. 20.10) that is similar to an otoscope, except that it has a speaker that generates a tone (80 dB SPL) across several frequencies (2000–4500 Hz) in a brief period (100 ms). A built-in microphone receives acoustic energy that is reflected off the tympanic membrane, and the reflected energy is then compared with the transmitted sound. This instrument operates on the 1⁄4 wavelength theory; i.e., a sound wave traveling in a tube that is closed at one end will be almost completely reflected when it strikes the closed end. The reflected wave will then cancel the transmitted wave at a distance one-fourth the wavelength from the closed end of the tube, in this case the tympanic membrane. The greater the sound reflection, the greater the likelihood of middle ear effusion. The level of sound reflected is indicated on the instrument as units of reflectivity from 0 to 9. The higher the reflectivity, the more likely the presence of fluid. Precise criteria may vary for different protocols; however, a reflectivity of ≤2 is a pass, 3–5 is considered at risk, and ≥6 fails the screening (Oyiboro et al., 1987; Schwartz and Schwartz, 1987).

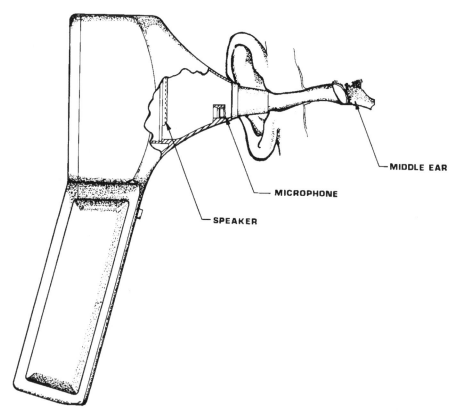

Figure 20.10. Acoustic Otoscope for measurement of acoustic reflectometry (sonar) and detection of middle ear disorders. A series of calibrated frequency sweeps are presented to the ear canal (no hermetic seal is required) and reflected sound is analyzed automatically. Graphic display provides guidelines for interpretation as normal versus abnormal (Courtesy of ENT Medical Devices, Wareham, MA).

In the 5 years or so since its introduction, several investigations have been reported concerning acoustic reflectivity. Initial reports advocated this procedure as a screening device claiming it was faster, and more sensitive and specific in its detection of middle ear effusion than tympanometry and pneumatic otoscopy (Oyiboro, et al., 1987; Schwartz and Schwartz, 1987; Wazen et al., 1988). The limitations of these early studies of reflectivity either were not confirmed by myringotomy, or else results were only evaluated for the presence/absence of fluid without regard to other tympanic membrane abnormalities (e.g., type C, type A_d, and type A_s). The reported test sensitivity and specificity of this procedure is unclear. Various studies report sensitivity for acoustic reflectivity to middle ear effusion ranging from 54 to 94%, and specificity from 59 to 89% (Lampe and Schwartz, 1989). One of the first reports that questioned the efficacy of reflectivity in pediatrics compared results of reflectivity with actual findings upon myringotomy (Macknin et al., 1987). These investigators performed reflectivity on 198 ears just before surgery, with at least three readings for each ear. Of the patients who had middle ear effusion, test sensitivity was 76% or less, and specificity was less than 60%, using a reflectivity cutoff of 5 units.

Combs (1988, 1989, 1991) investigated acoustic reflectivity and offered two important observations. First, a significant amount of false positives and false negatives with acoustic reflectivity, as conventionally measured, may be the product of a "double reflectivity." Combs speculates that this double reflectivity may be the result of tympanic membrane abnormalities such as scarring, or pockets of air in effusion which distorts the shape of the membrane. In such cases, the reflected sound is distorted into two reflected echoes. This phenomenon can be documented with a chart recorder, and may be diagnostically useful. A second observation resulted from Combs' inspection of all acoustic reflectivity instruments. He found that variance showed a SD of 0.4 reflectivity units across instruments. This finding demonstrates that care should be taken to routinely check the calibration of the instrument. In his most recent publication on the topic, Combs (1991) provides evidence that the shape of the tracings (curve) produced by the acoustic otoscope, with a recorder, and the angle formed by the dip in reflectivity, contribute to accurate differentiation of normal versus abnormal ears. By taking into account all possible data obtained with a relatively new device, the acoustic otoscope with recorder (AOR), sensitivity increases to 98.7% and specificity to 94.5% (Combs, 1991). Acoustic reflectivity appears to hold promise as a practical, expedient screening device for middle ear effusion.

USE OF TYMPANOMETRY IN SCREENING PROGRAMS

Tympanometry is increasingly included in auditory screening protocols (see Chapter 30). Several states, such as Minnesota, have established guidelines for using tympanometry in screening programs (Minnesota, 1990). Bonny (1989) reported on a school screening program that combined immittance measures and puretone audiometry. Results of 16,500 auditory screenings performed over a 5-year period indicated that tympanometry significantly enhanced the effectiveness of the screening. Of particular importance was detection of middle ear conditions that required medical treatment, but that did not reduce the puretone thresholds below the referral criterion. Screening tympanometry, even in the primary care physician's office, has been given an additional boost with the advent of commercially available hand-held tympanometric devices, such as the MicroTymp analyzer illustrated in Figure 20.8.

Other studies have cautioned that although tympanometry should be included as part of the screening program, mass one-time tympanometric screening may not be productive. Results of this line of research have shown that a one-time finding of an abnormal tympanogram are correlated with, but not diagnostic of, middle ear effusion and prevalence of middle ear effusion (Wolthers, 1990). Furthermore, more than one-half of all cases of otitis media with effusion may resolve simultaneously (Zielhus, 1989). This research suggests that only when positive screening results are obtained should the screening be followed up with repeated, and more frequent, screening.

Audiometric screenings are usually associated with pediatric populations; however, there is evidence to suggest that tympanometry is also a useful screening test for treatable hearing loss in the elderly (Davies et al., 1988). In addition to the expected high incidence of presbycusis, this study found that 30% of the elderly subjects evaluated had middle and external ear anomalies ranging from impacted cerumen to cholesteatoma. Audiometric screening including tympanometry can obviously be productive for this population, particularly in settings such as residential care facilities.

From the preceding review, it is clear that tympanometry has a secure role in clinical audiology. We concur with Lilly (1984) that "the time is past for audiologists and manufacturers to debate the relative merits of low-frequency versus middle frequency probe tones" and "to debate the relative merits of acoustic impedance, acoustic admittance. . ." (p. 307). The time has come for increasing the use of combinations of instrumentation, techniques, and immittance quantities in clinical aural immittance measurement to most effectively describe the middle ear function of given patients.

ACKNOWLEDGMENTS

Preparation of this chapter was supported, in part, by a scholarship for doctoral study provided to the second author by the United States Department of Defense (U.S. Army).

REFERENCES

Barr G. Letter: Pneumatic otoscopy and tympanometry. Br J General Pract 1990;40:124.

Bennett MJ. Acoustic impedance bridge measurements with the neonate. Br J Audiol 1975;9:117–124.

Bonny IC. Five years' experience of combined impedance and audiometric screening at school entry. Public Health 1989;103:427–431.

Cavanaugh RM. Pediatricians and the pneumatic otoscope: are we playing it by ear? Pediatrics 1989;84:362–364.

Combs JT. Single versus double acoustic reflectometry tracings. Pediat Infect Dis J 1989;8:616–620.

Combs JT. Predictive value of the angle of acoustic reflectometry. Pediat Infect Dis J 1991;10:214–216.

Cooper JC, Jr, Hearne EM, III, and Gates GA. Normal tympanometric shape. Ear Hear 1982;3:241–245.

Creten WL, Van de Heyning PH, and Van Camp KJ. Immittance audiometry: normative data at 200 and 660 Hz. Scand Audiol 1985; 14:115–121.

Davies JE, John DG, Jones AH, and Stephens SD. Tympanometry as a screening test for treatable hearing loss in the elderly. Br J Audiol 1988;22:119–121.

deJonge R. Normal tympanometric gradient: A comparison of three methods. Audiology 1986;25:299–308.

Funasaka S, and Kumakawa K. Tympanometry using a sweep-frequency probe tone and its clinical evaluation. Audiology 1989; 27:99–108.

Gates G, Avery C, Cooper J, Hearne E, and Holt G. Predictive value of tympanometry in middle ear effusion. Ann Otol Rhinol Laryngol 1986;95:46–50.

Geddes N. Tympanometry and the stapedial reflexes in the first five days of life. Int J Pediat Otorhinolaryngol 1987;13:293–297.

Grontved A, Krogh H, Christensen P, Jensen P, Schousboe H, and Hentzer E. Monitoring middle ear pressure by tympanometry. Acta Otolaryngol 1989;108:101–106.

Groothuis JR, Selle SHW, Wright PF, Thompson JM, and Altemeier WA. Otitis media in infancy: tympanometric findings. Pediatrics 1979;63:435–442.

Haggard MP, and Lutman ME. Appropriate attitudes to tympanometry. J Laryngol Otol 1990;104:172–174.

Hall JW. Contemporary tympanometry. Semin Hear 1987;8:319–327.

Hall JW III. Effects of age and sex on static compliance. Arch Otolaryngol 1979;105:601–605.

Hall JW III. The Acoustic Reflex in Central Auditory Dysfunction. In Pinheiro ML, and Musiek FE, Eds. Assessment of Central Auditory Dysfunction: Foundations and Clinical Correlates. Baltimore: Williams & Wilkins, 1985:103–130.

Hall JW III, and Ghorayeb BY. Diagnosis of middle ear pathology and evaluation of conductive hearing loss. In Jacobson JT, and Northern JL, Eds. Diagnostic Audiology. Austin, TX: PRO-ED, 1991.

Himmelfarb MZ, Popelka GR, and Shanon E. Tympanometry in normal neonates. J Speech Hear Res 1979;22:179–191.

Holte L, Cavanaugh R, and Margolis R. Ear canal wall mobility and tympanometric shape in young infants. J Pediat 1990;117:77–80.

Holte L, and Margolis RH. Screening tympanometry. Semin Hear 1987;8:329–337.

Holte L, Margolis RH, and Cavanaugh RM, Jr. Developmental changes in multifrequency tympanograms. Audiology 1991;30:1–24.

Jerger J, Jerger S, and Mauldin L. Studies in impedance audiometry. I. Normal and sensori-neural ears. Arch Otolaryngol 1972; 96:513–523.

Jerger JF. Clinical experience with impedance audiometry. Arch Otolaryngol 1970;92:311–324.

Jerger JF, Jerger S, and Mauldin L. Studies in impedance audiometry. I. Normal and sensorineural ears. Arch Otolaryngol 1972;96: 513–523.

Keith RW. Impedance audiometry with neonates. Arch Otolaryngol Head Neck Surg 1973;97:465–467.

Kobayashi T, Okitsu T, and Takasaka T. Forward-backward tracing tympanometry. Acta Otolaryngol 1987;435(Suppl):100–106.

Koebsell KA, and Margolis RH. Tympanometric gradient measured from normal preschool children. Audiology 1986;25:149–157.

Lilly DJ. Multiple frequency, multiple component tympanometry: New approaches to an old diagnostic problem. Ear Hear 1984; 5:300–308.

Macknin M, Skibinski C, Beck G, Hughes G, and Kinney S. Acoustic reflectometry detection of middle ear effusion. Pediat Infect Dis J 1987;6:866–868.

Marchant CD, McMillan PM, Shurin PA, Johnson CE, Turczyk VA, Feinsten JC, and Panek DM. Diagnosis of otitis media in early infancy by tympanometry and ipsilateral acoustic reflex thresholds. J Pediatr 1986;109:590–595.

Margolis R, and Heller J. Screening tympanometry: Criteria for medical referral. Audiology 1987;26:197–208.

Margolis R, and Popelka G. Interactions among tympanometric variables. J Speech Hear Res 1977;20:447–462.

Margolis R, and Smith P. Tympanometric asymmetry. J Speech Hear Res 1977;20:437–446.

Margolis RH, and Popelka GR. Static and dynamic acoustic impedance measurements in infant ears. J Speech Hear Res 1975;18:-435–453.

Metz O. The acoustic impedance measured on normal and pathological ears. Acta Otolaryngol (Stockh) 1946;63(Suppl).

Minnesota Department of Health. Letter: Tympanometry screening. Minn Med 1990;73:9.

Muchnik C, Hildesheimer M, Rubinstein M, and Gleitman Y. Validity of tympanometry in cases of confirmed otosclerosis. J Laryngol Otol 1989;103:36–38.

Naunton RF. A masking dilemma in bilateral conduction deafness. Arch Otolaryngol 1960;72:753–757.

Norton SJ, and Widen JE. Evoked otoacoustic emissions in normal-hearing infants and children: emerging data and issues. Ear Hear 1990;11:121–127.

Osterhammel D, and Osterhammel P. Age and sex variations for the normal stapedial reflex thresholds and tympanometric compliance values. Scand Audiol 1979;8:153–158.

Oyiborhoro J, Olaniyan S, Newman C, and Balakrishnan S. Efficacy of acoustic otoscope in detecting middle ear effusion in children. Laryngoscope 1987;97:495–498.

Reidel C, Wiley T, and Block M. Tympanometric measures of eustachian tube function. J Speech Hear Res 1987;30:207–214.

Rubenstein A, Ribler A, Emmer M, and Silman M. Effect of direction of pressure change on obtaining airtight seals in tympanometry. Scand Audiol 1989;18:125–126.

Schwartz D, and Schwartz R. Validity of acoustic reflectometry in detecting middle ear effusion. Pediatrics 1987;79:739–742.

Shanks JE. Tympanometry. Ear Hear 1984;5:268–280.

Shanks JE, and Lilly DJ. An evaluation of tympanometric estimates of ear canal volume. J Speech Hear Res 1981;24:557–566.

Shanks JE, and Wilson RH. Effects of direction and rate of ear-canal pressure changes on tympanometric measures. J Speech Hear Res 1986;29:11–19.

Stevens JC, Webb HD, Hutchinson J, Connell J, Smith MF, and Buffin JT. Click evoked otoacoustic emissions in neonatal screening. Ear Hearing 1990;11:128–133.

Stoney PJ, and Rogers JH. Attitudes to tympanometry. J Laryngol Otol 1989;103:657–658.

Thompson D, and Robinette L. Temporal characteristics of aural acoustic immittance instruments. Ear Hear 1988;9:290–294.

Tompkins SM, and Hall JW III. Comparison of two gradient methods in normal ears versus otitis media. J Am Acad Audiol 1990;1:49–50 [abstract].

Tower J, and Mains B. Pneumatic otoscopy and tympanometry in the detection of middle ear effusion. Clin Otolaryngol 1990; 15:121–123.

VanCamp KJ, Margolis RH, Wilson RH, Creten WL, and Shanks JE. Principles of Tympanometry. Rockville, MD: ASHA Press, 1986.

Wada H, Kobayashi T, Suetake M, and Tachizaki H. Dynamic behavior of the middle ear based on sweep frequency tympanometry. Audiology 1989;28:127–134.

Wazen J, Ferraro J, and Hughes R. Clinical evaluation of a portable, cordless, hand-held middle ear analyzer. Otolaryngol Head Neck Surg 1988;99:348–350.

Wiley T. Static acoustic admittance measures in normal ears: a combined analysis for ears with and without notched tympanograms. J Speech Hear Res 1989;32:688.

Wiley T, Oviatt D, and Block M. Acoustic immittance measures in normal ears. J Speech Hear Res 1987;30:161–170.

Wilson RH, Shanks JE, and Kaplan SK. Tympanometric changes at 226 Hz and 678 Hz across ten trials and for two directions of ear-canal pressure change. J Speech Hear Res 1984;27:257–266.

Wolthers OD. Tympanometric screening in children on admission to a pediatric ward: A preliminary study. Int J Pediat Otorhinolaryngol 1990;19:251–257.

Zielhus G, Rach G, and van den Broek P. Screening for otitis media with effusion in preschool children. Lancet 1989;1:311–313.

CHAPTER 21

The Acoustic Reflex

Jerry L. Northern and Sandra Abbott Gabbard

Interpretation of the stapedius muscle reflex is one of the most powerful diagnostic techniques available in clinical audiology. Scientists have long been aware that the stapedius muscles contract bilaterally to the presence of a sufficiently loud sound. Since publication of the classic monograph by Metz (1946), audiologists have realized the immense diagnostic value of this simple physiologic reflex. In his study of clinical patients, Metz carefully documented the role of stapedial muscle contraction in patients with conductive and sensory-neural hearing loss. He described acoustic reflex elicitation in patients with unilateral facial paralysis, and in patients with unilateral total deafness. Metz' early investigations stimulated hundreds of studies of the middle ear muscles and subsequently the clinical applications of acoustic reflex measurement.

In lower mammals bilateral contraction of both middle ear muscles, the stapedius and tensor tympani, occurs to loud sound. In humans, only the stapedius muscle contracts to acoustic stimuli and the tensor tympani contracts as a response to nonacoustic stimuli such as touch and pressure. In this chapter, reference to the acoustic reflex refers to contraction of the stapedius muscles unless otherwise indicated.

This chapter will review the fundamental anatomy and physiology of the stapedial muscles and neural pathways innervating the acoustic reflex. However, the focus of the material will be on acoustic reflex threshold measurements and specialized diagnostic application of various test techniques. Despite the fact that the acoustic reflex is relatively easy to measure with today's immittance meters, skillful interpretation of acoustic reflex results requires the utmost in audiologic acumen.

ANATOMY AND PHYSIOLOGY OF THE ACOUSTIC REFLEX

Functions of the Stapedius Muscle

The stapedius muscle is attached to the posterior side of the neck of the stapes and is the smallest muscle in the body. The reflex contraction after a loud acoustic stimulus causes the stapes footplate to swing outward and backward from the oval window. This action limits the motion of the ossicles and attenuates the vibration of the stapes footplate, thereby reducing the fluid motion of the inner ear. Historically, this action has been considered a mechanism that helps to protect the inner ear from damage due to loud sounds, especially at low frequencies (Wever and Lawrence, 1954).

Simmons (1964) challenges the classic "protection theory" (also known as the "intensity-control" theory) that asserts the stapedial muscle acts to safeguard the inner ear against overstimulation by intense sounds. Although intratympanic muscles exist in numerous species of mammals, Simmons questions where in nature one finds sounds loud enough to produce stapedial reflex contraction to protect the cochlea from acoustic trauma. He provides experimental data that show that middle ear muscles are active in a number of common daily events, many of which are totally unrelated to the presence of external acoustic input. Through research with electrodes implanted in cat middle ear muscles, Simmons describes three functions of reflex activity: (a) continual ongoing changes in muscle tonus, (b) contractions to acoustic stimuli, and (c) contractions associated with other motor events, such as chewing and vocalization.

The changes in muscle tonus are regulated by the animal's level of alertness, and according to Simmons' hypothesis, this modulation provides a means by which an auditory signal can be separated from background environmental noise, as well as a mechanism for allowing attention to continuous sound. The use of acoustic reflex contractions may help isolate novel stimuli to quickly identify whether a sound of unknown origin is from an internal physiologic noise or from an environmental source. The muscle contractions that occur with vocalizations, head movements, and chewing may serve to attenuate low frequency body noise while preserving the ear's sensitivity for high frequency external sounds.

The Neural Acoustic Reflex Pathways

Our current understanding of the acoustic stapedius reflex pathway is based primarily on experimental study of the rabbit (Borg, 1973, 1976).

The stapedius muscle is innervated by the facial nerve (cranial nerve VII) and the tensor tympani muscle is innervated by the trigeminal nerve (cranial nerve V). The neural network of the stapedial (acoustic) reflex is located in the lower brainstem and consists of both ipsilateral and contralateral routes. During loud acoustic stimulation, the ipsilateral pathway begins with impulses from cochlear sensory cells that are transmitted by acoustic nerves to the ipsilateral ventral cochlear nucleus. The majority of axons from the ventral cochlear nucleus, which are involved in the ipsilateral acoustic reflex, pass through the trapezoid body to the medial part of the facial motor nucleus, then down through the facial nerve to the ipsilateral stapedius muscle. Some nerve fibers pass from the ventral cochlear nucleus through the trapezoid body to the ipsilateral medial superior olivary complex. From the ipsilateral medial superior olive nucleus, impulses are transmitted to the medial part of the ipsilateral facial motor nucleus. Thus, the ipsilateral stapedius reflex consists of mainly three, but in some cases four, neurons (Djupesland, 1980).

The contralateral acoustic reflex arc always contains four neurons. From the acoustic nerve and the ventral cochlear nucleus, impulses are transmitted to the medial superior olive and across to the contralateral facial motor nucleus. The fourth neuron transmits the impulse from the contralateral facial motor nucleus to the contralateral stapedius muscle. When either ear is activated by an appropriately loud sound, both ipsilateral and contralateral stapedial muscles contract in reflex fashion as shown in Figure 21.1.

Thompson (1983) suggests that although Borg's (1973) description of the acoustic stapedius reflex pathway is the best currently available, the complexity of reciprocal connections among the many motor and sensory nuclei of the lower brainstem implies that more elaborate, multisynaptic pathways may be involved. The acoustic reflex response depends on adequate physiologic function of the entire reflex arc including the sensory receptors (cochlea), and afferent neurons (eighth nerve), interneurons (brainstem), efferent neurons (seventh nerve), and an effector organ (stapedial muscle). The specific site of pathologic involvement within the acoustic reflex arc is determined by comparing stapedial reflexes between crossed (contralateral) and uncrossed (ipsilateral) stimulation (Jerger and Jerger, 1983; Jerger, 1980).

A   IPSILATERAL STAPEDIUS REFLEX PATHWAYS

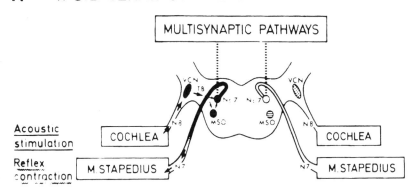

B   CONTRALATERAL STAPEDIUS REFLEX PATHWAYS

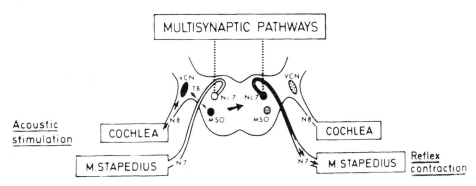

Figure 21.1 Schematic diagram of ipsilateral and contralateral multisynaptic stapedius reflex pathways. *N*8, acoustic nerve; *N*7, facial nerve. (From Borg, E. 1973. On the neuronal organization of the acoustic middle ear reflex; a physiological and anatomical study. Brain Res. 49, 101–123.)

ACOUSTIC REFLEX THRESHOLD

In the demonstration of the acoustic reflex, the immittance meter measures the sudden increase in ear canal sound pressure caused by the decrease in compliance (or increase in impedance) of the middle ear system as the muscles contract. The acoustic signal is introduced contralaterally through an earphone or ipsilaterally through the immittance probe tip. If the acoustic stimulus is loud enough to elicit the middle ear muscle reflex, the contraction of the stapedius muscle in the ear with the immittance probe tip will suddenly decrease the compliance of that tympanic membrane with presentation of the stimulus. Under some clinical circumstances the audiologist may be especially interested in the presence or absence of the acoustic reflex in the contralateral ear, although in other situations attention is focused on the reflex results in the ipsilateral ear. Comparison of ipsilateral and contralateral reflexes obtained from each ear can be particularly useful in many diagnostic situations. It is standard routine clinical practice to specify the acoustic reflex based on the stimulated ear.

The acoustic reflex threshold (ART) is the lowest intensity of an acoustic stimulus at which a minimal change in the middle ear compliance can be measured. Numerous researchers have documented that the necessary intensity range to elicit the acoustic reflex at threshold for normal-hearing subjects is 70 to 100 dB hearing level (HL) (Metz, 1946; Fria et al., 1975). The median threshold value for the contralateral stapedial reflex to puretone signals is approximately 85 dB HL and 65 dB HL for broad-band noise. Ipsilateral acoustic stimulation results in slightly lower acoustic reflex thresholds (Moller, 1962). The ART is generally established by an ascending and descending 5-dB increment bracketing procedure to determine the minimal intensity required to note a change in middle ear compliance (Silman and Gelfand, 1982). ART measurement is usually conducted at test frequencies of 500, 1000, 2000 and 4000 Hz. There is little threshold variability for the acoustic reflex for various stimuli among studies of normal listeners, suggesting that the ART is a relatively stable auditory system characteristic (Popelka, 1981a).

In determining the ART, the clinician must establish criteria for what minimal amount of compliance change is to be considered a response. Although this measurement can be determined visually from the immittance meter, considerable increase in objectivity and accuracy may be obtained by using a graphic recorder to determine the presence of minimal immittance change that is time locked to the presentation of an acoustic stimulus indicated by an event marker on the graph.

The ART is influenced by several signal and procedural variables including intensity, frequency, duration and bandwidth of the activating stimulus, size (or amplitude) of the acoustic reflex contraction and contralateral versus ipsilateral stimulation. Reflex amplitude increases as stimulus intensity is increased above the reflex threshold for 10 to 15 dB. Beyond this increase little additional amplitude change can be noted at higher stimulus intensities. Wilson (1979) reported that reflex magnitude for puretone stimuli is similar across frequencies, although the greatest mean reflex magnitude is observed with broad-band noise.

The duration of the activating signal should not be too short or too long. Silman and Gelfand (1982) suggest that activators lasting 1 to 2 sec are ideal, because with brief activators (i.e., 300 msec or less), the stimulus level must be increased in order to compensate for the reduction in stimulus on-time. Signals longer than 2 sec seem to have little affect on the ART.

The fact that the ART for broad-band noise is lower than the ART for pure tones suggests that a specific relationship exists between the activating stimulus bandwidth and the reflex threshold. In fact, the ART is reduced as bandwidth increases at each test frequency, and this tone-noise reflex threshold relationship forms the basis of the prediction of hearing sensitivity techniques using acoustic reflex measurements.

Early studies report that the ipsilateral acoustic reflex can be elicited at lower intensities than the contralateral acoustic reflex (Moller, 1961; Fria et al., 1975). Moller (1961) states that ipsilateral reflexes are between 2 dB and 16 dB more sensitive than contralateral reflexes. More recently, Leis and Lutman (1979) and Laukli and Meir (1980) note that the threshold differences between the two modes of acoustic stimulation are confounded by problems inherent in the calibration techniques used for ipsilateral and contralateral stimulation. Laukli and Meir (1980) were not able to establish that the ipsilateral reflex threshold is lower than the contralateral reflex threshold. In an exemplary study of the ipsilateral versus contralateral reflex problem, Jerger et al. (1978) used a special immittance measuring technique to record both types of acoustic reflex response simultaneously. This approach controlled for the presentation level and simply compared the reflex time course and amplitude ipsilaterally and contralaterally. With this procedure, Jerger et al. showed that differences noted between ipsilateral and contralateral reflex measurements were due to neuromuscular events rather than measurement, calibration, artifact and other variables (Hannley, 1983).

Special instrumentation has been described by Stach and Jerger (1984, 1987) that features a dual probe assembly for the simultaneous measurement of contralateral (crossed) and ipsilateral (uncrossed) acoustic reflexes. This advanced instrumentation includes a microprocessor for signal averaging and uses the same stimulus origin for both sets of reflexes elicited from the same transducer, thus controlling for differences that must be accounted for when the ipsilateral stimulus comes from a probe tip assembly and the contralateral signal is transduced by an earphone. Stach and Jerger point out that signal averaging of the acoustic reflex adds the advantage of improving the signal-to-noise ratio to the extent that minimal filtering of the signal is required, thus reducing temporal distortion of the reflex wave form and permitting minute analysis of onset latency, waveform rise, and decay times, etc.

Other variables that may influence the ART include drugs (including alcohol), subject gender (male or female) and patient age. Bauch and Robinette (1978) report that ethanol and barbiturates can elevate the ART, although the effect appears to be greater for alcohol. Acoustic reflexes may be observed in sedated patients, but the thresholds may be elevated above normal levels (Borg and Moller, 1968; Robinette et al., 1974). Studies of patients under general anesthesia indicate acoustic reflexes to be influenced by anesthesia technique and drug agent. Acoustic reflexes during general anesthesia follow the same pattern demonstrated by other observable reflexes such as deep tendon and pupillary reflexes (Mitchell and Richards, 1976). According to Borg (1976) barbiturates have varying influence on the stapedial reflex mechanism. Accordingly, the audiologist must be aware that any drug that can alter central nervous system responses may have a dilatory or inhibitive effect on the acoustic reflex (Northern, 1980).

For the newborn and the geriatric patient, age is a consideration in acoustic reflex measurements. Studies by Hall (1978), Jerger et al. (1978) and Hall and Weaver (1979) show that the ART to puretone stimuli tend to improve slightly with increasing age from 0 to 59 years, but demonstrate no change as a function of age for broadband noise stimuli. Contrary to the previous findings, Silman and Gelfand (1982) found no *significant* clinical change in ART measurements as a function of age. Wilson (1981) noted that the amplitude, or size, of the acoustic reflex diminishes with age.

At the other end of the age extreme, McCandless and Allred (1978) as well as Weatherby and Bennett (1980) reported that the immittance probe tone frequency that is used in testing infants has significant influence on the probability of eliciting acoustic reflexes in infants. Higher frequency probe tones, such as 660 Hz, result in an increased percentage of acoustic reflex responses and lower ART than noted with a 220 Hz probe tone with infants. Mahoney (1980) reports data, however, that indicate artifacts occur in infants and young children during contralateral acoustic reflex stimulation due to bone-conduction cross-over that is

evident because of high frequency probe tone interaction with test stimuli.

DIAGNOSTIC APPLICATIONS OF THE ACOUSTIC REFLEX MEASUREMENT

The diagnostic applications of the acoustic reflex considerably outweigh the contribution of tympanometry and static compliance in the acoustic immittance test battery (Jerger and Hayes, 1980; Northern, 1984). Acoustic reflex measurements, however, should not be examined in isolation from other audiologic tests and must be considered as an integral part of the total immittance test battery.

Interpretation of absence of an acoustic reflex threshold can be difficult because it can result from a number of pathologic conditions. For example, the absence of a right crossed (contralateral) acoustic reflex can result from (a) a severe sensory hearing loss on the right ear; (b) a substantial conductive loss on the right ear; (c) right eighth nerve tumor; (d) a lesion of the crossing fibers of the central portion of the reflex arc in the lower brainstem; (e) left facial nerve disorder; or (f) left middle ear disorder. For this reason the addition of uncrossed (ipsilateral) reflex measurement, tympanometry, and static immittance are important in reflex threshold interpretation (Stach and Jerger, 1991).

Conductive Hearing Loss

The immittance test battery provides information, which when combined with a complete audiometric evaluation, often portrays both a distinct clinical picture of the middle ear and the presence or absence of conductive hearing loss. However, the immittance test battery, and especially acoustic reflex findings, demonstrate greater sensitivity to middle ear pathology than traditional audiometric threshold tests. The presence of middle ear pathology may or may not result in a conductive hearing loss, and therefore the measurement of the acoustic reflex is vital in confirming the presence of middle ear pathology (Jerger and Hayes, 1980).

A valuable diagnostic implication of the acoustic reflex is the fact that the reflex is obscured when the probe is coupled to an ear with a middle ear disorder of even the slightest degree. Middle ear disorders typically prevent the tympanic membrane from showing a change in compliance when the stapedial muscles contract whether the disorder is otitis media, otosclerosis, or some other disease entity. Ipsilateral and contralateral reflexes are therefore absent bilaterally in the presence of even a mild bilateral conductive hearing loss. Conversely, if acoustic reflexes can be noted in the immittance probe ear, it is highly unlikely that a conductive hearing loss exists in that ear.

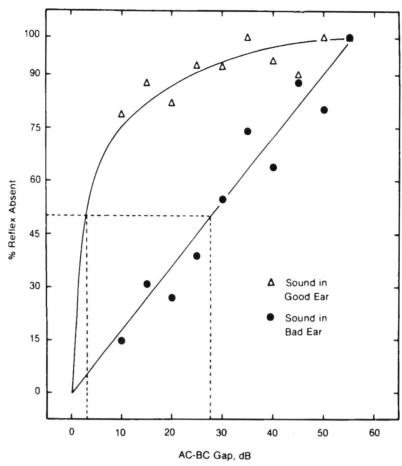

Figure 21.2 Percentage of absent acoustic reflexes as a function of air-bone gap in 154 patients with unilateral conductive hearing loss. (From Jerger, J. F., L. Anthony, S. Jerger, and B. Crump. 1974b. Studies in impedance audiometry. III. Middle ear disorders. Arch. Otolaryngol. 99, 165–171.)

The acoustic reflex function for 154 patients with unilateral conductive hearing loss and unilateral normal hearing is shown in Figure 21.2 (Jerger et al., 1974b). The patients who were selected had a hearing loss in one ear along with an air-bone gap and an abnormal tympanogram, whereas the opposite normal ear showed no air-bone gap with a normal tympanogram. Figure 21.2 shows acoustic reflex results (a) when the good ear was stimulated with sound and the probe was situated in the ear with the conductive loss, and (b) with sound stimulation of the conductive loss ear and the probe in the normal ear. The straight line function shows the effect of attenuation by the conductive loss ear when stimulating the conductive ear. The likelihood of an absent acoustic reflex increases as the magnitude of the air-bone gap increases. Thus, when the earphone is over the unilateral conductive loss ear, the reflex has only a small chance of being absent as long as the air-bone gap is less than 30 dB. When the air-bone gap exceeds 30 dB, the stimulating tone can no longer be perceived sufficiently loud in the conductive loss ear to cause the stapedial

muscle to contract. The acoustic reflex has a 50% chance of being present when the probe is in the normal ear with a 27 dB unilateral air-bone gap in the conductive loss ear as shown in Figure 21.2.

When the stimulating sound is presented to the normal-hearing ear, and the immittance probe tip is inserted into the ear with the air-bone gap, the acoustic reflex is absent even when the air-bone gap is very small. Inasmuch as the sound can easily be heard loudly enough by the normal ear, absence of the acoustic reflex on the probe ear must be caused by the air-bone gap or the mechanical problem of the affected ear. It may be seen in Figure 21.2 that an air-bone gap of only 10 dB is sufficient to obscure the acoustic reflex as much as 80% of the time. The 50% chance of acoustic reflex presence in the probe ear is coincident with an air-bone gap of less than 5 dB.

In the presence of a unilateral conductive loss, the contralateral reflex is obscured bilaterally when the hearing loss exceeds 30 dB HL. In fact, conductive hearing loss is the only type of *unilateral* hearing loss that will obscure the contralateral reflex bilaterally. The unilateral conductive loss will obscure the ipsilateral reflex only on the affected side. Thus, skillful interpretation of acoustic reflexes in unilateral hearing loss cases can suggest the degree and nature of hearing loss (see Fig. 21.3).

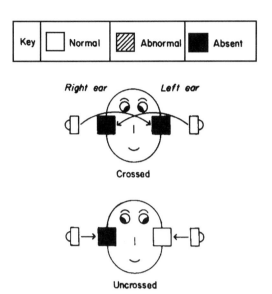

Figure 21.3. Ipsilateral and contralateral acoustic reflex results in a unilateral right ear conductive hearing loss, greater than 30 dB HTL. Note the bilateral absence of reflexes to contralateral stimulation, and unilateral absence of reflex to ipsilateral stimulation.

The acoustic reflex in patients with otosclerosis has a unique and characteristic pattern. According to Terkildsen et al. (1973) and Jerger et al. (1974b), although the tympanogram may often be within normal limits, it is sometimes a shallow type A and the acoustic reflex is generally not observed in either ear. Figure 21.4 illustrates the graphic recording of the acoustic reflex present in early otosclerosis as compared to a normal acoustic reflex tracing. In early otosclerosis there is a momentary negative deflection at the start of the reflex and again at the end of the reflex as the stimulating signal is shut off (Bel et al, 1976). Patients with fixated middle ear disorders, such as otosclerosis, have the only conductive hearing losses with normal tympanograms and absent reflexes.

Unfortunately there are exceptions to every rule. Not all middle ear pathologies inhibit the acoustic reflex. Northern (1977a) reported that an exception occurs in cases of ossicular disruption when the connection is maintained between the insertion point of the stapedius muscle on the stapes and the eardrum. In most cases of ossicular disruption the reflexes are absent in all conditions, with the exception of normal reflexes being present with ipsilateral stimulation of the good ear. However, the reflex may be absent with stimulation of the impaired ear (due to the magnitude of the conductive hearing loss), but intact with the probe

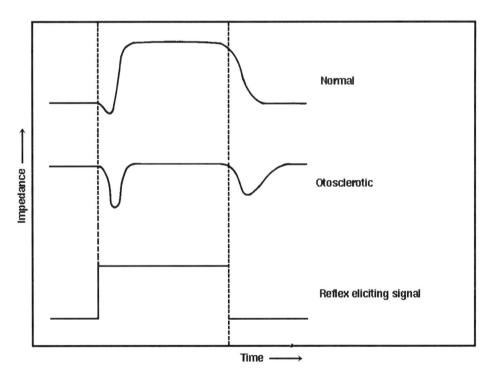

Figure 21.4. Time course of the acoustic reflex in a normal ear and in an otosclerotic ear. Note that both graphic patterns show negative deflection at onset, but only "otosclerotic" reflex shows negative deflection at conclusion. (From Jerger, J.F., and D. Hayes, 1980. Diagnostic applications of impedance audiometry; middle ear disorder, sensori-neural disorder, in J.F. Jerger and J. L. Northern, eds. *Clinical Impedance Audiometry*. American Electromedics, Acton, MA.)

in the impaired ear if the discontinuity involves only the crus of the stapes. A middle ear cholesteatoma that does not impinge on the eardrum or ossicular chain, as well as some ears with serous otitis media and negative middle ear pressure, may also produce normal reflex patterns. The chance of obtaining ipsilateral or contralateral acoustic reflexes is generally increased if the measurement is taken at the middle ear pressure value as noted by the point of maximum compliance of the tympanogram.

Sensory-Neural Hearing Loss

The differentiation of cochlear versus eighth nerve disorders has been a primary challenge in audiometric evaluation. The important diagnostic patterns of the acoustic reflex in sensory-neural differential diagnosis are based on (a) the relationship of the acoustic reflex hearing threshold level to the degree of hearing loss, (b) the time course of the reflex to sustained signals and (c) the relationship of the ipsilateral reflex to the contralateral reflex (Jerger and Hayes, 1980).

Cochlear Pathology

An early application of the acoustic reflex was in the evaluation of the cochlear phenomena of abnormal loudness growth. Metz (1952) found that the acoustic reflex is elicited at sensation levels of less than 60 dB SL in ears with cochlear lesions. Therefore, the comparison between the acoustic reflex threshold hearing level (HL) to the degree of hearing loss is referred to as the Metz test for loudness recruitment. A positive

Metz test result indicates that the acoustic reflex is observed when stimulating an ear at 60 dB or less above the puretone threshold. This is a strong indicator of a cochlear site of lesion.

Figure 21.5 shows the sensation level required for ART compared to the puretone threshold levels for the same frequencies. Median performance is shown for 515 patients who were diagnosed as having cochlear pathology (Jerger et al., 1972). The median acoustic reflex sensation level decreases from approximately 70 dB for patients with 20 dB sensory-neural hearing levels, to approximately 25 dB sensation level (SL) for patients with 85 dB losses. The acoustic reflex functions at 500, 1000, and 2000 Hz are quite similar and show a decrease in the sensation level of the ART as a function of increase in hearing loss. The acoustic reflex function at 4000 Hz does not follow the exact pattern of the other stimulus frequencies. Because the acoustic reflex is often absent for no clear reason at 4000 Hz, clinicians should be cautious in interpreting reflex findings at this test frequency. Note that 50% of the cases had acoustic reflexes with cochlear hearing losses of 85 dB as shown by the *dotted lines*. If a patient has an 85 dB HL threshold the clinician can expect to elicit acoustic reflexes at 25 dB SL or less in 50% of patients with cochlear hearing loss.

Figure 21.7 also shows that there is a 90% likelihood of observing the acoustic reflex as long as the cochlear hearing loss is less than 60 dB. As the cochlear loss increases above 60 dB, chances of observing the reflex de-

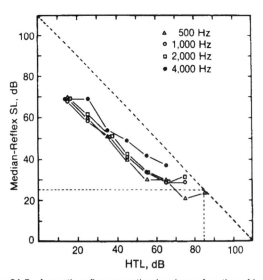

Figure 21.5. Acoustic reflex sensation level as a function of hearing loss severity in 515 patients with sensory-neural hearing loss. (From Jerger, J .F., S. Jerger, and L. Mauldin. 1972. Studies in impedance audiometry. 1. Normal and sensori-neural ears. Arch. Orolaryngol. 96, 513–523.)

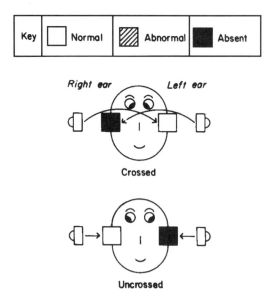

Figure 21.6. Ipsilateral and contralateral acoustic reflex results in a unilateral left ear profound sensory-neural hearing loss, and normal hearing in right ear. (From Jerger, J. F., and D. Hayes. 1980. Diagnostic applications of impedance audiometry; middle ear disorder, sensorineural disorder, *in* J. F. Jerger and J. L. Northern, eds. Clinical Impedance Audiometry. American Electromedics, Acton, MA.)

crease. Silman and Gelfand (1982) point out that acoustic reflexes should be observed at 125 dB HL or lower for cochlear hearing losses of 75 dB or less. Figure 21.6 represents the expected reflex pattern in an ear with a unilateral cochlear disorder in the left ear of 90 to 100 dB. Normal acoustic reflexes are present when stimulating the normal-hearing ear, although absence of the reflex to 105 dB or more is present when stimulating the hearing-impaired ear.

Retrocochlear Pathology

Careful interpretation of the acoustic reflexes can also supply diagnostic information about the presence or absence of acoustic or eighth nerve tumors. In achieving this goal, the commonly used parameters of the reflex are the reflex threshold level and the persistence of the reflex response on prolonged stimulation, referred to as the acoustic reflex decay test (Anderson et al., 1970a, 1970b). Jerger et al. (1987) report a series of case studies in which suprathreshold changes in the morphologic characteristics of the acoustic stapedius reflex were more sensitive to acoustic tumor identification than conventional reflex threshold or reflex decay measures.

Figure 21.7 from Jerger et al. (1974c) shows the relationship between degree of hearing loss and the likelihood of an absent reflex. Pathologic ears with eighth nerve involvement and normal hearing do not exhibit acoustic reflexes 30% of the time. The likelihood of absent reflexes quickly rises to 70% with a mild 30 dB loss.

The absence of acoustic reflex at 500, 1000, and 2000 Hz, in light of normal or near normal hearing levels, must be considered a suspicious finding until the presence of an acoustic tumor is ruled out.

The presence of acoustic reflexes in eighth nerve disorders is the exception rather than the rule as shown by many authors including Jerger et al. (1974a), Olsen et al. (1975), Johnson (1977), and Hirsch (1983). In most patients with acoustic tumors, the acoustic reflexes are absent when the involved ear is stimulated. However, when the ART is present in a patient under consideration for an eighth nerve lesion, the acoustic reflex decay test may be applied. Reflex decay is determined by presenting the stimulus test tone at 10 dB above the acoustic reflex HTL for 10 sec at 500 and 1000 Hz. Reflex decay may be measured for both contralateral and ipsilateral test conditions. Reflex decay occurs when the amplitude of the acoustic reflex declines by more than half its initial magnitude in less than 10 sec under continuous puretone stimulation (Anderson et al., 1969). According to Givens and Seidemann (1979), reflex decay is common in many normal ears at higher test frequencies such as 2000, 3000, and 4000 Hz; however, reflex decay is unusual at 500 and 1000 Hz. Therefore, the frequencies 500 and 1000 Hz are used for diagnostic purposes in the acoustic reflex decay test. Figure 21.8 illustrates the phenomenon of acoustic reflex decay. Despite the presence of an eighth nerve lesion there is a normal acoustic reflex when initially stimulated acoustically. However, when the signal is sustained for the decay test, the reflex response amplitude de-

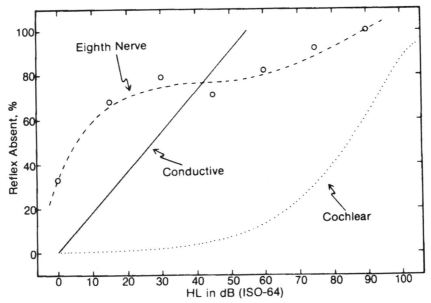

Figure 21.7. The relationship between degree of hearing loss and the likelihood of acoustic reflex absence in patients with conductive, cochlear and eighth nerve disorders. (From Jerger, J. F., E. Harford, J. Clemis, and B. Alford. 1974c. The acoustic reflex in VIIIth nerve disorders. Arch. Otolaryngol. 99, 409–413.)

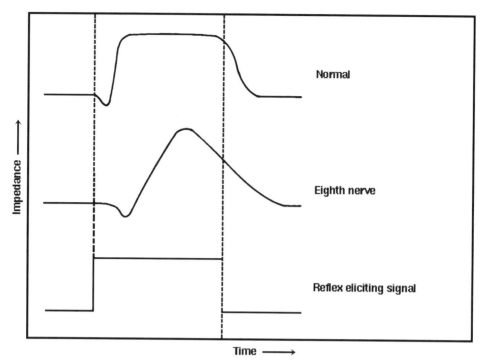

Figure 21.8. Time course of acoustic reflex in normal ear and in ear with eighth nerve disorder. Note that both show normal amplitude deflection when reflex-eliciting signal is first turned on, but that eighth nerve reflex amplitude gradually declines and finally disappears altogether within a 10-sec period. (From Jerger, J. F., and D. Hayes. 1980. Diagnostic applications of impedance audiometry; middle ear disorder, sensorineural disorder. *in* J. F. Jerger and J. L. Northern, eds. *Clinical Impedance Audiometry*, American Electromedics, Acton, MA.)

clines and disappears altogether within the 10-sec stimulus presentation.

The sensitivity of detection of eighth nerve disorders by both acoustic reflex measures has been widely confirmed in the literature and summarized by Sanders (1982, 1984). These studies reveal the accurate identification of eighth nerve pathology to be as high as 86 to 98% with acoustic reflex measurements. However, the audiologist must be aware that acoustic reflex measures indeed show a significant false positive rate for eighth nerve pathologies (Chiveralls, 1977; Jerger, 1983). The clinician must keep this in mind and use acoustic reflex measures as part of a test battery approach to identify retrocochlear pathologies.

Stach and Jerger (1991) discuss the limitations regarding the use of acoustic reflex latency as a diagnostic measure. Although acoustic reflex latency has been advocated as a diagnostic indicator for identifying eighth nerve lesions (Clemis and Sarno, 1980), Stach and Jerger point out that measurement of acoustic reflex latency is difficult, at best, because of typical limitations in commercially available immittance equipment. Response times of commercial instrumentation is generally too slow to accurately reproduce temporal characteristics of the acoustic reflex. Jerger et al. (1986) report that although latency abnormalities can gener-

ally be due to equipment artifact, acoustic reflex temporal characteristics have been found to be sensitive to brainstem disorder.

Brainstem Pathology

The application of acoustic reflex measurements to the identification of brainstem pathology has focused on a comparison of contralateral and ipsilateral reflex thresholds (Greisen and Rasmussen, 1970; Jerger and Jerger, 1975, 1983; Jerger, 1983). The absence of contralateral reflexes, with ipsilateral reflexes intact, may be seen in patients with confirmed brainstem pathology. These abnormalities are considered to be the result of the presence of a lesion in the area of the crossed brainstem pathways while the uncrossed brainstem pathways remain intact (see Fig. 21.9).

Hayes and Jerger (1981) point out that the acoustic reflex is mediated, in part, by neural structures that also form the initial component waves of the auditory brainstem response (ABR) (see Chapter 21): the acoustic nerve, cochlear nucleus and superior olivary complex. Thus, in-depth analysis of the ABR wave complex, with consideration of the presence or absence of crossed and uncrossed acoustic reflexes, will help in determining the specific site of lesion in patients with brainstem dysfunc-

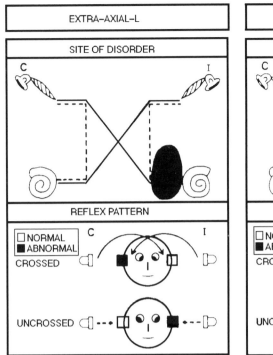
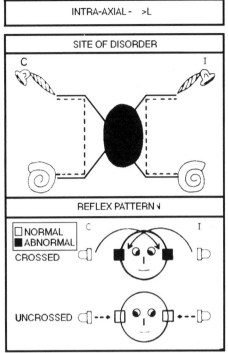

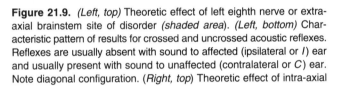

Figure 21.9. *(Left, top)* Theoretic effect of left eighth nerve or extra-axial brainstem site of disorder *(shaded area)*. *(Left, bottom)* Characteristic pattern of results for crossed and uncrossed acoustic reflexes. Reflexes are usually absent with sound to affected (ipsilateral or *I*) ear and usually present with sound to unaffected (contralateral or *C*) ear. Note diagonal configuration. *(Right, top)* Theoretic effect of intra-axial brainstem site of disorder. *(Right, bottom)* Characteristic pattern of results for crossed and uncrossed acoustic reflexes. Reflexes are usually absent to crossed stimulation and usually present to uncrossed stimulation. Note horizontal configuration. (From Jerger, S., and J. Jerger. 1977. Diagnostic value of crossed vs uncrossed acoustic reflexes: Eighth nerve and brain stem disorders. Arch. Otolarnygol. 103, 445.)

tion. If the lesion is higher in the auditory pathway, the acoustic reflex finding is likely to be within normal limits or involved in accordance with any hearing loss that might be present.

Facial Nerve Disorder

The acoustic reflex is also a valuable tool in the management of seventh nerve dysfunction (Alford et al., 1973; Citron and Adour, 1978). The acoustic reflex measurement is helpful in determining the site of lesion of the facial nerve disorder as either distal (away from) or proximal (toward the point of origin) of the stapedial branch of the seventh nerve. It is important, however, to identify or rule out the presence of middle ear pathology that may prevent the observation of the reflex.

In evaluation of facial nerve disorders, the acoustic reflex may be measured with ipsilateral or contralateral stimulation. Interpretation of facial motor disorder is a function of the efferent nerve pathway, so acoustic reflex results are interpreted for the immittance probe ear only. If the acoustic reflex is present at normal HL, the localization of pathology is likely to be distal to origin of the stapedius branch of the nerve; if the reflex is absent, the disorder is likely proximal to the nerve. If the reflexes are present but elevated, the disorder is

likely proximal to the nerve. According to Citron and Adour (1978), the acoustic reflex is an efficient indicator of impending nerve degeneration and predictor of recovery. Therefore, reflex testing over the course of several days or weeks may be appropriate. A patient with Bell's palsy may initially exhibit no acoustic reflexes, then present elevated reflexes and finally show normal reflex responses as the disorder gradually resolves to complete recovery.

Nonorganic Hearing Loss

Another application of acoustic reflex measurement pertains to the patient suspected of having a nonorganic or pseudohypacusic hearing loss. The discussions above have established that the greater the hearing loss, the less the likelihood there is of obtaining an acoustic reflex. It is highly unlikely to observe an acoustic reflex at a level less than 15 dB above the patient's threshold and impossible to obtain a reflex measure at a lower hearing level than the true hearing threshold (Olsen, 1991). The presence of an acoustic reflex suggests that true hearing loss is no more than 20 dB less than the reflex HL. These patients are especially good candidates for the prediction of hearing sensitivity techniques using the acoustic reflex described later in this chapter (Hall, 1978).

The Relationship of the Acoustic Reflex to Other Auditory Tests

Acoustic reflex measurements are not a test of hearing, and accordingly are not a substitute for puretone air-conduction or bone-conduction evaluations. Although immittance audiometry is used clinically to identify the nature of a patient's hearing impairment, behavioral puretone audiometry is still the procedure of choice to represent hearing thresholds. However, immittance measurement, because of its simplicity and objectivity, provides clinical information with greater accuracy, in less time, and often with less patient and clinician distress than traditional behavioral site of lesion procedures. According to Hall and Ghorayeb (1991), when patients show unequivocally normal acoustic immittance findings (with the exception of positive acoustic reflex decay), bone-conduction pure tone threshold measurement is absolutely superfluous and a waste of clinical time.

The short increment sensitivity index (SISI) and loudness balance procedures (alternate binaural loudness balance and monaural loudness balance) are part of a traditional psychoacoustic differential diagnostic test battery. They are used to localize pathology to the cochlea and rely on a patient's ability to detect small changes in signal intensity or to equate the loudness of various tones. Excellent agreement exists between behavioral tests of loudness recruitment and the Metz acoustic reflex recruitment test to identify cochlear hearing impairment. The Metz test is objective and quicker to administer than the complex listening tasks involved in the loudness balance techniques.

The relationship between uncomfortable loudness levels (UCL) and ART has been controversial and inconclusive in the literature. McLeod and Greenberg (1979) reported successful prediction of UCL by the ART. They examined levels utilizing speech and puretone stimulation. Greater variability exists for the speech stimulus that therefore may not have as strong a clinical application. In contrast, Ritter et al. (1979) demonstrated that ART correlate too poorly with the UCL measurements to permit an accurate prediction of loudness discomfort. The variability in agreement of the measures was dependent on the instructional pattern used for the UCL measure, the type of acoustic stimulus used and the degree of hearing loss of the patient.

Although the tone decay test (TDT) was devised as a technique to identify the presence of eighth nerve lesions, the use of the acoustic reflex in identifying retrocochlear tumors has several obvious advantages. Research with acoustic tumors suggests that "positive" acoustic reflex findings are more sensitive to the presence of retrocochlear pathology than the TDT (Sanders, 1982, 1984, 1988).

Significantly reduced speech discrimination scores have long been recognized as a sign of eighth nerve disorders. Hannley and Jerger (1981) examined the relationship between phonetically balanced rollover and the acoustic reflex in 52 patients with surgically confirmed acoustic neurinoma. Patients who presented with absent acoustic reflexes experienced significantly greater rollover of speech intelligibility at high intensities than did patients with all or some reflexes intact. The authors concluded that the status of the acoustic reflex bears a significant relationship to the amount of rollover produced by these patients.

An audiometric revolution in the identification of disorders involving specific structures in the brainstem has taken place in the past decade. The use of ABR audiometry and the acoustic reflex measure has enabled the clinical audiologist to predict site of lesion with much more confidence than traditional behavioral procedures have allowed. Hayes and Jerger (1981) have examined the patterns of acoustic reflex and ABR response abnormality. Their results demonstrate (a) the close correspondence between patterns of ART abnormalities of waves I, II, and III of the ABR and (b) the importance of a combined acoustic reflex and ABR diagnostic approach. Although acoustic reflex measurements and ABR provide valuable information individually, their most significant contribution to disorder identification may be in combination.

When the tympanogram shows negative middle ear pressure, it is necessary to attempt the acoustic reflex

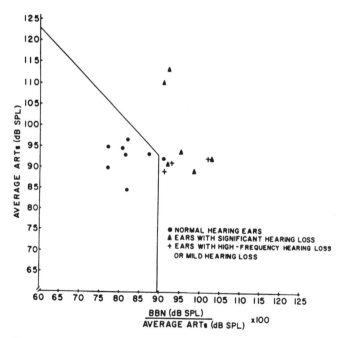

Figure 21.10. Acoustic reflex threshold data from 17 subjects with functional hearing loss are plotted on the modified bivariate plot of Silman et al., page 213, 1984.

measurement at the point of maximum compliance of the tympanic membrane (also known as the middle ear pressure value) in order to increase the chance of observing a change in the compliance of the middle ear system as the stapedial muscle contracts. However, there are a number of circumstances under which it is not likely to observe an acoustic reflex, and in fact, probably is not time efficient to even attempt the measurement. Under most conditions of a nonmobile middle ear as evidence by tympanogram, i.e., significant otitis media, tympanic membrane perforation, patent ventilation tubes in the tympanic membrane, etc., the acoustic reflex will generally not be seen. Often, during middle-ear surgery the stapedial muscle is cut, so that the postoperative acoustic reflex study will also be negative.

The use of other audiometric tests in addition to the immittance battery will depend on the clinical situation, including the needs of the referring sources, the clinic caseload, the interests of the clinical personnel, and consideration of time. It seems obvious, however, that the acoustic reflex measurements do provide valuable information concerning the nature of the patient's hearing loss in relationship to the contribution of other audiometric techniques. Interested readers would do well to review recent published materials by Jerger et al. (1983) and Sanders (1988).

SPECIAL APPLICATIONS OF THE ACOUSTIC REFLEX

Hearing Loss Prediction by the Acoustic Reflex

A unique application of acoustic reflex measurement was reported by Niemeyer and Sesterhenn (1974) to determine air-conduction hearing thresholds from stapedial reflex measurements. They noted that the ART for white noise was lower than the ART for puretones, and that the difference in dB between the two thresholds is related to the degree of sensory-neural hearing impairment. They verified their results on a large group of normal-hearing and hearing-impaired subjects, and concluded that their technique provided an objective means to predict hearing levels within 10 dB in just a few minutes without extensive equipment expenditures.

Jerger et al. (1974a) simplified the procedure into a test they called SPAR (sensitivity prediction with the acoustic reflex). Initially, the SPAR was an attempt to ascertain sensory-neural hearing loss within four categories of impairment (normal hearing, mild loss, severe loss, or profound loss). The Jerger technique called for establishment of puretone acoustic reflexes at 500, 1000, and 2000 Hz and broad-band noise threshold difference to predict the degree of hearing loss.

Jerger et al. (1978) subsequently published a modified version of the SPAR. In the revised SPAR procedure, if the noise-tone ART difference is less than 20

and the broad-band noise (BBN) reflex threshold is 95 dB sound pressure level (SPL) or less, a mild to moderate sensory-neural hearing loss is predicted. When the BBN threshold is more 95 dB SPL, a severe sensory-neural hearing loss is predicted. The revised SPAR takes into account the absolute reflex threshold for the 1000-Hz signal. If the ART at 1000 Hz is more than 95 dB HL, regardless of the BBN reflex threshold, a hearing loss is always predicted. Normal hearing sensitivity is predicted when the 1000 Hz ART is 95 dB SPL or less and the noise-tone reflex threshold difference is more than 20 dB. In the event that neither of these requirements is met, sensory-neural hearing loss is predicted and the BBN threshold must be considered.

The success of the SPAR procedure has inspired a number of innovative approaches to predict hearing loss with acoustic reflex measurements. These approaches may be divided into three general categories—SPAR, regression equations, and the bivariate plot system. All depend, in one fashion or another, on the noise-tone difference in ART and have been reviewed in detail by Hall (1978) and Popelka (1981b).

In general, the regression equations predict HL by assigning ART data for puretones and noise in differentially weighted equations. Rizzo and Greenberg (1979) developed a regression equation for HL prediction. For example, dB HL = $(0.216$ ART $HPN_{(SPL)}$ -0.078 ART 500 $Hz_{(HL)}$ $2 - 7.515)^2$ where HPN = high-pass noise of 1800 to 6000 Hz. These formulas are based on statistical regression techniques. The bivariate plot coordinate system simply differentiates those patients with normal hearing from those with sensory-neural hearing loss (Hall, 1978). For patients with a sensory-neural hearing loss ART cluster in the upper right portion of the graph as shown in Figure 21.10, whereas normal-hearing patients cluster in the lower area of the graph. Figure 21.10 shows an example of the bivariate-plot procedure as modified by Silman et al. (1984) with a group of 17 patients demonstrating functional hearing loss. It can be noted that all patients with confirmed hearing loss fall outside the normal range, and among the eight functional hearing loss patients with normal hearing, only one was eventually found to have an actual hearing loss of more than 30 dB HL.

Hearing loss prediction from the acoustic reflex is apparently influenced by a number of variables including chronologic age, minor middle ear abnormalities and audiometric configuration (Jerger et al, 1978). Predictive accuracy with the SPAR test is more successful in children (ages 0 to 10 years) and grows less accurate in older children and adults. In the Jerger et al. study, 100% of the children predicted to have normal hearing did, indeed, demonstrate normal audiograms. Severe hearing loss was accurately predicted in children 85% of the time. The prediction of moderate sensory-neural hearing losses was accurate in 54% of the children.

The prediction of hearing loss with the acoustic reflex is an important asset to those clinicians involved with hearing evaluations in children. At the other age extreme, successful use of predicting mild- and/or high-frequency hearing impairment in the older adult population has been described by Wallin et al. (1986). According to Hall (1978), there is reason for optimism about the potential of acoustic reflex-hearing level predictions. In difficult-to-test patients, acoustic reflex prediction methods clearly offer a rapid, efficient, economical, and objective estimate of hearing sensitivity.

Use of the Acoustic Reflex in Hearing Screening Programs

Immittance screening for the detection of middle ear pathology is a useful technique when implemented in conjunction with puretone audiometric screening (see Chapter 30). Many children with middle ear disorders who would benefit from medical referral have sufficiently good hearing to pass the traditional puretone hearing screening test. The use of immittance measurements in hearing screening programs increases the accuracy of identification of those children with treatable ear disorders and reduces the number of false referrals for children who really have normal hearing and no otologic problems.

The use of acoustic reflex in screening is based on the supposition that the presence of a reflex to a puretone stimulus at approximately 100 dB HL in the midfrequency range is indicative of normal middle ear physiology. That is to say, the presence of the acoustic reflex rules out the possibility of conductive pathology. However, it must be noted that the absence of an acoustic reflex does not necessarily mean that a medical problem exists because some 5% of the normal-hearing population have absent acoustic reflexes in the midfrequency range (Jerger, 1970; Brooks, 1978).

Early immittance screening protocols used tympanometry and acoustic reflex evaluation. Two national sets of guidelines for immittance screening were published (Harford et al., 1978; ASHA, 1979). Both sets of guidelines called for acoustic reflex screening at 100 dB HL with a contralateral stimulus or 105 dB SPL with ipsilateral stimulation at 1000 Hz.

Problems exist in establishing practical guidelines for acoustic immittance screening regarding pass-fail and referral criteria. There is controversy in the literature as to the necessity of acoustic reflex screening in immittance screening programs. Brooks (1976) states that acoustic reflex screening is a more sensitive test than tympanometry. Hoover et al. (1982) reported in a screening study of 91 preschool-aged children, using the 1979 ASHA guidelines for immittance screening. They reported good sensitivity findings with acoustic reflex screening (94%), but a low, unacceptable specificity rate of only 71%. Bess (1980), Cantekin et al. (1980), Lucker (1980), and Queen et al. (1981) reported that the utilization of ASHA's 1979 guidelines without modifications (particularly in use of the acoustic reflex) results in too many overreferrals. In the most recent ASHA guidelines for screening for hearing impairment and middle-ear disorders (1990), use of the acoustic reflex was purposefully left out of the recommended screening protocol. This decision to omit the acoustic reflex in screening programs was based on the numerous research reports that cite the unacceptably high false-positive, or low specificity, rate reported in the literature.

Hearing Aid Selection, Fittings, and Management

Acoustic reflex measurement has been suggested in the selection and fitting of hearing aids, especially with young children and mentally retarded patients. The acoustic reflex is an objective measure that can help the clinician take some of the "guesswork" out of hearing aid fitting. The clinician has numerical data with which to select an appropriate acoustic gain and frequency response as it relates to the configuration of the hearing loss, and maximum power output (MPO) settings on the aid, provided that no conductive element exists as part of the hearing impairment (see Chapter 43). The technique that is used for measuring the ART to hearing aid signals is shown in Figure 21.11.

McCandless and Keith (1980) discuss a number of techniques of determining sound saturation pressure level values. They suggest that the output of the aid should be at or slightly above the ART for puretones of 500, 1000, 2000, and 4000 Hz. Dudich et al. (1975) and others suggest that the output of the aid ideally should be set 5 to 8 dB lower than the ART, because they indicate that puretones produce higher reflex thresholds than do verbal stimuli. To avoid overamplification and loudness discomfort, the output of the hearing aid should be restricted to levels just below the point where speech and other stimuli elicit sustained muscle contraction, but allow for periodic reflex activity caused by short bursts of energy.

The hearing aid gain setting is perhaps more important for young children than it is for adults, because adults are able to manipulate the volume controls for the desired listening level. Ideally, gain corresponds to the hearing aid user's most comfortable loudness (MCL) level setting. Rappaport and Tait (1976) found that the highest speech discrimination scores are ob-

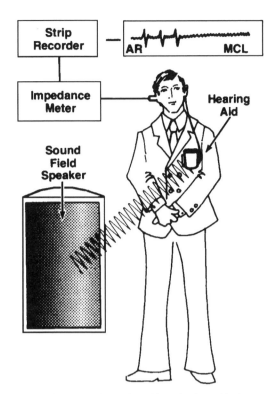

Figure 21.11. Diagram of hearing aid evaluation with the use of an impedance meter to measure acoustic reflexes. Adult hearing aid users tend to set the gain of their hearing aids at a most comfortable level (MCL), which is often just below elicitation of the acoustic reflex (AR). (From Northern, J. L. 1978b. Hearing aids and acoustic impedance measurements. Monogr. Contemp. Audio. 1:2.

tained where reflex activity is initiated. Keith (1979) reports that the ART procedure is successful for setting hearing aid gain for children because in quiet, the ART and MCL for speech are correlated. He found for subjects whose ART were less than 90 dB, the gain was adjusted exactly to the level of the ART, although for subjects whose ART were more than 90 dB HL, the gain was adjusted to just below their ART. Seventy-five percent of the hearing aid users reported that they were amplified to their most comfortable listening level.

Although additional research is needed in the area of hearing aid fittings as it relates to the ART, there are practical and useful techniques available for certain patients. For a thorough review of literature related to acoustic reflex applications with hearing aids, the reader is referred to Northern (1978b).

Nonacoustic Middle Ear Muscle Stimulation

Under certain circumstances, the neurootologic evaluation requires differential diagnosis between activity of the stapedius muscle and the tensor tympani muscles. The tensor tympani muscle response is elicited through the use of nonacoustic stimulation and may be noted

with an immittance meter. Elicitation of the tensor tympani muscle reflex is somewhat difficult to isolate from stapedius muscle activity, but is useful in clarifying the middle ear status in patients with severe hearing loss, retrocochlear lesions, ossicular fixations, and facial paralysis. Although the presence of the tensor tympani reflex is useful information, the absence of a response is ambiguous. Thorough discussions of nonacoustic middle ear responses are presented by Djupesland (1975), Fee (1981), and Stach and Jerger (1984).

Electrical Stimulation of the Stapedial Reflex

An innovative application of the acoustic reflex measurements to cochlear implant patients has been developed over the past few years by Jerger (1986). This study demonstrated that contralateral stapedial reflex contractions to intracochlear electrical stimulation in cochlear implant recipients may be used to evaluate various electrode configurations of multichannel cochlear implant devices. Jerger et al. (1988) suggest that the electrically elicited stapedius reflex growth function may provide a basis for estimating cochlear implant electrode dynamic range. Their results showed that the electrically elicited acoustic reflex threshold was in good agreement with the preferred listening level, and the acoustic reflex saturation level was usually well below the patient's uncomfortable listening level. These acoustic reflex applications may be especially valuable with the preoperative and postoperative evaluation of potential implant candidates who are too young to make adequate behavioral responses to cochlear implant settings.

ACOUSTIC REFLEX MEASUREMENTS IN SPECIAL POPULATIONS

The immense clinical value of the acoustic reflex is highlighted by a wide variety of applications in special populations (Northern, 1980). Interestingly, some authors have commented on applications of acoustic reflex measurement in speech disorders such as spastic dysphonia and stuttering (McCall, 1973; Hall and Jerger, 1976).

Measurement of the acoustic reflex is particularly useful in clarifying the presence of hearing impairment in special populations of children (see Chapter 29). In fact, no hearing evaluation in a child should be considered complete without acoustic immittance measurements. Children at risk for middle ear effusion, such as those with Down's syndrome, cleft lip and cleft palate, craniofacial disorders, and others who are otitis-prone are especially suited for evaluation with the acoustic reflex (Bluestone et al., 1973).

Very often immittance measurements in children who are difficult to test provide the best means of identifying the presence of hearing impairment (see Chapter 33). These children include the multiply handicapped (Keith et al., 1976), autistic children (Suria and Serra-Raventos, 1975), and retarded children (Lamb and Norris, 1970).

Review articles, with extensive bibliographies, on the use of immittance and acoustic reflex evaluations in children and infants and other distinctive population groups have been published by Northern (1977b, 1978a, 1980, 1981), Orchik and MacKimmie (1983), and Northern and Downs (1991).

REFERENCES

Alford B, Jerger JF, Coats A, Peterson C, and Weber S. Neurophysiology of facial nerve testing. Arch Otolaryngol 1973;97: 214.

American Speech-Language-Hearing Association. Guidelines for acoustic immittance screening of middle ear function. Asha 1979; 21:283–288.

American Speech-Language-Hearing Association. Guidelines for screening for hearing impairments and middle ear disorders. Asha 1990;32 (Suppl. 2):17–24.

Anderson H, Barr B, and Wedenberg E. Intraural reflexes in retrocochlear lesions. In Hambarger C, and Wasall J, Eds. *Disorders of the Skull Base Region.* Stockholm: Almquist and Wikesell, 1969:49–55.

Anderson H, Barr B, and Wedenberg E. Early diagnosis of the eighth nerve tumors by acoustic reflex tests. Acta_Otolaryngol Suppl 1970a;263:232–237.

Anderson H, Barr B, and Wedenberg E. The early detection of acoustic tumors by the stapedius reflex test. In Wolstenhome GEW, and Knight J, Eds. *Sensorineural Hearing Loss.* London: J.A. Churchill, 1970b:278–289.

Bauch C, and Robinette M. Alcohol and the acoustic reflex: effects of stimulus spectrum, subject variability and sex. J Am Aud Soc 1978;4:104–112.

Bel J, Causse P, Michaux P, Cezard R, Canut Y, and Tapon J. Mechanical explanation of the on-off effect (diphasic impedance change) in otospongiosis. Audiology 1976;15:128–140.

Bess FH. 1980. Impedance screening for children: a need for more research. Ann Otol Rhinol Laryngol 1980;89 (Suppl 68): part 2, 228–232.

Bluestone CD, Beery QC, and Paradise JL. Audiometry and tympanometry in relation to middle ear effusions in children. Laryngoscope 1973:83:594–604.

Borg E. On the neuronal organization of the acoustic middle ear reflex: a physiological and anatomical study. Brain Res 1973; 49:101–123.

Borg E. Dynamic characteristics of the intra-aural muscle reflex. In Feldman A, and Wilber L, Eds. *Acoustic Impedance and Admittance— The Measurement of Middle Ear Function.* Baltimore: Williams & Wilkins, 1976:236–299.

Borg E, and Moller AR. The effect of ethylalcohol and pentobarbital sodium on the acoustic reflex in man. Acta Otolaryngol 1968; 64:415.

Brooks D. School screening for middle-ear effusions. Ann Otol Rhinol Laryngol 1976;85(Suppl 25):223–228.

Brooks D. Acoustic impedance testing for screening auditory function in school children. Parts I and II. Maico Aud Lib Ser 1978;15.

Cantekin E, Bluestone C, Fria T, Stool S, Beery Q, and Sabo D. Identification of otitis media with effusion in children. Ann Otol Rhinol Laryngol 1980;89:(Suppl 68):part 2, 190–195.

Chiveralls K. A further examination of the use of the stapedius reflex in the diagnosis of acoustic neuroma. Audiology 1977;16:331–337.

Citron D, and Adour K. Acoustic reflex and loudness discomfort in acute facial paralysis. Arch Otolaryngol 1978;104:303–308.

Clemis JD, and Sarno CN. The acoustic reflex latency test: clinical applications. Laryngoscope 1980;90:601–611.

Djupesland G. Advanced reflex considerations. In Jerger J, Ed. *Handbook of Clinical Impedance Audiometry*, 1st ed. Dobbs Ferry, NY: American Electromedics, 1975:102–110.

Djupesland G. The acoustic reflex. In Jerger J, and Northern J, Eds. *Clinical Impedance Audiometry*, 2nd ed. Acton, MA: American Electromedics, 1980:65–82.

Dudich TM, Keiser M, and Keith RW. Some relationships between loudness and the acoustic reflex. Impedance Newsletter 4, 12-15. American Electromedics, Acton, MA, 1975.

Fee WE. Clinical applications of nonacoustic middle ear muscle stimulation. Arch Otolaryngol 1981;107:224–226.

Fria T, LeBlanc J, Kristensen R, and Alberti PW. Ipsilateral acoustic reflex stimulation in normal and sensorineural impaired ears: a preliminary report. Canad J Otol 1975;4:695–703.

Givens GD, and Seidemann MF. A systematic investigation of measurement parameters of acoustic reflex adaptation. J Speech Hear Disord 1979;44:534–542.

Greisen O, and Rasmussen PE. Stapedius muscle reflexes and otoneurological examinations in brain stem tumors. Acta Otolaryngol 1970;70:366–370.

Hall JW. Predicting hearing level from the acoustic reflex: a comparison of three methods. Arch Otolaryngol 1978;104:601–606.

Hall JW, and Jerger JF. Acoustic reflexes in spastic dysphonia. Arch Otolaryngol 1976;102:411–415.

Hall JW, and Weaver T. Impedance audiometry in a young population: the effect of age, sex and tympanogram abnormalities. J_Otolaryngol 1979;8:210–222.

Hall JW, and Ghorayeb BY. Diagnosis of middle ear pathology and evaluation of conductive hearing loss. In Jacobson J, and Northern J, Eds. *Diagnostic Audiology.* Austin, TX: Pro-Ed, 1991:161–168.

Hannley, M. Immittance audiometry. In Jerger J, Ed. *Hearing Disorders in Adults.* San Diego, CA: College-Hill Press, 1983.

Hannley M, and Jerger J. PB rollover and the acoustic reflex. Audiology 1981;20:251–258.

Harford E, Bess F, Bluestone C, and Klein J. *Impedance Screening for Middle Ear Disease in Children.* New York: Grune and Stratton, 1978.

Hayes D, and Jerger J. Patterns of acoustic reflex and auditory brainstem response abnormality. Acta Otolaryngol 1981;92:199–209.

Hirsch A. The stapedius reflex tests in retrocochlear hearing disorders. Audiology 1983;22:463–470.

Hoover K, Chermak G, and Doyle C. A comparative study of immittance screening procedures with preschool aged children. Am J Otol 1982;4:142–147.

Jerger JF. Clinical experience with impedance audiometry. Arch Otolaryngol 1970;92:311–324.

Jerger JF. Strategies for neuroaudiological evaluation. Semin Hear 1983;4:109–120.

Jerger JF, and Hayes D. Diagnostic applications of impedance audiometry: middle ear disorder, sensori-neural disorder. In Jerger JF, and Northern JL, Eds. *Clinical Impedance Audiometry.* Acton, MA: American Electromedics, 1980;109–127.

Jerger JF, Jerger S, and Mauldin L. Studies in impedance audiometry. I. Normal and sensorineural ears. Arch Otolaryngol 1972;96:513–523.

Jerger JF, Burney P, Mauldin L, and Crump B. Predicting hearing loss from the acoustic reflex. J Speech Hear Disord 1974a;39:11.

Jerger JF, Anthony L, Jerger S, and Crump B. Studies in impedance audiometry. III. Middle ear disorders. Arch Otolaryngol 1973b;99: 165–171.

Jerger JF, Harford E, Clemis J, and Alford B. The acoustic reflex in VIIIth nerve disorders. Arch Otolaryngol 1974c;99:409–413.

Jerger JF, Hayes D, Anthony L, and Mauldin L. Factors influencing prediction of hearing levels from the acoustic reflex. Monogr Contemp Audiol 1978;1:1–20.

Jerger JF, Jerger S, and Neely JG. The neurological evaluation. Semin Hear 1983;4:81–178.

Jerger JF, Fifer R, Jenkins H, and Mecklenburg D. Stapedius reflex to electrical stimulation in a patient with a cochlear implant. Ann Otol Rhinol Laryngol 1986a;95:151–157.

Jerger JF, Oliver TA, Rivera V, and Stach BA. Abnormalities of the acoustic reflex in multiple sclerosis. Amer J Otolaryngol 1986b; 7:163–176.

Jerger JF, Oliver TA, and Jenkins H. Suprathreshold abnormalities of the stapedius reflex in acoustic tumor: a series of case reports. Ear Hear 1986;3:131–139.

Jerger JF, Oliver TA, and Chmiel RA. Prediction of dynamic range from stapedius reflex in cochlear implant patients. Ear Hear 1988;9:4–8.

Jerger S. Diagnostic application of impedance audiometry in central auditory disorders. In Jerger JF. and Northern JL, Eds. Clinical Impedance Audiometry, 2nd Ed. Acton, MA: American Electromedics, 1980.

Jerger S. Decision matrix and information theory analyses in the evaluation of neuroaudiologic tests. Semin Hear 1083;4:121–132.

Jerger S, and Jerger J. Neuroaudiologic findings in patients with central auditory disorders. Semin Hear 1983;4:133–159.

Jerger S, Neely G, and Jerger J. Recovery of crossed acoustic reflexes in brain stem and auditory disorder. Arch Otolaryngol 1975; 101L:329–332.

Johnson E. An analysis of auditory test results in 500 cases of acoustic neuroma. Arch Otolaryngol 1977;103:152–157.

Keith RW. An acoustic reflex technique of establishing hearing aid settings. J Am Aud Soc 1979;5:71–75.

Keith RW, Murphy KP, and Martin F. Acoustic impedance measurement in the otologic assessment of multiply handicapped children. Clin Otolaryngol 1976;1:221–224.

Lamb LE, and Norris TW. Relative acoustic impedance measurement with mentally retarded children. Am J Ment Defic 1970;75:51–56.

Laukli E, and Meir IWS. Ipsilateral and contralateral acoustic reflex thresholds. Audiology 1990;19:469–494.

Leis BR, and Lutman ME. Calibrations of ipsilateral acoustic reflex stimuli. Scand Audiol 1979;8:93–99.

Lucker J. Application of pass/fail criteria to immittance screening. Asha 1980;22:815–816.

McCall G. Acoustic impedance measurement in the study of patients with spasmodic dysphonia. J Speech Hear Disord 1973;38:250–255.

McCandless GA, and Allfred PL. Tympanometry and emergence of the acoustic reflex in infants. In Harford ER, Bess FH, Bluestone CD, and Klein JO, Eds. Impedance Screening for Middle Ear Disease in Children. New York: Grune and Stratton, pp 57–68.

McCandless GA, and Keith R. Use of impedance measurements in hearing aid fittings. In Jerger JF, and Northern JL, Eds. Clinical Impedance Audiometry, 2nd ed. Acton, MA: American Electromedics, 1980.

McLeod HL, and Greenberg HJ. Relationship between loudness discomfort level and acoustic reflex threshold for normal and sensorineural hearing impaired individuals. J Speech Hear Res 1979; 22:873–883.

Mahoney, T. Acoustic reflex crossover artifacts in infants and young children. Arch Otolaryngol 1981;107:363–366.

Metz O. The acoustic impedance measured on normal and pathological ears. Acta Otolaryngol Suppl 1946;63:397–405.

Metz O. Threshold of reflex contractions of muscles of middle ear and recruitment of loudness. Arch Otolaryngol 1952;55:536–543.

Mitchell O, and Richard G. Effects of various anesthetic agents on normal and pathological middle ears. Ear Nose Throat J 1976;55:36–38.

Moller AR. Bilateral contraction of tympanic muscles in man. Ann Otol Rhinol Laryngol 1961;70:735–745.

Moller A. The sensitivity of contraction of the tympanic muscle in man. Ann Otol 1962;77:86.

Niemeyer W, and Sesterhenn G. Calculating the hearing threshold from the stapedius reflex threshold for different sound stimuli. Audiology 1974;13:421–427.

Northern JL. Impedance audiometry for otologic diagnosis. In Shambaugh G, and Shea JJ, Eds. Proceedings of the Shambaugh Fifth International Workshop on Middle Ear Microsurgery and Fluctuant Hearing Loss. Huntsville, AL: Strode, 1977a.

Northern JL. Acoustic impedance in the pediatric population. In Bess FH, Ed. Childhood Deafness: Causation, Assessment and Management. New York: Grune and Stratton, 1977b:135–152.

Northern JL. Impedance screening in special populations—state of the art. In Harford ER, Bess FH, Bluestone CD, and Klein JO. Eds. Impedance Screening for Middle Ear Disease in Children. New York: Grune and Stratton, 1978a:229–248.

Northern JL. Hearing aids and acoustic impedance measurements. Monogr Contemp Audiol 1978b;1:2.

Northern JL. Impedance measurements with distinctive groups. In Jerger J, and Northern J, Eds. Clinical Impedance Audiometry, 2nd ed. Acton, MA: American Electromedics, 1980.

Northern JL. Clinical applications of impedance audiometry. In Northern JL, Ed. Hearing Disorders. Boston: Little, Brown and Co., 1984.

Northern JL, and Downs MP. Hearing in Children, 4th Ed. Baltimore: Williams & Wilkins, 1991.

Olsen WO, Noffsinger D, and Kurdziel S. Acoustic reflex and reflex decay occurrence in patients with cochlear and VIII nerve lesions. Arch Otolaryngol 1975;101:622–625.

Olsen WO. Special auditory tests: a historical perspective. In Jacobson J, and Northern J, Eds. Diagnostic Audiology. Austin, TX: Pro-Ed, 1991:19–52.

Orchik DJ, and Mackimmie KS. Immittance audiometry. In Jerger JF, Ed. Pediatric Audiology, San Diego, CA: College-Hill Press, 1983: 45–70.

Popelka G. The acoustic reflex in normal and pathological ears. In Popelka G, Ed. Hearing Assessment with the Acoustic Reflex. New York: Grune and Stratton, 1981a:5–6.

Popelka G. First attempts at hearing assessment with acoustic reflex measures. In Popelka G, Ed. Hearing Assessment with the Acoustic Reflex. New York: Grune and Stratton, 1981b:23–45.

Queen S, Moses F, Wood S, Harryman D, and Couty C. The use of immittance screening by the Kansas City, Missouri public school district. Semin Speech Lang Hear 1981;2:119–122.

Rappaport B, and Tait C. Acoustic reflex threshold measurement in hearing aid selection. Arch Otolaryngol 1976;102:129–134.

Ritter R, Johnson RM, and Northern JL. The controversial relationship between loudness discomfort levels and acoustic reflex thresholds. J Am Aud Soc 1979;4:123–131.

Rizzo S, Jr, and Greenberg HJ. Predicting hearing loss from the acoustic reflex. Presented at Fiftieth Meeting of the Acoustical Society of America, Boston, 1979.

Robinette MS, Rhodes DP, and Marion MW. Effects of secobarbital on impedance audiometry. Arch Otolaryngol 1974;100:351.

Sanders JW. Diagnostic audiology. In Lass N, McReynolds L, Northern J, and Yoder D, Eds. Handbook of Speech-Language Pathology and Audiology. Toronto: B.C. Decker, Inc., 1988:1123–1142.

Sanders JW. Diagnostic audiology. In Northern JL, Ed. Hearing Disorders, 2nd Ed. Boston: Little, Brown and Company, 1984:25–40.

Silman S, and Gelfand S. The acoustic reflex in diagnostic audiology, Part 2. Audiology 1982;7:111–124.

Silman S, Gelfand SA, Piper N, Silverman CA, and Van Frank L. Prediction of hearing loss from the acoustic-reflex threshold. In Silman

S, Ed. *The Acoustic Reflex Basic Principles and Clinical Applications.* Orlando, FL: Academic Press, Inc., 1984:187–223.

Simmons FB. Perceptual theories of middle ear muscle function. Ann Otol Rhinol Laryngol 1964;73:724–739.

Stach BA, Jerger JF, and Jenkins HA. The human acoustic tensor tympanic reflex. Scand Audiol 1984;13:93–99.

Stach BA, and Jerger JF. Acoustic reflex averaging. Ear Hear 1984;5:289–296.

Stach BA, and Jerger JF. Techniques for acoustic-reflex measurement and analysis. Semin Hear 1987;8:359–367.

Stach BA. The acoustic reflex in diagnostic audiology: from Metz to present. Ear and Hear 1987;8:(Suppl 4):365–415.

Stach BA, and Jerger JF. Immittance measures in auditory disorders. In Jacobson JT, and Northern JL, Eds. *Diagnostic Audiology.* Austin, TX: Pro-Ed, 1991:113–140.

Suria D, and Serra-Raventos W. Acoustic impedance measurement and autistic children. Folia Phoniatr (Basel) 1975;27:387–388.

Terkildsen K, Osterhammel P, and Bretlau P. Acoustic middle ear muscle reflexes in patients with otosclerosis. Arch Otolaryngol 1973;98:152–155.

Thompson G. Structure and function of the central auditory system. Semin Hear 1983;4:1–13.

Wallin A, Mendez-Kurtz L, and Silman S. Prediction of hearing loss from acoustic-reflex thresholds in the older adult population. Ear Hear 1986;7:400–404.

Weatherby L, and Bennett M. The neonatal acoustic reflex. Scand Audiol 1990;9:103–110.

Wever EG, and Lawrence M. *Physiological Acoustics.* Princeton, NJ: Princeton University Press, 1954.

Wilson R. Factors influencing the acoustic immittance characteristics of the acoustic reflex. J Speech Hear Res 1979;22:480–499.

Wilson R. The effects of aging on the magnitude of the acoustic reflex. J Speech Hear Res 1981;24:406–414.

CHAPTER 22

Auditory Evoked Potentials: Overview and Basic Principles

John A. Ferraro and John D. Durrant

Auditory evoked potentials (AEP) have assumed an essential role in the clinical practice of audiology and several other professions. The technical capability to record electrical potentials generated at various levels of the nervous system in response to acoustic stimulation has produced a multitude of applications relevant to the hearing/ear/nervous system specialist. That these potentials can be recorded noninvasively with no discomfort to the patient, and often without sedation or anesthesia, further enhances their clinical applicability.

This chapter will provide a basic overview of the history, nomenclature, and characteristics associated with those AEP that have become popular in the clinical domain. Technical-, subject-, and examiner-related variables relevant to the recording and interpretation of these responses also will be addressed. The authors have chosen to take a practical approach to these issues with the aim of providing a source of clinically meaningful information and reference, and preparing the reader for the subsequent chapters of the Handbook which deal with specific AEP.

HISTORICAL PERSPECTIVES

A recording of the random and spontaneous bioelectric activity generated by the central nervous system in the absence of sensory stimulation is known as the electroencephalogram (EEG). The EEG in humans was first described by Berger (1929) as consisting of semirhythmic electrical patterns with varying frequencies and amplitudes, depending on the state of the subject. In the presence of sensory stimulation, these patterns undergo certain stimulus-related changes that can be extracted from the background EEG, the resultant being known as an evoked potential (EP).

The evolution of EP measurement as a clinical tool has occurred over a period of more than six decades. Subsequent to Berger's work, Loomis et al. (1938) described a triphasic response to sensory stimulation in the EEG pattern of sleeping patients. This was identified as the "K complex." Davis (1939), and Davis et al. (1939) went on to describe the K complex evoked by auditory stimulation in both awake and sleeping subjects. The re-

sponses were referred to as "V potentials" because they were most prominent when recorded from the vertex of the scalp (a locus defined by the intersection of a mid-sagittal plane and a coronal plane through the center of the ear canals).

As reported by the early investigators of these phenomena, the stimulus-related patterns described above were at best minute, and often unobservable within the much larger background of spontaneous EEG activity. It thus became necessary to devise techniques for extracting the low-level voltage changes evoked by sensory stimulation from this background. Development and application of the "signal averaging" or "summating" computer represented the most successful solution to this problem. Clark (1958) and Clark et al. (1961) reported the use of a computer that converted analog data (such as the EEG) into digital information that could be stored and manipulated by the computer. The principles applied to this process are that the changes in the EEG produced by a fixed and synchronous stimulus are consistent, whereas the background EEG itself is random. Furthermore, the result of repeated stimulation is that the algebraic sum of the consistent signals (i.e., the EP) grows in proportion to the number of signals summed, whereas the amplitude of the random noise (EEG) averages to zero. Thus, if several samples of neuroelectric activity containing both EP and background EEG are digitized, stored, and summed via the computer, the magnitude of the EP will be enhanced as the EEG becomes reduced toward zero. Despite certain caveats that will be described later in this chapter, the above principles underlie the measurement of all evoked potentials.

Early interests in AEP were directed toward those components thought to be of cortical origin and generated in a time period of between 50–500 milliseconds after stimulus onset (Davis and Yoshie, 1963; Davis et al., 1964; Walter et al., 1964; McCandless and Best, 1964). At about the same time, but to a lesser degree, AEP generated in the comparatively early time domain of between 15–50 milliseconds after stimulation were also under investigation (Geisler et al., 1958; Lowell, 1965; Ruhm et al., 1967; Goldstein and Rodman, 1967; Mendel and

Goldstein, 1969). Still others were investigating the gross response of the human auditory nerve, which occurred within the first few milliseconds after stimulus onset (Ruben et al., 1960).

Despite their promise, AEP in general did not enjoy widespread acceptance and application as clinical tools until the discovery of the auditory brainstem response (ABR). First reported by Sohmer and Feinmesser (1967) and later described by Jewett et al. (1970) and Jewett and Williston (1971), the ABR has become the most popular and widely used AEP for audiologic and otoneurologic purposes. Indeed, for a time after its discovery, the ABR dominated clinical attention to AEP. However, due in large part to the popularity of the ABR, interest in other AEP has been rekindled. This has led to dramatic developments, refinements, and expansions of the various applications of virtually all AEP during the past decade. These advancements will continue to evolve as our knowledge of the transduction and neural processes of hearing expands, and the techniques for measuring and analyzing the electrophysiologic events associated with these processes become more sensitive and/or sophisticated.

CLASSIFICATION AND NOMENCLATURE

There have been several approaches to classifying and naming AEP, but none has yet to be completely standardized. AEP classification and nomenclature systems are generally based on such aspects as the time domain within which the response occurs after stimulus onset, known as the "latency epoch" (i.e., short/early, middle, long/late) (Ruth and Lambert, 1991), anatomic origin (e.g., brainstem, cortical), stimulus-response relationship (i.e., transient versus sustained, exogenous versus endogenous), or electrode placement (i.e., near- versus far-field) (Jacobson and Hyde, 1985). A summary of the classification and nomenclature systems used for AEP, with examples of specific responses that fall under these various categories, is shown in Table 22.1.

The current classification of AEP according to latency epoch was adapted from the work of Picton et al. (1974, 1977), and Picton and Fitzgerald (1983). Figure 22.1, adapted from Michelini et al. (1982), displays a series of AEP analyzed on a logarithmic time-base according to their latency epochs. Figures 22.2 - 22.6 display the more clinically "popular" responses within each of these epochs with their names and specific components identified. Those AEP occurring within the first 10–15 milliseconds following stimulus onset are generally referred to as the "early" or "short" latency responses (SLR). The SLR include the ABR seen in Figures 22.1 and 22.2, and also several components preceding the ABR that are recorded via electrocochleography (ECochG) (Figure 22.3). Other SLR include the slow-negative$_{10}$ potential

(SN$_{10}$) (Davis and Hirsh, 1979), and the frequency following response (FFR) (Moushegian et al., 1973). The SN$_{10}$ appears as a negative trough approximately 10 milliseconds after stimulus onset, whereas the FFR is phase-locked to and thus mimics the frequency of a tonal stimulus. The clinical use of both the SN$_{10}$ and the FFR has been overshadowed by that of other AEP. The term "middle latency response" (MLR) is used with reference to those components in the latency epoch of 10–50 milliseconds. It is interesting to note that in the first edition of this Handbook, published in 1972 (i.e., shortly after the discovery of the ABR but before clinical development), the present MLR were referred to as the early AEP. Although the "abbreviation MLR" have come to denote the specific pattern of responses seen in Figures 22.1 and 22.4, other patterns occurring in this time domain also have been described. The most prominent of these is the 40 Hz steady state potential (SSP) (formerly called the 40 Hz event-related-potential ERP), shown in Figure 22.5. Finally, those components generated beyond 50–80 milliseconds post-stimulus onset are considered to be the "slow," or "long" latency responses (LLR), or "late" potentials. These include the N$_1$-P$_2$ complex seen in Figures 22.1 and 22.6, and the P$_{300}$ (or P$_3$) also shown in Figure 22.6.

As is apparent in Figures 22.2 - 22.6, the nomenclature assigned to specific responses and their components is inconsistent across the family of AEP. For example, the conventional method of identifying individual ABR peaks or waves is with Roman numerals (Jewett and Williston, 1971). However, as seen in Figure 22.3, ECochG components are labeled according what they actually represent (i.e., SP = summating potential, AP = auditory nerve action potential). N$_1$ and N$_2$ denote the first and second negative peaks of the AP. These components are virtually identical to waves I and II of the ABR.

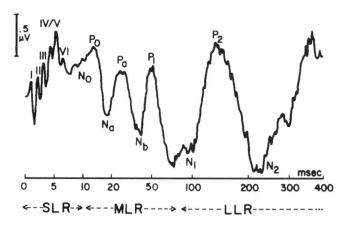

Figure 22.1. Auditory evoked potentials analyzed on a logarithmic time–base and categorized according to latency epoch as short- (SLR), middle- (MLR) and long- (LLR) latency responses. (From ASHA, 1988.)

Table 22.1.
AEP Classification Systems and Descriptions

Common Name	Physiologic Description	Anatomic Source	Latency Epoch	Latency Range *msec*	Stimulus-Response	Electrode-Response
Cochlear microphonic (CM)	Receptor	Hair cells	short/early	0	Sustained	Near field
Summating potential (SP)	Receptor	Hair cells	short/early	0	Sustained	Near field
Action potential (AP) (N₁, N₂) ECochG	Neurogenic	Auditory nerve	short/early	~2	Transient	Near and far field
Auditory brainstem response (ABR) (I to VII)	Neurogenic	Auditory nerve Brainstem	short/early	<10	Transient	Far field
Slow-negative (SN10)	Neurogenic	Brainstem	short/early	~10	Transient	Far field
Frequency following response (FFR)	Neurogenic	Brainstem	short/early	Tone duration	Sustained	Far field
Middle latency response (MLR) (No, Po, Na, Pa, Nb, Pb)	Neurogenic	Thalamus Auditory cortex	middle	8–50	Transient	Far field
Steady State potential (40 Hz)	Neurogenic	Brainstem-thalamus Auditory cortex	early? middle?	12–50	Transient? Sustained?	Far field
N₁-P₂ complex (P₁, N₁, P₂, N₂)	Neurogenic	Cerebral cortex (primary and association)	long	50–300	Transient	Far field
Late positive component (P300)	Neurogenic	Cerebral cortex (primary and association)	late	250–350	Perceptual	Far field
Contingent negative variation (CNV)	Neurogenic	Cerebral cortex (association)	late	300+	Perceptual	Far field

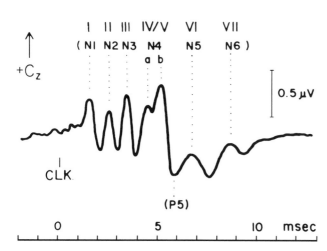

Figure 22.2. Auditory brainstem response (ABR) to click stimuli, labeled according to Jewett and Williston (1971) method (waves I - VII). **Clk.** indicates onset of click stimulus. Electrode configuration: vertex (**Cz**)-to-ipsilateral mastoid, ground at nasion (just above bridge of nose). Peak identifiers in parentheses: from Sohmer and Feinmesser (1967) who used an ipsilateral earlobe-to-bridge of nose configuration. (From ASHA, 1988.)

Labeling of the middle and long latency AEP is slightly more consistent, where the initials P (for positive) and N (for negative) denote component polarity. P or N labeling of an MLR is followed by alphabetical subscripts (Mendel and Goldstein, 1969), whereas numerical subscripts are generally used to denote the components of the LLR (Davis and Zerlin, 1966). To add to this confusion, the first components of the MLR, as shown in Figure 22.4, are identified with the subscript "0," which refers to zero, whereas the remaining components are identified in alphabetical order. Finally, the P_{300}, as shown in Figure 22.6, is named according to its polarity and general, absolute latency (time of occurrence after stimulus onset). Because it is the third positive peak of the LLR, the P_{300} is often labeled P_3.

The nomenclature of AEP and their components can also be assigned according to anatomic origin. Unfortunately, the use of this method has often been misleading. For example, the term auditory brainstem response is commonly used to denote an AEP whose first two components actually arise predominantly from the auditory nerve (Moller et al., 1981, Moller and Janetta, 1982). Of course, the naming or classification of AEP according to anatomic origin is based on the premise that these origins have been precisely identified. This is tenuous, considering that AEP recorded from the surface of the scalp are generated by literally thousands of neurons. However, it is generally agreed that the latency epoch of an AEP is reflective of the level of the auditory system contributing the bulk of electrical activity for a given response. Thus, the SLR arise from the auditory periphery

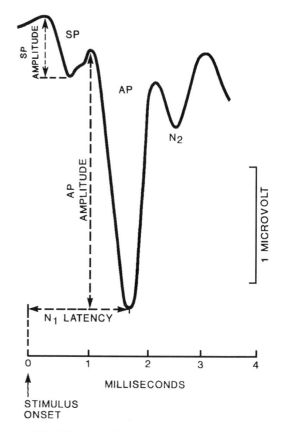

Figure 22.3. Electrocochleographic response to click stimuli recorded from the ear canal, with components defined and labeled. **SP** = summating potential; **AP** = action potential; N_1 and N_2 indicate first and second negative peaks of the AP. (Adapted from Ferraro et al., 1989.)

and pontine-to-midbrain level brainstem, whereas the LLR are cortically-generated. The MLR appear to arise from structures beyond the inferior colliculus to and including the primary auditory cortex (Kraus et al., 1982; Kileny et al., 1987; Kraus and McGee, 1988; Kraus and McGee, 1990). However, the precise origins of all AEP components except wave I of the ABR (or ECochG N_1) is still a controversial area.

A less common method used to classify AEP is according to stimulus-response relationship. Under this system responses may be classified as transient or sustained. For example, the ABR and other AEP evoked by clicks or tones with fast rise/fall times may be identified as transient because the response is dependent on a rapid change in the stimulus. Prolonged stimulation, such as that from long tone-bursts or quasi-steady-state signals, may produce a sustained response that lasts as long as the stimulus. Cochlear microphonic or summating potential ECochG responses to tone-bursts are examples of sustained responses.

AEP are also characterized as being "exogenous" or "endogenous" based on stimulus-response relationship.

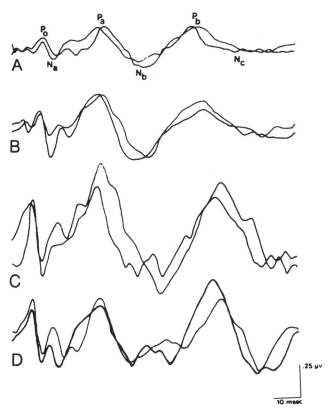

Figure 22.4. Middle latency responses from two premature infants (**A**), full term newborns (**B**), young children (**C**), and adults (**D**). Components labeled on top tracing (From Mendelson and Salamy, 1981.)

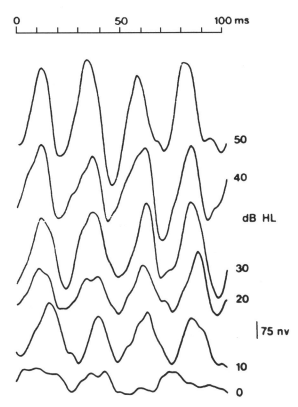

Figure 22.5. Intensity series of 40 Hz steady-state potentials elicited by 500 Hz tone-bursts from a normal subject. **O dB HL** = average behavioral threshold to 500 Hz tone-bursts based on clinic norms. (From Brown and Shallop, 1982.)

The SLR, MLR and the N_1-P_2 complex of the LLR are predominantly exogenous because they depend on the physical features of the stimulus. An endogenous (or perceptual) response is one that is largely independent of the physical features of the stimulus, but is sensitive to the "context" within which the stimuli are presented and the ability of the subject to recognize or attach meaning to this context. The P_{300} is an endogenous potential and can be elicited when two different stimuli are presented together in a "rare-frequent" ("oddball") paradigm (see subsequent section on P_{300}). The contingent negative variation (CNV) after the P_{300} is also endogenous (Walter et al., 1964), but has received comparatively less clinical attention in audiology/otoneurology.

Finally, AEP responses may be classified as near-field or far-field, depending on the location of the recording electrodes relative to the site of the response generator(s). As implied, near-field recordings are obtained when the electrodes are near or even on the neural generator(s). Under these conditions, slight changes in the location of the electrodes can have profound effects on the morphology of the resultant waveform. In far-field recordings the distance between the electrodes and generator(s) is comparatively large and placement site

becomes a less critical variable. Virtually all AEP recordings from the scalp may be considered far-field, whereas those made during intraoperative, direct nerve monitoring and electrocochleography are examples of near-field recordings. Although more rigorously defined in some areas of physics, a clear demarcation between near- and far-field conditions is not always apparent in AEP measurement.

This section would not be complete without calling attention to yet another confusing aspect associated with the nomenclature of AEP. Namely, certain responses may be referred to by more than one name. For example, the ABR is also called the brainstem auditory evoked potential (BAEP), brainstem auditory evoked response (BAER), auditory brainstem evoked potential (ABEP), brain stem response (BSR), etc. Indeed, we have counted no less than 10 different terms which are commonly used to refer to this particular AEP, although ABR, BAEP, and BAER appear to the most popular at this time. It is also customary to refer to specific AEP by their initials or with the use of acronyms. This is seemingly done for the sake of brevity regardless of where it occurs (e.g., in the literature, clinic reports, hospital charts, oral communica-

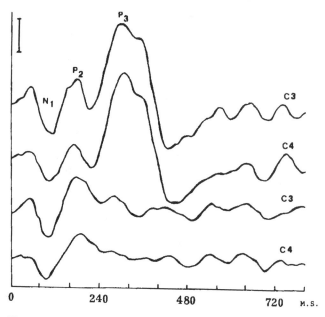

Figure 22.6. Long-latency responses from a normal subject. The **top two traces** include the N_1-P_2 complex (primarily exogenous components) and the P_{300} or P_3 (primarily endogenous component) elicited by presenting 1000 Hz and 2000 Hz tone-bursts in an "oddball" paradigm. The **two bottom traces** show the response elicited by the frequent stimulus (1000 Hz tone-burst) yielding only the N_1-P_2 complex. Calibration marker at the **left top** = 4.88 microvolts. C_3 and C_4 indicate primary recording sites (10-20 system). (From Musiek, 1991.)

tion). Unfortunately, the standardization of terms, abbreviations, and acronyms used to reference specific AEP is woefully lacking, as is a general consensus regarding which are the best to use, or most descriptive of the responses being measured. It is not the intent here to resolve this problem, but merely to acknowledge and call attention to its nagging presence.

TECHNICAL ASPECTS OF RECORDING AEP

There are several technical-, subject/patient-, and examiner-related variables associated with the recording and interpretation of AEP. The technical or physical variables generally pertain to the settings and/or characteristics of the various components used to elicit, record, store, and analyze AEP. Figure 22.7 is a simplified block diagram of the elements essential to these purposes. In general, these elements function to: generate, transduce, and deliver appropriate acoustic stimuli to the subject, and trigger the onset of the signal averaging process; conduct the electrophysiologic response to acoustic stimulation evoked from the subject to subsequent electronic components; amplify and filter the electrophysiologic response; perform signal averaging; display/store and produce a written record of the response for analysis/interpretation.

Stimulus-Related Variables

Stimulus Type

In general, AEP are elicited by either click or brief-tone acoustic stimuli, although other signals such as complex tones and speech are also used. Stimulus type, and specific stimulus variables such as spectrum, polarity, repetition rate, and level are dependent on the particular AEP being measured and the reason for testing (e.g., audiometric versus neurologic assessment).

The transducers used to deliver AEP stimuli are usually headphones or insert earphones, which circumvent certain problems associated with loudspeakers (e.g., variability in distance to the ear, sound propagation delays, environmental acoustics). Tubal, insert-type earphones, which are growing in popularity, use a flexible, silicon tube to convey the stimulus from the transducer to the ear. This, too, increases sound propagation time, thus delaying the onset of the AEP by a factor proportional to the length of the tubing. Bone vibrators can be used but have inherent problems or limitations. Namely, their frequency response characteristics are different than those of typically-used earphones; placement site and physical coupling to the head are somewhat variable; electromagnetic radiation (a major source of recording artifact) is higher for bone vibrators than for earphones; and masking of the non-test ear may be of concern at nearly all stimulus levels.

An important factor, especially for the short-latency AEP such as ECochG and ABR, is that the stimulus must elicit a synchronous response from a large population of neurons. This is best achieved with transient stimuli of rapid onset. Such stimuli activate a considerable portion of the cochlear partition because of their relatively broad spectra. One stimulus that meets these criteria and elicits robust AEP is the broad-band click (BBC). The BBC is produced by exciting the transducer with a rectangular voltage pulse. A pulse with a duration of 100 microseconds is commonly used because its spectrum is nearly flat up to 10,000 Hz (i.e., its first null occurs at 1/100 microseconds) (Durrant and Lovrinic, 1984). The upper frequency limit of the click output generally ranges from 5,000–10,000 Hz, depending on the frequency response characteristics of the transducer; the "flatness" of the spectrum depends on the resonances of the transducer. Thus, the waveform of the BBC acoustic output is different than that of the electrical input. This relationship is shown in Figure 22.8. When presented to a subject, the output is further modified by the frequency response of the outer and middle ears. Consequently, the spectrum of the actual stimulus reaching the cochlea is less than flat, and substantially narrower in bandwidth than the spectrum of the signal driving the transducer.

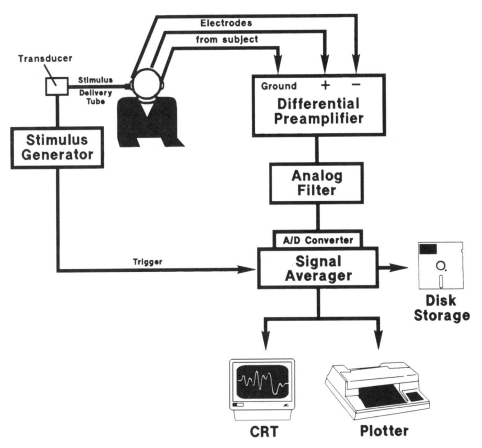

Figure 22.7. Basic components of an auditory evoked potential test unit (**A/D** = analog-to-digital; **CRT** = cathode ray tube).

The above factors combine to emphasize the contributions of higher frequency units when BBC are used to elicit AEP (Jerger et al., 1980; Gorga et al., 1985). The threshold of the BBC-elicited ABR, for example, has been shown to correlate most closely with the average of behavioral puretone thresholds in the 1–4 kHz range (Jerger and Mauldin, 1978). Inferences regarding low frequency auditory sensitivity, therefore, cannot be made directly from AEP elicited by BBC.

Generally speaking, filtered clicks and sinusoidal stimuli with longer rise times than BBC are used when "frequency-specific" information is desired from the AEP. The presentation of masking noise with these stimuli also has been used for this purpose. In addition, sinusoidal stimuli are used when the response is dependent on the entire duration of the stimulus rather than its onset.

Filtered clicks, as the term implies, are produced by sending the rectangular driving pulse used to produce the BBC through a band-pass filter before transduction. Although this produces a signal whose spectrum is narrower in bandwidth than the BBC, the filtered click does not have a discrete spectrum, as does the pure tone. The temporal characteristics of the filtered click, as well as its bandwidth, are determined by the filter characteristics.

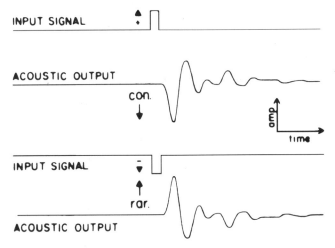

Figure 22.8. Electrical input signals to an earphone (Telephonics TDH-39) and corresponding acoustic outputs for condensation (**con.**) and rarefaction (**rar.**) clicks. (From ASHA, 1988.)

Responses from relatively narrow frequency regions also may be elicited by sinusoidal pulses, such as tone-pips and tone-bursts. The envelope of the tone-pip is characterized by a rise/fall time and no plateau, whereas the tone-burst contains a plateau of some duration. The tone-burst may be created using a variety of gating functions that shape the stimulus envelope (i.e. rise/fall time after linear, cosine, cosine-squared, or other mathematical functions). The shape of the gating function and relationship between duration of the rise/fall versus plateau determines the relative amount of energy concentrated near the frequency of the sinusoid versus energy "splattered" into surrounding frequencies (i.e., side lobes) (Gorga et al., 1988). One strategy for choosing stimulus envelope is to maintain a constant power spectrum by setting the temporal parameters according to the number of cycles of the underlying sinusoid. For example, a "2-1-2" envelope has a rise/fall equal to two cycles and a plateau duration equal to one cycle. 2-1-2 tone bursts at 2000 and 8000 Hz thus demonstrate the same power spectrum even although the 2000 Hz burst is four times longer in duration. Additional transients that have been applied in AEP measurement include single- and half-period sinusoids and pulses with Gaussian envelopes (Jacobson and Hyde, 1985).

For the acquisition of frequency-specific information, two important considerations for selecting stimulus type and parameters are 1) how long can the stimulus be without interfering with the recorded response, and 2) how much splatter of acoustic energy can be tolerated. The first problem arises from possible contamination from stimulus artifact (e.g., radiation from the transducer). At moderately high stimulus levels, at least, it is generally preferable that the stimulus last into the time epoch of the AEP components of interest (e.g., a few milliseconds or less for the SLR). This tends to exacerbate the second concern, that of splatter, although some envelopes yield less splatter than others. This will be most critical in cases of hearing loss with other than flat configurations. In these instances, the splattered energy rather than the energy of the test frequency may be detected by the cochlea. Although certain envelopes have been suggested to minimize this problem (Gorga et al., 1988), at high stimulus intensities the spread of excitation extends into the basal regions of the cochlea regardless of stimulus spectrum (Bekesy, 1960; Durrant et al., 1981). An alternative approach is to use notch-band masking. That is, a masker with energy above and below the main lobe of the stimulus spectrum is used to limit the response to the frequency region of interest (Stapells et al., 1985). Regardless of method, the frequency specificity of AEP elicited by low-frequency stimuli, and the practicality of the methods used to achieve this, continue to be debated. This is especially true for the SLR.

Stimulus Polarity

Stimulus "polarity" is defined by the dominant, initial direction of the transducer diaphragm, and is a variable especially important for SLR. If the electrical pulse produces an initial diaphragm movement that is outward, the acoustic output is considered to be a "condensation" click; if the deflection is inward a "rarefaction" click results (see Figure 22.8). The initial polarity of successive clicks in an averaging "run" may be fixed (condensation or rarefaction) or alternated. Alternating polarity is commonly used to suppress stimulus-induced electrical artifact (i.e., by phase cancellation over time). This is especially the case for the short latency components, wherein the artifact may extend into the waveform of the response. However, the use of alternating clicks may produce AEP waves/peaks that are less sharply defined than those elicited by condensation or rarefaction stimuli. This is because the initial displacement of the cochlear partition in response to a condensation pressure wave (initial stapes movement inward) is toward the scala tympani, whereas the direction of initial displacement to a rarefaction wave (initial stapes movement outward) is toward the scala vestibuli. Inasmuch as the auditory nerve is excited only during the latter motion, there will be a slight temporal disparity and resultant latency difference between the auditory nerve and brainstem components evoked by condensation versus rarefaction stimuli. Thus, alternating clicks may "smear" or broaden the waveform of the averaged response. Although the basis is not always apparent, this smearing may be exaggerated for some individuals, especially those with high-frequency, sensory-neural hearing loss. Finally, alternating polarity cannot be used when the desired AEP is dependent on stimulus phase. For example, alternating clicks or tones will cancel/inhibit the signal-averaged cochlear microphonic or FFR.

Given the above and if a choice must be made, it is usually preferable to use fixed as opposed to alternating polarity when recording the short latency AEP. However, if stimulus artifact precludes or distorts the definition of any components, most recording systems allow the examiner to store responses to condensation and rarefaction stimuli separately, then combine these "off-line" to derive the response to alternating stimuli.

Stimulus Repetition Rate

The rate at which AEP stimuli are presented must be slow enough to prevent significant adaptation of the response, but not so slow that clinical use is compromised due to excessive data collection time. Rates on the order of 10–40/second are common, again depending on the specific AEP desired, degree of adaptation tolerable and reason for testing. Figure 22.9 illustrates the effects of stimulus repetition rate on the ABR. For the SLR such as the ABR, a general observation is that component amplitudes decrease and absolute latencies increase when repetition rate is increased beyond 10 Hz or so (Suzuki et

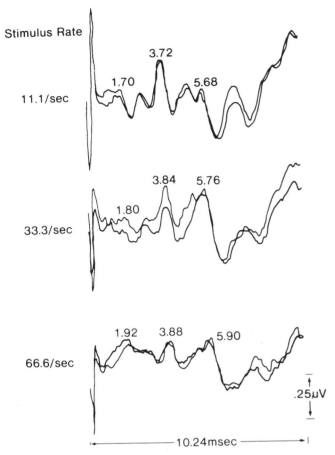

Figure 22.9. Effects of increasing stimulus (click) repetition rate on the ABR. (From ASHA, 1988.)

al., 1986). Up to 30–40 Hz, these changes are negligible if response detection is the primary application and the earliest waves are of little interest. For example, rates on the order of 30–35 Hz are very common in neonatal ABR screening protocols, where testing time is an important variable. For the MLR, stimulus rate tends to be lower (i.e., 5–10 Hz). This is because the MLR has a longer fundamental period than the SLR, the response itself takes longer to recover from stimulation, and there is a more pronounced reduction in component amplitudes with higher rates. The exception to this is the 40 Hz SSP-MLR, whose waveform is best elicited by stimuli presented at a rate of approximately 40 Hz. Finally, stimulus repetition rates for the LLR must be even lower (i.e., usually no more than 1 Hz) because of the still longer periods and recovery cycles of these potentials.

Certain abnormalities (e.g., multiple sclerosis, acoustic tumors) may be sensitive to stimulus repetition rate (Pratt et al., 1981; Yagi and Kaga, 1981; Keith and Jacobson, 1985). Thus, it may be appropriate to record the AEP using two distinctly different rates (i.e., low and high) when these conditions are suspected. However,

for most audiologic and otoneurologic applications, lower stimulus rates are favored because they facilitate optimal wave identification.

As a final note on this topic, stimulus repetition rates should be chosen so as to minimize phase-locking of 60 Hz electrical interference. This is accomplished by avoiding rates that are integer submultiples of 60 and whose interstimulus intervals are even multiples of the period of one-half cycle of 60 Hz (i.e., 8.333 milliseconds). Even multiples encourage phase-locking, whereas odd multiples facilitate phase cancellation because each averaging epoch will start at the opposite phase of the 60 cycle noise. Thus, good rate choices include 0.9, 5.2, 11.0, 17.1, and 40.0 Hz, whereas 1.0, 6.0, 10.0, 15.0, and 30.0 Hz are poor choices. Intermediate rates may work reasonably well because the line frequency is not always exactly 60 Hz. If stimulus-related sinusoidal artifact is a problem, slight variations in rate during a given run may help to cancel it.

Stimulus Calibration and Level

Stimulus calibration and the selection of units of stimulus level are more complex for AEP testing than for conventional audiometry. This is primarily because of the inability of most sound level meters (especially those in audiometer calibration sets) to accurately measure short duration stimuli. For clicks, the three most popular decibel (dB) references used to indicate intensity are: hearing level (HL) or normal hearing level (nHL); sensation level (SL); and peak-equivalent sound pressure level (peSPL).

As in conventional, puretone audiometry, dB HL (or nHL) for transient AEP stimuli relates to an average threshold from a group of normally hearing individuals, whereas dB SL is most often used to indicate the number of decibels above a threshold value. Unlike conventional audiometry, however, a reference standard (e.g., re: ANSI, 1969) has not yet been adopted for transient stimuli. Because of this, calibration values tend to be specific to the laboratory/clinic where "normal" thresholds were determined and/or a particular AEP test system. In addition, HL and SL usually refer to psychoacoustic thresholds to the click, but AEP detection levels also may be used. The lack of standardization is especially problematic when data from different laboratories and clinics, often using different recording systems, are compared.

Although nHL and SL are very useful for clinical reference, neither is indicative of a direct physical measurement of intensity. A method to provide such a reference involves using an oscilloscope to match the peak amplitude of a continuous sinusoid to that of a transient stimulus. The RMS SPL of the steady sinusoid equivalent to that of the transient can then be measured with a sound level meter, and this becomes the peak equivalent SPL (peSPL) of the transient. Common frequencies for the sinusoid used to establish peSPL are 1000, 2000 or 4000 Hz. The relationship between peSPL (using the above frequencies) and HL for clicks is such that zero dB HL corresponds to approximately 30 dB peSPL (Stapells et al., 1982). The use of peSPL as a reference for AEP transient stimuli makes it easier to check stimulus output and also to make comparisons across clinics/laboratories.

The need for accurate calibration is highlighted in AEP measurements due to the dramatic response-related effects produced by changing stimulus level. In general, reducing stimulus level is accompanied by three primary response characteristics: (a) a prolongation of component absolute latencies, (b) a reduction in component amplitudes; and (c) the eventual disappearance of components into the noise floor. The magnitude of these changes are variable depending on the particular AEP or AEP component. A more detailed description of the effects of stimulus level on AEP will be presented in the *Response Characteristics, Recording Parameters,* and *Clinical Applications* section of this chapter.

Subject Interface

The electrophysiologic response of a subject/patient to acoustic stimulation must be conveyed to subsequent electronic instrumentation with the use of electrodes. The reader is referred to Kriss (1982) for a detailed discussion of electrodes and underlying principles. For AEP applications, disk/cup surface electrodes made of gold or silver are typically used. Subdermal, needle electrodes also are used, but not for routine clinical applications. More recently, disposable electrodes consisting of a porous foam impregnated with conductive gel, and attached to an adhesive backing have become popular, especially for infant testing. For certain AEP techniques such as ECochG and intraoperative monitoring, a variety of electrode types, ranging from ball-tipped wires to foam ear plugs, have been used. The reader is referred to subsequent chapters in this text for a more thorough discussion of these (also see Ferraro et al., 1986; Stypulkowski and Staller, 1987; Ruth et al., 1988; Bauch and Olsen, 1990).

The transfer of current from biologic tissue to an electrode is dependent on good electrical contact between these two elements. In addition, this transfer will be impeded by factors associated with the electrode's characteristics (e.g., surface area and material), the tissue itself and anything in between (e.g., dirt, make-up, hair, fluid). In the case of surface electrodes, cleansing the skin and applying a conductive medium such as an electrolyte gel/paste/cream between the skin and the electrode will assist in achieving good contact and reducing impedances. Plating silver electrodes with chloride salt will also help. The electrode-skin interface also must

be mechanically stable, and the conductive medium will assist with this. It should be noted, however, that these substances are not adhesives, and it is usually necessary to use tape or other fastening materials to secure the electrode in position.

Most commercially available AEP test units allow for a quick assessment of the impedances between the skin and the various electrodes attached to it. To facilitate recording, these impedances should be minimized and balanced across electrode pairs. Although upper limit values recommended for electrode impedances tend to vary in the literature, skin-electrode impedances of less than 5000 ohms, with interelectrode impedance differences no greater than 2000 ohms, should facilitate good recordings. An exception to this has been noted with the various electrodes used for ECochG, where useful clinical responses can be obtained in the face of very high impedances (e.g., Coats, 1974, 1986; Durrant, 1986; Ferraro, et al., 1986, 1989; Stypulkowski and Staller, 1987).

Amplification and Filtering

Differential Preamplification

As indicated earlier in this chapter, the magnitudes of AEP recorded from the scalp are very small, generally in the microvolt and submicrovolt range. These analog signals must eventually be converted into digital form for signal averaging, and this conversion process operates within a certain range of magnitudes. The voltages picked up by the electrodes are usually not within this range and must therefore be amplified before analog-to-digital (A-D) conversion (i.e., "pre"amplified). In addition, although it is important to optimize the desired voltages, signals other than these should be excluded or rejected. These processes can be accomplished through "differential" preamplification. The differential preamplifier subtracts the input of one electrode from that of another by inverting one of the inputs, although leaving the other noninverted. This produces a combined output representative of the potential difference between the two electrodes. A "ground" or "common" connection to the subject also is needed and serves as an internal reference for the noninverted and inverted inputs. Several terms other than noninverting/inverting have been used to denote the inputs to the preamplifier. These may include positive(+)/negative(-) and primary/secondary. However, active/reference or active/inactive are inappropriate because both inputs are typically active.

The premise underlying differential recording is that the desired voltages occur between the two "active" electrodes and are seen in opposite phases by them, whereas remote and unwanted signals (i.e., background noise) are seen in-phase. When one of the inputs is inverted then added to the noninverted input, voltages of opposite phase (signal) will be enhanced although those of the same or common phase (noise) will be canceled. This is known as common mode rejection (CMR), and is usually specified in dB. In general, the higher the CMR, the better the signal-to-noise ratio (SNR) of the output. Ideally then, the CMR of a differential preamplifier should be infinite. Practically, however, values of 80–100 dB (i.e., 10,000–100,000:1) are common in commercially available instrumentation. In addition, CMR is degraded when electrode impedances are not well balanced because both inputs will have different amplitides of "noise."

Another important aspect of differential recording is the electrode "configuration" or "montage." This is defined by the location of the recording electrodes and their connections to the inputs of the preamplifier. For example, a common configuration for recording the ABR and several other AEP involves directing the signal from an electrode at the vertex of the scalp into the noninverting (positive) input of the preamplifier, and inverting the signal from an electrode attached to the ear lobe or mastoid process of the stimulated side. Another electrode, usually from the nasion (just above the bridge of the nose) or the contralateral ear lobe or mastoid process, provides the common input or ground. This vertex (+)-to-ipsilateral ear lobe/mastoid (-) configuration produces "vertex-positive" responses wherein waves/ peaks that are positive voltages at the vertex will be seen as upward or positive deflections. Reversing the noninverting and inverting inputs to the preamplifier will simply change the polarity of the recorded AEP by 180°, without affecting component amplitudes or morphology. Because of this, the selection of response polarity is a matter of personal preference. For example, some prefer to record ECochG using an ear canal-positive configuration. This will display the components of the whole nerve action potential, which are indeed negative potentials, as negative/downward deflections. Regardless of preference, electrode configuration always should be specified to avoid mislabeling the peaks and troughs of an AEP waveform.

Amplification parameters associated with differential recording are variable, depending on the AEP being sought and the proximity of the electrodes and/or their orientation to the cochlear/neural generators. For example, less gain is needed for cortical responses (e.g., the LLR), than for brainstem responses (e.g., the SLR) and, as a general rule, near-field recordings require less gain than far-field recordings.

Filtering

The differential recording and amplification of AEP is accompanied by at least some degree of filtering to further eliminate or reduce unwanted noise. The filters are often built in to the preamplifier and perform analog filtering within a certain frequency range, specified by "high-" and "low-pass" settings. The high-pass setting (or "low-frequency cut-off") is usually chosen to eliminate low-frequency electrical and electrophysiologic noise (including EEG) and direct current potentials that are irrelevant to the desired potentials but may alter the baseline waveform. Low-frequency noise also can distort or mask the morphology of the AEP. The low-pass setting (or "high-frequency cut-off") is used to reduce high frequency noise and to restrict the spectrum of the signal to the sampling limits of the A-D converter. The selection of specific high- and low-pass filter settings, therefore, is dependent on the spectrum of the AEP. Consequently, it is essential to pass those frequencies that comprise the fundamental components of the desired response. Inasmuch as these frequencies are variable across the family of AEP, filter settings will vary according to the particular response(s) being sought. It may also be necessary to restrict the filter band-pass to a "less-than-ideal" range to achieve an adequate ratio between the levels of the desired response and background noise (i.e., signal-to-noise ratio or SNR). The benefits of doing this must be weighed against the amount of distortion it causes in the resultant response waveform.

Although the use of analog filtering helps to improve SNR, analog filters also introduce artifacts such as phase shifts and ringing, which are specific to the characteristics of the particular filter in use. These problems are especially obvious when extremely narrow bandwidths and/or steep filter skirts are used. Because of this latter aspect, filter skirts of 6 or 12 dB/octave are commonly used for AEP applications.

The above-mentioned problems associated with analog filters can be avoided with the use of digital filtering, performed computationally by the computer after the signal averaging process (Boston and Ainslie, 1980; Domico and Kavanaugh, 1986). "Post-hoc" digital filtering has been suggested by several authors to help improve waveform morphology (Fridman et al., 1982; Moller, 1983; Spivak and Malinoff, 1990), and most AEP recording units use this to at least "smooth" the displayed response once it has been collected.

A prominent problem in the recording of AEP is the pickup of extraneous electrical noise via the electrodes, often in the form of a 60 Hz sinusoid. Although this can be avoided through the use of proper grounding and shielding of equipment (see section on *Environmental Variables*) many AEP units use a "notch-filter" to reduce 60 Hz artifact. This feature may be particularly helpful when testing is performed in "hostile" electrical environments (e.g., intensive care units and operating rooms), but should be used judiciously because the notch may cut into the response components of interest.

Artifact Rejection

As a final note regarding preaveraging steps, most signal averaging software includes an "artifact rejection" routine to prevent waveform contamination from large, spurious voltage changes during recording. These signals can arise from a variety of sources, including the subject. Typically, artifact rejection is designed to detect any signal larger in amplitude than a specified value within the sensitivity range of the A-D converter or a percentage thereof (e.g., 90% of full-scale deflection). When such a signal is detected during an averaging run, the entire sweep is excluded from the average. In noisy situations, the use of artifact rejection will prolong testing time or even preclude the signal averaging process. When this occurs, attempts should be made to reduce the noise (i.e., getting the subject to relax more, improving electrode impedances, and/or more aggressive filtering). However, when these attempts are unsuccessful and if the desired response is relatively large, it may be reasonable to deactivate the artifact rejection routine or reduce the amplifier gain to improve the efficiency of data collection. More averages may be required to achieve the desired SNR under these conditions (as discussed below).

The Signal Averaging Process

Analog-to-Digital Conversion

The next step after preamplification and analog filtering of the AEP is the signal averaging process, which is usually triggered at the onset of stimulus presentation. As indicated earlier (see Historical Perspectives), signal averaging is designed to extract the small voltage responses to sensory stimulation (i.e., the signal) from the much larger background of physical and biologic electrical noise. This is accomplished by first converting the amplitude of the analog signal received from the preamplifier/filter into binary values for computations by the computer. This process is known as A-D conversion. To do this, the analog waveform is sampled at discrete points during its epoch, as shown in Figure 22.10 (adapted from Coats, 1983). The rate at which this done is referred to as the "sampling rate," whereas the amount of time spent sampling each point is called the "dwell time." Sampling rate and dwell time are reciprocal measures. As also shown in Figure 22.10, increasing the sampling rate improves the accuracy with which the signal can be represented in the computer's memory.

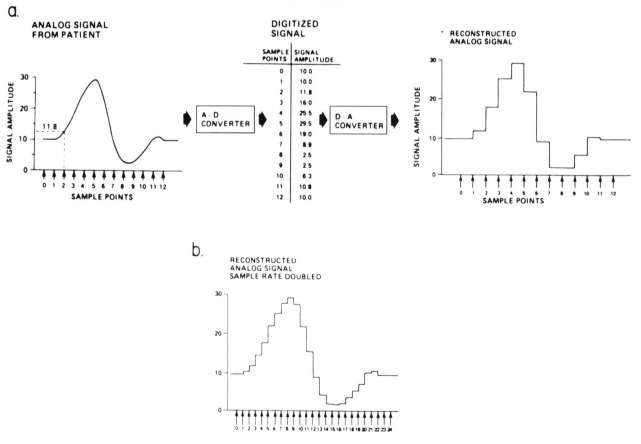

Figure 22.10. Digital sampling and reconstruction of an analog signal (**a**) and signal reconstructed at twice the sampling rate as a. (**b**) (From ASHA, 1988).

Thus, the factors associated with sampling rate will determine the temporal resolution of the waveform. The amplitude resolution of the signal is determined by the numeric precision of the A-D converter, which is defined by the number of "bits" representing full-scale. The larger the number of bits, the more precisely the amplitude will be represented and the greater the amount of SNR improvement realizable. Typical AEP units provide temporal resolution of at least 40 microseconds per data point, and 8- to 12-bit (2^8 - 2^{12}) amplitude resolution in selectable ranges of sensitivity of ± 1 - ± 500 microvolts.

Signal Averaging

Once digitized, the response undergoes the averaging process, in which discrete samples containing both signal (i.e., the AEP) and background noise (EEG and other electrical noises) are summed over time and stored in the memory banks, or "channels," of the computer. The underlying principles of signal averaging have already been discussed (see Historical Perspectives section), and are based on the concept that the signal is fixed and the noise is random in time. The improvement in SNR resulting from signal averaging has been shown to be proportional to the square root of the number of samples (N) averaged (Picton and Hink, 1974). Ideally, then, "noisy" responses could be improved by simply taking more samples, ad infinitum. In reality, however, the response may display "time jitter," wherein its temporal aspects vary slightly over time. In addition the background noise may deviate from a truly stationary, random distribution (e.g., the subject swallows, moves, etc.) If this occurs, the SNR will not be proportional to N. Thus, simply increasing the number of samples in an effort to improve SNR actually may produce the opposite effect. Generally speaking, the improvement in SNR seen with sample sizes of more than 2000–4000, say for the SLR, may be difficult to justify in light of the extended time taken to complete runs of these lengths. Typically, sample size will vary with the magnitudes of both the signal and the noise. That is, relatively small N will be required for cortically generated responses or direct nerve recordings, whereas several thousand may be needed to extract small, brainstem AEP/components.

Multi-Channel Recordings

It is often the case that the computer of an AEP unit (especially the more expensive ones) has more than one input channel to permit averaging of signals from two or more preamplifiers at the same time. This is done to permit simultaneous recording of AEP from more than one electrode configuration (e.g., vertex-to-ipsilateral ear lobe and vertex-to-contralateral ear lobe). Multi-channel recordings are often used to facilitate the labeling of a specific AEP (especially the ABR) when different AEP occurring in similar epochs to the same stimulus are desired (e.g., ECochG and ABR), or when additional channels are desirable for monitoring artifacts (e.g., eye blinks).

Waveform Display

Once the response has undergone the signal averaging process, the digitized average is reconverted to an analog waveform and usually displayed on the face of a cathode ray tube (CRT), liquid crystal diode display, or other video imaging/plotting device interfaced with the computer. Some AEP units, designed primarily for infant screening, do not provide a waveform display, but these have not been well-accepted, in part, because of this (Ferraro and Ruth, 1988). Most AEP units also provide a "cursor" that allows the examiner to label and/or measure the components of the displayed AEP. The flexibility to perform other on-screen waveform manipulations such as smoothing, inverting, memory transfer, etc. may also be available to the examiner. The number and variety of these "special" features vary considerably among different AEP units, often in accordance with their cost (see Ferraro and Ruth, 1988, 1990).

Once displayed, and after all on-screen manipulations have been performed, it is usually desirable to write out the waveform and/or print the results of the measurements made. This is accomplished via an internal or external digital printer or X-Y plotter connected to the computer. Disk storage also may be available for storing (usually) the original data, again depending on the level of sophistication (and cost) of the particular AEP unit.

Environmental Variables

Environmental variables associated with AEP testing assume many forms, and may certainly contribute to or even cause unacceptable recordings. To begin with, the tremendous amplification required for recording AEP makes them very susceptible to contamination from extraneous electrical noises. These can emanate from such sources as the room lighting or any nearby electronic equipment, including the AEP unit itself (e.g., it is bad practice to set the recording amplifiers on top of the CRT). Although subject to reduction through filtering and signal averaging, the magnitude of electrical noise in a given environment may still be too large for recording the desired AEP with acceptable SNR. Shielding of the testing area and equipment, and proper grounding can help, as can keeping the electrode leads as short as practical, close to the subject's body and routed well away from the offending sources. Even with these precautions, it still may be necessary to remove or unplug extraneous electrical devices in the immediate area of the patient. Of course, many of the steps identified above may not always be feasible, especially when the recordings are taking place in an intensive care unit (ICU), or operating room (OR). Under such conditions, it may be necessary to isolate and disengage specific "culprits", or record when they are not in use. In any event, ICU and OR are difficult recording environments, in part because there may be multiple ground paths to the subject. Although very important at all times, this is where the utmost in electrical safety is critical. All AEP units should be certified and periodically re-certified against excessive leakage current. Under no circumstances is it acceptable to use 3-to-2 prong adaptor/"cheater" plugs for powering such equipment, and the power plug should be of hospital/OR grade.

The level of background acoustic noise is also an important environmental variable, especially if this is high enough to mask the AEP stimuli. Such noises often occur in testing areas outside the clinic (e.g., ICU, OR, nurseries) and may come from both non-human and human sources. Obviously, attempts should be made to achieve maximal reduction of acoustic noise during testing, especially if low-level stimuli are going to be used. Certain stimulus delivery systems, such as tubal insert phones (Gorga et al., 1988; Schwartz et al., 1989) or circumaural earphone cushions sealed around the ear (Jacobson, 1990), can substantially attenuate these sounds and reduce them to acceptable levels. Awareness of ambient noise level is especially important for neonatal AEP screening and acceptable levels for this purpose have been recommended by Richmond et al. (1986).

SUBJECTIVE ASPECTS OF RECORDING AEP

Subject/Patient-Related Variables

There are a number of variables associated with AEP that pertain directly to the subject and are nonpathologic. The most obvious of those that have been identified are age, gender, and state of arousal or consciousness. Changes in body temperature can also affect AEP (i.e., prolong interwave intervals), but the magnitude of the changes necessary to produce clinically significant effects are generally brought about by pathologic conditions (e.g., drug-induced, hypothermic treatment, surgical anesthesia) (Stockard et al., 1978).

Age

It is well known that infant AEP differ substantially from those obtained from adults. For current clinical applications, this is especially relevant to the ABR, which may take from 18 to 24 months after birth to mature (Starr et al., 1977; Fria, 1980; Cevette, 1984; ASHA, 1988). Figure

22.11 (adapted from Salamy and McKean, 1976) displays a series of ABR tracings from subjects of different ages, ranging from newborn to adult. As can be seen from this figure, the morphologic and temporal characteristics of the ABR change dramatically with age. Especially noteworthy is the dynamic nature of the interpeak intervals in the immature response. These changes will be addressed more specifically in Chapter 25.

In general, age-related changes tend to reflect the maturational development of the cochlear and/or neural generators of the particular AEP being recorded. This development, in turn, proceeds in a peripheral-to-central direction. Thus, the electrocochleographic components of the SLR may be mature at or shortly after birth, whereas developmental-related changes in the LLR can occur over several years.

Inasmuch as the most dynamic age-related changes in AEP occur in the first few years of life, it is necessary to establish age-specific norms when working with infant populations. The effects of age on AEP in adults, however, are more controversial. For example, several studies have shown that the latency of wave V of the ABR increases systematically with age (e.g., Rowe, 1978; Jerger and Hall, 1980; Kelly-Ballweber and Dobie, 1984; Jerger and Johnson, 1988). Others have shown the effects of age alone on the ABR to be minimal into the sixth and seventh decades of life, especially when the ef-

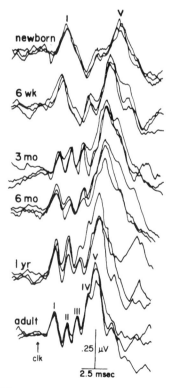

Figure 22.11. ABR from subjects of different ages as indicated. (From ASHA, 1988.)

fects of presbycusis are controlled (Beagley and Sheldrake, 1978; Rosenhamer et al., 1980; Otto and McCandless, 1982; Schwartz et al., 1991). Prolongation of LLR components has also been associated with aging (Goodin et al., 1978; Polich et al., 1985).

Gender

Differences between the AEP of males versus females have been investigated most thoroughly in the SLR. A general finding is that females tend to have slightly shorter component latencies than males (Beagely and Sheldrake, 1978; Michalewski et al., 1989; Rosenhamer et al., 1980; Jerger and Johnson, 1988). Because of this, the use of gender-specific norms has been advocated by some (Jerger and Hall, 1980; Jerger and Johnson, 1988). However, because the magnitude of latency differences due to gender alone appears to be somewhat variable and small (i.e., 200 microseconds or less), the necessity of establishing separate norms for males and females remains questionable. Interactions between age and gender on the ABR have also been found (Rosenhamer et al., 1980), but are not well established. When stimuli are presented at levels that accommodate differences in hearing level and audiometric configuration among subjects, the clinical relevance of both gender- and age-related changes on the adult ABR becomes less apparent. However, in the interest of minimizing false positives, it may still be necessary to give some consideration to these variables in cases of marginally long latencies in males and/or older subjects in general.

An even more controversial aspect of the gender difference is the basis for it. This was first suggested by Allison et al. (1983) to be simply a matter of differences in stature. That is, males have larger heads and, therefore, perhaps inherently longer neural pathways (causing longer conduction times). This, in turn, would suggest that latency corrections for head size might be appropriate. However, the correlation between head size and eighth nerve/pontine brainstem dimensions necessary to substantiate this theory has not been found (Sabo et al., 1991). In addition, Durrant et al. (1990) have reported that the head size factor can only account for a fraction of the variance represented by the intergender difference. Thus, latency corrections for head size, a priori, do not appear to be warranted except when the dimensions of the head are abnormally large (i.e., more than 2 SD from normal).

State of Arousal/Consciousness

AEP may be substantially influenced by the subject's level of arousal or state of consciousness during testing, and, in general, the subject must cooperate by remaining quiet and relatively motionless during data acquisition. Any bodily movement, especially of the head or lower jaw, produces myogenic potentials and/or electrical artifact from movement of the electrodes/leads and may even disrupt the electrode contacts. In the case of infants, the ultimate degree of cooperation is usually achieved only when the child is asleep (natural or induced). In adults, it is generally necessary (and sufficient) to instruct the patient to remain quiet and still during testing. Sedation may be required for certain pediatric or adult patients (e.g., young children, mentally retarded, developmentally delayed) who do not or cannot cooperate by remaining still.

Certain AEP undergo pronounced changes related to the subject's state of consciousness, although others remain relatively unaffected by this. In general, the SLR fall into the latter category (Amadeo and Shagass, 1973; Goff et al., 1977; Sohmer et al., 1978; Sanders et al., 1979; Marsh et al., 1974), and can be applied in situations where the subject may be asleep, unconscious, or comatose (e.g., neonatal screening, intraoperative and ICU monitoring). However, the MLR and LLR show considerable variability depending on whether the subject is awake or asleep (Mendel and Goldstein, 1971; Suzuki et al., 1983; Okitsu, 1984). Indeed, the LLR can be affected by an awake subject's level of attention (Picton and Hilyard, 1974; Schwent et al. 1976). Thus, the clinical applications of MLR and LLR require consideration of these effects and responses are most consistent and easily interpreted when the subject remains awake and alert during testing.

Examiner-Related Variables

As indicated in the beginning of this chapter, the use of AEP extends into several professions. Because of this, a diversity of backgrounds exists among the various specialists within these professions who perform AEP examinations. The competencies needed by these individuals to recommend, record, and interpret AEP, however, should transcend professional diversity. Certain groups (e.g., American Speech-Language-Hearing Association (ASHA)) have developed competency guidelines for these skills. Unfortunately these have not been standardized across professions, nor has the level of training necessary to acquire them.

As indicated above, ASHA (1990) has published a statement of competencies pertaining to AEP measurement and clinical applications. These guidelines identify the competencies, knowledge bases and skills necessary to (a) identify patients for whom AEP evaluations are appropriate; (b) identify and administer appropriate test procedures and strategies; (c) interpret findings; and (d) report findings and recommendations. The reader is strongly encouraged to refer to the ASHA statement not only for additional information on this issue, but also as an outline for training and professional development.

RESPONSE CHARACTERISTICS, RECORDING PARAMETERS AND CLINICAL APPLICATIONS

This section will describe the characteristics of the more clinically popular AEP, as seen in Figures 22.2 - 22.6, and provide brief statements regarding their respective clinical applications. More specific information on individual AEP is offered in subsequent chapters of the Handbook.

Table 22.2 provides a very general list of parameters commonly used to obtain single-channel recordings of the described AEP. It should be noted that these parameters tend to vary among investigators/clinicians and those listed are not all-inclusive. Electrode configuration has been omitted from the table because virtually all of the AEP listed, with the exception of ECochG, are conventionally recorded with a vertex (+)-to-ipsilateral ear lobe or mastoid process (-) configuration. A vertex-to-ear canal montage is also popular for the SLR, because of the enhancement of wave I this provides (see Ruth et al., 1988). Also for the SLR, an electrode placed high on the forehead (i.e., at the hairline) is often substituted for a true vertex electrode. Ground is usually at the contralateral ear lobe or mastoid, nasion, or back of the neck. For ECochG, the primary electrode is usually located in the ear canal or on the tympanic membrane for extratympanic recordings, or on the cochlear promontory for transtympanic recordings. Finally, the configuration for recording LLR often includes a vertex-to-contralateral ear lobe/mastoid montage, or vertex-to-tied earlobes/mastoids or -noncephalic reference.

Short Latency Responses

Electrocochleography

The stimulus-related responses of the cochlea and auditory nerve are recorded via ECochG. As shown in Figure 22.3, the components of the electrocochleogram most often used for clinical purposes include the cochlear summating potential (SP) and the whole nerve action potential of the auditory nerve. The cochlear microphonic (CM) can also be recorded, but has received far less clinical attention than the SP-AP complex.

Although ECochG has been available to the scientist/clinician practically since the time the CM was discovered by Wever and Bray (1930), its application for clinical purposes was overshadowed after the discovery of the ABR. This was primarily due to the audiometric advantages afforded by the ABR in comparison to non-invasive ECochG. Recently, however, and certainly due in part to the widespread popularity of the ABR, there has been renewed interest in ECochG for a variety of applications. Currently, these include: (a) the objective identification and monitoring of Meniere's disease/endolymphatic hydrops; (b) the enhancement of wave I and identification of the I-V interwave interval of the ABR in the presence of hearing loss or less-than-optimal recording conditions; and (c) the monitoring of cochlear and auditory nerve function during surgical procedures that involve the peripheral and central auditory systems and/or place them at risk for permanent damage (Ruth et al., 1988; Ferraro and Ferguson, 1989). The relevant features of the response used in the above applications include changes in the absolute and relative amplitudes of the SP and AP, and shifts in the latency of the N_1 component of the AP. Representative examples of these characteristics and more specific information on all aspects of ECochG are provided in Chapter 23.

Auditory Brainstem Response

As indicated numerous times in this chapter, the ABR is certainly the most clinically popular AEP. Because of this, the prefacing information presented here will be followed by two separate chapters of the Handbook devoted specifically to the ABR (Chapters 24 and 25).

Table 22.2.
Parameters to Obtain Single-Channel Recording of AEP

AEP	Stimulus Type	Stimulus Repetition Rate (no./Second	Preamplification Gain (X)	Low- and High-pass Filter Settings (Hz)	Averaging Window (milliseconds)	No. of Samples
SLR						
ECochG[a]	BBC/TB	9–11	20,000–100,000	1 to 10 and 3,000	5–10	1,000 to 2,000
ABR	BBC/TB	11–33	100,000–250,000	30 to 100 and 3,000	10–20	2,000 to 3,000
MLR						
MLR	BBC Tone-bursts	8–10	50,000–100,000	1 to 20 and 1,000	50–100	1,000 to 2,000
40 Hz SSP	Tone-bursts	40	50,000–100,000	1 to 20 and 1,000	50–100	1,000 to 2,000
LLR						
N1-P2	Tone-bursts	0.5–1.0	20,000–50,000	1 and 100	500	50 to 100
P300	Two different tone-bursts	0.5–1.0	20,000–50,000	1 and 100	500 to 750	100 to 200

[a]Extratympanic.

As shown in Figure 22.2, the ABR is characterized by a series of five to seven "waves" occurring within a millisecond or so of each other. In general, waves I, III, and V are considered to be the most important components of the ABR. As shown in Figure 22.12, the features of the response most often used for clinical purposes include the absolute latencies of the respective peaks of each wave, the time intervals between peaks (especially the I-V, I-III, and III-V interpeak intervals), the peak-to-trough amplitude of each wave, and the general morphology of the overall waveform. For audiometric applications, the visual detection level or so-called "threshold" of wave V is also of paramount importance.

Figure 22.13 displays component latency-intensity functions and corresponding ABR waveforms from a normal subject (recorded via surface electrodes). As stimulus intensity is lowered, absolute latencies increase, component amplitudes decrease, and all waves eventually disappear into the noise floor. Interpeak intervals are affected only slightly by changes in stimulus intensity in normal subjects. Generally, wave I is among the first components to disappear as stimulus intensity is reduced, whereas wave V persists the longest. Because of this, the threshold of the ABR is usually defined with reference to the lowest level at which wave V is still visually detectable.

There are numerous audiologic, otologic, and neurologic applications of the ABR and these will be addressed with representative examples in subsequent chapters. In general, the audiologic and otologic applications involve the examination of component absolute latencies and thresholds as a function of stimulus level.

Measurement of interpeak intervals are of particular interest in the identification, assessment, and monitoring of neurologic disorders. Overall waveform morphology and the presence/absence of components are important variables for all ABR applications. Component absolute amplitudes tend to be the weakest measures of the ABR because of their high variability (Thornton, 1975). The use of relative amplitude measures has been suggested (Starr and Achor, 1975), but the clinical use of these seem apparent only when wave V (or the IV-V complex) is very small in comparison to wave I (Durrant, 1986; Durrant and Wolf, 1991).

Middle-Latency Responses

Middle Latency Response

The MLR has received the most attention of those AEP occurring within the latency epoch of 10–100 milliseconds after stimulus onset. As shown in Figure 22.4, the overall response is characterized by two primary waves that tend to be larger, broader, and of lower fundamental frequency than those of the ABR. P_a is usually the most robust component of the MLR, and analogous in this sense to ABR wave V (Mendel and Wolf, 1983).

The basic measures of the MLR are similar to other AEP and include component absolute amplitudes and latencies, and "threshold." Much of the earlier work

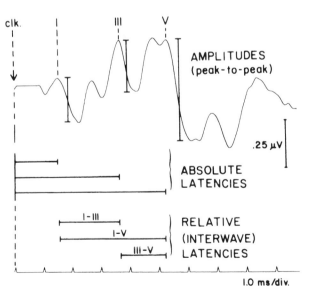

Figure 22.12. Basic amplitude and latency measures of the ABR. **Clk.** indicates onset of click. (From ASHA, 1988.)

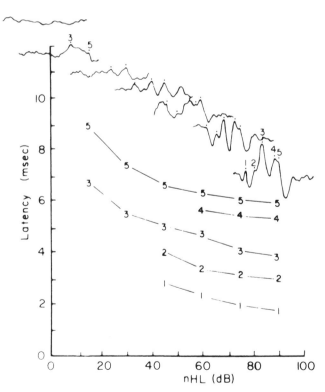

Figure 22.13. ABR latency-intensity functions and corresponding waveforms. (From ASHA, 1988.)

with the MLR focused on the use of threshold to estimate low-frequency hearing sensitivity (Thornton et al., 1977; McFarland et al., 1977). However, recent reports indicate that the MLR also may be helpful in evaluating the integrity of the central auditory nervous system (Harker and Backoff, 1981; Musiek et al., 1984; Jerger and Jerger, 1985; Kileny and Shea, 1986; Weber, 1987; Vedder et al., 1988; Musiek, 1991). As indicated earlier, the MLR is affected by the subject's state of consciousness and this has limited its clinical appeal. Additional information regarding the MLR is presented in Chapter 26.

40 Hz Steady State Potential

In 1981, Galambos et al. described a procedure for obtaining an MLR (or some components thereof) that involved presenting stimuli at a rate that would allow successive neural responses to "overlap." The most robust responses were observed when this rate was approximately 40 Hz, thus the name 40 Hz event-related-potential. Inasmuch as the resultant waveform is representative of continuous activity throughout the stimulation period, the term "steady state potential" (SSP) has more recently been applied to this particular AEP (Weber, 1987).

As seen in Figure 22.5, the 40 Hz SSP comprises approximately four cycles over a 100 millisecond epoch, and resembles a 40 Hz sinusoid. This overall pattern, and not a particular component or wave, is the relevant feature of the response. A phase delay in this waveform corresponds to a latency change/prolongation in the MLR.

Initially, the 40 Hz SSP promised to offer more frequency- specific information than the ABR in estimating low-frequency thresholds. The response was also larger than the conventional MLR (Galambos et al., 1981). Unfortunately, the 40 Hz SSP, like the MLR, is sensitive to subject state. Thus, its use in infants and children or in patients in natural or drug-induced sleep may be limited (Brown and Shallop, 1982; Kileny, 1983; Kileny and Shea, 1986).

Long Latency Responses

N_1-P_2 Complex

As shown in Figure 22.6, the N_1-P_2 complex, like the MLR, is characterized by two primary waves of relatively low fundamental frequency. The comparatively large amplitude of the complex in general allows it to be recorded using lower preamplifier gains and smaller sample sizes than the earlier AEP. When stimulus intensity is lowered, waveform characteristics change in a manner similar to that of other AEP. That is, component amplitudes decrease and absolute latencies increase. The magnitude of latency shift accompanying reduction

in stimulus level, however, is not as dramatic, proportionately, as that observed in the SLR.

Although the N_1-P_2 complex was among the first AEP to receive clinical attention, its use, like that of the MLR, has been overshadowed by the SLR. Again, this is primarily due to the susceptibility of the LLR to changes in subject state. Despite this, the N_1-P_2 complex has a long history in the audiometric arena, and was the benchmark response of "evoked response audiometry (ERA)" for several years (see Reneau and Hnatiow, 1975). Inasmuch as it is readily evoked by tone-bursts with relatively long rise-fall times and durations, frequency specificity can be achieved with the N_1-P_2 complex. In awake and cooperative subjects, the differences between N_1-P_2 and behavioral puretone thresholds are generally systematic and often as little as 10 dB (McCandless, 1967; Reneau and Hnatiow, 1975; Hyde et. al, 1986). The N_1-P_2 complex has been used successfully as an indicator of hearing sensitivity in difficult-to-test populations (e.g., mentally retarded, multiply handicapped) (Rose and Rittmanic, 1968; Nodar and Graham, 1968), and in the assessment of pseudohypacusis (McCandless and Lentz, 1968; Durrant and Wolf, 1991).

In addition to its audiometric applications, the N_1-P_2 complex can assist in the detection of lesions in the central auditory pathway (e.g., Shimazu, 1968; Peronnet and Michel, 1977; Knight et al., 1980; Jerger and Jerger, 1985; Musiek, 1986; Scherg and von Cramon, 1986). In these instances the primary manifestation of abnormality is a reduction in amplitude or absence of components. Latency prolongations and other morphological changes in the complex have also been reported in patients with central lesions (Shimizu, 1968; Musiek, 1991).

P_{300}

Unlike the other AEP described above, the P_{300} (or P_3) is considered to be an endogenous potential, generated in response to an "internally-generated event" brought about by the cognitive processing of sensory stimuli (Squires and Hecox, 1983; Musiek, 1991). As shown in Figure 22.6, the P_{300} is normally characterized by a single, large wave after the N_1-P_2 complex, with a peak latency of approximately 300 milliseconds. The response is usually recorded using an "oddball paradigm" of stimulus delivery. That is, a stimulus train containing two different stimuli (e.g., 1000 Hz and 2000 Hz puretones) is presented to the listener. Within the train, one stimulus (i.e., the frequent stimulus) is delivered 75 - 80% of the time, and the other (i.e., the rare stimulus) is interspersed randomly among the frequent stimuli to occur 25–20% of the time. The subject is asked to attend to the rare stimulus and count the number of times it occurs, and to ignore the frequent stimulus. The signal averaging computer, in turn, stores data epochs separately for the rare versus frequent stimuli. If the P_{300} appears (i.e., in the rare response epoch), it is an indication that the subject recognizes the difference between the rare and frequent stimuli. A variety of acoustic stimuli has been used to evoke the P_{300}, including speech (Squires and Hecox, 1983).

The most common use of the P_{300} has been in studies of aging, dementia and disorders of attention (Musiek, 1991). A general finding is that these conditions prolong the peak latency of the response, although the amount of prolongation is highly variable (Goodin et al., 1978; Polich et al., 1978; Kileny and Kripal, 1987). The P_{300} has been used to a lesser extent to identify subcortical lesions (Musiek, et al., 1987), monitor head-injured patients (Musiek, 1991), define attention disorders in children (Loisell et al., 1980) and depict auditory-language processing deficits after stroke (Squires and Hecox, 1983), and evaluate processing ability of patients who have cochlear implants (Oviatt and Kileny, 1991). Alterations of the P_{300} ranging from prolonged latency to the reduction or absence of a response have been observed in these applications.

SUMMARY

AEP measurement continues to be a powerful tool in the diagnosis, assessment and monitoring of audiologic, otologic, and neurologic disorders. This chapter provided an historical perspective of the development of AEP leading to current applications, described the current systems for classifying and naming AEP, discussed common variables associated with technical and subjective aspects of AEP recording, and described the salient features, recording parameters and applications of those AEP that are currently popular in the clinical domain. The goal of this presentation was to provide general, introductory information and to prepare the reader for subsequent chapters in the Handbook that pertain to specific AEP.

Various areas of AEP measurement necessarily were beyond the scope of this chapter but are worthy of the reader's interest. These include, for example, the use of electrical stimulation in eliciting EP. This area has gained increasing attention with the advent of cochlear implantation as an accepted treatment of deafness (e.g., see Simmons and Smith, 1983; Burton et al., 1989). Some of the more technically advanced areas of AEP measurement are dipole generator analysis and topographical or brain electrical activity mapping (TBM or BEAM). Although clinical use is still evolving, these are methods that promise to provide more focal information about site/level of lesion (see Finitzo and Pool, 1987). In general, it is expected that AEP measurement

methods and procedures will continue to develop and be refined as knowledge of the AEP generators expands and as clinical needs evolve.

REFERENCES

Allison T, Wood CC, and Goff WR. Brain stem auditory, pattern-reversal visual, and short-latency somatosensory evoked potentials: latencies in relation to age, sex, and brain and body size. Electroencephalog Clin Neurophysiol 1983;55:619–636.

Amadeo M, and Shagass D. Brief latency click-evoked potentials during waking and sleep in man. Psychophysiology 1973;10:244–250.

American Speech-Language-Hearing Association. The short latency auditory evoked potentials. A tutorial paper by the Audiologic Evaluation Working Group on Auditory Evoked Potential Measurements. Rockville, MD: ASHA, 1988.

American Speech-Language-Hearing Association. Competencies in auditory evoked potential measurement and clinical applications. Asha 1990;32(Suppl 2):13–16.

Bauch CD, and Olsen WO. Comparison of ABR amplitudes with TIP-trode and mastoid electrodes. Ear Hear 1990;1:463–467.

Beagley HA, and Sheldrake JB. Differences in brainstem response latency with age and sex. Br J Audiol 1978;12:69–77.

von Bekesy, G. Experiments in Hearing. New York: McGraw-Hill, 1960.

Berger H. Uber das elektroenkaphalogram des menschen. Arch Psychiatr Nervenkr 1929;87:527–570.

Boston R, and Ainslie PJ. Effects of analog and digital filtering on brainstem auditory evoked potentials. Electroenceph Clin Neurophysiol 1980;48:361–364.

Brown DD, and Shallop JK. A clinically useful 500 Hz evoked response. Nicolet Potentials 1982;1:9–12.

Cevette MJ. Auditory brainstem response testing in the intensive care unit. Semin Hear 1984;5:57–68.

Clark WA Jr. Average response computer (ARC–1), Quarterly Progress Report No. 49. Research Laboratory of Electronics, Massachusetts Institute of Technology. Cambridge, MA: MIT Press, 1958.

Clark WA Jr, Goldstein MH Jr, Brown RM, Molnar CE, O'Brien DF, and Zieman HE. The average response computer (ARC): a digital device for computing averages and amplitudes and time histograms of electrophysiological responses. Trans IRE 1961;8:46–51.

Coats AC. On electrocochleographic electrode design. J Acoust Soc Am 1974;56:708–711.

Coats AC. Instrumentation. In Moore EJ, Ed. Bases of Auditory Brainstem Evoked Responses. New York: Grune and Stratton, 1983.

Coats AC. Electrocochleography: Recording techniques and clinical applications. Semin Hear 1986;7:247–266.

Davis PA. The electrical response of the human brain to auditory stimuli. Am J Physiol 1939;126:475–476.

Davis H, Davis PA, Loomis AL, Harvey EN, and Hobart G. Electrical reactions of the human brain to auditory stimulation during sleep. J Neurophysiol 1939;2:500–514.

Davis H, and Yoshie N. Human evoked cortical responses to auditory stimuli. Physiologist 1963;6:164.

Davis H, Engegretson M, Lowell EL, Mast T, Satterfield J, and Yoshie N. Evoked responses to clicks recorded from the human scalp. Ann NY Acad Sci 1964;112:224–225.

Davis H, and Zerlin S. Acoustic relations of the human vertex potential. J Acoust Soc Am 1966;39:109–116.

Davis H, and Hirsh SK. A slow brainstem response for low-frequency audiometry. Audiology 1979;18:445–461.

Domico WD, and Kavanaugh KT. Analog and zero phase-shift digital filtering of the auditory brainstem response waveform. Ear Hear 1986;7:377–382.

Durrant JD. Combined ECochG–ABR versus conventional ABR recordings. Semin Hear 1986;7:289–305.

Durrant JD, Shelhamer M, Fria TJ, and Ronis ML. Examination of the sidedness of the brainstem auditory evoked potential. Presented at the Biennial Symposium of the International Electric Response Audiometry Study Group, Bergamo, Italy, 1981.

Durrant JD, and Lovrinic JH. Bases of Hearing Science, 2nd Ed. Baltimore: Williams & Wilkins, 1984.

Durrant JD, Sabo DL, and Hyre RJ. Gender, head size, and ABRs examined in a large clinical sample. Ear Hear 1990;11:210–214.

Durrant JD, and Wolf KE. Auditory evoked potentials. In Rintleman W, Ed. Hearing Assessment. Austin, TX: Pro-ed, 1991.

Ferraro JA, Murphy GB, and Ruth RA. A comparative study of primary electrodes used in extratympanic electrocochleography. Semin Hear 1986;7:279–287.

Ferraro JA, and Ruth RA. A comparison of commercial auditory evoked potential units: The economy units. Am J Otol 1988;(Suppl)9:57–62.

Ferraro JA, and Ferguson R. Tympanic EcochG and conventional ABR: A combined approach for the identification of wave I and the I-V interwave interval. Ear Hear 1989;10:161–166.

Ferraro J, Nunes R, and Arenberg IK. Electrocochleographic effects of ear canal pressure change. Am J Otol 1989;10:42–48.

Ferraro JA, and Ruth RA. A comparison of commercial auditory evoked potential units: The midpriced and luxury units. Am J Otol 1990;11:181–191.

Fria T. The auditory brainstem response: Background and clinical applications. Monogr Comtemp Audiol 1980;2:1–44.

Fridman J, John ER, Bergelson JB, Kaiser JB, and Baird JB. Application of digital filtering and automatic peak detection to brain stem auditory evoked potentials. Electroencephalogr Clin Neurophysiol 1982;53:405–416.

Galambos R, Makeig S, and Talmachoff PJ. A 40-Hz auditory potential recorded from the human scalp. Proc Natl Acad Sci USA 1981;78:2643–2647.

Geisler CD, Frishkopf LS, and Rosenblith WA. Extracranial responses to acoustic clicks in man. Science 1958;128:1210–1211.

Goff WR, Allison J, Lyons W, Fisher JC, and Conte R. Origins of short latency auditory evoked potentials in man. In Desmedt JE, Ed. Auditory Evoked Potentials in Man: Psychopharmacology Correlates in Evoked Potentials. Basel, Switzerland: Karger, 1977.

Goldstein R, and Rodman LB. Early components of averaged evoked responses to rapidly repeated auditory stimuli. J Speech Hear Res 1967;10:697–705.

Goodin D, Squires K, and Starr A. Long latency event-related components of the auditory evoked potential. Brain 1978;101:635–648.

Gorga MP, Worthington DW, Reiland JK, Beauchaine KA, and Goldgar DE. Some comparisons between auditory brainstem response thresholds, latencies, and the pure-tone audiogram. Ear Hear 1985;6:105–112.

Gorga MP, Reiland JK, and Beauchaine KA. Auditory brainstem responses from graduates of an intensive care nursery using an insert earphone. Ear Hear 1988;9:144–147.

Harker L, and Backoff P. Middle latency electric auditory responses in patients with acoustic neuroma. Otolaryngol Head Neck Surg 1981;89:131–136.

Hyde M, Matsumoto N, Alberti P, and Li Y. Auditory evoked potentials in audiometric assessment of compensation and medicolegal patients. Ann Otol Rhinol Laryngol 1986;95:514–519.

Jacobson JT, and Hyde ML. An introduction to auditory evoked potentials. In Katz J, Ed. Handbook of Clinical Audiology, 3rd Ed. Baltimore: Williams & Wilkins, 1985.

Jacobson JT, Jacobson CA, and Spahr RC. Automated and conventional ABR screening techniques in high risk infants. J Am Acad Audiol 1991;1:187–195.

Jerger J, and Mauldin L. Prediction of sensorineural hearing level from the brainstem evoked response. Arch Otolaryngol 1978;106:181–187.

Jerger J, and Hall J. Effects of age and sex on auditory brainstem response. Arch Otolaryngol 1980;106:387–391.

Jerger J, Neely J, and Jerger S. Speech, impedance and auditory brainstem audiometry in brainstem tumors. Arch Otolaryngol 1980;106, 218–223.

Jerger S, and Jerger J. Audiologic applications of early, middle and late auditory evoked potentials. Hear J 1985;38:31–36.

Jerger J, and Johnson K. Interactions of age, gender and sensorineural hearing loss on ABR latency. Ear Hear 1988;9:168–175.

Jewett DL, Romano MN, and Williston JS. Human auditory evoked potentials: Possible brain-stem components detected on the scalp. Science 1970;167:1517–1518.

Jewett DL, and Williston JS. Auditory-evoked far fields averaged from the scalp of humans. Brain 1971;94:681–696.

Keith R, and Jacobson J. Physiological responses in multiple sclerosis and other demyelinating diseases. In Jacobson J, Ed. The Auditory Brainstem Response. San Diego, CA: College Hill Press, 1985.

Kelly-Ballweber D, and Dobie R. Binaural interaction measured behaviorally and electrophysiologically in young and old adults. Audiology 1984;23:181–194.

Kileny P. Auditory evoked middle latency response: Current issues. Semin Hear 1983;4:403–413.

Kileny P, and Shea SL. Middle latency and 40 Hz auditory evoked responses in normal–hearing subjects: Click and 500-Hz thresholds. J Speech Hear Res 1986;29:20–28.

Kileny P, and Kripal J. Test-retest variability of auditory event-related potentials. Ear Hear 1987;8:110–114.

Kileny P, Paccioretti D, and Wilson A. Effect of cortical lesions on middle latency auditory evoked responses (MLR). Electroenceph Clin Neurophysiol 1987;66:108–120.

Knight RT, Hillyard SA, Woods DL, and Neville HJ. The effects of frontal and temporal parietal lobe lesions on the auditory evoked potential in man. Electroenceph Clin Neurophysiol 1980;50:112–124.

Kraus N, Ozdamar O, Hier D, and Stein L. Auditory middle latency responses (MLR's) in patients with cortical lesions. Electroenceph Clin Neurophysiol 1982;45:275–287.

Kraus N, and McGee T. Color imaging of the human middle latency response. Ear Hear 1988;9:159–167.

Kraus N, and McGee T. Clinical applications of the middle latency response. J Am Acad Audiol 1990;1:130–133.

Kriss A. Setting up an evoked potential (EP) laboratory. In Halliday AM, Ed. Evoked Potentials in Clinical Testing. New York: Churchill Livingstone, 1982.

Loisell D, Stamm J, Maitinsky S, and Whipple S. Evoked potential and behavioral signs of auditory-dysfunctions in hyperactive boys. Psychophysiology 1980;17:193–201.

Loomis AL, Harvey PN, and Hobart G. Distribution of disturbance patterns in the human electroencephalogram with special reference to sleep. J Neurophysiol 1938;1:413–430.

Lowell E. Early components of the AER in the hearing of young children. Acta Otolaryng Suppl (Stockh) 1965;206:124–126.

Marsh R, Frewen T, Sutton L, and Potsic W. Resistance of the auditory brain stem response to barbiturate levels. Otolaryngol Head Neck Surg 1984;92:685–688.

McCandless GA, and Best L. Evoked responses to auditory stimuli in man using a summing computer. J Speech Hear Res 1964;7:193–202.

McCandless GA. Clinical application of evoked response audiometry. J Speech Hear Res 1967;10:468–478.

McCandless GA, and Lentz WE. Amplitude and latency characteristics of the auditory evoked response at low sensation levels. J Auditory Res 1968;8:273–282.

McFarland WH, Vivion MD, Goldstein R. Middle components of the AER to tone-pips in normal-hearing and hearing-impaired subjects. J Speech Hear Res 1977;20:781–798.

Mendel MI, and Goldstein R. Stability of the early components of the averaged electroencephalic response. J Speech Hear Res 1969; 12:351–361.

Mendel M, and Goldstein R. Early components of the averaged electroencephalic response to constant level clicks during all night sleep. J Speech Hear Res 1971;14:829–840.

Mendelson T, and Salamy A. Maturational effects on the middle components of the averaged electroencephalic response. J Speech Hear Res 1981;24:140–144.

Michalewski HJ, Thompson LW, Patterson JV, Bowman TE, and Litzelman D. Sex differences in the amplitudes and latencies of the human auditory brain stem potential. Electroenceph Clin Neurophysiol 1980;48:351–356.

Michelini S, Arslan E, Prosser S, and Pedrielli F. Logarithmic display of auditory evoked potentials. J Biomed Engineer 1982;4:62–64.

Moller AR. Auditory Physiology. New York: Academic Press, 1983.

Moller AR, Janetta PJ, Bennett M, and Moller MB. Intracranially recorded responses from the human auditory nerve: New insights into the origin of brainstem evoked potentials (BSEP). Electroenceph Clin Neurophysiol 1981;52:18–27.

Moller AR, and Janetta PJ. Comparison between intracranially recorded potentials from the human auditory nerve and scalp recording auditory brainstem responses (ABR). Scand Audiol 1982;11:33–40.

Moushegian G, Rupert AL, and Stillman RD. Scalp-recorded early response in man to frequencies in the speech range. Electroenceph Clin Neurophysiol 1973;35:665–667.

Musiek F, Geurkink N, Weider D, and Donnelly K. Past, present, and future applications of the auditory middle latency response. Laryngoscope 1984;94:1545–1552.

Musiek F. Neuroanatomy, neurophysiology and central auditory assessment. Part II. The cerebrum. Ear Hear 1986;7:207–219.

Musiek F, Gollegly K, Verkest S, and Kibbe-Michal K. Auditory P-300 profiles for patients with cerebral lesions. Presented at the annual convention of the American Speech-Language-Hearing Association, New Orleans, LA, 1987.

Musiek F. Auditory evoked responses in site-of-lesion assessment. In Rintleman W, Ed. Hearing Assessment. Austin, TX: Pro-Ed, 1991.

Nodar RH, and Graham JT. An investigation of auditory evoked responses of mentally retarded adults during sleep. Electroenceph Clin Neurophysiol 1968;25:73–76.

Okitsu T. Middle components of the auditory evoked response in young children. Scand Audiol 1984;13:83–86.

Otto WC, and McCandless G. Aging and the auditory brain stem response. Audiology 1982;21:466–473.

Oviatt D, and Kileny P. Auditory event-related potentials elicited from cochlear implant recipients and hearing subjects. Am J Audiol 1991;1:48–55.

Peronnet F, and Michel F. The asymmetry of the auditory evoked potentials in normal man and in patients with brain lesions. In Desmedt JE, Ed. Auditory Evoked Potentials in Man: Psychopharmacology Correlates of Evoked Potentials. Basel, Switzerland: Karger, 1977.

Picton TW, and Fitzgerald PG. A general description of the human auditory evoked potentials. In Moore E, Ed. Bases of Auditory Brainstem Evoked Responses. New York: Grune & Stratton, 1983.

Picton TW, and Hillyard SA. Human auditory evoked potentials: Effects of attention. Electroenceph Clin Neurophysiol 1974; 36:191–200.

Picton TW, and Hink RF. Evoked potentials: How? What? & Why? Am J EEG Technol 1974;14:9–44.

Picton TW, Hillyard SH, Frauz HJ, and Galambos R. Human auditory evoked potentials. Electroenceph Clin Neurophysiol 1974; 36:179–190.

Picton TW, Woods DL, Baribeau-Braun J, and Healey TM. Evoked potentials in audiometry. J Otolaryngol 1977;6:90–118.

Polich J, Howard L, and Starr A. Effects of age on the P–300 component of the event-related potential from auditory stimuli: Peak definition, variation, and measurement. J Gerontol 1985;40:721–726.

Pratt H, Ben-David Y, Peled R, Podoshin L, and Scharf B. Auditory brainstem evoked potentials: Clinical promise of increasing stimulus rate. Electroenceph Clin Neurophysiol 1981;51:80–90.

Reneau JP, and Hnatiow GZ. Evoked Response Audiometry: A Topical and Historical Review. Baltimore: University Park Press, 1975.

Richmond KH, Konkle DF, and Potsic W. ABR screening in high risk infants: Effects of ambient noise in neonatal nursery. Otolaryngol Head Neck Surg 1986;94:552–557.

Rose DE, and Rittmanic PA. Evoked response tests with mentally retarded. Arch Otolaryngol 1986;88:495–498.

Rosehnamer HJ, Lindstrom B, and Lundborg T. On the use of click–evoked electric brainstem responses in audiological diagnosis II. The influence of sex and age upon the normal response. Scandinavian Audiology 1980;6:176–196.

Rowe MJ. Normal variability of the brain-stem auditory evoked response in young and old adult subjects. Electroenceph Clin Neurophysiol 1978;44:459–470.

Ruben RJ, Sekula J, Bordley JE, Knickerbocker GG, Nager GT, and Fisch U. Human cochlear responses to sound stimuli. Ann Otol Rhinol Otolaryngol 1960;69:459–476.

Ruhm H, Walker E, and Flanigin H. Acoustically evoked potentials in man; mediation of early components. Laryngoscope 1967;77:806–822.

Ruth R, and Lambert P. Auditory evoked potentials. Otolaryngol Clin North Am 1991;24:349–352.

Ruth RA, Lambert PR, and Ferraro FA. Electrocochleography: Methods and clinical applications. Am J Otol 1988;9:1–11.

Sabo DL, Durrant JD, Curtin H, Boston JR, and Rood S. Correlations of neuro-anatomical measures to brainstem auditory evoked potential latencies. Ear Hear 1992;13:213–222.

Salamy A, and McKean CM. Postnatal development of human brainstem potentials during the first year of life. Electroenceph Clin Neurophysiol 1976;40:418–426.

Sanders RA, Duncan PG, and McCullough DW. Clinical experience with brainstem audiometry performed under general anesthesia. Otolaryngology 1979;8:24–32.

Scherg M, and von Cramon D. Psychoacoustic and electrophysiologic correlates of central hearing disorders in man. Psychiat Neurol Sci 1986;236:56–60.

Schwent VL, Hillyard SA, and Galambos R. Selective attention and the auditor vertex potential. I. Effects of stimulus delivery rate. Electroenceph Clin Neurophysiol 1976;40:606–614.

Schwartz DM, Pratt RE, and Schwartz JA. Auditory brainstem responses in preterm infants: evidence of peripheral maturity. Ear Hear 1989;10:14–22.

Shimazu H. Evoked response in eighth nerve lesions. The Laryngoscope 1968;78:2140–2152.

Sohmer H, and Feinmesser M. Cochlear action potentials recorded from the external ear in man. Ann Otol Rhinol Otolaryngol 1967; 76: 427–435.

Sohmer H, Gafni M, and Chisin R. Auditory nerve and brainstem responses: Comparison of awake and unconscious subjects. Arch Neurol 1978;35:228–230.

Spivak LG, and Malinoff R. Spectral differences in the ABRs of old and young subjects. Ear Hear 1990;11:351–358.

Squires K, and Hecox K. Electrophysiological evaluation of higher level auditory processing. Semin Hear 1983;4:415–432.

Stapells D, Picton TW, and Smith AD. Normal hearing thresholds for clicks. J Acoust Soc Am 1982;72:74–79.

Stapells DR, Picton TW, Perez-Abalo M, Read D, and Smith A. Frequency specificity in evoked potential audiometry. In Jacobson JT, Ed. The Auditory Brainstem Response. San Diego, CA: College-Hill Press, 1985.

Starr A, and Achor J. Auditory brainstem responses in neurological diseases. Arch Neurol 1975;32:761–768.

Stypulkowski PH, and Staller SJ. Clinical evaluation of a new ECochG recording electrode. Ear Hear 1987;8:305– 310.

Suzuki T, Hirabayashi M, and Kobayashi K. Auditory middle responses in young children. Br J Audiol 1983;17:5–9.

Suzuki T, Kobayashi K, and Takagi N. Effects of stimulus repetition rate on slow and fast components of auditory brainstem responses. Electroenceph Clin Neurophysiol 1986;65:150–156.

Teas DC, Eldredge DH, and Davis H. Cochlear responses to acoustic transients and interpretation of the whole nerve action potentials. J Acoust Soc Am 1962;34:1438–1459.

Thornton A. Statistical properties of surface-recorded electrocochleographic responses. Scand Audiol 1975;4:91–102.

Thornton A, Mendel MI, and Anderson C. Effects of stimulus frequency and intensity on the middle components of the averaged electroencephalic response. J Speech Hear Res 1977;20:81–94.

Vedder JS, Barrs DM, and Fifer RC. The use of middle latency response in diagnosis of cortical deafness. Otolaryngol Head Neck Surg 1988;98:333–337.

Walter WG, Cooper R, Aldridge VJ, McCallum WC, and Winter AL. Contingent negative variation: An electric sign of sensorimotor association and expectancy in the human brain. Nature 1964; 203:380–384.

Weber B. Assessing low frequency hearing using auditory evoked potentials. Ear Hear 1986;8:(Suppl 4):49S–54S.

de Weerd JPC, and Stegeman DF. Technical and methodological considerations on the measurement of evoked potentials. In Colon EJ, and Visser SL, Eds. Evoked Potential Manual: A Practical Guide to Clinical Applications. The Netherlands: Kluwer Academic Publishers, 1990.

CHAPTER 23

Electrocochleography

Roger A. Ruth

Electrocochleography (ECochG) refers to the method of measuring stimulus-related electrophysiologic potentials of the most peripheral portions of the auditory system (i.e., the cochlea and auditory nerve). The stimulus-related electrical potentials associated with this part of the auditory pathway include the cochlear microphonic (CM), the summating potential (SP), and the compound action potential (AP) of the auditory nerve. Although in some cases these potentials can be measured by surface electrodes, such as those used to obtain the auditory brainstem response, more accurate and detailed studies of these events requires the placement of recording electrodes in closer proximity to the inner ear.

The earliest attempts to record from the human peripheral auditory system often involved the use of invasive or traumatic needle electrodes placed through the ear drum onto the promontory wall of the middle ear or in the skin of the external ear canal near the tympanic membrane. Due to a number of factors including the increased difficulty and time in placement of such electrodes, level of training required by the examiner (physician) and the potential discomfort experienced by the patient, ECochG measures never gained widespread acceptance as a clinical tool in the United States. The development over the past several years of a variety of so called noninvasive electrodes has largely been responsible for a resurgence of interest in the clinical application of ECochG. For example, a recent national survey found that about a quarter of the audiologists sampled included ECochG in their auditory evoked potential test battery (Jacobson, et al., 1988).

The current areas in which ECochG is believed to be clinical value to the audiologist and otologist include: (*a*) the assessment and monitoring of patients with Ménière's disease (i.e., endolymphatic hydrops); (*b*) the enhancement of wave I of the auditory brainstem response in patients who have substantial amounts of hearing loss or who are tested under less than optimal recording conditions; and (*c*) the intraoperative monitoring of the peripheral auditory structures (Ruth et al., 1988). This chapter will provide an overview of current recording techniques and clinical applications of ECochG.

REVIEW OF PERIPHERAL ELECTROPHYSIOLOGY

The manner in which the auditory system extracts sound energy from an individual's environment and relays it to the brain is highly complicated and only partially understood. Part of the problem arises from the small size of the inner ear and the fact that it is entirely encased in the hardest bone of the body making direct observation of this extraordinary mechanical wonder all but impossible. As such, much of its function must be viewed indirectly. One way of doing so is by observing the electrophysiologic response to stimulation. Although most of these electrical potentials are not considered essential for the actual process of hearing, they are viewed as by-products of auditory system function, and therefore potentially valuable in furthering our understanding of the normal and impaired ear. The three major classifications of stimulus-related electrical potentials that can be measured from the peripheral auditory system will be summarized. The reader requiring more extensive coverage of this topic is referred to other sources.

Cochlear Microphonic (CM)

Wever and Brey (1930) were the first to describe the CM in an animal model. The CM is an alternating current (AC) response that tends to mirror the waveform of low to moderately intense sound stimuli and is thought to reflect the displacement-time pattern of the cochlear partition (Dallos, 1973). When recorded from an electrode resting outside the inner ear proper, as is the case in all human studies, the CM appears to arise from outer hair cells in the basal most turn of the cochlea. Its role in the actual transduction process is uncertain; however, most investigators now believe that the CM is merely an epiphenomenon associated with activation of the hair cells.

The magnitude of the CM is dependent on hair cell output and is fairly linear over a sizable range of stimulus intensities. However, the absolute amplitude of the CM is of little value due to the dependence of the response on electrode type and placement. For example, the CM can be recorded in humans using noninvasive procedures (Elberling and Salomon, 1973) but, as with all neuroelectric responses, the CM decreases in amplitude as distance from the recording electrode to the generator site increases. Aberrations in the CM, such as diminished amplitude or waveform distortion, have been observed in some patients with cochlear pathology (Kumagami et al., 1982; Morrison et al., 1980). In our experience, the response variability and difficulty encountered in accurately interpreting the CM make this potential less suitable than others for most clinical ECochG applications (Ferraro and Ruth, 1985; Ruth et al., 1988).

Summating Potential

This cochlear potential was first described in two independent investigations by Davis et al. (1950) and Bekesy (1950). Unlike the CM the SP is a direct current potential. The SP may be viewed as a complex multicomponent response representing the sum of various nonlinearities associated with cochlear processing (Dallos et al., 1972). The SP tends to follow the envelope (i.e., on-off pattern) of the stimulus, rather than its waveform (Dallos, 1973). The polarity of the DC shift may be positive or negative depending on stimulus frequency, intensity, and the electrode recording site. When recorded with noninvasive electrodes in the ear canal or on the tympanic membrane the SP is generally characterized by a negative shift in baseline that persists for the duration of the evoking stimulus.

The SP has received a good deal of attention in recent years for its application to the assessment of Ménière's disease. The amplitude of the SP is often enlarged in patients with endolymphatic hydrops, particularly as compared to AP amplitude (Ruth et al., 1988). The reason for this finding is still unclear, but may reflect increased asymmetry in basilar membrane movement or increased nonlinearity in hydropic inner ears (Gibson et al., 1977). In any event, it is well established that an enlarged SP may be pathonomonic of Ménière's disease.

Action Potential

The whole-nerve or compound action potential of the auditory nerve was first recorded in humans undergoing ear surgery by Ruben et al. (1960). The AP represents the most popular stimulus-related potential measured by means of ECochG in humans. When using conventional ECochG electrodes the AP reflects the summed response of synchronous discharges from several thousand individual nerve fibers primarily located in the basal or high frequency region of the cochlea (Kiang, 1965). As with the CM, the AP is represented as an alternating current voltage. The waveform of

the AP is characterized by a relatively large negative deflection referred to as N_1. This component (N_1) is identical to wave I of the surface recorded ABR. Both N_1 of the ECochG and wave I of the ABR arise from the distal portion of the auditory nerve (Moller and Jannetta, 1983). The response often has a subsequent and smaller negative deflection referred to as N_2 that arises from the more proximal portion of the auditory nerve (the part of the nerve located between the porus acousticus and the brainstem) and corresponds to wave II of the surface recorded ABR.

Both amplitude and latency of the AP are dependent on the intensity of the evoking stimulus. For example, as stimulus intensity decreases latency of N_1 increases whereas N_1 amplitude decreases. The latency of N_1 is generally around 1.5 and 2.5 milliseconds depending on stimulus intensity and is thought to reflect the travel time of wave propagation in the cochlea. The amplitude of N_1 is thought to be related to the sheer number of neural elements activated by a sound stimulus; that is the higher the intensity the more fibers participate in the synchronous response forming N_1.

TECHNIQUES FOR RECORDING ECochG

ECochG may be defined as the measurement of stimulus-related electrical potentials associated with the inner ear and auditory nerve. Although some of these earliest potentials can be observed with surface type electrodes (i.e., waves I and II of the ABR), the resolution of the recordings is far greater when the measurement electrodes are placed closer to the response generators of the CM, SP, and AP. One can classify the electrodes used for ECochG recordings in humans as being either *invasive* or *noninvasive* depending on whether or not they penetrate skin of the ear drum or ear canal (see Table 23.1).

Invasive Electrodes

The major advantage of using an invasive ECochG electrode is the acquisition of clearer, more robust

Table 23.1.
ECochG Electrode Recording Techniques

Invasive
Transtympanic (TT-ECochG)
Promontory needle electrode
Round window ball electrode
Noninvasive
Extratympanic (ET-ECochG)
Foam plug ear canal electrode
Leaf-type ear canal electrode
Tympanic membrane (TM-ECochG)
Flexible tubing with foam or cotton ball at end

electrical responses from the auditory periphery. This results simply from the fact that the recording electrode is usually very near the generators of the response (hair cells and auditory nerve). As such, amplitude of the response is large in comparison to the background noise and thus presents a more favorable signal-to-noise ratio. An obvious disadvantage is the potential for some degree of discomfort to the patient. In addition, the electrode must be placed by a physician which limits its use to medical settings.

Transtympanic Needle ECochG Electrode

The most often used invasive ECochG electrode is the transtympanic (TT-ECochG) needle as shown in Figure 23.1 (*top*). The needle is generally insulated by a coating such as teflon except for 1 millimeter or 2 at its tip. Because of the relatively small surface area of contact, electrode impedance is generally higher than surface electrodes (ranging from 40 to 100 kohm). The transtympanic needle is placed, with the aid of an operating microscope, on the promontory wall of the middle ear near the round window niche. Before placement the tympanic membrane should be treated with a local anesthetic. After placement the needle must be secured so as to prevent slippage due to minor movements on the part of the patient.

ECochG recordings obtained with a transtympanic needle are often on the order of 20 to 40 microvolts in amplitude at moderate to high stimulus intensities (Ruth and Lambert, 1989). Given the relatively large amplitude of ECochG responses recorded in this fashion, fewer repetitions are required per average. For example, as few as 50 to 150 stimulus repetitions may be needed to resolve the response with this recording technique. Thus, at a stimulus presentation rate of 10 per second a recording can be obtained within 5 to 15 seconds. This is far less time than that required by most noninvasive ECochG or surface electrode ABR procedures. More importantly, the AP response may be observed down to stimulus levels approximating hearing threshold. The transtympanic needle is still used routinely in many European countries.

Round Window ECochG Electrode

Also shown in Figure 23.1 (*bottom*) is a silver-ball electrode used for round window ECochG measurements. This type of ECochG recording electrode has been used for decades as a way of monitoring cochlear responses in animals for various research purposes. Its use in humans is limited due to the fact that placement of the electrode requires that the ear drum be surgically lifted so that the round window is both visible and accessible to the surgeon. This type of recording is therefore generally reserved for those cases in which exposure of the middle ear is also needed for other purposes or for long term monitoring of the auditory system (i.e., intraoperative monitoring of the auditory nerve). In most cases round window ECochG recordings are similar to those obtained with the transtympanic needle in terms of amplitude and response clarity.

Noninvasive Electrodes

Noninvasive or nontraumatic ECochG recording techniques by definition are relatively painless, thus obviating the need for sedation or local anesthetics. In addition, these electrodes can be placed without the direct assistance of a physician. The availability of several types of noninvasive ECochG electrodes is largely responsible for the renewed interest in clinical ECochG measurements in the United States. There

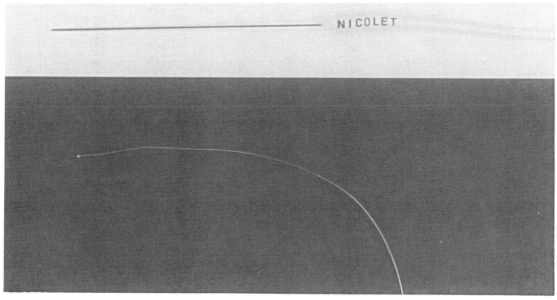

Figure 23.1. Invasive TT-ECochG electrodes.

are two major categories of noninvasive electrodes; extratympanic (ET-ECochG) and tympanic membrane (TM-ECochG).

Extratympanic ECochG Electrodes

Several versions of ET-ECochG electrodes are commercially available at the present time. Two of the more popular ET-ECochG electrodes are shown in Figure 23.2. The eartrode was first described by Coats in 1974. It consists of insulated silver wire with a ball tip glued to a small strip of flexible plastic. The eartrode electrode is placed by pinching the leaves of plastic together with fine forceps and inserting the device into the ear canal. It is held in place against the skin of the ear canal by pressure from the plastic leaf once the forceps are removed. Cerumen must be removed and the ear canal cleaned in the vicinity of the ball tip before placement. After a small amount of gel is placed on the ball tip, the eartrode is placed in the posterior-inferior quadrant of the ear canal. The depth of insertion may range from shallow (mid-canal) to deep (within a few millimeters of TM). The magnitude of the response will be larger for deeper insertions (Staller, 1986), however, positioning the eartrode closer to the TM usually creates some discomfort for

the patient and increases the risk of traumatizing the ear drum.

More recently a disposable foam plug electrode was introduced. The original version of this electrode consisted of a reticulated foam earplug materal saturated with gel. A plastic tube running through the center of the earplug served as a sound channel for stimulus delivery. The current version of the disposable foam plug electrode is the TIPtrode (see Fig. 23.2). The TIPtrode consists of a compressible foam covered by an extremely thin, pliable layer of gold foil. The electrode is coupled to an insert transducer by flexible, silicon tubing. These disposable foam plug electrodes are designed to compress upon insertion into the ear canal and expand to conform to its contour. The large surface area of contact with the canal skin allows for lower electrode impedance comparable to that of surface electrodes. The TIPtrode cannot be inserted beyond the mid portion of the ear canal and, as such, is considered a shallow ET-ECochG placement.

Tympanic Membrane ECochG Electrode

One of the more novel approaches to noninvasive ECochG involves the use of an electrode that rests directly on the tympanic membrane (TM-ECochG). The

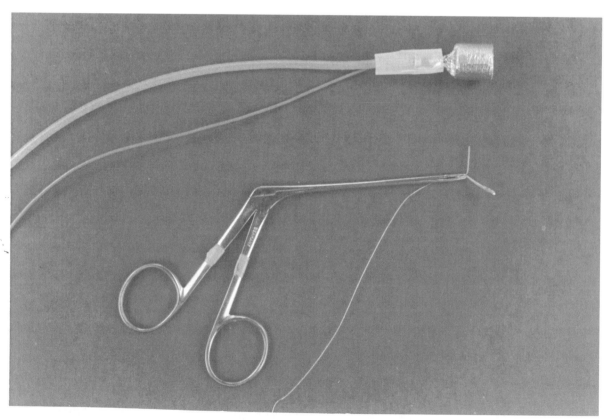

Figure 23.2. Noninvasive ET-ECochG electrodes.

TM electrode is considered noninvasive in as much as no anesthesia is required for its use. Such an electrode was first used for nontraumatic ECochG recordings 20 years ago by Cullen et al. (1972). These authors described the successful use of a wick electrode placed on the unanesthetized eardrum for the purpose of hearing sensitivity assessment in children. Despite their promising findings, the TM-ECochG recording technique they pioneered failed to gain widespread acceptance due in part to the intense interest throughout the world with the development and clinical application of the ABR. It was not until some years later that the TM-ECochG procedure was revisited first by Stypulkowski and Staller (1987) and subsequently by other investigators (Ruth et al., 1988; Ruth and Lambert, 1989; Ferraro and Ferguson, 1989; Ruth, 1990; Durrant, 1991; Arsenault and Benitez, 1991).

The TM-ECochG electrode used in our lab is shown in Figure 23.3. It is not commercially available at this time. However, it can be fashioned from the following materials with little effort: flexible lightweight Silastic tubing (American Scientific Products, American Hosp. Supply Corp., 1430 Waukegan Rd., McGraw Park, IL 60085), fine Teflon-coated silver wire (Medwire, AG5T, 121 South Columbia Ave., Mount Vernon, NY 10553) and a small piece of foam (cut from ear block material) or cotton wisp. The tip of the TM electrode consists of a 3-mm piece of foam or cotton through which a stripped end of the silver wire is threaded. The portion of the foam or cotton attached to the wire and the wire itself are encased in the flexible Silastic tubing. Preparation of the electrode involves injecting a small amount of standard electrode gel into the foam with a hypodermic needle or soaking the cotton wisp in saline. The electrode is inserted by holding the external canal open with pediatric nasal speculum and gently sliding the tubing until the tip makes contact with the ear drum. In our experience the TM electrode is tolerated well and most patients describe no significant discomfort with the electrode in place other than a sensation comparable to that of having water in their ears.

Ruth and Lambert (1989) compared ECochG recordings obtained from the TM electrode to those derived simultaneously from a TT needle electrode in a group of patients with Ménière's disease. Although smaller in magnitude, the TM-ECochG recordings were similar to the TT-ECochG responses in terms of overall waveform quality and identifiability of waveform components (SP and AP). Comparisons between TM-ECochG and ET-ECochG recordings reveal that the TM responses are less distorted, more sensitive and larger in amplitude than those measured from the ear canal (Stypulkowski and Staller, 1987; Ruth et al., 1988; Ferraro and Ferguson, 1989). An example of recordings obtained from ET-, TM-, and TT-ECochG electrodes are shown in Figure 23.4.

Recording Parameters

The stimulus and response parameters used to carry out ECochG testing are similar in many respects to those used for ABR recordings. The actual parameters used depend to some extent on the application and the particular components of the ECochG waveform in which the examiner is interested. For example, the AP and SP measurements used for evaluation of patients with endolymphatic hydrops require parameters that differ somewhat from those employed to monitor auditory function during surgeries involving the ear and auditory nerve that make use of the AP and CM components.

Table 23.2 illustrates the stimulus parameters typically used for clinical ECochG measurements. A high intensity broadband click is the most common ECochG stimulus; however, for some applications a tone burst may be desirable (i.e., examination of CM). An alternating polarity stimulus may be used to eliminate the CM and any electromagnetic artifact present. The CM is actually enhanced and the AP and SP diminished by obtaining separate responses to rarefaction and condensation stimuli and subsequently subtracting them from one another. Because as the AP

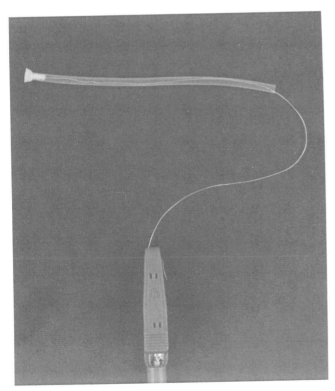

Figure 23.3. Tympanic membrane TM-ECochG electrode.

ECochG

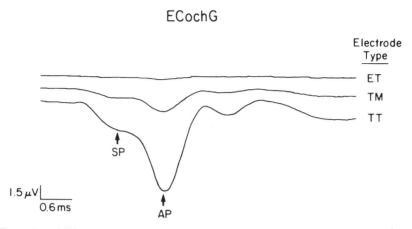

Figure 23.4. Examples of ECochG recordings obtained with an ET-ECochG, TM-ECochG and TT-ECochG electrode.

Table 23.2.
Stimulus Parameters

		For Optimal Recording of
Type	Broadband clicks Tone burst	AP/SP[a] CM/SP[a]
Polarity	Alternating Rarefaction/condensation	AP/SP CM
Rate	5 to 11/second 80 to 100+/second	AP/SP/CM SP
Intensity	75 to 95 dB HL Variable	AP/SP/CM AP threshold
Masking	Generally not necessary	

[a]SP may be measured using broad band clicks or tone bursts.

Table 23.3.
Strategies for Optimizing ECochG Recording

Enhance AP and SP and remove CM
Alternate polarity or add responses from rarefaction and condensation polarity stimuli

Enhance CM and remove SP and AP
Subtract responses from rarefaction and condensation stimuli

Enhance SP
Alternate polarity or add responses from rarefaction and condensation stimuli
Use fast stimulus rate (>80/second)

is rate sensitive (increasing latency and decreasing amplitude with increasing rate) observation of the SP can sometimes be improved by using a fast stimulus rate (i.e., >80/second). The AP can be viewed in isolation by subtracting a response obtained to a fast rate of stimulation from a response to a slow rate of stimulation. Table 23.3 summarizes the stimulus polarity and rate parameters used to enhance certain ECochG components.

The typical reponse recording parameters used for ECochG measurement are illustrated in Table 23.4. The primary electrode is located in the ear canal, on the ear drum or on the promontory wall of the middle ear. The secondary or reference electrode site can be the contralateral earlobe, mastoid, ear canal, or forehead. It is important to realize that when the primary electrode is plugged into the noninverting (+) channel of the differential amplifier the resulting AP response will be pointing down as in Figure 23.3. If the primary electrode is plugged into the inverting (−) channel of

the amplifier then the AP response will be pointing up. The responses obtained under these two recording conditions would be mirror images of one another. The analysis time is between 5 and 12 milliseconds. If one is interested in the earliest components only (AP, CM, and SP) without regard for brainstem responses, then 5 milliseconds would be sufficient. However, if ABR recordings are simultaneously acquired, then a longer analysis window is necessary. The number of repetitions and amplification factor required to resolve the response largely depend on electrode site; i.e., the closer to the generator source the fewer stimulus repetitions and the less amplification needed.

Electrode impedance is generally held below about 5000 ohm for surface recorded ABR measures. However, ECochG electrodes may have much higher impedance. Table 23.5 summarizes the range of impedance values associated with different types of electrodes.

CLINICAL APPLICATIONS

Probably most attention with regard to the clinical application of ECochG has been focused on the evaluation and monitoring of Ménière's disease or endolymphatic hydrops. This is largely due to the unique nature of the information provided by ECochG pertaining to cochlear function. However, ECochG does have other clinical uses, including enhancement of wave I in patients with substantial hearing loss and in the intraoperative monitoring of peripheral auditory structures at risk for damage secondary to surgically induced trauma. Each of these areas of clinical application will be summarized below.

Ménière's Disease and Endolymphatic Hydrops

Ménière's disease has been the focus of considerable attention because its initial description over 130 years ago. Despite a considerable research effort, however, the true nature of this unique cochlear and labyrinthine disorder continues to elude us. The classic triad of symptoms associated with Ménière's disease include fluctuating unilateral sensory-neural hearing loss, tinnitus, and episodic vertigo. Patients with these classic findings do not present a diagnostic dilemma. However, the hallmark of Ménière's disease is its variable

expression from one patient to the next or even within the same patient over time. As such, there many situations wherein the certainty of a diagnosis of Ménière's disease is less clear. It is in these patients for whom ECochG measures may offer some insight to the diagnostic process.

A number of studies have demonstrated distinctive ECochG patterns in patients with Ménière's disease as compared to normal ears. This difference is primarily in the form of an enlarged SP amplitude relative to the AP amplitude (see Fig. 23.5). It has been postulated that an increase in endolymphatic volume alters the mechanical characteristics of basilar membrane motion. Inasmuch as the vibratory asymmetry of the basilar membrane is thought to cause the SP, enhancement of this asymmetry by hydrops could explain the enlarged SP seen in Ménière's patients (Gibson et al., 1977). Consistent with this hypothesis is the finding by Durrant and Dallos (1974) that displacement of the basilar membrane toward the scala tympani tends to increase the magnitude of the SP. Further support for the notion that the enlargement of the SP is a physiologic manifestation of endolymphatic hydrops may be found in clinical studies that have observed reductions in SP amplitude folowing dehydration by administration of glycerol (Moffat et al., 1978; Coats and Alford, 1981).

The absolute amplitude of the SP and AP both show considerable variability across subjects. A more consistent amplitude feature is the SP-AP amplitude ratio (Eggermont, 1976). On the average an SP-AP ratio of 0.45 or greater is generally considered abnor-

Table 23.4.
Response Recording Parameters

Channels	One	
Electrode site		
Primary (+) (Noninverting)	Ipsilateral ear canal Tympanic membrane Promotory	
Secondary (−) (Inverting)	Contralateral earlobe Mastoid/ear canal/forehead Vertex	
Ground	Any other surface location	
Analysis time	5–12 milliseconds	
Filter bandwidth	High pass—1–30 Hz Low pass—1500–3000 Hz	
Repetitions	100–200 500–1500 1000–3000	TT-ECochG TM-ECochG ET-ECochG
Amplification	5–25 K 25–75 K 75–125 K	TT-ECochG TM-ECochG ET-ECochG

Table 23.5.
Electrode Impedance for ECochG Electrodes

	Electrode Impedance (kohm)
Surface electrode	1–5
ET-ECochG electrode	3–20
TM-ECochG electrode	10–50
TT-ECochG electrode	40–100

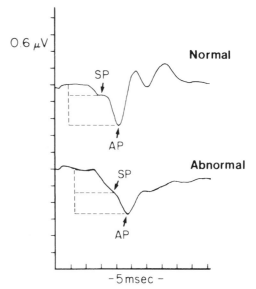

Figure 23.5. Normal and abnormal ECochG waveforms obtained using a TM-ECochG electrode. **SP,** summating potential; **AP,** action potential (from Ruth, 1990).

mal (i.e., SP amplitude $\geq 45\%$ of AP amplitude). However, Coats (1986) has noted that this ratio is not a simple linear relationship. That is, in normal subjects as the AP amplitude increases from 1 to 4 microvolts, the normal SP to AP ratio decreases from 0.4 to 0.25, respectively. Thus a single ratio differentiating normal from abnormal may be at times misleading. In order to compensate for this relationship Coats has proposed the use of an "AP-normalized SP" amplitude plot as shown in Figure 23.6. The **dashed line** represents the 95% confidence interval for a normal SP-AP amplitude relationship. Any values plotted above this line are considered abnormal (that is the SP amplitude is larger than expected given the value of the AP amplitude).

Most studies have found an abnormally enlarged SP-AP relationship in approximately two-thirds of the patients thought to have Ménière's disease (Gibson et al., 1977; Coats, 1981; Ferraro et al., 1983). The reason all Ménière's patients do not demonstrate this abnormality is unclear. It may reflect the fluctuant nature of the disorder or to the deterioration of outer hair cells known to occur in more advanced stages of Ménière's disease. It is apparent that the incidence of an abnormal SP-AP relationship is dependent on the extent of hearing loss and the presence of certain symptoms at the time of testing. For example, Ferraro et al., (1985) have noted a close correspondance between an enlarged SP-AP amplitude ratio and the presence of aural fullness or pressure and some degree of hearing loss at the time of the ECochG recording.

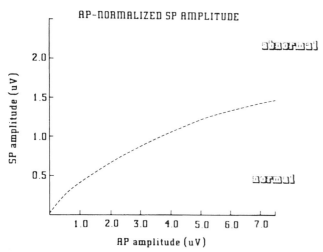

Figure 23.6. Method for plotting summating potential (**SP**) and action potential (**AP**) amplitudes after Coats (1986). **Dashed line** represents 95% confidence limit for normal SP-AP relationship (from Ruth, 1990).

Enhancement of Wave I of the ABR

Measurement of the elapsed time from ABR component waves I to V is generally considered the most important and sensitive ABR parameter for assessment of retrocochlear disorder (see Chapter 24). This is due to the fact that wave I serves as an indicator of the peripheral auditory output, whereas wave V represents brainstem activity. As such, the wave I to V interwave interval (IWI) is relatively insensitive to peripheral hearing loss and its abnormal prolongation is thought to be due to retrocochlear impairment. Of course, wave I must be clearly observed for the IWI to be calculated. In many patients with significant hearing impairment, the observation of a wave I may be problematic with routine surface or scalp electrode recording procedures. Hyde and Blair (1981), for example, reported that only 42% of 400 patients with sensory (cochlear) hearing loss had a reliable or identifiable wave I from surface recorded ABR. Cashman and Rossman (1983) reported similar results, with wave I present in only 32% of their cochlear impaired population and 14% of all patients with confirmed acoustic tumors. Thus, the most sensitive index of the ABR (i.e., IWI) may be immeasurable in a large portion of hearing impaired patients.

Placing a recording electrode closer to the source of wave I (distal auditory nerve) greatly increases the probably of observing this potential. Several investigators have reported increased detectability of wave I with a combined ECochG and surface recorded ABR approach (Harder and Arlinger, 1981; Walter and Blegvad, 1981; Yanz and Dodds, 1985; Ferraro, Murphy and Ruth, 1986; Ruth et al., 1988; Ferraro and Ferguson, 1989). Even a noninvasive canal electrode can increase the amplitude of wave I by as much as 65% compared to conventional scalp recordings (Ruth et al., 1988). In more severe high frequency hearing loss these shallow canal ET-ECochG electrodes may not be sufficient to resolve wave I. In such cases we have used a TM-ECochG electrode with great success (Ruth et al., 1988). Figure 23.7 illustrates the degree of wave I enhancement possible with a TM-ECochG electrode compared with a surface recording of the ABR in an individual with high frequency sensory-neural hearing loss. Note that the ABR obtained for this patient with a conventional scalp electrode array yielded only a wave V, with no wave I. The upper tracing shows a simultaneously recorded ABR using the TM electrode, instead of the earlobe location. In this case the TM-ECochG recording allows for a clear and repeatable wave I that may be used to calculate the I to V IWI.

Using the TM-ECochG recording technique

ABR

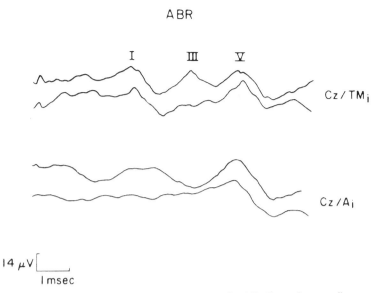

Figure 23.7. Simultaneous surface and TM-ECochG electrode recordings of the ABR in a hearing impaired patient.

Ferraro and Ferguson (1989) found that wave I was always present when hearing reserve was sufficient to allow for a definable wave V in the surface recording. In addition, they found that wave I threshold was identical to wave V threshold when the TM-ECochG electrode was used.

Intraoperative Monitoring of Peripheral Auditory Function

Virtually any surgical operation within the posterior fossa places the auditory nerve and its postoperative function at risk for permanent damage or impairment. In such cases the surgeon sould benefit from accurate, ongoing knowledge about the status of the ear, as this information could lead to reversal of adverse conditions by a change in surgical approach. Given that we routinely measure the electrophysiologic properties of the auditory system as part of the current audiologic diagnostic test battery, it seems reasonable to extend these observations to the operating room where they may provide more immediate information to the surgeon. However, certain general assumptions must be made regarding the use of neurophysiologic intraoperative monitoring (NIM) procedures.

The specific NIM procedures used must: (a) reflect properties of the system(s) at risk for permanent damage; (b) be sufficiently sensitive to detect surgically induced alterations in the system(s) at risk; and (c) exhibit changes in sufficient time to prevent or minimize permanent damage.

To a first approximation, the current otologic NIM techniques appear to meet these assumptions. During the past decade a number of investigators have demonstrated both the feasibility and benefit of NIM in a variety of otologic and neurosurgical cases. As such, auditory and facial nerve NIM has become an integral part of the modern otologic/neurotologic and neurosurgical surgical practice.

Due primarily to its ease of use the surface recorded ABR is most often used to monitor the auditory system during surgery (see Chapter 24). Intraoperative measurements can also been made using near-field recordings acquired with ET-ECochG and/or TT-ECochG electrodes, as well as from direct recording of the auditory nerve compound action potential (ANCAP). Regardless of technique all such measurements have one primary goal in common: *to forewarn the surgeon of possible injury to the auditory system or surrounding structures. A secondary goal is to predict postoperative hearing function.*

Any otologic surgery in which the ear is at risk for damage and preservation of hearing is intended should be considered for monitoring. The most frequently monitored procedures in an otologic/neurotologic practice include (a) acoustic tumor removal (suboccipital, middle cranial fossa, or retromastoid approaches); (b) vestibular nerve section; (c) facial nerve exploration; (d) endolymphatic sac decompression or shunt, and (e) microvascular decompression of cranial nerve VII or VIII.

The major sites of damage to the auditory system during a neurotologic operation are the cochlea, eighth nerve proper and its root entry zone at the brainstem. The most serious damage to the cochlea usually occurs as a result of disruption of normal blood supply to the inner ear via the internal auditory artery. This generally results in an abrupt loss of all measured auditory evoked potentials and unless immediately corrected will render the cochlea permanently impaired. The eighth nerve itself and its root entry zone at the brainstem can be damaged by stretch or compression injury due to excessive manipulation or improper retractor placement. This type of event, in the absence of end organ vascular occlusion, typically causes a more gradual change in measured auditory evoked potentials, which can often be reversed with proper action (i.e., retractor replacement). The eighth nerve may also be temporarily or permanently impaired by the heat produced from drilling the internal auditory meatus or as a byproduct of a laser used for tumor resection.

The most frequently used invasive ECochG electrode is the transtympanic (TT) insulated needle. It is placed by the surgeon through the tympanic membrane onto the cochlear promontory. Prass et al. (1987) have developed a technique for placing the transtympanic needle through the tragus to help stabilize the electrode. We have found this technique very helpful during intraoperative monitoring of ECochG. There are also several ET-ECochG electrodes available, including the compressible foam tip covered by an extremely thin pliable layer of gold foil. One advantage of this electrode is that it also serves to couple the stimulus delivery to the ear. In most cases we use both the transtympanic needle and the compressible gold foil electrode for our neurotologic intraoperative monitoring (Ruth et al. 1986).

Figure 23.8 shows a series of TT-ECochG recordings from a patient undergoing an acoustic tumor resection. Notice the high amplitude broad AP (wave I)

compared to the small wave V of the ABR. During NIM the ECochG is evaluated for any change in amplitude or latency of the AP component compared to simultaneously acquired ABR recordings. In addition, threshold of the ECochG may be determined at various points during the procedure. Figure 23.9 illustrates an intraoperative ECochG threshold search on the same patient. Stanton et al. (1989) have found threshold of the TT-ECochG to correlate highly with postoperative hearing function.

It is now apparent that no single monitoring technique is sufficiently sensitive in all cases. Rather a combination of responses sampled from the various levels of the auditory system is necessary to optimize early detection of injury. Figure 23.10 illustrates the simultaneous use of TT-ECochG and ABR in a patient undergoing acoustic tumor resection. Clear resolution of AP (wave I) is important because observation of this parameter can be used to detect cochlear injury. This includes monitoring for vascular compromize and differentiates it from damage to the nerve proper. In the case shown, although no wave I is present in the ABR recordings, a clear AP potential is observed in the TT-ECochG tracing. Using AP of the ECochG response and wave V from the ABR the I-V interwave interval can be easily calculated. In addition, the ECochG response can be resolved with fewer averages due to the improved signal-to-noise ratio with this recording technique compared to surface recordings. Table 23.6 summarizes several relevant features of these three recording techniques.

SUMMARY

Electrocochleography provides the audiologist with information regarding the functional status of the pe-

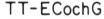

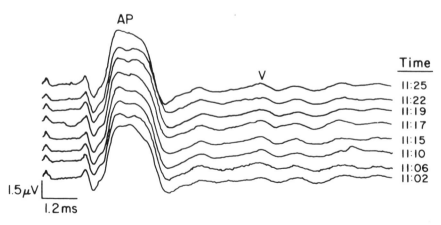

Figure 23.8. Intraoperative TT-ECochG recordings obtained from a patient undergoing removal of acoustic tumor.

TT-ECochG

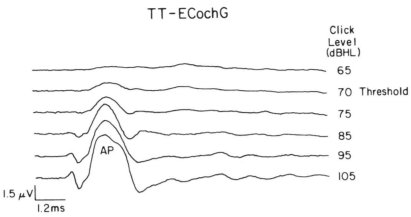

Figure 23.9. Intraoperative TT-ECochG threshold recordings obtained from the same patient as Figure 23.8.

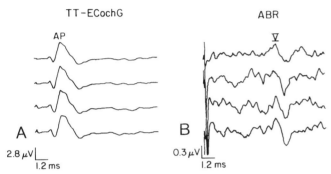

Figure 23.10. Simultaneous recording of intraoperative TT-ECochG and surface derived ABR in a patient undergoing resection of acoustic tumor.

Table 23.6.
Intraoperative EAP Recording Options

	Amplitude (μV)	No. Sweeps	Time (second) @ 20/second
Surface recorded ABR	0.1–0.5	500–1500	25–75
ET-ECochG	0.3–1.0	250–1200	12–60
TT-ECochG	10–20	40–100	2–5
Direct ANCAP	25–30	1–5	<1

ripheral most portions of the auditory system. Such information has been shown to be of value in a variety of clinical situations ranging from its use as a differential diagnostic tool to its application as a monitor of auditory function during neurotologic surgeries. The relatively recent development of noninvasive electrodes has spawned an increased interest in the clinical use of ECochG. Together with other auditory evoked potentials it gives the audiologist a unique perspective of this extraordinarily complex sensory system we call the "ear" and in some cases provides insights unavailable by other means.

REFERENCES

Arsenault MD, and Benitez JT. Electrocochleography: A method for making the Stypulowski-Staller electrode and testing technique. Ear Hearing 1991;12:358–360.

Bekesy LG. DC potentials and energy balance of the cochlear partition. J Acoust Soc Am 1950;22:29–35.

Coats AC. On electrocochleographic electrode design. J Acoust Soc Am 1974;56:708–711.

Coats AC. (1981). The summating potential and Meniere's disease. Arch Otolaryngol 1981;107:199–208.

Coats AC. The normal summating potential recorded from the external ear canal. Arch Otolaryngol 1986;112:759–768.

Coats AC, and Alford B. Meniere's disease and the summating potential: III. effect of glycerol administration. Archives of Otolaryngology 1981;107:469–473.

Cashman MZ, and Rossman R. (1983). Diagnostic features of the auditory brainstem response in identifying cerebellopontine angle tumors. Scand Audiol 1983;12:35–41.

Cullen JK, Ellis MS, Berlin CI, and Lousteau RJ. (1972). Human acoustic nerve action potential recordings from the tympanic membrane without anesthesia. Acta Otolaryngol 1972;74:15–22.

Dallos P. The auditory periphery: Biophysics and physiology. New York: Academic Press, 1973.

Dallos P, Schoeny ZG, and Cheatham MA. Cochlear summating potentials: descriptive aspects. Acta Otolaryngol 1972;(Suppl) 302:1–46.

Davis H, Fernandez C, and McAuliffe DR. The excitatory process in the cochlea. Proc Nat Acad Sci 1950;36:580–587.

Durrant JD. Extratympanic electrode support via vented earmold. Ear Hear 1991;11:468–469.

Durrant JD, and Dallos P. (1974). Modification of DIF summating potential components by stimulus biasing. J Acoust Soc Am 1974;56:562–568.

Eggermont JJ. (1976). Summating potentials in electrocochleography: Relation to hearing disorders. In Ruben RJ, Elberling C, and Salomon G, Eds. Electrocochleography. Baltimore: University Park Press, 1976:67–87.

Elberling C, and Salomon G. (1973). Cochlear microphonics recorded from the ear canal in man. Acta Otolaryngol 1973;75:489–495.

Ferraro JA, Best LG, and Arenberg IK. The use of electrocochleography in the diagnosis, assessment and monitoring of endolymphatic hydrops. Otolaryngol Clin North Am 1983;16:69–82.

Ferraro JA, Arenberg IK, and Hassanein RS. Electrocochleography and symptoms of inner ear dysfunction. Arch Otolaryngol 1985;111:71–74.

Ferraro JA, Murphy GB, and Ruth RA. A comparative study of the primary electrodes used in extratympanic electrocochleography. Semin Hear 1986;7:279–287.

Ferraro JA, and Ferguson R. Tympanic ECochG and conventional ABR: a combined approach for the identification of wave I and the I–V interwave interval. Ear Hear 1989;10:161–166.

Gibson WPR, Moffat DA, and Ramsden RT. Clinical electrocochleography in the diagnosis and management of Meniere's disorder. Audiology 1977;16:389–401.

Harder H, and Arlinger S. (1981). Ear canal compared to mastoid electrode placement in ABR. Scand Audiol 1981;13(Suppl): 55–57.

Hyde ML, and Blair RL. The auditory brainstem response in neuro-otology: perspectives and problems. J Otolaryngol 1981;10:117–125.

Jacobson J, Kileny P, and Ruth RA. Auditory evoked potentials: a survey of educational and practice patterns. ASHA 1988; 30:49–52.

Kiang NS. Discharge patterns of single nerve fibers in the cat's auditory nerve. Research monograph 35, Cambridge, MA: MIT Press, 1985.

Kumagami H, Nishida H, and Masaaki B. Electrocochleographic study of Meniere's disease. Arch Otolaryngol 1982;108: 284–288.

Moffat DA, Gibson WPR, and Ramsden R. Transtympanic electrocochleography during glycerol dehydration. Acta Otolaryngol 1978;85:158–166.

Moller AR, and Janetta PJ. Monitoring auditory functions during cranial nerve microvascular decompression operations by direct monitoring from the eighth nerve. J Neurosurg 1983;59: 493–499.

Morrison AW, Moffat DA, and O'Connor AF. Clinical usefulness of electrocochleography in Meniere's disease: An analysis of dehydrating agents. Otolaryngol Clin North Am 1980;11:703–721.

Prass RL, Kinney SE, and Luders H. Transtragal transtympanic electrode placement for intraoperative electrocochleographic monitoring. Otolaryngol Head Neck Surg 1987;97:343–350.

Ruben R, Sekula J, and Bordely JE. Human cochlear responses to sound stimuli. Ann Otorhinolaryngol 1960;69:459–476.

Ruth RA, and Lambert PR. Comparison of tympanic membrane to promontory electrode recordings of electrocochleographic responses in Meniere's disease. Otolaryngol Head Neck Surg 1989;100:546–552.

Ruth RA, and Lambert PR, and Ferraro JA. Electrocochleography: Methods and clinical applications. Am J Otol 1988; 9:1–11.

Ruth RA, Mills J, and Jane JA. Intraoperative monitoring of electrocochleographic and auditory brainstem responses. Semin Hear 1986;7:307–327.

Ruth RA, Mills JA, and Ferraro JA. Use of disposable ear canal electrodes in auditory brainstem response testing. Am J Otol 1988;9:310–315.

Ruth RA. Trends in electrocochleography. J Am Acad Audiol 1990;1:134–137.

Staller S. Electrocochleography in the diagnosis and management of Meniere's disease. Semin Hear 1986;7:267–277.

Stanton SG, Cashman MZ, Harrison RV, Nedzelski JM, and Rowed DW. Cochlear nerve action potentials during cerebellopontine angle surgery: Relationship of latency, amplitude and threshold measurements to hearing. Ear Hear 1989;10:23–28.

Stypulkowski PH, and Staller SJ. Clinical evaluation of a new ECoG recording electrode. Ear Hear 1987;8:304–310.

Walter B, and Blevgard B. (1981). Identification of wave I by means of an atraumatic ear canal electrode. Scand Audiol 1981;13(Suppl):63–64.

Wever EG, and Bray C. Action currents in the auditory nerve in response to acoustic stimulation. Proc Nat Acad Sci 1930; 16:344–350.

Yanz JL, and Dodds H. An ear-canal electrode for the measurement of the human auditory brainstem response. Ear Hear 1985;6:98–104.

CHAPTER 24

Auditory Brainstem Response: Neurodiagnostic and Intraoperative Applications

Frank E. Musiek, Steven P. Borenstein, James W. Hall III, and Mitchell K. Schwaber

In 1975 Starr and Achor published their findings on the use of the auditory brainstem response (ABR) as a diagnostic technique for patients with neurologic disease. They demonstrated that the ABR waveform was different for patients with various types of brainstem involvement as compared with a control group. Subsequent reports on the ABR and brainstem disorders including multiple sclerosis (MS) were published again showing the value of these brainstem potentials (Stockard et al., 1976; Robinson and Rudge, 1975). In 1977, Daly et al. reported on ABR results in four patients with acoustic nerve tumors. Their results, along with the study reported by Selters and Brackmann (1977), indicated that the ABR could be a valuable tool for detecting auditory nerve lesions. Levine, in 1979, and Grundy, in 1982, were among the first to introduce the use of the ABR to monitor hearing and neurologic activity during neurological surgery.

The aforementioned studies provided the foundation for subsequent studies that made the ABR a valid and popular test for assessing neurologic integrity of the auditory nerve and brainstem. This chapter highlights the more salient clinical information on the ABR as it pertains to neurodiagnosis and intraoperative monitoring.

NEURODIAGNOSIS USING AUDITORY BRAINSTEM RESPONSE

ABR Indices in Neurodiagnosis

Many ABR measurements (also termed indices) may be used for neurodiagnostic purposes. Each measurement may yield unique information; however, some measurements are clearly more sensitive and reliable than others. In this section we will consider normative values and will report on the ABR findings in cochlear, VIIIth nerve, and brainstem lesions for the ABR.

Latency measures of the ABR wavepeaks have excellent diagnostic potential. The three latency measures most often examined include: the absolute latency of wave V; the interaural latency difference (ILD) between ears of wave V; and the interpeak laten-

cies (IPL) between waves I and III, I and V, and III and V. These measures can be affected by numerous stimulus, recording, and subject variables. Therefore, it is important to realize that exact values correspond to a specific paradigm, and until large-scale standardized values have been developed, each clinic must establish its own criteria for normal, cochlear, or retrocochlear results. For normal subjects the absolute latencies of waves I, III, and V can vary considerably. However, the IPL seem to be consistent across labs and clinics. The I–III and III–V IPL are approximately 2 msec, and the I–V IPL generally is 4 msec (Beagley and Sheldrake, 1978). Some reports indicate that in normal subjects the I–III maybe slightly longer than the III–V. Standard deviations of approximately 0.2 msec have been reported for individual wavepeaks and IPL (Stockard and Rossiter, 1976; Chiappa et al., 1979). Therefore, if one uses a 95% confidence interval for normal results, the I–III and the III–V IPL would be abnormal if the latency exceeded 2.4 msec, and a I–V IPL would not be considered abnormal until it exceeded 4.4 msec.

The ILD is the comparison of absolute latencies between ears of wave V (Selters and Brackmann, 1977), or less often wave III (Moller and Moller, 1983). The ILD of normal subjects typically is <0.3 msec (Selters and Brackmann, 1977; Rowe, 1978), and therefore ILD >0.3 msec are often considered consistent with retrocochlear pathology (Thomsen et al., 1978; Clemis and McGee, 1979; Hyde, 1981; Terkildsen et al., 1981; Musiek et al., 1986).

Poor waveform morphology, or the presence-absence of waveforms, may indicate abnormality. However, the interpretation of abnormal wave morphology is subjective and may be influenced by several nonpathologic variables, such as poor electrodes or electrical and muscle artifact. Schwartz and Morris (1991) have discussed ways to circumvent some of these problems. However, poor waveform morphology alone should not be used to determine retrocochlear involvement. If the waveform morphology is abnormal due to the absence of certain waves, correct interpretation is more likely (this will be discussed later). In individuals with normal hearing, when using a high intensity stimulus, waves I and III should be present a high percentage of the time and the presence of wave V should be nearly 100%.

For diagnostic purposes, ABR generally are elicited at slow repetition rates (<20/second). An increase in the absolute latency of all wavepeaks and a decrease in waveform clarity occurs when the repetition rate increases (Picton, 1977; Weber and Fujikawa, 1977; Rosenhamer et al., 1981; Chiappa et al., 1979; Stockard et al., 1976). The effect of presentation rates varies in normal patients (Don et al., 1977; Weber and Fujikawa, 1977). However, despite this variability the trend is a consistent one that has promulgated the comparison of the latency shifts for high rates with those of low rates. It was and is thought that the higher rates of presentation may "stress" the system more and uncover subtle dysfunctions that are reflected as excessive latency delays or as an absence of a response.

Amplitude measures of the ABR are not clinically useful due to large intra- and inter-subject variability, although animal studies have shown that ABR amplitudes are more affected than latencies when specific brainstem lesions have been made (Wada and Starr, 1983). The amplitude measure of choice is the V–I amplitude ratio measure, which should be used conservatively by the experienced clinician, controlling for various recording and stimulus parameters (Musiek et al., 1984). The basis for using amplitude ratios is that wave V is consistently larger than wave I (Rowe, 1978; Chiappa et al., 1979; Musiek, Kibbe et al., 1984). However, there is no standard ratio for the following reasons: (a) because amplitude ratios have not been sufficiently studied regarding sensitivity and specificity, and (b) because factors such as filtering, type of signal averager used, electrode position, stimulus intensity, and stimulus rate all may affect amplitude measures (Rowe, 1978, 1981; Chiappa, 1983; Musiek et al., 1984). Therefore, each center should establish its own norms and criteria for abnormality. A study at our center (Musiek et al., 1984) showed that when the variables mentioned above were controlled, only 8% of the patients with normal hearing sensitivity demonstrated abnormal V–I amplitude ratios.

VIIIth NERVE LESIONS

Overview of Pathologic Aspects

Although there are several disorders that can affect the auditory nerve, such as infections, inflammation, demyelinization, and vascular dysfunction, the acoustic tumor is the most common.

The acoustic tumor is the popular name for a tumor that arises from the Schwann cells of the vestibular portion of the VIIIth cranial nerve. Hence, an acoustic tumor is often a vestibular schwannoma that, because of its close proximity, affects auditory nerve structure and function. Occasionally schwannomas arise from the facial or acoustic nerve (Nager, 1964). Approximately 80% of mass lesions of the cerebellopontine angle (CPA) are vestibular schwannomas. Based on clinical diagnoses it is estimated that these tumors occur in approximately 1/100,000 persons. However, the incidence at autopsy is much higher (Moberg et al., 1969; Morrison, 1975). The acoustic tumor arises in the internal auditory canal but often grows into the CPA where there is more room to accommodate its growth. Often there also can be bony erosion of the medial aspect of the internal auditory canal. The vestibular schwannoma is considered a benign tumor.

Unilateral hearing loss is the primary and most common symptom, and is found in approximately 90% of acoustic tumor patients. This symptom is often accompanied by an aural fullness. Even in rare cases where the audiogram does not demonstrate a puretone hearing loss, the patient may still complain that hearing in one ear is worse than in the other. The rate of vestibular symptoms is approximately 65%, with imbalance more common than vertigo (Jerger and Jerger, 1981). In acoustic tumor cases tinnitus often accompanies the hearing loss. Involvement of the fifth and seventh cranial nerves (from expansion of the acoustic tumor) can result in facial parasthesia.

When bilateral acoustic tumors occur, it is highly likely that neurofibromatosis 2 is the disorder. This is a genetic disorder thought to occur on chromosome number 22 (Gusella, 1991).

ABR Findings

Sensitivity-Specificity

Testing with the ABR has several advantages. It is relatively fast and it has good sensitivity and specificity for differentiating VIIIth nerve pathology from cochlear pathology (Selters and Brackmann, 1977; Musiek et al., 1983). The sensitivity or "hit rate" for detecting acoustic tumors is >90%, and the specificity is approximately 85 to 90% (Glasscock et al., 1979; Harker, 1980; Terkildsen et al., 1981; Jerger, 1983; Turner and Nielsen, 1984; Turner, 1991). These values change depending on the number and type of ABR measures (indices) examined. Theoretically, as more ABR measures are examined, sensitivity increases and specificity decreases, although no studies, to our knowledge, have been performed to document this. Test sensitivity and specificity can also be altered by the incidence of this disorder in the clinical practice population (Turner, 1991), as well as the proficiency of the clinician using the ABR.

Waveform Morphology (Wave Presence-Absence)

An ABR finding that can indicate an VIIIth nerve tumor is the complete absence of the primary ABR waves (I, III, and V). Although other lesion sites can result in a total absence of ABR waves, the possibility of a retrocochlear lesion should be strongly considered and further investigated. The absence of ABR waves with acoustic tumors has ranged from approximately 30% (Harker, 1980; Rosenhall et al., 1981; Musiek et al., 1986) to nearly 50% (Selters and Brackmann, 1977, 1979; Bauch et al., 1983). When wave I is present and waves III and V are absent, there is a strong possibility that an VIIIth nerve or low brainstem lesion exists (Terkildsen et al., 1981; Antonelli et al., 1987) (House and Brackmann, 1979; Musiek and Gollegly, 1985) (Table 24.1). The degree of hearing loss plays a major role in the presence/absence of ABR waves and will be discussed later.

Latency Indices

The absolute latency of wave V is significantly greater for VIIIth nerve tumors than for cochlear site-of-lesion (Musiek et al. 1987; Prosser and Arslan, 1987). However, in most clinical situations hearing loss is present, which will also prolong wave V latency. This makes a differential diagnosis difficult and thus limits the usefulness of this measure. The advantage of the wave V absolute latency measure is that it can be ob-

tained a high percentage of the time in various clinical populations.

The ILD has excellent sensitivity and specificity for VIIIth nerve tumor detection, and has low false positive rates and a sensitivity of more than 90% (Clemis and McGee, 1979; Selters and Brackmann, 1979; Hyde, 1981; Terkildsen et al., 1981; Bauch et al., 1982; Musiek, Josey, Glasscock, 1986). The ILD used to indicate an VIIIth nerve lesion vary from >0.2 to >0.4 msec (Bauch et al., 1982; Selters and Brackmann, 1977). An ILD of >0.3 msec is perhaps the most popular criteria for neurodiagnostic purposes (Musiek et al., 1986; Clemis and McGee, 1979; Hyde, 1981) (Figs. 24.1 and 24.2). However, confounding results may occur in the presence of both asymmetrical and symmetrical hearing loss. The ILD is the diagnostic measurement of choice when earlier waves are missing prohibiting the use of the IPL measure.

The most sensitive and most specific diagnostic indicator of VIIIth nerve tumors is the IPL, when waves I, III, and V can be obtained. However, IPL utility is less than that of the ILD or the absolute latency of wave V. Acoustic neuromas typically cause a greater increase in the I–III IPL than in the III-V IPL (Eggermont et al., 1980; Moller and Moller, 1983; Musiek et al., 1986). The I–III extension usually, although not always, results in an abnormal I–V interval. Occasionally the I–V IPL may be normal in the presence of an abnormal I-III IPL (Musiek et al., 1986). Therefore, all IPL should be examined when possible. It has been reported that when using standard recording techniques, <30% of acoustic tumor patients have all waves (I, III, and V) present (Musiek et al. 1986).

Stimulus Repetition Rate

Reports suggest that the use of high stimulus repetition rates does not enhance ABR sensitivity to detecting retrocochlear pathology (Chiappa, 1983; Campbell and Abbas, 1987). However, there have also been several reports of an abnormal prolongation in wave V latency in patients with VIIIth nerve or brainstem lesions at high repetition rates (Weber and Fujikawa, 1977; Yagi and Kaga, 1979; Gerling and Finitzo-Hieber, 1983; Paludetti et al., 1983; Campbell and Abbas, 1987). However, the criteria for determining the amount of latency shift between low and high stimulus repetition rates, which indicates retrocochlear involvement, have not been clearly delineated. Hecox (1980) suggested multiplying the difference between high and low repetition rates by 0.006 msec and adding 0.4 msec. Musiek and Gollegly (1985) calculated a 0.1 msec shift for every 10 clicks per second increase, and added a variance factor of 0.2 msec to define the limits of normal function.

Table 24.1.
Common ABR Wave Presence/Absence Interpretations[a]

ABR Pattern	Normal	Cochlear	VIIIn	Bs
No response (poor hearing)		+	+	+
No response (good hearing)			+	+
Wave 1 present only			+	+
Waves I and II present only				+
Waves I and III present only				+
Wave V present only (normal latency)		+		
Wave V present only (delayed latency)		+	+	+
Waves III and V present only (normal latency)		+		
Waves III and V present only (delayed latency)		+	+	+

[a] Assuming normal middle ear function

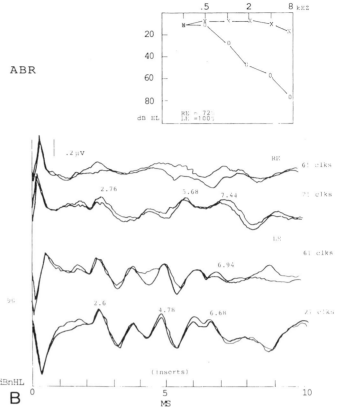

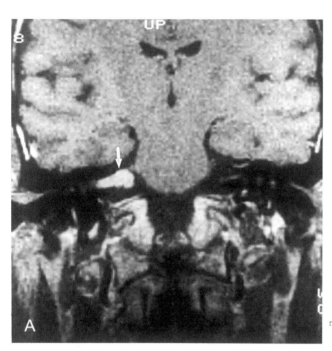

Figure 24.1. MRI and ABR for 44-year-old patient with progressive hearing loss for 5 years, tinnitus for 15 to 20 years, and a blocked sensation on the right side for several months. **A,** Coronal view of the MRI shows a 1.5-cm acoustic tumor (**arrow**). **B,** ABR (using in-serts) shows extended I–III and I–V interwave intervals, and an abnormal interaural latency difference for the right side (**clks** = clicks per second). Insert phones were used, resulting in a 0.9 msec delay in latency values.

It appears that cochlear pathology does not result in any greater latency shift of wave V at high repetition rates than that which is seen in the normal auditory system (Debruyne, 1986; Fowler and Noffsinger, 1983). Therefore, the use of repetition rate studies may be clinically useful to help separate cochlear from VIIIth nerve and brainstem lesions. However, an abnormal repetition rate result by itself should not be considered a strong sign of retrocochlear involvement and should be interpreted with caution.

Amplitude Ratios

As previously noted, reduced amplitude ratios may occur when there is an acoustic tumor and they may be useful in differentiating cochlear from retrocochlear pathology. Musiek et al. (1984) reported that 44% of patients with retrocochlear lesions (VIIIth nerve and brainstem involvement) demonstrated abnormal amplitude ratios, although all of the patients with cochlear lesions had amplitude ratios within normal limits. It should be kept in mind that the smaller wave V is, as compared with wave I, the more likely that a retrocochlear lesion may exist. This is es-

pecially true for ratios less than one. Although this index is more often used by the neurologic than the audiologic community, there can be interpretation problems with the index and thus it should be used as an adjunct to other ABR measures.

Laterality Effects

The laterality effect of VIIIth nerve tumors is one aspect of the ABR that especially requires the clinician to have an appreciation of the anatomy of the auditory system and the effects of the various pathologies previously discussed. Abnormal findings occur in the ipsilateral ear when there is a small, unilateral tumor, with no effect found when testing the contralateral ear. However, if the tumor has grown large enough (>2 cm) abnormal ABR results may occur bilaterally (Nodar and Kinney, 1980; Rosenhall et al., 1981; Shannon et al., 1981; Zapulla et al., 1982; Moller and Moller, 1983; Musiek and Kibbe, 1986). The reason for this contralateral effect may be due to the brainstem being displaced or compressed by the tumor, or due to the dysfunction of crossed pathways that contribute to generation of wavepeaks (Nodar and

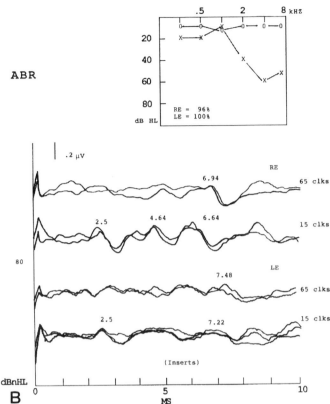

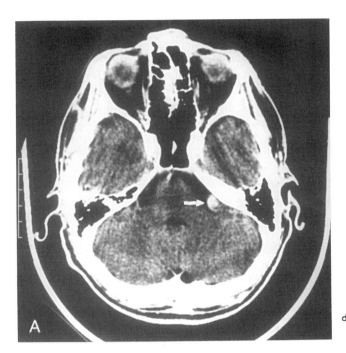

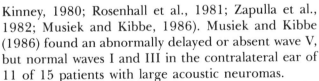

Figure 24.2. MRI and ABR for 55-year-old man with a 5-year history of hearing loss on the left side, and a several month history of balance problems. **A,** Transverse view of the MRI shows a 1-cm acoustic tumor (**arrow**) on the **left**. **B,** ABR shows a poor morphol-

ogy and reduced amplitude wave V. It also shows an abnormal I–V interwave latency and extended interaural latency difference for the left ear. Insert phones were used, resulting in a 0.9 msec delay in latency values.

Kinney, 1980; Rosenhall et al., 1981; Zapulla et al., 1982; Musiek and Kibbe, 1986). Musiek and Kibbe (1986) found an abnormally delayed or absent wave V, but normal waves I and III in the contralateral ear of 11 of 15 patients with large acoustic neuromas.

A variation of laterality effects was reported by Coelho and Prasher (1990) in a study that used two channel recordings. The patient in the study demonstrated normal ABR responses stimulating the ear ipsilateral to an acoustic neuroma, recording ipsilaterally. However, abnormalities were seen recording from the contralateral ear to both ipsilateral and contralateral stimulation.

BRAINSTEM LESIONS

Unlike VIIIth nerve lesions where there are a restricted number of disorders with which to contend, there are a wide variety of disorders associated with the brainstem that may affect auditory function in some manner. This may be one of the reasons that the ABR is not as sensitive in detecting brainstem involvement as it is in detecting VIIIth nerve lesions.

Anatomical Limitations of the ABR

It is not known which neural generators are responsible for each ABR wavepeak. However, it is fairly certain that wave I is generated by the distal portion of the VIIIth nerve (Moller and Jannetta, 1981). Because most acoustic tumors originate from the proximal (near brainstem) part of the VIIIth nerve, which in the human is approximately 2.5 cm, the presence of wave I does not rule out an VIIIth nerve tumor. There is also strong support for the concept that multiple generator sites are responsible for the later waves beyond wave II (which is generated by the proximal portion of the VIIIth nerve). The multiple generators responsible for wave V reside at levels of the lateral lemniscus and caudal auditory tracts. Although it is still open to discussion, it is thought that the midbrain (e.g., inferior colliculi) and caudal thalamic (e.g., medial geniculate bodies) structures are minimally involved in generation of wave V (Moller and Moller, 1985). This means that the ABR may not be sensitive to lesions confined exclusively to levels rostral to the lateral lemniscus. This theory is supported by clinical cases and animal data (Jerger et al., 1980; Wada and Starr,

1983; Musiek et al., 1988) (Fig. 24.3). Because the brainstem is compact, lesions are seldom isolated to the rostral brainstem and often involve or affect the mid to lower pons, resulting in ABR abnormalities.

Intra- and Extra-Axial Mass Lesions

An intra-axial neoplasm arises from brainstem tissue itself. The most common type of intra-axial brainstem tumor is the glioma (Huertas and Haymaker, 1969). An extra-axial neoplasm arises from outside the brainstem but directly affects the brainstem by compressing and or displacing it. The vestibular schwannoma is the most common extra-axial brainstem lesion. Meningiomas and gliomas are the second and third most common tumors of the brainstem region (Huertas and Haymaker, 1969). The meningioma is a slow-growing tumor that arises from the meninges of the brain. These can show up in various regions of the brain, including the CPA where they can mimic an acoustic tumor (Huertas and Haymaker, 1969). Meningiomas of the CPA often result in less auditory compromise than schwannomas (Granick et al., 1985). Gliomas arise from the glial cells that compose the connective tissue of the brain. They are more common than meningiomas overall but are not as common in the brainstem region (McLeod and Lance, 1989).

Symptoms of intra- and extra-axial lesions are dependent on the location and size of the lesion.

Common symptoms include: hearing loss (if caudal brainstem is affected), hearing difficulties (compromise of more complex processes), balance problems, headache, and facial parathesia.

Degenerative Processes

The most common degenerative disorder that affects the auditory pathways in the brainstem is multiple sclerosis (MS). There are many types of MS. The disease is chronic and usually progressive, and is caused by demyelinization with resultant sclerotic plaques affecting the peripheral and central nervous systems. MS is characterized by exacerbations that are accompanied by edema, which worsens the symptoms. When the exacerbation abates, the symptoms improve. These changes in symptoms often correlate with alterations in the ABR. The incidence of MS is higher in colder climates (40–60/100,000 cases in northern states; 6–14/100,000 cases in southern states) (Poser, 1979). Common symptoms of MS include muscle weakness, ocular problems and parathesae (Poser, 1979). The incidence of auditory symptoms depend on whether the auditory tracts are involved (Musiek et al., 1989). Though categorized here as a brainstem disorder, MS can affect the myelinated portion of the VIIIth nerve as well as the myelin in the cerebrum.

Another degenerative disorder that compromises the brainstem is olivopontocerebellar degeneration

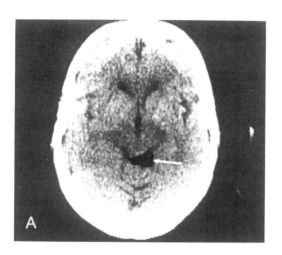

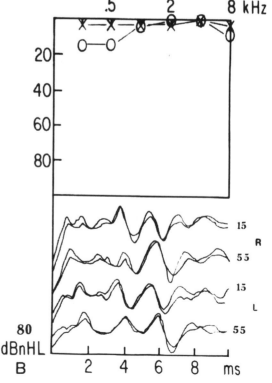

Figure 24.3. CT scan of a 30-year-old woman with a lesion of the inferior colliculus, consistent with a lipoma. **A,** Note a normal audiogram and **B,** ABR bilaterally. (**R** = right ear; **L** = left ear; **15** and **55** = click rates).

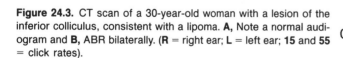

(OPCD), which is characterized by a marked atrophy of the medullary olives, pons and cerebellum. It is a rare disorder that is either inherited or acquired. The main symptoms of OPCD are ataxia and dysarthria, which may first appear at adolescence or as late as the sixth decade (Lynn et al., 1983).

Charcot Marie Tooth disease is an inherited disorder with a strong auditory link. This disorder causes slow atrophy of the distal muscles, hearing difficulties, weakness of the hands and/or feet (intrinsic muscles) and sensory loss (Musiek et al., 1982). Charcot Marie Tooth disease is categorized as a peripheral nerve disorder, which implicates the auditory nerve as the possible lesion site.

The leukodystrophies, primarily adrenoleukodystrophy, are degenerative disorders that involve the white matter (myelin) of the nervous system. Adrenoleukodystrophy is characterized by the progressive deterioration of the adrenal glands. These disease processes are mainly childhood disorders, and in some cases show abnormal ABR and other audiologic abnormalities (Shimizu et al., 1988).

Vascular Disorders

Some common pathologies of the cerebral blood vessels include atherosclerosis, intracerebral hemorrhage, aneurysms, arteriovenous malformations, ischemia, and stroke. A common vascular syndrome associated with auditory and vestibular dysfunction is vertebral-basilar syndrome (poor vascular supply via the vertebral and basilar arteries). Vascular loop syndrome

occurs when the anterior inferior cerebellar artery or one of its branches forms a loop in the CPA region, thus affecting the auditory, facial, or vestibular nerves. Symptoms associated with brainstem vascular problems can vary, depending on the extent, type, and location of the lesion.

ABR Findings

The sensitivity and specificity of the ABR to brainstem lesions is not well documented. The ABR is more sensitive to some types of brainstem lesions than to others. The ABR has a hit rate of more than 95% for intra-axial brainstem lesions, but a lower hit rate for other types of lesions (Fig. 24.4). Studies done on a variety of brainstem lesions show similar results. Chiappa (1983) reported that 19 of 24 patients (79%) with a variety of brainstem lesions had abnormal ABRs, Musiek et al., (1988) reported abnormal ABR in 17 of 23 patients (74%) with various brainstem lesions. House and Brackmann (1979) found abnormal ABRs in 15 of 20 patients (75%) with various extra-axial lesions of the low pons. The sensitivity of the ABR to brainstem involvement depends on the nature of the disorder, its location and the size of the lesion. Intra-axial lesions of the pons, because they arise from the pons itself, will usually compromise some of the primary auditory tracts. This in turn causes abnormal ABR results. Some degenerative disorders may not affect or may only slightly affect the auditory tracts in the pons, resulting in a smaller percentage of abnormal ABR.

There are two specificity issues central to ABR and

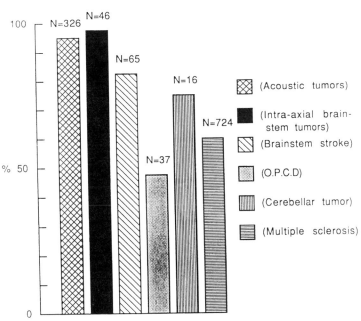

Figure 24.4. Percentage of abnormal ABR for selected disorders of the auditory nerve and brainstem based on multiple published studies. (**OPCD** = olivopontocerebellar degeneration). (Musiek and Baran, 1991, used with permission of publisher.)

brainstem involvement: (a) differentiating brainstem from cochlear involvement, and (b) differentiating brainstem from VIIIth nerve involvement. Generally, hearing sensitivity is not affected as much with brainstem lesions as with VIIIth nerve involvement, and therefore the chances are better for obtaining the earlier waves. This should enhance specificity but we know of no studies that support this assumption. Differentiating brainstem and VIIIth nerve lesions may not be critical in most audiological situations because they both require similar referral procedures.

Waveform Morphology and Latency Indices

The ability to differentiate VIIIth nerve from brainstem lesions using the ABR is difficult and warrants further investigation. This difficulty is compounded by the fact that many acoustic tumors also affect the brainstem, and some brainstem lesions affect the VIIIth nerve. Nevertheless, there are patterns of abnormality consistent with brainstem involvement. For example, Antonelli et al. (1987) reported that the incidence of wave I was more than 90% in patients with brainstem lesions, whereas the incidence of wave V was low (approximately 50% with low brainstem lesions and 15% for high brainstem lesions). In addition, an absent wave V (with waves I and III present) or an abnormally prolonged III-V IPL is indicative of a brainstem lesion (Table 24.1). For example, disorders that are more likely to effect the brainstem than the auditory nerve, such as MS, will have the III–V interval extended more often than the I–III interval (Fig. 24.5). However, a I–III latency abnormality could be consistent with either an acoustic tumor or a brainstem lesion, although it more likely represents an VIIIth nerve lesion (Starr and Hamilton, 1976; Chiappa, 1983; Lynn and Verma, 1985). In some cases of brainstem involvement IPL may help differentiate between lesions of the upper pons and midbrain

from those of the lower pons (Gilroy et al., 1977; Hashimoto et al., 1979; Antonelli et al., 1987). However, these reports are not conclusive and the ability to define the specific locus of brainstem abnormality is beyond the scope of the ABR in most situations.

Few data are available on the effects of brainstem lesions on the ILD. One study found the ILD to exceed 0.3 msec in only 56% of the patients with brainstem lesions who had bilaterally symmetrical hearing (Musiek et al., 1989) (Fig. 24.6). This sensitivity is much less than is seen in patients with VIIIth nerve tumors, and most likely occurs because brainstem lesions may affect both ipsilateral and contralateral brainstem auditory pathways, thus causing similar latency delays for each ear.

Stimulus Repetition Rate and Amplitude Ratios

The use and limitations of comparing latency shifts in wave V for low- and high-repetition rates for retrocochlear pathology have been discussed. With regard to brainstem pathology, there have been a few reports of abnormal prolongation for high repetition rates in patients with MS (Robinson and Rudge, 1975; Stockard and Rossiter, 1976; Antonelli et al. 1986; Musiek et al. 1989). Similarly, the limitations of using amplitude ratios have been discussed previously. Keeping these limitations in mind, a few investigations have shown that the V–I amplitude ratio helps to identify brainstem le-

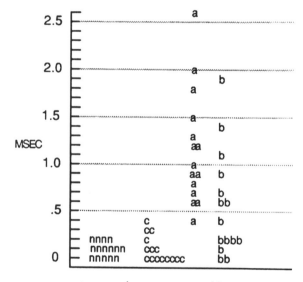

n= normal group   c= cochlear group
a= acoustic tumor group
b= brainstem group
* all values plotted to the nearest tenth
  of a msec.

Figure 24.6. Scattergram showing interaural latency differences (ILD) for cochlear, acoustic tumor and brainstem patients, as well as for control patients. (Musiek et al., 1989, used with permission of publisher.)

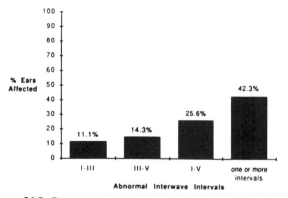

Figure 24.5. Percentage of patients with definite multiple sclerosis with abnormal interwave intervals on the ABR (n = 26). (Musiek et al., 1989, used with permission of publisher.)

sions (Stockard and Rossiter, 1976; Rosenhall et al., 1981). Also, wave I may become larger than normal in some patients with brainstem involvement, thereby reducing the V–I amplitude ratio (Starr and Achor, 1975; Musiek et al., 1982).

Jiang (1991) noted that amplitude ratios are more sensitive to detecting brainstem lesions than are other ABR measures, but results must be interpreted with the use of norms for specific intensities. Sand (1991) studied 45 patients with MS and calculated a "shape ratio" amplitude for the wave IV–V complex. He found this ratio to be more sensitive to MS than the traditional V–I ratio, and had high specificity. This measure deserves further investigation.

Laterality Effects

As was discussed with VIIIth nerve lesions, the laterality effects of the ABR with brainstem lesions also provide important information about the neuroanatomical and generator substrates for the ABR (Chiappa, 1983; Musiek, 1986; Musiek and Kibbe, 1986). In brainstem lesions the ABR abnormalities are most often found when stimulating the ear ipsilateral to the side of the lesion (Oh et al., 1981; Musiek and Geurkink, 1982; Chiappa, 1983), or in some cases bilaterally, particularly with midline lesions (Musiek et al., 1988) (Fig. 24.7). Midline lesions, and most likely concomitant bilaterally abnormal ABR, are most often due to intra- rather than to extra-axial lesions (Musiek and Baran, 1986). It is also more likely that the degen-

erative and vascular diseases may result in bilateral deficit. When stimulating only the ear contralateral to the lesion, ABR abnormality seldom occurs with lesions confined to one side of the brainstem (Brown et al., 1981; Oh et al., 1981; Musiek and Geurkink, 1982; Chiappa, 1983).

Effects of Cochlear Hearing Loss

The interpretation of the ABR can be confounded by the presence of cochlear hearing loss, primarily because cochlear hearing loss will affect almost all of the measures previously discussed (with the possible exception of the IPL), and therefore the sensitivity and specificity of the ABR.

Severe to profound high frequency sensorineural hearing loss and advancing age are two factors that often compromise ABR waveform morphology (Hyde, 1985). Therefore, the absence of ABR waves in such cases does not necessarily mean retrocochlear pathology, but neither does it rule out an VIIIth nerve tumor. Jerger (1983) showed that when the pure tone audiometric average of 1000, 2000, and 4000 Hz exceeds 65 dB HL, the ABR may be absent or difficult to interpret, even with a 90 dB nHL click stimulus. Musiek et al., (1987) found that when conventional ABR were conducted on individuals less than 66 years old who had cochlear hearing loss that did not exceed 65 dB at 1000 Hz, 70 dB at 2000 Hz, and 75 dB at 4000 Hz, wave presence was fairly high.

Using these criteria, in a group of 15 individuals

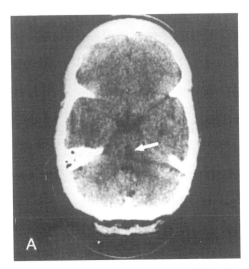

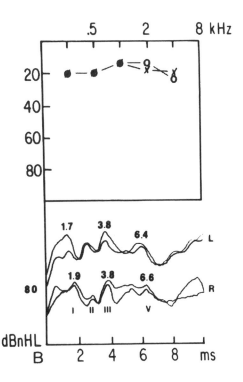

Figure 24.7. CT scan (*A*) of 57-year-old woman with a midline lesion of the caudal pons resulting from an infarct. Normal pure tone audiogram (*B*) as well as the ABR, which shows an extended III–V interval bilaterally but normal I, II, and III waves. This finding is consistent with waves I, II, and III being generated by the auditory nerve (I and II) and cochlear nucleus (III). (Musiek and Baran, 1991, used with permission of publisher.)

who had PTA 2 (average of 1000, 2000, and 4000 Hz) that ranged between 50 and 70 dB HL, wave I was present in 11 (73.3%), wave III was present in 12 (80%), and wave V was present in all 15 (100%). Consistent with this finding, in high-frequency cochlear impairment, waves I and III are often absent in the presence of wave V (Selters and Brackmann, 1977; Fowler and Noffsinger, 1983; Musiek et al., 1987). However, in many cases all waves, including wave V, may be absent due to the degree of high frequency hearing loss, and therefore the interpretation of retrocochlear pathology is equivocal.

It is generally agreed that as high frequency hearing sensitivity decreases, waveform morphology becomes poorer and the absolute latency for each wave increases (Coats and Martin, 1977; Galambos and Hecox, 1978; Rosenhamer, 1981; Hyde, 1985). This latency delay may be due to the time necessary for the traveling wave to stimulate an apical region of the cochlea that is capable of producing a synchronous response. The specific hearing loss frequencies of importance depend on the spectral energy of the click stimulus, which is in part due to the response properties of the transducer (Weber et al., 1981). For example, Bauch and Olsen (1986) found that loss of hearing at 3000 Hz is a key factor in the cause of abnormal ABRs, whereas other reports suggest that 4000 Hz is a more critical frequency (Selters and Brackmann, 1977; Rosenhamer, 1981).

Despite the fact that wave V is often present in cochlear hearing loss, sensitivity and specificity of the absolute latency of wave V are often confounded by two factors. First, because the amount of increased latency as a function of hearing loss varies considerably (Rosenhamer, 1981) predictability is compromised. Second, in many cases of high-frequency cochlear hearing loss the cochlear impaired ear behaves similarly to a normal ear with regard to absolute latencies, perhaps due to recruitment or to the capability to sufficiently stimulate the basal regions of the cochlea (Galambos and Hecox, 1978; Gorga et al., 1985).

Diagnosis in cases of severe hearing loss is made difficult because wave I is often absent whereas wave V remains present but delayed. Thus, when wave V is delayed the question becomes whether it is due to cochlear or to retrocochlear involvement. Formulas have been developed to correct for the degree of high frequency hearing loss. Prosser and Arslan (1987) developed a formula that took into consideration the latency of wave V in the pathologic ear for a 90 dB nHL click as a function of sensation level for pure tone thresholds in the 2 to 4 kHz range, as compared with wave V latency for a normal ear. In a study using this formula all patients with retrocochlear pathology

were correctly identified. However, further investigation of this approach is needed to verify these initial findings (Eberling and Parbo, 1987; Musiek et al., 1987).

The problems that confound interpretation of wave V absolute latencies also apply to use of the ILD in cases of asymmetrical hearing loss. Bauch and Olsen (1989) found that as hearing thresholds at 2, 3, and 4 kHz became asymmetrical between ears, the ILD increased. For example, they found that as the difference between ears ranged from 20 to 39 dB, 19% of patients with cochlear pathology yielded an abnormal ILD ($>$0.3 msec). Selters and Brackmann (1977, 1979) recommended a 0.1 msec latency correction factor for every 10 dB of hearing loss at 4000 Hz exceeding 50 dB HL in computing the ILD. Clemis and McGee (1979) recommended that a 0.3 msec ILD be used as a criterion for retrocochlear involvement for hearing losses $<$65 dB, and a 0.4 msec criterion for hearing losses $\geq$65 dB. Hyde (1981) reported a 14% false-positive rate for patients with presumed cochlear hearing loss when a 0.2 msec ILD criteria was used. It should be noted that these results apply for the use of an 80 to 90 dB nHL stimulus. Correction factors may prove helpful but also may be misleading. In some cases the correction factor may turn an abnormal finding into a normal finding, resulting in a false-negative interpretation.

It is generally agreed that when all wavepeaks are present, they are equally prolonged by cochlear hearing loss. Therefore IPL, unlike absolute latencies or ILD, are insignificantly affected by cochlear hearing loss (Eggermont et al., 1980; Rosenhamer, 1981; Chiappa, 1983). However, Keith and Greville (1987) reported a prolonged I-V IPL in notched-type cochlear hearing losses. Although this finding seems possible, further corroboration is necessary.

Another problem that occurs when cochlear hearing loss exists is that waveform morphology often is poor. This can result in difficulty in accurately selecting a peak for latency measurement, even when the necessary waves are present.

One solution to the absence of wave I when recording the ABR with scalp electrodes is to use electrocochleography (ECochG) (see Chapter 23). There are three common applications of EcochG: the diagnosis and monitoring of endolymphatic hydrops (Coats, 1981); intraoperative monitoring; and the enhancement of wave I for IPL measurements. The ECochG response can be recorded with a promontory electrode (Eggermont, 1976), an electrode on the tympanic membrane (Cullen et al., 1972; Stypulkowski and Staller, 1987), or an electrode placed in the ear canal near the tympanic membrane (Durrant, 1986). The promontory electrode provides the largest response because as the recording site moves closer to the cochlea, the generated neural-electrical activity becomes larger and the noise effects are reduced. However, using a tympanic membrane electrode, Ferraro and Ferguson (1989) recorded a wave I in eight hearing-impaired subjects who did not show a wave I when tested with standard ABR recording techniques. Musiek and Baran (1990) showed that foil-wrapped foam extra-tympanic electrodes in some cases may enhance the presence and amplitude of wave I. Ruth et al. (1988) also discussed the use of noninvasive ear canal electrodes to enhance wave I.

Another approach to identifying an otherwise absent wave I using standard ABR techniques is to use multi-channel recordings that use a horizontal electrode montage. In this situation, the active electrode is attached to the ipsilateral earlobe, the reference electrode is attached to the contralateral earlobe, and the ground electrode is attached to the forehead. Schwartz and Morris (1991) have also suggested that the amplitude and detection of wave I may be enhanced by slowing down the repetition rate (<10/second), by increasing the stimulus intensity 10 dB (usually to 90 dB nHL), or by using a condensation click in some patients.

Unilateral high frequency hearing loss makes the interpretation of the ILD difficult, and attempting to offset the effect of hearing loss can be problematic. However, if the patient has similar hearing in both ears at a lower frequency, it may be helpful to use tone pips centered at this frequency. This will allow a better comparison between ears for latency effects. This technique has been sensitive to VIIIth nerve lesions in clinical trials and should be considered in appropriate cases of asymmetrical hearing loss at some frequencies (Telian and Kileny 1989).

Because all ABR measures are not of equal diagnostic value and are not equally attainable, some interpretations can be difficult. Also, the ABR is more sensitive to acoustic tumors than to brainstem lesions of various etiologies. Therefore, the test strategy and the value of a specific index must be decided for each individual patient, taking into account presenting symptoms and the validity, reliability and time required for each measure. Because patients differ in their anatomy, the effects of pathology on anatomy and physiology, test results (both cochlear and retrocochlear) differ as well. In summary, the IPL and ILD are the most useful ABR measures. Absolute latencies, effects of repetition rate and amplitude ratios are useful in specific situations but should be used with caution and should be considered "soft" retrocochlear signs that require additional corroborative clinical evidence and/or follow-up.

IMAGING TECHNIQUES AND ABR IN NEURODIAGNOSTICS

Presently there is controversy over the use of ABR and/or modern imaging techniques in the workup for acoustic tumors. The main concern is whether patients suspected of having acoustic tumors should first be referred for magnetic resonance imaging (MRI) without the benefit of an ABR. The MRI with gadolinium enhancement has better sensitivity and specificity for acoustic tumors than does the ABR. However, it is approximately five to six times more expensive to perform an MRI than an ABR. Another factor to consider is the predictive value of a test, which is the probability of the tumor being present. The predictive value is directly associated with the prevalence of the disease (VIIIth nerve tumor). If the prevalence of the disease is low then the predictive value will probably be low (Hall, 1992). Because the prevalence of acoustic tumors is indeed extremely low, there should be some way of screening the general population to find individuals who are at risk for an acoustic tumor. The main symptom of an acoustic tumor is unilateral sensory-neural hearing loss. Based on the audiologic finding of asymmetric hearing loss as well as on other symptoms, some clinicians suggest proceeding directly to an MRI. However, the vast majority of people with unilateral or asymmetrical sensory-neural hearing loss do not have acoustic tumors. Conducting an ABR after defining a unilateral or asymmetric hearing loss would prove helpful. Those patients who failed or had a questionable ABR could then go on for imaging studies. This would improve the cost-benefit ratio of the MRI. Because the ABR is less expensive than the MRI, it would be preferable to screen out the non-tumor patients with an ABR rather than with the MRI (for further discussion of cost benefit ratio, see Chapter 13).

INTRAOPERATIVE MONITORING WITH AUDITORY EVOKED RESPONSES

Indications for Intraoperative Cochleovestibular Nerve Monitoring

Evoked responses, in general, can provide an early indicator of changes in neurophysiologic status of the peripheral and central nervous system during surgery. These changes may be due to a variety of physiologic and surgical factors, including hypotension, hypoxia, and either compression or retraction of cranial nerves or brain tissue. Early detection of a significant alteration in neurophysiologic status can potentially lead to effective medical or surgical correction of the problem with reversal of the pathophysiologic process.

Neurophysiologic intraoperative monitoring of the facial and cochleovestibular nerves and auditory brainstem is now regularly applied during various neurotologic surgical procedures (Table 20.1). In most cases, auditory system monitoring is most effective with a combined electrocochleography (ECochG) and ABR technique, as described below. As intraoperative experience with electrocochleography (ECochG) and ABR has accumulated over the past decade, indications for monitoring have evolved. Ideally, hearing should be monitored any time it is at risk during surgery. In practice, however, monitoring is attempted only with patients who have enough residual hearing to warrant preservation and during operations that pose significant risk to the patient's hearing. For instance, hearing loss is rare in chronic ear and stapes surgery, and it would be impractical to place a microphone near the ear every few minutes to record ABR intraoperatively. As a result, monitoring with auditory evoked responses (AER) is not typically attempted during chronic ear and stapes surgery, even though facial nerve monitoring is certainly indicated.

In contrast, the suboccipital approach for the removal of an acoustic neuroma is associated with only a 50–60% success rate of hearing preservation, even in the best of circumstances. Therefore, with a 40–50% chance of surgery-related hearing impairement, monitoring for hearing preservation is clearly indicated during acoustic neuroma removal. In addition to suboccipital acoustic tumor removal, intraoperative ECochG/ABR monitoring is commonplace during suboccipital vestibular nerve section and microvascular decompression of the cochleovestibular nerve (Hall, 1992; Hall and Schwaber, 1992; Kileny et al. 1988; Moeller and Jannetta, 1983). AER monitoring during these surgical procedures provides information regarding excessive retraction of the cochleovestibular nerve or excessive manipulation of the cochlear nerve during the procedure.

There are also reports describing the benefits of intraoperative ECochG measurement during inner ear surgery, such as endolymphatic sac decompression (Arenberg et al., 1989) and labyrinthotomy with streptomycin infusion (LSI). During endolymphatic sac decompression and LSI, we obtain the auditory evoked responses to document any changes of the summating potential (SP). As new vestibular surgical procedures evolve, our technique of monitoring can be applied. One such procedure is transmastoid posterior semicircular canal occlusion for benign paroxysmal positional vertigo. Although we have not performed this procedure yet, we anticipate doing so in the near future.

PATHOPHYSIOLOGIC CORRELATES IN AER MONITORING

In monitoring with AER, the integrity of the cochlea is essential. If serious cochlear impairment develops intraoperatively, AER will be markedly altered or even abolished. Surgery related compromise of blood supply to the cochlea produces "cochlear ischemia" and sensory hearing impairment). Obvious damage to the blood vessels is not necessary to produce cochlear deficit. Manipulation of labyrinthine blood vessels may result in vasospasm and subsequent interruption of blood supply to the cochlea and VIIIth nerve. The relationship between blood supply and cochlear function has been appreciated for more than 30 years. Perlman et al. (1959) showed in animal experiments that the cochlea could survive up to 5 minutes of interruption in blood supply. The cochlear microphonic (CM) and action potential (AP) disappeared within 30 seconds, but returned after blood supply was restored. Other mechanisms for cochlear damage resulting from surgery include fenestration of the labyrinth and disruption of cochear nerve fibers.

Maintenance of integrity of the auditory portions of the VIIIth nerve integrity intraoperatively is, of course, essential for postoperative preservation of hearing. As summarized in Table 24.2, damage to the auditory portion of the VIIIth nerve may result from direct trauma or from secondary mechanisms, such as interruption of blood supply. At this point, it is appropriate to make an important distinction in the objectives of intraoperative monitoring with AER among types of neurotologic surgery. Vestibular neurectomy by definition involves sectioning of the vestibular branch of the VIIIth nerve. The goal of intraoperative monitoring is to assure that the auditory branch, and usually the facial nerve, remain intact. In contrast, with other posterior fossa surgeries, such as tumor removal, the objective is to prevent intraoperative damage to the entire VIIIth nerve (vestibular and auditory portions), as well as the facial nerve.

TECHNIQUES

Intraoperative auditory evoked response monitoring in the O.R. can be very challenging. The test environment typically contains multiple sources of electrical activity that may interfere with evoked response measurment. The surgical protocol limits ready access to the patient. In addition, the patient's status is not always stable. In fact, momentary alterations in neurophysiologic status, and therefore auditory evoked response patterns, are commonplace. These neurophysiologic alterations may result from surgical manipulations, from anesthetic agents, and from changes in physiologic parameters (e.g., body temperature and blood pressure). The challenge is to differentiate as quickly as possible between causes of AER or facial nerve response alteration that are related to surgery versus all other causes. Evoked response interpretation may seriously influence surgical decisions and, ultimately, patient outcome. Whether a patient's hearing is preserved can depend to a large extent on prompt and accurate interpretation of intraoperative evoked response findings.

The most common cause of AER alterations, and the one of primary interest intraoperatively, is mechanically induced disruption of auditory system function (Table 24.2). Naturally, these alterations will be detected only during the intraoperative period when auditory nerve structures are being manipulated. Other intraoperative events, such as saline irrigation within the surgical field, may also produce neurophysiologic changes due, for example, to reduced focal temperature. In contrast, other AER changes due to

systemic factors (e.g., hypothermia or hypotension) can theoretically occur at any time during surgery, from induction of anesthesia to closing. The tester, therefore, should be informed of the surgeon's activities throughout the case and remain especially vigilant during manipulations such as retraction of structures (e.g., cerebellum), decompression of the endolympatic sac, or sectioning of the vestibular portion of the VIIIth cranial nerve.

Setting Up in the Operating Room (O.R.)

The location of equipment and tester in the O.R. (Fig. 24.8) will vary substantially depending on the layout and size of the room, location, and type of other equipment in the room, the other personnel involved in the case, and even the patient's surgical position (Hall, 1992). The clinician is advised to visit an O.R. in advance to develop a plan for equipment set up. Then, once the patient has been brought to the O.R. this

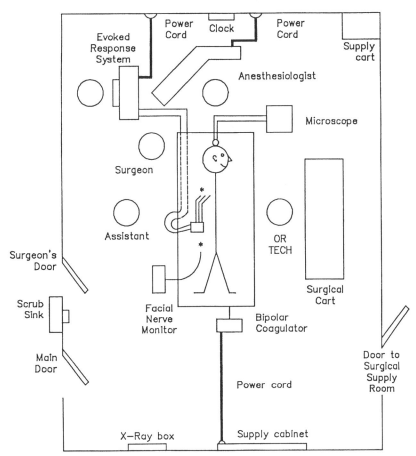

Figure 24.8. Schematic diagram of an O.R. (**OR**) layout showing location of evoked response equipment in relation to the patient, surgeons, anesthesiologists, O.R. technician, and surgical equipment (from Hall, 1992).

plan can be discussed with the surgeon(s), head O.R. nurse or technician, and the anesthesiologist. Features of a satisfactory equipment arrangement are, minimally, access to an appropriate electrical outlet, proximity to the patient and surgeon, location away from possible sources of electrical interference, location of equipment, tester, and evoked response electrode and stimulus cables away from main traffic areas. Convenient location of the electrode box, removed from the surgeons whenever possible, is particularly important to facilitate access to electrode leads in the event that changes are required during surgery. A remote electrode box location also may allow the clinician to disconnect electrodes from the equipment during or at the end of monitoring to move equipment or turn equipment power off. It may be necessary to set up evoked response equipment only after the operating table and patient have been moved into position for surgery and essential surgical equipment (e.g., microscope, coagulator, laser, TV monitor) are in place. Finally, the clinician should insist on having access to a stool or small chair during monitoring.

The O.R. typically contains multiple sources of electrical activity that may interfere with AER measurements, including the monopolar and bipolar cauteries, surgical lasers, microscopes, and even the EKG leads. Another electrical interference is the "twitch monitor," the electrical stimulator that anesthesiologists place on the wrist of the patient to determine the status of neuromuscular blockade. Even if electrical artifacts can be eliminated, the operating room is a very noisy environment, and it is extremely difficult, if not impossible, to monitor AER while the surgical drill is being used. Each of these factors must be taken into account during the monitoring process. The best way to deal with artifacts during surgery is to anticipate them before the case begins. The electrode wires, the boxes in which they are plugged, and the cables leading to the monitors should be isolated from other electrical cables as much as is practical. To prevent electrodes from being pulled out inadvertently, we tape our electrodes and cables into the desired position. We use subdermal needle electrodes for all intraoperative monitoring cases, which provides a somewhat secure placement of the electrodes as well as low electrode impedance (3K ohms). Also, needle electrodes significantly improve the signal-to-nose ratio for recording bioelectric potentials.

The location of the monitoring equipment depends primarily on which ear is to be operated. In either case, the monitors are located near the foot of the patient, so that the various electrode boxes are placed near the head and the cords run toward the foot of the patient. The cords and electrodes are placed immedi-

ately after the induction of general anesthesia. One of the unavoidable difficulties of intraoperative monitoring is the need to have the various monitoring electrodes and the sound tube immediately adjacent to a sterile field. Maintenance of a sterile field during surgery is essential and this can be accomplished in several different ways. One technique is to have the electrodes, the ear plug, and the sound tube gas sterilized so that they can be placed by the surgeon after the field has been prepped. Alternatively, the electrodes and sound tube can be placed before surgical preparation of the patient. The electrodes are then covered with Betadine prep solution. The ear plug, sound tube, and the electrodes are draped out of the sterile field by using a Betadine impregnated plastic drape. The surgeon then must make certain that this portion of the field is not violated during the procedure. While the surgeon is scrubbing in preparation for the operation, the audiologist obtains baseline values for the various parameters being monitored.

Measurement Parameters

Stimulus and acquisition parameters used in intraoperative monitoring with auditory evoked responses, and their respective rationale, are summarized in Table 24.3. The overall objective in the selection of these parameters is to optimize neurophysiologic recording of the pertinent auditory system in the O.R. environment. Specifically, the goal is to rapidly detect a robust and reliable response from the cochlea, the VIIIth nerve, and auditory regions of the brainstem, while

Table 24.2.
Rationale for Auditory Evoked Response ECochG/ABR Monitoring for Selected Neurotologic Surgical Procedures

Surgical Procedure	Neurophysiologic Monitoring Rationale
Removal of posterior fossa tumor	• Pressure cochlear integrity • Preserve eighth nerve integrity • Hearing preservation • Prevent brainstem trauma
Vascular decompression of 8th cranial nerve	• Preserve 8th nerve integrity
Vestibular neurectomy	• Preserve 8th nerve integrity • Hearing preservation
Middle fossa approach for decompression of 8th cranial nerve	• Preserve cochlear integrity • Preserve eighth nerve integrity • Hearing preservation
Endolymphatic sac decompression and shunt procedure	• Assess immediate effect on cochlear functional status • Determine indication for additional surgery • Preserve cochlear integrity

minimizing physiologic and electrical artifact. A flexible measurement technique is essential for consistently successful intraoperative evoked response recordings. Test conditions and physiologic status invariably changes, both from one patient to the next and within a single patient during surgery. It is often necessary to promptly modify the test protocol in response to these changes. In short, the only "correct" test protocol is the one that produces optimal evoked response results for a particular patient under test conditions encountered at the time of the monitoring (Hall, 1992).

A detailed discussion of the principles underlying the selection of the measurement parameters listed in Table 24.2 is beyond the scope of this chapter. The reader is referred to a recent text by Hall (1992) for this invaluable background information. However, several rather straightforward points should be kept in mind. First, the closer the recording electrodes are to the anatomic region of interest, the larger the response recorded. For example, if the region of interest is the cochlea, then the promontory is the preferred recording site. Any other electrode site (e.g., ear canal or ear lobe) is suboptimal. Our simplified promontory recorded technique for ECochG (Schwaber and Hall, 1990) is described later in this section. Second, selection of some test parameters can be made only at the time of monitoring. Stimulus polarity is a parameter that illustrates this point. Alternating polarity clicks are often used in recording ECochG clinically and in the O.R. That is, a response is averaged from a comparable number of rarefaction (negative) polarity and condensation (positive) polarity clicks, each polarity presented in an alternating fashion. Some patients, however, will show little or no ECochG for alternating polarity stimuli, yet produce a clear and reliable response with a single polarity (either rarefaction or condensation). Again, the overriding practical principle is to use whatever test strategy works for a given patient at a given time during surgery. Although intraoperative alterations in test protocol are often essential to obtain high quality data, unnecessary deviations from the customary test protocol should be avoided because it is possible that they will produce evoked response changes that are mistaken as evidence of impending damage to the auditory system.

In summary, each clinician is likely to develop a test strategy that is best suited for his/her intraoperative monitoring needs, objectives, and measurement conditions. Nevertheless, the overall goal during intraoperative monitoring with auditory evoked responses invariably remains the same regardless of the factors just noted—to record a response with all major waves clearly, reliably, and quickly throughout surgery.

Electrodes

AER systems and overall test protocols used intraoperatively (Table 20.2) are similar in many respects to those used in the clinic setting (Hall, 1992; Schwaber and Hall, 1990; Schwaber et al., 1991a, 1991b). However, one major distinction is the type and location of the recording electrodes. During intraoperative auditory monitoring, one inverting ("reference") electrode is, optimally, a transtympanic needle electrode, placed in the hypotympanic air cell system after the induction of anesthesia. The advantage of promontory electrode is that it is very close to the generator site for the summating potential (SP) and action potential (AP) of the ECochG and, therefore, wave I of the ABR. The promontory-recorded response is robust, often more than 5 microvolts in amplitude. In contrast, the response recorded with a scalp (e.g., earlobe) or ear canal (extratympanic) inverting electrode is typically one-tenth as large (<0.5 microvolts). Thus, the signal to noise ratio is greatly improved and much less signal averaging is required to detect a reliable response. This is a major advantage in the operating room because neurophysiologic information on the status of the cochlea, VIIIth nerve, and auditory brainstem is required on a minute-to-minute basis.

Most clinical investigators dismiss intraoperative transtympanic ECochG as impractical, citing technical problems in placing the needle and maintaining stable placement during otologic surgery. Schwaber and Hall (Hall, 1992; Schwaber and Hall, 1990; Schwaber et al., 1991a, 1991b), however, recently reported on the development of a simplified transtympanic electrode placement, using a standard subdermal needle held in place by a foam earphone. The promontory electrode is a sterile, stainless steel, uninsulated, subdermal needle electrode (Nicolet Biomedical Instruments, Madison, WI). This needle has a 12-mm shank and a 0.4-mm diameter, a 1-meter wire and a standard pin. In the O.R., all other auditory (and facial nerve) responses are also recorded with this type of needle electrode. An exception is that a TIPtrode is often used as an inverting electrode in a second ECochG/ABR channel (Table 24.2).

In the O.R., the patient is already under general anesthesia when the needle electrode is placed on the promontory by the otologist under an operating room microscope. The portion of the sterile subdermal needle electrode (between the shank and the wire) is grasped with bayonette forceps and the electrode is directed down the external auditory canal. The needle is inserted through the inferior-posterior portion of the tympanic membrane to rest on the promontory. Then, the electrode lead that begins just lateral to the tympanic membrane is secured temporarily by hand against the wall of the ear canal. The otologist takes a compressed ER-3A type foam insert or a gold-foil insert (TIPtrode) and places it within the ear canal in the customary fashion. The TIPtrode is sterile for intraoperative ECochG. Both the promontory electrode lead and transducer tube are secured with surgical tape to the patient's neck or chest. The entire promontory electrode placement procedure requires less than 1 minute in the operating room. In a series of more than 60 intraoperative monitoring cases, Schwaber and Hall (1990) found that no promontory electrode placed with this technique became dislodged during testing. In addition, there have been no known medical complications, such as chronic tympanic membrane or middle ear damage, resulting from promontory needle placement.

Combined ECochG, ABR, and Direct VIIIth Nerve Recording

The conventional ECochG and ABR recording techniques are still important for intraoperative monitoring during neurotologic surgery. The main disadvantages of the technique have already been noted. Because amplitude of wave V is relatively small, as recorded with the far field electrode array, the response often must be averaged from as many as 1000 or more stimuli to obtain an adequate signal-to-noise ratio. Whereas a clear response with stable latency throughout surgery is generally considered evidence of auditory integrity, interpretation of an alteration, or loss of the response is less straightforward.

A three-channel measurement technique, combining promontory ECochG, conventional ABR, and direct VIIIth nerve recordings is therefore sometimes preferable (Hall, 1992). There is substantial clinical experience confirming that combined ECochG, ABR, and VIIIth nerve recording is an effective intraoperative monitoring technique for preservation of hearing. Near field AER recordings, by definition, produce relatively large amplitude responses. The near field ECochG detected with a promontory electrode, therefore, provides the major clinical advantage of a large response, namely, a very favorable signal-to-noise ratio. A clear ECochG AP wave (ABR wave I) is observed with minimal signal averaging, as depicted in Figure 24.9. In most cases, AP amplitude is on the order of 5 to 10 uV with a promontory electrode, as compared to less than 0.5 uV with an ear canal electrode type (Schwaber and Hall, 1990). Furthermore, with the promontory electrode site a distinct AP is typically recorded even from patients with severe (60–75 dB HL) high frequency sensorineural hearing impairment, at maximum stimulus intensity levels. In

contrast, a reliable AP is rarely observed from patients with high frequency sensorineural hearing impairment greater than approximately 35 to 40 dB HL with ear canal electrode designs.

A secondary and related advantage is that a wave I or AP component may be recorded with the near field transtympanic technique when no response can be detected with surface electrodes, including ear canal types. One must keep in mind, however, that presence of an ECochG AP component, in isolation, appears to be an insufficient intraoperative measure of auditory function. Although disappearance of the component must be considered strong evidence of cochlear deficit, preservation of the AP component intraoperatively does not necessarily imply auditory integrity. Even complete sectioning of the VIIIth nerve resulting in profound hearing impairment does not invariably eliminate ECochG AP, provided cochlear blood supply remains intact (Hall, 1992; Ruben et al. 1963).

Recording a response directly from the VIIIth nerve as it exits the internal auditory canal or enters the brainstem offers similar advantages. In fact, this near field response may be larger by up to four or five times than the promontory ECochG AP and, therefore, also requires little or no signal averaging. Electrophysiologic data are collected almost instantaneously, permitting continuously prompt information for the surgeon. With conventional ABR measurement in the O.R., signal averaging over 1000 to 2000 stimulus repetitions may be required with a data collection time of 1 to 2 minutes. During this period the AER may not be stable but, rather, dynamic. The averaged response does not, consequently, reflect the status of the auditory system at any one time, whereas the response recorded directly, with at most several seconds of averaging, is essentially time specific.

A second and very important advantage of the direct VIIIth nerve recording is site specificity. Presumably, the technique provides information on status of the proximal portion of the nerve, between the porus of the internal auditory canal and the root entry zone near the brainstem. A major disadvantage of the technique is that an electrode cannot be placed directly on the nerve until the nerve is exposed, and then it often must be removed for periods of time during surgery so as not to interfere with dissection of tumor, transection of the vestibular portion of the nerve, or other manipulations. A fine silver wire with a cotton wick at the end is less obtrusive.

Waveform Analysis

ECochG

Although recent papers have described the application of automated analysis techniques in intensive care unit

Intraoperative ABR/ECochG

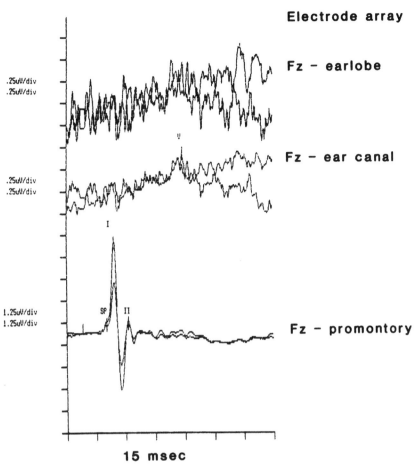

Figure 24.9. Combined ECochG/ABR waveforms recorded intraoperatively with a promontory versus ear canal inverting electrode. The noninverting electrode was located on the forehead (Fz site) for each waveform. Note the difference in the amplitude scale for the two sets of waveforms.

and operating room neurophysiologic monitoring (Bertrand et al., 1987), manual calculations of sensory evoked response latency and amplitude remain the conventional analysis approach at this time. The ECochG waveform, as described in detail in Chapter 23, consists of two or three major components, depending on certain stimulus parameters. With single polarity (rarefaction or condensation) stimuli, the CM, an oscillating waveform, is observed from stimulus onset until the appearance of the AP. The SP takes the form of either a distinct peak less than 1 msec before the AP, and usually less than half as large as the AP, or as a hump on the initial slope of the AP component.

A common ECochG analysis approach is calculation of SP and AP amplitude (in microvolts) from a common baseline, and then computation of an SP/AP amplitude relation (Hall, 1992). We routinely collect at least three separate ECochG averages for the test ear. After verifying response replicability (the major

components are present consistently across waveforms), we digitally add the separate waveforms and calculate SP and AP amplitude, and the SP/AP ratio, from the summed (composite) wavefrom. The same technique is always used for each ear.

In analyzing ECochG data, one must appreciate factors which can differentially influence the SP versus AP (Hall, 1992). In addition to stimulus polarity, the stimulus intensity and rate and the recording electrode site probably have the most pronounced effects on the SP/AP relation. As the recording electrode is moved closer to the cochlea, amplitude increases for the SP and for the AP, but the increase is relatively greater for the AP. Consequently, the SP/AP ratio invariably become smaller when recorded closer to the cochlea. For example, the upper limit for normal SP/AP ratio is 50% for an ear canal (TIPtrode) electrode versus 30% for a promontory electrode. The practical implications of this phenomenom are significant for clinical ECochG measurement and interpretation, particularly if various electrode types and sites are used. This is not a factor, of course, when recording ECochG intraoperatively with a single electrode site. An SP is characteristically not detected for stimulus intensity levels of less than 55 to 60 dB sound pressure level (SPL). The most stable SP/AP relation is found at very high stimulus intensity levels. With increasing stimulus rates (e.g., from a slow rate of 7.1/sec to a rapid rate of more than 100/sec), AP amplitude will decrease whereas SP amplitude shows little change. The result is a progressive increase in the SP/AP ratio with increasing rate. Thus, rate should be held constant intraoperatively for confident SP/AP interpretation.

Two final ECochG analysis parameters are AP latency and amplitude. Latency is usually calculated as the time (in msec) between stimulus onset and AP peak. Amplitude (in microvolts) is generally calculated either from a preceding baseline value to AP peak, or from AP peak to the immediately following trough. Another analysis parameter described in early ECochG studies, but rarely reported now, is a measure of the time in msec from the onset of the SP to the AP return to baseline (SP plus AP width).

ABR

During acoustic neuroma surgery, we monitor the ABR wave I (the AP of the ECochG) as well as later components (waves III and V). The ABR wave I component arises from the cochlear end of the VIIIth nerve (Moeller, 1981). This site is distal to the region at greatest surgical risk, because posterior fossa tumors generally arise from the cochleovestibular nerve near the porus acoustus (e.g., vestibular schwannomas or "acoustic tumors") or from within the cerebellopontine angle (e.g., meningiomas). We are nonetheless very interested in monitoring wave I (ECochG AP) as it provides valuable on-line information on the status of the cochlear circulation and cochlear integrity. Compromise of blood flow to the cochlea, which is a primary cause of surgery related hearing loss, is usually accompanied by the loss of wave I within 30 seconds. We constantly analyze wave I latency and amplitude intraoperatively for any sign of alteration. Changes in latency or amplitude data that cannot be explained by technical factors (e.g., earphone slippage, acoustic tube kinking) or other surgical events (e.g., drilling induced threshold shifts, irrigation fluid in the middle ear space) are interpreted as early signs of cochlear blood supply compromise (Hall, 1992; Hall and Schwaber, 1992; Schwaber and Hall, 1990; Schwaber and Hall, 1992.

We also closely monitor the ABR wave I to III latency interval (Fig. 3). Again, wave I is generated by distal VIIIth nerve whereas wave V arises from regions proximal to the surgical region (caudal auditory brainstem). Therefore, the wave I–III interval is an electrophysiologic index of VIIIth nerve integrity. The wave I–V latency interval is also routinely monitored in such cases. However, one must always keep in mind that this measure reflects status of not only the VIIIth nerve, but also more rostral brainstem structures. Consequently, a change in the wave I–V latency interval does not necessarily imply VIIIth nerve involvement.

With suboccipital vestibular procedures, including vestibular neurectomies, we monitor specifically the ABR wave I–III and wave I–V latency intervals. AEP monitoring in these cases provides important information regarding excessive retraction of the cochleovestibular nerve or excessive manipulation of the cochlear nerve during the procedure (Fig. 24.10). The actual monitoring process is quite similar for vestibular neurectomies and acoustic tumor removals. The two main differences are that the risk to cochlear blood supply and the surgical time window for concern is considerably greater with posterior fossa tumor removal.

Criteria for Intraoperative AER Alterations

There are few published guidelines for interpreting significance of intraoperative changes in AER findings (Table 24.3). In interpretation of AER data intraoperatively, regardless of the parameters analyzed or the criteria for abnormality used, it is assumed that potential nonsurgical causes of AER changes are first ruled out. Examples of these nonsurgical causes would include physiologic fluctuations (e.g., body temperature or blood pressure), equipment problems (e.g., electrode or transducer slippage), modifications in measurement parameters, and effects of anesthesia. We should point out, at this juncture, that there is a strong argument against reliance on only wave V absolute latency, or amplitude in intraoperative AER monitoring. Absolute wave V latency or amplitude reflects both central *and* peripheral (including middle ear and cochlear) auditory functioning, whereas interwave intervals (e.g., wave I–II, I–III, or I–V latencies) predominantly reflect VIIIth nerve through auditory brainstem integrity. A reduction in stimulus intensity level, for example, due to slippage of an insert earphone during surgery, would be likely to effect amplitude and latency of wave V but not the wave I–III or I–V latency interval, assuming a clear wave I remained present. The importance of recording a distinct wave I (ECochG AP component) is clear from this discussion.

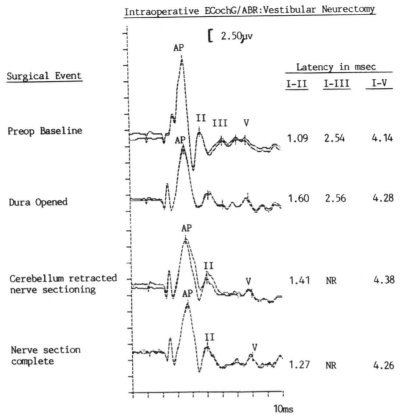

Figure 24.10. Example of trending of ECochG/ABR waveforms recorded intraoperatively over time during surgery. Selected surgical events are noted.

Patients with hearing sensitivity deficits, particularly in the high frequency region, may not have a detectable wave I with extratympanic recording electrode techniques. However, as noted above, a clear wave I can be recorded from most patients with a transtympanic electrode approach.

Optimally, one should record an evoked response component from the structure that is being operated on, and also for components immediately distal (peripheral to) and immediately proximal (central to) the anatomic region of surgery intraoperatively. For surgery where the cochlea will be at risk, then, it is best to monitor all ECochG components (CM, SP, AP). If the VIIIth nerve is at risk, it is appropriate to monitor the ECochG AP component (ABR wave I), along with ABR waves II, and III, and the wave I–II and I–III intervals. When the auditory brainstem is also at risk, all ABR components, including wave V, should be monitored. Perhaps the best approach for rapidly and consistently obtaining this information is the two or three channel measurement of ECochG/ABR, described above, with electrodes located on the promontory, the forehead and, on occasion, directly on the VIIIth nerve as it enters the brainstem. Assuming a promon-

tory electrode recording technique and a clear wave I component, we interpret ECochG/ABR intraoperatively using the following general criteria. We view a repeatable increase in major interwave latencies (I–III, III–V, or I–V) of more than 0.5 msec as an "alert." Once physiologic factors, such as decreased body temperature, are ruled out, the surgeon is informed that there is a small but definite change in the response. An interwave latency increase of more than 1.0 msec, or the loss of a clear and repeatable wave V or wave III and V, is more serious and is reported as a "warning." In contrast to response latency, amplitude tends to be considerably more variable intraoperatively. However, if amplitude of wave V as defined by the wave V/I ratio decreases by more than 50%, then this also is reported as a "warning." Naturally, waveforms illustrating such AER changes are stored on computer disk and documented (see Fig. 24.10). In addition, pertinent AER findings, along with corresponding surgical events and their time of occurrence, are documented in writing.

It is important to emphasize that latency and amplitude of ABR wave I (ECochG AP) is *not* sensitive to proximal VIIIth nerve or auditory brainstem dysfunc-

Table 24.3.
**Guidelines for Intraoperative Electrocochleography (ECochG)/Auditory Brainstem Response (ABR) Test Protocol
(Adapted from Hall, 1992)**

Parameter	Suggestion	Rationale/Comment
Stimulus:		
Transducer	ER-3A	Permits TIPtrode usage; secures transtympanic electrode placement; feasible in O.R. with otologic operations; does not invade surgical field or obstruct the surgical procedure
Type	Click	Produces robust response, but only evaluates basal turn of cochlea; tone bursts can be used
Duration	0.1 msec	For this onset response, an extended duration tone burst useful SP delineation; 2-1-2 cycle duration for tone bursts
Polarity	Alternating	ECochG: cancels out cochlear microphonic; single polarity used for CM detection
	Rarefaction	ABR: usually enhances waveform definition, but manipulate polarity if response is not optimal
Rate	7.1/second	Slow rate enhances N1 (AP) component; a very rapid rate (e.g., >91/second) is useful for SP delineation; modifying rate slightly may reduce some types of electrical interference; rate of 21.1/sec is appropriate if a robust AP (wave I) is present
Intensity	70–95 dB	Produces robust response (normally there is no ECochG SP for intensities below about 50 dB); intensity is decreased to estimate sensorineural hearing threshold levels
Masking	None	Masking is never necessary for ECochG (a detectable AP response is always from the test ear); very rarely required for ABR (only with markedly delayed wave V latency and absent wave I.
Presentation Ear	Monaural	
Mode	Air conduction	Bone conduction ECochG and ABR are possible, but not typically required in the O.R.
Acquisition Electrodes: Types	Needles	Sterile stainless steel, subdermal-type needle electrodes are used exclusively for ECochG and ABR recording in the O.R., including promontory site.
Arrays (Options ranked)[a]		
1.	Fz-prom	Noninverting electrode is at upper forehead, approximately at the hairline; technically at a point midway between vertex and nasion; this array typically yields a response of large amplitude (e.g., 4 to 20 Uv)
2.	Fz-IEAC	For example, with TIPtrode in the ipsilateral external ear canal; noninvasive (no advantage in O.R.), but amplitude rarely exceeds 0.6 Uv
3.	AC-prom	Customary ECochG electrode array; yields response of large amplitude and sometimes reduced electrical artifact interference
	Ground = Fpz	Low forehead ground electrode is convenient and is used for both ECochG and ABR
Impedance	<5 to 10 K ohm	Except for promotory electrode, impedance should be less than 5 K ohm; for promontory electrode, impedance should be less than 10 K ohm
Filter	10–1500 Hz	Encompasses response frequencies; lower high pass cut-off may be desirable for SP definition
	Notch	Not recommended; may introduce response distortion
Amplification	X75,000	Adequate for large ECochG response
Analysis time	5, 10, or 15 msec	Shorter time for ECochG and longer time for ABR or combined ECochG/ABR recording
Sweeps	<50 to> 1500	Often less than 50 sweeps are needed with promontory electrode; over 1500 for EAC electrode

[a]TT = transtympanic; EAC = external auditory canal; I and i = ipsilateral to stimulus; C and c = contralateral to stimulus; TM = tympanic membrane.

tion. There are repeated accounts of brainstem dysfunction or inactivity and marked VIIIth nerve dysfunction, including complete transection of the nerve, in the presence of a consistently recorded and normal appearing wave I or AP component. Hearing in these cases is, of course, entirely lost. In time, there is apparently retrograde degeneration of cochlear functioning, or delayed vascular disturbance, and the ABR wave I (ECochG AP) also disappears.

Steps in Monitoring

The most important step during monitoring is to trend evoked response findings. This is particularly important for AER, as opposed to facial nerve findings. Trending is the display of responses as a function of time. One approach is to display a representative baseline averaged waveform at the top of the evoked response system oscilloscope (screen) and then to also display the waveform being averaged (monitored) just below. One cursor is placed on a peak of interest (e.g., ABR wave V) in the baseline waveform and the other cursor is placed on this same peak in the ongoing average. The latency difference can then be continuously calculated. Amplitude values can be similarly calculated periodically during surgery. As the case proceeds, representative waveforms recorded at certain surgical events are displayed on the screen, along with the baseline and ongoing averaged waveform. To facilitate accurate analysis of evoked response waveforms, especially calculation of amplitude, it is important to display all waveforms with the same gain setting. Use of an automatic gain setting option often presents a very misleading display of waveforms because amplitudes displayed for each waveform are adjusted to be equivalent by the equipment. With automatic gain adjustment, substantial differences between waveforms, and changes in the amplitude among the waveforms over time, can easily go undetected.

CONCLUSIONS

Intraoperative monitoring of auditory system status during surgery putting the auditory system at risk is clinically feasible and useful. Although it is technically challenging to record quality ECochG/ABR data intraoperatively, accumulated clinical experience and the scientific literature clearly confirm that monitoring can result in rapid electrophysiologic measurement of cochlear, VIIIth nerve, and auditory brainstem function and early detection of dysfunction.

ACKNOWLEDGMENTS

In preparation of this chapter, Drs. F. Musiek and S. Bornstein contributed the portions on neurodiagnostic use of ABR whereas Drs. J. Hall and M. Schwaber contributed the portions on intraoperative monitoring.

REFERENCES

Antonelli A, Bellotto R, and Grandori F. Audiologic diagnosis of central versus VIII nerve and cochlear auditory impairment. Audiology 1987;26:209–226.

Antonelli A, Bellotto R, Bertazzoli M, Busnelli G, Nunez-Castro M, and Romagnoli M. Auditory brainstem response test battery for multiple sclerosis patients: Evaluation of test findings and assessment of diagnostic criteria. Audiology 1986;25:227–238.

Arenberg IK, Gibson WPR, Bohlen HKH, and Best L. An overview of diagnostic and intraoperative electrocochleography for inner ear disease. Insights Otolaryngology 1989;4:1–6.

Bauch C, and Olsen W. The effect of 2000-4000 Hz hearing sensitivity on ABR. Ear Hear 1986;7:314–317.

Bauch CD, and Olsen W. Wave V interaural latency differences as a function of asymmetry in 2000-4000 Hz hearing sensitivity. Am J Otol 1989;10:389–392.

Bauch C, Olsen W, and Harner S. Auditory brainstem response and acoustic reflex test: Results for patients with and without tumor matched for hearing loss. Arch Otolaryngol Head Neck Surg 1983;109:522–525.

Bauch C, Rose D, and Harner S. Auditory brainstem response results from 255 patients with suspected retrocochlear involvement. Ear Hear 1982;3:83–86.

Beagley HA, and Sheldrake JB. Differences in brainstem responses latency with age and sex. Br J Audiol 1978;12:69–77.

Bertrand O, Garcia-Larrera L, Artru F, Mauguiere F, and Pernier J. Brain-stem monitoring. I. A system for high-rate sequential BAEP recording and feature extraction. Electroencephalogr Clin Neurophysiol 1987;68:433–445.

Brown R, Chiappa K, and Brooks A. Brainstem auditory evoked responses in 22 patients with intrinsic brainstem lesions: Implications for clinical interpretations. Electroencephalogr Clin Neurophysiol 1981;5:38.

Campbell K, and Abbas P. The effect of stimulus repetition rate on the auditory brainstem response in tumor and nontumor patients. J Speech Hear Res 1987;30:494–502.

Chiappa K. Evoked Potentials in Clinical Medicine. New York: Raven Press, 1983:125–128, 145–150, 165–177.

Chiappa K, Gladstone K, and Young R. Brainstem auditory evoked responses. Studies of waveform variations in 50 normal human subjects. Arch Neurol 1979;36:81–87.

Clemis J, and McGee T. Brainstem electric response audiometry and the differential diagnosis of acoustic tumors. Laryngoscope 1979;89:31–42.

Coats A. The summating potential and Ménière's disease. I. Summating potential amplitude in Ménière and non-Ménière ears. Arch Otolaryngol 1981;107:199–208.

Coats A, and Martin J. Human auditory nerve action potentials and brainstem evoked responses. Arch Otolaryngol 1977;12:506–622.

Coelho A, and Prasher D. Brainstem potentials in the diagnosis of an acoustic neuroma. Scand Audiol 1990;257–262.

Cullen J, Ellis M, and Berlin C. Human acoustic nerve action potential recordings from the tympanic membrane without anesthesia. Acta Otolaryngol (Stockh) 1972;74:15–22.

Daly DM, Roeser R, Aung M, and Daly DD. Early evoked potentials in patients with acoustic neuroma. Electroencephalogr Clin Neurophysiol 1977;43:151–159.

Debruyne F. Influence of age and hearing loss on the latency shifts of the auditory brainstem response as a result of increased stimulation rate. Audiology 1986;25:101–106.

Don M, Allen A, and Starr A. Effect of click rate on the latency of auditory brainstem responses in humans. Ann Otol Rhinol Laryngol 1977;86:186–195.

Durrant J. Observations on combined noninvasive electrocochleography and auditory brainstem response recording. Semin Hear 1986;7:289–303.

Eberling C, and Parbo J. Reference data for ABRs in retrocochlear diagnosis. Scand Audiol 1987;16:49–55.

Eggermont J. Summating potentials in electrocochleography: Relation to hearing disorders. In Ruben R, Eberling C, Salomon G, Eds. Electrocochleography. Baltimore: University Park Press, 1976:67–87.

Eggermont J, Don M, and Brackmann D. Electrocochleography and auditory brainstem electric responses in patients with pontine angle tumors. Ann Otol Rhinol Laryngol 1980;89:1–19.

Ferraro J, and Ferguson R. Tympanic ECochG and conventional ABR: A combined approach for the identification of wave I and the I-V interwave interval. Ear Hear 1989;10:161–166.

Fowler C, and Noffsinger D. Effects of stimulus repetition rate and frequency on the auditory brainstem response in normal, cochlear-impaired, and VIII nerve/brainstem-impaired subjects. J Speech Hear Res 1983;26:560–567.

Galambos R, and Hecox K. Clinical applications of the auditory brainstem response. Otolaryngol Clin North Am 1978;11:709–722.

Gerling I, and Finitzo-Hieber T. Auditory brainstem response with high stimulus rates in normal and patient populations. Ann Otol Rhinol Laryngol 1983;92:119–123.

Gilroy J, Lynn G, Ristow G, and Pellerin R. Auditory evoked brainstem potentials in a case of "locked-in" syndrome. Arch Neurol 1977;34:492–495.

Glasscock M, Jackson C, Josey A, Dickins J, and Wiet R. Brainstem evoked response audiometry in clinical practice. Laryngoscope 1979;89:1021–1034.

Gorga M, Reiland J, and Beauchaine K. Auditory brainstem responses in a case of high frequency conductive hearing loss. J Speech Hear Disord 1985;50:346–350.

Grancik MS, Martuza RL, Parker SW, Ojemann RG, and Montgomery WW. Cerebello-pontine angle meningioma: Clinical manifestations and diagnosis. Ann Otol Rhinol Laryngol 1985;94:34–38.

Grundy B. Monitoring of sensory evoked potentials during neurosurgical operations: methods and applications. Neurosurgery 1982;11:556–575.

Gusella J. Acoustic neuromas. In Neurofibromatosis II. Proceedings of the NIH Consensus on Development Conference, December 11–13, 1991. Bethesda, MD: National Institutes of Health, 1991:24–25.

Hall JW III. Handbook of Auditory Evoked Responses. Needham, MA: Allyn and Bacon, 1992:385–418.

Hall JW III, and Schwaber MK. Intraoperative electrocochleography in vestibular surgery. In Jacobson GP, Ed. Handbook of Balance Testing. New York: B.C. Decker Publishers, 1992.

Harker L. ABR in cases of acoustic tumors. Presented at Symposium on Auditory Evoked Response in Otology and Audiology, Cambridge, MA, 1980.

Hashimoto I, Ishiyama Y, and Tozuka G. Bilateral recorded brainstem auditory evoked responses: Their asymmetric abnormality in lesions of the brainstem. Arch Neurol 1979;36:161–167.

Hecox K. ABR and brainstem involvement. Presented at the symposium on auditory evoked response in otology and audiology. Cambridge, MA, August 8–9, 1980.

House J, and Brackmann D. Brainstem audiometry in neurologic diagnosis. Arch Otolaryngol 1979;105:305–309.

Huertas J, and Haymaker W. Localization of lesions involving the statoacoustic nerve. In Haymaker W, Ed. Bing's Localization in Neurological Disease, 15th ed. St. Louis: CV Mosby, 1969:186–216.

Hyde M. Effect of cochlear lesions on the ABR. In Jacobson J, Ed. The Auditory Brainstem Response. San Diego, CA: College Hill Press, 1985:133–146.

Hyde M. The auditory brainstem response in neuro-otology: Perspectives and problems. J Otolaryngol 1981;10:117–125.

Jerger J, and Jerger S. Auditory Disorders: A Manual for Clinical Evaluation. Boston: Little, Brown, and Co., 1981.

Jerger J, and Mauldin L. Prediction of sensori-neural hearing level from the brainstem evoked response. Arch Otolaryngol 1978; 103:181–187.

Jerger J, Neely J, and Jerger S. Speech, impedance, and auditory brainstem response audiometry in brainstem tumors. Arch Otolaryngol 1980;106:218–223.

Jerger S. Decision matrix and information theory analysis in the evaluation of neuroaudiologic tests. Semin Hear 1983;4:121–132.

Jiang ZD. Intensity effect on amplitude of auditory brainstem responses in humans. Scand Audiol 1991;20:41–47.

Keith W, and Greville K. Effects of audiometric configuration on the auditory brainstem response. Ear Hear 1987;8:49–55.

Kileny PR, Niparko JK, Shepard NT, and Kemink JL. Neurophysiologic intraoperative monitoring: I. Auditory function. Am J Otol 1988;9:17–24.

Levine RA. Monitoring auditory evoked potentials during acoustic neuroma surgery. In Silverstein H, and Norrell H, Eds. Neurologic Surgery of the Ear, Vol. 2. Birmingham, AL: Aesculapius, 1979:287–293.

Lynn G, Cullis P, and Gilroy J. Olivopontocerebellar degeneration: Effects on auditory brainstem responses. Semin Hear 1983;4:375–384.

Lynn G, and Verma N. ABR and upper brainstem lesions. In Jacobsen J, Ed. The Auditory Brainstem Response. San Diego, CA: College Hill Press, 1985.

McLeod J, and Lance J. Introduction to Neurology. Melbourre: Blackwell Scientific Publications, 1989:178–190.

Moberg A, Anderson H, and Wedenberg E. In Hamberger CA, and Wersall J, Eds. Nobel Symposium 10: Disorders of the Skull Base Region. Stockholm: Almqvist and Wiksell, 1969.

Moeller AR, and Janetta PJ. Compound action potentials recorded intracranially from the auditory nerve in man. J Exp Neurol 1981;74:862–864.

Moeller AR, and Janetta PJ. Monitoring auditory functions during cranial microvascular decompression operations by direct recording from the eighth nerve. J Neurosurg 1983;59:493–499.

Moller A, and Moller M. Physiology of the ascending auditory pathway with special reference to the auditory brainstem response (ABR). In Pinheiro M, and Musiek F, Eds. Assessment of Central Auditory Dysfunction: Foundations and Clinical Correlates. Baltimore: Williams & Wilkins, 1985:43–66.

Moller M, and Moller A. Brainstem auditory evoked potentials in patients with cerebellopontine angle tumors. Ann Otol Rhinol Laryngol 1983;92:645–650.

Morrison AW. Management of sensorineural deafness. London: Butterworths, 1975.

Musiek FE. Auditory Evoked Responses in a Site of Lesion Assessment. In Rintelmann W, Ed. Hearing Assessment, 2nd Ed. Austin, TX: Pro-Ed Publishers, 1991:383–428.

Musiek FE. Auditory brainstem (evoked) response results in patients with posterior fossa tumors and normal pure-tone hearing. Arch Otolaryngol 1986:112–255.

Musiek FE, and Baran JA. Neuroanatomy, neurophysiology, and central auditory assessment: Part I: Brainstem. Ear Hear 1986;7: 207–219.

Musiek FE, and Baran JA. Canal electrode electrocochleography in patients with absent Wave I ABRs. Otolaryngol Head Neck Surg 1990;103:25–31.

Musiek FE, and Geurkink N. ABR and central auditory test results in patients with brainstem lesions. Laryngoscope 1982;92: 891–900.

Musiek F, Gollegly K. ABR in eighth nerve and low brainstem lesions. In Jacobsen J, Ed. The Auditory Brainstem Response. San Diego, CA: College-Hill Press, 1985:181–203.

Musiek F, Gollegly K, Kibbe K, and Reeves A. Electrophysiologic and behavioral auditory findings in multiple sclerosis. Am J Otol 1989;10:343–350.

Musiek F, Gollegly K, Kibbe K, and Verkest S. Current concepts on the use of ABR and auditory psychophysical tests in the evaluation of brainstem lesions. Am J Otol 1988;9(Suppl Contemporary Issues Clini Audiol):25–36.

Musiek F, and Johnson G. ABR interaural latency difference in patients with brainstem lesions and symmetrical hearing. Presented at the 22nd Annual Scientific Meeting of the American Neuro-otology Society, Denver, CO, April 1987.

Musiek F, Johnson G, Gollegly K, Josey A, and Glasscock M. The auditory brainstem response interaural latency difference (ILD) in patients with brainstem lesions. Ear Hear 1989;10:131–134.

Musiek FE, Josey AF, and Glasscock ME III. Auditory brainstem response in patients with acoustic neuromas: Wave presence and absence. Arch Otolaryngol 1986;112:186–189.

Musiek FE, and Kibbe K. Auditory brainstem response: Wave IV–V abnormalities from the large cerebellopontine lesions. Am J Otol 1986;7:253–257.

Musiek FE, Kibbe K, Rackliffe L, and Weider D. The auditory brainstem response I–V amplitude ratio in normal, cochlear, and retrocochlear ears. Ear Hear 1984;5:52–55.

Musiek F, Kibbe-Michal K, and Josey A. Selected auditory brainstem response indices in patients with cochlear and eighth nerve lesions matched for hearing loss. International ERA Study Group Symposium, August 25, 1987.

Musiek FE, Mueller R, Kibbe K, and Rackliffe L. Audiologic test selection in the detection of eighth nerve disorders. Am J Otol 1983;4:281–287.

Musiek FE, Weider DJ, and Mueller R. Audiological findings in Charcot-Marie-Tooth disease. Arch Otolaryngol 1982;108: 595–599.

Nager G. Association of bilateral VIIIth nerve tumors with meningiomas in von Recklinhausen's disease. Laryngoscope 1964A;74: 1220.

Nodar R, and Kinney S. The contralateral effects of large tumors on brainstem auditory evoked potentials. Laryngoscope 1980; 90:1762–1768.

Oh S, Kuba T, Soyer A, Choi I, Bonikowski F, and Vitek J. Lateralization of brainstem lesions by brainstem auditory evoked potentials. Neurology 1981;31:14–18.

Paludetti G, Maurizi M, and Ottaviani F. Effects of stimulus repetition rate on the auditory brainstem response. Am J Otolaryngol 1983;4:226–234.

Perlman H, Kimura R, and Fernandez C. Experiments on temporary obstruction of the internal auditory artery. Laryngoscope 1959;69:591–613.

Picton T, Woods D, Baribeau-Braun J, and Healey T. Evoked potential audiometry. J Otolaryngol 1977;6:90–119.

Poser CM. Diseases of the Myelin Sheath. In Merritt H, Ed. A Textbook of Neurology. Philadelphia: Lea & Febiger, 1979.

Prosser S, and Arslan E. Prediction of auditory brainstem wave V latency as a diagnostic tool of sensori-neural hearing loss. Audiology 1987;26:179–187.

Robinson K, and Rudge P. Auditory evoked responses in multiple sclerosis. Lancet 1975;24:1164–1166.

Rosenhall U, Hedner M, and Bjorkman G. ABR and brainstem lesions. Scand Audiol Suppl 1981;13:117–123.

Rosenhamer H. The auditory evoked brainstem electric response (ABR) in cochlear hearing loss. Scand Audiol Suppl 1981;13: 83–93.

Rowe M. Normal variability of the brainstem auditory evoked responses in young and old adult subjects. Electroencephalogr Clin Neurophysiol 1978;44:459–470.

Ruben R, Hudson W, and Chiong A. Anatomical and physiological effects of chronic section of eighth nerve in cats. Acta Otolaryngologica 1963;55:473–484.

Ruth R, Lambert P, and Ferraro J. Electrocochleography: Methods and clinical applications. Am J Otol 1988;9(Suppl):1–11.

Sand T. The choice of ABR click polarity and amplitude variables in multiple sclerosis patients. Scand Audiol 1991;20:75–80.

Schuknecht HF. Pathology of the Ear. Cambridge: Harvard University Press, 1974:425.

Schwaber MK, and Hall JW III. A simplified approach for transtympanic electrocochleography (ECochG). Am J Otol 1990; 11:260–265.

Schwaber MK, and Hall JW III. Monitoring auditory function intraoperatively with ABR and ECochG. In Kartush J, and Boucherd K, Ed. Intraoperative Monitoring in Otology and Head and Neck Surgery. New York: Raven Press, 1992:215–228.

Schwaber MK, Hall JW III, and Zealer DL. Intraoperative monitoring of the facial and cochleovestibular nerves in otologic surgery: Part I. Insights Otolaryngol 1991a;6:1–7.

Schwaber MK, Hall JW III, and Zealer DL. Intraoperative monitoring of the facial and cochleovestibular nerves in otologic surgery: Part II. Insights Otolaryngol 1991b;6:1–8.

Schwartz DM, and Morris MD. Strategies for optimizing the detection of neuropathology from the auditory brainstem response. In Jacobson JT, and Northern JL, Eds. Diagnostic Audiology. Austin, TX: Pro-ED, 1991:141–160.

Selters W, and Brackmann D. Brainstem electric response audiometry in acoustic tumor detection. In House W, and Luetje C, Eds. Acoustic Tumors, Vol 1. Baltimore: University Park Press, 1979:225–236.

Selters W, and Brackmann D. Acoustic tumor detection with brainstem electric response audiometry. Arch Otolaryngol 1977;103: 181–187.

Shannon E, Gold S, and Himmelfarb M. Auditory brainstem responses in cerebellopontine angle tumors. Laryngoscope 1981; 80:1477–1484.

Shimizu H, Moser H, and Naidu S. ABR and the audiologic findings in adrenoleukodystrophy: Its variant and carrier. Otolaryngol Head Neck Surg 1988;98:215–220.

Starr A, and Achor J. Auditory brainstem responses in neurological disease. Arch Neurol 1975;32:761–768.

Starr A, and Hamilton A. Correlation between confirmed sites of neurological lesions and abnormalities of far-field auditory brainstem responses. Electroencephalogr Clin Neurophysiol 1976;41:595–608.

Stockard JJ, Rossiter VS, and Weiderholt W. Brainstem auditory evoked responses in suspected central pontine myelinosis. Arch Neurol 1976;33:726–728.

Stypulkowski P, and Staller S. Clinical evaluation of the new ECochG recording electrode. Ear Hear 1987;8:304–310.

Telian SA, and Kileny PR. Usefulness of 1000 Hz tone-burst-evoked responses in the diagnosis of acoustic neuroma. Otolaryngol Head Neck Surg 1989;101:466–471.

Terkildsen K, Osterhammel P, and Thomsen J. ABR and MLR in patients with acoustic neuromas. Scandinavian Symposium on Brainstem Response (ABR). Scand Audiol 1981;(Suppl 13): 103–108.

Thomsen J, Terkildsen K, and Osterhammel P. Auditory brainstem responses in patients with acoustic neuromas. Scand Audiol 1978;7:179–184.

Turner R. Making clinical decisions. In Rintelmann W, Ed. Hearing Assessment, 2nd Ed. Austin, TX: Pro-Ed Publishers, 1991:679–738.

Turner R, and Nielsen D. Application of clinical decision analysis to audiological tests. Ear Hear 1984;5:125–133.

Wada S, and Starr A. Generation of auditory brainstem responses. III. Effects of lesions of the superior olive, lateral lemniscus and inferior colliculus on the ABR in guinea pig. Electroencephalogr Clin Neurophysiol 1983;56:352–366.

Weber B, and Fujikawa S. Brainstem evoked response (BER) audiometry at various stimulus presentation rates. J Am Aud Soc 1977;3:59–62.

Weber B, Seitz M, and McCutcheon M. Quantifying click stimuli in auditory brainstem response audiometry. Ear Hear 1981;2:15–19.

Yagi T, and Kaga K. The effect of the click repetition rate on the latency of the auditory evoked brainstem response and its clinical use for a neurological diagnosis. Arch Otorhinolaryngol 1979;222:91–97.

Zapulla R, Greenblatt E, and Karmel B. The effects of acoustic neuromas on ipsilateral and contralateral brainstem auditory evoked responses during stimulation of the unaffected ear. Am J Otol 1982;4:118–122.

CHAPTER 25

Auditory Brainstem Response:
Threshold Estimation and Auditory Screening

Bruce A. Weber

A hearing loss occurring early in life can have a major impact on speech and language development. Even a mild hearing loss during the first 3 years of life can adversely affect a child's development in areas that rely on auditory input (Alberti et al., 1983). The longer a hearing loss goes undetected, the greater is the likelihood that handicapping delays will occur. At least partially, such developmental delays can be offset by intensive education and training. However, the older the age of the child at the onset of therapy, the more difficult will be the task. To minimize the adverse effects of hearing impairment in young children, it is widely accepted that the loss should be identified as early as possible. The Joint Committee on Infant Hearing (1991), composed of representatives from pediatrics, nursing, otolaryngology, and speech and hearing, has recommended that newborns at risk for hearing loss be screened before hospital discharge. When this is not possible hearing testing should be performed by the time the child reaches 6 months of age.

As reviewed in Chapter 29, behavioral audiometric procedures have been developed for use with young infants. Although these are valuable clinical techniques, they possess major limitations when used with children less than 6 months of age. Behavioral hearing testing of very young infants usually relies on spontaneous responses, such as head turns or eye movements. Newborns and young infants have limited motor control so these responses cannot be elicited near threshold, even when some form of reinforcement is used. Routinely, the test stimuli are presented via a loudspeaker so behavioral audiometry with this age group does not provide direct information about the hearing status of individual ears. Because of these limitations in the behavioral hearing testing of young infants, audiologists have looked to auditory brainstem response (ABR) audiometry as the preferred technique for obtaining information about the hearing status of infants younger than about 6 months of age.

An overview of the ABR (or the Brainstem Auditory Evoked Response (BAER) as it is commonly termed in the pediatric literature) is presented in Chapter 24 and the principles will not be discussed in detail here. With ABR audiometry response to sound can be routinely recorded at low stimulus intensity levels from sleeping infants. Because the ABR test stimuli are presented through an earphone it is possible to obtain information about the hearing status of individual ears.

ABR audiometry, however, is not without its own shortcomings. A significant weakness is the limited range of stimuli that can be used. The ABR is an onset response that is elicited by the leading edge of the acoustic signal. With a more abrupt the stimulus onset, more neural fibers will respond in synchrony, and, in turn, a more clearly defined ABR will result (Hecox et al., 1976). The energy that occurs after stimulus onset does not play a major role in eliciting the ABR. As a result, abrupt onset acoustic clicks are the most common test stimulus and long duration stimuli, such as conventional pure tones or words, are not applicable to ABR testing.

Routinely, click stimuli are created by delivering a brief (e.g., 100 μsec) electrical pulse to an earphone. The pulse causes the earphone to vibrate and its resonant characteristics are the primary determiners of the spectrum of the resulting acoustic stimulus. The acoustic click created by most earphones has its greatest energy around 3000 Hz. Thus, ABR testing with click stimuli provides only a one point audiogram, with only information about the child's peripheral hearing status in the 2000-4000 Hz range. Efforts to use the ABR to obtain information about low frequency hearing will be discussed in some detail later in this chapter.

Despite its limitations, the ABR has been found to be a highly useful clinical procedure when behavioral audiometric procedures are not suitable or when the results of such testing are inconclusive. It has been consistently demonstrated that there is good agreement between ABR test results and behavioral pure tone thresholds at 2000-4000 Hz (Pratt and Sohmer, 1978; Gorga, et. al., 1985; Bauch and Olsen, 1986; Kileny and Magathan, 1987; van der Drift et al, 1987; Fjermedal and Laukli, 1989a). Hyde et al., (1990) conclude that, although the accuracy of the ABR is strongly dependent on the precise criteria that are chosen to define both hearing loss and ABR outcome, its accuracy is excellent for detecting average sensory-neural loss at 2000-4000 Hz more than 30 dB.

Because the ABR can be recorded from premature infants as young as 30 weeks conceptual age (Weber, 1982), the audiologist has a technique for estimating hearing status regardless of a child's age. Clearly, postponing audiometric testing until the child matures sufficiently to permit sensitive behavioral hearing testing cannot be justified.

APPLICATION OF THE ABR TO THRESHOLD ESTIMATION

The focus of this chapter is on the utilization of the ABR with infants and young children. However, it should be noted that there are older children and adults for whom ABR threshold estimation techniques are equally appropriate. This group would include individuals with severe mental retardation, closed head injuries, and whenever pseudohypoacusis is suspected. For convenience, in this chapter it will be assumed that the patient is a child. It should not be inferred that the

techniques and principles described here are limited to this group.

When ABR testing is performed to estimate hearing status, click stimuli are presented at different intensity levels to determine which levels elicit detectable responses. The resulting tracings are displayed in a manner similar to the one shown in Figure 25.1. Characteristically, the amplitude of the response decreases and latency of the component waves increases as stimulus intensity is lowered. Of major importance in ABR testing of children is the ABR threshold which is defined as the lowest stimulus intensity which elicits a detectable response. For the child shown in Figure 25.1, the ABR threshold was judged to be 20 dB nHL (0 dB nHL is customarily defined as the normal adult behavioral threshold for the click stimuli in the quiet testing environment).

When the ABR is used to estimate the hearing status of children it is not essential that all major component waves (I, III and V) be identifiable. It is necessary only to determine that the test stimulus elicited a detectable response and then measure the absolute latency (the time interval from stimulus onset to the point of peak amplitude) of a dominant ABR compo-

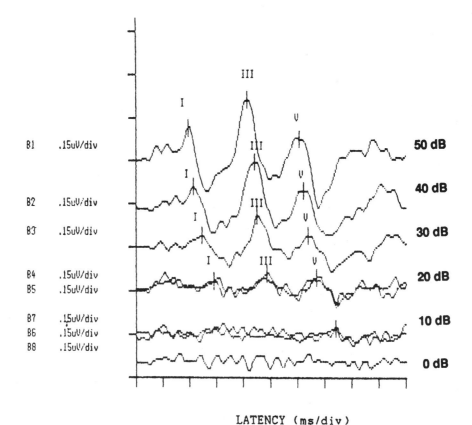

Figure 25.1. Auditory brainstem responses from a 2-year-old child. Response amplitudes are decreased and component wave latencies are prolonged as stimulus intensity is reduced. Threshold was judged to be 20 dB nHL, although there is a possible response at 10 dB nHL.

nent wave. In latency measurements, Wave V is routinely used because it is consistently the most robust and stable component of the ABR. As stimulus intensity is decreased, Wave V is usually the last wave to disappear. As will be discussed later in this chapter, comparing a child's Wave V latencies with clinic norms can provide useful information about the extent and type of hearing loss. ABR testing of young children is, thus, directed toward determining the response threshold for each ear and comparing the resulting ABR latencies with appropriate clinic norms. This focus on detecting responses at low stimulus intensity levels has resulted in test protocols which differ significantly from those used to detect a retrocochlear lesion. Typical test parameters for testing children are shown in Table 25.1.

Because the amplitude of the ABR decreases as stimulus intensity is reduced, it is usually necessary to average a large number of individual responses (usually 2000-4000) to detect an ABR at low intensity levels. A sleeping child may awaken at any moment, so a primary concern is obtaining the maximum amount of information in the shortest possible time. As a result, a click presentation rate around 30-40/sec is usually used because rates in this range do not significantly reduce the ability to detect ABRs at low intensity levels (Cox, 1985). Infants have longer ABR latencies than adults (Hecox and Galambos, 1974; Salamy et al., 1982). To ensure that portions of the young infant's response do not fall beyond the time period sampled by the averaging computer, the sampling epoch is often extended to 12-20 msec after stimulus onset. Such a long epoch is particularly important when testing is performed near threshold where ABR latencies are their longest.

In a typical ABR protocol for children, the examiner initiates testing at a moderate click intensity level (e.g., 50 dB nHL). Based on the presence or absence of a detectable response at this initial level, stimulus intensity is increased or decreased and a new stimulus trial is begun. Intensity level continues to be adjusted in a bracketing fashion until the ABR threshold is established. Unless the ABR is very clearly defined at a given intensity level, conventional practice is to obtain tracings on two identical stimulus runs. Good agreement between these two tracings increases examiner confidence that a response has occurred. If there is still question whether a response is present three or more replications may be appropriate. Control (no stimulus) tracings are also routinely recorded and compared with the tracings obtained when a click was presented to the child. Confidence that a response has occurred is high if: (a) there is good agreement between the tracings obtained at the same click intensity and (b) these tracings are clearly different from the control tracings.

Masking

In all aspects of audiometry it is essential that the test stimuli are not heard in the non-test ear. ABR testing is no exception and masking noise must be administered whenever stimulus cross-over to the non-test ear is suspected. Reports of interaural attenuation for click stimuli range from 45 to 75 dB (Elberling, 1978; Humes and Ochs, 1982). Using a relatively conservative 50 dB estimate of interaural attenuation, masking should be administered to the non-test ear whenever a stimulus is presented more than 50 dB above the ABR threshold of the non-test ear. Weber (1983) discusses this topic in some detail. In behavioral audiometry, the use of insert earphones significantly reduces the need for contralateral masking, particularly at lower frequencies. However, for click stimuli, insert earphones have little effect on the interaural attenuation (Van Campen, et al., 1990). As a result, crossover to the non-test ear must be a concern in ABR testing, regardless of type of transducer.

Sedation

Particularly when the test stimulus is near threshold, detection of the ABR can be thwarted by patient movement artifacts. It is important, therefore, that the child remains as quiet as possible. Although it is sometimes possible to record acceptable responses from an awake infant, it is clearly preferable if the child is sleeping throughout the test session. If the infant is younger than about 6 months of age (corrected for prematurity), the examiner can reasonably expect sufficient periods of natural sleep to permit ABR testing without the use of sedation. This is especially true if the child has been deprived of sleep and testing is scheduled to follow a normal feeding. After the age of about 6 months, however, natural sleep may be too unpredictable. Therefore, for older infants some form of sedative, often chloral hydrate administered orally, is usually required to insure adequate test conditions. Sedation does not adversely affect the amplitude, la-

Table 25.1.
Typical ABR Test Parameters for Estimating the Hearing Status of Infants

Stimulus:	Alternating polarity clicks
Stimulus rate:	33.3/sec
Number of stimuli averaged:	2000
Intensity level:	Varied to determine ABR threshold
Filter settings:	100–3000 Hz
Amplication:	X100,000
Analysis time:	10–15 msec

tency, or detectability of the ABR. The use of sedation, of course, does require the involvement of a physician acquainted with the child's medical history. Even with the use of sedation, ABR audiometry with older infants and children can be a time consuming procedure. If the child does not quickly fall into a satisfactory sleep state, test sessions in excess of two hours are not uncommon.

ABR TEST RESULTS

Central to the interpretation of ABR test results is an understanding of what information the ABR does, and does not, provide about a child's hearing status. As discussed above, a click stimulus has most of its energy concentrated between 2000 and 4000 Hz. Thus, when clicks are used little information is obtained about a child's low frequency hearing status.

Of equal importance is the distinction between the inferences that can be drawn from an ABR versus a behavioral response to the same stimulus. ABR testing examines only a limited portion of the auditory system. The presence of an ABR indicates that the test stimulus has elicited synchronous neural firings within the auditory system up to the level of the midbrain (Moller and Jannetta, 1983). Thus, a normal ABR threshold (e.g., clearly defined responses down to 20 dB nHL) does not insure normal processing of auditory stimuli at the cortical level. Similarly, the absence of an ABR does not insure that a peripheral hearing loss exists. Disorders, such as hydrocephalus and demylinating diseases, which reduce the synchrony of neural firings within the brainstem, may obliterate the ABR even though the peripheral auditory system is normal (Worthington and Peters, 1980; Kraus et al., 1984; Hall and Tucker, 1988). Because the ABR is a subcortical response, which is highly sensitive to disorders impacting the brainstem, it cannot not be viewed as a measure of hearing in the same manner as a conscious behavioral response. The ABR can be used to estimate a child's hearing status, but it is not a direct measure of hearing. Despite this limitation, as discussed above, there is good overall agreement between ABR click thresholds and behavioral hearing thresholds in the region of 2000-4000 Hz. Although audiologists must be cognizant of its limitations, the clinical value of ABR testing far exceeds its shortcomings.

Children with peripheral hearing losses in the 2000-4000 Hz range routinely demonstrate elevated ABR thresholds. The extent to which an individual child's threshold is elevated provides information about the degree of the child's hearing loss. In comparable test conditions, a child with an 80 dB ABR threshold is likely to have a greater hearing loss than a child with a 40 dB threshold. Even if ABR estimates of the magni-

tude of loss are in error by as much as 10 dB, the test results are still of significant value in determining the next appropriate step in the management of the child.

It is routinely possible to detect ABRs down to 20 dB nHL from a quietly sleeping, normal hearing child. When this occurs it is reasonable to conclude that the responses are consistent with normal peripheral hearing in at least the high portion of the speech range. It is not unusual to detect responses at even lower stimulus intensity levels. However, if the child is restless or if there is excessive electrical or acoustic interference during testing, the low amplitude ABRs may not be detectable near threshold. As a result, an elevated ABR threshold could be misleading. When test conditions are unavoidably only marginally acceptable, it is often necessary to use an alternative method for estimating the extent of hearing loss. This alternative form of analysis uses response latency to predict the extent to which a stimulus intensity is above the child's threshold. To perform this extrapolation, Wave V latency is measured at each stimulus intensity where a response was detected. As shown in Figure 25.2, these latencies are then plotted against the appropriate clinic norms based the child's age, adjusted for prematurity.

For the child shown in Figure 25.2, no detectable ABRs were present below 40 dB nHL. This could be explained, at least in part, by his restlessness through testing. Plotting the child's Wave V latencies at the levels where an ABR could be detected shows that they fall well within clinic norms. These test results are consistent with grossly normal peripheral hearing even though no ABR could be detected below 40 dB nHL. In contrast, the child shown in Figure 25.3 also demonstrated no detectable ABRs less than 40 dB. For this child, however, all Wave V latencies are prolonged beyond clinic norms. The extent of this prolongation

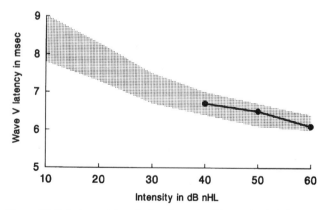

Figure 25.2. Latency-intensity function of a 12-month-old infant. Although no response is detectable below 40 dB nHL, Wave V latencies fall within normal limits. The shaded area reflects ±1 SD from mean response latencies for normal hearing 12-month-old infants.

provides information about the degree of hearing loss. For this child, a 40 dB nHL stimulus produced an ABR Wave V latency that is essentially the same as was recorded from normal hearing individuals when the stimulus was presented at a level of 10 dB nHL. This suggests that the child's hearing deviates from the clinic norms by approximately 30 dB. This relationship also holds at 50 dB, where the child's Wave V latency equals normal ABR latencies for a 20 dB nHL stimulus. Both extrapolations estimate that the child in Figure 25.2 has a 30 dB hearing loss in the frequency range tested. Generally, at stimulus intensity levels above 60 dB there is a poorer relationship between ABR latency and extent of hearing loss. As a result, high intensity levels are not routinely used in threshold extrapolations. It must be cautioned that not all hearing impairments produce consistent latency prolongations across intensity levels. This topic will be discussed in greater detail in the next section.

Whenever response latencies are used to estimate hearing status, it is essential that comparisons are made using appropriate age norms. With age, ABR latencies shorten due to a maturation process that includes such factors as myelination, cochlear maturation, increased synaptic efficiency, and synchrony of neural firing (Cox, 1985; Musiek, et al., 1987). Because this maturation process lasts up to the age of about 2 years, this factor must be taken into consideration whenever ABR latencies are used to predict the extent of a young infant's hearing loss. For infants under the age of 24 months, each clinic should have latency norms for different ages, preferably at 2-month intervals. Table 25.2 shows a portion of the clinic norms that the author uses with young infants. It can be seen that with increased maturation ABR Wave V latency shortens and variability across children decreases. Responses from children older than two years of age can be compared with adult latency norms without risk of significant error.

EFFECTS OF DIFFERENT TYPES OF PERIPHERAL HEARING LOSS

All hearing impairments do not influence the ABR equally. Typically the latency-intensity (L-I) functions are different for conductive and sensory-neural losses. A conductive hearing loss routinely extends latencies approximately equally across intensity levels (Finitzo-Hieber and Friel-Patti, 1985). As a result, the consistently prolonged ABR latencies create a L-I function that parallels those of normal hearing individuals. The latencies for the child shown in Figure 25.3 are consistent with a purely conductive hearing loss. When there is a consistent separation between clinic norms and a child's Wave V latencies, degree of hearing loss can be estimated with some confidence.

In contrast with the uniform ABR latency prolongation which are routinely produced by conductive impairments, a sensory-neural hearing loss may result in a variety of L-I functions. The configuration of the child's sensorineural hearing loss has a significant influence on the slope of the L-I function (Gorga, et al., 1985; Keith and Greville, 1987). For individuals with a high frequency sensorineural loss, Wave V latencies tend to be prolonged at lower stimulus intensity levels, yet they approach or reach normal values at higher intensities. Figure 25.4 shows the L-I function of a child with a high frequency sensory-neural loss. The Wave V latencies are well beyond normal limits at 40 dB and 50 dB, but fall within the normal range at 70 dB and 80 dB.

Extended ABR latencies at the lower stimulus inten-

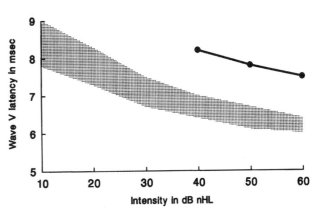

Figure 25.3. Latency-intensity function of an infant with a conductive hearing loss. Wave V latencies are approximately equally prolonged at all stimulus intensity levels.

Table 25.2.
Mean Wave V Latencies in msec from Infants at Selected Ages; Intensity Levels (nHL) Are Based on Adult Behavioral Thresholds to the Click Stimuli; are shown in parentheses

Intensity	Newborn	3 Months	6 Months	12 Months	24 Months
70 dB	6.9 (0.74)	6.6 (0.38)	6.4 (0.36)	6.1 (0.28)	5.8 (0.19)
60 dB	7.3 (0.81)	6.8 (0.41)	6.5 (0.29)	6.3 (0.31)	6.0 (0.19)
50 dB	7.7 (0.79)	7.0 (0.37)	6.8 (0.35)	6.6 (0.30)	6.2 (0.24)
40 dB	8.0 (0.93)	7.6 (0.46)	7.0 (0.38)	6.8 (0.38)	6.5 (0.28)
30 dB	8.2 (0.98)	7.9 (0.52)	7.5 (0.44)	7.2 (0.40)	6.9 (0.40)

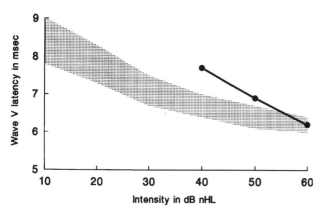

Figure 25.4. Latency-intensity function of an infant with a sensory-neural hearing loss. Commonly Wave V latencies are prolonged near threshold, but approximate normal values at higher intensity levels.

sity levels can be explained by increased transmission time along the cochlear partition (Borg, 1981). Because of the child's impairment in the high frequency (basal) region of the cochlea, an extended transmission time occurs before a more apical portion of the basilar membrane is excited by the stimulus. The normal ABR latencies at high intensity levels may reflect that the stimulus reached a level that exceeded the thresholds of the impaired high-frequency fibers in the basal region of the cochlea. Thus, the latency of the ABR appears to be related to the cochlear region that is predominately responsible for generating the response (Gorga et al., 1985). Yamada, et al., (1979) found that, for all but the steepest sloping high-frequency hearing losses, Wave V latencies fell within normal limits at high intensity levels. Flat sensory-neural losses tend to result in L-I functions that parallel normal values (Keith and Greville, 1987).

Wave V latencies across stimulus intensity are clearly influenced audiogram configuration and though a child's L-I function may provide some gross information about shape of the hearing loss, this must be approached with great caution. There is considerable variability in L-I functions across individuals with highly similar audiograms (Gorga et al., 1985). Because of the complexitiy of the relationship between Wave V latency and puretone thresholds, no L-I shape can be viewed as clinically diagnostic of a specific type or configuration of hearing loss. It should also be noted that when there is unequal prolongation of Wave V across stimulus intensity, it is difficult to use the L-I function to confidently predict even the magnitude of hearing loss in the 2000-4000 Hz range.

Bone Conduction Testing

A modification in ABR testing provides a direct estimate of a child's sensory-neural status and thus help

differentiate between a conductive and a sensory-neural hearing loss. Bone conduction (BC) and air conduction ABR thresholds can be compared, just as the two thresholds are compared in conventional puretone audiometry. Oscillator location has been shown to have a significant influence on the amplitude and latency of the BC ABR (Yang et al., 1987; Stuart et al., 1990) To produce a BC click stimulus, a bone conduction oscillator is substituted for the earphone. Because of the increased mass of the oscillator, the resulting BC click has a lower dominant frequency (around 1500 versus 3000 Hz for air conduction clicks) (Weber,1983). Due to the increased energy necessary to drive the BC oscillator, when conventional test equipment is used, the maximum output level for BC clicks is usually around 60 dB nHL. Even before this maximum output is reached, a large amplitude stimulus artifact originating from the oscillator may obliterate the ABR. Compared with ABRs elicited by AC clicks at the same intensity levels, BC ABRs have essentially the same waveform morphology, but have approximately 0.5 msec longer latencies in adults and older children. This is likely due to increased travel time along the cochlear partition for the lower frequency BC stimulus. Due to maturation differences, this prolongation in BC ABR latencies appears to be less pronounced in young infants (Hooks and Weber,1984). Air and bone conduction ABRs from a newborn infant are shown in Figure 25.5.

Just as in behavioral audiometry, similar ABR thresholds for both AC and BC clicks suggests a sensory-neural hearing loss, although lower thresholds for BC clicks are consistent with a conductive impairment. However, due to the greater low frequency energy in BC clicks, lower BC thresholds may also be a reflection of the contour of the child's hearing loss. Rather than indicating the presence of a conductive loss. That is, lower BC thresholds may be due to better hearing at 1500 Hz (the region stimulated by the BC clicks) than at the high frequency region stimulated by AC clicks. To overcome this problem, Hicks (1980) has advocated examining the level of bone conducted high-pass noise necessary to mask an air conduction click presented 5 dB above the ABR threshold. This technique is similar to the behavioral sensory-neural acuity level (SAL) originally described by Jerger and Tillman (1960).

ESTIMATING LOW FREQUENCY HEARING STATUS

Because of its abrupt onset, the acoustic click is an ideal stimulus for eliciting a detectable ABR near a child's peripheral hearing threshold. However, as mentioned earlier, most of the energy in the click is routinely in the 2000-4000 Hz range. Thus, click stimuli

AIR CONDUCTION   BONE CONDUCTION

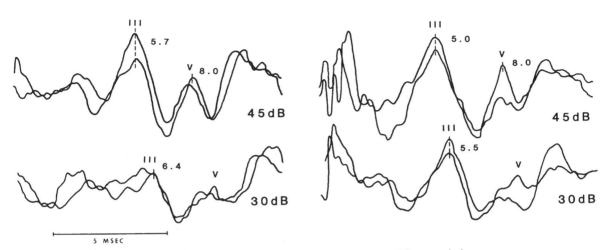

Figure 25.5. Air conduction and bone conduction ABRs recorded
from a preterm infant in the neonatal intensive care unit.

provide information about a child's peripheral hearing only in the high-frequency portion of the speech range. Because ABR testing with clicks results in only a one point audiogram, it is not possible to distinguish among rising, flat, and falling hearing losses (Eggermont, 1982). Sensory-neural hearing losses are characteristically most severe in the high frequencies, so the click ABR threshold may overestimate the magnitude of the overall loss in the speech frequencies. In contrast, a significant low frequency hearing loss may go undetected.

Ideally, it would be desirable to obtain ABR thresholds for frequencies at octave intervals to approximate the information obtained by behavioral audiometry. Unfortunately, the time necessary to obtain a single ABR threshold for each ear often exceeds 30 minutes, so a full audiogram is not practical. At a minimum, however, some information about a child's low frequency hearing status is needed to compliment the results obtained with click stimuli. Clinicians frequently conclude that a single measure of low frequency hearing is the most practical compromise. It is generally accepted that the single most valuable addition to click test results would be information about hearing status at 500 Hz because it is in the lower portion of the speech range (Fjermedal and Laukli, 1989b).

Considerable effort has been expended in an effort to find an effective evoked potential technique for obtaining information about a child's hearing status around 500 Hz. The most straightforward approach would appear to be a simple substitution of a 500 Hz tone burst for the conventional click stimulus. Unfortunately, the situation is more complicated than it first appears. Care must be taken to ensure that the onset of a tone burst is not so rapid that contaminating high frequency switching transients are introduced. Such transients can be minimized by gradually gating the onset of the tone burst. However, a long stimulus rise time produces a signal that possesses a less abrupt wave front. Because the ABR is an onset response, this more gradual wavefront produces less synchronous neural firings within the auditory system and, in turn, routinely results in a poorly defined response that cannot be detected consistently at low stimulus intensity levels.

The use of low frequency tone bursts thus creates a dilemma for the examiner: gradual stimulus onset ensures good frequency specificity, but the resulting stimulus is not effective in eliciting a clear ABR. The alternative is to use an abrupt stimulus onset. This improves the quality of the response, but introduces contaminating high frequency energy into the test stimulus. Obviously, the examiner cannot interpret ABRs with confidence when the low frequency test stimulus also contain high frequency energy.

Several alternative ABR techniques have been used by investigators in an attempt to ensure the frequency specificity of the test stimulus while maximizing the likelihood of a response at low intensity levels (Weber, 1987). Masking techniques used in conjunction with clicks and puretones are frequently used. In this approach, ipsilateral high-pass or notched masking noise is presented along with the test stimulus. The masking noise is introduced to eliminate the effects of the unwanted high frequency energy in the test stimulus. As shown in Figure 25.6, the ABR to masked tone bursts is characterized by a very slow wave that may persist past 10 μ sec after stimulus onset. To maximize the de-

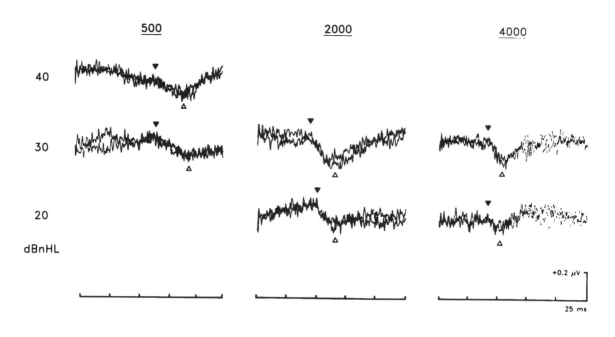

A03791 (6 mos)

Figure 25.6. Auditory brainstem responses recorded from a 6-month-old infant in response to 500, 2000, and 4000 Hz tone bursts presented in notched noise. Responses to low intensity stimuli show only a Wave V (**filled triangles**) followed by a nega-tive-going deflection (**open triangles**). Early components of the response are not discernible. Note that the response to the lowest frequency tone burst is the least clearly defined. (From Stapells and Kurtzberg 1991, with permission.)

tection of this response, the recording bandpass filters are opened to 30-3000 Hz and the sampling epoch is extended to at least 15 msec. Using this technique, Stapells (1989) reported some success with low frequency tone bursts. However, the resulting ABRs were not clearly defined at low to moderate to stimulus intensity levels. Fjermedal and Laukli (1989b) combined wide filter settings and high pass ipsilateral masking and reported difficulty recording detectable responses at low intensity levels. The authors concluded that a correction factor of 30-40 dB would be needed to predict behavioral thresholds for low frequencies. Laukli et al. (1988) performed ABR testing on 35 noncooperative children after they had been anesthetized. They concluded that the use of a 500 Hz tone burst with high-pass masking noise is not a reliable technique for routine assessment of low frequency peripheral hearing. It appears that, as the high frequency portion of the cochlear partition is masked, the clarity of the ABR decreases markedly. Poor response clarity for low frequency stimuli can be explained by the slowing in the velocity of cochlear excitation that occurs as it travels toward the apex. As the velocity of excitation decreases, less neural fibers fire in synchrony. A reduction in synchrony of neural firing, in turn, results in a poorly defined response.

Using tone bursts embedded in notched noise, Stapells et al. (1990) obtained quite good agreement

(e.g., 11.6 dB at 500 Hz) between ABR and behavioral hearing thresholds. A more recent report (Stapells and Kurtzberg, 1991) is also promising. In contrast, the findings of Beattie and Spence (1991) do not support the use of notched noise with frequencies as low as 500 Hz. Questions have also been raised about the validity of masking procedures with pathologic cochleas (Gorga and Worthington, 1983).

Because of its limited success to date, the research into the use of ipsilateral masking noise has not had an major impact on the design of commercial ABR test equipment. As a result, clinical ABR equipment routinely does not permit the presentation of the test stimulus in the presence of shaped ipsilateral masking. This is unlikely to change until more encouraging reports are forthcoming.

The quest continues for a sensitive and robust electrophysiologic measure of low frequency hearing status that can be used with the sleeping child. It should be noted that there are evoked potentials other than the ABR that have been examined for their usefulness in providing information about low frequency hearing. These longer latency responses are discussed in Chapter 26.

APPLICATION OF THE ABR TO HEARING AID FITTING

Just as behavioral audiometric techniques are often unsatisfactory for assessing the hearing of very young and difficult-to-test children, the same behavioral techniques may also be of limited value in evaluating the benefits a hearing aid provides to a hearing-impaired infant. It is not surprising, therefore, that there has been interest in using the ABR to assist in the fitting of a hearing aid and in assessing its benefit. Two approaches have been most widely used. Kileny (1982) and Mahoney (1985) have reported a technique that compares aided vs. unaided ABR thresholds. In the aided condition a specified input is delivered from an earphone suspended over the hearing aid microphone. Hearing aid gain is manipulated until a recognizable waveform is evident and benefit is described in terms of the difference between the aided and unaided ABR thresholds. In an alternative approach, the gain, output, and compression characteristics of the hearing aid are adjusted until an infant's aided ABR latencies closely approximate normal latency values. Hecox (1983) has used normalization of an infant's aided L-I function as indication of appropriate hearing aid gain.

The clinical application of ABRs to hearing aid fitting has been limited because of the complexity of the procedural problems encountered (Seitz and Kisiel, 1990). First, the abrupt click stimulus, which is so important in eliciting a clear ABR, can produce ringing in the hearing aid. The resulting high amplitude electromagnetic artifacts originating from the hearing aid may persist sufficiently long so that it obliterates much or all of the ABR. The use of tone bursts, with their longer duration, results in even greater artifact problems (Kileny, 1982). A second procedural problem relates to the compression circuits in the hearing aid. Gorga et al. (1987) contend that the compression circuits respond too slowly to be reflected in the ABRs to click stimuli. As a result, there are serious questions concerning how well ABR measures provide an accurate picture of a hearing aid's performance. Beauchaine and Gorga (1988) caution against the application of the ABR to pediatric hearing aid selection. Because of the procedural problems involved and the concerns about the validity of the technique, this ABR application is receiving very limited clinical use at this time.

USE OF THE ABR IN NEWBORN HEARING SCREENING

The need for early detection of hearing loss to minimize its impact on speech, language, and intellectual development was discussed at the beginning of the chapter. Because of the importance of early identification, an increasing number of states have created legislative mandates to carry out statewide hearing screening programs (Blake and Hall, 1990; Brooks, 1990). Although this legislation has not always been supported with adequate funding, it does indicate the growing awareness of the importance of early detection of a hearing impairment.

Certainly, there is no earlier time to screen for a hearing loss than before the neonate leaves the newborn nursery. Legitimate arguments can be made for postponing screening until after the infant is discharged from the nursery (Swigonski et al., 1987), however, the overriding concern is that a hearing impaired infant will not return for outpatient testing. Because hearing screening in the newborn nursery maximizes the likelihood that all at risk infants will be tested, it is the approach recommended by the Joint Committee (1991). In recent years there has been a significant growth in the number of hospitals which now provide this service.

Although a variety of test procedures have been used in newborn hearing screening, ABR audiometry, because of its accuracy and cost effectiveness, has now clearly emerged as the technique of choice (Weber, 1988). However, due to the time and costs involved, it is routinely not practical to perform ABR hearing screening on all newborns. Therefore, a decision must be made regarding which babies are at greatest risk; with efforts focused on this group. Commonly, a high risk register, containing such factors as congenital perinatal infections and birth weigh less than 1500 grams, is used to determine which babies should receive screening (Joint Committee, 1991). Rather than concentrating on specific risk factors, however, some audiologists prefer to screen all babies whose health problems have caused them to be transferred to a neonatal intensive care unit (NICU). Whichever approach is used to identify the target group, not all babies with a congenital hearing impairment will be tested. In a retrospective study, Papas (1983) noted that less than half (46%) of the hearing impaired children examined, would have fallen on a high risk register as newborns. Thus, at least half of the congenitally hearing-impaired babies appear normal and at low risk at the time of birth. It is essential, therefore, that newborn hearing screening programs have some mechanism, (e.g., an informational booklet and questionnaire for the baby's mother), for serving babies who do not appear to be at high risk for hearing loss. Even if a baby does not receive an ABR screening in the newborn nursery, the family should receive information about normal development of auditory behavior and know how to arrange for a hearing evaluation if concerns arise.

Typical newborn hearing screening test parameters are very similar to those used in threshold estimation with older infants and children. The screening is routinely performed as close to time of discharge as possible to allow for greatest maturation and to increase the likelihood that testing can be performed with a minimum of electrical interference from incubators, infusion pumps, and monitors. Click stimuli are presented through a monaural earphone and the screening level ranges from 30 to 40 dB nHL. When an ABR is not detected at the screening level most protocols call for probing at higher intensity levels in an attempt to estimate the extent of the hearing loss. If a newborn fails the ABR screening it is possible to use bone conduction click stimuli in an effort to help differentiate between conductive and sensory-neural hearing impairments (Hooks and Weber, 1984; Yang et al., 1987).

In many ways, the NICU is the worst imaginable location for ABR hearing screening. Obstacles include high ambient noise levels and contaminating electrical interference. The babies have immature auditory systems and they are sick, often with neurologic deficits that influence the ABR. In addition, there are such logistical problems as scheduling the ABR screening to coincide with the baby's quiet state and avoiding interfering with the caregiving activities of other hospital staff. Despite all these difficulties, ABR hearing screening has been shown to be feasible and an effective method for early detection of hearing loss.

The Joint Committee (1991) recommends that the pass criterion be a response from each ear at an intensity level of 40 dB nHL or less. The sensitivity (correctly identifying a significant hearing impairment) and specificity (correctly passing a normal hearing baby) of ABR screening depend greatly on the intensity level at which hearing is screened. Raising the screening level, (e.g., from 30 dB to 40 dB) will reduce the test's sensitivity and increase its specificity. Hyde et al. (1990) calculated the performance of ABR screening for different screening levels and definition of hearing loss. They concluded that ABR screening accuracy is excellent for detecting sensory-neural hearing loss at 2000 and 4000 Hz in excess of 30 dB and recommend that the choice of screening level be determined by such factors as prevalence of hearing loss in the tested population and the quantitative costs associated with test overhead and outcome error. Turner (1991) discusses in detail the issue of costs and performance of early identification programs.

In addition to the relatively large general purpose ABR equipment small more dedicated portable ABR units are also available. The former must be wheeled to the nursery, whereas the latter can be easily carried. Although portable ABR systems are less flexible than the more sophisticated general purpose units (Ferraro and Ruth, 1988), their basic operation is essentially the same. With either the conventional or portable ABR equipment, the audiologist assumes the primary role in administering, analyzing, and interpreting the results of each screening test. In contrast to this conventional form of ABR screening, there is an automatic ABR screener (ALGO-1) that requires little examiner participation. After the recording electrodes have been attached to the baby's scalp, and when test conditions (background noise level, patient movement artifacts, and electrical interference) are satisfactory, the screener automatically begins presenting 35 dB click stimuli. The baby's responses are accumulated in computer memory and compared with an internal template of a newborn ABR. If the baby's ABR sufficiently matches the template, the screener stops testing and indicates a "PASS." However, if the automatic screener does not detect a satisfactory agreement after a maximum of 1500 click presentations the screener displays a "REFER." A multicenter comparison of conventional and automated ABR screening revealed outcome agreement in 489 of 507 ears tested (Kileny, 1988). In some NICU environments test time may be significantly extended because noise and/or electrical interference levels are too high to meet the screener's acceptance criteria. A special test area may be needed. The use of an automated screener is attractive to screening programs in which threshold measurements and neurologic interpretation are not factors (Jacobson et al., 1990). It is particularly suited for programs that use volunteers in high volume testing within the full term nursery.

Follow-up of Screening Failures

Of the newborns who receive an ABR screening in the NICU, from 3 to 10% will fail the test, depending on the pass criterion used. Failure of an ABR screening test should not be viewed as confirming the presence of a handicapping hearing loss. Caution is required because a screening failure may be due to such factors as poor test conditions, a neurologic disorder, or a transient conductive hearing loss. As a result, each baby who fails the newborn screening requires retesting to determine if a permanent sensory-neural hearing loss is indeed present. Follow-up of the babies who have failed the screening test is a critical aspect of a screening program. Unfortunately, it is often one of the weakest components of the program because of the problems encountered in tracking babies after hospital discharge. Despite the difficulties encountered, effective follow-up is essential to any screening program because the original ABR screening test is of no value if it does not result in earlier intervention than would have been achieved otherwise. Thus, all effective ABR screening programs have a tracking mechanism to arrange for additional ABR and/or behavioral hearing testing. Follow-up testing on an outpatient basis allows time for increased maturation and improved health status.

Commonly, follow-up testing of the relatively small group of screening failures usually occurs when the babies reach an age of 3 to 6 months, corrected for prematurity. The younger age is preferred by programs that elect to use ABR testing without sedation as the primary follow-up procedure. The older age is more common with programs that require good head-turning responses for behavioral follow-up testing.

There is increasing evidence of the presence of emerging (delayed onset) and progressive hearing loss in infants (Bergstrom, 1988). As a result, follow-up testing should not be limited to babies who failed the original NICU screening test. Screening programs are now being expanded to include infants who pass the initial ABR screening, but who continue to be at risk for hearing loss because of such factors as family history, potentially ototoxic medications, meningitis, persistent fetal circulation, and cytamegalovirus. Emerging and progressive hearing impairments may help explain the relatively infrequent instances in which a baby passes the ABR newborn hearing screening, but later is found to have a significant handicapping sensorineural hearing loss. Despite its limitations the ABR has been found to be the most effective technique available today for the early detection of hearing impairment in newborns.

CONCLUSIONS AND FUTURE DIRECTIONS

The ABR is now well established as a valuable clinical tool for use with young and difficult to test children. In the evaluation of very young infants it has two primary advantages over behavioral audiometric procedures: (a) the response is very stable and can be recorded at low stimulus intensity levels; and (b) no active participation is required, so the infant's level of interest and understanding are not critical factors. The primary shortcoming of the ABR technique is the limited amount of information which a click stimulus provides about a child's hearing status. The ABR does not assess the status of the auditory system above the level of the brainstem and it provides information only about peripheral hearing status in the high portion of the speech range (2000-4000 Hz). No completely satisfactory clinical technique has yet been devised for using the ABR to obtain information about a child's low frequency hearing status. It remains to be seen if such a technique will be forthcoming or if this responsibility will be assumed by longer latency evoked potentials (see Chapter 26) or by newer recording techniques such as evoked otoacoustic emissions

(Bonfils et al., 1989; Lonsbury-Martin and Martin, 1990).

REFERENCES

Alberti PW, Hyde ML, Riko K, Corbin H, and Abramovich S. An evaluation of BERA for hearing screening in high-risk neonates. Laryngoscope 1983;93:1115–1121.

Bauch CD, and Olsen W. The effect of 2000-4000 Hz hearing sensitivity on ABR results. Ear Hear 1986;7:314–317.

Beattie RC, and Spence J. Auditory brainstem response to clicks in quiet, notch noise, and high pass noise. J Am Acad Audiol 1991;2:76–90.

Beauchaine KA, and Gorga MP. Applications of the auditory brainstem response to pediatric hearing aid selection. Semin Hear 1988;9:61–73.

Bergstrom L. Infectious agents that deafen. in Hearing Impairment in Children, Bess FH, Ed. Parkton, MD: York Press, 1988:33–56.

Blake PE, and Hall JW. The status of state-wide policies for neonatal hearing screening. J Amer Acad Audiol 1990;1:67–74.

Bonfils P, Uziel A, and Narcy P. The properties of spontaneous and evoked acoustic emissions in neonates and children: A preliminary report. Arch Otorhinolaryngol 1989;246:249–251.

Borg E. Physiological mechanisms in auditory brainstem-evoked response. Scand Audiol 1981(Suppl 13):11–22.

Brooks WS. Status of nationwide hearing screening programs and procedures. Poster Presentation at annual meeting of the American Academy of Audiology, New Orleans, LA, 1990.

Cox LC. Infant assessment: Developmental and age-related considerations. In Jacobson JT, Ed. The Auditory Brainstem Response. San Diego: College-Hill Press, 1985:297–316.

Eggermont JJ. The inadequacy of click-evoked auditory brainstem responses in audiological applications. Ann NY Acad Sci 1982; 388: 707–709.

Elberling C. Compound impulse response for the brain stem derived through combinations of cochlear and brain stem recordings. Scand Audiol 1978;7:147–15?

Ferraro JA, and Ruth RR. A comparison of commercial auditory evoked potential units: The economy units. Am J Otol 1988;9(Suppl):57–62.

Finitzo-Hieber T, and Friel-Patti S. Conductive hearing loss and the ABR. In Jacobson JT, Ed. The Auditory Brainstem Response. San Diego, CA: College-Hill Press, 1985:113–129.

Fjermedal O, and Laukli E. Pediatric auditory brainstem response and pure–tone audiometry: threshold comparisons. Scand Audiol 1989a;18:105–111.

Fjermedal O, and Laukli E. Low-level 0.5 and 1 KHz auditory brainstem responses. Scand Audiol 1989b;18:177–183.

Gorga MP, Worthington DW, Reiland JK, Beauchaine KA, and Goldgar DE. Some comparisons between auditory brain stem response thresholds, latencies, and pure-tone audiogram. Ear Hear 1985;6:105–112.

Gorga MP, Beauchaine KA, and Reiland JK. Comparison of onset and steady-state responses of hearing aids: implications for use of the auditory brainstem response in the selection of hearing aids. J Speech Hear Res 1987;30:130–136.

Hall JW, and Tucker DA. Auditory brainstem response in the evaluation of peripheral versus central nervous system dysfunction in the pediatric intensive care unit. Semin Hear 1988;9:47–60.

Hecox K. Role of auditory brainstem response in the selection of hearing aids. Ear Hear 1983;4:51–55.

Hecox K, and Galambos R. Brain stem auditory evoked response in human infants and adults. Arch Otolaryngol 1974;99:30–33.

Hecox K, Squires NK, and Galambos R. Brainstem auditory e-voked responses in man. I. Effect of stimulus rise fall time and duration. J Acoust Soc Am 1976;60:1187–1197.

Hicks G. Auditory brainstem response, sensory assessment by bone conduction masking. Arch Otolaryngol 1980;106:392–395.

Hooks RG, and Weber BA. Auditory brain stem responses of premature infants to bone-conducted stimuli: A feasibility study. Ear Hear 1984;5:42–45.

Humes L, and Ochs M. Use of contralateral masking in the measurement of the auditory brainstem response. J Speech Hear Res 1982;25:528–535.

Hyde ML, Riko K, and Malizia K. Audiometric accuracy of the click ABR in infants at risk for hearing loss. J Am Acad Audiol 1990;1:59–66.

Jacobson JT, Jacobson CA, and Spahr RC. Automated and conventional ABR screening techniques in high-risk infants. J Am Acad Audiol 1990;1:187–195.

Joint Committee on Infant Hearing. 1990 Position statement. ASHA. 1991;33(Suppl 5):3–6.

Keith WJ, and Greville KA. Effects of audiometric configuration on the auditory brainstem response. Ear Hear 1987;8:49–55.

Kileny PR. Auditory brainstem responses as indicators of hearing aid performance. Ann Otol 1982;91:61–64.

Kileny PR, and Magathan MG. Predictive value of ABR in infants and children with moderate to profound hearing impairment. Ear Hear 1987;8:217–221.

Kileny PR. New insights on ABR hearing screening. Scand Audiol Suppl 1988;(Suppl 30):81–88.

Kraus N, Ozdamar O, Stein L, and Reed N. Absent auditory brain stem response: peripheral hearing loss or brainstem dysfunction? Laryngoscope 1984;94:400–406.

Laukli E, Fjermedal O. and Mair IWS. Low-frequency auditory brainstem response threshold. Scand Audiol 1988;17:171–178.

Lonsbury-Martin BL, and Martin GK. The clinical utility of distortion-product otoacoustic emissions. Ear Hear 1990;11:144–154.

Mahoney TM. Auditory brainstem response hearing aid application. In Jacobson JT, Ed. The Auditory Brainstem Response. San Diego, CA: College-Hill Press, 1985:349–370.

Moller AR, and Jannetta PJ. Interpretation of brainstem auditory e-voked potentials: Results from intracranial recordings in humans. Scand Audiol 1983;12:125–133.

Musiek FE, Verkest SB, and Gollegly KM. Effects of Neuro maturation on auditory evoked potentials. Sem Hear 1988;9:1–13.

Pappas DG. A study of the high-risk registry for sensorineural hearing impairment. Otolaryngol Head Neck Surg 1983;91:41–44.

Pratt H, and Sohmer H. Comparison of hearing threshold deter-mined by auditory pathway electric responses and behavioural responses. Audiology 1978;17:285–292.

Salamy A, Mendelson T, and Tooley WH. Developmental profiles for the brainstem auditory evoked potential. Early Hum Dev 1982;6:331–339.

Seitz MR, and Kisiel DL. Hearing aid assessment and the auditory brainstem response. In Sandlin R, Ed. Handbook of Hearing Aid Amplification, Vol. II: Clinical Considerations and Fitting Practices. Boston: College Hill Press, 1990:203–223.

Stapells DR. Auditory brainstem response assessment of infants and children. Semin Hear 1989;10:229–251.

Stapells DR, and Kurtzberg D. Evoked potential assessment of auditory system integrity in infants. Clin Perinatol 1991;18:497–518.

Stapells DR, Picton TW, Durieux-Smith A, Edwards CG, and Moran LM. Thresholds for short-latency auditory-evoked potentials to tones in notched noise in normal-hearing and hearing-impaired subjects. Audiology 1990;29:262–274.

Stuart A, Yang EY, and Stenstrom R. Effect of temporal area bone vibrator placement on auditory brainstem response in newborn infants. Ear Hear 1990;11:363–369.

Swigonski N, Shallop J, Bull MJ, and Lemons JA. Hearing screening of high risk newborns. Ear Hear 1987;8:26–30.

Turner RG. Modeling the cost and performance of early identification protocols. J Am Acad Audiol 1991;2:195–205.

Van Campen LE, Sammeth CA, and Peek BF. Interaural attenuation using Etymotic ER-3A insert earphones in auditory brain stem response testing. Ear Hear 1990;11:66–69.

Van der Drift JFC, Brocaar MP, and van Zanten GA. The relation between the pure-tone audiogram and the click auditory brainstem response in cochlear hearing loss. Audiology 1987;26:1–10.

Weber BA. Comparison of auditory brain stem response latency norms for premature infants. Ear Hear 1982;3:257–262.

Weber BA. Masking and bone conduction testing in brainstem response audiometry. Semin Hear 1983;4:343–352.

Weber BA. Assessing low frequency hearing using auditory evoked potentials. Ear Hear 1987;8(Suppl):49–54.

Weber BA. Screening of high-risk infants using auditory brainstem response audiometry. In Hearing Impairment in Children Bess, FH, Ed. Parkton, MD: York Press, 1988:112–132.

Worthington DW, and Peters GL. Quantifiable hearing and no ABR: Paradox or error? Ear Hear 1980;1:281–285.

Yamada O, Kodera K, and Yagi T. Cochlear processes affecting Wave V latency of the auditory evoked brain stem response. Scand Audiol 1979;8:67–70.

Yang EY, Rupert AL, and Moushegian G. A developmental study of bone conduction auditory brain stem response in infants. Ear Hear 1987;8: 244–251.

CHAPTER 26

Middle Latency Auditory Evoked Potentials

Nina Kraus, Paul Kileny, and Therese McGee

It is generally accepted that there are two main reasons for the use of electrophysiologic tests of auditory function: (*a*) to determine signal detection threshold; and (*b*) to make inferences concerning the functional and structural integrity of the auditory pathway's neural components. The contemporary, clinical audiologist is confronted with a wide variety of auditory disorders that frequently necessitate a test battery approach. It is important to remember that there is a wealth of information to be obtained by using all possible components of the auditory evoked response and not limit neurodiagnostic testing to the auditory brainstem response (ABR). The purpose of this chapter is to lay the foundations for the understanding of the principles and applications of the middle latency response (MLR) with special emphasis on those applications where the MLR may be the preferred clinical tool.

DEFINITIONS AND HISTORIC PERSPECTIVE

The MLR is the series of waveforms occurring from 10 to 80 milliseconds (ms) after the onset of an auditory stimulus. The bioelectric events associated with auditory stimulation of the auditory pathway include very early components resulting from electrical events in the cochlea (such as the summating potential and the cochlear microphonic), as well as components with latencies of several hundred milliseconds associated with cortical and cognitive functions. Within the continuum of components comprising the scalp-recorded "auditory evoked response," the MLR follows the auditory brainstem response (ABR) and precedes the late auditory evoked potentials.

Geisler et al., (1958) were the first investigators to describe the MLR to clicks in awake subjects. They identified "an early response with onset latency of about 20 ms" characterized by a vertex-positive peak with a latency of approximately 30 ms. They reported that the threshold of this electrophysiologic phenomenon coincided with the subject's psychophysic threshold to the same stimuli. Geisler et al. hypothesized that this response was generated by the neural discharge of the afferent pathway to the auditory cortex. It is interesting to note that a close examination of

their recordings also reveals a consistently appearing vertex positive peak with a latency of 10 ms or less, representing the earliest display of the ABR. However, this component was overshadowed by the consistency and amplitude of the P30, and the authors did not refer to it in this early report.

Picton et al. (1974) described the various components of the human auditory evoked potentials including the MLR. The MLR is characterized by several scalp or vertex negative and positive peaks, including N18 (Na), P30 (Pa), and P50 (Pb or P1). Overall, the MLR is widely distributed over frontocentral scalp areas and can be recorded with an electrode montage identical to that used for recording the ABR.

The approximate interpeak latency of the most prominent peak of the ABR (wave V) and Pa is 25 ms. When a stimulus is presented at 40 times/second, these waves overlap, producing the 40 Hz response described later in this chapter. A more recently described auditory evoked response component within the 10–80 ms post-stimulus time (TP41) occurs at an approximate latency of 45 ms. The scalp distribution of this wave is very localized, being centered over the temporal lobe. Cacace et al. (1990) proposed that TP41, combined with some later peaks, constitutes a sequence of components focused over and probably originating in the auditory cortex. These components have yet to be investigated thoroughly in terms of their relationship to stimulus characteristics and the effects of neurological or hearing impairments. MLR components recorded from over the vertex and over the temporal lobe are shown in Figure 26.1.

MLR GENERATING SYSTEM

Myogenic Responses

In addition to the neural generators (discussed below), several scalp muscles produce sonomotor reflexes that may contribute to the MLR. At relatively high stimulus intensities, several reflexes originating from scalp musculature occur within a post-stimulus latency range of 7–50 ms (Picton et al., 1974). These are the postauricular reflex, the temporalis reflex, and the inion and frontalis reflexes. The scalp distribution of the temporalis, inion, and frontalis reflexes and the fact

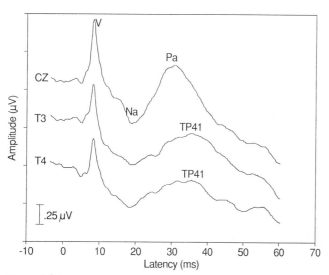

Figure 26.1. MLR recorded simultaneously from vertex (**Cz**) and from over the left (**T3**) and right (**T4**) temporal lobes. Wave V of the ABR is evident at all three sites. Pa (30 ms) is present at Cz. Wave TP 41 (35 ms) is present at T3 and T4. Responses were elicited by click stimuli (11.1/second) to the right ear.

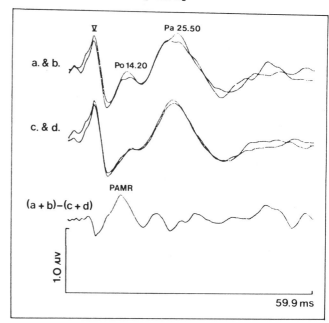

Figure 26.2. Effects of reference electrode placement on the myogenic contribution to the MLR (PAMR) **a** and **b** mastoid reference; **c** and **d** lower neck reference; **lower trace** is the result of subtracting the second from the **first trace** emphasizing the PAMR (reproduced from Kileny, 1983, with permission).

that they depend to a great extent on muscle tension make it easy to distinguish them from the neurogenic MLR.

The postauricular reflex is maximal over the upper mastoid regions and thus is recorded on a mastoid electrode, the usual placement for the inverting electrode (Fig. 26.2). This reflex appears to be independent of general muscle tension, and has a latency of approximately 12 ms (Bochenek and Bochenek, 1976), making it visible in recordings in which the sweep duration exceeds 12 ms. Inasmuch as the postauricular reflex dominated their recordings, Bickford et al. (1964) concluded that the MLR was a purely myogenic rather than mixed or neurogenic scalp-recorded response.

In 1977, Harker et al. demonstrated that succinylcholine-induced muscle paralysis had no effect on MLRs recorded from a single subject (Dr. Lee Harker). They stated that the reason for the discrepancy with the Bickford et al. (1964) study was that the small number of averaged sweeps (150) was not sufficient to enhance the smaller-amplitude neurogenic MLRs but only the relatively large amplitude myogenic responses, which were subsequently abolished by curare. In 1983, Kileny et al. recorded MLRs in 12 patients after the administration of a nondepolarizing muscle relaxant (pancuronium) and the induction of narcotic (fentanyl) anesthesia in preparation for open-heart surgery. The responses were elicited by clicks presented at a moderate intensity level (60 dB nHL) usually not associated with a postauricular muscle reflex. Anesthesia by fentanyl and muscle paralysis

induced by pancuronium brought about minimal changes in MLR configuration and peak latencies, as shown in Figure 26.3. These findings ruled out a major myogenic contribution to the most consistent and robust component of the MLR, the Pa.

Neural Generators

The MLR generating system involves the interaction of many brain structures that include auditory specific structures central to the midbrain, as well as structures outside the primary auditory pathway such as the reticular formation and multi-sensory divisions of the thalamus.

Auditory Thalamo-Cortical Pathway

In human research, hypotheses regarding a temporal lobe origin for wave Pa are derived from studies reporting a polarity reversal across the Sylvian fissure (Vaughan and Ritter, 1970; Cohen, 1982; Celesia, 1968; Wood and Wolpaw, 1982a, 1982b, Lee et al., 1984) and from others showing intracranial responses at the latency of Pa (Chatrian et al., 1960, Ruhm et al., 1967, Lee et al., 1984). The contribution of the primary auditory cortex was questioned by Celesia and Pulletti (1971), who failed to detect a temporal correspondence between the scalp-recorded MLR and responses recorded from the exposed human primary auditory cortex. One of the authors (Kileny) also had the opportunity to record responses from the exposed human temporal cortex. These responses, illustrated in Figure 26.4 were obtained with surface electrodes placed in a close bipolar configuration on the posterior half of the superior temporal gyrus. As illustrated, a negative polarity peak (with respect to the noninverting electrode) with a midpoint latency of approximately 30 ms was obtained with this recording.

Dipole source analysis (Scherg and von Cramon, 1986) in normal and lesioned subjects provides evidence for a temporal lobe contribution to each of the MLR waves. For wave TP41, a generator located in the temporal lobe and oriented radially to the scalp has been suggested based on source analysis (Scherg and von Cramon, 1986), results from patients with cortical lesions (Knight et al., 1988) and neuromagnetic studies (Hari et al., 1987). For wave P1, neuromagnetic studies (Makela and Hari, 1987), correspondences between magnetic and electrical fields (Scherg et al., 1989), and data from patients with auditory pathway lesions (Scherg and von Cramon, 1986; Scherg et al., 1989) point to a temporal lobe source.

Case studies of patients with cortical lesions have largely supported a temporal lobe or thalamo-cortical origin for Pa. In patients with unilateral temporal lobe lesions, the most consistent finding has been a reduction in wave Pa amplitude over the lesioned temporal lobe in comparison to the intact hemisphere (Kraus et al., 1982; Kileny et al., 1987; Scherg and von Cramon, 1986; Pool et al., 1989). Wave Pa is usually disrupted

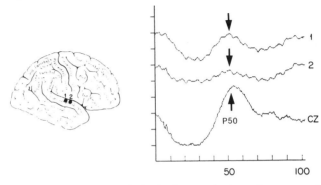

EXTRACRANIAL & CORTICAL INTRAOPERATIVE AEP

Figure 26.4. MLR recorded simultaneously from the exposed human temporal cortex and scalp (**Cz**). A P50 peak was recorded at all electrode locations. This is comparable with a delayed Pa peak due to halothane anesthesia.

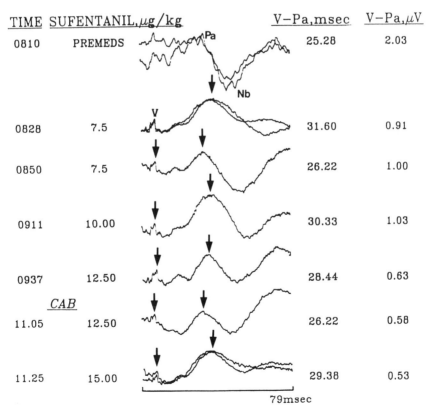

TIME	SUFENTANIL, μg/kg		V–Pa, msec	V–Pa, μV
0810	PREMEDS		25.28	2.03
0828	7.5		31.60	0.91
0850	7.5		26.22	1.00
0911	10.00		30.33	1.03
0937	12.50		28.44	0.63
CAB				
11.05	12.50		26.22	0.58
11.25	15.00		29.38	0.53

79msec

Figure 26.3. Paralysis by means of a nondepolarizing neuromuscular blocking agent (pancuronium) and anesthesia by means of an artificial narcotic (Fentanyl) have minimal effects on the MLR. Premeds: Premedication before anesthesia consisted of diazepam; **CAB:** Coronary artery bypass.

but not necessarily absent when bilateral temporal lesions are present (Graham et al., 1980; Ozdamar et al., 1983; Parving et al., 1980; Rosati et al., 1982; Woods et al., 1987). The persistence of wave Pa after some bilateral temporal lobe lesions suggests either that the temporal lobe generators were only partially damaged by the lesions or that the thalamus or the projections from thalamus may contribute substantially to the response. Woods (1987) has argued that only those temporal lobe lesions that have also damaged the thalamo-cortical pathway produce wave Pa abnormalities. Also feasible is that the intact Pa observed in some patients with bitemporal lobe lesions reflects the contributions of generating sources outside the auditory pathway.

Animal research provides the strongest evidence for a generating system consisting of contributions and interactions from multiple sources. In certain animals, MLR components from different generating systems are well separated topographically (Kaga et al., 1980; Buchwald et al., 1981; Chen and Buchwald, 1986; Farley and Starr, 1983; Arezzo et al., 1975; Kraus et al., 1988a; Comperatore and Patterson, 1988). In the guinea pig, two distinct MLR morphologies have been identified, one recorded over the temporal cortex and the other recorded over the posterior midline (McGee et al., 1983). These waves, referred to as "temporal" and "midline" components, appear to be mediated by distinct generating systems because they differ in response characteristics and course of development (Kraus et al., 1988).

In animals, MLR components obtained over the temporal lobe have been shown to be affected by lesions of the auditory cortex (Celesia, 1968; Kaga et al., 1980; Chen and Buchwald, 1986; Kraus et al., 1988). Reversible inactivation of axonal transmission with lidocaine has been used to investigate the neural structures underlying the MLR. Pharmacologic inactivation of auditory cortex did not disrupt waveform morphology although amplitude changes were observed (Kraus et al., 1988). Inactivation of the medial geniculate body (MGB) significantly affected auditory cortex and surface temporal responses (McGee et al., 1991).

The thalamo-cortical pathway appears to play an important role in the generation of the temporal response. Contributions from primary sensory portions of the thalamo-cortical pathways have been distinguished from contributions from association or extralemniscal portions of the system in an animal model (McGee et al., 1992). The primary (ventral) division of the medial geniculate body appears to be linked to the responses recorded over the temporal lobe in the guinea pig. The nonprimary, polysensory (caudo-medial) division of the nucleus appears to be linked to

both midline and temporal responses. Interestingly, primary and nonprimary pathway contributions to the MLR can also be distinguished functionally on the basis of their rate functions (Kraus et al., 1988) and their distinctive responses to binaural stimuli (Littman et al., 1992). Viewed together, these data suggest that both primary and non-primary components of the auditory thalamo-cortical pathway contribute to the MLR.

Reticular Formation

In children, wave Pa is affected by arousal state and thus by inference is tied to the reticular formation (Osterhammel et al., 1985; Collett et al., 1988; Kraus et al., 1989). Buchwald and colleagues (Buchwald et al., 1981; Hinman and Buchwald, 1983; Erwin and Buchwald, 1986) suggest that wave P1 is generated by thalamic nuclei that receive essential input from the midbrain reticular activating system. This wave is also affected by sleep stage (Erwin and Buchwald, 1986). The 40 Hz response, consisting partially of MLR activity, has also been tied to the reticular formation and is affected by sleep (Galambos et al., 1981).

Several lines of evidence point to the reticular formation as an important contributing source to the generation of the auditory middle latency response. Wave Pa is affected by arousal state (sleep) and is thus tied by inference to the reticular formation (Osterhammel et al., 1985; Dieber et al., 1989; Collett et al., 1988; Kraus et al., 1989). In the guinea pig model, pharmacologic inactivation of the mesencephalic reticular formation affects MLR waves reflecting both primary and nonprimary auditory pathway activity, functioning not unlike a power supply to both systems (Kraus et al., 1992).

Buchwald and colleagues (reviewed in Buchwald, 1990) provide considerable experimental evidence that human MLR wave P1 is generated by thalamic nuclei receiving essential input from the midbrain reticular activating system. In the cat, ablation experiments and correlations between intracranial and surface recordings point to the ascending RF as a generating source for a component occurring at 22 ms (Buchwald, 1981; Hinman and Buchwald, 1983). Both this wave and human P1 show decreases in amplitude during slow wave sleep with increases during REM sleep (Chen and Buchwald, 1986; Erwin and Buchwald, 1986a). Furthermore, human and cat waves share similar rate/recovery cycles (Erwin and Buchwald, 1986b) and appear to be generated by cholinergic neurons (Dickerson et al., 1986; Buchwald et al., 1991).

Further linking the RF to the MLR are data suggesting that the RF exerts modulatory influences on the MLR both during sleep and during classical conditioning and appears to include neurons capable of reducing thalamic inhibitory responses (Molnár et al., 1986, 1988). Additionally, the 40 Hz response, consisting partially of MLR activity, is affected by sleep and has thus been tied to the reticular formation (Galambos et al., 1981).

Midbrain

Evidence exists for both cortical and subcortical contributions to wave Na, which is sometimes considered a slow component of the ABR (the SN10). Subcortical origins have been postulated on theoretical grounds (Dieber et al., 1988), the resistance of Na to cortical lesions (Kileny et al., 1987), and the existence of a large negative wave at the latency of Na that is recorded at the level of the inferior colliculi (Hashimoto, 1982).

In animal models, aspiration of the inferior colliculi in the guinea pig resulted in an amplitude reduction of the slow negative component following the ABR (Caird and Klinke, 1987). Lidocaine injection into the inferior colliculus of the guinea pig affected all waves both at surface and depth locations. The disruption of local inferior colliculus activity correlated with changes in a surface wave that may be an animal analogue of wave Na. Thus, the midbrain appears to be important to the generation of wave Na (McGee et al., 1991).

SUMMARY

The multiple generators that contribute to the MLR include the auditory thalamo-cortical pathway, the mesencephalic reticular formation, and the inferior colliculus. The distinction between contributions from primary sensory versus association or extralemniscal portions of the thalamo-cortical pathway is evolving. A challenge is to understand how the activity from these regions combines to produce the fairly simple morphology of the middle latency response. Another challenge is to separate the contributions from these sources in humans, topographically and functionally so that dysfunction of components of the system can be identified clinically.

Clinically, the ability to topographically differentiate primary from nonprimary pathway activity using surface responses may hold promise for increasing the accuracy with which the MLR may identify discrete lesions of the respective pathways. In addition, the ability to detect subtle central auditory processing deficits may be enhanced. For example, "primary" auditory pathway abilities can be thought of as including such

functions as word recognition, discrimination, and figure-ground perception. Multimodal or "nonprimary" skills might include auditory attention, auditory-visual integration and auditory sequencing.

MATURATION AND SLEEP EFFECTS

For practical reasons, electrophysiologic testing is performed while children are asleep. However, numerous studies have demonstrated that the MLR is obtained inconsistently in children (Engel, 1971; Skinner and Glattke, 1977; Okitzu, 1984; Hirabayashi, 1979; Suzuki et al., 1983a, 1983b; Kileny, 1983; Kraus et al., 1985; Stapells et al., 1988; Collett et al., 1988) and it has been suggested that this inconsistency is sleep related. This inconsistency has been, although need not continue to be, a major factor limiting the clinical use of the MLR in children.

Although some amplitude and latency changes with sleep state may be observed in adults (Osterhammel et al., 1985; Okitsu, 1984; Osterhammel et al., 1985; Brown, 1982), there is general agreement that sleep does not impede MLR recording in adults as it does in children. However, the occurrence of the MLR (detectability) is not haphazard. A series of studies has revealed that a systematic process, linked to how sleep affects the generating system, underlies the maturational changes observed in the MLR. From birth to adolescence, the detectability of MLR waves recorded during sleep increases monotonically (Kraus et al., 1985). A trend of increased MLR detectability with age has also been observed in the more controlled context of an animal model (Kraus et al., 1987a; 1987c; 1988).

It appears that MLR in children are consistently present during certain stages of sleep, undetectable during other stages of sleep, and that detectability during those stages improves with age (Kraus et al., 1989). Figure 26.5 shows the percent detectability of wave Pa as a function of sleep state. Pa detectability was consistently high during wakefulness, stage 1 and REM sleep, but poor during stage 4, and variable during stages 2 and 3. This has the important clinical implication that if sleep state can be tracked during a test session, and MLR is recorded only during favorable periods, then the MLR may be a reliable measure for clinical use in children.

Data on the MLR generating system combined with the data on MLR development indicate that generators involving the auditory thalamo-cortical pathway are responsible for the robust MLR typically seen in adults (Kraus et al., 1988). Other inconsistently active generators such as the reticular formation also contribute to the response. Without the thalamo-cortical

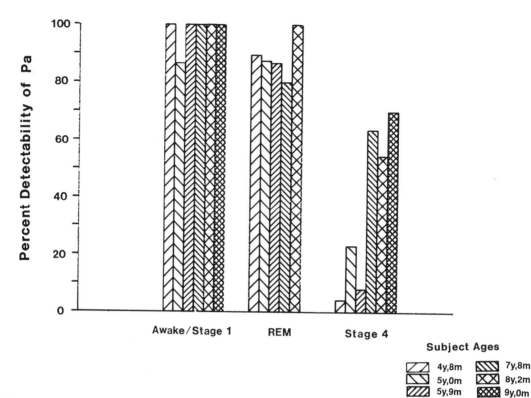

Figure 26.5. Percent detectability of Wave Pa as a function of sleep state in six normal children, ages 4 to 9 years. Each **bar pattern** denotes an individual child. Detectability of Pa was high during wakefulness, stage 1, and REM sleep, and lower during stage 4. During stage 4, Wave Pa was more likely to be present in the older children. (Reproduced from Kraus et al. 1989, with permission.)

contribution, the response comes and goes depending on the patient's level of alertness.

Under this premise, in adults the thalamo-cortical system imparts stability to the response, making the MLR consistently detectable regardless of sleep stage. In children, this system is only partially developed, not reaching maturity until puberty. The observed MLR is then dominated by the other, more labile generators. There is evidence that myelinization of the human thalamo-cortical pathway and sensory cortex continues until puberty (Yakovlev and Lecours, 1967; reviewed by Courchesne, 1990). The systematic development of MLR components observed in humans is consistent with such a maturational process (Kraus et al., 1985). Therefore development of the temporal lobe and the auditory thalamocortical pathway may account for increases in detectability with age.

The division of generators into an early developing labile generating system and another later developing stable system is supported by an animal model (Kraus et al., 1987, 1988). In gerbils, certain waves within the MLR latency period develop early while another set of components matures later in life. It is the later developing waves that have been linked closely to the thalamo-cortical pathway. The early developing waves have been linked to the function of the reticular formation (Kraus et al., 1988; Kraus et al., 1992).

Because the EEG and MLR frequency spectra overlap more in children than in adults, there has been speculation that the EEG may mask out the MLR in children, making it less detectable (Suzuki et al., 1983a; Kraus et al., 1987b). However, during stage 4, when the MLR is not detectable, the dominant EEG frequency is very low, less than 5 Hz. When this activity is filtered out, the MLR is still not detectable. Thus, it is our view that the changes seen in MLR truly reflect the development of MLR generators (Kraus et al., 1988, 1989), and the EEG changes reflect coincident neural development.

Clinical Implications

At Northwestern University, MLRs are recorded for clinical purposes from infants and children while sleep state is simultaneously monitored by observing ongoing EEG. With this arrangement, it appears that reliable 500 Hz MLR thresholds can be obtained. There are difficulties in the clinical application of this procedure: (*a*) The procedure is equipment-intensive, requiring an EEG system as well as an evoked potential system. (b) The clinician must be able to visually recognize the on-line EEG pattern characteristic of unfavorable periods, thus requiring considerable expertise.

However, the EEG of favorable and unfavorable periods is sufficiently disparate that computerized signal analysis techniques or a reasonably simple circuit probably could be used to detect favorable from unfavorable periods. Figure 26.6 shows two 10 second epochs of EEG from a 5-year-old child. One was recorded during a time period when the MLR was easily detectable; the other is from a time period when no MLR could be obtained. Differences are visually obvious, with the unfavorable period having a predominance of high amplitude, low frequency waves (delta activity). McGee et al., (1993) have proposed that favorable and unfavorable periods be detected by analyzing the EEG with a software algorithm, which computes the "delta ratio," a measure of the degree of delta activity in an EEG epoch.

The validation of the delta ratio as a parameter sensitive to the characteristics of favorable EEG activity is ongoing. Inasmuch as it is amenable to incorporation in a software algorithm or a hard-wired circuit, it could be the basis for on-line determination of periods favorable for reliable recording of the MLR and later potentials.

In summary, MLR components appear to be consistently obtained during wakefulness, stage 1, and REM sleep in young children. Reliable MLRs can be obtained in children with ongoing monitoring of sleep stage. Although the monitoring of sleep stages is impractical in most clinical settings, a means to automatically signal the clinician when the patient enters a sleep stage unfavorable for MLR is being developed by two of the authors (Kraus and McGee). Because every auditory evoked potential protocol for the assessment of hearing requires recording of the ABR, the clinician could obtain the ABR when conditions were unfavorable for the MLR and concentrate MLR recording during optimal periods.

CLINICAL APPLICATIONS

The MLR is used clinically in the electrophysiologic determination of hearing thresholds in the lower frequency range, the assessment of cochlear implant function, the assessment of auditory pathway function, the localization of auditory pathway lesions and intraoperative applications.

Assessment of 500–1000 Hz Thresholds

For assessing higher frequency sensitivity in cases of peripheral hearing loss, the auditory brainstem response (ABR) is the test of choice when behavioral methods cannot be used. The ABR, however, is highly dependent on neural synchrony and is best elicited by stimuli, such as clicks, with a rapid onset. Lower frequency stimuli (500–1000 Hz) inherently have a slower onset and therefore elicit a poorly defined ABR. The response is small and may be undetectable in clinical situations. Inasmuch as the MLR is less dependent than the ABR on neural synchrony (Vivion et

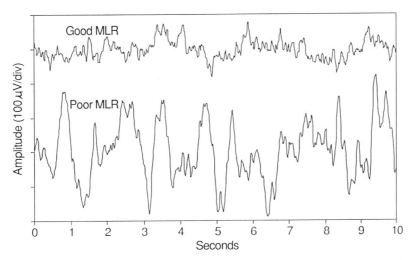

Figure 26.6. Two 10-sec epochs of EEG from a 5-year-old child. The **top record** was obtained when the MLR was present. The **bottom record** was obtained when the MLR was absent.

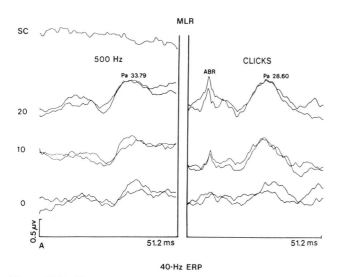

Figure 26.7. Silent control (**SC**) and MLR evoked by 500 Hz tonebursts and clicks presented at 20, 10, and 0 dB nHL from a normal hearing subject. (Reproduced from Kileny and Shea, 1986, with permission.)

al., 1980), it can be valuable in the assessment of low frequency sensitivity. MLRs in response to clicks and tones in a normal hearing subject are shown in Figure 26.7. The MLR reflects the subject's normal hearing at 500 Hz. Figure 26.8 illustrates the use of the MLR as a test of low frequency hearing sensitivity in a patient with a moderate to severe sloping hearing loss. No ABR was obtained to either click or 500 Hz stimuli. The MLR provided the only electrophysiologic indication that this patient had hearing in the lower frequencies.

It has been demonstrated in adults that the MLR will accurately reflect low frequency hearing thresholds (Zerlin and Naunton, 1974; Musiek and Geurnink, 1981; Scherg and Volk, 1983). The MLR in children is of chief interest, however, because an accurate electrophysiologic measure of low frequency hearing thresholds is essential to the appropriate management of hearing loss in children too young to be tested by behavioral audiometric methods. The infor-

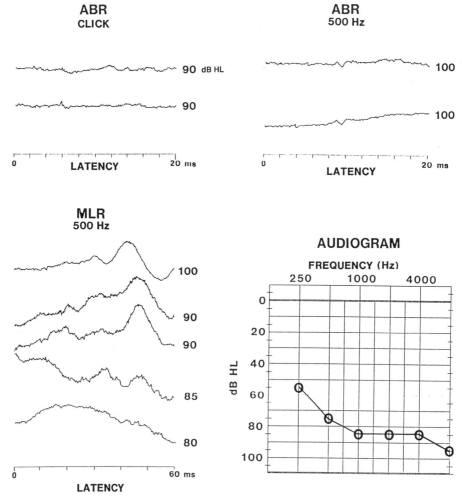

Figure 26.8. ABR and MLR recorded from a patient with moderate to severe sloping sensorineural hearing loss. ABR was absent with either click or 500 Hz stimuli. The MLR threshold of 85 dB nHL reflects this patient's hearing in the lower frequencies.

mation obtained is particularly important for children who have residual hearing only in the low frequencies. For other children, knowledge of low frequency thresholds can be critical to the appropriate fitting of a hearing aid. Since for practical reasons electrophysiologic testing is performed during sleep, the response must be reliable in sleeping children. As discussed above, it is important that sleep state be monitored during recording in pediatric populations.

Assessing Threshold When Neural Synchrony Is Impaired

Because the ABR is highly dependent on neural synchrony within the brainstem auditory pathway, dam-

age can result in an abnormal or absent response. This occurs even when the peripheral hearing mechanism is functional, e.g., in infants sustaining diffuse neurologic damage as a consequence of perinatal asphyxia, hyperbilirubinemia, or head trauma (Worthington and Peters, 1980; Kraus et al., Özdamar, Stein, Reed 1985). Nevertheless, the MLR can often be recorded in these patients. An example is illustrated in Figure 26.9. Although the ABR is absent, the click-evoked MLR reflects the patient's audiologic threshold of 30 dB HL. Kavanaugh et al., (1989) obtained click-evoked MLRs in four hearing-impaired, multiply handicapped patients lacking ABRs. Although the peripheral hearing mechanism or the brainstem pathway may have been deficient in the synchrony necessary to

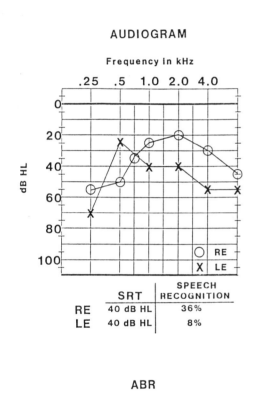

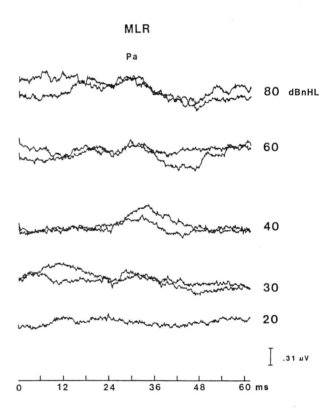

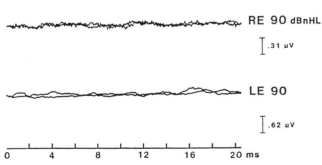

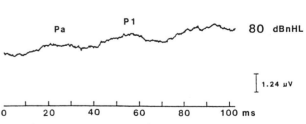

Figure 26.9. Damage to the brainstem in the vicinity of the generators of the ABR may result in an abnormal or completely absent response, even when behavioral hearing thresholds show only a mild or moderate hearing loss. The MLR may still be present in these patients, accurately reflecting this 30 dB HL threshold.

produce an ABR, the MLR provided information about hearing sensitivity at all frequencies important for understanding speech.

Cochlear Implants (Figs. 26.10–26.12)

Over the past 5 to 10 years, cochlear implants have become the standard of care for partial hearing restoration in profound sensorineural hearing loss in adults and children. The introduction of this new management modality has also created the need for the adaptation of well-known auditory diagnostic and neurodiagnostic procedures to the realm of electrical stimulation. There is as much need for the establishment of electrical thresholds by means of evoked potential measures as there is for the establishment of acoustic thresholds. The introduction of electrical evoked potential techniques brought with it a complexity of problems far in excess of those encountered with acoustic stimulation. Recording problems such as the unwanted spread of the electrical stimulus artifact to the recording electrode, problems with directing the electrical stimulus to the desired neural structures, and other difficulties have underscored the need for the understanding and careful control of recording parameters, such as filter settings, filter slopes, and amplification.

One of the inherent advantages of the MLR over the ABR in electrical evoked potential applications is the relatively remote time frame of wave Pa from the onset of the electrical artifact when compared to the relevant component of the ABR. Because of this, the ABR is far more likely to be contaminated and distorted by the spread of the electrical artifact than is the MLR. This was primarily the rationale behind studies comparing electric MLR to behavioral thresholds (Kileny and Kemink, 1987) and an intrasubject comparison of electric and acoustic MLR characteristics (Kileny et al., 1989).

Another advantage of the MLR over the ABR in electrical stimulation applications is the possibility of eliciting the response with relatively long-duration pulses, such as 2.5 ms per phase (analogous to the possibility of evoking the acoustic MLR with relatively long-duration tone-bursts), resulting in the utilization of a lower current level to elicit a response. Figure 26.10 shows the overall configuration of the electrically evoked MLR was similar to the acoustically evoked MLR. A notable difference is the earlier latency of the electrical Pa when compared to the acoustic Pa. These comparisons were done in patients who were unilaterally deaf, allowing the comparison of an electrically evoked MLR from the deaf ear to an acoustically evoked MLR from the normal-hearing ear.

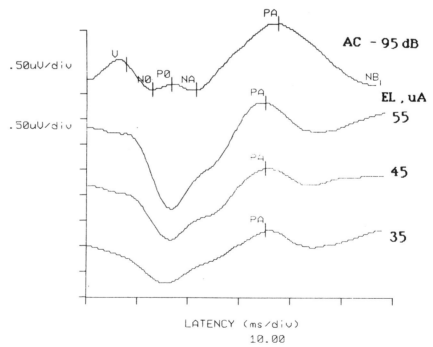

Figure 26.10. Comparison of acoustic MLR evoked by 95 dB nHL clicks delivered to a subject's normal hearing ear to electric MLR evoked by 2.5 ms/phase charge balanced biphasic rectangular pulses delivered to the subject's deaf ear by means of a needle electrode placed over the round window before labyrinthectomy. (Reproduced from Kileny et al., 1989, with permission.)

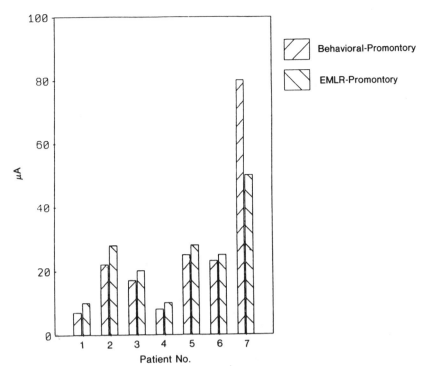

Figure 26.11. Relationship between behavioral and electric middle latency responses evoked by transtympanic promontory stimulation in seven patients. (Reproduced from Kileny and Kemink, 1987, with permission.)

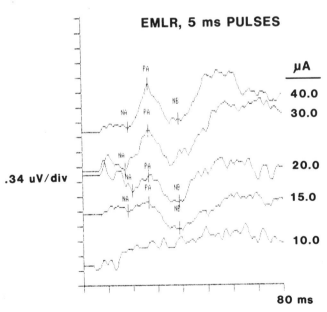

Figure 26.12. Electric MLR intensity series obtained preoperatively with transtympanic promontory stimulation from a patient subsequently implanted with a Cochlear Corporation multi-electrode implant.

In threshold determinations, it was found that MLR thresholds closely approximated behavioral thresholds in most cases (Fig. 26.11). For clinical use in patients less than 13 or 14 years of age, the electric MLR, like the acoustic MLR, must be coupled with the simultaneous monitoring of sleep state (Fig. 26.12).

Intraoperative Applications

Due to its susceptibility to anesthetic agents, the MLR is not the auditory evoked response component of choice for monitoring the integrity of the auditory pathway during surgical procedures. The MLR is significantly affected by a variety of anesthetic agents, especially halogenated agents, although it has been established that it can be reliably maintained under a nitrous oxide with a narcotic such as fentanyl or sufentanil anesthesia. Thus, the MLR has been used intraoperatively during open-heart surgery and cochlear implant surgery. An investigation of the MLR in open-heart surgery indicated that the response is particularly sensitive to changes in blood pressure or perfusion pressure (Kileny et al., 1985).

The cortical origins of the MLR may make it a useful intraoperative tool when it is necessary to monitor cortical function. In addition, at times it may be reasonable to choose the MLR over the ABR for monitoring purposes because of its latency characteristics, as would be the case when electrical stimulation is used to elicit the response. In this situation, the prolonged latency of the MLR makes it less sensitive to contamination by the spread of the electrical stimulus artifact than the ABR.

Neurodiagnostic Applications

The MLR has been shown to reflect damage to the auditory thalamo-cortical pathway. With unilateral auditory cortex lesions, the amplitude of wave Pa is diminished or absent over the lesioned hemisphere (Kraus et al., 1982; Scherg and von Cramon, 1986; Kileny et al., 1987). Testing requires the use of a coronal montage with electrodes at Cz and over each temporal lobe (halfway between Cz and the mastoid). An example of the response using a coronal electrode montage with a patient having left temporal lobe damage is shown in Figure 26.13.

The hemispheric asymmetry in these cases has sparked speculation that the scalp topography of the MLR holds clinical information. Fueling the speculation is the availability of brain mapping systems that

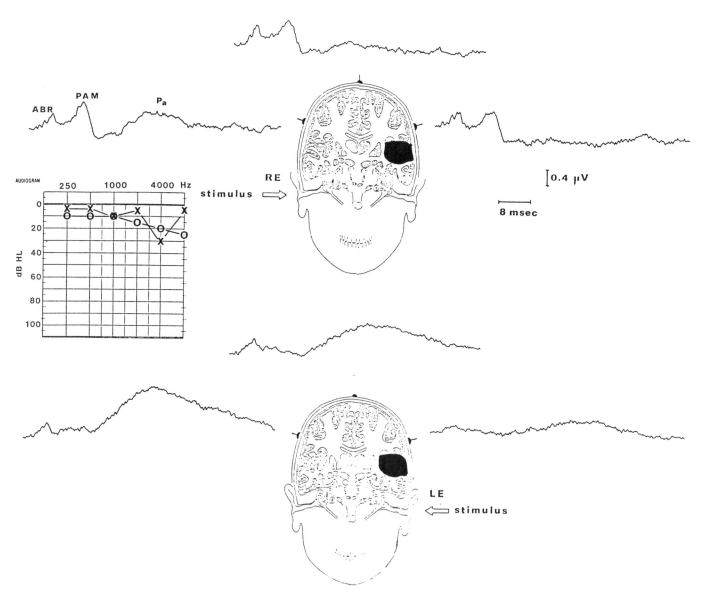

Figure 26.13. Coronal distribution of wave Pa in a patient with a left temporoparietal lesion and severe Wernicke's aphasia. Pa was largest over the intact hemisphere relative to vertex, and absent over the lesioned hemisphere regardless of the ear stimulated. The patient's puretone audiogram is shown on the left. **PAM** refers to posterior auricular muscle reflex. (Reproduced from Kraus et al., 1982, with permission.)

WAVE Pa

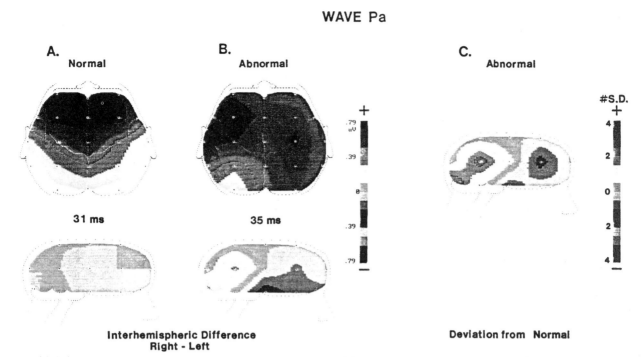

**Interhemispheric Difference
Right - Left**

Deviation from Normal

Figure 26.14. Top view of the scalp topography at the latency of Wave Pa showing a normal (**top, left**) and an abnormal response (**top, middle**). When right hemispheric Pa values are subtracted from left hemispheric values, the resulting map is green, indicating little interhemispheric differences in normal subjects (**bottom, left**). The interhemispheric Pa amplitude difference is illustrated for an abnormal-looking map (**bottom, right**). When these differences are compared to the normal population using the z statistic, this subject's data falls outside two standard deviations at several electrode locations (**right**). (Reproduced from Kraus and McGee, 1988, with permission.)

allow recording and visualization of the scalp topography in a clinically practical manner (Kraus and McGee, 1988; Jacobson and Grayson, 1988; Pool et al., 1989). For Wave Pa, the analysis of interhemispheric symmetry holds promise as a strategy for assessing abnormal response patterns. Figure 26.14 shows a top view of the scalp topography at the latency of Pa showing a normal (**top, left**) and an abnormal response (**top, middle**). When right hemispheric Pa values are subtracted from left hemispheric values, the resulting map is green, indicating little interhemispheric difference in normal subjects (**bottom, left**). The interhemispheric Pa amplitude difference is illustrated for an abnormal-looking map (**bottom, middle**). When these differences are compared to the normal population using the z statistic, this subject's data fall outside 2 SD at several electrode locations (**right**).

There are indications that alternative electrode configurations will yield additional human MLR components. Specifically, using a noncephalic reference, a positive component at about 45 ms (TP41) can be recorded over the temporal area (Knight et al., 1988; Cacace et al., 1990). Although research on the topography of the MLR is just beginning, many see mapping as a potentially valuable clinical technique.

Wave P1 (or Pb) has also been investigated as an index of auditory pathway dysfunction. This wave is thought to reflect activity of the reticular activating system that modulates attention to sensory stimuli (Buchwald et al., 1981; Hinman and Buchwald, 1983; Erwin and Buchwald, 1986). Abnormalities of this MLR component have been associated with Alzheimer's disease (Buchwald et al., 1989), autism (Buchwald et al., 1992) schizophrenia (Erwin et al., 1988), and stuttering (Hood et al., 1990). P1 is also affected by handedness (Hood et al., 1989), which may suggest some modulatory influence from the cortex.

Summary of Clinical Uses

Clinical uses of the MLR include the electrophysiologic determination of hearing thresholds for low frequencies, the assessment of hearing thresholds at all sound frequencies in patients with abnormal ABR due to neurologic damage to the brainstem, and in the pre- and post-operative management of patients with cochlear implants. The MLR can be used in the localization of auditory pathway lesions, the diagnosis of syndromes that compromise the MLR generating system and intraoperative monitoring.

ISSUES OF RECORDING PARAMETERS/PROCEDURES (FIGS. 26.15 AND 26.16)

Stimulus Rate

Wave Pa is generally obtained at a stimulation rate of 10/sec (Picton et al., 1974), while TP41 and P1 are more rate sensitive and are obtained at rates of 1–2/sec (Cacace et al., 1990; Erwin and Buchwald, 1986). For Pa, there is a general trend toward increasing amplitude with slower stimulation rates (Picton et al., 1974; McFarland et al., 1975). In experimental animals, some MLR waves also follow this trend (Buchwald et al., 1981; McGee et al., 1983; Knight et al., 1985; Kraus et al., 1987).

Clinical Implications

There has been speculation that slowing down the stimulation rate may make Pa more detectable in children. Jerger et al. (1987) describe a rate-dependent peak at about 50 ms in human infants which they suggest is a developmentally early version of Pa. It is observed at rates of 1–2/sec but seldom observed at rates of more than 4/sec. Also possible is that this peak represents component P1 which is extremely rate sensitive even in adults (Erwin and Buchwald, 1986b). Our own experience is that slowing the rate enhances neither the detectability nor amplitude of wave Pa in children consistently. Nevertheless, one can take the clinically conservative approach of reducing rate for cases in which the MLR is difficult to detect.

HIGH-PASS FILTER EFFECTS

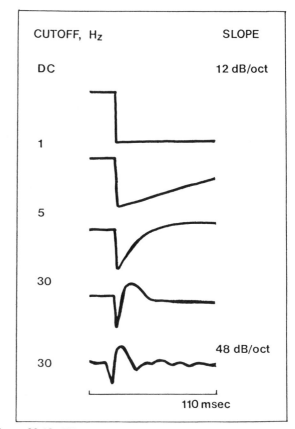

Figure 26.16. Effects on a step function of varying high-pass filter cut-off and filter slope.

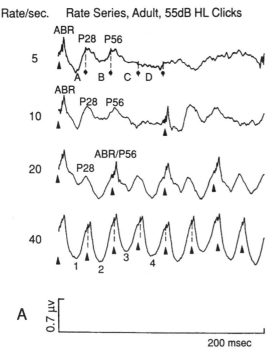

A

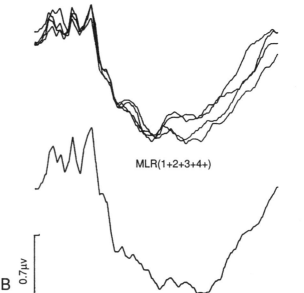

B

Figure 26.15. A, MLR rate series demonstrating the development of the 40-Hz response. **Arrows** indicate the timing of the stimulus at various rates. **B,** Comparison of the result of the summation of four consecutive 25-ms segments of a "standard" MLR (**bottom**) to four superimposed 25-ms segments of a 40-Hz response.

The 40 Hz Response

An exception to the trend of improved amplitude with slower rate occurs at a stimulation rate of 40/sec. This rate produces larger amplitude responses than are observed at slower rates (Galambos et al., 1981; Suzuki et al., 1984; Stapells et al., 1984; Kileny and Shea, 1976). This effect may be due, in part, to a superimposition of ABR and MLR waves, which are typically 21–25 msec apart in adults. Suzuki and Kobayashi (1984) found that in children, an amplitude maximum occurred at rates of 20–30/sec, corresponding with an average ABR-Pa latency difference of 31 msec observed in those children.

However, the 40 Hz response may be more than just a superimposition of waves. A 40 Hz response can also be elicited by visual and somatosensory stimuli. Furthermore, in adults, 40 Hz responses are more affected by sleep than the ABR or MLR. This indicates that, at least in adults, the 40 Hz response may be influenced by generators in addition to those of the ABR and MLR.

Recording Filters

Low Filter Setting

Suzuki and colleagues (1983, 1984) reported that MLR variability in both children and adults can be reduced when EEG activity below 20 Hz is filtered out, although settings higher than 20 Hz caused unacceptable amplitude reductions in the child MLR. In a study of 217 children, Kraus et al. (1987a) examined MLR detectability, amplitude, and latency using two filtering conditions: (a) 3–2000 Hz with a 6 dB/octave slope and (b) 15–2000 Hz with a 12 dB/octave slope. In all age groups studied, the detectability of waves Na and Pa was better with highpass filter settings of 15 Hz than with lower settings. These results are consistent with the hypothesis that large amplitude, low frequency EEG activity obscures MLRs in children. Although a high-pass filter setting of 10–15 Hz can enhance MLR in children, it does not solve the problem of response lability. Even with optimum filter settings, response detectability varies, as has been discussed.

The amplitude of MLR waves increases as filter settings are lowered from 30 to 3 Hz, in human adults (McGee et al., 1988) and in developing experimental animals (Kraus et al., 1987). In children, no trends are obvious.

High Filter Setting and Filter Slope

Two other technical issues arise with filtering. One concerns the high filter setting. The spectral energy for the MLR lies below 100 Hz, and no significant changes in the morphology or latency of Pa are seen with settings greater than 300 Hz (McGee et al., 1988). However, when the appropriate equipment is available, it is often desirable to open the filters to 2000–3000 Hz to allow simultaneous recording of the ABR (Suzuki et al., 1981; Özdamar and Kraus, 1983).

The second issue concerns the slope of the response filter. Scherg (1982), and Kraus et al. (1987) demonstrated that steep (24–48 dB/octave) analog filtering causes distortion of the MLR and the emergence of nonphysiologic peaks. That is, in patients with no MLR, the steep filters produce an MLR-like artifact. This artifact may be a distorted ABR and for this reason correlates with the presence of hearing. However, the ABR is better recorded with the filter settings usually recommended. In recording the MLR, analog filtering of 6 or 12 dB/octave yields an undistorted waveform (see Fig. 24.16).

RECOMMENDED PARAMETERS FOR CLINICAL APPLICATIONS

Tonal Thresholds

The primary differences between an MLR protocol and a typical ABR protocol are the wider filter settings and longer time base required for the MLR. The equipment settings for recording the MLR are summarized in Table 26.1. For the assessment of hearing sensitivity, a protocol involving both the ABR and MLR has been described (Kraus and McGee, 1990).

Table 26.1.
Stimulus and Recording Parameters for Middle Latency Response

Electrodes
  G1: Cz
  G2: ipsi mastoid or earlobe
  Ground: forehead

Stimuli
  Monaural rarefaction clicks
  Monaural tone bursts
    Envelope: 4-1-4 ms (500 Hz); 2-1-2 ms (1000 Hz), linear ramp
    2-0-2 ms, Blackman ramp

Recording parameters
  Time base: 60, 80, or 100 ms
  Low filter:
    Adults: 3–15 Hz
    Children: 10–15 Hz
  High filter: 300 Hz or 2–3 kHz (to include ABR)
  Filter slope: 6 or 12 dB/octave or digital filtering
  Rate: 11/second

Simultaneous ABR and MLR recording
  Computer capabilities to:
    1. record with a dual time base or
    2. record time window suitable for the MLR, at a sampling rate fast enough for ABR; expand initial segment to view ABR

Because many patients potentially have neurologic problems, the click-evoked ABR is used to assess brainstem function. The click-evoked ABR is also used to assess hearing for the higher frequencies. The ABR and the MLR are obtained in response to 500 and 1000 Hz tone bursts as a measure of hearing sensitivity for the lower frequencies. The ABR and MLR are recorded simultaneously, either on separate channels, or using a single channel, with a recording system having a fast sampling rate (<20 μsec/pt), and the capability to expand the initial portion of the 60–100 ms recording epoch.

Clinical experience over the past 10 years has indicated this procedure to be effective in predicting degree and configuration of hearing loss. An approach involving threshold estimation of threshold using a mathematical model (McGee et al., 1988) is likely to allow further refinement of the clinical protocol and more precise prediction of hearing thresholds.

Assessment of Auditory Pathway Function

Because of the multiple neural sources contributing to the MLR, it is necessary to observe the topography of the response to detect abnormalities in the generating system. The most parsimonious electrode montage (coronal) consists of active electrodes at Cz and over the temporal lobes (Kraus et al., 1982). The activity from these sites is referenced to the earlobe ipsilateral to the stimulated ear (Fig. 26.17). Normal and ab-

normal topographies are described above. Recording parameters are the same as in Table 26.1. Monaural, 70 dB click stimuli are used.

SUMMARY AND CONCLUSIONS

The MLR provides a clinical electrophysiologic tool that extends our assessment of the auditory system beyond the brainstem to the thalamo-cortical auditory pathway. Its clinical applications range from threshold determination (electric and acoustic) to the determination of site of lesion and intraoperative monitoring. The MLR is less dependent than the ABR on neural synchrony. As such, the MLR has advantages in the clinical assessment of low frequency hearing, since those nerve fibers show poorer synchrony. Also, in clinical cases where neural synchrony is impaired, the MLR may remain robust while the ABR is absent.

The MLR is a multicomponent response, receiving contributions from both the primary and the nonprimary auditory pathway. The MLR generators from these two pathways appear to have different developmental time courses, with the nonprimary generators dominating the response in young children. Complicating clinical use is the finding that the nonprimary generators are sleep stage dependent. If children are to be tested while sleeping, sleep state must be monitored, and the MLR must be recorded during favorable states.

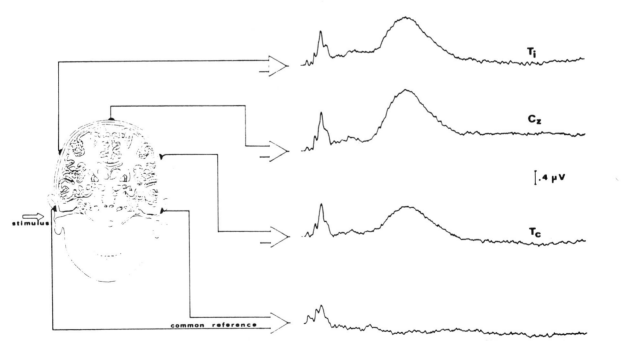

Figure 26.17. Recording configuration used for obtaining the coronal distribution of the MLR. Responses are recorded simultaneously from vertex (**Cz**) and temporal (**TI** and **TC**) electrodes referenced to the ipsilateral mastoid. The coronal distribution characteristic of normal subjects in whom Pa amplitude is largest at the vertex, symmetrical between temporal lobe recording sites and absent between the mastoids is demonstrated. (Reproduced from Kraus et al., 1982, with permission.)

The combined use of ABR and MLR in clinical assessment provides the advantages of both responses. Although some adjustments must be made in the equipment settings, the similarity of electrode placement and stimulus paradigm makes the recording of both measures clinically practical. Thus, it is reasonable to make the MLR an integral component in the audiologist's clinical armamentarium. The incorporation of additional electrophysiogic measures in routine clinical practice is consistent with the concept of a comprehensive evaluation approach to assess auditory pathway function. Such an evaluation combines various electrophysiologic measures with audiometry, tympanometry, and behavioral assessment of auditory function, with tests being selected according to the patient's symptomatology. As the ABR, MLR, later cortical potentials, and otoacoustic emissions become more familiar to clinicians, a comprehensive evaluation approach becomes feasible. We expect that such an approach will allow a better delineation of auditory disorders than is now available, vastly improving our clinical diagnostic capabilities.

REFERENCES

Arezzo J, Pickoff A, and Vaughan HG. The sources and intracerebral distribution of auditory evoked potentials in the alert rhesus monkey. Brain Res 1975;90:57–73.

Bickford et al. MLR is totally myogenic bochenek and bochenek (1976). PAM is at 12 ms.

Buchwald J, Erwin R, Van Lancker D, Schwafel T, and Tanguay P. Midlatency auditory evoked responses: P1 abnormalities in adult autistic subjects. Electroenceph Clin Neurophysiol 1992;84:164–171.

Buchwald JS, Erwin RJ, Read S, Van Lancker D, and Cummings JL. Midlatency auditory evoked responses: Differential abnormality of P1 in Alzheimer's disease. Electroenceph Clin Neurophysiol 1989;74:378–384.

Buchwald JS, Hinman C, Norman RS, Huang CM, and Brown KA. Middle- and long-latency auditory evoked potentials recorded from the vertex of normal and chronically lesioned cats. Brain Res 1981;205:91–109.

Cacace AT, Satya-Murti S, and Wolpaw JR. Human middle-latency auditory evoked potentials: Vertex and temporal components. Electroenceph. Clin. Neurophysiol 1990;77:6–18.

Caird DM, and Klinke R. The effect of inferior colliculus lesions on auditory evoked potentials. Electroenceph Clin Neurophysiol 1987;68:237–240.

Celesia GC. Auditory evoked response. Arch Neurol 1986;19:430–437.

Celesia GG, and Puletti F. Auditory input to the human cortex during states of drowsiness and surgical anesthesia. Electroenceph Clin Neurophysiol 1971;31:603–609.

Chatrian GE, Peterson MC, and Lazerte JA (1960). Responses to clicks from the human brain: Some depth electrographic observations. Electroenceph Clin Neurophysiol 1960;12:479–489.

Chen BM, Buchwald JS. Midlatency auditory evoked responses: Differential effects of sleep in the cat. Electroenceph Clin Neurophysiol 1986;65:373–382.

Cohen MM. Coronal topography of the middle latency auditory evoked potential in man. Electroenceph Clin Neurophysiol 1982;53:231–236.

Collett L, Duelaux R, Challand MJ, and Revol M. Effect of sleep on middle latency response (MLR) in infants. Brain Dev 1988;10:169–173.

Courchesne E. Chronology of postnatal human brain development: Event related potential, positron emission tomography, myelinogenesis and synaptogenesis studies. In Rohrbaugh J, Parasuraman R, and Johnson R, eds. Event Related Brain Potentials. New York: Oxford University Press, 1990:210–241.

Dieber MP, Ibanez V, Fischer C, Perrin F, and Manguiere F. Sequential mapping favors the hypothesis of distinct generators for N1 and P1 middle auditory evoked potentials. EEG Clin Neurophysiol 1988;71:187–197.

Engel R. Early waves of the electroencephalic auditory response in neonates. Neuropaediatrie 1971;3:147–154.

Erwin R, and Buchwald JS. Midlatency auditory evoked responses: Differential recovery cycle characteristics. Electroenceph Clin Neurophysiol 1986;64:417–423.

Erwin R, Buchwald JS. Midlatency auditory evoked responses: Differential effects of sleep in the human. Electroenceph Clin Neurophysiol 1986;65:383–392.

Erwin R, Mauhinney-Hec M, and Gur RE. Midlatency auditory evoked responses in schizophrenics. Neuroscience 1988;14:339(Abstr).

Farley GR, and Starr A. Middle and long latency auditory evoked potentials in cat. II. Component distributions and dependence on stimulus factors. Hear Res 1983;10:139–152.

Galambos R, Makeig S, and Talmachoff PJ. A 40 Hz auditory potential recorded from the human scalp. Proc Natl Acad Sci 1981;78:2643–2647.

Galambos R. Tactile and auditory stimuli repeated at high rates (30–50 per sec). produce similar event-related potentials. Ann NY Acad Sci 1981;388:722–728.

Geisler CD, Frishkopf LS, and Rosenblith WA. Extracranial responses to acoustic clicks in man. Science 1958;128:1210–1211.

Graham J, Greenwood R, and Lecky B. Cortical deafness: A case report and review of the literature. J Neurol Sci 1980;48:35–49.

Hari R, Pelizzone M, Mäkelä JP, Hällström J, Leinonen L, and Lounasmaa OV. Neuromagnetic responses of the human auditory cortex to on- and offsets of noise bursts. Audiology 1987;26:31–43.

Harker LE, Hosick E, Voots RJ, and Mendel M. Influence of succinylcholine on middle component auditory evoked potentials. Arch Otolaryngol 1977;103:133–137.

Hashimoto I. Auditory evoked potentials from the human midbrain: Slow brain stem responses. Electroenceph Clin Neurophysiol 1982;53:652–657.

Hinman CL, and Buchwald JS. Depth evoked potential and single unit correlates of vertex midlatency auditory evoked responses. Brain Res 1983;264:57–67.

Hirabayashi M. The middle components of the auditory electric response. I. On their variation with age. J Otolaryngol Jpn 1979;82:449–456.

Hood LJ, Martin DA, and Berlin CI. Auditory evoked potentials differ at 50 milliseconds in right- and left-handed listeners. Hear Res 1990;45:115–122.

Hood LJ, Martin DA, and Berlin CI. Auditory evoked potentials differ at 50 milliseconds in right and left-handed listeners. Hearing Res 1990;45:115–122.

Jacobson GP, and Grayson AS. The normal scalp topography of the middle latency auditory evoked potential Pa component following monaural click stimulation. Brain Topography 1988;1:29–36.

Jerger J, Chmiel R, Glaze D, and Frost JD. Rate and filter dependendence of the middle latency responses in infants. Audiology 1987;26:269–283.

Kaga K, Hink R, Shinoda Y, and Suzuki J. Evidence for a primary cortical origin of a middle latency auditory evoked potential in cats. Electroenceph Clin Neurophysiol 1980;50:254–266.

Kavanagh KT, Gould H, McCormick G, and Franks R. Comparison of the identifiability of the low intensity ABR and MLR in the mentally handicapped patient. Ear Hear 1989;10:124–130.

Kileny PR, Kemink JL, and Miller JM. An intrasubject comparison of electric and acoustic middle latency responses. Am J Otol 1989;10:23–27.

Kileny P, and Berry DA. Selective impairment of late vertex and middle latency auditory evoked responses. In Menches G, and Gerber S, Eds. The Multiply Handicapped Hearing Impaired Child. New York: Grune and Stratton, 1983.

Kileny PR, and Kemink JL. Electrically evoked middle-latency auditory potentials in cochlear implant candidates. Arch Otolaryngol Head Neck Surg 1987;113:1072–1077.

Kileny P, Paccioretti D, and Wilson AF. Effects of cortical lesions on middle-latency auditory evoked responses (MLR). Electroenceph Clin Neurophysiol 1987;66:108–120.

Kileny P, and Shea S. Middle-latency and 40-Hz auditory evoked responses in normal-hearing subjects: Click and 500-Hz thresholds. J Speech Hear Res 1986;19:20–28.

Knight RT, Brailowsky S, Scabini D, and Simpson GV. Surface auditory evoked potentials in the unrestrained rat: Component definition. Electroenceph Clin Neurophysiol 1985;61:430–439.

Knight RT, Scabini D, Woods DL, and Clayworth C. The effects of lesions of superior temporal gyrus and inferior parietal lobe on temporal and vertex components of the human AEP. Electroenceph Clin Neurophysiol 1988;70:499–509.

Kraus N, and McGee T. Clinical implications of primary and non-primary pathway contributions to the middle latency response generating system. Ear Hear 1993;14:36–48.

Kraus N, and McGee T. Color imaging of the human middle latency response. Ear Hear 1988;9:159–167.

Kraus N, and McGee T. Clinical applications of the middle latency response. J Am Acad Audiol 1990;1:130–133.

Kraus N, McGee T, Littman T, and Nicol T. Reticular formation influences on primary and non-primary auditory pathways as reflected by the middle latency response. Brain Res 1992;587:186–294.

Kraus N, McGee T, and Comperatore C. MLRs in children are consistently present during wakefulness, stage 1 and REM sleep. Ear Hear 1989;10:339–345.

Kraus N, Özdamar Ö, Hier D, and Stein L (1982). Auditory middle latency responses in patients with cortical lesions. Electroenceph Clin Neurophysiol 1982;54:247–287.

Kraus N, Özdamar Ö, Stein L, and Reed N. Absent auditory brain stem response: Peripheral hearing loss or brain stem dysfunction? Laryngoscope 1984;94:400–406.

Kraus N, Smith DI, and McGee T. Rate and filter effects on the developing middle latency response. Audiology 1987;26:257–268.

Kraus N, Smith DI, and McGee T. Midline and temporal lobe MLRs in the guinea pig originate from different generator systems: A conceptual framework for new and existing data. Electroenceph Clin Neurophysiol. 1988;70:541–558.

Kraus N, Smith DI, McGee T, Stein L, and Cartee C. Development of the auditory middle latency response in an animal model and its relationship to the human response. Hear Res 1987;27:165–176.

Kraus N, Smith D, Reed N, Stein L, and Cartee C. Auditory middle latency responses in children: Effects of age and diagnostic category. Electroenceph Clin Neurophysiol 1985;62:343–351.

Lee YS, Lueders H, Dinner DS, Lesser RP, Hahn J, and Klem G. Recording of auditory evoked potentials in man using chronic subdural electrodes. Brain Res 1984;107:115–131.

Littman T, Kraus N, McGee T, and Nicol T. Binaural stimulation reveals functional differences between midline and temporal components of the middle latency response in guinea pigs. Electroenceph clin Neurophysiol 1992;84:362–372.

Makela JP, and Hari R. Evidence for cortical origin of the 40 Hz auditory evoked response in man. Electroenceph Clin Neurophysiol 1987;66:539–546.

McFarland WH, Vivian MD, Wolf KE, and Goldstein R. Reexamination of effects of stimulus rate and number on the middle components of the averaged electroencephalic response. Audiology 1975;14:456–465.

McGee T, Kraus N, and Manfredi C. Toward a strategy for analyzing the human MLR waveforms. Audiology 1988;27:119–130.

McGee T, Kraus N, Littman T, and Nicol T. Contributions of medial geniculate body subdivisions to the middle latency response. Hear Res 1992;61:147–154.

McGee TJ, Kraus N, and Wolters C. Viewing the audiogram through a mathematical model. Ear Hear 1988;9:153–156.

McGee T, Kraus N, Comperatore C, and Nicol T. Subcortical and cortical components of the MLR generating system. Brain Res 1991;544:211–220.

McGee T, Kraus N, Killion M, Rosenberg R, and King C. Improving the reliability of the auditory middle latency response by monitoring EEG delta activity. Ear Hear 1993;14:76–84.

McGee T, Özdamar Ö, and Kraus N (1983). Auditory middle latency responses in the guinea pig. Am J Otolaryngol 1983;4:116–122.

Molnár M, Karmos G, Csépe V, and Winkler I. Intracortical auditory evoked potentials during classical aversive conditioning in cats. Biol Psych 1988;26:339–350.

Musiek FE, and Geurkink NA. Auditory brainstem and middle latency evoked response sensitivity near threshold. Ann Otol 1981;90:236–240.

Okitzu T. Middle components of auditory evoked response in young children. Scand Audiol 1984;13:83–86.

Osterhammel PA, Shallop JK, and Terkildsen K. The effect of sleep on the auditory brainstem response (ABR) and the middle latency response (MLR). Scand Audiol 1985;14:47–50.

Özdamar Ö, and Kraus N (1983). Auditory middle latency responses in humans. Audiology 1983;22:34–49.

Özdamar Ö, Kraus N, and Curry F. Auditory brainstem and middle latency responses in a patient with cortical deafness. Electroenceph Clin Neurophysiol 1983;53:275–287.

Parving A, Solomon G, Elbering C, Larsen B, and Lassen NA. Middle components of the auditory evoked response in bilateral temporal lobe lesions. Scand Audiol 1980;9:161–167.

Picton TW, Hillyard SA, Krausz HI, and Galambos R. Human auditory evoked potentials. I. Evaluation of components. Electroenceph Clin Neurophysiol, 1974;36:179–190.

Pool K, Finitzo T, Chi-Tzong-Hong, Rogers J, and Pickett RB. Infarction of the superior temporal gyrus: A description of auditory evoked potential latency and amplitude topology. Ear Hear 1989;10:144–152.

Rosati G, Bastiani PD, Paolino E, Prosser A, Arslan E, and Artioli M. Clinical and audiological findings in a case of auditory agnosia. J Neurol 1982;227:21–27.

Ruhm H, Walker E, and Flanigan H. Acoustically-evoked potentials in man: Mediation of early components. Laryngoscope 1967;77:806–822.

Scherg M. Distortion of the middle latency auditory response produced by analogue filtering. Scand Audiol 1982;11:57–69.

Scherg M, and Von Cramon D. evoked dipole source potentials of the human auditory cortex. Electroenceph Clin Neurophysiol 1986;65:344–360.

Scherg M, and Volk SA. Frequency specificity of simultaneously recorded early and middle latency auditory evoked potentials. Electroenceph Clin Neurophysiol 1983;56:443–452.

Scherg M, and Von Cramon D. Two bilateral sources of the late AEP as identified by a spatio-temporal dipole model. Electroenceph clin Neurophysiol 1985;62:32–44.

Scherg M, Hari R, Hänäläinen M. (in press). Frequency-specific sources of the auditory N19-P30-P50 response detected by a multiple source analysis of evoked magnetic fields and potentials. In Williamson S, Ed. Advances in Biomagnetism. New York: Plenum Publ. Corp., 1990.

Scherg M, Vajsar J, and Picton T. A source analysis of the late human auditory evoked potentials. J Cogn Neurosci 1989;1: 336–355.

Skinner P, and Glattke TJ. Electrophysiologic responses and audiometry: State of the art. J Speech Hear Dis 1977;42:179–198.

Stapells D, Galambos R, Costello J, and Makeig S. Inconsistency of auditory middle latency and steady-state responses in infants. Electroenceph Clin Neurophysiol 1988;71:289–295.

Stapells DR, Linden D, Suffield JB, Hamel G, and Picton TW. Human auditory steady state potentials. Ear Hear 1984;5: 105–113.

Suzuki T, and Kobayashi K. An evaluation of 40-Hz event-related potentials in young children. Audiology 1984;23:599–604.

Suzuki T, Hirabayashi M, and Kobayashi K. Effects of analog and digital filtering on auditory middle latency responses in adults and young children. Ann Otol 1984;93:267–270.

Suzuki T, Hirabayashi M, and Kobayashi K. Auditory middle latency responses in young children. Br J Audiol 1983b;17: 5–9.

Suzuki T, Hirabayashi M, and Kobayashi K. Frequency composition of auditory middle responses. Br J Audiol 1983a;17:1–4.

Suzuki T, Yasuhito H, and Kiyoko H. Simultaneous recording of early and middle components of auditory electric response. Ear Hear 1981;2:276–282.

Vaughan HG, Jr, Ritter W. The sources of auditory evoked responses recorded from the human scalp. Electroenceph Clin Neurophysiol 1970;28:360–367.

Vivion MC, Hirsh JE, Frye-Osier H, and Goldstein R. Effects of stimulus rise-fall time and equivalent duration on middle components of AER. Scand Audiol 1980;9:223–232.

Wood CC, and Wolpaw JR. Scalp distribution of human auditory evoked potentials. II. Evidence for overlapping sources and involvement of auditory cortex. Electroenceph Clin Neurophysiol 1982b;54:25–38.

Woods DL, Clayworth CC, Knight RT, Simpson GV, and Naeser MA. Generators of middle- and long-latency auditory evoked potentials: Implications from studies of patients with bitemporal lesions. Electroenceph Clin Neurophysiol 1987;68:132–148.

Worthington DW, and Peters JF. Quantifiable hearing and no ABR: paradox or error? Ear Hear 1980;5:281–285.

Yakovlev PL, and Lecours AR. The myelogenetic cycles of the regional maturation of the brain. In Regional Development of the Brain in Early Life. Philadelphia: Davis, 1967:3–70.

Zerlin S, and Naunton RF. Early and late averaged electroencephalic responses at low sensation levels. Audiology 1974;13: 366–378.

CHAPTER 27

Auditory Event-Related Potentials

Nina Kraus and Therese McGee

At poststimulus latencies of more than 50 msec, evoked potentials primarily reflect the activity of the thalamus and cortex, structures that involve the discriminative, integrative and attentional functions of the brain. Multiple structures and systems contribute to each auditory evoked potential (AEP) component. For example, responses from a primary sensory pathway may be modulated by the reticular and limbic systems, which in turn may generate additional components. Long latency responses also tend to be less modality-specific and need not depend on intact earlier potentials. Since the generators reflect brain areas which integrate input, similar responses can be obtained to auditory, visual or somatosensory stimuli. The longer latency AEPs are called event-related or late potentials.

A characteristic of event-related potentials is that they are affected less by the physical properties of the stimulus and more by the functional use that the organism has for the stimulus. That is, the response may be determined less by stimulus frequency or intensity and more by attention paid to the stimulus, a task associated with the stimulus, or stimulus change. The distinction between stimulus characteristics and functional use allows a distinction to be made between components. Evoked potentials that are primarily influenced by the stimulus characteristics are called "exogenous" components, while potentials which are highly dependent on attention or cogitive tasks are called "endogenous" components (Sutton et al., 1967; Donchin et al., 1978). The auditory brainstem response (ABR) clearly is exogenous while some of the later potentials, such as the N400, are clearly endogenous. For other potentials, the distinction is a matter of degree, where functional use of the signal is not essential but does affect response amplitude.

For some late potentials, variations in the task or recording paradigm result in significant changes in the response. Unlike the ABR and middle latency response (MLR), in which the peaks can be listed and the variations with stimuli or sleep stage can be described as latency or amplitude changes in a well-defined peak, a finite listing of peaks is controversial (Lovrich et al., 1988). As the paradigm changes or the subject's attentional state changes, waveform morphology varies such that an entirely different set of components can be recorded.

A focus of current research on late potentials has been to investigate the relationship between their characteristics and information processing such as encoding, selecting, memory, and decision making. Experimental designs are often borrowed from the domain of cognitive psychology. This research represents a convergence of paradigms and conceptual frameworks between psychological and physiologic research (Hillyard and Kutas, 1983; Rosler et al., 1986).

For the ABR and MLR, understanding of neural coding and response generators is quite detailed. Clinical applications are guided by an understanding of the underlying physiology, and animal models play a large role in the development of clinical techniques and the interpretation of results. In contrast, understanding of the generation of cortical responses is more limited. Clinical applications may center on correlating surface potential waveform changes with pathologic conditions or with stimulus variations, sidestepping altogether an understanding of physiologic cause and effect.

For clinical purposes, one must determine what paradigms would be sensitive to the clinical disorder of interest, and define the specific set of waveforms elicited by that paradigm. Then begins the process of developing norms, designing clinical test protocols, and establishing clinical validation. It is to be expected that a paradigm designed to consider acoustic processing of speech would differ from one designed to examine auditory attention or semantic processing, although the paradigms may result in waves which overlap in time. Both clinically and theoretically, one may envision more standardization in the future. It is also quite probable that future research will uncover as yet unknown responses.

Considering the complexity of the brain and the enormous number of possible permutations of simultaneous processes, it is hardly surprising that an altered stimulus/task paradigm would stimulate different brain centers and give rise to an altered summation of field potentials. Those variations do, however, make difficult the task of summarizing the cortical potentials in a finite list of peaks and valleys. We will discuss here the major auditory paradigms and their associated responses. This chapter is organized into the major headings: (a) description of responses, (b) responses to speech stimuli, (c) generating systems, (d) maturation, and (e) clinical applications. The study of the late evoked responses has been chronicled in literally thousands of articles. We provide here an overview.

The classic late auditory evoked potentials can be observed in the EEG at a poststimulus latency between 70 and 500 msec (Davis, 1939). Table 27.1 outlines major response components. The sequence usually described is N1, P2, N2 and P3 among others. P1 (sometimes referred to as Pb) can be considered either as a component of the middle latency response or the late AEPs. Waves are often denoted by polarity and latency (e.g., N100), and a number of subcomponents within the sequence have been reported. Event-related potentials are generally elicited either by a single repeating stimulus or by an "oddball" paradigm in which a deviant, or rarely occurring stimulus is presented within a series of frequent, or standard stimuli. One can readily comprehend the oddball paradigm by referring to

Table 27.1
Listing of Late Auditory Evoked (AEP) or Event-Related Potentials

Response	Abbreviation	Latency (msec)
N1, N1b (N100), N1c (N150)		80–250
P2		200
N2		200–400
Sustained negativity		Duration of stimulus
Cortical auditory evoked potential	CAEP	100–800 (infants)
Elicited with oddball paradigm		
Mismatch negativity	MMN	150–275
Nc		400–700
Processing negativity	Nd	60–700
P300, P3a, P3b		250–350
Cortical discriminative response	CDR	200–900 (infants)
N400		400

Figure 27.1. In this procedure, comparisons are made between the averaged responses to standard and deviant stimuli.

The mismatch negativity (MMN) component has particular relevance to audiology because it is an objective, neurophysiologic reflection of the processing of stimulus differences. It may provide a useful clinical measure of auditory discrimination. AEPs reflecting semantic, cognitive processing and attention include the N400, P300, and processing negativity.

The late auditory potentials are followed by the contingent negative variation (CNV), a slow, negative potential that usually depends upon the association between two successive stimuli. Stimulus conditions that produce the CNV are similar to Pavlovian conditioning. This response, which has gained widespread acceptance by psychologists is beyond the scope of this chapter.

DESCRIPTION OF RESPONSES

N1

In response to auditory stimuli in an awake subject, a negative wave, N1, occurs at a latency of about 100 msec. Several different processes generate waves associated with N1. Some components are mainly controlled by the physical and temporal features of the stimulus and by the general state of the subject, whereas others depend on discrimination, memory, and cognition (Näätänen and Picton, 1987).

N1b is largest at the vertex (midline) and has a latency of 100 msec, while N1c, shows a positive peak at 100 ms and negative trough at 150 ms, and is best recorded over the temporal lobes. They occur in response to the physical and temporal features of the stimulus (Wolpaw and Penry, 1975; McCallum and Curry, 1980). An N1a component was originally described by McCallum and Curry (1979, 1980). However, Perrault and Picton (1984) were unable to dissociate N1a from N1b in a variety of conditions and

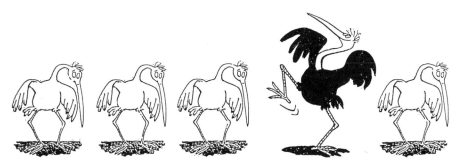

Figure 27.1. Schematic representation of the oddball paradigm. A stimulus sequence in which a deviant (rare) stimulus occurs within a series of homogeneous, or standard (frequent), stimuli.

suggested that N1a and N1b represented the same cerebral process. Another stimulus-bound component is the "sustained potential," a negative baseline shift that lasts for the duration of the stimulus. Most of the evoked potentials discussed here are generated by neurons that respond chiefly to stimulus onset. The sustained potential, as one might suspect, reflects activity from auditory cortex neurons which sustain a response for the duration of the stimulus.

Mismatch Negativity

N1 can be elicited by a stimulus train consisting of the repetition of identical stimuli. If a "deviant" stimulus (which is physically different from the aforementioned train of identical stimuli) is inserted in the stimulus train, the N1 will still be elicited but an additional negativity appears, lasting another 100 msec. This is called the "mismatch negativity" or MMN (Näätänen et al., 1978). The MMN reflects central processing of very fine differences in acoustic stimuli. It can occur when the difference between the standard and deviant stimuli is as small as 8 Hz or 5 dB, even when stimulus differences are near psychophysical threshold (Näätänen, 1992; Sams et al., 1985; Kraus et al., 1993a; Sharma et al., 1993). MMN has been obtained in response to frequency, intensity, duration, spatial and phonemic changes (Sams et al., 1985, 1990; Näätänen 1990; Näätänen et al., 1987, 1989; Snyder and Hillyard, 1976; Novak et al., 1990; Kaukoranta et al., 1989; Paavilainen et al., 1989; Aaltonen et al., 1987; Ritter et al., 1979). Consequently, it appears that the MMN reflects a neuronal representation of the discrimination of numerous auditory stimulus attributes. If this response reflects the ability to discriminate between acoustic stimuli, then it may not only be of research interest but may have clinical value because speech perception, by its very nature, depends on a neuronal response to stimulus change.

The MMN is passively-elicited, not requiring attention (Näätänen et al., 1991; Novak et al., 1992) or a behavioral response. It has been obtained during sleep in infants (Alho et al., 1990) and adults (Nielsen-Bohlman et al., 1988), and during sleep and barbiturate anesthesia in animal models (Csépe et al., 1987). This suggests that the MMN is an automatic, preattentive response to stimulus change. Thus, the MMN is a potential clinical tool for the objective evaluation of patients for whom communication is difficult or compromised, or for whom auditory discrimination is in question (at-risk infants, children with language or learning disorders, cochlear implant users, adults with aphasia or dementia) (Näätänen, 1992; Korpilahti et al., 1992; Kraus et al., 1993b).

A large volume of data indicates that the MMN is a robust phenomenon in adult subjects (Näätänen, 1992, review). More recently, the MMN has been shown to be robust in children (Kraus et al., 1992; 1993a; Csépe et al., 1992). The MMN has been shown to be robust in grand averaged group data. It can also be robust in individual subjects but requires statistical procedures to ensure response validity (Lang et al., 1992; Kraus et al., 1993a, 1993b). The apparent stability of the MMN in individuals is promising for eventual clinical application because the absence of a response can legitimately be considered abnormal. Representative MMNs are shown for one adult and one child in Figure 27.2. The MMN can be seen in the response to the deviant stimulus at

REPRESENTATIVE SUBJECTS

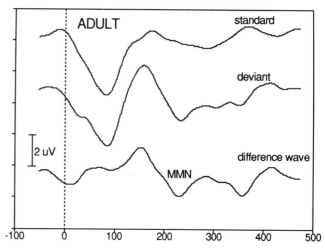

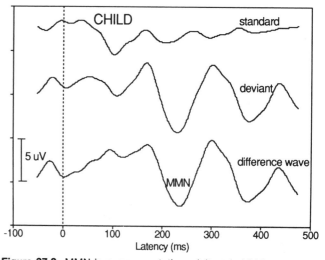

Figure 27.2. MMN in a representative adult and child in response to synthesized speech stimuli /ga/ and /da/. The MMN is evident in response to the deviant stimuli and in the difference waveform, obtained by subtracting the ERP to the standard stimulus from the ERP to deviant stimuli (Reprinted from Kraus et al., Ear Hear 1992;13:158-164).

about 235 msec. The MMN also is evident in the difference waves, obtained by subtracting the response to the standard stimulus from the response to the deviant stimulus.

Processing Negativity

The "processing negativity" (Nd) is a broad, negative, attention-related response which also occurs within, and extends after, the N1 time frame, increasing the amplitude of the N1 component (Hink et al., 1978; Donald and Little, 1981; Okita 1981; Hillyard and Kutas, 1983). Selective attention to stimuli elicits a large negative potential. To separate this component from the N1 component, typically the response to the unattended stimulus is subtracted from the response to the attended stimulus and the difference is termed the "Nd" (Näätänen, 1975; Hillyard and Picton, 1979; Hansen and Hillyard, 1980). The Nd appears to be related to memory and cognition. Initially, this early attention effect was viewed as an augmentation of the evoked N1 wave to attended-channel stimuli (Hillyard et al., 1973), but recent studies have shown that the negativity can extend well beyond the normal time course of the N1 and is primarily endogenous in nature (Näätänen and Michie, 1979; Okita, 1979; Hansen and Hillyard, 1980). The Nd has been resolved into two distinct phases. The second lasts up to several hundred milliseconds and is more frontally distributed than the first (Hansen and Hillyard, 1980). In the monkey, auditory cortex, single unit activity with response properties similar to the Nd has been described (Benson and Heinz, 1978).

P2 and N2

The P2 is a positive wave, also called P200. Classically, the N2 is a negativity following the P2, but this negativity is influenced by the long duration negative components attributed above to the N1 time frame, as well as those occurring after the P2 such as the MMN, the sustained potential, N400 and the CNV (Picton et al., 1986).

There are two distinct components at the N2 latency. One component is affected by stimulus intensity and is best recorded from the scalp; the other is unchanged by intensity manipulations and is best recorded from the nasopharynx (Perrault and Picton, 1984). The amplitude of the first process is affected by attention, temporal probability of the deviant stimulus, stimulus modality and intensity. As such, it might reflect a response to stimulus evaluation. The second process is the MMN.

Wave P2, P300 and P4 may occur during the latency range of N2 include P300 (Squires et al., 1975)

and P4 (Stuss and Picton, 1978). Both N2 and P300 latency increase when the target is more difficult to discriminate, indicating that they may be part of a series of evoked potentials that reflect a functional sequence of neural events following the discrimination of infrequent target tones. Presumably they do not directly reflect sensory discrimination because accurate discrimination and initiation of a motor response can precede these potentials (Goodin and Aminoff, 1984).

P300

Originally described by Sutton et al. (1965), the P300 response depends on attention to and discrimination of stimulus differences. It is elicited in an "oddball paradigm," in which an unexpected stimulus occurs in a series of expected stimuli (Fig. 27.4). The unexpected event can even be the omission of an expected stimulus. Typically, a task is associated with the rare stimulus, such as having the subject count the number of times the rare event occurred (Courchesne, 1978; Kurtzberg et al., 1979; Woods, 1980). The P300 (or P3) can be elicited by visual, auditory, or somatosensory stimuli. P300 is a large response, requiring averaging of only 20-30 presentations of target stimuli (Polich and Starr, 1984). Most commonly, the auditory P300 is elicited by tones, but other acoustic stimuli including speech can be used (Klinke et al., 1968; Picton

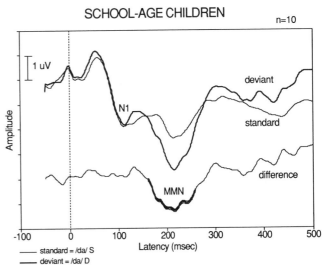

Figure 27.3. MMN in response to just–perceptibly different speech stimuli (variants of the synthesized phoneme /da/). Grand average event–related potentials obtained in response to the standard stimulus /da/S (top) and to the deviant stimulus /da/D (bottom). The grand average difference wave was obtained by subtracting the ERP to the standard stimulus from the response to the deviant stimulus. The thick portion of the difference wave indicates the range during which the difference between the standard and deviant waveforms were significantly different from zero. (Reprinted with permission from Kraus et al. EEG Clin Neurophysiol 1993a;88:123-130).

et al., 1974; and Squires et al., 1975). Using speech stimuli, Kurtzberg and coworkers (1984a, 1984b, 1988) have elicited a P300-like response which they call the cortical discriminative response (CDR).

P300 can be further divided into waves P3a and P3b. P3a occurs in response to large stimulus differences whether or not the subject is actively attending to the stimulus sequence, although P3b occurs only when the subject is actively discriminating between stimuli (Squires et al., 1975; Roth, 1973; Polich, 1989). In general, P300 is best recorded from central areas of the scalp (Polich and Starr, 1983), but at least three types of P3 have been identified, differentiated by scalp topography and type of task (Courchesne, 1978).

A considerable body of research has been concerned with paradigms that elicit a P300 in normal subjects. These efforts have focused on a delineation of the cognitive processes reflected in the components and subcomponents. Processes of attention, auditory discrimination, memory and semantic expectancy appear to be involved in the generation of P300 (Picton and Hillyard, 1988). It has been suggested that P300 may be a neural correlate of sequential information processing, short-term memory, and/or decision making (Squires et al., 1976, 1977; Ford et al., 1980; Donchin, 1981; Harrison et al., 1986).

N400

The N400 is an endogenous potential that appears to reflect semantic processing of language. Like the P300, N400 is not modality specific, and can be elicited by auditory, visual and sign language stimuli (McCallum et al., 1984; Herning et al., 1987; Kutas et al., 1987). Because it appears to assess language function, N400 could be a valuable part of an auditory processing battery. As with other late auditory potentials, N400 should not be considered a single phenomenon, rather as a family of waves underlying several psychological processes.

The N400 eliciting task involves the perception of semantic incongruity. For example, the sentence "I take coffee with cream and dog" would elicit an N400. A semantically appropriate sentence, "I take coffee with cream and sugar," would not elicit an N400. The latter sentence elicits a slow positive response (Kutas and Hillyard, 1980a; 1980b; Kutas et al., 1987). The more complex or unexpected the stimulus, the larger the N400 response.

Other semantic tasks can elicit an N400: Reading isolated words that are semantically incongruous with a preceding phrase (Neville et al., 1986), discrepant word contexts (Harbin et al., 1984; Bentin et al., 1985; Polich, 1985), and naming pictures (Stuss et al.,

1984). Words will elicit a larger N400 than pictures (Noldy-Cummum and Stelmack, 1987).

N400 was not elicited by words that were physically deviant on a visual task such as words in larger type (Kutas and Hillyard, 1980b, 1984). Kutas et al., (1987) observed visual N400 in congenitally deaf adults to sign stimuli and argue on that basis, that the response represents conceptual processing of the word's meaning rather than phonological processing of the acoustic aspects of the stimulus. That the N400 indexes a linguistic process was further demonstrated by Besson and Macar (1987) who failed to find N400 to deviations involving nonlinguistic expectancies such as geometric patterns of increasing or decreasing size, scale notes of increasing or decreasing frequency and well known melodies.

However, Rugg (1984a; 1984b) found that rhyming and nonrhyming words are differentiated by a negative component after the nonrhyming words in the same way that related and unrelated word pairs are differentiated by the N400. Possibly this weakens the hypothesis that N400 is tied to semantic processes. Also possible is that the N400 response to semantic expectancy and the response to rhyming are non-identical.

Stuss et al., (1988) speculate that two distinct processes are involved, one associated with detection of a stimulus and a second associated with the evaluation of complex or anomalous stimuli. Stuss et al. (1983) describe an N400 for both semantic (naming) and nonsemantic (mental rotation) tasks, but the tasks elicited different scalp distributions suggesting that N400 differs for different tasks. Some processes may be common to both semantic and nonsemantic processing, whereas other processes are specific to the semantic interpretation. They describe a biphasic negative wave. The Nx wave of this complex may represent the initial registration of the stimulus, while the Ny component may occur due to further processing, perhaps involving access to long-term memory.

RESPONSES TO SPEECH STIMULI

Although the information presented above was obtained largely in response to tonal or click stimuli, comparable potentials can be elicited with speech (Rugg et al., 1984a, 1984b). The MMN can be obtained in response to speech stimuli that are at psychophysical threshold (Sams et al., 1985; Näätänen et al., 1986; Kraus et al., 1993a; Sharma et al., 1993). Figure 27.4 illustrates the MMN obtained in response to variants of the phoneme /da/ that are just-perceptibly different. The MMN is evident in the response to the deviant stimulus and is clearly seen in the 200 msec region of the difference wave. The dark-

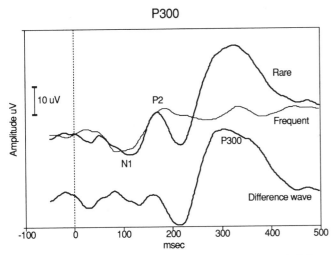

Figure 27.4. ERP recorded in response to rare (/da/, probability = 15%, thick line) and frequent (/di/, thin line) synthesized speech stimuli. P300 is evident in response to rare stimuli to which the subject attended and detected accurately. N1 and P2 occur in response to both stimuli.

ened portion of the difference wave denotes the region during which the responses to standard and deviant stimuli were significantly different.

A group for whom an objective measure of central auditory processing is of interest is cochlear implant users. The wide range of speech perception abilities exhibited by cochlear implant recipients may depend in part upon differences in the central auditory processing abilities of implant users. MMNs to synthesized speech stimuli have been obtained in cochlear implant users and can be similar to those obtained in normal hearing individuals (Kraus et al., 1993b).

Kurtzberg and colleagues (1984a, 1984b, 1988, 1989) have described a series of cortical auditory evoked potentials (CAEP) that are determined by the physical features of speech stimuli. A component of the N1 complex, N110, occurs during detection of speech and nonspeech stimuli. An auditory discrimination task is associated with another component, N140, a response obtained by computing the difference between waves generated by standard versus deviant speech stimuli. The topography of N140, which begins concurrently with N110, shares the central maximum of N110 but extends laterally over the posterior scalp. Thus, there appears to be more extensive cortical activation when stimuli are presented with specific processing requirements such as discrimination as compared to stimulus detection (Lovrich et al., 1988).

The psychophysical phenomenon associated with the discrimination of specific acoustic features of speech known as "categorical perception" (Lieberman et al., 1967) has been investigated with evoked poten-

tials studies (Molfese, 1979; Sharma et al., 1993). Consistent with the notion that speech stimuli are processed differently by the left and right cerebral hemispheres (Geschwind and Levitsky, 1968), hemispheric asymmetries have been noted in AEPs to speech stimuli such as second formant transitions (Molfese and Molfese, 1979). Whether the eliciting stimulus had been analyzed by the subject for phonetic or acoustic cues also affected symmetry (Brown et al., 1973).

Novick et al., (1985) demonstrated that AEPs are sensitive to semantic processing of verbal stimuli. They reported differences between acoustic analysis of nonsense syllables versus words as well as tasks requiring assessment of the word's meaning. Differences in the latency range of 50 to 140 msec, were noted between tasks requiring simple detection and discrimination of acoustic features. Up to 200 msec, responses were sensitive to acoustic processing necessary for stimulus identification, while a negativity between 150 and 400 msec was associated with meaning and semantic processing. Boddy (1981), Brown et al., (1976), and Molfese (1979) also describe AEPs that appear to reflect semantic processes. The cortical discriminative response (CDR), elicited by speech stimuli and N400 which reflects semantic processing, are discussed elsewhere in this chapter.

GENERATORS

An incomplete knowledge of the generating system does not preclude clinical use. For example, the auditory brainstem response generating system is only partially understood, yet the potentials are widely used clinically. Understanding of generating systems underlying the later latency potentials is even less complete; nevertheless these potentials have been clinically applied. Theoretically, we expect that clinical use of late potentials would be enhanced if we understood the generating systems better, but the complexity of those systems may make this goal difficult to achieve, at least in the immediate future. Analysis of the generator systems broadens our understanding of how the normal brain works. Applying that knowledge, however incomplete, to damaged systems seems worthwhile despite its frustrations.

N1

Based on the analysis of scalp topography (Vaughan and Ritter, 1970; Wood and Wolpaw, 1982; Scherg and von Cramon, 1986), effects of lesions in humans (Peronnet and Michel, 1977; Knight et al., 1980; Michel et al., 1980; Woods et al., 1987), and neuromagnetic recordings (Hari et al., 1980; Elberling et al., 1982), a superior temporal cortex generator appears to contribute heavily to N1 (Näätänen, 1984). Using dipole source analysis, Scherg et al., (1989) predicted three auditory cortex sources for N1: (a) the auditory koniocortex (primary auditory cortex), generating a vertically oriented dipole at 100 msec (N1b), (b) the supratemporal plane anterior to the koniocortex generating a vertically oriented dipole, contributing to both N1 and the sustained potential, and (c) the temporal cortex contributing a laterally oriented dipole at 150 msec (N1c) (Arezzo et al., 1975; Perrault and Picton, 1984; Scherg and von Cramon, 1985, 1986).

Näätänen and Picton (1987) demonstrated a frontocentral, slightly contralateral distribution for N1b. The scalp distribution (Vaughan and Ritter, 1970; Scherg and von Cramon, 1985, 1986) and magnetic recordings (Elberling et al., 1982; Hari et al., 1980) indicate that N1b derives from the auditory cortex on the supratemporal plane. Cortical recordings (Celesia, 1976; McCallum and Curry, 1979) and data from patients with cortical lesions (Knight et al., 1988) indicate that N1c is probably generated in the association auditory cortex and the superior temporal gyrus (temporal and parietal cortex).

Activity from the motor and premotor cortices are also thought to contribute to components in the N1 time frame. Based on magnetic studies (Hari et al., 1980) and intracranial recordings in humans (Velasco et al., 1985) and monkeys (Arezzo et al., 1975), this source is associated with a process that facilitates motor activity, perhaps being generated in the frontal cortex, but having influences from the reticular formation and the ventrolateral nucleus of thalamus, cingulate cortex, and hippocampus (Näätänen and Picton, 1987).

Processing Negativities

The auditory cortex appears to be a major generating source for the MMN (Kaukoranta et al., 1989; Näätänen et al., 1989; Näätänen and Picton, 1987; Sams et al., 1991; Scherg and Picton, 1990; Giard et al., 1990; Javitt et al., 1992; Krous et al., 1993d), with contributions from auditory thalamus and hippocampus (Csépe et al., 1987). Dipole analysis has demonstrated two distinct and partially overlapping sources for MMN, corresponding to the subcomponents which differentially respond to the size of the stimulus deviation (Scherg et al., 1989). The processing negativity appears to have two components, a temporal component with a variable scalp distribution that derives from auditory sensory and association cortex, and a frontal, attentional component.

P2 and N2

In general, the temporal lobes and the limbic system contribute heavily to the late potentials. P2 appears to have major generators within the auditory cortex (Vaughan and Ritter, 1970; Hari et al., 1980; Elberling et al., 1982). N2 appears to receive major contributions from subcortical limbic generators (Näätänen et al., 1982; Renault et al., 1982; Ritter et al., 1982), and Perrault and Picton (1984) postulate a neocortical contribution to one of the N2 subcomponents. Skinner and Lindsley (1971) have also demonstrated a role of the reticular activating system in the region of the inferior thalamic peduncle in modulating auditory and visual late evoked potentials.

P300 (Human Studies)

In humans, intracranial recordings of P300 have suggested that its generation involves multiple subcortical sites (Wood et al., 1980). Regions of the limbic system, particularly the hippocampus, have been postulated as generators both on the basis of surface electromagnetic recordings (Okada et al., 1983) and intracranial recordings (Halgren et al., 1980; McCarthy et al., 1982; Squires et al., 1983). Large P300-like potentials manifesting steep voltage gradients and polarity reversals across recording sites were recorded from the limbic system and single unit activity from these structures was correlated with the behavior of P300.

Thalamic contributions to P300 have been proposed based upon intracranial recording in humans (Wood et al., 1980). Pathways involving the mesencephalic reticular formation, medial thalamus, and prefrontal cortex are thought to contribute to the P300 based on the role of these structures in the regulation of selective attention (Yingling and Skinner, 1977; Yingling and Hosobuchi, 1984). Topographic mapping, intracranial recordings, and neuromagnetic field data have indicated that the frontal cortex (Courchesne, 1978; Desmedt and Debecker, 1979; Wood and McCarthy, 1986), centroparietal cortex (Vaughan and Ritter, 1970; Simson et al., 1977a, 1977b and 1977c; Goff et al., 1978; Pritchard, 1981) and the auditory cortex (Richer et al., 1983) contribute to the P300.

P300 (Animal Models)

In response to omitted stimuli, a positivity in the 200-500 msec latency range can be recorded in the cat. The response depends on stimulus probability, and shows decreased amplitude and increased latency as a function of aging (Wilder et al., 1981; Buchwald and Squires, 1982; Harrison and Buchwald, 1985). Wilder et al. (1981) demonstrated a long latency component that was present only when the evoking stimulus was relevant to a task. The amplitude of this component varied inversely with stimulus probability and was independent of stimulus modality. Using this model, O'Connor and Starr (1985) reported that cat P300 showed polarity reversals, sometimes more than once, as the electrode was advanced into the hippocampus. The cat P300, which was positive at the dura, appeared as a negative component within a few millimeters of the surface over wide areas of the marginal and suprasylvian gyri, indicating a cortical in addition to the hippocampal contribution to the generation of the cat P300.

Bilateral ablation of primary auditory cortex did not affect cat P300 (Harrison et al., 1986). This finding was interpreted to rule out primary auditory cortex in the generation of the P300 and contributions from several other pathways were postulated. These included auditory association cortex receiving direct input from the nonprimary divisions of the medial geniculate body, multimodal association cortex receiving input from the intralaminar and centre median nuclei of thalamus (the "medial auditory pathway" described by Irvine and Phillips, 1982) or systems that are primarily subcortical.

Katayama et al., (1985) correlated surface and intracranial AEPs during the same classical conditioning task in both humans and cats. In humans, a negative wave that depended on stimulus relevance, in the same latency range as P300, was noted at all thalamic and mesencephalic recording sites that included the center median nuclei, nucleus parafascicularis, and periaqueductal gray. Similar negative waves were also observed over wide areas of the thalamus of cats including specific and nonspecific thalamic nuclei. Larger wave amplitudes were found in thalamus as compared to white matter, further supporting a thalamic origin.

By lesioning the septal area, Harrison et al. (1988) assessed the role of the septohippocampal system in the generation of the cat P300. Destruction of the septohippocampal projection, a major afferent input to the hippocampus, with marked depletion of hippocampal AChE, led to the transient postoperative persistence of the cat P300 followed by its disappearance. Harrison and colleagues suggest that the cat P300 does not depend on intact septal cells, since it persisted transiently. The response may, however, critically depend upon the cholinergic terminals in the hippocampus (Woolf et al., 1984; Amaral and Kurz, 1985).

N400

Little is known of the generators of N400. Inasmuch as this wave underlies several psychological processes,

it is to be expected that the generating system is dynamic and involves interactions from multiple brain areas. N400 is larger over the right than the left hemisphere (Kutas and Hillyard, 1982; Fischler et al., 1983; Kutas et al., 1988). Picton and Hillyard (1988) speculate that this may be related to clinical evidence that patients with right hemispheric damage have difficulty understanding the contextual framework of narratives, in appreciating humor, and in interpreting metaphors.

In studies of the scalp topography of speech elicited potentials, semantic processing elicited a posterior extension in later components, indicating that a more extensive portion of language cortex is engaged in semantic classification than in verbal identification (Lovrich et al., 1988). Blood flow and metabolism studies indicate that the frontal cortex is activated during semantic processing and that this area may also contribute to a speech-elicited negativity in the N400 time-frame.

MATURATION

Developmental changes during infancy have been extensively investigated (Davis and Onishi, 1969; Kurtzberg et al., 1988). Certain components have been shown to have an orderly maturational sequence and to show adult-like scalp topography at approximately two years, with the midline responses maturing before the lateral responses (Kurtzberg et al., 1984; Kurtzberg et al., 1988).

For practical reasons, the clinical assessment of babies with AEPs is best performed while the baby is sleeping. It has long been known that AEPs are affected by sleep (Weizman et al., 1965; Shucard et al., 1987). In general, clinical use of these potentials has been limited because cyclic changes in sleep state cause substantial variability in the responses.

Some groups, however, have demonstrated that certain AEPs are reliable as long as procedures are in place to monitor and control for sleep state. Some investigators routinely exclude data obtained in quiet sleep (stages 3 and 4) (Novak et al., 1989). An MMN-like response has been recorded during sleep in infants (Alho et al., 1990) and sleep has been shown to systematically affect this response in an animal model (Csépe et al., 1987, 1988). Moreover, cortical evoked potentials during REM sleep have been found to be similar to those recorded during wakefulness (Kurtzberg et al., 1984; Ellingson et al., 1974). Since infants have a high percentage of REM sleep (Roffwarg et al., 1966), they are particularly likely to spend a significant amount of time in sleep stages favorable for ERP recording. Certain analyzes of the EEG may facilitate

AEP recording during sleep in babies (Kraus and McGee, 1993; McGee et al., 1993).

Developmental changes in late potentials do not involve changes in a single parameter, like a gradual latency or amplitude shift, as a function of age (Courchesne, 1990; Eggermont, 1989). Rather, it appears that various passively elicited event-related potentials develop at different rates. Development of P1, N1, P2, and P3b waves appears to continue beyond the first ten years of life. On the other hand, the MMN and a P3a-like response are evident early in life (Kurtzberg et al., 1986; Courchesne, 1990; Kraus et al., 1992, 1993; Csépe et al., 1992).

The N1-P2 complex is ubiquitous in adults, but there is some question as to its developmental sequence in children (Courchesne, 1990). As the N1 wave is thought to consist of at least three distinctively generated subcomponents (Näätänen and Picton, 1987), these components are likely to have distinctive developmental time courses as well. According to Courchesne (1990), it is not until preadolescence and puberty that the familiar auditory N1/P2 vertex potential begins to be clearly seen. Both Goodin et al. (1978) and Martin et al. (1988) report that N1 and P2 are unreliably obtained in 6 year olds, but become easier to identify in older children.

Representative responses to the repetitive stimulus /ga/ from several children are compared to the adult response in Figure 27.5. In school-age children, a positive wave at the latency of P1 often dominates the early portion of the ERP. N1 peak latency is not as well defined as the adult response and occurs later. The reduced amplitude of P2 in children also impedes the identification of the "N1/P2 complex" that is so characteristic of the adult response (Courchesne, 1990; Csépe et al., 1992; Kraus et al., 1992c). In contrast, Johnson (1989) reported adult-like latencies and amplitudes for N1 and P2 in school-age children.

The MMN appears to be robust in school-age children occurring at adult latencies, with MMN magnitude generally larger in children (Kraus et al., 1992, 1993; Csépe et al., 1992). This may be an indication that the MMN reflects processes that are particularly salient in children.

The peak-to-offset portion of the MMN may be related to the P3a or passively-elicited component of the P300 ERP, which unlike the classic P300 is nontask related. It may also be associated with the early developing P300-like response to speech stimuli that is present at birth (Kurtzberg et al., 1986). Other studies have shown that from early childhood to young adulthood, there is a P3a-like positivity of about 300-360 msec that is elicited by auditory targets, auditory high-probability nontargets, and auditory novel, unexpected

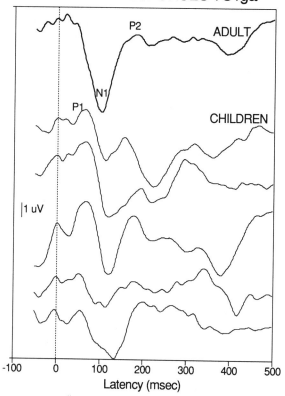

Figure 27.5. Representative responses to the synthesized phoneme /ga/ from several school-age children are compared to the adult response. Note the large P1 and the later and more variable latency of N1 in the children in comparison to the adult (Reprinted from Kraus et al. J Am Acad Audiol 1993c;in press).

sounds (Courchesne, 1990). That P3a-like component does not change in latency from childhood to adulthood. Also, there is a component of similar latency, in an animal model, dependent on the locus coeruleous (Pineda et al., 1988), that may be an analog of the P3a. In contrast, strong developmental differences between adults and children are reported for the task-related P3b component of the P300 response. Latency of P3b decreases systematically throughout childhood, reaching asymptote beyond puberty (Goodin et al., 1978; Martin et al., 1988; Polich et al., 1985; Courchesne, 1990; Finley et al., 1985; Johnson, 1989). The negativity at 400 msec seen in the response to deviant stimuli is likely related to the Nc response described by Courchesne (1978), which is known to be larger in children and inconsistently obtained in adults.

CLINICAL APPLICATIONS

N1, MMN, P2, N2, and Associated Components

Once used as a measure of hearing thresholds (Suzuki and Taguchi, 1965; Rapin et al., 1966; Davis et al.,

1967), the late potentials were replaced by the ABR in the early 1970s for that purpose. In cases where the ABR is elevated in threshold or absent due to brainstem dysfunction (Worthington and Peters, 1980; Kraus et al., 1984) the late potentials still provides a valuable measure of hearing threshold (Gravel et al., 1989).

Late components need not depend on intact earlier potentials. Late AEPs have been observed when ABRs are absent or very abnormal in patients with neurologic disease (Starr et al., 1977; Satya-Murti et al., 1983). Patients with diffuse brain damage primarily due to anoxia showed normal ABRs but abnormal or absent late potentials (Kileny and Berry, 1983). Cortical evoked potentials can be observed in the absence of an intact peripheral auditory system, as evidenced by their occurrence in cochlear implant users (Oviatt and Kileny, 1991; Kileny et al., 1991; Kraus et al., 1993b).

The late potentials have been seen as a tool for identifying brain lesions and localizing brain function and specifically assessing auditory function. Patients with various brain lesions show abnormal late potentials (Curry et al., 1986). Abnormal late potentials have also been observed in psychologic disorders such as schizophrenia (Hink and Hillyard, 1978). Distinctive evoked potentials have been reported in autistic children (Novick et al., 1980; Martineau et al., 1981). Deficits of selective attention such as hyperactivity and autism also are reflected in evoked potential changes (Loiselle et al., 1980; Satterfield et al., 1987; Ciesielki, Courchesne and Elmasian, 1990). Children with Down Syndrome showed longer N1 latencies (Squires et al., 1979) and higher amplitude P2 (Dustman and Callner, 1979). Jirsa (1990) noted longer P2 latencies in children 8 to 11 years old with auditory processing disorders.

Deficient auditory perception has been associated with certain auditory-based learning problems (Elliott and Hammer, 1988; Elliott et al., 1989; Tallal et al., 1980, 1985). The MMN, which reflects auditory sensory processing, by inference, may be linked to auditory perceptual deficits (Krams et al., 1993e; Korpilahti et al., 1992). Cochlear implant users are another group for whom an objective measure of central auditory function is of interest (Kraus et al., 1993b).

The wide range of speech perception abilities exhibited by cochlear implant recipients may depend in part on differences in the central auditory processing abilities of implant users. MMNs to synthesized speech stimuli have been obtained in cochlear implant users and can be similar to those obtained in normal hearing individuals (Kraus et al., 1993b). Figure 27.6 shows the grand average difference waveforms for eight

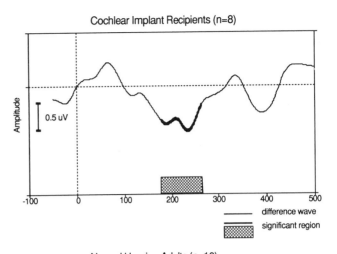

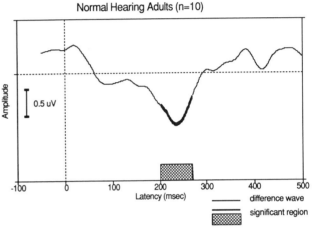

Figure 27.6. MMN in cochlear implant subjects. Grand average MMN difference waveforms for eight "good" cochlear implant subjects (top) and ten normal-hearing adults (bottom). The bolder trace represents the grand average waveform obtained by subtracting the response to the standard stimulus /da/ from the response to the deviant stimulus /ta/. The bottom trace shows the t-scores and the significant MMN range (Reprinted with permission from Kraus et al. Hear Res 1993b;65:118-124).

"good" implant subjects and ten normal hearing controls. The MMN is remarkably similar in the two groups. Preliminary data suggest that "good" and "poor" implant users have distinctive MMNs. The specific relationship between the MMN and behavioral auditory sensory processing is yet to be determined. The characteristics of the MMN suggest its potential clinical use with patients for whom communication is difficult or compromised and for whom auditory discrimination and memory are in question (e.g., at-risk infants, children with language or learning disorders, cochlear implant users, adults with dementia or aphasia). Inasmuch as it does not require conscious attention to the stimuli, the MMN may provide an objective measure of the discrimination of stimulus differences. Consequently, it may permit an objective analysis of sensory processing and discrimination.

There has been some speculation that evoked potentials recorded from infants could have diagnostic or even predictive value in auditory processing. In infants, hemispheric response asymmetries to acoustic stimuli showed sex differences, indicating that evoked potentials are sensitive to possible processing differences even at the earliest stages (Molfese and Molfese, 1979). Neville et al. (1982a, 1982b) have used late potentials to assess the impact of altered early environments upon later cognitive and linguistic development. Kurtzberg and her colleagues have extensively studied infant CAEP and CDR responses. These will be discussed in the P300 section.

P300

Kurtzberg and colleagues studied speech-evoked CAEPs and CDRs in infants at risk for language dysfunction due to low birth weight, perinatal asphyxia, or respiratory distress. A total of 21% showed abnormal CAEPs, and all of these had absent CDRs. Of 55 infants with normal CAEPs, 15 had absent CDRs. CAEP to speech sounds of at-risk babies were significantly less mature than those of normal newborns. The trend was similar, but not significant for tonal stimuli. By 3 months of age, both groups of babies had similar AEPs, but later behavioral tests of language function showed that the early CAEPS and CDRs were predictive of language function (Kurtzberg et al., 1984a and 1984b). They conclude that CAEPs and CDR to speech sounds accurately reflected the infants' capacity for processing stimuli important for development of speech and language (Kurtzberg et al., 1988).

In children, low amplitude P300 has been linked to hyperactivity, schizophrenia, autism and reading disability with few changes in P300 latency (Squires et al., 1983; Ciesielki et al., 1990). P300 abnormalities have also been linked to attentional disorders in hyperactive children (Loiselle et al., 1980), auditory processing disorders (Jirsa, 1990), Down syndrome (Lincoln et al., 1985), and psychiatric disorders (Diner et al., 1985). Finley et al. (1985) used P300 to differentiate functional from organic cognitive disorders in children.

In adults, P300 has been studied in patients with Parkinson's disease (Hansch et al., 1982), chronic renal failure (Cohen et al., 1983), chronic alcoholism (Pfefferbaum et al., 1979), senile dementia (Goodin et al., 1978a, 1978b; Pfefferbaum et al., 1980), cerebrovascular lesions, head trauma, brain tumors (Ebner et al., 1986; Michalewski et al., 1986; Musiek et al., 1989), schizophrenia (Roth et al., 1980; Baribeau-Braun et al., 1983), and aphasia (Selinger and Prescott, 1989). Amplitude reductions and prolonged

latencies have been observed in patients with Alzheimer's disease (Brown et al., 1982; Syndulko et al., 1982; Chayasirisobhon et al., 1985; Goodin et al., 1978b). Tests of memory function derived from P300 latency measures have been applied to conditions where deficiencies of recognition and storage have been implicated (Goodin et al., 1978a, 1978b; Ford et al., 1979).

Unlike other AEPs, P300 shows little asymmetry in patients with asymmetric hemispheric lesions. In patients with temporal lobe lesions, Musiek et al. (1989) noted no significant effects of site of brain lesion either with ear of stimulation or location of the recording electrode. Similarly, no differences in amplitude for affected versus nonaffected hemisphere were seen in groups of patients with head trauma or brain tumors (Olbrich et al., 1986). Johnson and Fedio (1987) did show laterality effects in patients with unilateral temporal lobectomy using C4 and C3 electrode sites.

P300 is not adversely affected by hearing loss, as long as the subject can perceive the stimulus, thus peripheral hearing loss should not impede the use of this measure (Musiek et al., 1989). However, P300 shows a great deal of intersubject variability in latency and amplitude. Picton and Hillyard (1988) observed that the P300 may correlate more with the degree of global cognitive dysfunction than with any specific diagnosis, since the response is abnormal with a wide range of disorders affecting cognition. One proposed use of P300 is to monitor effects of therapy, since a decrease in latency is concomitant with increased cognitive capability (Goodin et al., 1983; Polich and Starr, 1983). This uses the P300 in one of its most stable conditions, that of within-subject measurements.

P300 has been proposed as a communication aid for individuals who cannot use any motor system for communication (e.g., locked-in syndrome patients) (Farwell and Donchin, 1988). The alphabet was presented visually and a P300 elicited when the subject focused attention on a particular letter as it occurred in flashing rows and columns of a matrix. Subjects could communicate at 2.3 characters/minute. Such a system for stimuli presented auditorily might be faster.

N400

There are obvious clinical uses for N400 in the evaluation of language processing. Thus far, it has been found that normal readers have larger amplitude visual N400 than disabled readers (Kutas and Van Petten, 1987; Stelmack et al., 1988). However, Neville et al. (1988) found that language-impaired children display nearly normal responses to semantic anomalies, but abnormal responses to grammatical anomalies.

CONCLUSIONS

Auditory evoked potentials occur as a series of "waves" that are generated from all levels of the auditory system. Almost all evoked potential waves represent activity from multiple contributing sources. These contributions tend to become more numerous and more complex the later the potentials occur in time.

The information that can be gained from the appropriate application of evoked potentials is critical to the accurate diagnosis and effective management of many hearing-impaired and neurologically impaired patients. The ability of these potentials to reflect processes of detection, coding, discrimination, attention, and semantic understanding holds tremendous promise.

Clinical use of the later potentials is not routine, but many studies have identified AEP abnormalities associated with specific diagnoses. From a practical standpoint, technologic advances have made the use of late AEP more clinically feasible. Although the generating networks underlying the late potentials are not well understood, these potentials can be clinically applied using, e.g., the types of paradigms described by Kurtzberg and colleagues and by our group. In the former studies, deviations in responses correlate with specific developmental abnormalities and can be predictive of future language function.

Measures such as the MMN and N400 may have considerable clinical value that has only recently been considered. In the assessment of auditory pathway function, paradigms using speech stimuli may allow the testing of specific properties of the brain's analysis of speech. Correspondences between the MMN and speech perception may add another dimension to the assessment of auditory-based learning problems in school-age children, individuals with attentional disorders, and cochlear implant users.

An obvious clinical issue is whether AEP findings can influence the course of treatment or rehabilitation. It is well known that ABR results affect surgical decisions, hearing aid choice, or other rehabilitative options. If late AEP abnormalities can be correlated with auditory processing deficits, then we can change events in the patient's life to make the processing problem less handicapping. Realistically, there will be aspects of "auditory processing" for which this will be possible, although other subcategories of processing will defy our efforts. As we gain a deeper appreciation of the complexity of the auditory system and the brain, we become increasingly skeptical of using any test in isolation. For example, using the ABR without audiometric information is very likely to lead to a confusion of peripheral auditory damage with neurologic

disorders. Similarly, equating a normal ABR with normal "hearing" ignores the possibility of auditory processing disorders.

As the ABR, MLR, and later cortical potentials have become more familiar to clinicians, the concept of a comprehensive evaluation approach to assess auditory pathway function has emerged. This evaluation combines various electrophysiologic measures with audiometry, tympanometry, otoacoustic emissions and behavioral assessment of auditory function, with tests being selected according to the patient's symptomatology. Broad diagnoses such as "peripheral hearing loss" or "auditory processing disorders" now include various types of physiologic damage. The appropriate application of late AEPs may allow a categorization of discriminative versus attentional disorders. More research is needed to ascertain the location of generators, and to correlate the evoked potential characteristics and patterns with the symptomatology and disorders they represent.

The administration and interpretation of such an evaluation requires considerable clinical expertise. Economic considerations preclude simply performing all available tests. Appropriate decisions must be made as to which responses will be most clinically meaningful. To facilitate the comprehensive approach, there is a need for a more sophisticated way of thinking about the clinical application of auditory evoked potentials. For example, with the ABR, clinicians have worked hard to simplify the procedures and the concepts. Irrelevant neural activity is filtered or averaged away and abnormalities are expressed in narrowly-defined latency differences. Although the ABR is produced by multiple generators, the generators are often considered simple and sequential for clinical interpretations.

The role of AEPs in the clinical assessment of auditory stimulus detection is well accepted. However, it is increasingly important to assess how the brain as well as the ear contributes to hearing. Of interest is the processing of complex stimuli with features that are essential to the perception of natural speech. Ongoing, is the development of clinical applications of cortical, event-related potentials to the assessment of auditory discrimination, semantics, attention and various cognitive aspects of auditory processing. To make the best clinical interpretations, we must consider broader contexts.

Acknowledgments

Modified in part from Kraus, N., and McGee T. Electrophysiology of the Human Auditory System, In Popper A, and Fay R, Eds. The Mammalian Auditory System: Neurophysiology, Vol. II. New York:

Springer-Verlag, 1992. We thank Trent Nicol and Cindy King for their efforts in the preparation of this manuscript. Supported by NIH R01-DC 00264

REFERENCES

Aaltonen O, Niemi P, Nyrke T, Tuhkanenen M. Event-related brain potentials and the perception of a phonetic continuum. Biol Psychol 1987;24:197–207.

Alho K, Sainio K, Sajaniemi N, Reinikainen K, Näätänen R Event-related brain potential of human newborns to pitch change of an acoustic stimulus. Electroenceph Clin Neurophysiol 1990; 77:151–155.

Amaral DG, and Kurz J. Analysis of the origin of the cholinergic and noncholinergic septal projections to the hippocampal formation of the rat. J Comp Neurol 1985;240:37–59.

Arezzo J, Pickoff A, and Vaughan HG. The sources and intracerebral distribution of auditory evoked potentials in the alert rhesus monkey. Brain Res 1975;90:57–73.

Baribeau-Braunn J, Picton TW, and Gosselin J-Y. Schizophrenia: A neurophysiological evaluation of abnormal information processing. Science 1983;219:874–876.

Benson D, and Heinz R. Single unit activity in the auditory cortex of monkeys selectively attending right and left ear stimuli. Brain Res 1978;159:307–320.

Bentin S, McCarthy G, and Wood CC. Event-related potentials, lexical decision and semantic priming. Electroenceph Clin Neurophysiol 1985; 60:343–355.

Besson M, Macar F, and Pynte J. Is N400 specifically related to the processing of semantic mismatch? Soc Neurosci Abstr 1984;10: 841. (Abstr).

Besson M, and Macar F. An event-related potential analysis of incongruity in music and other non-lingual contexts. Psychophysiology 1987;24:14–25.

Boddy J. Evoked potentials and the dynamics of language processing. Biol Psychol 1981;13:125–140.

Brown WS, Marsh JT, and Smith JC. Contextual meaning effects on speech evoked potentials. Behav Biol 1973;9:755–761.

Brown WS, Marsh JT, and Smith JC. Evoked potential waveform differences produced by the perception of different meanings of an ambiguous phrase. Electroenceph Clin Neurophysiol 1976; 41:113–123.

Brown WS, Marsh JT, and Larue A. Event-related potentials in psychiatry: Differentiating depression and dementia in the elderly. Bull LA Neurol Soc 1982;47:91–107.

Buchwald JS, and Squires NS. Endogenous auditory potentials in the cat. In: Woody C, Ed. Conditioning: Representation of Involved Neural Function. New York: Plenum Press, 1982: 503–515.

Celesia GG. Organization of auditory cortical areas in man. Brain 1976;99:403–414.

Chayasirisobhon S, Brinkman S, Gerganoff S, Gershon S, Pomara N, and Green V. Event-related potential in Alzheimer Disease. Clin Electroenceph 1984;16:48–53.

Ciesielki K, Courchesne E, and Elmasian R. Effects of focused selective attention tasks on event-related potentials in autistic and normal individuals. Electroenceph Clin Neurophysiol 1990;75: 207–220.

Cohen MM. Coronal topography of the middle latency auditory evoked potential in man. Electroenceph Clin Neurophysiol 1982;53:231–236.

Cohen SN, Syndulko K, Rever B, Kraut J, Coburn J, Tourtellotte WW. Visual evoked potentials and long latency event-related potentials in chronic renal failure. Neurology 1983;33:1219–1222.

Courchesne E. Neurophysiological correlates of cognitive development: Changes in long-latency event-related potentials from childhood to adulthood. Electroenceph Clin Neurophysiol 1978;45:468–482.

Courchesne E. Chronology of postnatal human brain development: Event related potential, positron emission tomography, myelinogenesis and synaptogenesis studies. In Rohrbaugh J, Parasuraman R, and Johnson R, Eds. Event Related Brain Potentials. New York: Oxford University Press, 1190:210–241.

Csépe V, Karmos G, and Molnár M. Evoked potential correlates of stimulus deviance during wakefulness and sleep in cat-animal model of mismatch negativity. Electroenceph Clin Neurophysiol 1987;66:571–578.

Csépe V, Karmos G, and Molnár M. Evoked potential correlates of sensory mismatch process during sleep in cats. In Koella WP, Obál F, Schulz H, and Visser P, Eds. Sleep '86. Stuttgard: Gustav Fischer, Verlag, 1988:281–283.

Csépe V, Dieckmann B, Hoke M, and Ross B. Mismatch negativity to pitch change of acoustic stimuli in preschool and school-age children. EPIC X Abstr 1992.

Curry SH, Woods DL, and Low MD. Applications of cognitive ERPs in Neurosurgical and Neurological Patients. Cerebral Psychophysiology: Studies in Event-Related Potentials. EEG Suppl. 38. McCallum WC, Zappoli R, and Denoth F, Eds. Amsterdam: Elsevier, 1986:469–484.

Davis H, and Onishi S. Maturation of auditory evoked potentials. Int Audiol 1969;8:24–33.

Davis H, Hirsch SK, Shelnutt J, and Bowers C. Further validation of evoked response audiometry (ERA). J Speech Hear Res, 1967;10:717–732.

Davis PA. Effects of acoustic stimuli on the waking human brain. J Neurophysiol 1939;2:494–499.

Desmedt JE, and Debecker J. Wave form and neural mechanism of the decision P350 elicited without pre-stimulus CNV or readiness potential in random sequences of near threshold auditory clicks and finger stimuli., Electroenceph Clin Neurophysiol 1979;47:648–670.

Diner B, Holcomb P, and Dykman R. P-300 in a major depressive disorder. Psychiat Res 1985;15:175–185.

Donald MW, and Little R. The analysis of stimulus probability inside and outside the focus of attention, as reflected by the auditory N1 and P3 components. Can J Psychol 1981;35:175–187.

Donchin E. Surprise! ... Surprise? Psychophysiology 1981;18: 493–513.

Donchin E, Ritter W, and McCallum C. Cognitive psychophysiology: the endogenous components of the ERP. In Callaway E, Tueting P, and Koslow S, Eds. Brain Event-Related Potentials in Man. New York: Academic Press, 1978:424–437.

Dustman RE, and Callner DA. Cortical evoked responses and response decrement in nonretarded and Down's syndrome individuals. Am J Ment Defic 1979;83:391–397.

Ebner A, Haas J, Lucking C, Schily M, Wallesch C, and Zimmerman P. Event-related brain potentials. P300 and neuropsychological deficit in patients with focal brain lesions. Neurosci Lett 1986;64:330–334.

Elberling C, Bak C, Kofoed B, Lebech J, and Saermark K. Auditory magnetic fields from the human cerebral cortex: Location and strength of an equivalent current dipole. Acta Neurol Scand 1982;65:553–569.

Elliott L, and Hammer M. Longitudinal changes in auditory discrimination in normal children and children with language-learning problems. J Speech Hear Dis 1988;53:467–474.

Elliott L, Hammer M, and Scholl M. Fine-grained auditory discrimination in normal children and children with language-learning problems. J Speech Hear Res 1989;32:112–119.

Farwell LA, and Donchin E. Talking off the top of your head: Toward a mental prosthesis utilizing event-related brain potentials. Electroenceph Clin Neurophysiol 1988;70:510–523.

Finley WW, Faux SF, Hutcheson J, and Amstutz L. Long-latency event-related potentials in the evaluation of cognitive function in children. Neurology 1985;35:323–327.

Fischler I, Bloom PA, Childers DG, Roucos SE, and Perry Jr. NW. Brain potentials related to stages of sentence verification. Psychophysiology 1983;20;400–409.

Ford JM, Mohs RC, Pfefferbaum A, and Kopell BS. On the utility of P3 latency and RT for studying cognitive processes. In Kornhuber HH, and Deecke L, Eds. Motivation, Motor and Sensory Processes of the Brain. Progress in Brain Research, Vol. 54, Amsterdam: Elsevier 1980:661–667.

Ford JM, Roth WT, Mohs RC, Hopkins WF, and Kopell BS. Event-related potentials recorded from young and old adults during a memory retrieval task. Electroenceph Clin Neurophysiol 1979;47:450–459.

Geschwind N, and Levitsky W. Human brain: Left-right asymmetries in temporal speech region. Science 1968;161:186–187.

Giard M, Perris F, Pernier J, and Bouchet P. Brain generators implicated in the processing of auditory stimulus deviance: A topographic event-related potential study. Psychophysiology 1990; 27:627–640.

Goff ER, Allison T, and Vaughan Jr HG. The functional neuroanatomy of event-related potentials. In Callway E, Tueting P, and Koslow SH, Eds. Event-related potentials in Man. New York: Academic Press, 1978:1–79.

Goodin DS, Aminoff MJ. The relationship between the evoked potential and brain events in sensory discrimination, and motor response. Brain 1984;107:241–251.

Goodin DS, Squires KC, Henderson BH and Starr A. Age-related variations in evoked potentials to auditory stimuli in normal human subjects. Electroenceph Clin Neurophysiol 1978a;44: 447–458.

Goodin DS, Squires K, and Starr A. Long latency event-related components of the auditory evoked potential in dementia. Brain 1978b;101:635–648.

Goodin DS, Squires KC, and Starr A. Variations in early and late event-related components of the auditory evoked potential with task difficulty. Electroenceph Clin Neurophysiol 1983;55: 680–686.

Gravel J, Kurtzberg D, Stapells D, Vaughan H, and Wallace I. Case studies, Semin Hear 1989;10:272–287.

Halgren E, Squires NK, Wilson CL, Rohrbaugh JR, Babb TL, and Crandall PH. Endogenous potentials generated in the human hippocampal formation and amygdala by infrequent events. Science 1980;210:803–805.

Hansch EC, Syndulko K, Cohen SM, Goldberg ZI, Potvin AR, and Tourtellotte WW. Cognition in Parkinson disease: An event-related potential perspective. Ann Neurol 1982:599–607.

Hansen JC, and Hillyard SA. Endogenous brain potentials associated with selective auditory attention. Electroenceph Clin Neurophysiol 1980;49:277–290.

Hansen JC, and Hillyard SA. Selective attention to multi-dimensional auditory stimuli in man. J Exp Psych Human Percept Perform 1982;9:1–19.

Harbin TJ, Marsh GR, and Harvey MT. Differences in the late components of the event-related potential due to age and to semantic and non-semantic tasks. Electroenceph Clin Neurophysiol 1984;59:489–496.

Hari R, Aittoniemi K, Jarvinen ML, Katila T, and Varpula T. Auditory evoked transient and sustained magnetic fields of the human brain. Exp Brain Res 1980;40:237–240.

Harrison J, and Buchwald J. Aging Changes in the cat P300 mimic the human. Electroenceph Clin Neurophysiol 1985;62:227–234.

Harrison J, Buchwald J, and Kaga K. Cat P300 present after primary auditory cortex ablation. Electroenceph Clin Neurophysiol 1986;63:180–187.

Harrison JB, Buchwald JS, Kaga K, Woolf NJ, and Butcher LL. ¥Cat P300' disappears after septal lesions. Electroenceph Clin Neurophysiol 1988;69:55–64.

Henry KR. Auditory brainstem volume conducted responses. Origins in the laboratory mouse. J Am Aud Soc 1979;4:173–178.

Herning RI, Jones RT, and Hunt JS. Speech event related potentials reflect linguistic content and processing level. Brain Lang 1987;30:116–129.

Hillyard SA, and Kutas M. Electrophysiology of cognitive processing. Annu Rev Psychol 1983;34:33–61.

Hillyard SA, and Picton TW. Event-related brain potentials and selective information processing in man. In Desmedt JE, Ed. Progress in Clinical Neurophysiology, Vol 6. Basel: Karger 1979;1–50.

Hillyard SA, Hink RF, Schwent VL, and Picton TW. Electrical signs of selective attention in the human brain. Science 1973;182:177–180.

Hink RF, Hillyard SA, and Benson PJ. Electrophysiological measures of attentional processes in man as related to the study of schizophrenia. J Psychiatr Res 1978;14:155–65.

Irvine DRF, and Phillips DP. Polysensory ¥association' areas of the cerebral cortex. Organization of acoustic input in the cat. In: Woolsey CN, ED. Cortical Sensory Organization: Multiple Auditory Areas Clinton, NJ: Humana Press 1982:111–156.

Javitt D, Schroeder C, Steinschneider M, Arezzo J, Vaughan J. Demonstration of mismatch negativity in monkey. Electroenceph Clin Neurophysiol 1992;83:87–90.

Jirsa R, and Clontz K. Long latency auditory event-related potentials from children with auditory processing disorders. Ear Hear 1990;11:222–232.

Johnson R. Developmental evidence for modality-dependent P300 generators: A normative study. Psychophysiology 1989;26: 651–667.

Johnson R, and Fedio P. Task related changes in P-300 scalp distribution in temporal lobectomy patients. In Johnson R, Rohrbaugh J, and Parasuraman R, Eds. Current Trends in Evoked Potential Research. Electroenceph Clin Neurophysiol 1987(Suppl 40):699–704.

Kaga K, Hink R, Shinoda Y, and Suzuki J. Evidence for a primary cortical origin of a middle latency auditory evoked potential in cats. Electroenceph Clin Neurophysiol 1980;50:254–266.

Katayama Y, Tsukiyama T, and Tsubokawa T. Thalamic negativity associated with the endogenous late positive component of cerebral evoked potentials (P300): Recordings using discriminative aversive conditioning in humans and cats. Brain Res Bull 1985;14:223–226.

Kaukoranta E, Sams M, Hari R, Hämäläinen M, and Näätänen R. Reactions of human auditory cortex to changes in tone duration: indirect evidence for duration-specific neurons. Hear Res 1989;41:15–22.

Kileny P, and Berry DA. Selective impairment of late vertex and middle latency auditory evoked responses. In Menches G, and Gerber S, Eds. The Multiply Handicapped Hearing Impaired Child. New York: Grune and Stratton, 1983.

Kileny P. Use of electrophysiologic measures in the management of children with cochlear implants: brainstem, middle latency and cognitive (P300) responses. Am J Otol 1991;12:37–42.

Klinke R, Fruhstorfer H, and Finkenzellar P. Evoked responses as a function of external and stored information. Electroenceph Clin Neurophysiol 1968;25:119–122.

Knight RT, Hillyard SA, Woods D, and Neville H. The effects of frontal and temporal-parietal lesions on the auditory evoked response in man. Electroenceph Clin Neurophysiol 1980;50: 112–124.

Knight RT, Scabini D, Woods DL, and Clayworth C. The effects of lesions of superior temporal gyrus and inferior parietal lobe on temporal and vertex components of the human AEP. Electroenceph Clin Neurophysiol 1988;70:499–509.

Korpilahti P, Ek M, and Lang H. The defect of 'pitch MMN' in dysphasic children. EPIC X Abstr 82, 1992.

Kraus N, and McGee T. Clinical implications of primary and non-primary components of the MLR generating system. Ear Hear 1993;14:36–48.

Kraus N, McGee T, Sharma A, Carrell T, and Nicol T. Mismatch negativity event-related potential to speech stimuli. Ear Hearing 1992;13:158–164.

Kraus N, McGee T, Micco A, Sharma A, Carrell T, and Nicol T. Mismatch negativity in school-age children to speech stimuli that are just perceptibily different. Electroenceph Clin Neurophysiol 1993a;88:123–130.

Kraus N, Micco A, Koch D, McGee T, Carrell T, Wiet R, Weingarten C, and Sharma A. The mismatch negativity cortical evoked potential elicited by speech in cochlear-implant users. Hear Res 1993b;65:118–124..

Kraus N, McGee T, Carrell T, Sharma A, Micco A, and Nicol T. Speech-evoked cortical potentials in children. J Am Acad Audiol 1993c;in press.

Kraus N, McGee T, Littman T, Nicol T, and King C. Non-primary thalamic contributions to the mismatch negativity generating system. Neurosci Abstr 1993d;223:10.

Kraus N, McGee T, Ferre J, Hoeppner J, Carrell T, Sharma A, Nicol T. Mismatch negativity in the neurophysiologic/behavioral evaluation of auditory processing deficits, Ear Hear.

Kraus N, Özdamar Ö, Stein L, and Reed N. Absent auditory brain stem response: Peripheral hearing loss or brain stem dysfunction? Laryngoscope 1984;94:400–406.

Kurtzberg D, Vaughan HG, and Kreuzer JA. Task-related cortical potentials in children. Prog Clin Neurophysiol 1979;6:216–223.

Kurtzberg D, Hilpert P, Kreuzer J, and Vaughan HG. Differential maturation of cortical auditory evoked potentials to speech sounds in normal fullterm and very low-birthweight infants. Dev Med Child Neurol 1984a;26:466–475.

Kurtzberg D, Vaughan HG, Courchesne E, Friedman D, Harter MR, and Putnam LE. Developmental aspects of event-related potentials. Ann NY Acad Sci 1984b;425:300–318.

Kurtzberg D, Stone CL, and Vaughan HG Jr. Cortical responses to speech sounds in the infant. In Cracco RQ, and Bodis-Wollner I, Eds. Frontiers of Clinical Neuroscience, Vol 3, Evoked Potentials. 1986:513–520.

Kurtzberg D, Stapells DR, and Wallace IF. Event-related potential assessment of auditory system integrity: Implications for language development. In Vietze P, and Vaughan HG Jr, Ed. Early Identification of Infants with Developmental Disabilities. Philadelphia: Grune and Stratton, 1988:160–180.

Kutas M, and Hillyard SA. Event-related brain potentials to semantically inappropriate and surprisingly large words. Biol Psychol 1980a;11:99–115.

Kutas M, and Hillyard SA. Reading senseless sentences: Brain potentials reflect semantic incongruity. Science 1980;207:203.

Kutas M, and Hillyard SA. The lateral distribution of event-related potentials during natural sentence processing. Neuropsychologia 1982;20:579–590.

Kutas M, and Hillyard SA. Event-related brain potentials to grammatical errors and semantic anomalies. Mem Cogn 1983;11: 539–550.

Kutas M, and Hillyard SA. Event-related brain potentials (ERPs) elicited by novel stimuli during sentence processing. In Karrer R, Cohen J, and Tueting P, Eds. Brain and Information: Event-Related Potentials. Ann NY Acad Sci 1984;425:236–241.

Kutas M, Neville HJ, and Holcomb P. A preliminary comparison of the N400 response to semantic anomalies during reading, listening and signing. In Ellington RJ, Murray NMF, and Halliday AM, Eds. The London Symposia, EEG Suppl 39, 1987:325–330.

Kutas M, Van Petten, and Besson M. Event-related potential asymmetries during the reading of sentences. Electroenceph Clin Neurophysiol 1988b;69:218–233.

Lang A, Aaltonen O, and Eerola O. Normal variation of the mismatch negativity (MMN). EPIC Abstr 87, 1992.

Lieberman AM, Cooper FS, Shankweiler DP, and Studdert-Kennedy M. Perception of the speech code. Psychol Rev 1967;74:431–461.

Lincoln A, Courchesne E, Kilman B, and Galambos R. Neuropsychological correlates of information processing by children with Down's syndrome. Am J Ment Def 1985;89:403–414.

Loiselle DL, Stamm JA, Maitinsky S, and Whipple SC. Evoked potential and behavioral signs of attentive dysfunctions in hyperactive boys. Psychophysiology 1990;17:193–201.

Lovrich D, Novick B, and Vaughan Jr. HG. Topographic analysis of auditory event-related potentials associated with acoustic and semantic processing. Electroenceph Clin Neurophysiol 1988;71: 40–54.

Martin L, Barajas J, Fernandez R, and Torres E. Auditory event-related potentials in well-characterized groups of children. Electroenceph Clin Neurophysiol 1988;71:375–381.

Martineau J, Garreau B, Barthelemy C, Callaway E, and Lelord G. Effects of vitamin B6 on averaged evoked potentials in infantile autism. Biol Psychiat 1981;16:625–639.

McCallum WC, and Curry SH (1979). Hemisphere differences in event related potentials and CNVs associated with monaural stimuli and laterized motor responses. In Lehmann D, and Callaway E, Eds. Human Evoked Potentials: Applications, and Problems. New York: Plenum, 1979:235–250.

McCallum WC, and Curry SH. The form and distribution of auditory evoked potentials and CNVs when stimuli and responses are lateralized. In: Kornhuber HH, and Deecke L, Eds. Progress in Brain Research, Vol 54. Motivation, Motor and Sensory Processes of the Brain: Electrical Potentials, Behaviour and Clinical Use. Amsterdam: Elsevier, 1980;767–775.

McCallum WC, Farmer SF, and Pocock PK. The effects of physical and semantic incongruities on auditory event-related potentials. Electroenceph Clin Neurophysiol 1984;59:477–488.

McCarthy G, Wood CC, Alison T, Goff WR, Williamson PD, and Spencer DD. Intracranial recordings of event-related potentials in humans engaged in cognitive tasks. Soc Neurosci Abst 1982;8:976 (Abstr).

McGee T, Kraus N, Killion M, Rosenberg R, and King C. (in press). Improving the reliability of the auditory middle latency response. Ear Hear 1993; in press.

Michalewski H, Rosenberg C, and Starr A. Event related potentials in dementia. In Cracco R, and Bodis-Wollner I, Eds. Evoked potentials. New York: Alan R. Liss, Inc., 1986:521–528.

Michel F, Peronnet F, and Schott B. A case of cortical deafness: clinical and electrophysiological data. Brain Lang 1980;10: 367–377.

Molfese DL. Cortical involvement in the semantic processing of coarticulated speech cues. Brain Lang 1979;7:86–100.

Molfese DL, and Molfese VJ. Hemisphere and stimulus differences as reflected in the cortical responses of newborn infants to speech stimuli. Dev Psychol 1979;15:505–511.

Musiek FE, and Geurkink NA. Auditory brainstem and middle latency evoked response sensitivity near threshold. Ann Otol 1981;90:236–240.

Näätänen R. Selective attention, and evoked potentials in humans—a critical review. Biol Psychol 1975;2:237–307.

Näätänen R. In search of a short–duration memory trace of a stimulus in human brain. In Pulkkinen L, and Lyytinen P, Eds. Essays in Honour of Martti Takala, Jyväskylä Studies in Education, Psychology and Social Science, Jyväskylä: University of Jyväskylä, 1984.

Näätänen R, Gaillard AWK, and Mäntysalo S. Early selective attention effect on evoked potential reinterpreted. Acta Psychol 1978;42:313–329.

Näätänen R, and Michie PT. Early selective attention effects of the evoked potential. A critical review and reinterpretation. Biol Psychol 1979;8:81–136.

Näätänen R, Simpson M, and Loveless NE. Stimulus deviance and evoked potentials, Biol Psychol 1982;14:53–98.

Näätänen R, and Picton T. The N1 wave of the human electric and magnetic response to sound. Psychophysiology 1987;24:375–425.

Näätänen R, Paavilainen P, Alho K, Reinikainen K, and Sams M. The mismatch negativity to intensity changes in an auditory stimulus sequence. In Johnson R, Rohrbaugh RW, Parasuraman R, Eds. Current Trends in Event-Related Potential Research, EEG Suppl 40. Amsterdam: Elsevier, 1987:129–130.

Näätänen R, Paavilainen P, Reinikainen K. Do event-related potentials reveal the mechanism of auditory sensory memory in the human brain? Neurosci Lett 1989;98:217–221.

Näätänen R. The role of attention in auditory information processing as revealed by event–related brain potentials and other brain measures of cognitive function. Behav Brain Sci 1990;13:201–233.

Näätänen R. Mismatch negativity outside strong attentional focus: A commentary on Woldorff et al., (1991) Psychophysiology 1991;28: 478–454.

Näätänen R. In: Attention and Brain Function, Lawrence Erlbaum Assoc, Hillsdale, New Jersey, 1992:136–200.

Neville HJ, Kutas M, and Schmidt A. Event-related potential studies of cerebral specialization during reading. I. Studies of normal adults. Brain Lang 1982a;16:300–315.

Neville HJ, Kutas M, and Schmidt A. Event-related potential studies of cerebral specialization during reading. II. Studies of congenitally deaf adults. Brain Lang 1982b;16:316–337.

Neville HJ, Kutas M, Chesney G, and Schmidt AL. Event-related brain potentials during initial encoding and recognition memory of congruous and incongruous words. J Mem Lang 1986;25:75–92.

Neville HJ, Holcomb PJ, Coffey SA, and Tallal P. Semantic and grammatical processing in normal and language-impaired children: An ERP study. Int Neuropsychol Soc 1988:(Abstr 1).

Nielsen-Bohlman L, Knight RT, Woods DL, and Woodward K. Differential processing of auditory stimuli continues during sleep. Neurosci Abstr 1988.

Noldy-Cullum N, and Stelmack R. Recognition memory for pictures and words: the effect of incidental and intentional learning on N400. In Johnson Jr R, Rohrbaugh JW, and Parasuraman R, Eds. Current Trends in Event-Related Potentials Research, EEG Suppl 40, 1987:350–354.

Novak G, Ritter W, and Vaughan H. The chronometry of attention-modulated processing and auditomatic mismatch detection. Psychophysiology 1989;29:412–430.

Novak GP, Kurtzberg D, Kreuzer JA, and Vaughan Jr. HG. Cortical responses to speech sounds and their formants in normal

infants: maturational sequence and spatiotemporal analysis. Electroenceph Clin Neurophysiol 1989;73:295–305.

Novak G, Ritter W, Vaughan H, and Wiznitzer M. Differentiation of negative event-related potentials in an auditory discrimination task. Electroenceph Clin Neurophysiol 1990;75:255–275.

Novick B, Lovrich D, and Vaughan Jr. HG. Event-related potentials associated with the discrimination of acoustic and semantic aspects of speech. Neuropsychologia 1985;23:87–101.

O'Connor TA, and Starr A. Intracranial potentials correlated with and event-related potential, P300, in the cat. Brain Res 1985;339:27–38.

Okada YC, Kaufman L, and Williamson SJ. The hippocampal formation as a source of the slow endogenous potentials. Electroenceph Clin Neurophysiol 1983;55:417–426.

Okita T. Slow negative shifts of the human event-related potential associated with selective information processing. Biol Psychol 1981;12:63–75.

Oviatt DL, and Kileny PR. Auditory event-related potentials elicited from cochlear implant recipients and hearing subjects. Am J Audiol 1981;1:48–55.

Paavilainen P, Karlsson M, Reinikainen K, and Näätänen R. Mismatch negativity to changes in the spatial location of an auditory stimulus. Electroenceph Clin Neurophysiol 1989;73:129–141.

Peronnet F, and Michel F. The asymmetry of the auditory evoked potentials in normal man and in patients with brain lesions. In Desmedt JE, Ed. Auditory Evoked Potentials in Man. Psychopharmacology Correlates of EPs. Prog Clin Neurophysiol, Vol 2. Basel: Karger, 1977:130–141.

Perrault N, and Picton TW. Event-related potentials recorded from the scalp and nasopharynx. I. N1 and P2. Electroenceph Clin Neurophysiol 1984;59:177–194.

Pfefferbaum A, Horvath T, Rothe W, and Kopell B. Event related potential changes in chronic alcoholics. Electroenceph Clin Neurophysiol 1984;47:637–647.

Pfefferbaum A, Ford J, Roth W, and Kopell B. Age-related changes in auditory event-related potentials. Electroenceph Clin Neurophysiol 1980;49:266–276.

Picton TW, and Hillyard SA. Endogenous event-related potentials. In: Picton TW, Ed. Human Event-Related Potentials, EEG Handbook, Rev series Vol 3. Amsterdam: Elsevier Science Publishers, 1988.

Picton TW, Hillyard SH, Krausz HI, and Galambos R. Human auditory evoked potentials I. Evaluation of components. Electroenceph Clin Neurophysiol 1974;36:179–190.

Picton TW, Gerri AM, Champagne SC, Stuss DT, and Nelson RF. The effects of age and task difficulty on the late positive component of the auditory evoked potential. In McCallum WC, Zappoli R, and Denoth E, Eds. Event Related Potentials of the Brain. Electroenceph Clin Neurophysiol Suppl 38. Amsterdam: Elsevier, 1986:132–133.

Pineda J, Foote S, and Neville H. The effects of locus coeruleus lesions on a squirrel monkey late positive component: A preliminary study. Electroenceph Clin Neurophysiol 1988;73:129–141.

Polich J. Semantic categorization and event-related potentials. Brain Lang 1985;26:304–321.

Polich J, Howard L, and Starr A. Aging effects on the P300 component of the event-related potential from auditory stimuli: peak definition, variation, and measurement. J Gerontol 1985;40:721–726.

Polich J. Frequency, intensity and duration as determinants of P300 from auditory stimuli. J Clin Neurophysiol 1989;6:277–286.

Polich J, and Starr A. Middle, late and long latency auditory evoked potentials. In Moore E, Ed. Bases of Auditory Brainstem Evoked Responses. New York: Grune & Stratton 1983:345–361.

Pool K, Finitzo T, Chi-Tzong-Hong, Rogers J, and Pickett RB. Infarction of the superior temporal gyrus: A description of auditory evoked potential latency and amplitude topology. Ear Hear 1989;10:144–152.

Pritchard WS Psychophysiology of P300. Psychol Bull 1981;89:506–540.

Probst R, Coats AC, Martin GK, and Lonsbury-Martin BL. Spontaneous, click- and toneburst-evoked otoacoustic emissions from normal ears. Hear Res 1986;21:261–271.

Rapin I, Schimmel H, Tourk L, Krasnegor NA, and Pollack C. Evoked responses to clicks and tones of varying intensity in waking adults. Electroenceph Clin Neurophysiol 1966;21:335–344.

Renault B, Rogot R, Lesevre N, and Remond A. Onset and offset of brain events as indices of mental chronometry. Science 1982;215:1423–1425.

Richer F, Johnson RA, and Beatty J. Sources of late components of the brain magnetic response. Soc Neurosci Abstr 1983;9:656.

Ritter W, Simson R, Vaughan Jr. HG, and Friedman DA. A brain event related to the making of a sensory discrimination. Science 1979;203:1358–1361.

Ritter W, Simson R, Vaughan HG, and Macht M. Manipulation of event-related potential manifestations of information processing stages. Science 1982;218:909–911.

Robinson K, and Rudge P. Abnormalities of the auditory evoked potentials in patients with multiple sclerosis. Brain 1979;100:19–40.

Roffwarg H, Muzio J, and Dement W. Ontogenetic development of the human sleep-dream cycle. Science 1966;152:604–619.

Rösler F, Sutton S, Johnson Jr. R, Mulder G, Fabiani M, Plooij-Van Gorsel E, and Roth W. In McCallum WC, Zappoli R, and Denoth F, Eds. Cerebral Psychophysiology: Studies in Event-Related Potentials. EEG Suppl 38. Amsterdam: Elsevier, 1986:51–92.

Roth W. Auditory evoked responses to unpredictable stimuli. Psychophysiology 1973;10:125–138.

Roth WT, Horvath TB, Pfefferbaum A, and Kopell BS. Event-related potentials. Electroenceph Clin Neurophysiol 1980;48:127–139.

Rugg MD. Event-related potentials and the phonological processing of words and non-words. Neuropsychologia 1984a;22:435–443.

Rugg MD. Event-related potentials in phonological matching tasks. Brain Lang 1984b;23:225–240.

Sams M, Paavilainen P, Alho K, and Näätänen R. Auditory frequency discrimination and event-related potentials. Electroenceph Clin Neurophysiol 1985;62:437–448.

Sams M, Kaurkoranta E, Hämäläinen M, and Näätänen R. Cortical activity elicited by changes in auditory stimuli: different sources for the magnetic N100m and mismatch responses. Psychophysiology 1991;28:21–29.

Sams M, Aulanko R, Aaltonen O, and Näätänen R. Event-related potentials to infrequent changes in synthesized phonetic stimuli. J Cogn Neurosci 1990;2:344–355.

Satterfield JH, Schell AM, and Backs R. Longitudinal study of AERPs in hyperactive and normal children: relationship to antisocial behavior. Electroenceph Clin Neurophysiol 1987;67:531–536.

Satya-Murti S, Wolpaw JR, Cacace AT, and Schaffer CA. Late auditory evoked potentials can occur without brain stem potentials. Electroenceph Clin Neurophysiol 1983;56:304–308.

Scherg M, Vajsar J, and Picton T. A source analysis of the late

human auditory evoked potentials. J Cogn Neurosci 1989;1:336–355.

Scherg M, and Volk SA. Frequency specificity of simultaneously recorded early and middle latency auditory evoked potentials. Electroenceph Clin Neurophysiol 1983;56:443–452.

Scherg M, and Von Cramon D. Two bilateral sources of the late AEP as identified by a spatio-temporal dipole model. Electroenceph Clin Neurophysiol 1985;62:32–44.

Scherg M, and Von Cramon D. Evoked dipole source potentials of the human auditory cortex. Electroenceph Clin Neurophysiol 1986;65:344–360.

Selinger M, and Prescott T. Auditory event-related potentials probes and behavioral measures of aphasia. Brain Lang 1989;36:377–390.

Sharma A, Kraus N, McGee T, Carrell T, and Nicol T. Acoustic vs. phonetic representation of speech stimuli as reflected by the mismatch negativity event-related potential. Electroenceph Clin Neurophysiol 1993;88:64–71.

Shucard DW, Shucard JL, and Thomas DG. Auditory event-related potentials in waking infants and adults: A developmental perspective. Electroenceph Clin Neurophysiol 1987;68:303–310.

Simson R, Vaughan Jr. HG, and Ritter W. The scalp topography of potentials in auditory and visual go/no go tasks. Electroenceph Clin. Neurophysiol 1977a;43:864–875.

Simson R, Vaughan Jr. HG, and Ritter W. The scalp topography of potentials in auditory and visual discrimination tasks. Electroenceph Clin Neurophysiol 1977b;42:528–535.

Simson R, Vaughan Jr. HG, and Ritter W. The scalp topography of potentials in auditory and visual go/no go tasks. Electroenceph Clin Neurophysiol 1977c;43:864–875.

Skinner JE, and Lindsley DB. Enhancement of visual and auditory evoked potentials during blockade of the non-specific thalamo-cortical system. Electroenceph Clin Neurophysiol 1977;31:1–6.

Skinner P, and Glattke TJ. Electrophysiologic responses and audiometry: State of the art. J Speech Hear Dis 1977;42:179–198.

Snyder E, and Hillyard S. Long-latency evoked potentials to irrelevant, deviant stimuli, Behav Biol 1976;16:319–331.

Squires NK, Donchin E, Squires KC, and Grossberg S. Bisensory stimulation: inferring decision-related processes from the P300 component. J Exp Psychol Hum Percept Performance 1977;2:299–315.

Squires NK, Galbraith GC, and Aine CJ. Event-related potential assessment of sensory and cognitive deficits in the mentally retarded. In Lehmann D, and Callaway E, Eds. Human Evoked Potentials: Applications and Problems. New York: Plenum Press, 1979:397–413.

Squires NK, Halgren E, Wilson C, and Crandall P. Human endogenous limbic potentials: cross–modality and depth/surface comparisons in epileptic subjects. In Gaillard AWK, and Rittaer W, Eds. Tutorials in ERP Research: Endogenous Components. Amsterdam: North-Holland, 1983:217–232.

Squires NK, Squires KC, and Hillyard SA. Two varieties of long-latency positive waves evoked by unpredictable auditory stimuli in man. Electroenceph Clin Neurophysiol 1975;38:387–401.

Squires KC, Wickens C, Squires NK, and Donchin E. The effect of stimulus sequence on the waveform of the cortical event-related potential. Science 1976;193:1142–1146.

Stapell Stelmack RM, Saxe BJ, Noldy-Cullum N, Campbell KB, and Armitage R. Recognition memory for words and event-related potentials: A comparison of normal and disabled readers. J Clin Exp Neuropsychol 1988;10:185–200.

Stuss DT, and Picton TW. Neurophysiological correlates of human concept formation. Behav Biol 1978;23:135–162.

Stuss DT, Sarazin FF, Leech EE, and Picton TW. Event-related potentials during naming and mental rotation. Electroenceph Clin Neurophysiol 1983;56:133–146.

Stuss DT, Leech EE, Sarazin FF, and Picton TW. Event-related potentials during naming. Ann NY Acad Sci 1984;425:278–282.

Stuss DT, Picton TW, and Cerri AM. Electrophysiological manifestations of typicality judgment. Brain Lang 1988;33:260–272.

Sutton S, Braren M, Zubin J, and John ER. Evoked-potential correlates of stimulus uncertainty. Science 1965;150:1187–1188.

Sutton S, Tueting P, Zubin J, and John ER. Information delivery and the sensory evoked potentials. Science 1967;155:1436–1439.

Suzuki T, and Taguchi K. Cerebral evoked response to auditory stimuli in waking man. Ann Otol Rhinol Laryngol 1965;74:128–139.

Syndulko K, Hansch MA, Cohen SN, Pearce JW, Goldberg Z, Montan B, Tourtellotte WW, and Potvin AR. Long-latency event-related potentials in normal aging and dementia. In Courjon J, Mauguière F, and Revol M, Eds. Clinical Applications of Evoked Potentials in Neurology. New York: Raven Press, 1982;279–285.

Tallal P, Stark R, Kallman C, and Mellitis D. Developmental dysphasia: The relation between acoustic processing deficits and verbal processing. Neuropsychologia 1980;18:273–284.

Tallal P, Stark R, and Mellitis F. The relationship between auditory temporal analysis and receptive language development: Evidence from studies of developmental language disorder. Neuropsychologia 1985;23:314–322.

Vaughan Jr. HG, and Ritter W. The sources of auditory evoked responses recorded from the human scalp. Electroenceph Clin Neurophysiol. 1970;28:360–367.

Velasco M, Velasco F, and Olvera A. Subcortical correlates of the somatic, auditory and visual vertex activities in man. I. Bipolar EEG responses and electrical stimulation. Electroenceph Clin Neurophysiol 1985;61:519–529.

Wilder MB, Farley GR, and Starr A. Endogenous late positive component of the evoked potential in cats corresponding to P300 in humans. Science 1981;211:605–607.

Woldorff M, and Hillyard S. Modulation of early auditory processing during selective listening to rapidly presented tones. Electroenceph Clin Neurophysiol 1991;79:170–191.

Wolpaw JR, and Penry JK. A temporal component of the auditory evoked response. Electroenceph Clin Neurophysiol 1975;39:609–620.

Wood CC, Allison T, Goff WR, Williamson PD, and Spencer DB. On the neural origin of P300 in man. In Kornhuber HH, and Deecke L, Eds. Motivation, Motor and Sensory Processes of the Brain. Progress in Brain Research, Vol 54. Amsterdam: Elsevier, 1980:51–56.

Wood CC, and Wolpaw JR. Scalp distribution of human auditory evoked potentials. II. Evidence for overlapping sources and involvement of auditory cortex. Electroenceph Clin Neurophysiol 1982;54:25–38.

Wood CC, and McCarthy G. A possible frontal lobe contribution to scalp P300. In Rohrbaugh JW, Johnson Jr R, and Parasuraman R, Eds. Research Reports: 8th International Conference on Event-Related Potentials of the Brain 1986:164.

Woods DL, Clayworth CC, Knight RT, Simpson GV, and Naeser MA. Generators of middle- and long-latency auditory evoked potentials: Implications from studies of patients with bitemporal lesions. Electroenceph Clin Neurophysiol 1987;68:132–148.

Woods D, Alho K, and Algazi A. Intermodal selective attention. I. effects on eventrelated potentials to lateralized auditory and visual stimuli. Electroenceph Clin Neurophysiol 1992;82:341–355.

Woldorff M, Hackley S, and Hillyard S. The effects of channel-selective attention on the mismatch negativity wave elicited by deviant tones. Psychophysiology 1991;28:30–42.

Woods D. Auditory selective attention in middle-aged and elderly subjects: an event-related brain potentials study. Electroenceph Clin Neurophysiol 1992;84:456–468.

Woolf NJ, Eckenstein F, and Butcher LL. Cholinergic systems in the rat brain. I. Projections to the limbic telencephalon. Brain Res Bull 1984;13:751–784.

Worthington D, and Peters J. Quantifiable hearing and no ABR: Paradox or error? Ear Hear 1980;5:281–285.

Yingling CD, and Hosobuchi Y. A subcortical correlate of P300 in man. Electroenceph Clin Neurophysiol 1984;59:72–76.

Yingling CD, and Skinner JE. Gating of thalamic input to cerebral cortex by nucleus reticularis thalami. In Desmedt JE, Ed. Attention, Voluntary Contraction and Event-Related Cerebral Potentials. Prog Clin Neurophysiol, Vol 1. Basel: Karger, Basel, 1977:70–96.

CHAPTER 28

Evaluation of Balance System Function

Neil T. Shepard and Steven A. Telian

Estimates of the number of persons in the United States seeking a physician visit each year for disequilibrium or true vertigo range as high as 7 million per year (Ambulatory Medical Care Survey, 1981). Approximately 30% of the U.S. population has experienced episodes of dizziness by age 65 (Roydhouse, 1974). The problem of balance disorders in the U.S. can only become greater as the country's population ages.

The majority of patients afflicted with an acute balance disorder recover spontaneously with only symptomatic treatment from the medical community (Igarashi, 1984; Pfaltz, 1983). For reasons that are poorly understood some of these patients develop chronic balance system problems requiring significant investments from a variety of medical and surgical specialist to evaluate and manage their disorder.

The balance system is more complex than the auditory system, primarily because of the motor component. Thus, the evaluation and interpretation of disorders in this system are also more complex. A single chapter cannot comprehensively describe the function and clinical assessment of the balance system, as well as the management of balance disorder patients. Entire texts have been written on the subject, to which the interested reader is referred (Baloh and Honrubia, 1989; Barber and Stockwell, 1980; Barber and Sharpe, 1988). The purpose of this chapter is to familiarize the audiologist with the tools currently available for the assessment of balance disorders and to introduce appropriate management alternatives. It is not the intent of this chapter to detail methods and interpretation of the procedures, but to provide the basis for understanding how this information may be helpful in the evaluation and management of the balance disorder patient.

FUNCTIONAL GOALS OF THE BALANCE SYSTEM

From a functional point of view the balance system has three primary goals:

1. To rapidly correct any inadvertent displacement of the body's center of mass from its equilibrium position over the base of support (the feet when standing) to prevent a fall from occurring

2. To provide accurate perceptions of the position of the body in its environment and perceptions of direction and speed of movement

3. To control the eye movements in order to maintain a clear visual image of the external world while the individual, the environment, or both are in motion.

Clearly the vestibular labyrinth has a critical role in accomplishing the goals of the system. It would be erroneous, however, to conceive of the system as consisting only of the vestibular end organ. A more accurate representation of the balance system involves multiple sensory inputs (vision, proprioception, and vestibular) with coordinated, automatic muscle outputs (muscles of postural control). This input/output system involves stimulus-coded response pairing, such that a combination of stimuli produces a particular, stereotyped muscle response. This characterization is true for both the maintenance of upright posture, as well as the control of eye movements to maintain a clear visual image. Understanding the complexity and integrated nature of the balance system would suggest that while the evaluation of vestibular end-organ function is necessary, it is often not sufficient to characterize a patient's status.

Before beginning the description of the evaluation of these patients, the rationale behind the various test procedures needs to be presented.

VESTIBULO-OCULAR AND OCULAR MOTOR SYSTEMS

A thorough review of the anatomy of the vestibular end organ and neural pathways is available elsewhere (Ryu, 1986; Harada, 1988) and only a brief overview will be presented. Figure 28.1 shows a schematized illustration of the membranous labyrinth, including the vestibular and auditory structures of the inner ear. This membranous structure is housed within the bony labyrinth in the petrous portion of the temporal bone, where it is secured by connective tissue and is bathed in perilymph. Endolymph is contained within the membranous structure where the specialized sensory neuroepithelial tissue is located. The vestibular apparatus consists of two groups of specialized sensory receptors: (a) the three semicircular canals—lateral (or

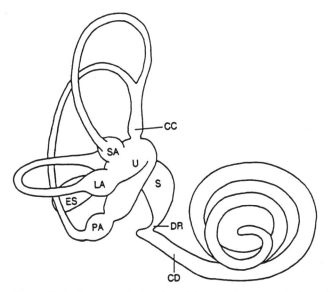

Figure 28.1. A schematic drawing of the membranous labyrinth of the human inner ear. *CD*—cochlear duct; *DR*—ductus reuniens; *S*—saccule; *U*—utricle; *PA*—ampulla of the posterior semicircular canal; *LA*—ampulla of the lateral (horizontal) semicircular canal; *SA*—ampulla of the superior semicircular canal; *CC*—common crus; *ES*—endolymphatic sac. (With permission from Kileny P. Evaluation of Vestibular Function. In Katz J, Ed. Handbook of Audiology. 3rd ed. Baltimore: Williams & Wilkins, 1985.).

horizontal), posterior, and superior, each of which originates from the utricle and terminates in a dilated end (ampulla) that also attaches to into the utricle; and (*b*) the two otolithic organs—the utricular macula and the saccular macula. The semicircular canals are oriented in approximate orthogonal planes to the other ipsilateral canals. While the two horizontal canals are in parallel planes, the two superior and the two posterior are in planes approximately orthogonal to each other. The canals are organized into functional pairs. The two members of each pair are in parallel planes of orientation. The three functional pairs are: (*a*) the two horizontal canals; (*b*) the ipsilateral superior canal and the contralateral posterior canal; and (*c*) the posterior canal on the ipsilateral side and the contralateral superior canal. The otolith organs also function in a paired format with the two utriculae maculae in approximately the horizontal plane and the saccular maculae in the vertical plane.

Contained within the ampulla of each semicircular canal and in the otolithic organs is an arrangement of hair cells that constitute the neuroepithelial transduction mechanism for the vestibular end organ. These hair cells are situated on a mound of supporting cells in the ampulla called the crista ampullaris, and within the maculae of the otolithic organ. Covering the hair cell projections (stereocilia and kinocilium) within the ampulla is a gelatinous membrane, the cupula. The cu-

pula, having the same specific gravity as the endolymph, is not responsive to slow static position changes of the head in the gravitational field. The gelatinous covering over the hair cells of the maculae of the otolithic organs has calcium carbonate crystals called otoconia embedded in its fibrous network. The presence of the otoconia increases the specific gravity significantly above that of endolymph. Thus the maculae are responsive to the linear acceleration force of gravity as the head is placed in different positions.

In both the semicircular canals and the otoliths, the activated hair cells modulate the firing rate of the corresponding nerve fiber. If the stereocilia are bent toward the kinocilium, an increase (excitation) in the spontaneous firing rate results. A decrease (inhibition) in spontaneous firing rate results from shearing action away from the kinocilium. The hair cells on the crista ampullaris are arranged such that the kinocilium for each cell is oriented in the same direction relative to the utricle. This is referred to as morphologic polarization. This polarization within the horizontal canals causes an excitation of neural activity when cupular movement creates a deviation of the stereocilia toward the utricle ("utriculopetal" endolymph flow) and inhibition of neural activity for shearing of the stereocilia away from the utricle ("utriculofugal" flow). The situation is reversed for the superior and posterior canals, with utriculopetal flow resulting in inhibition and utriculofugal flow causing excitation of the spontaneous firing rate. Therefore, stimulation of any of the three functional pairs by angular acceleration in their plane of orientation causes an increase in neural function on the side toward the direction of acceleration and a decrease of neural function on the contralateral side. This same paired action scheme occurs in the otolithic organs, however the morphologic polarization of the hair cells is significantly more complicated, allowing for sensitivity to linear acceleration in any direction.

The asymmetrical neural activity rate from the vestibular portion of the eight cranial nerves is interpreted by the central nervous system as either angular or linear acceleration. In addition, the asymmetry resulting from action of the semicircular canals causes a compensatory reflex eye movement in the plane of the canals being stimulated (Ewald's law (Baloh and Honrubia, 1989)). This compensatory reflex movement of the eye, called the vestibulo-ocular reflex (VOR), is opposite that of the direction of acceleration. To lesser extent this reflex also occurs for linear acceleration, mediated by the otolithic organs. Since the dominant system utilized for evaluating balance disorder patients is the VOR from the horizontal semicircular canals, we will concentrate on this response.

Figure 28.2 schematically illustrates the VOR from stimulation of the horizontal semicircular canals. In this example the subject was seated in a normal upright position and accelerated to the right rotating about the long axis of the body. Since the membranous horizontal canals are connected to the bony labyrinth within the petrous portion of the temporal bone, they also accelerate to the right. The endolymph, however, does not move immediately to the right but lags behind the membranous canal because of viscoelastic and inertial forces created by the capillary fluid mechanics effect of the canal. This effectively produces a relative flow of endolymph in the direction opposite that of the acceleration. Therefore, the cupula in the right canal is deflected toward the utricle while that in the left is deflected away from the utricle. This action results in an excitation of neural firing rate on the right and an inhibition on the left. The individual perceives rotation to the right and, assuming no visual input (darkness or eyes closed), a compensatory eye movement to the left (mediated by the VOR) is produced. This compensatory movement of the eyes is interrupted by fast jerk movements of the eyes back in the direction of the acceleration. This fast saccadic eye movement is not part of the VOR but a resetting reflex stimulated by the position of the eye within the orbit. If the acceleration continues, the VOR starts again to produce the slow component eye movement opposite the direction of acceleration. An individual viewing the eyes of the subject or recording their movement notes a jerking motion to the right and a slower motion to the left on a repeated basis. This eye movement is called jerk nystagmus and named by the direction of the fast component. In this example, the nystagmus would be right beating. If the acceleration is stopped and the subject simply continues to spin to the right at a constant velocity, the perception of motion and the jerk nystagmus would slowly decrease over a 20- to 25-second interval with loss of perceived angular motion and nystagmus. Therefore, without visual input the subject is unable to perceive constant velocity and will detect only changes in velocity, i.e. acceleration or deceleration. If the subject rotating to the right, at a constant velocity for 60 seconds is suddenly brought to a stop, a reversal of the action shown in Figure 28.2 would occur. The subject would now perceive intense rotation to the left and would demonstrate left-beating nystagmus, even though perfectly still. The sudden deceleration produces effective endolymph flow to the right. It will again take 20–25 seconds for the perception of motion and the left-beating nystagmus to dissipate. It is known that the cupula returns to its equilibrium position in 6–10 seconds. The prolongation of motion perception and nys-

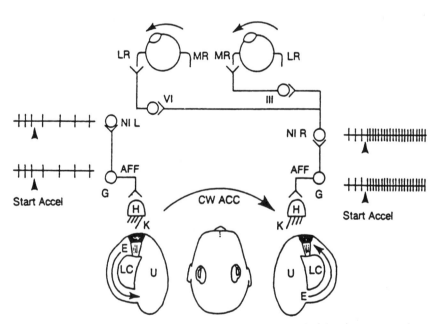

Figure 28.2. A schematic representation of the functioning of the horizontal semicircular canals under the condition of angular acceleration (*ACC*) in the clockwise (*CW*) direction. *LC*—Lateral semicircular canal; *E*—endolymph; *U*—utricle; *K*—kinocilium; *H*—hair cell of the lateral crista; *AFF*—Afferent nerve fiber; *G*—spiral ganglion cells; *NI R(L)*—vestibular nuclei, right and left; *III*—oculomotor nerve, cranial nerve III; *VI*—abducens nerve, cranial nerve VI; *LR*— lateral rectus muscle; *MR*—medial rectus muscle. Indications of firing rate changes on the primary afferent nerve fibers and at the level of the vestibular nuclei are given in the spike trains the right and left sides of the figure. (Adapted from Kileny P. Evaluation of Vestibular Function. In Katz J, Ed. Handbook of Audiology. 3rd ed. Baltimore: Williams & Wilkins, 1985.).

tagmus beyond the expected time frame due to neural firing rate asymmetry in the vestibular portion of the VIIIth cranial nerve (the primary afferent inputs) is caused by action believed to occur in the vestibular nuclei known as the velocity storage integrator (Cohen, et. al., 1981). Interaction between the primary afferent neural firing patterns from the otolith organs and the semicircular canals apparently take place through the velocity storage integrator.

As shown in Figure 28.2, the VOR of the horizontal canals is mediated by a simple three-neuron arc involving the vestibular nuclei and cranial nerves III and VI. Stimulation of the vertical canal pairs also produce a VOR along analogous brainstem pathways. Oblique (or rotatory) nystagmus can be seen with stimulation of the horizontal canal pair and one of the vertical pairs. The central nervous system pathways from the vestibular nuclei to the extraocular muscles use the cranial nerves III, IV, and VI, the medial longitudinal fasciculus, and collateral neural inputs from the reticular formation in the brainstem. A detailed description of these brainstem and cerebellar pathways and the neurophysiology of the VOR are discussed thoroughly elsewhere (Baloh and Honrubia, 1989; Ryu, 1986; Schwarz, 1986; Harada, 1988).

The principal functional purpose of the VOR is the control of eye position during transient head movements in order to maintain a stable visual image. In addition to this dynamic control system, several other neural pathways are involved with eye movement control, independent of head movement. Control of smooth pursuit, saccade, and optokinetic eye movements assist in maintaining clear visual images and contribute to one's perception of speed and direction of body motion. The smooth pursuit system allows for tracking of a visual target with a smooth continuous movement of the eye. This mechanism provides for stable image projection to the retinal fovea (that region providing for maximum sensitivity and therefore maximum clarity of the image). To utilize smooth pursuit, the trajectory of the target must be predictable, and the frequency of movement must be less than approximately 1.5 Hz. Constraints on maximum peak velocity and acceleration of the target also apply. While the vestibulocerebellum (flocculus, nodulus, and posterior vermis) plays a dominant role in smooth pursuit, the remainder of the cerebellum, portions of the brainstem, and cortical areas also participate under certain conditions (Lisberger, Morris and Tychsen, 1987; Robinson, 1968; Zee, 1984; Zee, 1990).

As indicated above, the saccadic system of eye movement control provides the fast component during the production of jerk nystagmus. The primary functional goal of the saccadic movements is to reposition a visual target of interest onto the fovea with a single rapid eye motion (Leigh and Zee, 1982). To accomplish this task, supratentorial processes must participate to calculate the strength of the neural signal to be delivered to the extraocular musculature needed to stimulate a rapid, single, and accurate movement of the eyes. In addition to the cortical activity, both the pontine reticular formation and the vestibulocerebellum participate in modulating the parameters of movement; i.e., the velocity of the saccade, the latency to onset of the saccade, and the accuracy of the saccade (Cohen and Buttner-Ennever, 1984; Cohen et al., 1985; Zee and Robinson, 1978). When a target of interest falls outside the operating parameters of the smooth pursuit system, the saccade system provides for the tracking ability substituting jerk movements for the smooth movements. These catch-up jerk motions are effective when the target gets ahead of the subject's eye movements. The difference between the position of the target on the retina and the desired position on the fovea is known as "retinal slip." It provides one of the cues hypothesized in the calculation of the saccade movement parameters (Zee and Robinson, 1978).

A combination of smooth pursuit and saccade mechanisms, the optokinetic response, may be produced by repeated movements across a subject's visual field, the subject moving in a stationary visual field, or a both. The optokinetic response is a perception of movement and produces optokinetic jerk nystagmus (OKN) similar in character to that of the VOR. Right-beating OKN results from objects crossing from right to left in a subject's visual field. While there is some indication of a separate "optokinetic control system," eye movement experts generally agree that the smooth pursuit and saccade control centers involving the same brainstem and cerebellar pathways mentioned above are the predominant control mechanisms (Rahko, 1984; Ventre, 1985; Zasorin et al., 1983; Honrubia et al., 1989). The main functional purpose of the optokinetic system is to provide for clear visual images during sustained head movements (Leigh and Zee, 1982). The perception of motion that can be generated with optokinetic stimulation is so powerful that the vegetative symptoms of motion sickness (nausea, emesis, etc.) can be generated without actual movement of the subject. This response is exploited commercially in amusement park rides that simulate motion. The production of nystagmus and the perceptions of motion may suggest some direct interaction between the vestibular system and the optokinetic system. It has been demonstrated that this does occur, not at the level of the periphery, but through the velocity storage integrator in the vestibular nuclei and vestibulocerebellar region (Kubo et al., 1981; Zee et al., 1981; Waespe et al., 1983). While the range of frequency, velocity, and acceleration over which optokinetic responses are stimulated is broad compared to the VOR or smooth pursuit systems, many errors in perception would occur if this were the only perceptual system of motion available. The integration of optokinetics, smooth pursuit, saccade movements, and the VOR for control of accurate visual perceptions will be discussed later.

POSTURAL CONTROL SYSTEM

The major functional goal of the postural control system is to evaluate a deviation of the center of mass from its equilibrium position and to produce an appropriate corrective reaction. There is no specific sensory system for position of the center of mass. Therefore, we rely on three sensory input mechanisms to provide the information needed: the visual, somatosensory (predominantly changes in ankle angle when standing and walking), and the vestibular apparatus. The integration of the sensory orientation information acts to stimulate automatic coordinated muscle contractions to produce the desired postural response, repositioning the center of mass. This stimulus-coded response pairing appears to produce stereotyped muscle responses for a given input combination for the majority of normal individuals (Nashner, 1979, 1983, 1987; Nashner and Berthoz, 1978; Allum and Pfaltz, 1985; Horak and Nashner, 1986). Yet, it is hypothesized that a large number of muscle response combinations could be used for any given stimulus and environmental context. Therefore, the goal of rapid reaction time is best served by a limited set of response actions that are contingent on the stimulus and environmental context, eliminating the need to consciously consider

and select the optimal responses (Nashner and McCoullum, 1985). Even though all three sensory inputs are available to provide orientation information, the somatosensory input from changes in the ankle angle while standing seem to be the dominating cue that triggers the automatic muscle responses (Allum, 1983; Diener et al., 1984; Keshner et al., 1987; Nashner and Grimm, 1978). Visual and vestibular end-organ inputs participate more by modulating the response as opposed to stimulating it, unless the somatosensory input is disrupted or the automatic response is inherently destabilizing (Allum and Pfaltz, 1985). The change in ankle angle is mediated through the muscle stretch receptors in the ankle, the afferent pathways involving the spinal cord and brainstem/cerebellum, to motor cortex projections, followed by the efferent responses returned through the spinal column tracks to the appropriate musculature (Keshner et al., 1988; Woollacott et al., 1988). This is referred to as the long-loop, automatic response pathway.

In addition to the stimulus-coded response mapping of this system, the response is contingent on the environmental context. The system can be characterized as context dependent, or feed forward. This term implies that the stereotyped response pattern is selected prior to a perturbation, based on the current environmental context. This is illustrated in Figure 28.3 where a subject standing on a flat surface (larger than the foot) is subjected to a sudden posteriorly directed perturbation of the support surface. This induces a forward sway to which an automatic response is generated. The processed, electromyographic response from the major lower limb musculature is plotted as a function of time. In Figure 28.3**A**, a distal to proximal progression of muscle response starting with the gas-

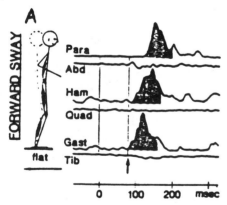
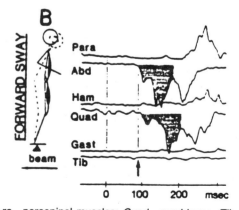

Figure 28.3. A, Induced forward sway of the subject with rectified surface EMG responses shown from the various muscle groups. **B,** Same size of perturbation inducing forward sway, but the subject is now standing on a beam instead of a flat, firm surface. *Abd*—abdominal musculature; *Gast*—gastrocnemius; *Ham*—hamstring; *Pa-* *ra*—paraspinal muscles; *Quad*—quadriceps; *Tib*—tibialis anterior. (Adapted from Horak FB, and Nashner LM. Central programming of postural movements: Adaptation to altered support-surface configurations. J Neurophysiol 1986;55(6):1369–1381.)

trocnemius occurs putting the subject back into position by pivoting around the ankle joint. This response uses force exerted by the toe and ball of the foot against the floor as part of the mechanics to reposition the center of mass. In Figure 28.3**B**, the same posterior surface perturbation is provided resulting in the same closing (dorsiflexion) maneuver of the ankle angle and similar inputs to the visual and vestibular organs. However, this time the subject is standing on a beam that does not allow for toe or heel contact with the support surface. As is shown, the muscle response is entirely altered, with simultaneous contraction of the hamstrings and paraspinal muscles resulting in a rotational motion at the hip joint. This represents a different stimulus-response pair despite the same provocative stimulus used in Figure 28.3**A** due to a different environmental context.

Feedback information is certainly used by the postural control system, yet the system does not respond as an immediate feedback network. In point of fact, the context dependency and automatic, stereotyped stimulus-response pairing of the system can provide a destabilizing response instead of appropriate action. For example, after the subject from Figure 28.3**A** has experienced five of the illustrated posterior perturbations without falling, causing forward sway and appropriate corrective action, on the next trial the toe and heal portions are lowered during the perturbation, leaving the subject standing on a beam as in Figure 28.3**B**. If the system was immediate feedback the muscle response shown in Figure 28.3**B** would be expected. Instead the response from Figure 28.3**A** is again recorded on the first trial, an initially destabilizing response that is followed by the appropriate response of Figure 28.3**B** to prevent a fall. Repeated trials of this same event produce a progressive change in muscle response from that shown in Figure 28.3**A** to that of 28.3**B** by the 4th or 5th trial with the others showing combinations of both muscle responses (Nashner, 1987). This example demonstrates the last major characterization of the postural control system, responsiveness as an adaptive learning system with significant plasticity (modifiable, not "hard wired") in function.

INTEGRATED BALANCE SYSTEM

To this point we have considered the function of the three major components of the total balance system; the vestibular end organs and the vestibulo-ocular reflex, the oculomotor system, and the postural control system. These systems do not, however, function as independent entities but as an integrated unit. Take, for example, the vestibular system's ability to provide perceptions of motion and control of eye movement during head movement. The semicircular canals function as integrating accelerometers that are relatively independent of frequency from 0.1–5.0 Hz. The vast majority of routine head movements fall within this range. The system continues to be responsive to accelerated head movements above and below this frequency range but shows a decreasing magnitude of response to frequencies below 0.1 or above 5.0 Hz (Schwarz, 1986; Baloh and Honrubia, 1989; Wall, 1990). Passive head movements in manmade vehicles many times produce zero acceleration conditions with constant velocities (such as a smooth airplane flight) or nonzero accelerations at frequencies far outside the typical operating range. Yet in these situations we usually have no difficulty in describing the direction, speed, or orientation of our movement provided we have visual input from the stationary world (optokinetics). This system effectively expands the range of frequency and magnitude of movements we can perceive with reasonable accuracy. While proprioceptive inputs such as pressure sensations, vibrations, or even wind against our skin assist in orientation, it is a combination of the vestibular apparatus and the optokinetic system that principally provide for our perceptions with respect to gravity and our stationary world.

The VOR control of eye movement while the head is in motion produces a gain (eye velocity divided by head velocity) of near 1 from approximately 1–5 Hz. Below 1 Hz, and especially below 0.1 Hz, the gain is substantially lower (0.3–0.6) when measured in the dark. However, in the light, the gain is essentially 1.0 (implying accurate and stable visual imaging of the target) from stationary to 5.0 Hz. The smooth pursuit system functions from stationary to just under 1 Hz providing a gain (eye velocity divided by target velocity) of 1.0, with poorer gains as frequency is increased above 1 Hz. Therefore, while each mechanism alone could not provide for accurate maintenance of stable gaze, the combination compensates for the ineffectiveness of systems in specific frequency regions. Thus, in a lighted situation, the ability to perform accurate foveal imaging of a visual target across a head movement frequency range from stationary to 5 Hz uses smooth pursuit initially, then a combination of smooth pursuit and VOR, and finally VOR alone. As with optokinetics, the range of function of the vestibular system is augmented by integration of the two systems. The adverse effects of using only one system is illustrated when a pathologic process destroys both vestibular end organs, creating a condition known as oscillopsia. This allows the perception of the stationary world to oscillate or bounce whenever the head is in motion within a frequency range above 0.01 Hz. Since most normal head motion takes place between 0.1 and 5.0 Hz, this condition can be most disruptive. The smooth pursuit system can accommodate the visual needs of the patient with increasing effectiveness as the frequency of motion decreases below 0.1 Hz.

As previously discussed, the dominant sensory input cue for triggering automatic corrective positioning of the center of mass when standing is the change in ankle angle. However, utilization of the visual and vestibular end-organ inputs must increase beyond simple modulation of the response if somatosensory input is compromised. For example, the patient with severe, bilateral vestibular end-organ weakness may step from a flat, firm surface onto a soft, uneven grassy area without significant difficulty in the light but, at night, is likely to fall. When visual information is available, it provides the information needed to compensate for the lack of accurate somatosensory information from the ankle. Yet at night the patient falls because all three systems are disrupted to some degree. If the patient had functioning vestibular end organs, then the removal of the visual information in the dark and the disruption of the somatosensory cue by traversing the uneven grassy area is less threatening. Another example from balance function testing involves a subject standing on a platform that suddenly tilts the toes up. The initial automatic muscle response that is stimulated by the change in ankle angle is the same as if the subject undergoes forward sway. This is now a destabilizing contraction of the gastrocnemius. After an additional delay of approximately 30–40 milliseconds, a stabilizing muscle response from the antagonistic muscle (the tibialis anterior) helps reposition the center of mass and prevent a fall backwards. This stabilizing response is hypothesized to be a vestibulospinal response correcting the initial somatosensory automatic response. Multiple examples of this continuous revaluing of the various input cues to the postural control system are seen routinely in daily living. In a normal subject, the vestibular apparatus probably serves as an internal reference against which the inputs from vision and somatosensory are compared to guide future decisions in the same stimulus-context situation (Barin, 1987).

LABORATORY EVALUATION OF BALANCE SYSTEM

The purpose of balance function studies encompasses three major goals. The most traditional is that of site-of-lesion localization concerning what sensory input elements, motor output elements, or neural pathways may be involved in producing the reported symptoms. Localization of lesion site (peripheral versus central, involvement in motor output systems, etc.) typically

shape recommendations concerning what medical/ surgical specialties need to be involved with the further evaluation and management of the patient. Second, assessment of the patient's functional ability to use the system inputs in an integrated fashion with the appropriate outputs is completed. This involves maintenance of stance after induced sway, and coordination of head and eye movements during gaze activities. The third assessment goal is to determine whether the patient may be an appropriate candidate for physical therapy rehabilitation. A wide variety of studies is used to assess the balance system in the broadest sense. Although the use of new, expensive technology has led to a better understanding and assessment of the balance system, the principles of these studies can be accomplished, if only qualitatively, even if these units are unavailable. With a sufficient understanding of the basic physiology of the normal balance system, the assessment of balance function can be accomplished even by laboratories of limited size and financial capability.

As both the history and laboratory studies are being performed and interpreted, generalizations regarding pathologic processes involved in balance disorders are important. Vertigo of acute onset usually results from pathology associated with the vestibular nerve or the vestibular labyrinth. In the acute phase, the nystagmus may be present despite attempted visual fixation suppression by the smooth pursuit system. This simply reflects the strength of the nystagmus rather than indicating pathology of the central pursuit system, assuming the nystagmus intensity increases when visual fixation is removed. As a lesion of peripheral vestibular origin becomes chronic, the nystagmus is typically observed only when visual fixation is eliminated. Processes effecting the vestibulo-ocular, vestibulospinal, or extravestibular (visual or somatosensory) portion of the balance system can produce a wide range of complaints, from mild unsteadiness when standing to severe vertiginous episodes. A report of intense vertigo with sudden onset is less likely when the peripheral vestibular system is not involved; however, small lesions of the central vestibulo-ocular pathways may mimic peripheral disorders (Cy Huang, 1985; Zee, 1990).

A complete neuro-otologic history is probably the single most important component in the diagnostic evaluation of the balance disorder patient. It is our opinion that balance function study results must be interpreted in light of the presenting symptoms and medical history. Discussion of specific historical information needed and its interpretation is provided elsewhere (Baloh and Honrubia, 1989). In general, the information should include the onset of symptoms and their characteristics at onset, the progression of symptoms over time, nature and duration of typical spells, predisposing factors in the past medical history, and past or current use of medications and other on-going management strategies.

Electronystagmography and Oculomotility Studies

Electronystagmography (ENG) is a process that provides a means of tracking eye movements behind closed lids or in a darkened environment. Changes in eye position are indicated by the polarity of the natural corneal-retinal potential relative to each electrode (Barber and Stockwell, 1980). Since the vestibular apparatus contributes to the control of eye movements, the latter are utilized to examine the function of the peripheral vestibular end organs and their central vestibulo-ocular pathways. This process is performed using ENG. Historically, ENG has become synonymous with vestibular function evaluation, but is now simply a subset of a more complete test battery. The ENG typically consists of a series of subtests during which eye movement recordings are made to assess the function of the vestibular end organs, the central vestibulo-ocular pathways, and oculomotor process independent of vestibular input. In addition to the Barber and Stockwell (1980) text, the reader is referred to other references discussing specific issues related to ENG testing and interpretation of the results (Barber and Sharpe, 1988; Baloh and Honrubia, 1989; Stockwell, 1983; Furman et al., 1988; Jacobson and Henry, 1989; Jacobson and Means, 1985; Wetmore, 1986).

ENG is useful for all patients with balance disorders. Spontaneous, eyes closed, unprovoked eye movements (spontaneous nystagmus) and eye movements provoked by changes in the orientation of the vestibular end organs relative to gravity (positional nystagmus) are recorded. Rapid positioning into specific head positions (Hallpike maneuvers) are performed to provide evidence for one specific condition—benign paroxysmal positional vertigo. A measure of the responsiveness of one horizontal semicircular canal relative to the other is typically performed through thermal caloric irrigations. The irrigations can be accomplished by open or closed-loop water irrigations in the external auditory canal or through air insufflation. The purpose of the irrigations is to produce a change in the temperature of the endolymph within each horizontal canal sequentially. This causes asymmetric central activity resulting in VOR nystagmus. Quantification of the eye movement recordings resulting from the irrigations are compared to produce the indications of relative sensitivity of the horizontal canal system. One must note that because of differential effects of pathologic processes, the horizontal canal may not be representative of the status of the vertical canals. In addition, an apparent weakness on one side could be from labyrinthine, VIIIth cranial nerve, or vestibular nuclei origin. In spite of these limitations and the potential of producing severe vertigo, this is currently the only direct method of selective determination of unilateral sensitivity. Major variations in the traditional methods for caloric stimulation have been proposed that provide for simultaneous stimulation of both external canals (Furman et al., 1988; Brookler, 1976, 1990) or the use of fixed temperatures with increasing length of time for the irrigation (Kumar, 1981).

All of the above measures exploit the VOR and rely on the integrity of the oculomotor pathways for normal performance. Thus, it is critical to evaluate these pathways independently by the use of the oculomotility studies. The oculomotor control systems discussed earlier are typically assessed during an ENG evaluation to provide information about the brainstem and cerebellar oculomotor pathways, independent of the vestibular end-organ function. The recent introduction of computerized ENG recording systems provide for the opportunity to significantly improve the traditional oculomotor studies. They allow for testing across a full physiologic range of function, as well as a quantitative analysis of the resulting eye movements. With the quantification capabilities comes better test reliability and the opportunity to analyze eye movement parameters that were previously impractical, such as latency and peak velocity of saccade movements. The typical procedures are designed to evaluate functions of gaze, smooth pursuit tracking, saccade movement, and optokinetic nystagmus. Abnormalities on these studies (with the exception of certain types of lateral gaze nystagmus (see Stockwell, 1983; Baloh and Honrubia, 1989; Barber and Stockwell, 1980) are indicative of central vestibulo-ocular pathway involvement. In general, the pathways involved are in the brainstem (pontine reticular area) and the vestibulocerebellum. It is important to realize that many other areas in the brainstem, cerebellum, and cortex can and do participate in the oculomotor activities evaluated. Therefore, great specificity of lesion site within these central pathways is not usually possible and probably presumptive. One notable exception is that of internuclear ophthalmoplegia (Shepard et al., 1990a). Functions of smooth pursuit and fixation suppression of the VOR, gaze holding in the primary eye position or lateral gaze, and adaptive changes in the amplitude and direction of the VOR are dependent on the integrity of the flocculus (a portion of the vestibulocerebellum). The action of the velocity storage integrator, especially as it relates to otolith and optokinetic interaction with the vestibular end organ, depends on both the vestibular nuclei and the nodulus region of the vestibulocerebellum. The dorsal vermis of the cerebellum contributes significantly to saccade accuracy, whereas the latency and velocity of saccades are determined by the function of the pontine brainstem. In situations where a prolonged latency for saccade action is the only abnormality of oculomotor function, the possibility of cortex motor planning deficiencies should also be entertained. The reader is referred to a sample of an extensive literature in the area of oculomotor function and pathophysiology for detailed discussion of the above (Hain et al., 1988; Optican et al., 1986; Thurston et al., 1987; Abel and Barber, 1981; Bogousslavsky and Meienberg, 1987; Gresty et al., 1984; Koenig et al., 1986; Leigh and Zee, 1982; Zee and Leigh, 1983; Yee et al., 1982; Ranalli et al., 1988).

In most studies of physiologic functioning, the sensitivity to subtle pathologic processes can be increased by testing function over a broad range of normal activity. In the case of smooth pursuit, this is achieved by stressing the pursuit system using progressively higher frequencies and target speeds. Unfortunately, this tends to highlight age-related deterioration of performance. This problem is sufficient to require age-related normative data for interpretation of smooth pursuit function. This is not to indicate that saccadic pursuit in a 70-year-old patient is normal, but that it may be explained by aging phenomena rather than primary central vestibulo-ocular pathway involvement. It may indicate abnormal function that may be preventing the patient's ability to compensate for a peripheral lesion. Thus, it may be related to the symptoms being reported by the patient.

With the oculomotility testing in place, we can now return to the interpretation of the eye movements recorded during spontaneous, position, and caloric testing. The finding of spontaneous or positional nystagmus of clinical significance (Stockwell, 1983) suggests possible lesion sites in the peripheral or central vestibular pathways, or both. The probability of peripheral versus central involvement is determined based on the characteristics of the nystagmus recorded. In most cases, the pathologic eye movements from are considered nonlocalizing but are more suggestive of peripheral system involvement when the appropriate oculomotor studies are normal. Caloric nystagmus measures peripheral responsiveness and becomes a major determinant of peripheral dysfunction. Normal caloric responses are necessary but not sufficient to rule out a peripheral vestibular lesion. This is

primarily because the caloric stimulus is only representative of one point on the frequency/intensity function over which the system operates.

The ENG is a physiologic test and does not measure the functional abilities of the patient. However, the results often help explain the symptoms that the patient has been experiencing. Discerning abnormal from normal or artifactual eye movement is predominantly a pattern recognition task requiring experience as well as formally acquired knowledge. Understanding the limitations of ENG interpretation significantly improves the appropriate use of this tool. This is especially true since the ENG is still the most frequently used modality for balance function evaluation (Kileny and Kemink, 1986; Kileny et al., 1980; Takemori et al., 1979; Weissman et al., 1989). The principal limitation is that a normal ENG evaluation is not sufficient to indicate normal balance function. Many aspects of the balance system that contribute to patient symptoms are not evaluated with the ENG. When the ENG study is suggestive of peripheral vestibular system involvement, this should not be interpreted as indicating a lesion of the labyrinth unless other supporting evidence such as cochlear hearing loss is present. ENG and other tests of balance function cannot differentiate among involvement of the labyrinth, cranial nerve VIII, or the vestibular nucleus. Lesion localization by evoked potentials analogous to the auditory brainstem response remains investigational (Elidan et al., 1987a, 1987b). A problem is also encountered when caloric irrigations produce no response from either periphery. This finding should not be interpreted as complete loss of peripheral vestibular function. The caloric stimulus is only a single low-frequency, low-intensity point on the spectrum of canal function (Fernandez and Goldberg, 1971; Honrubia et al., 1982; Kamerer and Furman, 1988; Schwarz, 1986). Consequently, absent caloric responses are often seen in patients who have not suffered a complete loss of function (Telian et al., 1990b). Finally, the ENG evaluation does not provide for testing of the capacity for integration of all sensory input information used by the balance system, nor does it test the patient's ability to handle conflicting information. This information is needed to assess the overall state of functional capacity.

To demonstrate the use of integrated test results, two patients will be presented and followed through each of the evaluation procedures discussed.

Patient RT

An 84-year-old male presents with gradual onset of constant unsteadiness over the last 1½ years, predominantly while attempting to walk or stand. He denies vertigo, lightheadedness, or other forms of disequilibrium.

Symptoms are typically worse in the morning and improve with activity throughout the day. The patient had peripheral neuropathy from significant pitting edema in the ankle area and diabetes. Past medical history was remarkable for a lumbar laminectomy performed in 1989, with ongoing pain in the right leg. Tinnitus, aural fullness, and hearing loss were all denied.

Patient FL

This was a 71-year-old male with sudden onset of symptoms following a motor vehicle accident 30 years ago. Symptoms were described as spells of vertigo with nausea that had recurred frequently over the 30 years, with a significant increase in intensity and frequency over the last 2 months. The spells occurred in two forms. The first were spontaneously occurring events, not provoked by particular head positions or movements, that had occurred twice in the last 2 months. These last for several hours with spontaneous resolution. The second variety were spells that occurred at least one time per day lasting for a few seconds. They were provoked by a variety of specific head positions and/or head movements. Constant tinnitus and aural fullness were reported bilaterally, with tinnitus greater on the right and aural fullness greater on the left. No perceived loss of hearing was noted but fluctuant hearing was reported on the left. Other than the accident, the past medical history was noncontributory.

As examples of ENG studies, we will examine the results of our two patient examples. Patient RT showed no evidence for abnormal eye movements for spontaneous or positional testing. No abnormalities were noted for Hallpike maneuvers. The four bithermal (44 and 30°C) alternating caloric irrigations produced no significant asymmetry in response. Oculomotor testing showed no abnormal eye movements for vertical, lateral, or straight gaze. Optokinetic nystagmus responses were normal as were the saccade results recording each eye individually. Figure 28.4 illustrates the patient's performance on smooth pursuit tracking at the lowest and highest frequencies evaluated. The analysis of saccade velocities, saccade accuracies and latencies are shown in Figure 28.5. This patient's pursuit abilities deteriorated as the frequency (and target peak speed) were increased. The smooth pursuit became more disrupted with saccadic catch-up eye movements. However, the performance is considered appropriate for the patient's age, and does not suggest a primary lesion in the central vestibulo-ocular pathways. For this patient, the ENG results are inadequate to explain his complaints, but do help rule out significant peripheral or central vestibular system involvement.

Patient FL demonstrated both spontaneous and positional eyes closed right-beating nystagmus, shown in Figure 28.6. The positional nystagmus was accentu-

ated in the right ear dependent position, was present in 6 of 11 positions tested with slow component velocities ranging from 2–6°/sec. The positional and spontaneous nystagmus was intense enough to be clinically significant (Stockwell, 1983). The positional nystagmus was oblique in nature, with the right-beating horizontal component associated sporadically with a down-beating vertical component. As with patient RT, the caloric testing revealed no abnormalities relative to peripheral sensitivity or nystagmus production. Oculomotor gaze testing and optokinetic nystagmus were normal. Examples of smooth pursuit testing and individual eye saccade recordings are shown in Figures 28.7 and 28.8, respectively. The pursuit results were interpreted to indicate abnormal function of the pursuit system within the central vestibulo-ocular pathways, consistent with age-related changes. The saccade evaluation was normal. Therefore, patient FL had ENG findings that should be considered abnormal, with the direction fixed nystagmus suggestive of peripheral vestibular system involvement in light of the oculomotor findings. Localization to the right or left is unclear but the direction of the nystagmus suggests a right side weakness or a left side irritative lesion. The ENG results begin to explain this patient's complaints, but are not definitive findings. Further support for a diagnosis of peripheral involvement would be desirable.

Rotational Chair Sinusoidal Harmonic Acceleration Test (SHA)

Vestibular function, like the auditory system, has frequency-specific characteristics over which it functions. Calorics provide for the equivalent of a low-frequency, low-acceleration stimulus. The use of rotational chair testing has developed as a means for stimulating the horizontal semicircular canal over a broader range of frequencies and accelerations. This technique allows for a more complete investigation of the VOR with a relevant physiologic stimulus. Control of the stimulus input is also superior to that of thermal calorics. While sinusoidal harmonic acceleration (SHA) testing is also a physiologic rather than a functional evaluation, it provides information about the vestibulo-ocular system that is not obtained from the ENG. Because it expands our investigation of the vestibular system function, it is useful for all patients with chronic balance disorders. This evaluation is critical in individuals whose calorics are either significantly reduced, absent, or ambiguous due to asymmetrical anatomy. This study can be especially useful in pediatric patients and others with mental age under 10, and in patients requiring pre and post-treatment evaluation. Serial ves-

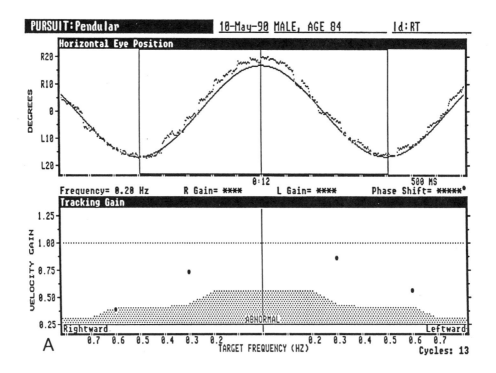

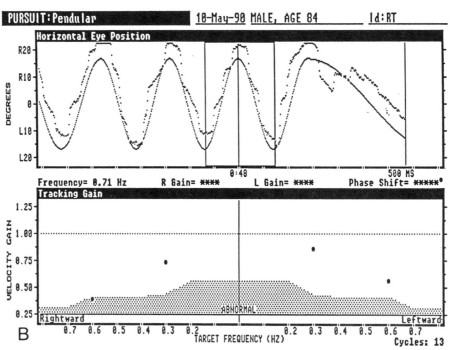

Figure 28.4. Results from smooth pursuit tracking test for patient RT. **A,** Plot of amplitude of the conjugate, horizontal eye movements in degrees versus time in the *top panel* for a target frequency of 0.2 Hz. The *bottom panel* plots velocity gain (velocity of the eye movements divided by the velocity of the target) versus frequency of target movement for rightward and leftward excursions. **B,** Same as **A** but for a target frequency of 0.71 Hz. (From ICS Medical Corporation. With permission.)

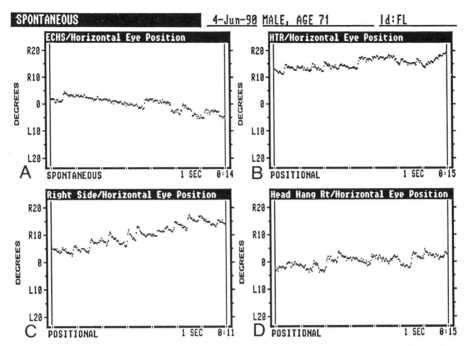

Figure 28.5. Results from patient RT for random saccade testing with conjugate eye recordings. These results were interpreted as normal. **A,** Amplitude of eye movement (*dotted line*) superimposed over the amplitude of target movement (*solid line*) as a function of time. **B,** Maximum saccade velocity for each saccade movement analyzed is plotted versus the subtended arc movement of the eyes in degrees. This shown for eyes moving in the rightward and leftward directions. The *stippled area* represents abnormal velocities. The percentage figures indicate the number of saccade move-ments with normal velocities. **C,** A plot of a measure of the accuracy of each saccade movement versus the subtended arc movement of the eyes in degrees. 100% indicates eye movement equal to target movement. Display of the conjugate eye movements arranged as in **A. D,** Plot of the latency to initiation of each of the saccade movements versus the subtended arc movement of the eyes in degrees. Display of the conjugate eye movements arranged as in **A.** (From ICS Medical Corporation. With permission.)

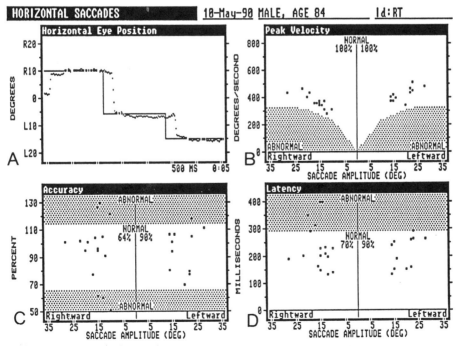

Figure 28.6. Plots of conjugate eye movement amplitude versus time showing examples of right beating nystagmus from patient FL. **A,** Eyes closed head straight, sitting position. **B,** Eyes closed head turned right, sitting position. **C,** Eyes closed head straight, patient laying on his right side (right decubitus). **D,** Eyes closed head turned right with hyperextension of the neck from the supine position. (From ICS Medical Corporation. With permission.)

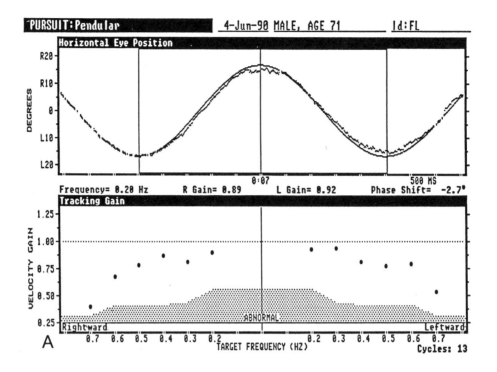

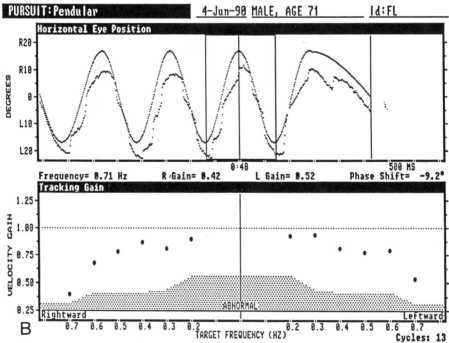

Figure 28.7. Results of the smooth pursuit tracking test for patient FL. **A**, Target movement frequency of 0.2 Hz. **B**, Target movement frequency of 0.71 Hz. See Figure 28.4 legend for details. (From ICS Medical Corporation. With permission.)

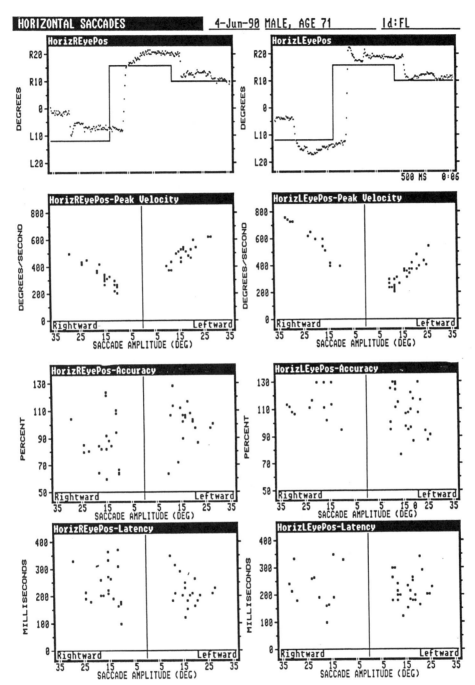

Figure 28.8. Results of the random saccade testing for patient FL shown with individual eye recordings. The left-hand column shows amplitude of movement, velocity, accuracy, and latency of the saccade movements for the right eye. The right-hand column gives the same information for the left eye. See Figure 28.5 for detailed descriptions of the individual plots. These results were interpreted as normal. (From ICS Medical Corporation. With permission.)

tibular testing is also appropriate when ototoxic drugs are given.

The commercially available devices provide for computer-controlled movement, recording of eye activity, and analysis of eye movements relative to chair (head) movement. The typical mode of chair movement is sinusoidal, hence the name *sinusoidal harmonic acceleration*. The acceleration stimulus that activates the VOR is repeated for multiple cycles at a given frequency with the slow-component eye movements averaged and analyzed by comparison to head movement. For general discussions of the theory of operation and use of the rotational chair the reader is referred to Hirsch, 1986, and Wall, 1990. Further consideration of specific applications, variations on the standard sinusoidal technique, interpretation of results, and examples in various patient populations are presented elsewhere (Baloh et al., 1982; Hamid et al., 1986; Hess et al., 1985; Honrubia et al., 1984a, 1984b; Istill et al., 1983; Wall, Black and Hunt, 1984; Peterka et al., 1990a, 1990b). Three specific parameters are evaluated (Figure 28.9):

1. *Phase* relates the timing between the sinusoidal input of head velocity and the sinusoidal behavior of the slow-component eye velocity. This measure can be related directly to a time constant value, i.e., the length of time following a sudden stop that it takes for the VOR response (and cortically perceived sensations) to dissipate.

2. *Gain* is the ratio of the average peak slow-component eye velocity to the average peak head velocity (output divided by input).

3. *Asymmetry* is a measure of the difference in average peak slow-component eye velocity resulting from acceleration to the right versus acceleration to the left, expressed in percentage.

In general, abnormal findings from this evaluation indicate peripheral vestibular dysfunction. The nature of the rotational stimulus does allow for testing of vestibular-visual interactions such as enhancement and suppression of the VOR with appropriate visual input during rotation. These latter measures relate specifically to the central vestibulo-ocular pathways.

Information about function at frequencies above that measured by calorics can be obtained without the need for a rotating chair, at least qualitatively, by having patients passively moving their heads in time to an auditory stimulus that changes frequency. The resulting eye movement can be recorded on standard ENG equipment (Goebel, 1990). The use of patient head shaking has also been developed to obtain information in the frequency range from 1–6 Hz quantitatively (O'leary and Davis, 1990) and as a bedside tool for qualitative assessment (Hain et al., 1987).

Figure 28.10 shows the rotational chair results from patient RT. Phase and gain are given in Figure 28.10**A** with the asymmetry information in Figure 28.10**B**. The results indicate phase and gain values within a normal range across all test frequencies. Abnormal asymmetry was noted at 1.28 Hz only suggesting a preponderance for right-beating nystagmus (left slow component) at that particular frequency. This has marginal clinical significance suggesting peripheral involvement. Therefore, we still lack significant findings to explain his symptoms. In contrast, Figure 28.11 shows the SHA testing results on patient FL. These results demonstrate an abnormal increase in phase at 0.01 and 0.08 Hz that results in a calculated time constant of approximately 7–8 seconds, significantly outside the normal range and strongly suggestive of peripheral vestibular system involvement. Gain values are normal, but there is a left greater than right asymmetry at all frequencies except 1.28 Hz. There was no spontaneous nystagmus recorded just prior to chair movement and the asymmetry is interpreted as a bias toward right-beating nystagmus. In other words, a consistently stronger response was obtained for rotations to the right than for those to the left. While these results do not localize the lesion to one periphery, they substantially support our earlier impression of peripheral system involvement (labyrinthine, VIIIth cranial nerve, or vestibular nucleus) consistent with either a left paresis or right irritative lesion.

SINUSOIDAL HARMONIC ACCELERATION TESTING

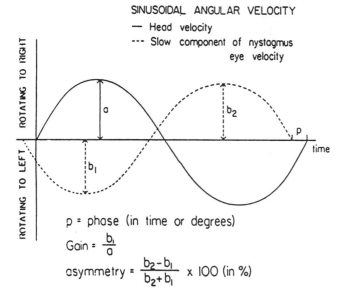

Figure 28.9. Shows pictorial and formulated definitions of the three major parameters used for analyzing sinusoidal harmonic acceleration testing. See text for further details.

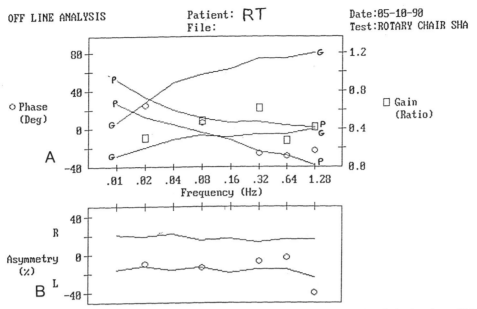

Figure 28.10. Results of the rotational chair testing on patient RT. **A,** Plot of both phase (*circles*) and gain (*squares*) versus frequency of the sinusoidal chair rotation with peak velocity of 50°/sec for each frequency tested. Phase values are given in degrees on the left ordinate with the gain on the right ordinate. The lines give the ± two standard deviation limits for phase (P-P) and gain (G-G). **B,** Plot of asymmetry versus test frequency. The lines represent ± two standard deviation limits. (From Neurokinetics, Inc. With permission.)

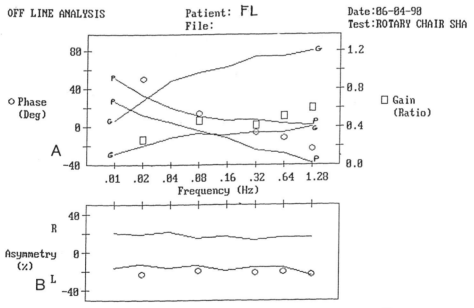

Figure 28.11. Results of the rotational chair testing on patient FL. See Figure 28.10 legend for descriptions of plots in portions **A** and **B**.

Postural Control Evaluation—Dynamic Posturography

ENG and rotational chair evaluations deal with isolated parts of the balance system and do not assess the system as a whole. The use of posturography has been proposed to provide quantitative assessment of postural stability during quiet and perturbed stance, thereby assessing integrated function of the balance system. Clinical observations and recordings of static postural control have been used for many years (Black et al., 1978; Wolfson et al., 1986; Yoneda and Tokumasu, 1983). This has provided some information about the function of the integrated balance system for maintenance of stance, but no assessment of reactions to controlled and systematic disruption in foot somatosensory cues or sensory conflict situations.

Another argument for expansion of the postural control evaluation is the suggestion that some gait abnormalities and unexplained falls, especially in the elderly, are related to changes in postural control seen with aging (Woollacott, 1988; Alexander et al., 1990; Gu et al., 1990). The concept of dynamic postural testing is rapidly gaining acceptance for clinical use. This provides for measurement of body sway during two distinct protocols. One assesses coordinated lower limb and upper body reactions to induced forward and backward sway (movement coordination), and the other analyzes the maintenance of stance during a variety of changing sensory input conditions (sensory organization) (Figure 28.12) (Black and Nashner, 1984; Black et al., 1988; Black et al., 1983; Nashner, 1983; Shepard, 1989). The patient stands on dual force-plate systems that provide the measures of reaction forces, allowing calculation of center of mass movements during the testing conditions. The dynamic aspects of the testing (movement coordination) (Voorhees, 1990) involve introduction of sudden anterior or posterior translations of the patient's support surface. During the sensory organization portion, conflicting sensory inputs are achieved through techniques whereby patient sway is synchronized to available visual and somatosensory cues as illustrated in Figure 28.12. A moving visual field synchronized with sway in the sagittal plane is not of functional use in maintaining stance. In fact, it will conflict with the information being obtained by the vestibular apparatus and the foot somatosensory cues. Stabilization of the ankle angle is accomplished by tilting the force plate down or up coincident with sway.

Assessment of postural control abilities are valuable whenever a complete evaluation of the balance system is needed. The specific findings seem highly population dependent. For example, normal findings are common in patients with peripheral lesions that show no signs of pathologic nystagmus or significant asymmetries on the SHA testing, and who report only motion-provoked symptoms. In contrast, patients with ongoing complaints of disequilibrium can demonstrate abnormalities that document continued dysfunction even when the ENG and rotational chair testing results show only minimal abnormalities. In point of fact, there is no way to reliably predict the outcome of dynamic posturography given the ENG and SHA findings. The reverse is also true, indicating that posturography is not a suitable screening tool to determine the need for the other evaluations. Like rotational chair, dynamic posturography provides adjunctive information about balance system function that is not available through other modalities.

The results from movement coordination are used to indicate potential pathology in the long-loop pathway (Vorhees, 1990). This may involve peripheral afferent or efferent pathways or lesions in the spinal column, brainstem/cerebellar complex, or motor cortex. A variety of musculoskeletal and/or biomechan-

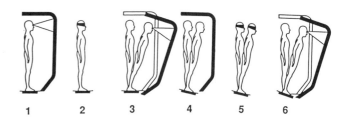

Sensory Condition

Figure 28.12. Six test conditions for the sensory organization portion of dynamic posturography. In the first three conditions, accurate foot somatosensory cues are available to the patient in all of the tests. The first and second conditions are simply eyes open and eyes closed. Condition 3 provides for orientationally inaccurate visual information in that if the patient sways anterior/posterior, the visual surround moves with the patient (sway referenced). In conditions 4, 5, and 6, inaccurate foot somatosensory cues are provided by tilting the platform equal to the patient's sway in the sagittal plane (sway referenced). Then, for each of these latter three conditions, eyes open, eyes closed, and sway referenced visual surround are presented, respectively. (From Shepard NT. The clinical use of dynamic posturography in the elderly. Ear Nose Throat J 1989;68:940–957, with permission.)

Figure 28.13. Results of dynamic posturography testing for patient RT are shown. The *bar graph* at the top plots a percentage equilibrium score for each of the six sensory organization test conditions (see Figure 28.12). A score of 100 indicates no sway in the sagittal plane with "Fall" indicating that sway reached a magnitude equal to the theoretical limits of sway for the patient in the sagittal plane. The *composite graph* is numerical average of the scores from the other six conditions. The *left panel* of the center three shows a ratio analysis of the six conditions relative to four of the most frequent abnormal patterns. *SOM*—somatosensory dysfunction; *VIS*—visual dysfunction (typically combined with vestibular dysfunction); *VEST*—vestibular dysfunction; *PREF*—visual preference pattern. See the text for discussion of these and other patterns.

The *middle panel* in the center row plots a measure horizontal shear force (an indication of body segment movement strategy) on the abscissa against the equilibrium scores on the ordinate for each of the six test conditions. The *right panel* of the center row shows a measure of alignment of the center of gravity (COG) in the sagittal and lateral planes for each of the six conditions tested. The *bar graphs* in the bottom (from movement coordination portion of the testing) row plot latency to onset of recover action to induced forward sway (*left graph*) and induced backward sway (*right graph*). The latencies are given in milliseconds for left and right leg for two sizes of platform translations. See the text for interpretation of these results. (From NeuroCom International, Inc. With permission).

EQUITEST SUMMARY
University of Michigan Medical Center
Vestibular Testing Center
Department of Otolaryngology

Patient: MALE, AGE 84
Age: 84
ID: RT

Referred By:
Sway-Referenced Gain: 1.00   Operator ID:

File: RT05100.EQT
Date: May 10 1990
Time: 14:41

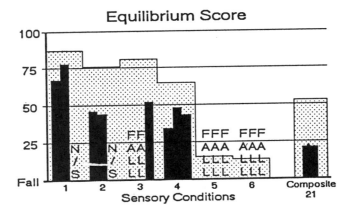

Equilibrium Score

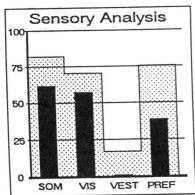

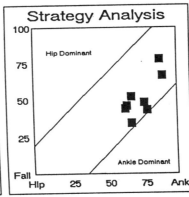

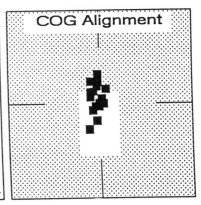

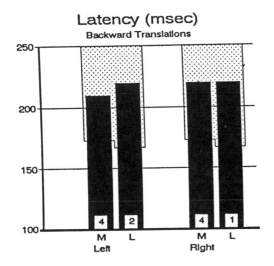

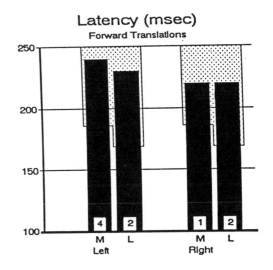

ical factors can influence the findings and need to be sought out in the history and physical examination. Additional information about weight bearing and strength responses to induced sway are obtained and influence the major factor in long-loop integrity, the latency to onset of reaction to the induced sway. The information acquired with movement coordination may help one better understand the source and nature of the patient's balance dysfunction.

The sensory organization test can be suggestive of pathology involving the vestibular system but does not distinguish between peripheral and central lesions. This portion of posturography determines whether the patient is unable to make proper use of appropriate input cues in maintaining quiet stance (sensory dysfunction). It also demonstrates which conflict cues are inappropriately selected when they should be ignored (sensory preference). This is primarily a test of functional abilities, not a site-of-lesion evaluation. Again, the data are interpreted by pattern recognition. The more common patterns are abnormalities on test conditions 5 and 6 (vestibular dysfunction pattern); 4, 5, and 6 (visual and vestibular dysfunction pattern); 3 and 6 (visual preference pattern); 3, 5, and 6 (visual preference and vestibular dysfunction pattern); and 2, 3, 5, and 6 (somatosensory and vestibular dysfunction pattern).

In addition to providing information about the patient's ability to use the available sensory information, posturography may identify environmental conditions in which the patient is at risk for a fall. This information is also used to assist in deciding who should be referred for physical therapy rehabilitation, determine prognosis in therapy, and monitoring of therapy progress (Smith-Wheelock et al., 1990; Shepard et al., 1990b).

As with rotational chair, qualitative assessment of the postural control system is possible even if equipment acquisition is prevented by financial constraints (Horak, 1987; Shumway-Cook and Horak, 1986). Various means of quantifying anterior/posterior sway may be substituted for the force plate. Of course, there are increased uncertainties in interpretation under these conditions.

A summary of the dynamic posturography findings for patient RT is shown in Figure 28.13. The results demonstrate significant difficulty with the maintenance of stance under all sensory input conditions, especially when visual conflict information is presented (condition 3) and when he is forced to rely on vestibular cues alone (conditions 5 and 6). These findings are suggestive of both vestibular and extravestibular system involvement. The results suggest that he is unable to utilize vestibular information alone for main-

taining stance and improves when provided with accurate visual foot somatosensory cues. It also indicates difficulty suppressing visual conflicts in favor of proper somatosensory cues. The increased sway and fall reactions on all conditions reflect a more global problem than just the selection of sensory input information. This impression is confirmed by the significantly prolonged latencies for reaction to induced forward or backward sway. This is a strong indication of long-loop pathway involvement and consistent with the poor performance on sensory organization. Not shown in Figure 28.13 are normal weight-bearing and normal strength responses to the perturbations inducing sway. In summary, this patient shows no significant indications for central or peripheral vestibular system involvement, but significant abnormalities of postural control with indications for severe involvement in the long-loop pathways. Given his residual lower limb pain and possible significant peripheral neuropathy, his symptoms may be explained by these factors. The patient was referred for balance retraining rehabilitation therapy to help improve use of available sensory inputs and reduce the risk for falls. He was counseled about safety issues in his living environment.

In contrast, Figure 28.14 shows the entirely normal posturography findings of patient FL. These results suggest that this patient is functionally compensated for the peripheral lesion and that the motion-provoked symptoms are not disturbing postural control abilities. This patient was also referred for therapy where habituation exercises for relief of his sensitivity to motion and head positions would be emphasized .

Central Compensation

One final issue that needs discussion is what information these tests provide about the progress the patient is making toward recovery following some type of balance system insult. A unique feature of the central system is the ability to compensate for peripheral system asymmetries, provided the lesion is stable over time or deteriorating very slowly (Igarashi, 1984; McCabe and Sekitani, 1972; Takahashi et al., 1984). The compensation process results from active neuronal processes in the cerebellum and the brainstem. The process of reestablishment of symmetric firing rates at the level of the vestibular nuclei is accomplished without modulating the neural input to the vestibular nuclei from the peripheral system. From empiric data and animal studies, it appears that the compensation process is enhanced by head movement but inhibited by preexisting or concurrent central vestibular dysfunction (Igarashi et al., 1978 and 1979;

EQUITEST SUMMARY

University of Michigan Medical Center
Vestibular Testing Center
Department of Otolaryngology

Patient: MALE, AGE 71
Age: 71
ID: FL

Referred By:
Sway-Referenced Gain: 1.00   Operator ID:

File: FL06040.EQT
Date: Jun 04 1990
Time: 13:12

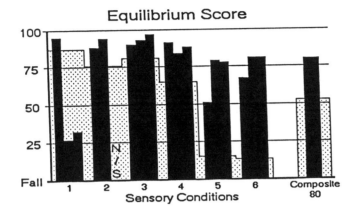

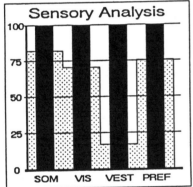

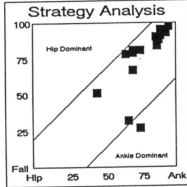

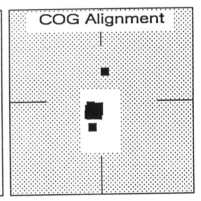

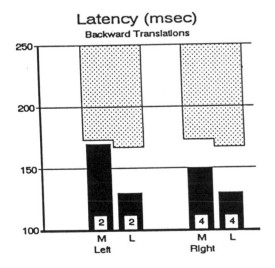

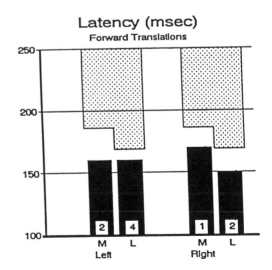

EquiTest ® Version 4.00 Copyright © 1990 NeuroCom ® International Inc. - All Rights Reserved
TEST NOTES: User Data Range: 70 - 85; Data from version 3.02

Figure 28.14. Results of dynamic posturography testing for patient FL. All results were interpreted as normal.
See Figure 28.13 for detailed explanation of the various plots.

Mathog and Peppard, 1982). Medications that cause central nervous system suppression, such as those typically used for acute symptoms of vertigo, may be counterproductive especially when used for extended periods of time (Peppard, 1986; Zee, 1985; Pykko et al., 1984; Ryu et al., 1984). There are some suggestions that elderly individuals are less likely to achieve complete compensation (Norré and Beckers, 1988; Stelmach and Worringham, 1985; Woollacott et al., 1986). Typically, the lack of physiologic compensation in the VOR is indicated by clinically significant spontaneous and/or positional nystagmus, a caloric directional preponderance, or asymmetries from the SHA testing. While the ENG and SHA results often agree, there is not 100% correlation, and both are helpful in addressing this issue in a given patient. A third dimension of compensation is derived from posturography, which addresses functional compensation relative to maintenance of stance. Enhancing this compensation process is one of the chief goals of vestibular rehabilitation therapy.

MANAGEMENT STRATEGIES FOR THE BALANCE DISORDER PATIENT

Management of the balance disorder patient may simply involve short-term use of vestibular suppressant medication for acute symptoms, or a more complex multidisciplinary approach. For further discussion of the medical/surgical management of these disorders, the reader is referred elsewhere (Graham et al., 1984; Hughes, 1981; Kemink and Graham, 1985; McElveen et al., 1988; Paparella and Sajjadi, 1988; Seltzer and McCabe, 1986; Kemink et al., 1989; Zee, 1988). Customized physical therapy rehabilitation programs for balance disorders are relatively new, although the rationale behind these techniques has been known for many years (Cawthorne, 1946; Cooksey, 1946; Brandt and Daroff, 1980; Hecker et al., 1974). A thorough review of the neurophysiologic basis for this therapeutic approach and treatment principles are presented by the key proponents of this technique (Shumway-Cook and Horak, 1990). Typically, the therapy programs involves two specific areas of concentration. The first is the use of habituation exercises in an effort to reduce or eliminate motion-provoked symptoms. The second area of concentration is that of balance retraining and correction of other functional deficits. More specifically, this involves direct attempts to modify the patient's postural control in order to correct particular deficits detected on by posturography and physical therapy clinical evaluations (Smith-Wheelock, Shepard and Telian, 1990a; Leigh, 1988; Tangeman and Wheeler, 1986).

The efficacy of therapy programs of this type is being investigated with randomized prospective clinical trials. Preliminary findings suggest that this technique is an effective management tool for a broad range of balance disorder patients. The results of a 2-year prospective observational clinical trial at the University of Michigan suggested reduction of symptoms in 85% of 152 patients. Using a disability rating scale, 80% of the 152 patients gave lower disability scores post-therapy compared to their scores pretherapy (Telian et al., 1990a; Telian et al., 1990b; Shepard et al., 1990b; Shepard et al., 1990c; Smith-Wheelock et al., 1990b). Statistical analysis of the results from the observational study suggested profiles of patients who have excellent, fair, or poor prognosis for therapy outcome.

This brief overview of the function and assessment of the balance system provides a sense of the difficulty of accurate clinical evaluation and the management of the balance disorder patient. Significant opportunities exist for basic science and clinical investigative work addressing these complex issues.

REFERENCES

Abel S, and Barber HO. Measurement of optokinetic nystagmus for otoneurological diagnosis. Ann Otol Rhinol Laryngol 1981;Suppl 79 90:1–12.

Allum JH. Organization of stabilizing reflex responses in tibialis anterior muscles following ankle flexion perturbations of standing man. Brain Res 1983;264:297–301.

Allum JH, and Pfaltz CR. Visual and vestibular contributions to pitch sway stabilization in the ankle muscles of normals and patients with bilateral peripheral vestibular deficits. Exp Brain Res 1985;58:82–94.

Alexander NB, Shepard NT, Gu MJ, and Schultz A. Postural control in young and elderly adults when stance is perturbed I: Kinematics. J of Gerontology: Medical Sciences 1992;47(3); M79–M87.

Baloh RW, and Honrubia V. Clinical Neurophysiology of the Vestibular System. Philadelphia: FA Davis, 1989.

Baloh RW, Yee RD, Jenkins HA, and Honrubia V. Quantitative assessment of visual-vestibular interaction using sinusoidal rotatory stimuli. In Honrubia V, and Brazier MAB, Eds. Nystagmus and Clinical Approaches to the Patient with Dizziness. New York: Academic Press 1982:231–237.

Barber HO, and Sharpe JA, Eds. Vestibular Disorders. Chicago, IL: Year Book Medical, 1988.

Barber HO, and Stockwell CW. Manual of Electronystagmography. St. Louis, MO:CV Mosby, 1980.

Barin K. Human postural sway responses to translational movements of the support surface. Boston, MA: Proceedings of the Ninth Annual Conference of the IEEE Engineering in Medicine and Biology Society, 1987:0745–0747.

Black FO, and Nashner LM. Vestibulo-spinal control differs in patients with reduced versus distorted vestibular function. Acta Otolaryngol (Stockh) 1984;Suppl 406:110–114.

Black FO, Shupert CL, Horak FB, and Nashner LM. Abnormal postural control associated with peripheral vestibular disorders. Prog Brain Res 1988;76:263–275.

Black FO, Wall C, and Nashner LM. Effects of visual and support surface orientation references upon postural control in vestibular deficient subjects. Acta Otolaryngol 1983;95:199–210.

Black FO, Wall C, and O'Leary DP. Computerized screening of the human vestibulospinal system. Ann Otol 1978;87:853–860.

Bogousslavsky J, and Meienberg O. Eye movement disorders in brain-stem and cerebellar stroke. Arch Neurol 1987;44:141–148.

Brandt T, and Daroff RB. Physical therapy for benign paroxysmal positional vertigo. Arch Otolaryngol 1980;106:484–485.

Brookler KH. The simultaneous binaural bithermal: A caloric test utilizing electronystagmography. Laryngoscope 1976;86:1241–1250.

Brookler KH. Electronystagmography. Neurol Clin 1990;8(2):235–259.

Cawthorne T. Vestibular Injuries. Proc Royal Soc Med 1946;39:270.

Cohen B, and Buttner-Ennever JA. Projections from the superior colliculus to a region of the central mesencephalic reticular formation (cMRF) associated with horizontal saccadic eye movements. Exp Brain Res 1984;57:167–176.

Cohen B, Matsuo V, Fradin J, and Raphan T. Horizontal saccades induced by stimulation of the central mesencephalic reticular formation. Exp Brain Res 1985;57:605–616.

Cohen B, Volker H, Raphan T, and Dennett D. Velocity storage, nystagmus, and visual-vestibular interactions in humans. Ann NY Acad Sci 1981;374:421–433.

Cooksey FS. Rehabilitation in Vestibular Injuries. Proc Roy Soc Med 1946;39:273.

Diener HC, Dichgans J, Guschlbauer B, and Mau H. The significance of proprioception on postural stabilization as assessed by ischemia. Brain Res 1984;296(1):103–109.

Elidan J, Langhofer L, and Honrubia V. The neural generators of the vestibular evoked response. Brain Res 1987a;423:385–390.

Elidan J, Langhofer L, and Honrubia V. Recording of short-latency vestibular evoked potentials induced by acceleration impulses in experimental animals: Current status of the method and its applications. Electroencephalogr Clin Neurophysiol 1987b;68:58–69.

Fernandez C, and Goldberg JM. Physiology of peripheral neurons innervating semicircular canals of the squirrel monkey. II. Response to sinusoidal stimulation and dynamics of peripheral vestibular system. J Neurophysiol 1971;34:661–673.

Furman JMR, Wall C, and Kamerer DB. Alternate and simultaneous binaural bithermal caloric testing a comparison. Ann Otol Rhinol Laryngol 1988;97:359–364.

Goebel J. ENG—Advantages of multi channel recordings. Presented as part of Diagnostic & Rehabilitative Aspects of Balance & Movement Disorders. Denver, CO: Oct 17–21, 1990.

Gresty M, Page N, and Barratt H. The differential diagnosis of congenital nystagmus. J Neurol Neurosurg Psychiatr 1984;47:936–942.

Graham MD, Sataloff RT, and Kemink JL. Titration streptomycin therapy for bilateral Ménière's disease: A preliminary report. Otolaryngol Head Neck Surg 1984;92(4):440–447.

Gu MJ, Schultz AB, Shepard NT, and Alexander NB. Postural control in young and elderly adults when stance is perturbed. II: Dynamics. Journal of Biomechanics. 1993. In Press.

Hain TC, Fetter M, and Zee DS. Head shaking nystagmus in patients with unilateral vestibular lesions. Am J Otolaryngol 1987;8:36–47.

Hain TC, Zee DS, and Maria B. Tilt-suppression of the vestibulo-ocular reflex in patients with cerebellar lesions. Acta Otolaryngol 1988;105:13–20.

Hamid MA, Hughes GB, Kinney SE, and Hanson MR. Results of sinusoidal harmonic acceleration test in one thousand patients: Preliminary report. Otolaryngol Head Neck Surg 1986;94(1):1–5.

Harada Y. The Vestibular Organs—S.E.M. atlas of the inner ear. Nishimura: Kugler & Ghedini, 1988.

Hecker HC, Haug CO, and Herndon JW. Treatment of the vertiginous patient using Cawthorne's vestibular exercises. Laryngoscope 1974;84(11):2065–2072.

Hess K, Baloh RW, and Honrubia V. Rotational testing in patients with bilateral peripheral vestibular disease. Laryngoscope 1985;95:85–88.

Hirsch BE. Computed sinusoidal harmonic acceleration. Ear Hear 1986;7(3):198–203.

Honrubia V, Baloh RW, and Khalili R. Subjective and oculomotor responses during interaction of smooth pursuit with optokinetic and vestibular stimuli. Abstracts of the Twelfth Midwinter Research Meeting. St. Petersburg, FL: Association for Research in Otolaryngology, 1989.

Honrubia V, Jenkins HA, Baloh RW, Lau CGY. Evaluation of rotatory vestibular tests in peripheral labyrinthine lesions. In Honrubia V, and Brazier MAB, Eds. Nystagmus and vertigo: Clinical approaches to the patient with dizziness. New York: Academic Press, 1982:57–67.

Honrubia V, Jenkins HA, Baloh RW, Yee RD, and Lau CGY. Vestibulo-ocular reflexes in peripheral labyrinthine lesions: I. Unilateral dysfunction. Am J Otolaryngol 1984a;5:15–26.

Honrubia V, Jenkins HA, Minser K, Baloh RW, and Yee RD. Vestibulo-ocular reflexes in peripheral labyrinthine lesions. II. Caloric testing. Am J Otolaryngol 1984b;5:93–98.

Horak FB. Clinical measurement of postural control in adults. J Am Phys Ther 1987;67(12):1881–1885.

Horak FB, and Nashner LM. Central programming of postural movements: Adaptation to altered support-surface configurations. J Neurophysiol 1986;55(6):1369–1381.

Huang C, and Yu Y. Small cerebellar strokes may mimic labyrinthine lesions. J Neurol Neurosurg Psychiatr 1985;48:263–265.

Hughes GB. A new decade of surgery for vertigo. Am J Otolaryngol 1981;2(4):391–401.

Igarashi M. Vestibular compensation: An overview. Acta Otolaryngol (Stockh) 1984;Suppl 406:78–82.

Igarashi M, Levy JK, Reschke M, Kubo T, and Watson T. Locomotor dysfunction after surgical lesions in the unilateral vestibular nuclei region in squirrel monkeys. Arch Otorhinolaryngol 1978;221:89–95.

Igarashi M, Levy JK, Takahashi M, Alford BR, and Homick JL. Effect of exercise upon locomotor balance modification after peripheral vestibular lesions (unilateral utricular neurotomy) in squirrel monkeys. Adv Oto-Rhino Laryng 1979;25:82–87.

Istil Y, Hyden D, and Schwartz DWF. Quantification and localization of vestibular loss in unilaterally labyrintectomized patients using a precise rotatory test. Acta Otolaryngol 1983;96:437–445.

Jacobson GP, and Henry KG. Effect of temperature on fixation suppression ability in normal subjects: The need for temperature- and age-dependent normal values. Ann Otol Rhinol Laryngol 1989;98:369–372.

Jacobson GP, and Means ED. Efficacy of a monothermal warm water caloric screening test. Ann Otol Rhinol Laryngol 1985;94:377–381.

Kamerer DB, and Furman JMR. Rotational responses of patients with bilaterally reduced caloric responses. Paper presented at Barany Society Meeting. Uppsala, Sweden, 1988.

Kemink JL, and Graham MD. Hearing loss with delayed onset of vertigo. Am J Otol 1985;6(4):344–348.

Kemink JL, Telian SA, Shepard NT, and Graham MD. Surgery of the vestibular system: Preoperative diagnostic considerations and surgical alternatives. In Johnson JT, Blitzer A, Ossoff R, and Thomas JR, Eds. Instructional Courses; American Academy of Otolaryngology Head and Neck Surgery. St Louis, MO: CV Mosby, 1989:119–130.

Keshner EA, Allum JHJ, and Pfaltz CR. Postural coactivation and adaptation in the sway stabilizing responses of normals and patients with bilateral vestibular deficit. Exp Brain Res 1987; 69:77–92.

Keshner EA, Woollocott MH, and Debu B. Neck, truck, and limb muscle responses during postural perturbations in humans. Exp Brain Res 1988;71:455–466.

Kileny P, and Kemink J. Artifacts and errors in the electronystagmographic (ENG) evaluation of the vestibular system. Ear Hear 1986;7(3):151–156.

Kileny P, McCabe B, and Ryu JH. Effects of attention-requiring tasks on vestibular nystagmus. Ann Otol 1980:89;9–12.

Koenig E, Dichgans J, and Dengler W. Fixation suppression of the vestibulo-ocular reflex (VOR) during sinusoidal stimulation in humans as related to the performance of the pursuit system. Acta Otolaryngol (Stockh) 1986;102:423–431.

Kubo T, Igarashi M, Jensen D, and Wright W. Eye-head coordination and lateral canal block in squirrel monkeys. Ann Otol 1981;90:154–157.

Leigh J. Management of oscillopsia. In Barber HO, and Sharpe JA, Eds. Vestibular Disorders. Chicago: Year Book Medical Publishers, 1988:201–211.

Leigh RJ, and Zee DS. The diagnostic value of abnormal eye movements: a pathophysiological approach. Johns Hopkins Med J 1982;151:122–135.

Lisberger SG, Morris EJ, and Tychsen L. Visual motion processing and sensory-motor integration for smooth pursuit eye movements. Ann Rev Neurosci 1987;10:97–129.

Mathog RH, and Peppard SB. Exercise and recovery from vestibular injury. Am J Otolaryngol 1982;3:397–407.

McCabe BF, and Sekitani T. Further experiments on vestibular compensation. Laryngoscope 1972;83(3):381–396.

McElveen JT, Shelton C, Hitselberger WE, and Brackmann DE. Retrolabyrinthine vestibular neurectomy: A reevaluation. Laryngoscope 1988;98:502–506.

Nashner LM. Organization and programming of motor activity during postural control. In Granit R, and Pompeiano O, Eds. Progress in Brain Research. Vol 50. Elsevier/North Holland Biomedical Press, 1979:177–184.

Nashner LM. Analysis of movement control in man using the movable platform. In Desmedt JE, Ed. Motor Control Mechanisms in Health and Disease. New York: Raven Press, 1983:607–619.

Nashner LM. A paper on advances in diagnosis and management of balance disorders: A systems approach to understanding and assessing orientation and balance disorders. Portland, OR: NeuroCom Int, 1987.

Nashner L, and Berthoz A. Visual contribution to rapid motor responses during postural control. Brain Res 1978a;150:403–407.

Nashner LM, and Grimm RJ. Clinical applications of the long loop motor control analysis in intact man: Analysis of multiloop dyscontrols in standing cerebellar patients. Neurophysiology 1978b;4:300–319.

Nashner LM, and McCoullum G. The organization of human postural movements: A formal basis and experimental synthesis. Behav Brain Sci 1985;8:135–172.

Norre ME, and Beckers A. Benign paroxysmal positional vertigo in the elderly. Treatment by habituation exercises. J Am Geriatr Soc 1988;36:425–429.

O'Leary DP, and Davis LL High-Frequency autorotational testing of the vestibulo-ocular reflex. Neurol Clin 1990;8(2):297–312.

Optican LM, Zee DS, and Miles FA. Floccular lesions abolish adaptive control of postsaccadic ocular drift in primates. Exp Brain Res 1986;64:596–598.

Paparella MM, and Sajjadi H. Endolymphatic sac revision for recurrent Ménière's disease. Am J Otol 1988;9(6):441–447.

Peppard SB. Effect of drug therapy on compensation from vestibular injury. Laryngoscope 1986;96:878–898.

Peterka RJ, Black FO, and Schoenhoff MB. Age-related changes in human vestibulo-ocular reflexes: Sinusoidal rotation and caloric tests. Vestibular Research—Equilibrium & Orientation 1990a; 1(1):49–60.

Peterka RJ, Black FO, and Schoenhoff MB. Age-related changes in human vestibulo-ocular and optokinetic reflexes: Pseudorandom rotation tests. Vestibular Research—Equilibrium & Orientation 1990b;1(1):61–72.

Pfaltz CR. Vestibular compensation. Physiological and clinical aspects. Acta Otolaryngol 1983;95:402–406.

Pykko I, Schalen L, Jantti V, and Magnusson M. A reduction of vestibulo-visual integration during transdermally administered scopolamine and dimenhydrinate. Acta Otolaryngol (Stockh) 1984;Suppl 406:167–173.

Rahko T. Optokinetic nystagmus. Acta Ophthalmologica 1984; Suppl 161:153–158.

Ranalli P, Sharped JA, and Fletcher WA. Palsy of upward and downward saccadic, pursuit, and vestibular movements with a unilateral midbrain lesion: Pathophysiologic correlations. Neurology 1988;38(1):114–122.

Robinson DA. The oculomotor control system: a review. Proceedings of the IEEE. 1968;56(6):1032–1049.

Roydhouse N. Vertigo and its treatment. Drugs 1974;7:297–309.

Ryu JH. Anatomy of the vestibular end organ and neural pathways. In Cummings C, Fredrickson J, Harker L, Krause C, and Schuller D, Eds. Otolaryngology—Head and Neck Surgery. Vol. 3. St. Louis, MO: CV Mosby, 1986:2609–2629.

Ryu JH, Babin RW, Liu C, and McCabe BF. Effects of ketamine on the adaptive responses of second-order vestibular neurons of the cat. Am J Otolaryngol 1984;5:262–265.

Schwarz DWF. Physiology of the vestibular system. In Cummings C, Fredrickson J, Harker L, Krause C, and Schuller D, Eds. Otolaryngology—Head and Neck Surgery. Vol. 3. St. Louis, MO: CV Mosby, 1986:2679–2718.

Seltzer S, and McCabe BF. Perilymph fistula: The Iowa experience. Laryngoscope 1986;94:37–49.

Shepard NT. The clinical use of dynamic posturography in the elderly. Ear Nose Throat J 1989;68:940–957.

Shepard NT, Telian SA, and Smith-Wheelock M. Balance disorders in multiple sclerosis: Assessment and rehabilitation. Semin Hear 1990a:11:292–305.

Shepard NT, Telian SA, and Smith-Wheelock M. Habituation and balance retraining therapy a retrospective review. Neurolog Clin 1990b;8(2):459–476.

Shepard NT, Telian SA, Smith-Wheelock M, and Raj A. Vestibular and balance rehabilitation therapy. J Otolaryngol Head Neck Surg 1993;102(3):198–205.

Shumway-Cook A, and Horak FB. Assessing the influence of sensory interaction on balance. Suggestion from the field. J Am Phys Ther 1986;66(10):1548–1550.

Shumway-Cook A, and Horak FB. Rehabilitation strategies for patients with vestibular deficits. Neurolog Clin 1990;8(2):441–458.

Smith-Wheelock M, Shepard NT, and Telian SA. Physical therapy program for vestibular rehabilitation. Am J Otol 19901;12(3): 218–225.

Smith-Wheelock M, Shepard NT, Telian SA, and Boismier T. Balance retraining therapy in the elderly. In: Proceedings of the Otolarynologic Cherry Blossom Conference, Clinical Otolaryngologic Care of the Geriatric Patient. B.C. Decker (Mosby-Year Book), Philadelphia, PA, 1992.

Stelmach GE, and Worringham C. Sensorimotor deficits related to postural stability. Implications for falling in the elderly. Clin Geriatr Med 1985;1(3):679–691.

Stockwell CW. ENG Workbook. Baltimore: University Park Press, 1983.

Takahashi M, Uemura T, and Fujishiro T. Recovery of vestibulo-ocular reflex and gaze disturbance in patients with unilateral loss of labyrinthine function. Ann Otol Rhinol Laryngol 1984;93:170–175.

Takemori S, Moriyama H, and Totsuka G. The mechanism of inhibition of caloric nystagmus by eye closure. Adv Oto-Rhino-Laryng 1979;25:208–213.

Tangeman PT, and Wheeler J. Inner ear concussion syndrome: Vestibular implications and physical therapy treatment. Topics Acute Care Trauma Rehabil 1986;1(1):72–83.

Telian SA, Shepard NT, Smith-Wheelock M, and Kemink JL. Habituation therapy for chronic vestibular dysfunction: Preliminary results. J Otolaryngol Head Neck Surg 1990;103(1)89–95.

Telian SA, Shepard NT, Smith-Wheelock M, and Hoberg M. Bilateral vestibular paresis: Diagnosis and treatment. J Otolaryngol Head Neck Surg 1991;104(1):67–71.

Thurston SE, Leigh RJ, Abel LA, and Dell'Osso LF. Hyperactive vestibulo-ocular reflex in cerebellar degeneration: Pathogenesis and treatment. Neurology 1987;37:53–57.

Ventré J. Cortical control of oculomotor functions. I. Optokinetic Nystagmus. Behav Brain Res 1985;15:211–226.

Voorhees RL. Dynamic posturography findings in central nervous system disorders. J Otolaryngol Head Neck Surg 1990;103: 96–101.

Waespe W, Cohen B, and Raphan T. Role of the flocculus and paraflocculus in optokinetic nystagmus and visual-vestibular interactions: Effects of lesions. Exp Brain Res 1983;50:9–33.

Wall C. The sinusoidal harmonic acceleration rotary chair test—theoretical and clinical basis. Neurol Clin 1990;8(2):269–285.

Wall C, Black FO, and Hunt AE. Effects of age, sex, and stimulus parameters upon vestibulo-ocular responses to sinusoidal rotation. Acta Otolaryngol (Stockh) 1984;98:270–278.

Weissman BM, DiScenna AO, Ekelman BL, and Leigh RJ. Effect of eyelid closure and vocalization upon the vestibulo-ocular reflex during rotational testing. Ann Otol Rhinol Laryngol 1989;98: 548–550.

Wetmore SJ. Extended caloric tests. Ear Hear 1986;7(3):186–190.

Wolfson LI, Whipple R, Amerman P, and Kleinberg A. Stressing the postural response. A quantitative method for testing balance. J Am Geriatr Soc 1986;34:845–850.

Woollacott MH. Posture and gait from newborn to elderly. In Amblard B, Berthoz A, and Clarac F, Eds. Posture and gait. Development, adaptation and modulation. The Netherlands: Elsevier, 1988:3–12.

Woollacott MH, von Hosten C, and Rösblad B. Relation between muscle response onset and body segmental movements during postural perturbations in humans. Exp Brain Res 1988;72: 593–604.

Woollacott MH, Shumway-Cook A, and Nashner LM. Aging and posture control: Changes in sensory organization and muscular coordination. Int Aging Human Dev 1986;23(2):97–114.

Yee RD, Baloh RW, Honrubia V, and Jenkins HA. Pathophysiology of optokinetic nystagmus. In Honrubia V, and Brazier MAB, Eds. Nystagmus and vertigo: Clinical approaches to the patient with dizziness. New York: Academic Press, 1982:251–275.

Yoneda S, and Tokumasu K. Frequency analysis of body sway in the upright posture. Statistical study in cases of peripheral vestibular disease. Acta Otolaryngol (Stockh) 1986:102:87–92.

Zasorin NL, Baloh RW, Yee RD, and Honrubia V. Influence of vestibulo-ocular reflex gainon human optokinetic responses. Exp Brain Res 1983;51:271–274.

Zee DS. New concepts of cerebellar control of eye movements. Otolaryngol Head Neck Surg 1984;92:59–62.

Zee DS. Perspectives on the pharmacotherapy of vertigo. Arch Otolaryngol 1985;111:609–612.

Zee DS. The management of patients with vestibular disorders. In Barber HO, and Sharpe JA, Eds. Vestibular Disorders. Chicago, IL: Year Book Medical Publishers, 1988:254–274.

Zee DS. The cerebellum in vestibular disorders. Paper presented as part of Dizziness Update '90. University of Toronto, Oct 25–27, 1990.

Zee DS, and Leigh RJ. Disorders of eye movements. Neurol Clin 1983;1(4):909–928.

Zee DS, and Robinson DA. A hypothetical explanation of saccadic oscillations. Ann Neurol 1978;5:405–414.

Zee D, Yamazaki A, Butler P, and Gucer G. Effects of ablation of flocculus and paraflocculus on eye movements in primate. J Neurophysiol 1981;46(4):878–899.

CHAPTER 29

Otoacoustic Emissions: An Emerging Clinical Tool

Susan J. Norton and Lisa J. Stover

Otoacoustic emissions (OAEs) are sounds generated within the normal cochlea, either spontaneously or in response to acoustic stimulation. The first measurements of OAEs were reported in 1978 by David Kemp from the Institute for Laryngology and Otology (ILO) in London, England. Kemp's original reports were greeted with a mixture of excitement and skepticism. Much of the early work was concerned with replicating Kemp's findings. In fact, over the past 14 years, Kemp's original observations have been confirmed by several laboratories in Europe, Asia, and the United States. Otoacoustic emissions are now thought to reflect the activity of active biological mechanisms within the cochlea responsible for the exquisite sensitivity, sharp frequency selectivity, and wide dynamic range of the normal auditory system. There is significant indirect evidence that these mechanisms are the outer hair cells (OHCs) at least in the mammalian cochlea (e.g., Kiang, Moxon and Levine, 1970; Khanna and Leonard, 1986a,b; Liberman and Dodds, 1984a,b; Sellick, Patuzzi and Johnstone, 1982). It is well documented that when OHCs are absent or damaged, (1) auditory sensitivity is reduced by 40–60 dB (Fig. 29.1A), (2) the "tips" of tuning curves are elevated or absent (Fig. 29.1B), and (3) responses to auditory stimuli as a function of stimulus level grow abnormally (Fig. 29.1C). Also, absence of OHCs is associated with a lack of otoacoustic emissions, supporting the hypothesis that OHCs are responsible for OAE generation.

Numerous observations support a cochlear origin for OAEs. (1) OAEs are independent of synaptic transmission and are preneural. That is, if 8th nerve activity is blocked either chemically (Arts, Norton and Rubel, 1990) or physically by severing it (Siegel and Kim, 1982; Martin, Lonsbury-Martin, Probst and Coats, 1987), OAEs can be measured while neural responses to sound are absent. (2) OAEs are unaffected by stimulus rate, unlike neural responses. (3) Evoked otoacoustic emissions are frequency dispersive (i.e., the higher the emission frequency, the shorter its latency) and their amplitudes grow nonlinearly with stimulus level. (4) OAE tuning or suppression curves are very similar to psychophysical and 8th nerve tuning curves. (5) OAEs are vulnerable to noxious

agents, such as ototoxic drugs, intense noise and hypoxia, which are known to affect the cochlea. (6) Finally, they are absent in frequency regions with cochlear hearing losses greater than 40–50 dB, and present where hearing sensitivity is normal. Thus, although there are many unanswered questions concerning cochlear function in general and OAEs in particular, there is growing interest in OAEs as an objective, noninvasive measure of cochlear status in clinical populations.

The availability of commercial devices for measuring OAEs makes it imperative that the clinician have a basic understanding of OAEs. This chapter will review current knowledge about OAEs, with particular emphasis on their potential use as either a screening or diagnostic tool in audiology. The reader should keep in mind, that unlike most of the information in the HOCA, our knowledge of OAEs is at the "clinical trials stage," and we do not yet know all the strengths and weaknesses of the clinical application of OAEs. Also, like electrical evoked potentials (i.e., ABR) OAEs are not per se essential to hearing but reflect the integrity of elements and/or processes that are.

TYPES OF OAE PHENOMENA

There are two basic OAE phenomena: 1) spontaneous otoacoustic emissions (SOAEs) and 2) evoked otoacoustic emissions (EOAEs). Spontaneous otoacoustic emissions occur in the absence of external stimulation, whereas evoked otoacoustic emissions occur during or after external acoustic stimulation. There are several subclasses of EOAEs based primarily on the stimuli used to evoke them. These include: 1) transient evoked otoacoustic emissions; 2) acoustic distortion product emissions; and 3) stimulus frequency emissions.

Spontaneous Otoacoustic Emissions

Basic Description. Spontaneous otoacoustic emissions (SOAEs) are more or less continuous narrowband signals emitted by about 50% of human ears even in the absence of external acoustic stimulation. Their existence was first postulated by Gold in 1948, but the first extensive measurements were reported by

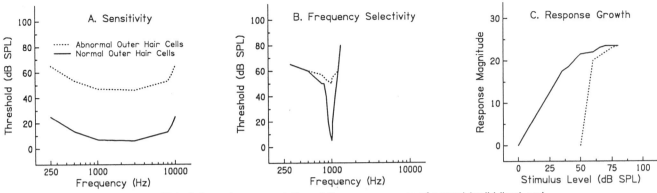

Figure 29.1. Schematic representation of the consequences of normal (*solid lines*) and abnormal (*dotted lines*) outer hair cell functioning.

Kemp (1979) and Zurek (1981). Subsequently, several surveys have been completed (e.g., Tyler and Conrad-Ames, 1981; Fritze, 1983; Schloth, 1983; Rabinowitz and Widin, 1984; Wier, Norton and Kincaid, 1984; Strickland, Burns and Tubis, 1985; Bonfils, 1989; Bilger, Matthies, Hammel and Demorest, 1990).

SOAEs are relatively simple to measure (Fig. 29.2). A probe containing a sensitive, low-noise microphone is placed in the external ear canal. The shape of the probe is similar to those used in immittance testing, and immittance tips are frequently adapted for use in measuring OAEs. The probe does not have to be hermetically sealed in the ear canal, but a good fit is desirable to eliminate as much external noise as possible from entering the external ear canal. The microphone, preamplifier and filter should all be "low noise." The subject should be seated quietly in a comfortable reclining chair with good head and neck support. The output of the microphone is generally led to a preamplifier and high-pass filter. It is usually necessary to filter out body noise and external noise below 300–400 Hz. The output of the preamplifier/filter is then subjected to frequency domain analysis (i.e., a Fast Fourier Transform or FFT) by using either a dedicated spectrum analyzer or FFT software and a computer. Data can be stored on high-quality tape or disk; i.e., the ear canal sound pressure can be recorded in the time domain, and the spectral analysis done later or "off-line." It is more usual in clinical settings to do on-line FFTs. Figure 29.3 shows SOAEs from two different ears.

Both were acquired with only 8 averages by using a dedicated spectrum analyzer. SOAEs generally appear quite rapidly when viewing the amplitude spectrum, but one must be cautious that a "peak" is not an harmonic of 60-cycle. There is general agreement that SOAEs in humans are concentrated in the frequency region from 1–3 kHz, but they have been observed be-

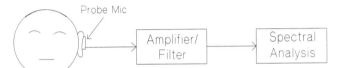

Figure 29.2. Schematic diagram of a representative system for measuring spontaneous otoacoustic emissions from human ears.

tween 0.5 and 9.0 kHz. They range in amplitude from about −25 dB SPL up to 20 dB SPL, with the majority falling between −10 and +10 dB SPL. Whether this is due to filtering by the middle ear or some intrinsic limitation of the mechanisms responsible for generating SOAEs is not clear. Audible SOAEs up to 50 dB SPL have been reported in dogs (Ruggero, Kramek and Rich, 1984) and cats (Norton and Rubel, 1992) and occasionally in humans (Wilson and Sutton, 1981; Mathias, Probst, Min and Hauser, 1991).

It has been noted by several investigators that SOAEs vary in their stability. Some are always present and show little variability in amplitude and frequency within and across recording sessions. Others are unstable. In some individuals, it is necessary to require sitting for 15 minutes or more, with the probe in, before SOAEs stabilize. Others demonstrate "linked SOAEs" (Burns, Strickland, Tubis and Jones, 1984; Champlin and Norton, 1987). In an ear with multiple SOAEs, the amplitudes of different emissions seem to vary inversely. That is, when one is present, another will be absent and vice versa. This can occur spontaneously, or if one is suppressed by external tones. Still other SOAEs appear for brief periods of time during and after acoustic stimulation.

Clinical Data. SOAEs occur in about 50% of normal hearing humans, including newborn babies (Burns, Arehart and Campbell, 1990). SOAEs are generally not observed in frequency regions with sensori-

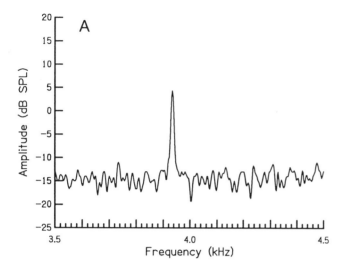

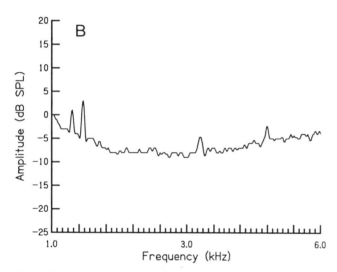

Figure 29.3. Examples of spontaneous otoacoustic emissions recorded from normal-hearing human ears. **A.** An ear with one SOAE. **B.** An ear with multiple SOAEs.

neural hearing loss exceeding 30 dB. They have been observed to occur on the steeply sloping edge of a hearing loss and in ears with unusual audiograms, such that there are small islands of normal hearing (and probably normal outer hair cells). Most people with spontaneous otoacoustic emissions are unaware of their SOAEs. After Kemp's (1979) initial reports, many clinicians were hopeful that SOAEs might be the objective basis of tinnitus. Unfortunately, several studies have indicated that only a small percentage of persons with tinnitus have recordable SOAEs that can be linked to their tinnitus (Wilson, 1980; Tyler and Conrad-Ames, 1981; Zurek, 1981; Hazell, 1984; Penner and Burns, 1987; Penner, 1990).

Penner (1990) analyzed several studies in which the coexistence of SOAEs and tinnitus with similar pitches

in the same ear was judged to be evidence that the tinnitus and SOAE were linked. The overall incidence was 4.4%, with 95% confidence intervals of 2.02% to 7.61%. Previously, Penner and Burns, 1987 proposed that in order for SOAEs and tinnitus to be causatively linked the following should be true: (*a*) the tinnitus should disappear when the SOAE is suppressed; (*b*) the iso-masking contour for the tinnitus must not be flat; and (*c*) a tone matching the tinnitus in pitch should be near the SOAE in frequency. In a study of 121 members of a tinnitus self-help group, Penner (1990) found that 2.42% had SOAEs and tinnitus that met these criteria. Using 95% confidence limits, she concluded that between 1.11% and 9.05% of tinnitus sufferers had SOAE-caused tinnitus.

TRANSIENT EVOKED OTOACOUSTIC EMISSIONS

Basic Description. Transient evoked otoacoustic emissions (TOAEs) also referred to as click evoked OAEs (COAEs) are frequency dispersive responses following a brief acoustic stimulus, such as a click or tone burst. Because this was the first emission type reported in the literature by Kemp (1978), the term *evoked otoacoustic emissions* (EOAE) is often applied specifically to transient evoked emissions. They are also known as *Kemp echoes, cochlear echoes* and *delayed evoked otoacoustic emissions.* TOAEs are obtained by using synchronous time-domain averaging techniques similar to those used to measure auditory evoked potentials as shown in Figure 29.4. In addition to a sensitive low-noise miniature microphone, as used for measuring SOAEs, the probe contains a miniature sound source for delivering the stimulus. Responses to several stimuli (e.g., 500–2000) are averaged to improve the signal-to-noise ratio. The ear canal sound pressure is amplified by a factor of 100–10,000, and high-pass filtered at 300–400 Hz. It is then digitized at a rate of 40–50 kHz. Figure 29.5 shows the averaged waveform (n=1600) of an emission evoked by an 80 microseconds-μsec, 40 dB spectrum level click, bandlimited to 400–5000 Hz. The first 2.5 msec of the response have been eliminated to remove the stimulus. One of the

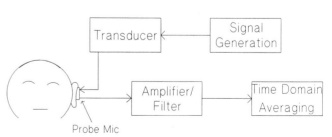

Figure 29.4. Schematic diagram of a representative system for measuring transient evoked otoacoustic emissions.

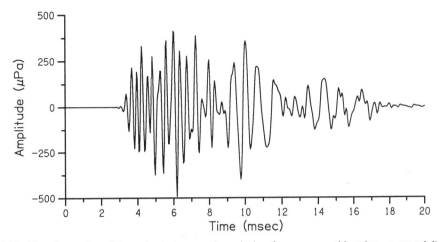

Figure 29.5. Waveform of a click evoked otoacoustic emission from a normal-hearing young adult.

most important characteristics of the respoıse is that it is frequency dispersive—high frequenies emerge sooner (i.e., have a shorter latency) than low frequencies. This frequency dispersion is consistent with frequency coding along the basilar membrane; i.e., high frequencies are coded basally, whereas low frequencies are coded apically. The latencies of emission components are roughly twice that of forward travel time for any given frequency. This supports the hypothesis that an emission of a particular frequency originates from the cochlear location tuned to that frequency. It is important to note that if we had used a different time window or filtering or a different stimulus, emission components would be present at higher and lower frequencies, depending on the parameters chosen. The measured response is determined by the evoking stimulus and recording parameters as well as the status of the peripheral auditory system.

Transient evoked emissions are measurable in essentially all normal-hearing persons with normal middle ears and normal cochleas (e.g., Kemp, 1978; Johnsen and Elberling, 1982; Grandori, 1985; Kemp, Bray, Alexander, and Brown, 1986; Probst, Coats, Martin and Lonsbury-Martin, 1986; Norton and Neely, 1987; Bonfils, Piron, Uziel and Pujol, 1988). In response to tone bursts as shown in Figure 29.6 the emissions are quite frequency specific. If, as in the ear shown in Figure 29.7, there are spontaneous emissions, one or more SOAEs can be "synchronized" by a transient evoking stimulus and strong components will appear at the SOAE frequencies throughout the evoked emission averaged waveform. In general, however, the frequency content of a transient evoked emission is determined by the spectrum of the evoking stimulus. This is true for both the level and bandwidth of the stimulus. There is some confusion about the "frequency specificity" of transient evoked emissions. This

arises, at least in part, because of the properties of transient stimuli. Figure 29.8 shows the amplitude spectra of a click, a tone burst, and two continuous puretones each with a peak equivalent or overall level of 75 dB SPL. Although the peak levels are equivalent in the time domain, their spectra and bandlevels are quite different. The shorter the stimulus duration, the broader the spectrum and the less energy at any one frequency. Because emissions can be evoked at most, if not all, locations in the normal cochlea, the broader the stimulus spectrum the broader the emission spectrum. That is, if there is more than one frequency in the stimulus, emissions will be evoked at more than one frequency. Each emission, however, is frequency specific in that the frequency of a given emission is specific to the frequency of the evoking stimulus. If clicks and tone bursts are equated for band levels, the emissions within the bandwidth of the tone burst are nearly identical (Stover and Norton, 1992).

Another important characteristic of evoked otoacoustic emissions is that their amplitude grows nonlinearly as a function of stimulus level. Figure 29.9 shows the input-output function for a 1500 Hz tone-burst evoked emission from the ear of a normal-hearing young adult. This function has the form of a saturating nonlinearity. Threshold is the lowest level at which the response waveform and spectrum are judged to be visually different from those of the baseline, no stimulus, condition. In this case, threshold is 9 dB peSPL. Above threshold, the amplitude of the emission grows steadily until a stimulus level of 39 dB peSPL and then saturates. That is, further increases in stimulus level result in no further increases in emission amplitude.

Clinical Data. Much of the clinical work related to OAEs has focused on click evoked emissions. This is

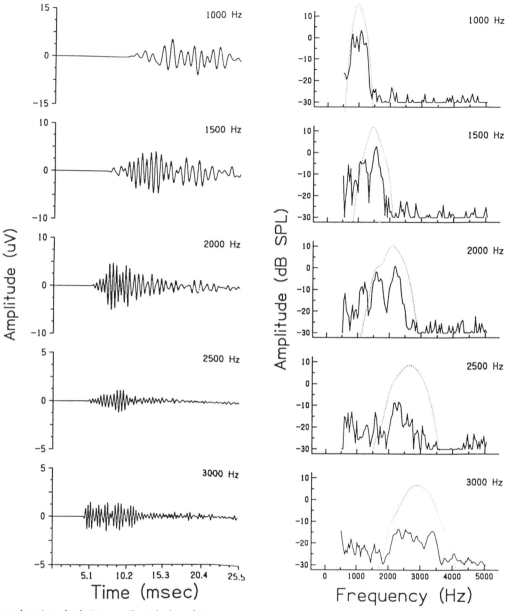

Figure 29.6. Tone-burst evoked otoacoustic emissions from a normal-hearing young adult. All stimuli were presented at 27 dB SPL. The response waveforms are shown on the left. The stimulus has been eliminated from the trace. The response (*solid lines*) and stimulus (*dotted lines*) spectra are shown on the right. Note that the stimulus spectra are not drawn to scale.

primarily because they provide broad band, cochlea-wide information. In clinical situations, this means the most information in the shortest time. The widespread application of transient evoked emissions is also due to the availability of commercial hardware and software, the ILO88, which is optimized for measuring click evoked OAEs. In the presence of hearing loss, transient evoked OAEs have been shown to decrease in incidence as hearing thresholds increase (e.g., Kemp, 1978; Kemp et al., 1986; Bonfils et al., 1988; Bonfils and Uziel, 1989; Collet, Gartner, Moulin, Kauffmann, Disant and Morgon, 1989). Generally, if the hearing

loss exceeds 40–50 dB, an emission cannot be evoked to a transient stimulus. Kemp et al. (1986) reported that the upper limit is 30 dB HL. This is true if one uses "the default" condition on the ILO88, which is an 80 dB peSPL, 80 μsec click. If one uses higher stimulus levels, the limit appears to be about 50 dB HL. Figure 29.10 shows the input-output functions for three subjects, two with sensory neural hearing loss, and the mean amplitudes for a group of 37 normal-hearing young adults. S1 is a normal-hearing 8-year-old child with very robust emissions, which are considerably higher in amplitude than the average

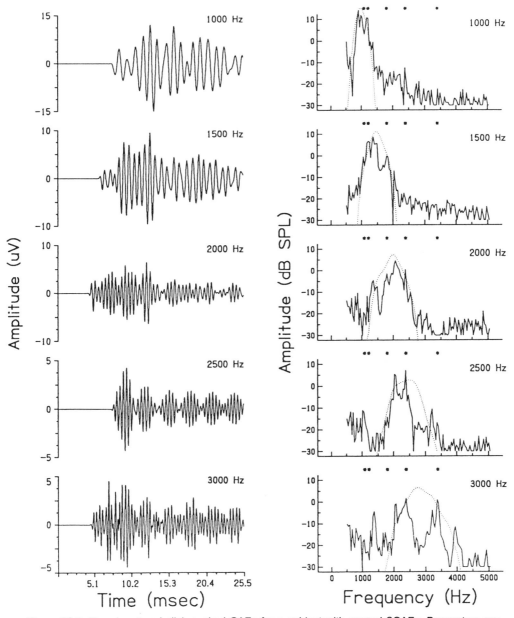

Figure 29.7. Tone-burst and click evoked OAEs for a subject with several SOAEs. Parameters are the same as for Figure 29.6. *Solid circles* indicate the frequencies of SOAE.

young adult. This finding is consistent with the observation that transient evoked OAE amplitudes decrease as a function of age even in normal-hearing persons (Norton and Widen, 1990). S2 is a 10-year-old child with a 40-dB sensory neural hearing loss. In response to high level stimuli, the amplitudes of his emissions are actually above the normal adults but decrease rapidly and are not detectable for stimuli lower than those shown. For S3, the EOAE amplitude is always below normal and disappears rapidly. Figure 29.11 shows tone-pip evoked emissions from a 20-year-old hearing-impaired subject with a rising audiogram. All stimuli were presented at 80 dB peSPL. EOAEs are absent for

tone pips between 500 and 1000 Hz, but present for stimuli above 1500 Hz.

Figure 29.12 displays similar information for an 11-year-old child with a rising sensory neural hearing loss. The output of the ILO88 is shown. The area labeled "Cochlear Response" is the EOAE waveform, whereas the area labeled "Response" shows the response spectrum in outline form, and an estimate of noise in the response is shown by the solid area. The click evoked response has energy from 1000 to about 3500 Hz. The stimulus in this case only went to 3800 Hz. The transient evoked response provided a good snapshot of the audiogram configuration for the subjects shown in

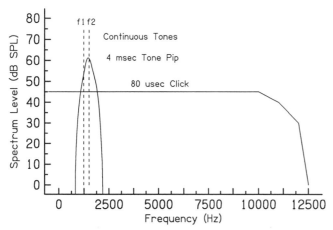

Figure 29.8. Schematic spectra for stimuli commonly used to evoke otoacoustic emissions.

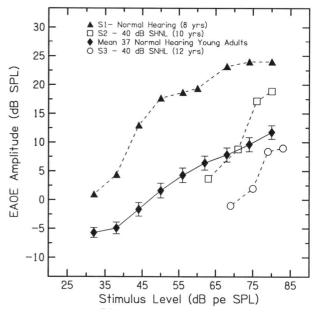

Figure 29.10. Input-output functions for click evoked otoacoustic emissions for normal-hearing and hearing-impaired humans.

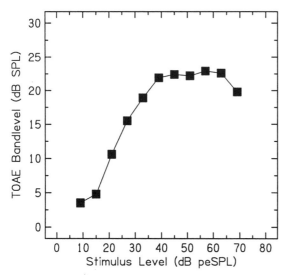

Figure 29.9. Input-output function for a 1500 Hz tone-burst evoked otoacoustic emission from the ear of a normal-hearing adult human.

Figure 29.11 and in 29.12, but there is no information about thresholds. The relationship between audiometric threshold and OAEs in response to suprathreshold stimuli is not yet well defined. There is good correlation between psychophysical thresholds and transient evoked emission thresholds for the same stimuli (Stover and Norton, 1992). In general, responses to suprathreshold stimuli decrease as sensitivity decreases. As seen in these subjects, however, when dealing with mild to moderate losses, EOAEs may appear to be within normal limits for high level stimuli. Thus, it is not clear what the optimal stimulus parameters are for clinical application. It may depend on the particular question being asked. If one is interested in sensitivity, one may need to measure emissions at sev-

eral stimulus levels and determine emission threshold. If interested only in cochlear reserve or integrity (i.e., is there any response?) one may be able to use a single, high-level stimulus.

As noted above, TOAEs also decrease in magnitude with age in normal-hearing persons. They are extremely robust in normal-hearing, full-term newborn babies, as seen in Figure 29.13. In contrast, Figure 29.14 shows the response from a newborn later confirmed as having a moderately severe (70 dB HL) sensory neural hearing loss. There is no measurable EOAE. Current results from some large clinical trials (Maxon, Norton, White and Brehens, 1991) indicate that transient OAEs can be a rapid, sensitive tool for detecting hearing loss in both normal and at risk newborns. In a cooperative, sleeping infant COAEs to one stimulus level can be measured in both ears in about 10 minutes, compared with about 20 minutes for screening ABR. The primary difference in terms of testing time is the additional preparation needed for ABR. Another advantage of EOAEs for screening is that they examine a broader frequency range than ABR; however, particularly with neurologically at risk populations, it must be remembered that EOAEs are preneural. EOAEs, therefore, could be normal if the cochlea were normal in cases of central auditory system dysfunction. For this population, EOAEs and ABR can be used together to help identify the site of lesion.

Similarly, EOAEs can be used to separate retrocochlear and cochlear effects in patients with acoustic

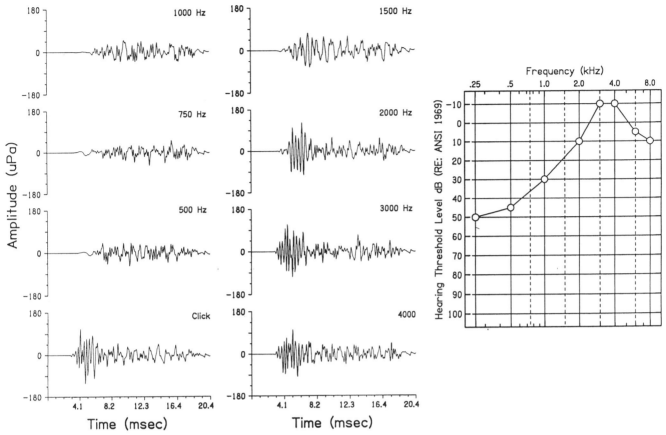

Figure 29.11. Tone-burst and click evoked OAEs in response to 80 dB peSPL stimuli from a young adult with the sensory neural hearing loss shown.

neuromas and adults with diseases known to affect the central nervous system, such as multiple sclerosis. EOAEs also show consistent decreases after intense sound exposure (Kemp, 1982; Norton and Hayes, 1990).

In cases of middle ear pathology, EOAEs may not be measurable because they are not effectively transmitted by the middle ear. Generally, if the air-bone gap for pure tone thresholds exceeds 30–35 dB, EOAEs cannot be measured. EOAEs can be measured in ears with patent pressure-equalization (PE) tubes if the air-bone gap is small and the middle ear cavity healthy. In testing newborns, debris including wax and vernix in the external ear canal can reduce and block EOAEs (Chang, Vohr, Norton and Lekas, 1992). Collapsed canals can also interfere with emission measurements.

ACOUSTIC DISTORTION PRODUCTS

Basic Description. Acoustic distortion products (ADPs) result from the interaction of two simultaneously presented puretones (the primaries). In humans, the most prominent distortion product is the cubic dif-

ference tone. Specifically, if two tones of frequencies F1 and F2 (F2 > F1) are presented externally, a third tone of frequency 2F1-F2 will be produced internally. ADPs are technologically the easiest types of emissions to measure, being relatively artifact free and requiring no post hoc processing. As shown in Figure 29.15, two separate channels of signal generation, as well as attenuation and transduction, are required for the primary tones. The eliciting tones are presented to the ear through a probe microphone assembly similar to those used in measuring other types of emissions except that there are two stimulus delivery ports. Care must be taken that the two channels are electrically isolated before being acoustically mixed in the ear canal. The ear canal sound pressure is averaged to reduce the noise floor and spectrally analyzed for the levels of the primaries and the distortion product(s). Figure 29.16 shows the spectrum of the sound pressure measured in the ear canal and includes both the primaries, F1 and F2, and the cubic difference tone ADP at 2F1-F2. The threshold (the lowest level of the primaries at which the ADP can be distinguished from the noise floor) as well as the magnitude of the ADP depends on the frequency ratio (F2/F1) and relative levels (L1 and L2)

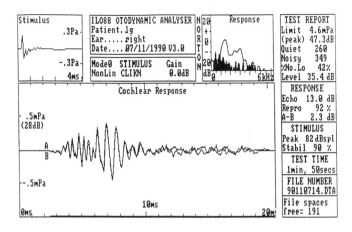

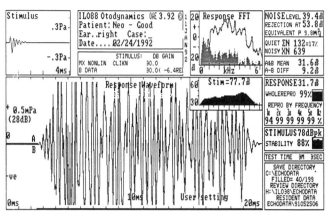

Figure 29.13. Click evoked OAE recorded from a normal-hearing, full-term newborn.

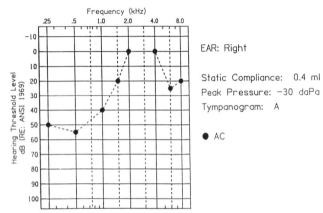

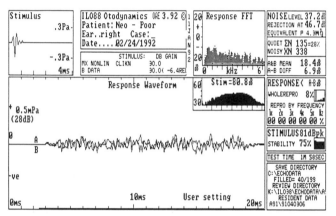

Figure 29.12. Click evoked OAE recorded using the ILO88 hardware and software. The audiogram for the patient's right ear is also shown.

Figure 29.14. Click evoked OAE recorded from a full-term newborn later diagnosed as having a moderately severe SNHL.

of the primaries in a complex fashion. Figure 29.17 shows ADP input-output functions for two normal-hearing subjects at four frequency (F2/F1) ratios. The functions for the two subjects are quite different for stimuli less than 60 dB SPL, but nearly identical for those above 70 dB SPL. Nulls or notches, such as those seen for F2/F1 equal to 1.25 for the squares, are thought to be due to the complex interaction of ADPs generated by different processes at low and high levels. In animal studies, responses generated by stimuli below 60 dB SPL are quite vulnerable to ototoxic drugs (Brown, McDowell and Forge, 1989; Mills, Norton and Rubel, 1992) and hypoxia (Schmiedt and Adams, 1981; Rubel and Norton, 1991), whereas those generated by higher level stimuli are significantly less vulnerable. The implications of this observation for human testing are not yet clear.

ADP behavior, primarily in terms of threshold but also in overall amplitude, is significantly affected by SOAEs closely related to the ADP frequency. Wier, Pasanen and McFadden (1988) reported that ADP amplitude for low-level stimulation is greater within 50

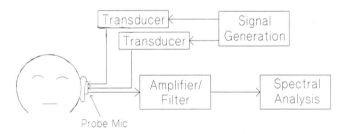

Figure 29.15. Schematic representation of a system used to measure acoustic distortion product emissions.

Hz of a spontaneous emission. At higher levels, the relationship between ADP output and SOAE was less clear. van Dijk and Wit (1990) describe the interaction between SOAEs and ADPs as a synchronization of the spontaneous emission to the distortion product frequency. Whatever the mechanism is, when interpreting ADPs, one must always be aware of any spontaneous emissions in the person being tested.

Clinical Data. Acoustic distortion products generally are absent in ears with sensory neural hearing loss greater than about 50–60 dB (e.g., Harris, 1990; Lonsbury-Martin and Martin, 1990; Ohlms, Harris, Franklin and Lonsbury-Martin, 1990; Spektor, Leonard, Kim, Jung and Smurzynski, 1991). Like

transient evoked emissions, the dynamic range of ADPs is highly dependent on the stimulus levels used. Clinically, the primaries are manipulated in one of two ways. Either the frequencies are changed while level is kept constant or the frequency is kept constant while the level is changed. The first results in what has been called a "distortion product audiogram," whereas the second gives an input/output (I/O) function. It should be noted that the "distortion product audiogram" does not include the concept of threshold as does the conventional audiogram. The ADP threshold can only be determined from an I/O function.

There is as yet no clear consensus on the best stimulus parameters for clinical use. The frequency ratio F2/F1 is a critical factor in ADP generation. Based on high level stimulation, the optimal ratio (i.e., the ratio yielding the greatest magnitude ADP) is approximately 1.22 (Harris, Lonsbury-Martin, Stagner, Coats and Martin, 1989). If, however, one is looking for the lowest or most sensitive threshold, a frequency ratio closer to 1.15 is optimal (Brown and Norton, 1990). The relative levels, L1 and L2, of the two primaries also have an effect on ADP output. The optimal level relationship between the primaries is L2 10 to 15 dB less than L1, however, this is affected by the overall level of the primaries as well as their frequency ratio. Finally, although numerous studies have shown that ADP generation takes place close to the cochlear place of the higher frequency primary, F2, the data in the

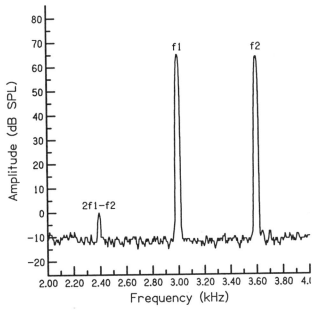

Figure 29.16. Spectra of ear canal sound pressure from the ear of a normal-hearing adult. F1 and F2 are the stimuli and 2F1-F2 is the ADP emission generated by the cochlea.

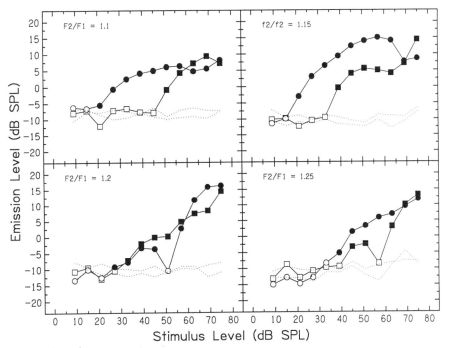

Figure 29.17. ADP input-output functions for two normal-hearing adults. F2 is 2000 Hz. Different F2/F1 ratios are shown across the panels. Within each panel the *dotted lines* indicate the noise floor. The *open symbols* indicate measurements at the ADP frequency and that were below the noise floor, i.e., no emission was detected. *Solid symbols* indicate that an emission was observed.

literature have reported results relative to F1 (Brown and Gaskill, 1990), F2 (Brown and Norton, 1990), the geometric mean of F1 and F2 (Lonsbury-Martin, Harris, Stagner, Hawkins and Martin, 1990), or the frequency of the distortion product, itself (Harris et al., 1989).

Because of the variability in evoking stimuli parameters, the diagnostic significance of ADP behavior is not yet clear. The interpretation of ADP data is further impeded because it is not yet clear what feature of ADP behavior is most informative. ADP "audiograms" supply information across a wide frequency range but usually only at one or two levels. I/O functions can provide information about the threshold and growth behavior of ADPs but for fewer frequencies within a given time period (i.e., a typical clinical test session). It is not even apparent within I/O functions which parameter is most informative; threshold, maximal amplitude, or saturation point (if indeed the functions saturate).

In spite of these problems in interpretation, there are a number of reports in the literature that link ADPs with auditory sensitivity. Brown and Gaskill (1990) report a close, reverse correspondence between ADP amplitude to moderate level stimulation and N1 threshold across the frequency range from 1–16 kHz in guinea pigs. Specifically, they report that ADP amplitude is greater when N1 threshold is lower (better) and that both reflect the overall audibility curve of guinea pigs. Similar results were reported for humans (Gaskill and Brown, 1990) with statistically significant negative correlations between auditory threshold and ADP amplitude in half of the ears tested. A number of case studies have also been reported in which ADP

amplitude is correlated with audiometric threshold in people with sensory neural hearing loss (e.g., Lonsbury-Martin and Martin, 1990; Martin, Ohlms, Franklin, Harris and Lonsbury-Martin, 1990).

Figure 29.18 shows an "ADP audiogram" for a subject with a high frequency hearing loss. In this case, the subject has normal audiometric thresholds in the left ear and a notch at 6 kHz in the right ear. The primaries were presented at 65 dB SPL. In the right ear, ADPs show a notch, similar to the audiogram. The left ear shows a broad decrease between about 2 and 4.5 kHz but is still generally within the range observed in normal-hearing subjects, indicated by the *dotted lines*. The significance of the decreased ADP amplitudes in the presence of normal hearing is not clear. This could indicate early damage to the ADP generator that is not yet sufficient to cause threshold shifts, or it could represent normal variability. As the stimulus level is increased, the ADP audiogram is in better agreement with audiometric thresholds, as shown in Figure 29.19.

ADP emissions are also present and robust in normal newborns (Lafreniere, Jung, Smurzynski, Leonard, Kim and Sasek, 1992), although there have been no large clinical trials testing their sensitivity to hearing loss in this population.

STIMULUS FREQUENCY EMISSIONS

Basic Description. Stimulus frequency emissions (SFEs) are the most frequency specific and probably the least clinically applicable of emission types. They reflect the response of the cochlea to puretone input, occurring simultaneously with and at the same fre-

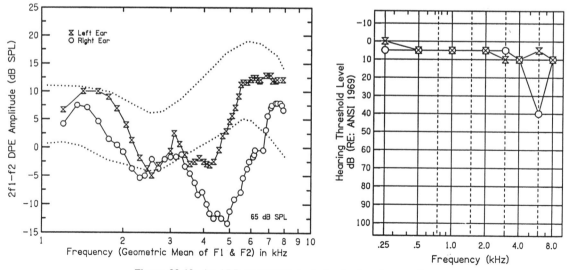

Figure 29.18. An ADP audiogram and standard audiogram for
a human subject. After Lonsbury-Martin & Martin, 1990.

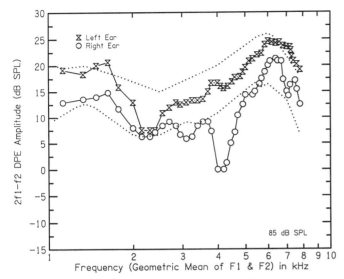

Figure 29.19. An ADP audiogram for the same subject as shown in Figure 29.18. Stimuli are at 85 dB SPL.

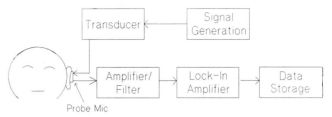

Figure 29.20. Schematic diagram of a system used to measure stimulus frequency emissions.

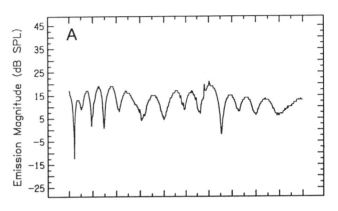

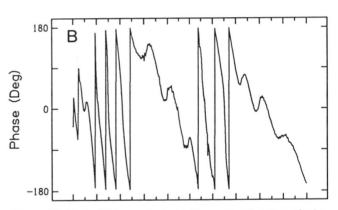

Figure 29.21. A. SFE magnitude. **B.** Phase as a function of stimulus frequency from the ear of a normal-hearing young adult. The stimulus was swept continuously from 1000–3000 Hz at 27 dB SPL.

quency of the eliciting stimulus. When a tone is presented to the ear, the sound pressure measured in the ear canal is the sum of both the tone presented and the retrograde output of the cochlear amplifier, the SFE. All other types of evoked OAEs previously discussed have been separated from the evoking stimulus either temporally (TOAEs and COAEs) or spectrally (ADPs). The lack of temporal or spectral separation requires more sophisticated equipment and processing to measure SFEs. They are not currently practical for clinical use and will be presented only briefly.

As shown in Figure 29.20, to measure SFEs, a tonal signal is presented to the ear through a probe microphone assembly system, as in measuring other types of emissions. Often the tone is swept across a certain frequency range. The SFE is extracted from the recorded ear canal sound pressure by using vector subtraction (Kemp and Chum, 1980). This requires a lock-in amplifier to specify the ear canal sound pressure both in terms of amplitude *and* phase. It also requires that the system of stimulus generation, delivery and measurement is linear in both amplitude and phase.

Figure 29.21 shows the SFE magnitude and phase for a 27-dB SPL swept tone. The SFE is characterized by a pattern of "dips" and "peaks" indicating the relative strength of the SFE. The SFE pattern across frequency is idiosyncratic, that is it is unique for each ear tested. Certain similarities, however, can be seen across subjects. In general, the frequency separation between adjacent peaks (or dips) increases with increasing frequency (Zwicker and Schloth, 1984). As seen in Figure 29.22 the SFE pattern flattens, or loses definition, as the evoking stimulus increases. SFEs seem to relate

closely with auditory sensitivity. Specifically, comparing auditory threshold microstructure (thresholds at closely spaced frequencies) with the SFE pattern reveals that threshold minima are found at frequencies where a SFE maxima occurs (Wilson, 1980; Zwicker and Schloth, 1984). As with other types of OAEs, SFEs are absent in ears with cochlear hearing loss exceeding 40–50 dB.

If the amplitude of tone sweeps is measured by using a spectrum analyzer, perturbations can be seen at lower levels that are closely related to the SFE. A

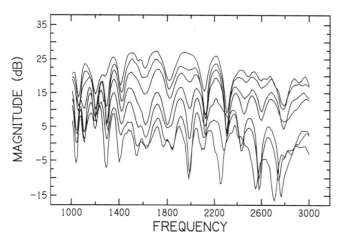

Figure 29.22. SFE magnitude as a function of stimulus frequency for several stimulus levels ranging from 9–69 dB SPL in 6 dB steps from the ear of a normal-hearing young adult.

number of reports in the literature have reported such amplitude data as SFEs. The phase must also be known, however, to perform the vector subtraction, as amplitude alone is not sufficient to define the nonlinearity, or the emission.

ISSUES IN THE CLINICAL IMPLEMENTATION OF OTOACOUSTIC EMISSIONS

Because OAEs can be measured noninvasively and are sensitive to cochlear status, they are potentially a valuable addition to clinical audiology. To some extent this potential is already being realized. There are a number of reports in the literature of various types of emissions measured in ears with hearing loss of cochlear origin. Potential clinical uses include: (*a*) screening for peripheral auditory system dysfunction in newborn babies and infants; (*b*) separating the cochlear and neural components of sensorineural hearing loss; (*c*) monitoring the effects of noxious agents, such as ototoxic drugs and intense sound on the cochlea; and (*d*) assessing fluctuating hearing loss, with or without therapeutic regimens. To optimize the clinical utility of OAEs, one needs to decide whether a particular application requires knowledge of the sensitivity as well as the integrity of the OAE generator(s). This requires better understanding of emission generation and cochlear mechanics. In addition, it requires a careful definition of the questions relative to a given patient population. For example, if one is interested in dividing neonates into two groups—those with hearing thresholds better than 30 dB HL and those with hearing thresholds worse than 30 dB HL— screening with a single moderate level click stimulus may be adequate. If, however, one is monitoring the effects of ototoxic drugs on the cochlea and wants to detect changes in cochlear status before threshold

shifts, one may need to measure input-output functions at several frequencies. In a more general sense, one needs to determine which aspects of OAEs relate best to subthreshold versus threshold versus suprathreshold performance.

Finally, evoked otoacoustic emissions should be viewed as an additional, objective audiological technique and may be most powerful when used in conjunction with neural sound evoked potentials and immittance measurements. Ideally, sophisticated engineering will allow us to measure external and middle ear impedance simultaneously, all types of OAEs, and sound-evoked neural potentials.

REFERENCES

Arts HA, Norton SJ, and Rubel EW. Influence of perilymphatic tetrodotixin and calcium concentration on hair cell function. 1990. Paper presented at the Midwinter Meeting of the Association for Research in Otolaryngology.

Bilger RC, Matthies ML, Hammel D, and Demorest M. Genetic implications of gender differences in prevalence of spontaneous otoacoustic emissions. J Speech Hear Res 1990;33:418–432.

Bonfils P. Spontaneous otoacoustic emissions: clinical interest. Laryngoscope 1989;99:752–756.

Bonfils P, Piron JP, Uziel A, and Pujol R. A correlative study of evoked otoacoustic emission properties and audiometric thresholds. Arch Otorhinolaryngol 1988;245:53–56.

Bonfils P, and Uziel A. Clinical applications of evoked acoustic emissions: Results in normally hearing and hearing-impaired subjects. Ann Otol Rhinol Laryngol 1989;98:326–331.

Bray P, and Kemp DT. An advanced cochlear echo technique suitable for infant screening. Br J Audiol 1987;21:191–204.

Brown AM, and Gaskill SA. Measurement of acoustic distortion reveals underlying similarities between human and rodent mechanical responses. J Acoust Soc Am 1990;88:840–849.

Brown AM, McDowell B, and Forge A. Acoustic distortion products can be used to monitor the effects of chronic gentamicin treatment. Hear Res 1989;42:143–156.

Brown SJ, and Norton SJ. The effects of contralateral acoustic stimulation on the acoustic distortion product 2f1-f2. 1990. Paper presented at the Midwinter Meeting of the Association for Research in Otolaryngology.

Burns EM, Arehart KM, and Campbell SL. Prevalence of spontaneous otoacoustic emissions in neonates. 1990. Paper presented at the Midwinter Meeting of the Association for Research in Otolaryngology.

Burns EM, Strickland EA, Tubis A, and Jones K. Interactions among spontaneous otoacoustic emissions. I. Distortion products and linked emissions. Hear Res 1984;16:271–278.

Champlin CA, and Norton SJ. The effects of pure tones on different spontaneous oto-acoustic emissions in the same ear. 1987. Paper presented at the Midwinter Meeting of the Association for Research in Otolaryngology.

Chang KW, Vohr BR, Norton SJ, and Lekas MD. External and middle ear status related to evoked oto acoustic emissions in neonates. Arch Otolaryngol Head Neck Surg 1993;119:276–282.

Collet L, Gartner M, Moulin A, Kauffmann I, Disant F, and Morgon A. Evoked otoacoustic emissions and sensorineural hearing loss. Arch Otolaryngol Head Neck Surg 1989;115:1060–1062.

Fritze W. Registration of spontaneous cochlear emissions by means of fourier transformation. Arch Otorhinolaryngol 1983;238:189–196.

Gaskill SA, and Brown AM. The behavior of the acoustic distortion product, 2f1-f2, from the human ear and its relationship to auditory sensitivity. J Acoust Soc Am 1990;88:821–839.

Gold T. Hearing II. The physical basis of the action of the cochlea. Proceedings of the Royal Academy B 1948;135:492–498.

Grandori F. Nonlinear phenomenon in click- and tone-burst-evoked otoacoustic emissions from human ears. Audiology 1985;24:71–80.

Harris FP. Distortion-product otoacoustic emissions in humans with high frequency sensorineural hearing loss. J Speech Hear Res 1990;33:594–600.

Harris FP, Lonsbury-Martin BL, Stagner BB, Coats AC, and Martin GK. Acoustic distortion products in humans: systematic changes in amplitude as a function of f2/f1 ratio. J Acoust Soc Am 1989;85:220–229.

Hazell JW. Spontaneous cochlear acoustic emissions and tinnitus. Clinical experience and the tinnitus patient. 1984; Laryngol Otol (London) (Suppl 9):106–110.

Johnsen NJ, and Elberling C. Evoked otoacoustic emissions from the human ear. Scand Audiol 1982;11:69–77.

Kemp DT. Stimulated acoustic emissions from within the human auditory system. J Acoust Soc Am 1978;64:1386–1391.

Kemp DT. Evidence of mechanical non linearity and frequency selective wave amplification in the cochlea. Arch Otorhinolaryngol 1979;224:37–45.

Kemp DT. Cochlear echoes: implications for noise-induced hearing loss. In Hamernik RP, Hendersen D, and Salvi R, Eds. New Perspectives on Noise-Induced Hearing Loss. New York: Raven Press, 1982:189–207.

Kemp DT, Bray P, Alexander L, and Brown AM. Acoustic emission cochleography-practical aspects. Scand Audiol 1986;25 (Suppl):71–83.

Kemp DT, and Chum R. Properties of the generator of stimulated acoustic emissions. Hear Res 1980;2:213–32.

Khanna SM, and Leonard DG. Measurement of basilar membrane vibrations and evaluation of cochlear condition. Hear Res 1986a;23:37–53.

Khanna SM, and Leonard DG. Relationship between basilar membrane tuning and hair cell condition. Hear Res 1986b;23:55–70.

Kiang NY, Moxon EC, and Levine RA. Auditory nerve activity in cats with normal and abnormal cochleas. In Wolstenholm GFW, and Knight J, Eds. Sensorineural Hearing Loss. Ciba Symposium. London: Churchill-Livingston, 1970:241–273.

Lafreniere D, Jung MD, Smurzynski J, Leonard G, Kim DO, and Sasek J. Distortion-product and click-evoked otoacoustic emissions in healthy newborns. Arch Otolaryngol Head Neck Surg (In Press).

Liberman MC, and Dodds LW. Single-neuron labeling and chronic cochlear pathology. II. Stereocilia damage and alterations of spontaneous discharge rates. Hear Res 1984a;16:43–53.

Liberman MC, and Dodds LW. Single-neuron labeling and chronic cochlear pathology. III. Stereocilia damage and alterations of threshold tuning curves. Hear Res 1984b;16:55–74.

Lonsbury-Martin BL, Harris FP, Stagner BB, Hawkins MD, and Martin GK. Distortion product emissions in humans. I. Basic properties in normally hearing subjects. Ann Otol Rhinol Laryngol 1990;99:3–42.

Lonsbury-Martin BL, and Martin GK. The clinical utility of distortion product otoacoustic emissions. Ear Hear 1990;11:144–154.

Mathias A, Probst R, Min N, and Hauser R. A child with an unusually high-level spontaneous otoacoustic emission. Arch Otolaryngol Head Neck Surg 1991;117:674–676.

Martin GK, Lonsbury-Martin BL, Probst R, Scheinin SA, and Coats AC. Acoustic distortion products in rabbit ear canal. II. Sites of origin revealed by suppression contours and pure-tone exposures. Hear Res 1987;28:191–208.

Martin GK, Ohlms LA, Franklin DJ, Harris EP, and Lonsbury-Martin BL. Distortion product emissions in humans. III. Influence of sensorineural hearing loss. Ann Otol Rhinol Laryngol 1990;99:30–42.

Maxon AB, Norton SJ, White K, and Brehens T. Evoked otoacoustic emissions in neonatal screening and follow-up: Clinical trials. Mini seminar presented at the ASHA Convention, 1991.

Mills DM, Norton SJ, and Rubel EW. Varying endocochlear potential by furosemide reveals different components in distortion product otoacoustic emission. ARO Abstracts 1992.

Norton SJ, and Hayes JM. Effects of prior stimulation on otoacoustic emission. Presented at the IVth International Conference on the Effects of Noise on the Auditory System, Beaune, France, 1990.

Norton SJ, and Neely ST. Tone-burst evoked otoacoustic emissions from normal-hearing subjects. J Acoust Soc Am 1987;81:1860–1872.

Norton SJ, and Rubel EW. Unpublished observations, 1992.

Norton SJ, Schmidt AR, and Stover LJ. Tinnitus and otoacoustic emissions: is there a link? Ear Hear 1990;11:159–166.

Norton SJ, and Widen JE. Evoked otoacoustic emissions in normal-hearing infants and children: emerging data and issues. Ear Hear 1990;11:121–127.

Ohlms LA, Harris FP, Franklin DJ, and Lonsbury-Martin BL. Distortion product emissions in humans. III. Influence of sensorineural hearing loss. Ann Otol Rhinol Laryngol 1990;99:30–42.

Penner MJ. An estimate of the prevalence of tinnitus caused by spontaneous otoacoustic emissions. Arch Otolaryngol Head Neck Surg 1990;116:418–423.

Penner MJ, and Burns EM. The dissociation of SOAE's and tinnitus. J Speech Hear Res 1987;30:396–403.

Probst R, Coats AC, Martin GK, and Lonsbury-Martin BL. Spontaneous, click-, and toneburst-evoked otoacoustic emissions from normal ears. Hear Res 1986;21:261–275.

Rabinowitz WM, and Widin GP. Interaction of spontaneous otoacoustic emissions and external sound. J Acoust Soc Am 1984;76:1713–1720.

Rubel EW, and Norton SJ. Vulnerability of oto acoustic emissions are a function of stimulus level. 1991. Paper presented at the Midwinter Meeting of the Association for Research in Otolaryngology.

Ruggero MA, Kramek B, and Rich NC. Spontaneous otoacoustic emissions in a dog. Hear Res 1984;13:293–296.

Schmiedt RA, and Adams JC. Stimulated acoustic emissions in the ear canal of the gerbil. Hear Res 1981;5:295–305.

Scholth E. Relation between spectral composition of spontaneous otoacoustic emissions and fine structure of threshold in quiet. Acustica 1983;53:250–256.

Sellick PM, Patuzzi R, and Johnstone BM. Measurement of basilar membrane motion in the guinea pig using the Mossbauer technique. J Acoust Soc Am 1982;72:131–141.

Siegel JH, and Kim DO. Efferent neural control of cochlear mechanics? Olivocochlear bundle stimulation affects cochlear biomechanical nonlinearity. Hear Res 1982;6:171–182.

Spektor Z, Leonard G, Kim DO, Jung MD, and Smurzynski J. Otoacoustic emissions in normal and hearing impaired children and normal adults. Laryngoscope 1991;101:965–974.

Stover LJ, and Norton SJ. Comparisons among different emission types. 1992. Paper presented at the Midwinter Meeting of the Association for Research in Otolaryngology.

Strickland EA, Burns EM, and Tubis A. Incidence of spontaneous otoacoustic emissions in children and infants. J Acoust Soc Am 1985;78:931–935.

Tyler RS, and Conrad-Ames D. Spontaneous acoustic cochlear emissions and sensorineural tinnitus. Br J Audiol 1981;16:193–194.

van Dijk P, and Wit HP. Synchronization of spontaneous otoacoustic emissions to a 2f1-f2 distortion product. J Acoust Soc Am 1990;88:850–856.

Wier CC, Norton SJ, and Kincaid GE. Spontaneous narrow-band oto-acoustic signals emitted by human ears: A replication. J Acoust Soc Am 1984;76:1248–1250.

Wier CC, Pasanen EG, and McFadden D. Partial dissociation of spontaneous otoacoustic emissions and distortion products during aspirin use in humans. J Acoust Soc Am 1988;84:230–237.

Wilson JP. Model for cochlear echoes and tinnitus based on an electrical correlate. Hear Res 1980;2:527–532.

Wilson JP, and Sutton GJ. Acoustic correlates of tonal tinnitus. Tinnitus 1981;82–107.

Zurek PM. Spontaneous narrowband acoustic signals emitted by human ears. J Acoust Soc Am 1981;69:514–523.

Zwicker E, and Schloth E. Interrelation of different otoacoustic emissions. J Acoust Soc Am 1984;75:1148–1154.

SPECIAL POPULATIONS

CHAPTER 30

Evaluating Infants and Young Children

William R. Hodgson

In the 1985 edition of this book, I indicated considerable progress in pediatric audiology during the past few years. Improvements were cited in various techniques including those for evaluation of very young children. Problem areas mentioned were lack of awareness in the medical community that efficient audiological evaluation could be carried out with very young children. Consequently, we still find children who are not evaluated audiometrically and therefore are either not identified or are misdiagnosed.

At the present time, the following progress and problems seem noteworthy: Electrophysiological testing (auditory brainstem response) has been improved and emerges as the test of choice for very young infants; behavioral procedures, such as Visual Reinforcement Audiometry, have been validated in terms of signal parameters and test protocols and have become computer-based. Concern continues about late identification of hearing impaired children and there may be inadequate treatment for those who are identified. Some of this concern is based on what we have learned about the effects of minimal hearing loss on language and school performance in these groups: children with chronic otitis media, as well as children with unilateral and high frequency hearing losses.

This chapter discusses the progress which has been made and the efforts continuing to solve the problems mentioned above. As an introduction, some guidelines for effective evaluation of infants and young children are suggested: The simplest methods which will obtain desired results are best. The audiologist must be flexible but maintain control of the evaluation. Appropriate test procedures must be determined by the responses the child is capable of making. A battery of tests is preferable to any single procedure, and cross-checking of test results from several tests is important for confirmation.

An effective evaluation requires information about the child, parents, and problem. Information taking starts with the Case History, and this process will be discussed first.

CASE HISTORY

Audiologic evaluation and habilitation require control of behavior. To control behavior, the audiologist must understand the child, the parents, and the problem. These needs are facilitated through taking a case history, with these purposes in mind: (a) gathering information which will be helpful in evaluation and in planning habilitation, (b) revealing misconceptions which parents may hold that must be removed prior to successful habilitation, and (c) involving the parents in the process of habilitation, without which successful remediation will not take place. As as adjunct, the history- taking period provides an opportunity to establish rapport with parents and child. Development of this harmonious working relationship is needed for evaluation and habilitation.

Taking of a case history may be facilitated through use of a Preliminary Information or Case History form. This form can be filled out by the parents before the evaluation. The length and content of such forms vary from clinic to clinic but for economy probably should be brief and aim to elicit most pertinent information to identify the patient, determine exactly what the parents wish from the evaluation, and get other health- and behavior-related information that will help in the evaluation. A sample case history form is shown in Figure 30.1.

The most common error I have observed in beginning students using (or misusing) the case history form is to ask questions which the patient has already answered in the case history form. This practice does not enhance rapport! Rather, the student should read and attend to the answers before the interview and inquire about questions left unanswered, about unclear answers, and about those provocative answers which suggest the need for followup. These guidelines permit case history taking to proceed efficiently, to provide needed information, and to enhance a comfortable working relationship.

TEST ENVIRONMENT

Test signals should be frequency-specific and sufficiently narrow and varied to assess hearing sensitivity across the range important for speech. For testing in sound field, frequency- modulated (warble) tones are popular. If bands of noise are used, they should be sufficiently narrow to permit exploration of the contour of the child's hearing.

THE UNIVERSITY OF ARIZONA HEARING CENTER

PRELIMINARY INFORMATION (CHILD). Please return to above address. (To be filled out by parent, relative, or guardian.)

I. IDENTIFYING INFORMATION:　　　　　　　　　　　　Today's date_____

Child's Name_____ Date of Birth_____ Age_____

Home address_____ Home phone_____
　　　　　　(Street)

_____Work phone_____
　　(City)　　　　　　(State)　　　　(Zip)

Father's name_____ Occupation_____ Age_____

Mother's name_____ Occupation_____ Age_____

Brothers and sisters (give names and ages)_____

Who referred you to this Clinic?_____

Parents' chief concerns_____

II. GENERAL HISTORY:

What is your child's problem? When did you first notice it? What do you think caused it?_____

Has anyone else in your family ever had a speech or hearing problem during childhood?_____

III. HEALTH HISTORY:

Were there any significant probems during the pregnancy, the delivery, or following the birth of the child?　Yes____　No____

If yes, please explain:_____

Has this child had any serious illnesses, accidents, or hospitalizations? Include recent medical history_____

Has this child had repeated ear infections?　Yes____　No____

If yes, please describe when they started, how many, the last one:_____

This child's general health is: Excellent_____ Good_____ Fair_____ Poor_____

Please explain any health concerns:_____

IV. DEVELOPMENTAL HISTORY:

At what age, in months, did your child sit alone _____, walk alone _____, use first words _____,

use sentences _____. Describe any unusual slow behavior_____

While keeping your child's current age in mind, please rate the following:

Motor coordination and balance: (skipping, hopping, running)	Excellent	Good	Fair	Poor
Eye/Hand coordination: (drawing, coloring, writing)	Excellent	Good	Fair	Poor
General behavior at home:	Excellent	Good	Fair	Poor
Ability to play with other children:	Excellent	Good	Fair	Poor
Ability to keep attention on an activity:	Excellent	Good	Fair	Poor
Ability to play appropriately with toys or games:	Excellent	Good	Fair	Poor
Ability solve problems:	Excellent	Good	Fair	Poor
Ability to follow directions:	Excellent	Good	Fair	Poor
Ability to speak clearly:	Excellent	Good	Fair	Poor

V. EDUCATIONAL HISTORY:

School and Address:_____

School Placement:_____
　　　　　　(grade)　　　　　　　　(teacher)

Progress in School?　　　Excellent　　Good　　Fair　　Poor

Any grades repeated?_____

VI. PREVIOUS EVALUATIONS and/or TRAINING: (when, where, by whom, and results_____

_____

Signature of person answering questions

_____

Relationship to this child

Figure 30.1. Sample Case History form. To save space in this text, the spaces ordinarily provided for the parents to answer questions have been condensed.

Noisemakers (non-electronic sound generators i.e., bells, whistles, drums, etc.) have been used to elicit reflexive responses in infants. They are simple and inexpensive and can be used effectively by an experienced examiner. Nevertheless, it must be remembered that they give qualitative rather than quantitative information. Broad spectral characteristics and the fact that sound levels cannot be accurately reported limit findings obtained with their use to general rather than specific results. For definitive results, it is necessary that test signals be controllable and reproducible. The test space should meet ANSI requirements for ambient noise levels (ANSI, 1977). Ear-specific assessment should be made whenever possible. Otherwise (as when testing in sound field) a statement can only be made about hearing in the better ear.

IDENTIFICATION AUDIOMETRY

Concern about early detection of heairng loss in infants led to experimentation with mass auditory screening of neonates. Many procedures were tried. Portable sound generators were used to deliver a high frequency warble tone or band of noise at a high output level, seeking to awaken the infant or to elicit an auropalpebral or startle reflex. Audomated procedures, such as the crib-o-gram (Simmons and Russ, 1974) aimed to screen hearing by placing a motion-sensitive transducer on the crib to detect infant movements associated with presentation of auditory signals.

Problems with the efficiency of neonatal hearing screening led to the formation in 1969 of a Joint Committee of the American Academy of Opthalmology and Otolaryngology, the American Academy of Pediatrics, and the American Speech and Hearing Association. Concerned about the high number of false negatives and positives which can occur in a behavioral screening program, the committee developed and recommended use of a high-risk register to highlight those neonates who have an increased probability of impaired hearing (Northern & Downs, 1978). Infants with any of the attributes described in the following register should be followed until a definitive statement about hearing status can be made.

1. A family history of childhood hearing impairment.
2. Congenital perinatal infection (e.g., cytomegalovirus, rubella, herpes, toxoplasmosis, syphilis).
3. Anatomic malformations involving the head or neck (e.g., dysmorphic appearance including syndromal and nonsyndromal abnormalities, overt or submucous cleft palate, morphologic abnormalities of the pinna).
4. Birth weight less than 1500 gm.
5. Hyperbilirubinemia at levels exceeding indications for exchange transfusion.
6. Bacterial meningitis, especially Haemophilus influenzae.
7. Severe asphyxia which may include infants with Apgar scores of 0 to 3 who fail to institute spontaneous respiration by 10 min and those with hypotonia persisting to 2 hr of age. (ASHA, 1982)

The Committee recommended follow-up audiologic screening for infants at risk for hearing loss, preferably by age 3 months but no later than 6 months. If (1) the infant fails the screening, (2) the results are equivocal, or (3) there is a family history of delayed onset of hearing loss, degenerative disease or intra- uterine infections, the Committee recommended medical and audiologic diagnosis.

Gerkin (1984), reviewing these risk factors and their relation to hearing loss, concluded that a high-risk register should be the basic tool in infant screening and early identification. Reviewing evidence on the effectiveness of behavioral screening, the ASHA Committee on Infant Hearing concluded that "there are no data to indicate that newborn behavioral screening programs are sufficiently sensitive and specific" (ASHA, 1989, p. 90), and endorsed use of the high- risk register. At the same time, the Committee recommended ABR screening as the procedure of choice for followup on infants detected by the high-risk register.

Current practices in neonatal hearing screening programs were described by Brooks (1990). Her nationwide survey of hospitals with neonatal intensive care units indicated that 76% employ only an electrophysiologic method for initial screening, 12% used only behavioral techniques, and 12% used both.

AUDITORY ASSESSMENT

The ASHA Committee on Infant Hearing has developed guidelines for the audiologic assessment of neonates, infants, toddlers, and young children (ASHA, 1989). In their deliberations, the committee recognized the need for procedures that were both multiple and nonduplicative and that sampled various dimensions of auditory function. At the same time they took into considered the need for cost containment in health care delivery. Noting that ABR testing has been refined to the point where both frequency-specific and bone-conducted thresholds can be obtained in addition to estimates of sensitivity obtained with traditional air-conducted click stimuli, the committee (ASHA, 1989) recommended ABR in particular for those children too young or too disabled for reliable assessment with behavioral techniques. At the same time, they cautioned that the use of any test alone is to be discouraged. Corroboration of results from a given test should be sought using information gained from the case history, parent comments, observations of behavior, and — of course — other tests. Thus while ABR testing grows in importance, there is still room for behavioral testing, as discussed below, as a quicker, cheaper procedure for establishing or corroborating hearing loss. Pediatic evaluation, especially of the youngest children, may require ongoing assessment, rather than the single evaluation session which is usually required for older children and adults. Serial evaluations are often important to confirm and extend initial impressions. As time passes and the child beomes capable of more sophisticated responses, more detailed and precise information may result from subsequent evaluations.

Procedures used in the assessment of a child at a given time are determined by the responses the patient is capable of making. The evaluation should be oriented toward obtaining the most pertinent information as quickly as possible, using the most sensitive test to which the child can respond. The sophistication of the child's response will depend on several factors:

1. MENTAL AGE - a determinant of ability to learn new responses, as well as in indicator of the responses already present (for example, the language requisite for speech audiometry).
2. CHRONOLOGIC AGE - relating primarily to adequate neuromuscular coordination.
3. NEUROLOGIC STATUS - relating both to motor and perceptual ability to make the required response.
4. HEARING LEVEL - an important determinant of experience in auditory response and the ease with which the child learns to respond to new auditory signals.
5. WILLINGNESS TO PERFORM - influenced by the child's motivation, fears, the rapport established by the clinician and the skill with which the clinician operates.
6. PRIOR EXPERIENCE - with auditory testing on the child's part.
7. TEST ENVIRONMENT - the quality and flexibility of the equipment, the appearance of the room and the toys or other motivational devices that are available to interest the child.

AGE 0 THROUGH 4 MONTHS

Along with ABR using clicks and frequency specific stimuli, information may be gained from behavioral observation, case- history and parent information, and cautious use of acoustic immitance, particularly with use of a 660 Hz probe tone. Behavioral auditory assessment, particularly during the early months of this age range, is primarily limited to behavioral observation audiometry, involving elicitation of reflexive responses to relatively intense auditory signals. The more useful responses are the auropalpebral reflex (APR), the startle reflex and arousal (observable by generalized body movement). The APR is seen as an eyeblink, or a tightening of the eyelids if they are already closed. The startle response consists of a small "jump" of the infant's body immediately following the stimulus. It is important that the infant be uncovered so that the entire body can be seen. Both the APR and the startle reflex tend to disappear quickly upon repeated presentation of the stimulus. An infant lying quietly may be aroused to make generalized movements by auditory signals. Unfortunately for our purposes, infants who are awake are seldom still and the examiner must be careful not to interpret random activity as responses. Possibly neonates, but more often infants later in the 0 - to 4-month range, will halt motor activity on the presentation of an auditory signal.

The responses described above can also be elicited by visual and tactile stimuli, and the examiner must avoid such stimulation. Some problems may be avoided by testing the infant in a state of light sleep. This procedure reduces the probability of false positive responses. Of course, this conclusion joins the audiologist with parents in a vexing problem: trying to get the baby to sleep. When possible it is helpful to observe the infant's responses both when sleeping and awake.

Table 30.1 provides an estimate of the levels required, and associated variability, to elicit certain responses at ages under discussion, as well as for older children, discussed below. Levels required for response to speech are substantially lower than those required for tones, and generally occur with less variability.

Assessment of hearing sensitivity during the first 4 months is generally qualitative, not quantitative. An experienced observer should be able to identify normal infants who have normal hearing. Among unresponsive infants it is difficult to differentiate those who have hearing loss from those with other problems. However, there is a good possibility that those with severe or profound hearing loss, characterized by consistent failure to respond to sound or by consistent response only to intense sound, can be correctly identified.

Table 30.1
Expected Level Required for Response and Standard Deviation (SD) Asssociated with Unconditioned Auditory Behavior in Normal Infants[a]

Age	Stimulus			Expected Response
	Noisemakers (Approx. dB SPL)	Warbled Puretones (db HL)	Speech (dB HL)	
0–6 wk	50–70	78 (SD = 6)	40–60	Eye widening, eye blink, stirring or arousal from sleep, startle
6 wk–4 mo	50–60	70 (SD = 10)	47 (SD = 2)	Eye widening, eye shift, eye blinking, quieting, beginning rudimentary head turn by 4 months
4–7 mo	40–50	51 (SD = 9)	21 (SD = 8)	Head turn on lateral plane toward sound; listening attitude
7–9 mo	30–40	45 (SD = 15)	15 (SD = 7)	Direct localization of sounds to side, indirectly below ear level
9–13 mo	25–35	38 (SD = 8)	8 (SD = 7)	Direct localization of sounds to side, directly below ear level, indirectly above ear level
13–16 mo	25–30	32 (SD = 10)	5 (SD = 5)	Direct localization of sound on side, above and below
16–21 mo	25	25 (SD = 10)	5 (SD = 1)	Direct localization of sound on side, above and below
21–24 mo	25	26 (SD = 10)	3 (SD = 10)	Direct localization of sound on side, above and below

[a] Adapted from Northern J, and Downs M. Hearing in Children. Baltimore: Williams & Wilkins, 1978.

AGE 5 MONTHS THROUGH 24 MONTHS

Some neonates show crude orientation responses to auditory stimuli (Wertheimer, 1961). There may be eye movement toward the sound source (cochleo-oculogyric reflex), and the head may turn also. However, localization responses can be expected to develop in normal infants only by 5 to 6 months of age. At first localization efforts are crude and limited by the infant's ability to control head movements. By 6 months the normal infant should make reasonably clear localization movements, and these orientation responses are valuable in assessing auditory sensitivity of children developmentally between 5 months and 2 years of age. This testing generally is called Visual Reinforcement Audiometry (VRA; Liden and Kankkunen, 1969).

The usual arrangement for most localization audiometry is to place the child between two loudspeakers in a sound-treated room as shown in Figure 30.2. If the child responds by turning toward the loudspeaker when a signal is produced, an estimate of hearing sensitivity can be obtained by varying the intensity of the signal with subsequent presentations until the lowest level at which the child will respond is found. Although various sounds have been used, probably the best are warble tones or narrow bands of noise because they are easily controlled and provide information about sensitivity at different frequencies. If narrow bands of noise are used, the bandwidth should be quite narrow, otherwise significant energy above or below the center of the band may cause errors in children who have uneven audiometric contours.

Reinforcement of localization responses is usually needed because children tend to lose interest and stop responding to such sounds fairly quickly. One simple method is to mount animated mechanical toys near the loudspeakers. Inexpensive battery-powered toys can be rewired so that they can be operated from the examiner's control room. We have used at various times a dancing bear, a drummer boy and a bartender who mixed and consumed his own drink. After receiving a temperance lecture from the mother of one client, the audiologist put tape over the sign "bartender" painted on the toy and called him a "soda jerk". This change in title did not affect the quality of response noted in the children.

Each time the child responds to an auditory stimulus by looking toward the loudspeaker, the toy is activated briefly to reinforce the response. With such reinforcement, most children will respond long enough for determination of minimal response levels at various frequencies. The noise made by the toys is of no consequence, since it is not activated until after the child has responded to the test signal. Some children, especially the very young, may be frightened by the action of these toys. Since most animated toys also have lights, it is convenient to have a three-way switch which will permit lights only, action only, or both.

Moore et al (1977) investigated the capacity of an animated toy animal to reinforce head-turn responses in infants 4 months, 5 to 6 months and 7 to 11 months of age. They found significantly increased responses, relative to those of subjects of the same age who did

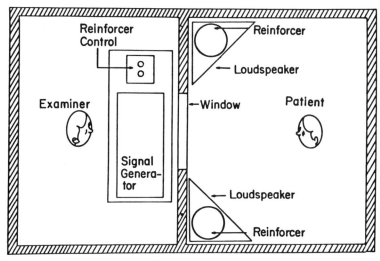

Figure 30.2. Arrangement for localization audiometry.

not see the animated toys after each response, only in the two older groups. This study supports the utility of localization audiometry in the age range being discussed.

A child who has a bilateral severe or profound hearing loss will probably not have learned to localize, or perhaps even to repond consistently to sound. Therefore, in localization audiometry, as with most techniques, it is more difficult to assess the child with hearing loss than the child who has normal hearing. If confusion in localization is noted, it is best to use only one loudspeaker in testing. This way, the child learns that all sounds come from a single source, and the task is made simpler. When using this technique, some provision should be made to distract the child's attention away from the loudspeaker between signals. Otherwise, the child could look at the loudspeaker all the time. A distraction can be provided by mounting a third animated toy on the wall of the sound room across from the child. Activating this toy distracts attention away from the loudspeaker between signals. Alternatively, an assistant seated in front of the child may mainain minimal attention until just before the signal is presented.

In their initial report of Visual Reinforcement Audiometry, Liden and Kankkunen (1969) did not limit responses to orientation. They accepted (a) reflexes, such as the APR, (b) investigatory responses (c) orientation responses and (d) spontaneous responses, such as a smile or vocalization. Because small loudspeakers were close to the child's ear, a clear head- shadow effect was produced. In addition, a plug was placed in the ear canal of the nontest ear and the ear was covered with a sound-attenuating muff. These precautions permit monaural testing for children in whom

the difference in sensitivity between ears is not as great as the attenuation provided by the head-shadow effect plus the plug and muff.

Because of the probability of improvement in response with maturation, Matkin (1977) suggested the term "minimal response level" be used instead of "threshold" during the testing of children in this age range. He reported, using visual reinforcement audiometry, minimal response levels to warble tones at about 25 dB hearing level (HL) by normal-hearing infants 6 to 11 months of age; at about 20 dB HL by children 13 to 17 months old; at about 15 dB HL for those 18 to 23 months of age; and near 10 dB HL at 24 to 29 months.

AGE 25 THROUGH 36 MONTHS

To evaluate children in this age range, ASHA guidelines say behavioral techniques along with acoustic immittance measures are usually sufficient but ABR additionally may be needed if validity or adequacy of behavioral results are questionable or if there is questionable neurologic integrity of the brainstem. (ASHA, 1989). Additionally, ASHA points out, word recognition testing completes the evaluation. Play audiometry is the test of choice for the majority of children within this age range, defined as any test in which the child is taught a play response to the stimulus (for example, dropping a block into a bowl when the tone is heard). Visual or tangible reinforcement of the response is a part of the procedure.

An early example of play audiometry was reported by Dix and Hallpike (1947). In their "peep-show" technique, the child is taught to press a button upon the presentation of a simultaneous light and sound. An interesting picture is illuminated only if the button is pushed immediately after the stimulus presentation. When the child is responding well, the auditory signal is presented alone. Each appropriate response is reinforced, and the process continues until threshold is determined.

By the age of 2 years, some children can be evaluated using play audiometry, and the probability of successful evaluation increases as the child approaches the age of 3 years. Thompson and Weber (1974) were successful in teaching the traditional procedure for play audiometry to only 2% of children under 24 months of age, but were successful with 70% of a group between 24 and 29 months, 90% of those between 30 and 35 months, 96% of the 36 to 41 months group and 100% of children between 42 and 59 months of age.

The goals in play audiometry are to obtain frequency-specific (pure-tone) thresholds under earphones from both ears by air conduction and to also obtain bone conduction thresholds if a hearing loss is indicated. Testing is routinely completed by obtaining speech thresholds and word recognition scores. Immittance measures are indicated if history or test results suggest a conductive disorder.

In play audiometry the initial task often is to assess and attentuate the child's fear and to establish a good working relationship. O'Neill et al (1961) utilized a period of semistructured play prior to audiometric evaluation (a) to establish rapport with the child, (b) to observe reaction to gross sounds in order to get an idea of the level of response, (c) to establish the idea of responding to sound in a play audiometry setting and (d) to help the examiners select procedures and responses suited to the child's ability and interests. These four points are crucial to play audiometry and cannot be ignored. Of course, individual children will require varying amounts of attention to each of the points. The key to the procedure is astute observation of the child's behavior and appropriate reaction by the examiner. Skill and experience are required, as well as thorough knowledge of the behavior of children and of the test equipment.

Once the child is in the test room and a test procedure is decided upon, the next action which may cause an emotional crisis is placing the earphones on the child's head. Many children will not object, especially if the audiologist has done the preliminary work well, in which case the headset can be positioned without fuss. For children who are reluctant to accept the earphones, the examiner can - to show the child what is expected - briefly wear the headset and illustrate the expected response. This action, valid as a training procedure, is usually not very successful as a motivational

device. The child who is reluctant to accept the headset will usually be content to let the examiner wear it indefinitely. In some extreme situations it may help to let the problem child observe the testing of another cooperative child to convey the idea that there is nothing painful about the test and that it is fun. You might call this the Tom Sawyer approach to hearing evaluation. However, the most efficient approach to the child who will not accept earphones may be first to obtain responses in sound field. Thereby a general idea of hearing sensitivity will be obtained while the child is becoming more accustomed to, interested in and less fearful of the test. Usually it is not helpful to try to sneak the earphones onto the child's head but rather to leave them in plain sight during the sound field conditioning and, eventually, without making a big thing of it, to place them on the child. Once the earphones are on, the child should be kept busy to reduce the tendency to remove them.

Because there is always the possibility that a young child will stop responding before the evaluation is completed, it is important to work quickly and to get the most important information first. The recommendation to work quickly must be interpreted with caution. Although working too slowly may permit the child's attention to wander, proceeding too rapidly may confuse the child and encourage false responses. One is left with the lame recommendation to observe the rate at which a given child can work and proceed accordingly. For example, in play audiometry if the child is responding by dropping a block in response to the signal, another block should be placed in the child's hand as soon as the previous one has been dropped, to keep the child involved.

The clinician must guard against accepting false responses. The criterion for the temporal relationship between signal and response must be observed rigidly, and responses outside that relationship must be ignored. Only levels at which responses are repeatable should be accepted. Because threshold is usually defined as the level at which 50% response occurs, a further check may be made by presenting signals 5 dB above the apparent threshold. At that level, 100% response should occur.

Because the examiner must work quickly, it is essential to be completely familiar with the instruments used in testing. Only minimal attention can be given to operation of the equipment. Attention must focus on the behavior of the child. Because the inexperienced clinician must concentrate on the operation of the audiometer, efforts at testing children may be quite unrewarding until manipulation of dials and switches becomes automatic.

Even if the clinician works quickly, some children

will stop responding before the evaluation is completed. If this seems likely, it is usually better to obtain thresholds for the midfrequencies (500, 1000 and 2000 Hz) than to get a complete audiogram for one ear only. For some restless children, whose behavior indicates that they may cooperate for only a short time, it may be preferable first to obtain thresholds for speech. It may be better to have speech thresholds for each ear than one or two puretone thresholds for one ear. This philosophy should not be an excuse for obtaining less than complete results, and any report of a partial examination should be so labeled.

When the child gets restless and responses become unreliable, changing the method of response may introduce enough variety to renew interest. That is, if the child has been dropping blocks in response to the signal, one might change to pegs in a pegboard or some other game. However, the game used for responding should not be too interesting in itself. For example, when attractive small animal toys were once supplied for children to drop into a box, the toys were so interesting that most children wanted to examine each one before responding. The toys provided good material for interest and motivation, but were not appropriate for actual testing.

Children who are interested in some other activity during testing may not respond to an audible sound. Therefore, it is important to avoid distracting stimuli and to have children ready to respond when the auditory signal is presented. This set may be facilitated by the audiologist or an assistant saying "Ready" or "Listen" or by the audiologist's own attentive listening attitude.

The child with a marked hearing loss may have difficulty learning the expected response because of lack of experience responding to sound. Since the child will have limited language or none at all, instructions must be by pantomime and demonstration. It is, of course, essential that the signal be audible during the conditioning process. In puretone testing, an intense 500-Hz tone is most likely to be audible. If difficulty in conditioning is encountered, two procedures have been suggested which may be helpful.

Visually Reinforced Operant Conditioning Audiometry (VROCA) involves use of an interesting visual signal to reinforce auditory responses. The illuminated pictures and animated toys mentioned earlier are appropriate. Tangible Reinforced Operant Conditioning Audiometry (TROCA, Lloyd, Spradlin, and Reid, 1968) involves providing an edible or other tangible reinforcement each time the child makes a specified response in the presence of the acoustic signal and withholding reinforcement when the child responds in the absence of the signal. Bricker and Bricker (1969)

presented a step-by-step program for operant audiometry. This technique may be useful with difficult-to-test individuals of all ages. It should be remembered that, as in any audiometric technique, operant audiometry is justified when it obtains responses more quickly, precisely or inexpensively than other methods. It is also important to note that all of the precautions necessary for valid audiometry must be followed.

Conditioning through use of a vibro-tactile signal may also be helpful. As described by Thorne (1962) the vibrations of a 250- or 500-Hz signal sent through the bone oscillator can be easily felt when the audiometer is set to maximum output for bone conduction. For a child with profound hearing loss, this tactile stimulus may implement conditioning. Once the response is established, response to air-conducted tones can again be investigated. If the child responds readily to tactile signals at 250- and 500-Hz but responds to neither bone-conducted signals at 2000- or 4000-Hz nor to air-conducted tones, it is likely that there is no measurable hearing.

The generalization that play audiometry is appropriate for children 25 through 36 months will have many exceptions. Under clinical conditions, successful conditioning of 2-year-olds may be difficult. However, if a three-year-old cannot be tested with play audiometry by a skilled clinician, there may be some other problem instead of or in addition to a hearing loss. Children who are developmentally between three and five years of age may respond better by play audiometry, or may prefer to respond by touching their ear in response to the signal, and testing becomes reminiscent of that used with adults. Remember that the test method is only a means to an end, and the procedure which elicits the best responses is the method of choice.

MASKING

When testing children, the use of masking to prevent the participation of the nontest ear is as necessary as it is in valid audiometry with adults. The same principles apply. In most cases, elaborate explanations to the child about the noise are unnecessary. If the child has sufficient language, the examiner may explain that there will be a noise in one ear which the child should ignore and continue to respond to the test signal only. If, because of the age or language level of the child, such an explanation is not possible, the examiner should simply introduce the noise into the nontest ear. It will probably help if a level between minimum and maximum masking is chosen, and once introduced, left on continually and without change in level. The fact that the signal does not change makes it easier to recondition the child and permit the test to continue. However, in some instances, when the examiner is just managing to maintain the test procedure (a situation not entirely foreign to audiologists), masking may not be possible. In such cases the examiner should report this fact so that the audiogram can be interpreted accordingly. Fortunately, immitance measures will often provide information about middle-ear status in cases where masking cannot be used to establish bone-conduction thresholds on either ear. Normal tympanograms and acoustic reflex thresholds at expected levels suggest that the hearing loss is sensory neural in nature and abnormal tympanogrms with absent or elevated reflexes suggest that at least part of the observed hearing loss is conductive.

SPEECH THRESHOLD TESTING

Just as is the case in good audiometry with adults, the audiologist will want to obtain speech thresholds to confirm puretone results and to give a direct measure of hearing for speech. When possible, signals used for obtaining thresholds of intelligibility with children should meet the same criteria as those used with adults. That is, the words presented should be highly intelligible and of equal difficulty.

In general, the test can be performed by selecting a few words within the child's vocabulary. If the child can repeat the words, the test can proceed in approximately the same manner as for adults. If not, pictures or objects must be found to represent the words. "Cowboy", "birthday (cake)" and "airplane" are good possibilities. The child points to the picture in response to hearing the word, and the intensity is varied until threshold is determined. Remember that if the test is limited to three or four words the child's task will be very easy and the resultant threshold may be closer to a threshold of detection than an ordinary speech reception threshold (SRT) would be. The test should be conducted under earphones so that each ear can be tested separately, but it may be done in sound field if the child will not wear the headset.

Martin and Coombes (1976) described an attractive procedure for obtaining speech thresholds in young children. Test words are names of parts of a colorful clown, who awards the child with candy if the part named is pressed by the child. The investigators reported success in obtained speech thresholds from children as young as 2 1/2 years.

If the child does not know words which meet the criteria of intelligibility and equality of difficulty usually required for threshold tests, other words or phrases within his vocabulary can be substituted ("Find mama", "let's go bye-bye", "Where is your nose?"). In all of the procedures one must avoid giving visual clues which will help the child identify the words. Since this testing usually requires the flexibility afforded by live voice, a two-room test environment is necessary if the intensity of the signal is to be carefully controlled.

If language limitations prevent establishment of SRT's, thresholds of detection for speech may be established with a procedure similar to that used in pure tone play audiometry. The child is conditioned to drop a block (or to make other appropriate responses) when the speech signal is heard. It seems to have become conventional to use [b÷-b÷-b÷] as the speech signal. By varying the intensity, threshold is established. These speech awareness thresholds are as reliable as SRTs and are reached at an intensity about 10 to 12 dB less than that required for SRT (Egan, 1948). If speech awareness thresholds are obtained, they should be labeled as such.

For some children, speech thresholds can be obtained when puretone thresholds cannot. For example, an older retarded child may have enough language to mediate speech thresholds, but cannot be conditioned easily to respond to play audiometry. These results are not complete because they do not give information about hearing sensitivity as a function of frequency. However, air-conducted speech thresholds give information about hearing sensitivity, and bone-conducted speech thresholds give some diagnostic information about sensory-neural status.

WORD RECOGNITION TESTING

Although it is important to obtain SRTs for purposes of rehabilitation and comparison with puretone findings, word recognition scores provide a different type of measure that in many cases is more important than the SRT. A measure of word recognition ability at an optimal presentation level is used to determine the degree of clarity with which the child hears speech. Different criteria are used in the selection of materials for word recognition than speech reception testing. Word recognition tests are usually lists of words whose phonetic composition covers the range of sounds in the language, with approximately the same proportion as the sounds occur in the language. There are several word recognition tests for children. The phonetically balanced PB-K lists (K for "kindergarten") developed by Haskins (1949) are most like the PB word lists used with adults. These lists can be used with children who have enough language and intelligible speech to repeat the words of the test. Unfortunately, receptive language level affects discrimination scores. The role of word familiarity is discussed elsewhere. Children with congenital hearing losses usually exhibit retarded language development which reduces scores. Results obtained under these circumstances must be interpreted with caution. Jerger and Jerger (1982) reported the development of the Pediatric Speech Intelligibility Test and its administration to children 3 to 6 years of age. This test consists of both monosyllabic words and sentences and in its taped version can be presented either in quiet or in a background of competing sentences.

With very young or language-limited children, picture tests may be used. Such tests include the Discrimination by Identification of Pictures (DIP) Test (Siegenthaler and Haspiel, 1966), the Word Intelligibility by Picture Identification (WIPI) Test developed by Ross and Lerman (1970) and the Northwestern University Children's Perception of Speech (NU-CHIPS) Test (Katz and Elliott, 1978). In these closed set tests, the child listens while looking at a set of pictures, one of which represents the stimulus word. Pointing to the proper picture consitutes a correct response.

Certain variables affect these scores. Lerman et al (1965) reported that some pictures may not be correctly identified as representing the stimulus word. Additionally, because the possible responses in picture tests are limited to a few words, the tests are easier than those that require the child to repeat the word. Hodgson (1973) administered the WIPI to normal-hearing children between 5 and 9 years of age. In one condition, the WIPI was presented in the usual way as a picture test. In the other, WIPI words were presented as an open set test, without the picture, and the subjects repeated the words they heard. The words were presented with ipsilateral noise to prevent 100% correct responses. The mean score was better by 10% for the closed set test. Jones and Studebaker (1974) concluded that a closed set test may be more informative when used with older children with severe hearing loss. They presented closed and open set tests to 23 such children. They found the closed set test correlated better with tests of auditory sensitivity and teacher ratings.

For young children with severe or profound losses, Erber (1980) developed the Auditory Numbers Test (ANT), which requires the differentiation of spoken numbers. Tests are also available for nonverbal children. The Sound Effects Recognition Test (SERT) utilizes a recording of familiar environmental sounds as test signals (Finitzo-Hieber et al, 1980).

Matkin (1977) recommends the PB-K lists for children with receptive language age (RLA) between 6 and 12 years. He advocates the WIPI or NU-CHIPS if RLA is from 4 to 6 years. Matkin recommends the ANT or an informal procedure if RLA is less than 4

years. In the latter, pictures or objects are used to represent words within the child's vocabulary to which pointing responses can be elicited. He also suggested that informal test scores be reported as the ratio of correct responses out of number of trials, rather than in percentage, as formal tests are reported.

An age effect has been reported in discrimination testing with young children with both open and closed set tests. Siegenthaler and Haspiel (1966) found improvement in scores obtained with a closed set test across an age range from 3 to 8 years. Smith and Hodgson (1970) presented PB-K lists to normal and to hearing-impaired children ages 4 to 8.5 years. For both groups scores improved with age.

SUMMARY

The astute clinician will combine behavioral and physiologic procedures as needed to obtain and confirm test results. Behavioral procedures should be keyed to exploiting the most sensitive procedures possible, based on the responses of which the child is capable. Successful evaluation requires the clinician (a) to know the developmental responses to sound expected in normals, (b) to have a thorough familiarity with audiometric instrumentation and procedures and (c) to be able to interpret results by integrating information based on the pattern of behavior elicited by an appropriate test battery.

To summarize age-appropriate test procedures, ABR is the procedure of choice for infants up to 4 months of age. Supplementary and corroborative information can be gained from behavioral observation audiometry, eliciting reflexive responses with relatively intense signals. Used with caution, immittance measures may give information about the status of the middle ear. The emerging acoustic reflex may also contribute. However, in this age range, normal tympanogrms may be obtained in abnormal ears and should not be used without other confirming evidence.

In the age range 5 through 24 months visual reinforcement audiometry provides quick identification of normal hearing and minimal response levels to estimate hearing loss. Frequency-specific signals can and should be used, but information obtained in sound field usually pertains only to the better ear. ABR information will often be helpful, especially when behavioral meausres cannot provide ear-specific information. For children who have acquired language, a good approximation of overall sensitivity for either ear may be obtained through speech reception thresholds. Word recognition ability can be estimated via tests designed for use with young children. Immitance measures provide information about the status of the middle ear. Children between 25 and 36 months of age developmentally (and older difficult-to-test children) may be evaluated via conditioned play audiometry. Air and bone conduction thresholds may be obtained for either ear. Speech reception and word discrimination scores may be routinely administered, using tests appropriate for the age range and receptive language level. Immitance measures contribute information about the status of the middle ear.

For children in each age range, reliance should not be placed on any single test. Rather, as many measures as possible should be obtained or repeated until a complete and precise picture of auditory function results.

REFERENCES

American National Standards Institute. American national standard for permissible ambient noise during audiometric testing. ANSI S3. 1-1977, New York.

American Speech-Language-Hearing Association. Joint committee on infant hearing position statement. ASHA 1982;24:1017–1018.

American Speech-Language-Hearing Association. Guidelines for audiologic screening of newborn infants who are at risk for hearing impairment. ASHA 1989;31:89–92.

American Speech-Language-Hearing Association. Guidelines for the audiologic assessment of neonates, infants, toddlers, and young children. ASHA (in press).

Bricker D, and Bricker W. A programmed approach to operant audiometry for low-functioning children. J Speech Hear Disord 1969;34:312–320.

Brooks W. Status of nationwide neonatal hearing screening programs and procedures. Paper presented at the meeting of the American Academy of Audiology, New Orleans, 1990.

Dix M, and Hallpike C. The peep-show; a new technique for pure tone audiometry in young children. Br Med J 1947;1:791–723.

Egan J. Articulation testing methods. Laryngoscope 1948;58:995–991.

Erber N. Use of the auditory numbers test to evaluate speech perception abilities of hearing-impaired children. J Speech Hear Disord 1980;45:527–532.

Finitzo-Hieber T, Gerling I, Cherow-Skalka E, and Matkin N. A sound effects recognition test for the pediatric audiological evaluation. Ear Hear 1980;1:271–276.

Gerkin K. High risk register for deafness. ASHA 1984;26(3):17–27.

Haskins H. A phonetically balanced test of speech discrimination for children [Unpublished Master's thesis]. Northwestern University, 1949.

Hodgson W. A comparison of WIPI and PB-K discrimination test scores. Paper presented at American Speech and Hearing Association Convention, Detroit, 1973.

Jerger S, and Jerger J. Pediatric speech intelligibility test: performance intensity characteristics. Ear Hear 1982;3:325–334.

Jones K, and Studebaker G. Performance of severely hearing-impaired children on a closed-response, auditory speech discrimination test. J Speech Hear Res 1974;17:531–540.

Katz D, and Elliott L. Development of a new children's speech discrimination test. Paper presented at American Speech and Hearing Association Convention, San Francisco, 1978.

Lerman J, Ross M, and McLauchlin R. A picture-identification test for hearing-impaired children. J Aud Res 1965;5:273–278.

Liden G, and Kankkunen A. Visual reinforcement audiometry. Acta Otolaryngol (Stockh) 1969;67:281–292.

Lloyd L, Spradlin J, and Reid M. An operant audio-metric procedure for difficult-to-test patients. J Speech Hear Disord 1968;33:236–245.

Matkin N. Assessment of hearing sensitivity during the preschool years, In Bess F, Ed. Childhood Deafness. New York: Grune and Stratton, 1977.

Martin F, and Coombes S. A tangibly reinforced speech reception threshold procedure for use with small children. J Speech Hear Disord 1976;41:333–338.

Moore J, Wilson W, and Thompson G. Visual reinforcement of head-turn responses in infants under twelve months of age. J Speech Hear Disord 1977;42:328–334.

Northern J, and Downs M. Hearing in Children. Baltimore: Williams and Wilkins, 1978.

O'Neill J, and Oyer H, and Hillis J. Audiometric procedures used with children. J Speech Hear Disord 1961;26:61–66.

Ross M, and Lerman J. A picture identification test for hearing-impaired children. J Speech Hear Res 1970;13:44–53.

Siegenthaler B, and Haspiel B. Development of two standardized measures of hearing for speech by children. Co-operatiave Research Program, Project No. 2372, United States Office of Education, Washington, DC, 1966.

Simmons F, and Russ F. Automated newborn hearing screening, the crib-o-gram. Arch Otolaryngol 1974;100:1–7.

Smith K, and Hodgson W. The effects of systematic reinforcement on the speech discrimination responses of normal and hearing-impaired children. J Aud Res 1970;10:110–117.

Thompson G, and Weber B. Responses to infants and young children to behavior observation audiometry (BOA). J Speech Hear Disord 1974;39:140–147.

Thorne B. Conditioning children for pure tone testing. J Speech Hear Disord 1962;27:84–85.

Wertheimer M. Psychomotor coordination of auditory and visual space at birth. Science 1961;134:1692.

CHAPTER 31

Hearing and Middle-Ear Screening of School-Age Children

Kathryn A. Barrett

A "hearing impairment is defined as a deviation or change for the worse in either auditory structure or auditory function, usually outside the range of normal" (ASHA, 1981). The goal of any school hearing screening program should be to accurately and efficiently identify those students whose hearing is impaired resulting from either conductive and/or sensory-neural pathology. Although some ear pathologies (e.g., middle ear effusion) might not produce a significant hearing loss, screening for these pathologies should be a part of the screening program because they may interfere with the child's physical well-being, thus possibly hindering the potential to learn.

According to Harker and Van Wagoner (1974), "The goal of screening should be the detection of disease, not just the detection of those diseases which at the time of test are accompanied by hearing loss." Several authors have noted the ineffectiveness of puretone sweep screening alone in identifying children with otitis media and have suggested the use of immittance screening as a viable tool to complement the puretone screening program (Brooks, 1973, 1985; Harker and Van Wagoner, 1974; Anderson, 1978; Downs, 1978; Lidén and Renvall, 1980; Renvall and Lidén, 1980; McKenzie et al., 1982; FitzZaland and Zink, 1984; ASHA, 1985; 1990). The advantage of an effective puretone and immittance screening program would not only be the detection of otitis media but the prevention of chronic otitis media (Lidén and Renvall, 1980). The "Guidelines for Identification Audiometry" (ASHA, 1985) indicate that the most effective approach for identifying individuals who need audiologic or otologic services is to use both puretone testing and acoustic immittance measurements.

The role of the educational audiologist in the screening process is important despite the relative simplicity of both the hearing and middle-ear screening procedures. Administration of the screening procedures requires the expertise of a trained technician; however, the need for organization and strict audiologic supervision cannot be overemphasized. Puretone-immittance screening is the primary means of identifying those children needing additional audiologic and/or medical assessment.

Identification is only the beginning in any audiologic management program. After this, audiologic and/or medical assessments can be completed, followed by appropriate educational/audiologic/medical management of the child.

The purpose of this chapter is to provide audiologists with information regarding the process and concerns of hearing and middle-ear screening of school-age children.

JUSTIFICATION FOR HEARING AND MIDDLE-EAR SCREENING

Incidence of Hearing Loss

General Statistics

According to Leske (1981), one of every 1000 newborns has a congenital hearing impairment. Authur and Sherwood (1980) stated that among children ages 5 to 19 years old, three in 4000 are deaf and one in 200 is hard of hearing. The National Speech and Hearing Survey examined 38,568 school children from grades 1 to 12 (Leske, 1981). Of these children, less than 1% were found to have bilateral hearing impairments with hearing levels for speech more than 25 dB. A unilateral loss was found in 1.9% of the sample, resulting in a total estimate of 2.6% hearing impairment in children from grades 1 to 12. Eagles et al. (1973) reported that 5% of school children have hearing levels (HL) in one or both ears, at one or more frequencies, beyond the normal range of hearing. To take these statistics one step further, Ross and Giolas (1978) suggest that a child with a loss of 15 dB HL or more in the speech frequencies in the better ear is at risk for the hearing loss to have an adverse effect on some aspect of her or his performance. The educational implications resulting from hearing impairment lend even more support for hearing and middle-ear screening of school-age children. The educational implications of hearing loss are discussed in Chapter 39.

Conductive Versus Sensory-Neural

None of the above statistics differentiate between type of hearing loss. However, if it is assumed that middle ear pathology or occlusion of the ear canal often results in a hearing loss, the following statistics give some insight into the percentage of conductive hearing loss in school-age children. The results of the Health Examination Survey 1963 to 1970 were reported by Leske (1981). Otoscopic findings in more than 7000 children, 6 to 11 years old, revealed 20% with at least one abnormal eardrum. In a similar sized group of youths, 12 to 17 years, there was 15% abnormality. In addition, 14% of the children and 10% of the youths had occlusion of the auditory canal, usually by cerumen. Overall, there were 34% of the younger group and 25% of the older group with presumed conductive hearing loss.

Using serial tympanometry to screen 553 five-year-old children, Hallett (1982) found that 35% of the children screened had evidence of middle-ear disease in both ears and 26% of the children had evidence of unilateral middle-ear disease on each occasion tested. Gimsing and Bergholtz (1983) reported abnormal tympanograms in 11% of the ears screened in 1120 seven- and ten-year-old children. The incidence of failure was twice as great in the younger children than in the older children, 15 and 8%, respectively. They further reported that 36% of the ears that failed tympanometry had a hearing loss exceeding 20 dB at 500 Hz.

In 1984, FitzZaland and Zink reported the puretone hearing and immittance screening results on a cohort of 3510 kindergarten and first grade children. The results revealed that 3.9% of the children screened had hearing and/or middle-ear function beyond the normal range (3.5%-conductive hearing loss and reduced middle ear function, 0.3%-purely sensory-neural hearing loss, and 0.1%-mixed hearing loss).

Sensitivity of Puretone and Immittance Screening

Several authors have reported results indicating an increased sensitivity to the detection of middle ear disease when using a combined method of puretone screening and immittance measures and/or otoscopy. Brooks (1973) reported 81.5% agreement between a puretone sweep method using 500, 1000, 2000, and 4000 Hz at 25 dB and a combined method using acoustic reflexes and a single frequency puretone (4000 Hz). The puretone sweep screening failed to identify 7.4% of middle ear abnormality (low compliance and flat pressure compliance curves) on 543 children, 5 to 6 years old.

Harker and Van Wagoner (1974) reported the results of puretone and immittance screening of 710 children (preschool to grade 12). Of those tested, 9.7% passed puretone but failed immittance, all of whom were in the preschool and kindergarten to third grade group with the exception of one.

In 1974, McCandless and Thomas reported the agreement between otoscopy, immittance and puretone screening on a group of 730 children ranging from 3 to 15 years of age. The overall agreement between puretone screening and otoscopy was 61%, whereas the agreement between immittance and otoscopy was 93%.

Lidén and Renvall (1980) reported the referral percentages of several screening tests from five separate investigations (n = 5886 7-year-old children). Otoscopic examination referred 5.8%, ipsilateral stapedial reflex greater than or equal to 110 dB SPL referred 7.6%, tympanometry referred 6.4%, and puretone screening at 500, 3000, and 4000 Hz referred 1.9, 1.5, and 2.1%, respectively. They concluded that tympanometry combined with a puretone screen at 500 and 4000 Hz was better than puretone screening alone in detecting middle ear disease.

Although the primary justification for using immittance screening in conjunction with puretone screening is its increased sensitivity in detecting middle-ear disease, immittance measures have other advantages when used to screen school-age children. According to ASHA (1979) sound attenuating environments are not necessary when using immittance; therefore, excessive ambient noise levels are not a serious factor in immittance screening. Other advantages of immittance are (a) test procedures are rapid, (b) test results are not subject to the student's lack of understanding instructions, (c) procedures are minimally limited by age, and (d) immittance screening can be used to obtain results on difficult-to-test individuals.

In contrast to the above findings, Aniansson (1986) reported the findings of puretone and immittance screening, which included a rescreen of initial failures in 6–8 weeks, on 7863 seven-year-old children. The criteria for failure were responses to puretones ≥25 dB at 500, 1000, 2000, 3000, 4000, 6000, or 8000 Hz and tympanogram peak pressure ≤200 mm H_2O for tympanometry. The results revealed that repeated puretone screening identified 86% of the children with middle-ear disorder although 14% were found by tympanometry. He concluded that cost analysis does not justify the use of tympanometry as a screening tool to identify middle-ear disorder. Also, because of its variability, tympanogram peak pressure is not recommended for use as a criterion for medical referral (Margolis and Heller, 1987; ASHA, 1990).

The Committee on School Health (1987) recommends that immittance measures should not be used in mass screening programs for the detection of hearing loss or middle ear effusion. Their recommendation is based on the premise that immittance measures are used to detect middle ear effusion, not hearing loss, and that clinical findings suggest that middle ear effusion usually resolves spontaneously within 2–3 months. However, immittance measures may be used in the school setting to aid in the diagnosis of individual children who are high risk for or who are suspected of having otitis media with effusion. Further, Bluestone et al. (1986) concludes that until more information is available, the "... continuation of existing screening programs (or initiation of programs) designed to identify asymptomatic otitis media with effusion in special populations known to be at high risk for the complications and sequelae of otitis media ..." is recommended. These populations include "... infants and children with cleft palate, Down syndrome, and other craniofacial abnormalities, American Indians, Alaskan Eskimos, residential students in schools for the deaf, and the mentally retarded ...". They advise caution before proceeding with mass screening of infants and children that are not high risk.

Summary of the Literature Review

Although opinions and interpretations vary regarding screening of children for middle-ear and hearing problems in school settings, much of the evidence suggests that puretone screening supplemented by immittance screening is an effective and efficient means of detecting hearing impairment and otitis media. Although not unanimously accepted for mass screening, using immittance screening measures for the detection of middle ear disorders is generally accepted for populations at risk for these disorders. Immittance and puretone screening should be implemented using carefully considered protocols for testing and referral. It also requires calibrated equipment, well-trained personnel, strict audiologic supervision, and an organized plan for follow-up.

PURPOSE OF A HEARING AND MIDDLE-EAR SCREENING PROGRAM

Guidelines have been proposed to help evaluate whether or not any screening program is likely to be effective in detecting disorders or risk factors in "seemingly healthy persons" (Cadman et al., 1984). Following these proposed guidelines will aid in determining whether or not a screening program should be implemented and/or target areas where the program is likely to be ineffective. These guidelines consider research findings, such as, (a) demonstration that the program will be effective, (b) availability of efficacious treatments, (c) data suggesting that the burden of suffering warrants screening and (d) availability of effec-

tive screening measures. These guidelines also consider organization and administrative factors, such as, (e) Does the program reach those who would benefit?, (f) Can the health system cope with the program? and (g) Do persons with positive screenings comply with advice and interventions?

Cross (1985) discussed criteria for evaluating existing screening programs, specifically in schools. They are as follows:

(a) Disease aspects: high prevalence, high incidence, adverse consequences.
(b) Treatment aspects: available, effective, early intervention benefit.
(c) Screening test: high sensitivity, high specificity, simple, brief, and acceptable to the person being screened.
(d) Screener/tester: well-trained.
(e) Target population: population in which the undetected disease is prevalent or in which early intervention is beneficial.
(f) Referral and treatment: those who obtain positive screening results must receive definitive evaluation and, if indicated, appropriate treatment.
(g) Cost/benefit ratio.
(h) Program maintenance: improvement of efficiency via periodic review.

Lescouflair (1975) indicated that the purpose of any hearing screening program is twofold: to identify and to refer with a goal of total prevention. More specifically, he states that a hearing screening program should (a) identify even minimal hearing losses, (b) identify the presence of active middle ear disease, (c) refer abnormal cases to a physician, and (d) refer cases in need of such services for appropriate rehabilitation. Lescouflair describes several determinants of failure in hearing screening programs. These determinants include: (a) poorly defined goals and objectives, (b) ineffectiveness of referral and follow-up procedures, (c) ineffectiveness of coverage (i.e., programs that reach only a portion of the school children), and (d) ineffectiveness of test procedures (i.e., poor test environment or poorly trained personnel).

According to Northern and Downs (1974), several important benefits can be obtained by an effective and well organized hearing screening program.

(a) Prevention—A potentially handicapping hearing loss, if detected at an early age, often can be remedied through medical treatment.
(b) Maintenance of adequate audition—An undetected hearing loss may have an adverse effect on educational achievement.
(c) Habilitation—Those children whose hearing

losses are identified and further diagnosed as permanent have the availability of audiologic and educational habilitation techniques that should lead to improved educational achievement.

A fourth benefit of an effective hearing screening program is the increased awareness of hearing and hearing loss by the school faculty and staff. A hearing screening program that is efficient and effective in identifying hearing impairment resulting in audiologic/medical remediation and, if necessary, educational assistance promotes a positive rapport between hearing screening and school personnel.

The goal of any hearing screening program is to accurately and efficiently identify hearing impairment by maximizing the number of correct identifications (sensitivity) while minimizing the false positives (specificity). Using a combined puretone and immittance screening protocol, students with questionable hearing or middle ear function can be identified quickly and referred for follow-up testing.

HEARING SCREENING METHODS

Screening Versus Testing

The goal of hearing testing is differential diagnosis, whereas, the goal of hearing screening is identification. Although hearing and middle-ear screening does not yield a diagnosis, the standards and procedures used are just as critical as those used in evaluating hearing impairment and middle-ear disorder.

Individual Hearing Screening Methods Using Puretones as Signals

Test Measures and Criteria

Currently, most school screening programs use individual screening methods because they are more accurate than group screening methods in identifying hearing loss (House and Glorig, 1957; Newby, 1979). The sweep check method has become more or less the standard screening procedure (Anderson, 1978). The sweep procedure involves setting the attenuator of a puretone audiometer at a predetermined intensity level and each frequency is presented at that level. A response, most often a raised hand, is required if the tone is heard. The sweep test method enables children to be screened individually at a fairly rapid rate.

Various frequencies and stimulus levels to be used in puretone sweep screening have been proposed over the past 30 years (House and Glorig, 1957; Darley, 1961; Melnick et al., 1964; Downs, 1978; and Katt and Sprague, 1981). The current ASHA guidelines, "Guidelines for Screening for Hearing Impairment

and Middle-Ear Disorders" (ASHA, 1990) are to be used in conjunction with the "Guidelines for Identification Audiometry" (ASHA, 1985). Methods and procedures specific to hearing screening are referred to in the ASHA (1985) guidelines, whereas, methods and procedures specific to middle-ear screening are referred to in the ASHA (1990) guidelines. ASHA (1985) recommends individual puretone sweep screening using a manual rather than an automatic method for testing. When acoustic-immittance measures are incorporated in the screening program ASHA (1985) recommends puretone screening at the frequencies of 1000, 2000, and 4000 Hz. Screening at 500 Hz should be included if acoustic-immittance measures are not part of the screening program and if ambient noise levels permit screening at this frequency. All frequencies are to be screened at 20 dB HL (re ANSI-1989).

Puretone Rescreening Criteria

Failure to respond to one or more frequencies regardless of ear requires rescreening preferably within the same session (ASHA, 1985).

Puretone Referral Criteria

Failure to respond to one or more frequencies on two consecutive screenings regardless of ear should result in a referral for further evaluation by an audiologist (ASHA, 1985).

IMMITTANCE SCREENING

Test Measures and Criteria

Bess et al. (1978) recommend a combination of tympanometry and acoustic reflex when screening middle-ear function using an air pressure range of −400 to +100 daPa with a 220 Hz probe tone for tympanometry, although, an air pressure range of −300 to +100 daPa and a probe tone up to 300 Hz are acceptable. Acoustic reflexes should be screened using a puretone of 1000 to 3000 Hz at an intensity level of 105 dB HL contralaterally or 105 dB SPL ipsilaterally. More recent recommendations for screening using acoustic immittance measures do not include acoustic reflex measurements because of its limited efficacy for detecting middle ear disorders (McKenzie et al., 1982; ASHA, 1990).

According to Renvall and Lidén (1980) and Lidén and Renvall (1980), stapedial reflexes give a higher percentage of false-positive results when screening for the detection of middle ear disease. Roberts (1976) proposed that by disregarding absent acoustic reflexes when occurring with normal tympanograms, immittance abnormalities would correlate better with otoscopy. Lidén and Renvall (1980) reported their criteria for failure as middle ear pressure values of less than or equal to −150 daPa or a flat tympanogram and/or hearing thresholds higher than 20 dB (re ISO 1964) at 500 and 1000 Hz. All children failing the screening should be rescreened in 4 to 6 weeks; if they continue to fail, otologic referral is indicated.

The "Guidelines for Screening for Hearing Impairment and Middle-Ear Disorders" (ASHA, 1990) recommend three acoustic immittance measures: (a) compensated static acoustic admittance, (b) equivalent ear canal volume, and (c) tympanogram width. The use of three different immittance measures for screening in an effort to increase the specificity of the test thus reducing over-referrals is justified. However, there are few acoustic immittance screening instruments that provide these three measures quickly and efficiently. In addition, current data on tympanogram width suggests that it may be a useful measure in acoustic immittance screening (ASHA, 1990), however, there is a paucity of clinical data available on the effects of middle ear disorders on tympanogram width.

It is not the intent of this chapter to define the concepts underlying acoustic-immittance measures. However, the fundamental concepts of acoustic immittance are covered in Chapter 19.

Immittance Rescreening Criteria

Immittance rescreening following an initial failure in an effort to decrease the rate of overreferrals has been recommended (Lewis et al., 1975; Brooks, 1976). Variations in immittance results have been demonstrated by Lewis et al. (1975). Although the flat tympanogram is relatively stable, the normal and negative pressure tympanograms can vary from day to day. Thus the need for rescreening any children who fail the initial immittance screening or who are at risk is indicated to assure appropriate referrals. However, according to Northern (1980), it is better to have a few overreferrals than not to identify a child who could benefit from additional evaluation.

Several authors suggest time limits for rescreening varying from 1 to 2 weeks (Lucker, 1980) to open-ended (Lewis et al., 1975). Rescreening using predetermined time limits or limits determined at the discretion of the audiologist enables children in need of medical/audiologic services to be referred within a reasonable length of time whereas decreasing the number of false-positive referrals. A reasonable approach would be to set time limits not to exceed 4 to 6 weeks for the second screen. A third screening may be considered given that spontaneous recovery of middle-

ear effusion may take as long as 3 to 6 months (Cross, 1985).

Immittance Referral Criteria

Minimizing the false-positive referral rate can also be accomplished using referral criteria that have been shown to be both sensitive and specific in identifying middle ear disease. For example, using a pressure of −100 daPa or less and an absent acoustic reflex as their referral criteria, McCandless and Thomas (1974) reported a 4 to 6% false-positive rate.

Bess et al. (1978) and Bess (1980) suggested that any student with an absent acoustic reflex at 1000 Hz presented contralaterally at 105 dB HL and abnormal tympanograms being either flat or rounded or having a pressure more negative than −200 daPa on retest (4 to 6 weeks after the initial screening) should be referred for evaluation.

In 1990, ASHA recommended immittance screening referral criteria based on the 90% range of values for children and adults for compensated static admittance, equivalent ear canal volume, and tympanogram width. Table 31.1 presents suggested interim norms (means and 90% ranges) for compensated static admittance (peak Y), equivalent ear-canal volume (V_{ec}), and tympanogram width (TW) (ASHA, 1990). These norms are based on data provided by Margolis and Heller (1987). The data were obtained with an acoustic immittance screening instrument that used a 226-Hz probe tone and a pump speed of 200 daPa/s. The instrument automatically compensated for ear-canal volume by subtracting the admittance at 200 daPa from the peak values. The normative values for children were obtained on children 3 to 5 years old.

Referral criteria for immittance screening recommended by ASHA (1990) are:

(a) Flat tympanogram and equivalent ear canal volume exceeding the normal range: suggestive of tympanic membrane perforation.
(b) Low compensated static admittance on two successive screenings within a 4- to 6-week interval.
(c) Tympanogram width exceeding the normal range on two successive screenings within a 4- to 6-week interval.

Table 31.1
Interim Immittance Screening Normative Values (ASHA, 1990)

	Peak Y (mmho or cm³)		V_{ec} (cm³)		TW (daPa)	
	Mean	90% Range	Mean	90% Range	Mean	90% Range
Children	0.5	0.2–0.9	0.7	0.4–1.0	100	60–150
Adults	0.8	0.3–1.4	1.1	0.6–1.5	80	50–110

Serial Immittance Measures

Another controversy surrounding the use of acoustic-immittance measures to screen for middle-ear disorders is that current recommended screening models or paradigms fail to identify children with recurrent or chronic otitis media (Hallett, 1982; McKenzie et al., 1982; Bluestone et al., 1986; Lous, 1987). Several studies have reported high spontaneous recovery rates of middle-ear effusion. For example, Cross (1985) concluded that 50% of children between the ages of 5 to 8 years will have middle-ear effusion and most will spontaneously recover within 3 to 6 months. Further 1.5 to 5% of children will have persistent effusions for more than 6 months. Gimsing and Bergholtz (1983) found that 52% of the 7-year-old and 80% of the 10-year-old children with abnormal tympanograms at the initial screening had spontaneously recovered at an 8- to 16-week follow-up. Hallett (1982) suggested that serial tympanometry on the same cohort of children is more likely to identify those children with chronic or recurrent middle-ear disorders than one time screening for all children then rescreening only those who fail the first screening. McKenzie et al. (1982) concluded from their findings that serial immittance measures demonstrated resolution of middle ear problems resulting in a substantial drop in the overreferral rate.

Although serial acoustic immittance screening on the same cohort of children is more likely to identify children with chronic or recurrent middle-ear effusion, serial screening in public schools is impractical given the lack of adequately trained personnel and available funding. Serial screening on children at risk for chronic middle-ear effusion may be a more practical approach to the problem rather than serial screening of all children between the developmental age of 3 years and the third grade and special populations. Downs and Northern (in Bluestone et al., 1986) provided guidelines for identifying children at risk for chronic middle-ear effusions. These guidelines are: (a) first bout of otitis media in the first year of life, (b) family history of recurrent otitis media with effusion, (c) attendance at day-care centers in the first 2 years of life, and (d) more than three episodes of acute otitis media.

OTHER IMPORTANT CONCERNS FOR HEARING AND MIDDLE-EAR SCREENING

Several other factors warrant consideration when implementing a hearing and middle-ear screening program for school-age children. These factors include population to be screened, selection and training of screening assistants, selection and calibration of equipment, screening site, screening time limits, instructions to students, and hearing screening forms and letters communicating with family and physician and/or audiologist for appropriate follow-up.

Population

Puretone Screening

Darley (1961) recommends that newly established programs should screen all students. Thereafter, screen grades kindergarten to 3, all new students, students returning to school after a serious illness, students with special adjustment problems and teacher referrals. He also suggested that students in grades 4 to 12 be screened no less frequently than every 3 years. ASHA (1985) recommends annual screening of all children functioning at a developmental level of 3 years through the third grade and all high risk students.

Although the recommendations for the population to receive hearing screening vary somewhat, all emphasize the need for annual screening in the early grades and special students. It seems reasonable that annual screenings should include all students in grades kindergarten, 1, 2, 3, all new students, all students enrolled in special education programs, all high-risk students, and all teacher referrals.

Immittance Screening

Bess et al. (1978) and Bluestone et al. (1986) recommend that the following children receive annual immittance screening: (a) children with known sensory-neural hearing losses, (b) children who are developmentally delayed or mentally handicapped, (c) children with cleft palate or other craniofacial anomalies, (d) native American children, and (e) children with Down syndrome. According to ASHA (1990), immittance screening should be performed annually on children functioning at a developmental age of 3 years through the third grade and on children at risk for hearing loss and/or middle-ear disorders.

Personnel and Training

Puretone Screening

Screening assistants may be volunteers selected from parent groups, local churches or service organizations, high school or college students, or salaried personnel hired specifically for hearing screening. Training is necessary when recruiting individuals whose abilities and knowledge of hearing and hearing loss vary. These individuals should be required to attend a short, intensive workshop in preparation for hearing screening. According to the Hearing Conservation Guide by the North Carolina Department of Public

Instruction (1983) the workshop curriculum should include the following: (a) basic physics of sound, (b) basic anatomy and physiology of the auditory mechanism, (c) etiology of hearing disorders, (d) importance of hearing conservation, (e) identification of hearing loss, (f) hearing screening procedures and equipment, (g) record keeping procedures, (h) care and biologic calibration of equipment, and (i) special testing techniques for younger or exceptional children. The workshop also should include a supervised practicum in which each assistant is required to perform a minimum of 10 hearing screening tests. Screening assistants who have attended previous workshops should be required to attend at least the practicum and screening procedure portions of the workshop to become reacquainted with the procedures and methods.

Immittance Screening

All immittance screening programs should be supervised by an audiologist with training and experience in immittance screening techniques and interpretation of the results (Bess et al., 1978; ASHA, 1990). Support personnel should receive training commensurate with the task they are expected to perform, i.e., immittance screening. According to Bess et al. (1978), a need exists for training programs to assure that personnel are appropriately trained. Support personnel may be recruited from the same resources as the personnel for puretone screening.

Equipment and Calibration

Puretone Audiometers

The equipment used in a hearing screening program should be manually operated puretone audiometers or screening audiometers for individual screening and should meet ANSI S3.6-1989 specifications. According to Darley (1961) the equipment should be checked for calibration every 4 months. ASHA (1985) recommends complete calibration of the screening equipment annually with checks of SPL outputs at least every 3 months; however, a biologic check should be performed at the beginning of each screening day and periodically throughout the day.

Immittance Instruments

Equipment used for acoustic immittance screening should be capable of measuring acoustic admittance in millimhos (or impedance in ohms), although alternative methods of expressing acoustic admittance can be used, for example, cubic centimeters (ASHA, 1990).

The calibration of the immittance instruments should comply with the ANSI standard on aural acoustic immittance instruments (ANSI S3.39-1987).

Calibration should be performed on a routine basis and should include the intensity and frequency of the probe tone, manometer pressure and reflex-activating stimulus (if applicable) (Bess et al., 1978). Although not addressed in the current guidelines (ASHA, 1990), the "Guidelines for Acoustic Immittance Screening of Middle Ear Function" (ASHA, 1979) recommends that during periods of screening, the equipment should be calibrated before the initial screening and again midway during the screening day.

Screening Site

Although ambient noise levels are not of primary concern when screening using immittance measures, they are crucial when screening using puretones. Darley (1961) recommends that hearing screening be performed in a quiet environment, preferably in a sound-treated room. However, most schools do not have sound-treated facilities. ASHA (1985) suggests that school environments may be appropriate if the noise levels do not exceed the proposed maximum allowable limits for ambient noise (ANSI-1969). The limits are frequency specific and are as follows: 4000 Hz-62 dB sound pressure level (SPL); 2000 Hz-54.5 dB SPL; 1000 Hz-49.5 dB SPL; and 500 Hz-41.5 dB SPL.

When selecting a location for hearing screening, the use of a sound level meter to clearly define the noise levels in the environment is preferable but may not always be available; in addition, noise levels within a school setting will vary from time to time during the school day. Therefore, a carpeted area removed from the main traffic flow would be the most desirable location. Possible screening sites include media centers and resource or music rooms. A biologic check of several subjects with normal hearing in the selected screening location should be performed to assure that ambient noise levels are not an interfering factor. At times, however, regardless of location, it may be necessary to cease testing for a short period of time when ambient noise levels become intolerable (e.g., while a class is passing by the screening location). Locations that are unsuitable for screening include areas adjacent to restroom facilities, cafeterias, playgrounds, or student commons areas.

Instructions to Students

Puretone Screening

The standard instructions of "raise your hand when you hear the beep or tone" will usually suffice for students from the first grade on. However, kindergarten students may need additional preparation before the actual screening as the puretone hearing screening procedure may be a new experience for them.

Anderson (1978) suggests that teachers, volunteers, or technicians incorporate training techniques into routine daily activities of the class before the screening day. He also suggests that the screener introduce the equipment and test procedure to these younger students as a group using some of the more willing students as volunteers, thus alleviating fears of the equipment and test procedure. It is good practice to ask groups of young students some simple questions about their ears, such as, "Where are your ears?" "How many ears do you have?" and "What do you do with your ears?" These questions will alert the students to the part of the body with which you will be working, in addition to providing positive reinforcement at the onset of the hearing screening, as most kindergarteners are eager to inform you of the correct answer. This type of additional training also may be needed for the mentally handicapped.

Immittance Screening

Although a behavioral response is not required to screen middle-ear function using immittance measures, younger students may not be familiar with immittance screening procedures. Introducing and demonstrating the immittance screening equipment and procedure in the classroom prior to screening should help allay any fears.

Time Needed for Screening

A third grader can be screened in less than 1 minute for puretones and within seconds for immittance; however, younger students may require more time (ASHA, 1985). When screening a class of 25 to 30 students using five to six trained hearing screening assistants and, at least, one trained immittance screening assistant, the following schedule is fairly accurate, provided the students understand the instructions: Kindergarten: 15 to 20 minutes; grades 1 and 2: 10 to 15 minutes; grades 3 and up: 8 to 10 minutes.

Knowledge of such time limits is essential when developing a screening schedule for an entire school. Using these time limits, approximately 600 children can be screened in a standard school day using five to six trained screening assistants.

Puretone and Immittance Screening Forms and Letters

Hearing and immittance screening records should be included in the students' permanent school records. Many schools include the screening results of each student on the student's health record. An alternative method is a cumulative puretone and immittance screening form for each student screened (Fig. 31.1). This form should include identifying information and

be designed to accommodate both the date and screening results for each occasion the child's hearing or middle ear is screened. Color coding and/or printing the form on 90-lb index paper allows for easy identification of the form in the students' cumulative record.

A second form that is useful in the hearing screening process is a teacher instruction and absentee form that provides each teacher, whose class is to be screened, with instructions for completing the identification portion of the cumulative audiologic record and teacher responsibilities on the screening day. The absentee section on this form is completed by the teacher on the day of the screening and returned to the screening supervisor.

Another form necessary to expedite the screening follow-up process is the rescreening list. All students who were referred for follow-up screening as determined by the results of the initial hearing or middle-ear screening or who have a cold or known middle-ear disorder are listed on this form.

A student referral list is a necessary form for hearing and middle-ear screening. All students not passing the rescreening(s) are listed on this form. These students are referred to an audiologist and/or physician for evaluation.

A hearing and middle-ear screening results sheet is completed by a screening assistant at the end of the screening day. This form provides each teacher with instructions on sending letters to parents regarding the outcome of the hearing and middle-ear screening and appropriate recommendations. This form also lists the names of (a) students who need to return for rescreening, (b) referrals for evaluation, and (c) students who were absent on the day of the screening.

Each parent whose child was screened should receive a letter informing them of their child's hearing and middle-ear screening results. This letter also should include the child's name and screening date. The letter to parents of children who passed the hearing and middle-ear screening should inform the parents of the purpose and results of the screening and an invitation for questions or concerns they may have regarding the hearing and middle-ear screening procedure (see Fig. 31.2). The letter to parents of children whose hearing or middle-ear function is in question should inform the parents of the need for good hearing and the purpose of the hearing and middle-ear screening program. In addition, the letter should, without implying failure (Anderson, 1978; ASHA, 1985), inform the parents that their child may need additional testing and include information on whom to contact for this additional testing (see Figs. 31.3–31.5). The letters to parents are given to the

CUMULATIVE AUDIOLOGICAL RECORD

Name: _____

Birthdate: _____

Schools: _____

_____

Parents: _____

Address: _____

_____

Phone: (H) (____) _____ (W) (____) _____

Date	Tchr Grade		1000 20dB	2000 20dB	4000 20dB	1000 20dB	Opt. 500 20dB	Pass	Refer	Pass	Recheck	Refer	Comments	Audiological Evaluation
		Pure Tone Screening								Immittance				
		R												
		L												
		R												
		L												
		R												
		L												
		R												
		L												
		R												
		L												
		R												
		L												
		R												
		L												
		R												
		L												
		R												
		L												
		R												
		L												
		R												
		L												
		R												
		L												

Figure 31.1. Form for hearing and immittance screening record.

NAME OF PROGRAM

Date: _____

Student's Name: _____

Dear Parent(s) or Guardian:

Hearing is very important to your child's ability to listen, to learn and to progress satisfactorily in school. For this reason, your school takes a special interest in the hearing ability of all students and periodically checks their hearing.

Your child has been given a routine hearing screening in school. This screening also includes a check for possible ear problems in children in grades K, 1, 2, 3 and special students. *We are happy to inform you that your child passed the screening.* Hearing may change at any time; therefore, please contact your child's school, at any time, if you suspect that your child is having difficulty hearing.

If you have any questions regarding your child's hearing screening results or about the Hearing Screening Program, please contact your child's school.

Figure 31.2 Letter to the parents of children who pass the hearing and middle-ear screening.

teachers to be distributed to the students at the end of the school day. Letters given to the students before the end of the school day run the risk of being lost or misplaced.

All paperwork associated with the hearing and middle-ear screening program is handled by screening assistants trained specifically for this task. This relieves the teacher of extra work with the exception of completing the identifying information on the cumulative audiologic record.

If a child referred for an audiologic evaluation has not received an evaluation or an appointment for the evaluation within 2 to 4 weeks after the initial referral letter was sent, a second letter is then sent home to the parents. Should the second letter produce no response within 4 weeks, a third notice is then mailed to the parents. Parents who fail to respond to the third letter may then be contacted by a designated representative of the child's school to obtain the necessary parental permission for evaluation, transportation, and release of information for further evaluation. The school rep-

NAME OF PROGRAM

Date:_____

Student's Name:_____

Dear Parent(s) or Guardian:

Hearing is very important to your child's ability to listen, to learn and to progress satisfactorily in school. For this reason, your school takes a special interest in the hearing ability of all students and periodically checks their hearing.

Your child has been given a routine hearing screening in school. This screening also includes screening for possible ear problems in children in grades K, 1, 2, 3 and all special students. *Although your child passed the hearing screening, our results show that your child may need medical attention with regard to his/her ears. It is recommended that your child be seen by a pediatrician, otolaryngologist (ear, nose and throat physician) or your family physician.* Most of the time ear problems in children can be helped with medical attention.

Below are the results of the screen tests for you to give to the physician. These results will aid in determining the course of treatment, if needed, for your child. If you have any questions regarding your child's screening test results or recommendations, please feel free to contact:

_____

SCREENING RESULTS

HEARING					MIDDLE EAR		
SCREENING LEVEL: 20 dB HL					SCREENING MEASURES**		
E A R	FREQUENCY (Hz)				PEAK Y (mmhos)	V_{EC} (daPa)	TW* (daPa)
	500*	1000	2000	4000			
R							
L							
IMPRESSIONS:							

**Peak Y = compensated static admittance; V_{EC} = equivalent ear canal volume; TW = tympanogram width
*optional

PLEASE INFORM YOUR CHILD'S SCHOOL OF THE DOCTOR'S RESULTS

Figure 31.3. Letter to parents of children who pass the hearing screening and have questionable results on the middle-ear screening

resentative can then schedule the evaluation and arrange transportation for the child.

SUGGESTED SCREENING PROGRAM FOR SCHOOL-AGE CHILDREN

A combined screening protocol has been recommended by several authors (McKenzie et al., 1982; FitzZaland and Zink, 1984; Brooks, 1985; Margolis and Heller, 1987; Bonny, 1989; and ASHA, 1979, 1985, 1990). The following is an outline of a sug-

NAME OF PROGRAM

Date:_____

Student's Name:_____

Dear Parent(s) or Guardian:

Good hearing is very important to your child's ability to listen, to learn and to progress satisfactorily in school. For this reason, your school takes a special interest in the hearing ability of all students and periodically checks their hearing.

Your child has been given a routine hearing screening in school. This screening also includes screening for possible ear problems in children in grades K, 1, 2, 3 and all special students. *The hearing screening results show that your child may have some difficulty in hearing. Although the screening test is not a conclusive hearing evaluation, it is recommended that your child receive a complete audiologic (hearing) evaluation.* This evaluation will determine the exact extent of your child's hearing difficulty, if any.

Most hearing difficulties found in children are not permanent and many times can be corrected. However, a hearing loss can affect your child's educational progress. By receiving a hearing evaluation, the extent and type of hearing difficulty can be assessed and recommendations made.

In order to schedule this evaluation for your child, please contact:

_____

_____

_____

Figure 31.4. Letter to parents of children whose hearing is in question.

gested screening program for school-age children. This program uses a combined hearing and immittance screening method, as recommended by ASHA (1990). This suggested program incorporates the ASHA (1985) protocol for hearing screening and the ASHA (1990) protocol for immittance screening. School systems vary in their organization and size; therefore, this program is presented as a guide for implementing a screening program and modifications should be considered for different populations and situations.

I. System-wide organization
  A. Selling the hearing and middle-ear screening program via in-service workshops
    1. System-wide administrative staff
    2. Principals
    3. Teachers
  B. System-wide screening schedule
    1. Preliminary screening schedules
      a. Screen one school per week
      b. Take into account pupil holidays and teacher workdays
    2. Confirm screening date with each principal
    3. Once confirmation is obtained, issue a system-wide screening schedule to each principal

NAME OF PROGRAM

Date:_____

Student's Name:_____

Dear Parent(s) or Guardian:

Hearing is very important to your child's ability to listen, to learn and to progress satisfactorily in school. For this reason, your school takes a special interest in the hearing ability of all students and periodically checks their hearing.

Your child has been given a routine hearing screening in school. This screening also includes screening for possible ear problems in children in grades K, 1, 2, 3 and all special students. *Our screening results show that your child may have some difficulty in hearing and may need medical attention with regard to his/her ears. Although the screening test is not a conclusive hearing evaluation, it is recommended that your child be seen by:*

1. a pediatrician, otolaryngologist (ear, nose and throat physican) or your family physician.

2. an audiologist for a complete audiological (hearing) evaluation.

Below are the results of the screening tests for you to give to the physician. These results will help determine the course of treatment, if needed, for your child. Most of the time ear problems in children can be helped with medical attention. In order to schedule the hearing evaluation for your child, please contact:

SCREENING RESULTS

HEARING					MIDDLE EAR		
SCREENING LEVEL: 20 dB HL					SCREENING MEASURES**		
E A R	FREQUENCY (Hz)				PEAK Y (mmhos)	V_EC (daPa)	TW* (daPa)
	500*	1000	2000	4000			
R							
L							
IMPRESSIONS:							

**Peak Y = compensated static admittance; V_{EC} = equivalent ear canal volume; TW = tympanogram width
*optional

PLEASE INFORM YOUR CHILD'S SCHOOL OF THE DOCTOR'S RESULTS

Figure 31.5. Letter to parents of children who have questionable hearing and middle-ear screening results

C. Recruit contact person in each school
   1. Speech/language pathologist in the elementary school
   2. Guidance counselor or speech/language pathologist in the middle and high schools
D. Prepare forms
   1. Individual cumulative audiologic record form
   2. Teacher instruction and absentee form
   3. Second screening form
   4. Referral list form

5. Letters to parents
   a. Passing form letters
   b. Referral form letters
6. Hearing screening results form for teachers
II. Individual school organization
   A. Reconfirm screening date with principal at least 1 month prior to screening date
   B. Meet with and discuss duties of the contact person at each school
      1. Scheduling classes for screening
         a. Screen grades kindergarten, 1, 2, 3, for pure-tones and immittance
         b. Screen all high risk students, teacher referrals and all students in special education for pure-tones and immittance
         c. Kindergarten: 15 to 20 min/class (best if screened early in the day)
         d. First and second grades: 10 to 15 min/class
         e. Third grade and up: 8 to 10 min/class
         f. Consideration of recess and lunch periods
      2. Recruiting screening assistants
         a. Five or six for actual screening
         b. Minimum of two for paperwork
   C. Training workshops for screening assistants
      1. Assistants from several schools can attend one workshop
      2. Lecture (see "Personnel and Training")
      3. Practicum
         a. Orientation to equipment
         b. Provide copy of screening instructions for each assistant
         c. Require a minimum of 10 practice screenings
   D. Location of screening site
      1. Joint effort of audiologist, contact person, and principal
      2. Carpeted area away from main traffic flow, restrooms, and cafeteria
      3. Record ambient noise levels, if possible, or check a group of normals
      4. Ample space and electrical outlets (if needed) for five to six screening locations
   E. Distribution of forms and schedules
      1. Two weeks before scheduled screening date
      2. All teachers whose classes are to be screened
      3. All teachers who are referring students
III. Screening day
   A. Biologic calibration of screening equipment
   B. Training of kindergarten students
   C. Screen classes according to schedule
   D. Screening assistants obtain list of absentees from teacher
   E. Each student gives screener his/her cumulative audiologic record form for recording results
   F. Screening procedure
      1. History: otalgia (ear pain) or otorrhea (ear discharge)
         a. Parent questionnaire
         b. Ask student

2. Visual inspection of the ear
  a. Structural defects of the ear, head and neck
  b. Ear canal abnormalities
  c. Eardrum abnormalities (optional): otoscopy should be performed by an individual with training and experience in this procedure.
3. Puretone
  a. Frequency (Hz): 500 (optional), 1000, 2000, and 4000
  b. Intensity level: 20 dB
4. Immittance
  a. Compensated static acoustic admittance
  b. Equivalent ear canal volume
  c. Tympanogram width

G. Referral criteria
1. Reports of otalgia or otorrhea: immediate medical referral
2. Visual inspection: medical referral
  a. Structural anomalies of the ear, head and neck
  b. Ear-canal abnormalities
  c. Eardrum abnormalities
3. Puretone
  a. no response at one or more frequencies regardless of ear
  b. If student has no cold or known middle ear pathology, send to another screener for rescreening
  c. Colds or known middle ear pathologies are noted on the Cumulative Audiologic Record and the student should be rescreened in 2 to 4 weeks
  d. No response to one or more frequencies on two consecutive screenings–audiologic referral
4. Immittance
  a. Initial Screen
    (1) Pass: normal acoustic immittance measures
    (2) Abnormally low compensated static acoustic immittance and large ear canal volume: medical referral
    (3) Abnormally low compensated static acoustic immittance: rescreen in 4 to 6 weeks
  b. Rescreening results
    (1) Abnormally low compensated static acoustic immittance: medical referral
    (2) Pass immittance measures: monitor
5. Combination puretone and immittance criteria for referral
  a. Passes puretone and continues to obtain abnormal results on immittance rescreen: direct medical referral (see Fig. 31.3)
  b. No response to one or more frequencies on the puretone rescreening and passes immittance screen: refer for audiologic evaluation (see Fig. 31.4)
  c. Abnormal puretone and immittance screening results: refer for audiologic and medical evaluation (see Fig. 31.5)

  d. Possible third screen based on the discretion of the audiologist
  e. A flow chart showing the steps in puretone and immittance screening is found in Figure 31.6.

H. Completion and routing of forms
1. After being screened, each student gives her or his cumulative audiologic record to the assistant doing the paperwork
2. At the end of the day, teachers are given a completed Hearing Screening Result form, the letters to parents for each student screened and the cumulative audiologic record for each student who passed the screening
3. The referral list and cumulative audiologic records of the students being referred for audiologic evaluation are sent to the audiologist within the school system. If the system does not provide audiologic services to students, all forms are returned to the student's cumulative school record and any further information regarding the student's hearing should be noted on the cumulative audiologic record. *Follow-up is important!*
4. The rescreening list and cumulative audiologic records for students to be rescreened are kept by the contact person until each student has been rescreened.
  a. If the student passes the rescreening, the cumulative audiologic record is returned to the student's cumulative school record and the appropriate letter is sent to the parent(s)
  b. If the student does not pass the rescreening, the cumulative audiologic record is sent to the audiologist within the system and the appropriate letter is sent to the parent(s)

SUMMARY

Hearing screening of school-age children is justified on the basis of prevalence of hearing loss in school-age children, educational handicaps resulting from hearing loss, and the prognosis of rehabilitation with respect to early intervention.

The primary purpose of hearing screening is the identification of hearing impairment; however, additional benefits are obtained by screening school-age children. These benefits include increased awareness of hearing and hearing loss by school staff, as well as, according to Northern and Downs (1974), the maintenance of good hearing, prevention of handicapping losses and needed habilitation for children with permanent losses.

Various methods of hearing screening are available for school-age children, such as group and individual as well as speech and puretone. Presently, the puretone individual screening method is the standard pro-

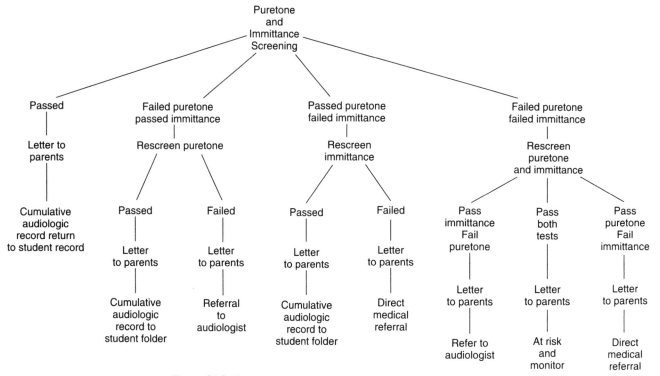

Figure 31.6. Puretone and immittance screening—flow chart.

cedure for screening the hearing of school-age children.

Procedures for puretone screening vary in the literature, but the test frequencies should include 1000, 2000, and 4000 Hz at a minimum. The intensity level for screening at these frequencies should not exceed 20 dBHL. Ambient noise levels should be determined, if possible, when deciding on a screening location. If not, testing a group of normal hearing individuals would aid in determining if ambient noise levels were too high for that particular screening location.

The use of immittance screening in conjunction with puretone screening is recommended because puretone screening may be ineffective in identifying children with middle ear disease. Benefits of immittance screening include: (*a*) identification of children with middle ear disease, (*b*) ambient noise is not a factor in obtaining reliable and valid results, (*c*) test procedures are rapid, (*d*) test results are objective, (*e*) testing is minimally limited by age, and (*f*) testing can be done with difficult-to-test students.

Immittance screening should include protocols and measures with high sensitivity and specificity to increase correct identifications and to reduce overreferrals. Controversies regarding these issues may be reduced by using serial tympanometry and/or immittance rescreenings.

Other considerations when screening hearing and

middle ear function in school-age children include screening protocol, test measures, referral criteria, population to be screened, personnel and training, equipment and calibration, screening site, instructions to students, time needed for screening, screening forms and letters.

A combined screening program for hearing and middle ear disease in school-age children is recommended. Continued evaluation and documentation of the sensitivity and specificity of puretone and, in particular, immittance screening measures is important. Individuals administering hearing and middle-ear screening programs are in an optimal position for ascertaining this information and are encouraged to do so.

A suggested program using a combined method has been outlined. Concerns regarding the need for serial tympanometry to identify children with chronic or recurrent middle-ear effusion, overreferrals and the lack of clinical data supporting the use of tympanogram width as a immittance screening measure should be considered when developing any screening program.

Administratively, differences in the organization and size of school systems, as well as availability of referral sources also should be considered. Modifications in administration, procedure, and screening protocol should be made as needed to adapt to specific conditions, situations, and future research findings.

REFERENCES

American National Standards Institute. Specifications for audiometers, ANSI S3.6-1969. New York, 1989.

American National Standards Institute. Specifications for instruments to measure aural acoustic impedance and admittance (aural acoustic immittance). ANSI S3.39-1987. New York, 1988.

American Speech-Language-Hearing Association (ASHA) Committee on Audiometric Evaluation. Guidelines for acoustic immittance screening of middle ear function. Asha 1979;21: 283–288.

American Speech-Language-Hearing Association (ASHA) Executive Board. On the definition of hearing handicap. Asha 1981;23:293–297.

American Speech-Language-Hearing Association (ASHA) Committee on Audiologic Evaluation. Guidelines for identification audiometry. Asha 1985;27:49–52.

American Speech-Language-Hearing Association (ASHA). Guidelines for screening for hearing impairment and middle-ear disorders. Asha 1990;(Suppl. 2)32:17–24.

Anderson CV. Hearing screening for children. In Katz J, Ed. Handbook of Clinical Audiology, 2nd Ed. Baltimore: Williams & Wilkins, 1978:48–60.

Aniansson G. Screening diagnosis of secretory otitis media. Scand Audiol 1986;(Suppl)24:65–69.

Authur D, and Sherwood S. Effectiveness of a teacher referral system in hearing screening programs. Hear Aid J 1980;33:40–41.

Bess FH. Impedance screening for children. A need for more research. Ann Otol Rhinol Laryngol 1980;(Suppl 68)89:228–232.

Bess FH, Bluestone CD, Harrington DA, Klein JO, and Harford ER. Use of acoustic impedance measurement in screening for middle ear disease in children. Ann Otol Rhinol Laryngol 1978;87:288–292.

Bluestone CD, Fria TJ, Arjona SK, Casselbrant ML, Schwartz DM, Ruben RJ, Gates GA, Downs MP, Northern JL, Jerger JF, Paradise JL, Bess FH, Kenworthy OT, and Rogers KD. Controversies in screening for middle ear disease and hearing loss in children. Pediatrics 1986;77:57–70.

Bonny IC. Five years' experience of combined impedance and audiometric screening at school entry. Public Health 1989;103: 427–431.

Brooks DN. Hearing screening—a comparative study of an impedance method and puretone screening. Scand Audiol 1973;2: 67–72.

Brooks D. School screening for middle ear effusions. Anal Otol Rhinol Laryngol 1976;(Suppl 2)85:223–228.

Brooks DN. Acoustic impedance measurement as a screening procedure in children: Discussion paper. J R Soc Med 1985;78: 119–121.

Cadman D, Chambers L, Feldman W, Sackett D. Assessing the effectiveness of community screening procedures. JAMA 1984; 251:1580–1585.

Committee on School Health. Impedance bridge (tympanometer) as a screening device in schools. Pediatrics 1987;79:472.

Cross AW. Health screening in schools. Part I. J Pediat 1985; 107:487–494.

Darley FL, Ed. Identification audiometry. J Speech Hear Disord Monogr 1961;(Suppl 9).

Downs MP. Auditory screening. Otolaryngol Clin North Am 1978;11:611–629.

Eagles EL, Wishik SM, Doerfler LG, Melnick W, and Levine HS. Hearing sensitivity and related factors in children. Laryngoscope 1973;(Monogr Suppl):73.

FitzZaland RE, and Zink GD. A comarative study of hearing screening procedures. Ear Hearing 1984;5:205–210.

Gimsing S, and Bergholtz LM. Audiological screening of school children—preliminary results. Scand Audiol (Suppl)1983;17: 65–67.

Hallett CP. The screening and epidemiology of middle-ear disease in a population of primary school entrants. J Laryngol Otol 1982;96:899–914.

Harker L, and Van Wagoner R. Application of impedance audiometry as a screening instrument. Acta Otolaryngol (Stockh) 1974;77:198–201.

House HP, and Glorig A. A new concept of auditory screening. Laryngoscope 1957;67:661–668.

Katt D, and Sprague H. Determining the puretone frequencies to be used in identification audiometry. J Speech Hear Disord 1981;46:433–436.

Lescouflair G. Critical view on audiometric screening in school. Arch Otolaryngol 1975;101:469–473.

Leske MC. Prevalence estimates of communicative disorders in the U.S.: Language, hearing, and vestibular disorders. Asha 1981;23:229–237.

Lewis H, Dugdale A, Canty A, and Jerger J. Open-ended tympanometric screening: a new concept. Arch Otolaryngol 1975;101:722–725.

Lidén G, and Renvall U. Impedance and tone screening of school children. Scand Audiol 1980;9:121–126.

Lous J. Screening for secretory otitis media: evaluation of some impedance screening programs for long-lasting secretory otitis media in 7-year-old children. Int J Pediat Otorhinolaryngol 1987;13:85–97.

Lucker JR. Application of pass-fail criteria to middle ear screening results. Asha 1980;22:839–840.

Margolis RH, and Heller JW. Screening tympanometry: criteria for medical referral. Audiology 1987;26:197–208.

McCandless GA, and Thomas GK. Impedance audiometry as a screening procedure for middle ear disease. Trans Am Acad Ophthalmol Otolaryngol 1974;78:98–102.

McKenzie E, Magian V, Stokes R. A study of the recommended pass/fail criteria for impedance audiometry in a school screening program. J Otolaryngol 1982;11:40–45.

Melnick W, Eagles EL, and Levine HS. Evaluation of a recommended program of identification audiometry with school age children. J Speech Hear Disord 1964;29:3–13.

Newby HA. Public school hearing conservation programs. In Audiology, 4th Ed. Englewood Cliffs, NJ: Prentice-Hall, 1979: 292–320.

North Carolina Department of Public Instruction, Division for Exceptional Children. Hearing Conservation Guide. Raleigh, 1983.

Northern JL. Impedance screening-an integral part of hearing screening. Ann Otol Rhinol Laryngol 1980;(Suppl 68)89: 233–235.

Northern JL, and Downs MP. Identification audiometry. In Hearing in Children. Baltimore: Williams & Wilkins, 1974: 93–133.

Reger SN, and Newby HA. A group puretone hearing test. J Speech Hear Disord 1947;12:61–66.

Renvall U, and Lidén G. Screening procedure for detection of middle ear and cochlear disease. Ann Otol Rhinol Laryngol 1980;(Suppl 68)89:214–216.

Roberts M. Comparative study of puretone, impedance and otoscopic hearing screening methods. Arch Otolaryngol 1976;102: 690–694.

Ross M, and Giolas TG. Introduction. In Ross M, and Giolas TG, Eds. Auditory Management of Hearing Impaired Children. Baltimore: University Park Press, 1978:1–13.

CHAPTER 32

Auditory Processing Disorders

Jack Katz and Lorin Wilde

An important and yet somewhat controversial aspect of audiology is the area of auditory processing (AP). Despite the heavy demand for services, some audiologists feel uncomfortable in evaluating, interpreting and remediating this problem. Among other concerns, audiologists often mention the lack of coursework and knowledge about AP as factors limiting their participation. It is therefore the purpose of this chapter to help fill this gap. Among other aspects it will include suggested approaches which we feel will make the work more relevant and important both to those who have AP dysfunctions and to the audiologists who provide the services.

WHAT IS AP AND WHAT IS AN AP DISORDER?

Generally speaking, AP is "what we do with what we hear." This implies that AP is the building that we do upon the auditory signal to make the information functionally useful. AP involves not simply the perception of sounds but more importantly how we clarify, locate, attend, analyze, store and retrieve the information. It deals with how we apply our knowledge to better understand the message and how we integrate and associate auditory information with visual and other sensory inputs.

Schoeny and Hasenstab (1983) enumerated auditory skills that the listener requires in order to maintain normal conversational abilities. They include 1) auditory sensitivity, 2) auditory localization, 3) sensory differentiation/auditory awareness, 4) responsiveness to sound, 5) auditory discrimination, 6) attention and vigilance, as well as 7) auditory synthesis and generalization.

An AP deficit is present when the individual is not able to make full use of the heard signal. It becomes a significant problem when the person is not able to reach full potential because of these AP deficiencies. AP skills may be viewed on a continuum from good to poor and an AP problem cannot be ruled out simply because there is an additional handicap such as hearing impairment. An AP deficit is not dependent upon a person's age or intelligence. The presence of mental retardation or other cognitive impairments does not preclude a potential AP problem. The question is whether AP skills are significantly depressed and whether they significantly restrict the individual.

WHAT AREAS OF DIFFICULTY ARE ASSOCIATED WITH AP DYSFUNCTION?

For many years AP has been associated with learning disabilities (LD), especially reading problems (Monroe, 1932; Orton, 1964; Sawyer, 1981). Difficulty with phonics and limitations in reading comprehension are both associated with AP dysfunction (Boder, 1973; Fried et al., 1981; Kavale, 1981; Shankweiler and Liberman, 1989). In addition, spelling (Bannatyne and Wichiarajote, 1969) and foreign language skills (Sparks et al., 1991) are often depressed in those with AP disorders.

Those with poor communicative skills are also considered at risk for AP difficulties. These limitations include, but are not limited to, articulation problems (Mange, 1960; Stovall et al., 1977), especially in younger children, as well as both receptive and expressive language disorders (Tallal, 1976; Burns and Canter, 1977; Lubert, 1981; Lasky and Cox, 1983; Young, 1983; Sloan, 1986). Other areas of interest relate AP to behavioral, emotional and other problems. Research has been directed toward AP dysfunction associated with schizophrenia (Yozawitz et al., 1979), Attention Deficit Disorder (ADD) (Ludlow et al., 1983; Keller, 1992), prison populations (Katz, Singer and Fanning, 1988) and those with Alzheimer's disease (Grimes et al., 1985).

Audiologists are often concerned that the AP problems they see might actually be the ramification of a more general disorder. For example, if a child has problems associated with an ADD, do the poor scores on audiologic tests simply reflect poor attention and motivation? If memory difficulties are demonstrated in both the auditory and visual domains, does this represent a generalized memory problem, and not simply an auditory problem?

It is not surprising that a variety of other problems also may be present when central auditory dysfunction exists. It is our feeling, however, that auditory skills generally do not improve unless they are specifically addressed. For example, while we have observed better behavioral controls in hyperactive children who are on medication such as Ritalin, the auditory skills measured by most of our tests are unaffected.

INFLUENCES

Heredity

Because AP is not a single entity and is associated with the many problems discussed above, it is not surprising that AP difficulties might result from a variety of etiological factors. Some major considerations are mentioned below. Of the factors associated with AP dysfunction, probably the most potent is familial characteristics. In children with AP dysfunction, it is common to find one of the parents to have had similar difficulties in their youth. This is generally assumed to be due to genetic factors (Kinsbourne, 1983; Willeford and Burleigh, 1985). In a sophisticated statistical analysis of identical and fraternal twins, LaBuda and DeFries (1988) found 40% of observed reading disability to be associated with genetic factors and 35% with environmental factors.

One factor that is closely associated with genetic influences is CNS organization. Hier et al. (1978) found gross differences in the CT brain scans of children with developmental dyslexia compared to a control population. This was most notable in the receptive language region of the left hemisphere and in the right visual-spatial region.

In addition, microscopic variations in brain structures have been shown. Kemper (1984) found abnormal development (verrucous dysplasia) in regions of the left hemispheres in the brains of two out of three dyslexic individuals. This abnormality is associated with improper neuronal migration during fetal development.

Gender Differences

Another observation is that AP problems, as is the case with LD, are more prevalent in males than females (DeFries et al., 1990). Geschwind and Behan (1982) proposed a testosterone hypothesis to explain the high incidence of males with developmental problems that might be associated with a smaller corpus callosum. The corpus callosum, which is associated with reading and spelling ability, is noticeably different in males and females. The splenium (i.e., posterior portion), that carries auditory and visual transmission between the hemispheres, was found to be generally larger and more bulbous in females (DeLacoste-Utamsingh and Holloway, 1982; Witelson, 1989). Therefore, females may be able to integrate auditory and visual information from the two hemispheres more effectively than males.

Familial Handedness

There has been a long-standing observation that reading and other cognitive disabilities are more common in left handers. For example, learning disabilities have been noted to be ten times more common in left handers than right handers. (Geschwind and Behan, 1982).

Kraft (1984) emphasized the importance of evaluating family history of handedness, as well as degree of assessed hand preference, when exploring brain organization and language specialization of the left hemisphere. A familial history of left-handedness has been associated with a lower than expected right- ear advantage for dichotic verbal stimuli.

Peripheral Hearing Loss

By definition, hearing loss cannot be the primary factor in a learning disability. However, major auditory processing and learning problems can be found in children with peripheral hearing losses. In these cases, it is necessary to evaluate if the clients perform at levels commensurate with their hearing and intelligence. It is very easy to overlook concomitant AP factors when an individual has a significant hearing loss. In fact, cochlear damage itself may have an adverse influence on the CNS (Salvi et al., 1992).

Otitis Media

One of the characteristics that is most closely associated with LD and AP dysfunction is a history of otitis media during early life. The first year-and- one-half is considered by many to be the most critical period (Northern and Downs, 1991). The number of bouts, their duration and age of onset are considered important factors (Teele et al., 1984).

The germinal article relating early otitis media to communicative problems was Holm and Kunze (1969). In a well controlled study they found auditory skills to be significantly depressed in those with histories of middle ear pathology compared to the control group. In contrast, performance on visual and other cognitive tasks generally were not significantly different for the two groups. Prospective studies have confirmed the findings of Holm and Kunze and provided further detail (Teele et al., 1990; Friel-Patti and Finitzo, 1990).

Socioeconomic Status

A variety of reasons may account for the finding of poorer AP skills in those of lower socioeconomic status (SES) (Menyuk, 1986). Although it is not clear if heredity, nutrition, incidence or treatment of middle ear problems, lack of stimulation, or some other factor is the major cause of this finding, the fact that there is such a discrepancy between SES groups complicates the evaluation, interpretation and management when poor performance is seen.

ASSESSMENT

Audiologists play an important role in the evaluation of AP functions. Although audiologic tests can assess the performance of the auditory system from the outer ear to the cortex, it is more useful to the client when they are viewed from the standpoint of management of the disability rather than simply site-of-dysfunction.

Behavioral AP tests challange the auditory system by providing difficult listening tasks for the individual in a carefully controlled environment (Willeford, 1977). They not only help to identify those who have impaired AP skills but also can indicate in what ways the person differs from the average listener of the same age. Because the limitations and strengths of those with AP problems may vary considerably, it is important to assess a variety of auditory functions. The pattern of impairment may then be examined to suggest appropriate management approaches.

Presently many central auditory tests are available to the audiologist; however, there are practical constraints (e.g., expense, the subject's attention span) that limit the number of tests that may be used with any individual client (Spitzer, 1983). Therefore, it is necessary to develop a strategy that provides both breadth of functions and sufficient depth as a check on reliability.

Behavioral Testing

The initial concern is to differentiate problems primarily associated with the peripheral system from those generally associated with CNS. Hypothesis forming begins with the case history. Willeford and Burleigh (1985) provide case history forms that help the audiologist obtain a base of information dealing with hearing and AP concerns.

Peripheral Evaluation

Evaluation for AP problems should begin with the basic audiometric battery to rule out peripheral hearing loss as either the primary or a contributing factor. This is important because 1) learning problems can be produced by peripheral hearing loss alone, 2) hearing threshold information is needed for the central battery because most tests require sensation level settings, and 3) central test results may be ambiguous in the presence of a hearing loss.

The basic battery should include puretone

threshold tests (air conduction and possibly bone conduction), word recognition (in quiet) and immittance (tympanometry and acoustic reflex) measurements. A puretone hearing screening (e.g., at 20–25 dB re: ANSI-1969) alone, or even in conjunction with tympanometry is inadequate.

Central Auditory Evaluation

The behavioral test battery that is used varies considerably depending on the goals and orientations of the audiologist. Those who attempt to play an active role in the management process will probably choose a somewhat different set of tests than those who focus on the assessment of weaknesses at various levels of the auditory system. At present there are more central evaluation procedures in use than there are tests to differentiate cochlear from retrocochlear pathology. Perhaps this is as it should be, because there are many more areas and functions to assess in the central system compared to the peripheral system.

Detailed information regarding many of the tests that are currently used in the evaluation of AP dysfunction are described in Section III of this text. For example, Masking Level Difference (MLD) is discussed in chapter 15, speech-in-noise tests and dichotic digits in chapter 16, Binaural Fusion and the SSW test in chapter 17, and the Competing Sentence Test and Preschool Sentence Identification (PSI) test in chapter 18. Also, Stecker (1992) provides a comprehensive account of the most widely used and studied AP procedures.

Age is an important factor when choosing and analyzing behavioral tests of central function. Some generalizations can be made regarding test performance as a function of age. Normal performance on most AP tests improves with age from young childhood to the pre-teen years. From then on through the middle adult years there is generally little variation in normal performance. While individual differences are noted in older age groups, group performance begins to deteriorate by the 60s. Major signs of central auditory dysfunction are typical for 70-year-olds. One can assume severely depressed performance on AP tests for individuals 80 years of age and older.

For monotic tests considerable variability generally exists at each age level. Therefore, scores should be considered abnormal only if markedly depressed in one or both ears, or if considerable asymmetry is noted between the ears. A right-ear-advantage for speech is not necessarily expected in the monotic presentation mode.

Dichotic speech test results show a maturational effect with increasing age, and reflect varying performance relationships between the ears, even in normal groups. In the preschool years normal children generally have similar scores in each ear. The most rapid improvement in the early school years is seen in right-ear performance. By 10 or 11 years, on many tests, left ear scores gradually approach the performance of the right. This variation in the left ear may be associated, at least in part, with maturation of the corpus callosum or other commissural pathways. On dichotic tests the major abnormality in children with learning disabilities is usually seen in the left ear. These and other signs will be discussed in the section on categorization of AP dysfunction.

Physiological Testing

Physiologic tests provide a vehicle for observing central auditory nervous system (CANS) function. Recent advances enable the non-invasive view of previously inaccessible human brain activity. Lauter (in press) provides a comprehensive review of brain-monitoring technology as applied to the study of AP.

This section will briefly overview the procedures that offer the most promise for the study of auditory processing. Acoustic reflex (AR), another physiological procedure, is covered in Chapter 21.

Evoked Potentials

Audiologic use of evoked potentials is generally associated with time-locked responses to auditory stimuli. The most commonly used of these procedures is auditory brainstem response (ABR) (Chapter 24). Because the lower brainstem is associated with binaural functions such as localization of sound and speech-in-noise skills, ABR has promise for the study of AP. However, ABR as it is traditionally used has not provided a clear relationship between neural substrates and AP. Lauter (1992) suggests that using ABR to assess variability for repeated EP rather than the traditional absolute latencies. This measure can demonstrate marked ear asymmetries that match dichotic test results.

Although relatively little information is now available, middle and long latency responses are more likely to provide insights into cerebral AP dysfunction (see Chapters 26 and 27). The later responses include both stimulus-related exogenous potentials and event-related endogenous potentials. Endogenous potentials are generated when the listener is actively involved in a cognitive decision about the stimuli. Therefore, it reflects higher level functions (Musiek and Bornstein, 1992).

The P300 potential may be useful in correlating psychoacoustic and electrophysiologic measures of selective auditory attention (Musiek, 1986a). The P300 (the "expectancy" wave) generally appears in response to a novel stimulus embedded in a train of frequently occurring stimuli. This "oddball" paradigm obviously involves memory and can be designed in several ways. Musiek and Bornstein (1992) caution that the relationship between P300 and auditory behaviors needs further investigation. Because endogenous responses are not modality specific, they suggest that comparisons can be made using different modalities to determine a specific AP problem from a more general attention deficit disorder.

Jirsa and Clontz (1990) investigated whether long latency components could be used to differentiate children identified as having AP disorders on behavioral tests from a matched control group. Their electrophysiologic measures were amplitude and latency of the most prominent negative and positive peaks, N_1 and P_2, and P300. The central test battery consisted of the Selective Auditory Attention Test (SAAT), the Pitch Pattern Sequence test and the Competing Sentence test of the Willeford battery. While there was no clear relationship between electrophysiological and behavioral findings, significant latency differences between the experimental and control groups were found. Fourteen of the eighteen subjects in the disordered group, but no controls, had abnormally delayed latencies for P300.

Another approach that has considerable promise is otoacoustic emissions (OAE). OAE are thought to be related to the mechanical activity of outer hair cells in response to stimulation by the descending olivocochlear bundle (OCB) (Chapter 28). Pickles (1988) indicates the functional significance of the OCB to be 1) improving the detection of signals in noise, 2) protecting the cochlea from noise damage, 3) controlling the mechanical state of the cochlea, and 4) playing a role in attention. It appears likely that efferent pathways participate in the auditory analysis of complex signals (Musiek, 1986b).

Imaging Techniques

New approaches are available to carefully define structure and function of the CNS. Presently, few audiologists are utilizing these techniques, however, it is likely that they will play a greater role in the future. Several promising techniques are described below.

Quantitative Electroencephalography (qEEG)

This approach offers a method for quantifying the traditionally qualitative aspects of electroencephalography. Using this methodology topographical maps can be made of brain activity. The promise of this computer-based technique is in the study of cerebral function under both resting and active states (Lauter, 1992a). Contributions from qEEG, under the name of brain electrical activity mapping (BEAM), has been reported to be useful in the diagnosis of dyslexia (Duffy et al., 1980).

Magnetoencephalography. Electrical activity of the human brain produces a magnetic field outside the head. Because it measures this activity, magnetoencephalography (MEG) can be used to study human auditory information processing in well-controlled tasks such as listening to a novel sound embedded in a standard repetitive signal (Sams and Hari, 1991). The promise for MEG is that it provides excellent localization of active cortical areas because of its sensitivity in both the spatial and temporal domains.

Magnetic Resonance Imaging. Magnetic Resonance Imaging (MRI) provides high-resolution anatomical imaging. When used in conjunction with MEG it can verify location of intracranial currents. For example, comparison can be made of auditory cortex responses to ipsilateral versus contralateral stimulation (Papanicolaou et al., 1990). With respect to speech and hearing, Lauter (in press) indicates that it may be valuable for the identification of individual differences such as hemispheric asymmetry.

Positron Emission Tomography. Positron Emission Tomography (PET) and photon emission computerized tomography (SPECT) are indicators of brain metabolism or blood flow. They involve the use of isotopes, introduced into the subject's cardiovascular system, which limits the types of experiments that are currently possible. However, interesting results have been observed, such as tonotopic organization of the human primary auditory cortex (Lauter, et al., 1985).

In summary, brain monitoring procedures have yielded methods relatively free of social and cultural biases which increase the sophistication of the questions that can be asked. Although audiologists have not traditionally had such tools at their disposal, their availability and acceptance for medical and other purposes is growing. Therefore, audiologists are encouraged to attain multidisciplinary support in applying these technologies to the study of auditory processing.

CATEGORIZATION OF AP DYSFUNCTION

Currently, there is no standard taxonomy for AP disorders. However, it would be advantageous, for both diagnosis and management, to categorize AP problems by test results and symptom clusters. Categories provide an organization for thinking about the area of study and for dealing with it more effectively (Dalby and Gibson, 1981; Fried et al., 1981). Teachers and therapists can devise appropriate strategies based on the type of disorders that exist and make intelligent assumptions about the problems that the client encounters. Parents and clients also benefit because through categorization the problem can be made more understandable. A taxonomy is not static. It encourages refinements and further study.

The categorization system presented here is a summary of the model proposed by Katz and Smith (1991) and Katz (1992). Based on knowledge that was obtained from site-of-lesion research, it provides an anatomical-physiological model for understanding AP without assuming any specific cause.

In this taxonomy the functional analysis of the central auditory system is based on various localizing Staggered Spondaic Word (SSW) test signs. The SSW test was initially devised to study site-of-dysfunction in adults with known brain lesions. A wide variety of indicators were established based on extensive research (Katz, 1968; Arnst and Katz, 1982). The SSW results are especially useful in distinguishing involvement of the auditory reception (AR) centers, in either hemisphere, from other cerebral lesions. Other criteria are used for identifying anterior cerebral lesions as well as involvement of the corpus callosum (Katz and Smith, 1991).

Children labeled LD who demonstrated the same SSW signs as brain-damaged patients were studied to see if there were similar test clusters and similar associated behaviors (e.g., receptive language problems in those with posterior temporal signs). The initial purpose was to determine if the CNS problems that are assumed to underlie the abnormal SSW signs in brain-damaged individuals also might be dysfunctional in those with AP disorders. The test performance for the LD-AP population was quite similar, although less severe, compared to that found in brain-damaged cases. In addition, the associated behaviors appeared consistent with the apparent site-of-dysfunction. This led to further understanding of how each category relates to academic performance and the typical findings on central tests.

AP Categories

It should be noted that the following four categories are not mutually exclusive. Rather, in a study of 120 subjects (6 to 12 years of age) with LD, more than 50% were classified as falling into two or more major AP categories (Katz et al., 1992). In this study two tests of AP, in addition to the SSW, were used. One test was Phonemic Synthesis (PS): simple words are presented one sound at a time and the listener is to say the word that is formed (Katz and Harmon, 1982). This test places heavy emphasis on the ability to decode phonemically, remember the sounds, keep them in order, blend them into a single syllable formulation and, if possible, to relate this to a known word. The other test was Speech-in-Noise (Olsen et al., 1975). In this procedure word recognition scores for Hirsh W-22 recordings are compared for a quiet versus an ipsilateral speech spectrum noise condition (S/N = +10 dB) for each ear. The difference between the quiet and noise condition scores was used as the measure of the subject's ability to block out background noise, with primary consideration given to the poorer ear. All of the symptoms and signs described below are not found in any one child. It is interesting, however, when interpreting test results using the category system, parents often see problem areas, that they associated with other factors, in a new light.

Decoding Category. This AP category includes those who evidence problems processing at the phonemic level. They generally have poor phonic ability and difficulty with both reading and spelling. Often there is history of a speech problem in the early school years with poor articulation of /r/ and other sounds. These children often have receptive language problems, as seen, for example, on the Peabody Picture Vocabulary test.

Table 32.1 shows results obtained for a 9-year-old child on the audiometric battery. These test results are typical of those found in cases with decoding problems.

Tolerance-Fading Memory (TFM) Category. Generally, individuals who are LD and who are classified as TFM demonstrate two important characteristics. In approximately 75% of the cases, there is evidence of both difficulty in blocking out background noise and

poor short term memory. Those who have TFM problems have poor understanding under noisy conditions and often react negatively to the presence of loud sounds. The memory aspect can be demonstrated on digit or sentence recall tasks. When young, these people are often distractable and may be hyperactive (although a significant percentage are hypoactive). The hyperactive ones call attention to themselves in class, especially when there are background noises or other distractions. The academic picture for these youngsters is not as bad as for the decoding group. In "pure" cases, spelling and phonic skills are normal, especially if the child has good visual skills. However, associated difficulties arise in reading comprehension. Problems in both oral and written expression, as well as poor handwriting, are typical.

Table 32.2 shows results obtained on the audiometric battery for a 10-year-old classified as having a TFM problem.

Integration Category

The term "Integration" is used here to refer to the bringing together of modalities, especially auditory-visual, and combining left and right hemisphere functions. Our information about this category and the following one is much more limited than for the two previous categories. Integration problems are primarily associated with Type A patterns on the SSW test. It appears that there is more than one type of Integration subgroup. The most typical and most prominent of these subgroups is called Type 1. Those in this subgroup generally have the most severe learning deficit of any of the AP categories. Often they are labeled "dyslexic" because they have extremely poor reading and spelling skills. The Type 1 cases resemble the De-

Table 32.1

The following results were obtained for a 9-year-old child on the audiometric battery. These test results are typical of those found in cases with Decoding problems. The asterisks (*) show the scores that contributed to the diagnosis of an AP decoding problem.

	Right ear		Left ear	
Puretone Speech Average A/C	10 dB HL		7 dB HL	
Puretone Speech Average B/C	8 dB HL		7 dB HL	
Tympanogram Type	A		A	
Acoustic reflex thresholds	85-100 dB		80-90 dB	
Word recognition score	100 %		96 %	
Word recognition (quiet - noise)	32 %		44 %	
SSW test	*R-NC*	*R-C*	*L-C*	*L-NC*
Corrected-SSW scores	2	20*	21	8*
(Normal limits)	(4)	(9)	(16)	(3)
Response bias	Order effect low/high*; 2 Reversals			
Phonemic Synthesis		14*		
(Normal limits)		(17)		

Table 32.2

The following results were obtained on the audiometric battery for a 10-year-old classified as having a TFM problem. The asterisks (*) show the scores that contributed to the diagnosis of an AP TFM problem.

	Right ear		Left ear	
Puretone Speech Average A/C	8 dB HL		5 dB HL	
Puretone Speech Average B/C	10 dB HL		2 dB HL	
Tympanogram Type	A		A	
Acoustic reflex thresholds	85-90 dB		85-95 dB	
Word recognition score	92 %		100 %	
Word recognition (quiet - noise)	60 %*		34 %	
SSW test	*R-NC*	*R-C*	*L-C*	*L-NC*
Corrected-SSW scores	4	4	25*	–3
(Normal limits)	(3)	(8)	(14)	(3)
Response bias	Order effect low/high*; 5 Reversals			
Phonemic Synthesis		20		
(Normal limits)		(17)		

coding group because of their poor phonic skills and difficulty on tests of phonemic abilities. The Type 2 Integration cases are quite similar to individuals in the TFM group and their academic successes are somewhat greater than the Type 1 cases.

One characteristic that is seen in Integration cases is that they occasionally have extremely long delays in responding. The delays may be so long that the listener or tester might assume that no answer is forthcoming. Table 32.3 shows these results obtained on the audiometric battery for a 14-year-old who was classified as having a Type 1 Integration problem.

Organization Category. Those who fall into this category have great difficulty with organizing and sequencing information. The problems generally overlap with one or more of the other categories; however, it may be found by itself in older children or adults. While some of these individuals learn (or are taught) to organize themselves and to use lists, their work spaces are generally messy (Lucker, 1980) and they may make a somewhat disheveled appearance. Because they must expend a great deal of effort in monitoring themselves to keep things straight, organization group cases fatigue easily when listening. They may take chancy shortcuts to reduce the strain of listening or may become easily frustrated, especially when tired. It is not clear what academic difficulties are found with this category of deficit when seen in isolation; spelling might be one of them, especially reversing the order of letters.

Table 32.4 shows results obtained on the audiometric battery for an 8-year-old who was classified as having an Organization problem.

Table 32.3

The following results were obtained on the audiometric battery for a 14-year-old who was classified as having a Type 1 Integration problem. The asterisks (*) show the scores that contributed to the diagnosis of an AP integration problem.

	Right ear		Left ear	
Puretone Speech Average A/C	0 dB HL		2 dB HL	
Puretone Speech Average B/C	DNT		DNT	
Tympanogram Type	A		A	
Acoustic reflex thresholds	85-90 dB		85-90 dB	
Word recognition score	96 %		96 %	
Word recognition (quiet - noise)	24 %		28 %	
	R-NC	R-C	L-C	L-NC
SSW test				
Corrected-SSW scores	-2	1	11	-4
(Normal limits)	(3)	(3)	(9)	(3)
Response bias		Type A pattern*		
Phonemic Synthesis		10*		
(Normal limits)		(22)		

Table 32.4

The following results were obtained on the audiometric battery for an 8-year-old who was classified as having an Organization problem. The asterisks (*) show the scores that contributed to the diagnosis of an AP Organization problem.

	Right ear		Left ear	
Puretone Speech Average A/C	12 dB HL		12 dB HL	
Puretone Speech Average B/C	8 dB HL		8 dB HL	
Tympanogram Type	A$_s$		A$_s$	
Acoustic reflex thresholds	90-105 dB		85-105 dB	
Word recognition score	92 %		88 %	
Word recognition (quiet - noise)	40 %		40 %	
	R-NC	R-C	L-C	L-NC
SSW test				
Corrected-SSW scores	2	10	18	-4
(Normal limits)	(5)	(13)	(18)	(4)
Response bias		16 Reversals*		
Phonemic Synthesis		14 with four reversals*		
(Normal limits)		(16)		

Reporting Test Results

The strengths and weaknesses revealed on the AP test battery can be translated into meaningful recommendations based on the above information. Another approach is to use a handicap scale that is designed to identify AP difficulties (e.g., Fisher, 1976; Smoski et al., 1992) as an aid in designing appropriate strategies for remediating the problems. The AP scale also can be used following therapy or classroom management as a measure of the effectiveness of the intervention.

MANAGEMENT APPROACHES

Once individual strengths and weaknesses have been identified, appropriate management procedures can follow. For example, speech-in-noise and competing-message test abnormalities, associated with individuals who experience difficulty under noisy conditions, signals a need for management strategies aimed at reducing distractions and improving the signal-to-noise ratio.

One helpful classroom technique is to use the chalkboard to write outlines and show new vocabulary, because children who have AP dysfunction may be much stronger in the visual modality. Even if they are weak visually, the written information will remain on the board long after the auditory counterpart has faded from memory. Such compensatory strategies are especially appropriate because the individual as well as the rest of the class will generally benefit from these adaptations. Another example of an AP adaptation that provides a general benefit is the use of classroom amplification systems. These devices are now available in many schools.

Classroom Amplification Systems

Project MARRS (Mainstream Amplification Resource Room Study) considered the value of sound field amplification in mainstreamed classrooms for the purposes of aiding children with minimal hearing losses and learning disabilities (Ray et al., 1984). By use of loudspeaker(s), the teacher's voice was amplified to provide a signal approximately 10dB above the noise level of the room. Data were collected on more than 1000 children in grades 4 through 6. Children in classrooms equipped with the amplification system were compared with those of the same grade who were in standard classrooms. The children in the experimental classrooms received no special services, while those in the control classrooms continued to receive resource room and other types of support.

The target children in this study were those children who had 1) hearing thresholds of 15 to 35dB HL, 2) academic difficulties, and 3) average intelligence. The target children who had benefit of sound field amplification exceeded the target children in the control classrooms in their academic progress. This difference was noted on the standard achievement tests given each of the three years of the study for students at each of the three grade levels.

Ray et al. (1984) point out that the MARRS system was also more cost effective than the standard approaches because fewer personnel were needed to achieve equal or better academic gains, and because the initial and continuing costs were less. Academically and legally, the system is more defensible because it maintains the learning disabled children in the least restrictive environment. Information may be obtained from the MARRS staff for setting up this system (Project MARRS, Wabash & Ohio Valley Special Education District, Box E, Norris City, IL 62869-0905). Similar systems are now available from other sources or the component parts can be assembled inexpensively.

Individual Auditory Aids

Assistive Listening Device (ALD)

Typically, classrooms are not ideal listening environments and therefore create a major problem for those with hearing and AP impairments (see Chapter 41; Hart, 1983). Assistive listening devices such as FM auditory trainers, which are useful in improving classroom listening conditions, are covered in detail in Chapter 42. Although the major use of FM auditory trainers is for the hard-of-hearing, similar devices are often recommended for those with AP problems. In part they improve the signal-to-noise ratios to the listener; however, the personal system has the further

benefit of bringing the teacher's clear speech, from a lapel or, better yet, from a boom microphone directly to the listener's ears. Thus, there is not only an improved signal-to-noise ratio, but also a higher fidelity speech signal. This ratio may be improved further by using more substantial earphone cushions.

Blake et al. (1991) reported that the attending behaviors of LD children improved significantly during FM auditory trainer use over similar periods when no ALD was used. Another approach to determine the effectiveness of ALDs is to evaluate their effect on speech recognition tasks in noise (Nast, Katz and Oleksy, unpublished study). A group of 15 children who were found to have AP dysfunction, including limited skills on speech-in-noise tasks, were tested in both quiet and noise (speech babble). For those conditions yielding at least a 10% deficit in noise compared to the quiet condition, the ALD was found to provide significantly better discrimination in noise for both monosyllabic words and sentences.

Although both the Tolerance-Fading Memory and the phonemic Decoding group cases stand to benefit from the use of an ALD, the former generally show the most dramatic improvements. Inasmuch as ALDs have the potential for improving attention and discrimination in the classroom, two cautions are appropriate. Most importantly, any auditory trainer that is not specifically designed for a normally hearing user must be modified to limit the maximum output level of the device. Most companies already have specific devices for those with AP dysfunction and normal hearing. A second concern is that the device may not help or might further restrict the child under quiet conditions or in certain classroom activities. Therefore, an ALD for children with AP problems should be provided for specific noise conditions and classroom activities and not simply used on a full-time basis.

Unilateral Earplugs

A simpler aid than sound field amplification or ALD devices is the use of an earplug to reduce the adverse influence of an offending ear (Willeford and Burleigh, 1985). The concept is that, in some cases, an individual's poor perception in one auditory channel may interfere with the better channel from the other ear. While the reduction of sound to one ear in a normally hearing and normally perceiving individual may be considered a disservice, it might be an effective treatment in certain cases with severe problems in only one ear.

Green and Kotenko (1980) have used unilateral earplugs to aid schizophrenic and brain damaged individuals. Later on Green (1983) used a similar approach with LD children. An earplug was recommended if there was a significant difference in auditory comprehension when the poorer ear was plugged than when both ears were unoccluded.

Many audiologists have had positive feedback when recommending unilateral earplugs for clients with major AP problems in a single ear. Recently, we had such a case: after brain surgery, an adult had a severe deficit in the right ear on the SSW test. A profound behavioral change was noted following the use of an earplug in the right ear. Improvement was reported for the ability to listen to speech in a background of noise as well as in the individual's personality and attitude.

When a unilateral earplug or other device is recommended, it is a good approach to recommend auditory training to help the person improve speech-in-noise skills. Training to decrease dependence on an ear plug is felt to be especially prudent when dealing with children. Training for AP problems will be reviewed in the next section.

Bilateral Ear Plugs

Because many individuals are highly distracted or hyper-sensitive to background noise, quite often they have difficulty concentrating on reading and doing other quiet activities in noise. For example, many children and adults complain that they cannot concentrate on homework because of even faint street sounds or TV. At such times a pair of ear plugs can be very helpful (Willeford and Burleigh, 1985).

Sound Reduction

A logical approach that will help many individuals in classrooms is to provide good room acoustics. This topic is covered in Chapter 40. Hart (1983) provides an architectural approach to deal with the problem of poor classroom acoustics.

Auditory Training and Strategies

It is our belief that recommendations should be based on the individual's needs and the problem situations faced, rather than simply a generic approach (Barnett et al., 1982). Although preferential seating and classroom amplification systems will probably benefit almost any child with an AP problem, other general recommendations may not. For example, speaking slowly would be likely helpful to someone with a decoding problem but potentially disadvantageous to someone with good decoding who has a memory problem. The test battery and the category system de-

scribed above, have been most helpful in developing strategies that address the specific problems. Strategies refer to suggestions, such as preferential seating or to tape-record classroom presentations when a student cannot take proper notes. Training refers to direct therapy, e.g., to aid the person in improving phonemic concepts, desensitization in dealing with background noise, auditory memory work and other trainable skills.

It is reasonable to offer a child both auditory training and the use of an assistive device. This approach is based on two factors, those who learn in a noisy classroom tend to have lower achievement than those in a quiet classroom, therefore those with speech-in-noise difficulty should be considered for listening aids. However, when tested under noisy conditions those who are often exposed to noise show less deterioration in understanding than those who are taught in quiet (Bronzaft and McCarthy, 1975). That is, although they perform less well academically they appear to be getting training in listening in noise. In normal life activities there are many occasions when noise cannot be avoided and therefore the ALDs that help children learn better in class may not benefit them on the outside. Rather than deny the child the vital help at school, it is advisable simply to provide some additional help for improving auditory performance.

Training for Improved Auditory Skills

People, especially children, have the potential to improve their auditory processing skills. While this may not be true in some extreme cases and in the elderly, it is probably true in the vast majority of cases seen by audiologists. The situation is especially promising when we work with young children (Bronfenbrenner, 1975; Mullin and Lange, 1984). It has been noted that young children appear to improve at a faster rate than older children and their gains appear to be more completely and perhaps more permanently incorporated (Katz and Burge, 1971). However, we have found the results of auditory therapy to be highly beneficial to older children and young adults as well.

There is much more information available about diagnostic aspects of AP than in the area of remediation (Katz and Cohen, 1985). This is no doubt because remedial studies require a great deal of time and have many potential confounding variables. Nevertheless, a number of therapeutic approaches have been applied to the rehabilitation of AP problems. Some deal with the processing of phonemic information and therefore would relate most directly to the decoding problems. Others deal with auditory figure-ground or with memory skills as seen in those with TFM problems. In addition, sequencing training may be especially useful for those with organizational difficulties and dichotic or auditory-visual training might benefit those who demonstrate limitations in integration.

Training at the phonemic level

Training materials, such as the Auditory Discrimination in Depth program, can have had an important effect in helping children to obtain a better understanding of speech sounds and how they can be analyzed and manipulated (Lindamood and Lindamood, 1969). Other programs, such as Phonemic Synthesis: Blending Sounds into Words, have been very effective in auditory training for those who are poor decoders (Katz and Harmon, 1982). Results show considerable improvement not only in Phonemic Synthesis ability but also in better decoding skills on the Lindamood Auditory Conceptualization (LAC) test (Katz, 1983).

Kahler (1983) evaluated 60 children on the test of PS at the beginning of first grade. Those who scored in the upper half were not considered to be at risk. Those who scored in the lower half were felt to be at risk for reading disability. Half of the lower group was given the PS training program. At the end of the academic year both the upper PS (not at risk) group and the PS trained group were on grade level for reading on the California Achievement Test (CAT). Their scores were not significantly different from one another. On the other hand the non-treated low PS group was significantly poorer than the other two groups on the CAT and scored below grade level. This study provides important data to suggest that PS training may be useful in averting reading impairment in first grade children. A review of the literature dealing with PS training and spontaneous improvement in articulation ability also provides encouraging results (Katz, 1983).

Other types of auditory training have been found to be useful. Alexander and Frost (1982) found training with decelerated speech (i.e., time-expanded 60-80 ms transitions) to be effective in developing improved discrimination in language delayed children. They improved in labeling of /ba/ versus /da/ over performance on the same syllables delivered at a normal rate. A matched control group that received syllables only at the normal rate showed significantly less improvement. It is of interest to note that Totter (1979) used time-expanded speech and found that severely retarded subjects improved in their comprehension without any special training.

Winitz and his colleagues (1963, 1965) demonstrated that training improves discrimination abilities and that these skills can generalize to other speech sounds. Based on the category system presented here,

this skill would relate primarily to the deficiencies of the poor phonemic decoders.

Training to desensitize those who have difficulty in noise

Very little empirical data are available to support the use of speech-in-noise training. However, many years of clinical experience provide us with a strong conviction that such training can help individuals deal with background noises. In one protocol, speech-in-noise training starts with relaxation before the introduction of noise. Speech materials are first presented from a loudspeaker in quiet and then background noise (e.g., cafeteria noise or speech babble) is increased in small units with about 10 items (e.g., monosyllabic words) at each level through a second speaker. When a noise level is reached at which the individual begins making more mistakes or shows increased hyperactivity the background noise is *eliminated* for the next set of 10 items and then the level is gradually increased again. Giving the patient control over the noise channel appears to be a useful strategy.

Over the years we have noted impressive gains in the ability to tolerate background noise and in the percentage of correct responses under noisy conditions following therapy. These individuals, especially younger children, seem to make better use of listening cues (e.g., listening from another room). However, unlike PS training, there is a tendency for this skill to regress when re-evaluated six months later. Therefore, weekly practice at home for at least 15 minutes is recommended to keep these skills sharp.

In the past few years considerable attention has been focused on Auditory Integration Training for hypersensitivity to noise. This treatment, developed by Dr. Guy Berard, has been recommended for autistic individuals and others who have hyperacute hearing. However, empirical evidence is not yet available.

Memory and sequencing training have also been applied to those with AP dysfunction

Memory training (Butler, 1983) is especially helpful for those in the TFM group. Another skill that can aid many individuals with AP difficulties is sequencing training (Aten, 1972). This is especially appropriate for those in the Organization group. Typically these services are provided by speech-language pathologists and resource room teachers.

SUMMARY AND CONCLUSIONS

The audiologist has an important part to play in the evaluation and management of individuals with auditory processing (AP) disorders. AP dysfunction is closely associated with many disabilities, no doubt because the auditory system is spread widely throughout the CNS and therefore is closely associated with a variety of other functions. Despite the complexity of AP and the individual differences noted in those with AP problems, auditory limitations can be divided into four basic categories. This system provides an understanding of how AP relates to learning and communication skills and also how to manage and remediate the difficulties. A transdisciplinary approach is likely to yield the best results. However, it appears clear that the best diagnosis and remedial plan may not be effective unless there is cooperation from the family, school, and of course the individual.

REFERENCES

Alexander DW, and Frost BP. Decelerated synthesized speech as a means of shaping speed of auditory processing of children with delayed language. Percept Mot Skills 1982;55:783–792.

Arnst D, and Katz J. The SSW Test: Development and Clinical Use. San Diego, College-Hill Press, 1982.

Aten J. Auditory memory and auditory sequencing, pp 108–135. Proceedings of the First Annual Memphis State Symposium on Auditory Processing and Learning Disabilities. Memphis: Memphis State University Press, 1972:108–135.

Bannatyne AD, and Wichiarajote P. Relationship between written spelling, motor functioning and sequencing skills. J Learning Disabilities 1969;2:6–18.

Barnett D, Nichols A, and Gould D. The effects of open-spaced versus traditional self contained classrooms. Lang Speech Hear Serv Schools 1982;13:138–143.

Blake R, Field B, Foster C, Platt F, and Wertz P. Effect of FM auditory trainers on attending behaviors of learning disabled children. Lang Speech Hear Serv Schools 1991;22:111–114.

Boder E. Developmental dyslexia: a diagnostic approach based on three atypical reading-spelling patterns. Dev Med Child Neurol 1973;15:663–687.

Bronfenbrenner U. Is early intervention effective? In: Guttentag, M, and Struening E, Eds. Handbook of Evaluation Research. Beverly Hills, CA: Sage Publishers, 1975.

Bronzaft AL, and McCarthy DP. The effect of elevated train noise on reading ability. Environ Behav 1975;7:517–527.

Burns MS, and Canter GJ. Phonemic behavior of aphasic patients with posterior cerebral lesions. Brain Lang 1977;4:492–507.

Butler KG. Language processing: selective attention and mnemonic strategies. In Lasky E, and Katz J, Eds. Central Auditory Processing Disorders: Problems of Speech, Language and Learning, Baltimore: University Park Press, 1983:297–318.

Dalby JT, and Gibson D. Functional cerebral lateralization in subtypes of disabled readers. Brain Lang 1981;14:34–48.

DeFries JC, Wadsworth SJ, and Gillis JJ. Gender differences in cognitive abilities of reading-disabled twins. Ann Dyslexia 1990;40: 216–228.

DeLacoste-Utamsingh C, and Holloway RL. Sexual dimorphism in the human corpus callosum. Science 1982;216:1431–1432.

Duffy FH, Denckla MB, Bartels PH, and Sandini G. Dyslexia: regional differences in brain electrical activity by topographic mapping. Ann Neurol 1980;7:412–420.

Fisher LI. Fisher Auditory Problems Checklist. Cedar Rapids, IA: Grant Woods Education Agency, 1976.

Fowler C. "Perceptual centers" in speech production and perception. Percept Psychophys 1979;25:375–388.

Fried I, Tanguay PE, Boder E, Doubleday C, and Greensite M. De-

velopmental dyslexia: electrophysiological evidence of clinical subgroups. Brain Lang 1981;12:14–22.

Friel-Patti S, and Finitzo T. Language learning in a prospective study of otitis media with effusions in the first two years of life. J Speech Hear Res 1990;33:188–194.

Geschwind N, and Behan PO. Left-handedness: association with immune disease, migraine, and developmental disorder. Proceedings of the National Academy of Sciences (USA) 1982;79: 5097–5100.

Green P. Increasing speech comprehension and recall by means of an earplug. Alberta Psychol 1983;12:16–17.

Green P, and Kotenko V. Superior speech comprehension in schizophrenics under monaural versus binaural listening conditions. J Abnorm Psychol 1980;89:339–408.

Grimes AM, Grady CL, Foster NL, Sunderland T, and Patronas NJ. Central auditory function in Alzheimer's disease. Neurology 1985;35:352–358.

Hart PJ. Classroom acoustical environments for children with central auditory processing disorders. In Lasky E, and Katz J, Eds. Central Auditory Processing Disorders: Problems of Speech, Language and Learning. Baltimore: University Park Press, 1983:343–352.

Hier DB, LeMay M, Rosenberger PB, and Perlo VP. Developmental dyslexia: evidence for a subgroup with reversal of cerebral asymmetry. Arch Neurol 1978;35:90–92.

Holm VA, and Kunze LH. Effects of chronic otitis media on language and speech development. Pediatrics 1969;43:833–839.

Jirsa RE, and Clontz KB. Long latency auditory event-related potentials from children with auditory processing disorders. Ear Hear 1990;1:222–232.

Kahler LB. Phonemic synthesis: a predictive measurement of early reading success. Paper presented at American Speech-Language-Hearing Association convention, Cincinnati, OH, 1983.

Katz J. The SSW test: an interim report. J Speech Hear Disord 1968;33:132–146.

Katz J. Phonemic synthesis. In Lasky EZ, and Katz J, Eds. Central Auditory Processing Disorders: Problems of Speech, Language and Learning. Baltimore: University Park Press, 1983:269–296.

Katz J. Classification of central auditory disorders. In Katz J, Stecker NA, and Henderson D, Eds. Central Auditory Processing: A Transdisciplinary View. Chicago: Mosby Year Book, 1992.

Katz J, and Burge C. Auditory perception training for children with learning disabilities. Menorah Med J 1971;2:18–29.

Katz J, Chertoff M, and Sawusch JR. Dichotic training. J Aud Res, 1984;24:251–264.

Katz J, and Cohen CF. Auditory training for children with perceptual difficulties. J Childhood Comm Disord 1985;9:65–81.

Katz J, and Harmon CH. Phonemic Synthesis: Blending Sounds into Words. Allen, Texas: Developmental Learning Materials, 1982.

Katz J, Kurpita B, Smith P, and Brandner S. A study of auditory processing in children: Categorizing AP results. SSW Reports 1992;14:1–6.

Katz J, Singer S, and Fanning J. Central auditory processing and communicative disorders in youthful offenders. New York State Speech-Language-Hearing Association Convention. Buffalo, NY, April 1988.

Katz J, and Smith P. A ten minute look at the CNS through the ears: using the SSW test. In R Zappulla, LeFever FF, Jaeger J, and Bilder R, Eds. Windows on the Brain: Neuropsychology's Technical Frontiers. Ann N Y Acad Sci 1991;620:1–19.

Kavale K. The relationship between auditory perceptual skills and reading ability: meta-analysis. J Learn Disabil 1981;14:539–546.

Keller W. Auditory processing disorder or attention deficit? In J Katz, NA Stecker, and Henderson D, Eds. Central Auditory

Processing: A Transdisciplinary View. Chicago: Mosby Year Book, 1992.

Kemper TL. Asymmetrical lesions in dyslexia. In N Geschwind, and Galaburda AM, Eds. Cerebral Dominance: The Biological Foundations. Cambridge, MA: Harvard University Press, 1984:75–89.

Kinsbourne M. Pediatric aspects of learning disorders. In Lasky E, and Katz J, Eds. Baltimore: University Park Press, 1983:49–68.

Kraft RH. Lateral specialization and verbal/spatial ability in preschool children: age, sex and familial handedness differences. Neuropsychologia 1984;22:319–335.

LaBuda MC, and DeFries JC. Genetic and environmental etiologies of reading disability: a twin study. Ann Dyslexia 1988;38: 131–153.

Lasky EZ, and Cox LC. Auditory processing and language interaction: evaluation and interaction strategies. In Lasky E, and Katz J, Eds. Central Auditory Processing Disorders: Problems of Speech, Language and Learning. Baltimore: University Park Press, 1983:243–268.

Lauter JL. Windows to the brain: what contemporary imaging devices can reveal about speech and hearing. Workshop sponsored by Department of Speech and Hearing Sciences, University of Arizona, Tucson, AZ, February 18, 1989.

Lauter JL. Processing asymmetries for complex sounds: Comparisons between behavioral ear advantages and electrophysiological asymmetries based on quantitative electroencephalography. Brain and Cognition 1992a;19:1–20.

Lauter JL. Imaging techniques and auditory processing. In Katz J, Stecker NA, and Henderson D, Eds. Central Auditory Processing: A Transdisciplinary View. Chicago, IL: Mosby Year Book, 1992b.

Lauter JL. Visions of the brain: noninvasive brain monitoring techniques and their applications to the study of human speech and language. In Winitz H, Ed. Human Communication and Its Disorders: Current Approaches to the Study of Language Development and Disorders, Vol. 4. Timonium, Md.: York Press (in press).

Lauter JL, Herscovitch P, Formby C, and Raichle M. Tonotopic organization in human auditory cortex revealed by positron emission tomography. Hear Res 1985;20:199–205.

Lindamood CH, and Lindamood PC. Auditory Discrimination in Depth. Boston: Teaching Resources, 1969.

Lubert N. Auditory perceptual impairments in children with specific language disorders: a review of the literature. J Speech Hear Disord, 1981;46:3–9.

Lucker JR. Diagnostic significance of the Type A pattern of the Staggered Spondaic Word (SSW) Test. Audiol Hear Educ 1980;6:21–23.

Ludlow CL, Cudahy EA, Bassich C, and Brown GL. Auditory processing skills of hyperactive, language-impaired, and learning disabled boys. In Lasky EZ, and Katz J, Eds. Central Auditory Processing Disorders: Problems of Speech, Language and Learning. Baltimore: University Park Press, 1983:163–184.

Mange C. Relationships between selected auditory perceptual factors and articulatory ability. J Speech Hear Res 1960;3: 367–374.

Menyuk P. Predicting speech and language problems with persistent otitis media. In Kavanaugh J, Ed. Otitis Media and Child Development, Parkton, MD: York Press, 1986:83–98.

Monroe M. Children Who Cannot Read. Chicago: University of Chicago Press, 1932.

Mullin LL, and Lange VA. Does the ability of kindergarten children to retain auditory and visual stimuli improve with training? Lange Speech Hear Serv Schools 1984;15:210–215.

Musiek FE. Neuroanatomy, neurophysiology, and central auditory assessment. Part II: The cerebrum. Ear Hear 1986a;7:283–294.

Musiek FE. Neuroanatomy, neurophysiology, and central auditory assessment. Part III: Corpus callosum. Ear Hear 1986b;7: 349–358.

Musiek FE, and Bornstein S. Auditory event related potentials in central auditory disorders. In Katz J, Stecker N, and Henderson D, Eds. Central Auditory Processing: A Transdisciplinary View. Chicago: Mosby Year Book, 1992.

Nast K, Katz J, and Oleksy N. Evaluation of speech recognition performance in noise using an FM auditory trainer, 1992 (unpublished study).

Northern JL, and Downs MP. Hearing in Children, 4th ed. Baltimore: Williams & Wilkins, 1991:18–27.

Olsen W, Noffsinger D, and Kurdziel S. Speech discrimination in quiet and in white noise by patients with peripheral and central lesions. Acta Otolaryngol 1975;80:375–382.

Orton ST. Reading Writing and Speech Problems in Children. New York: WW Norton & Company, 1964.

Papanicolaou C, Baumann S, Rogers R, Saydjari C, Amparo E, and Eisenberg H. Localization of auditory response sources using magnetoencephalography and magnetic resonance imaging. Arch Neurol 1990;47:33–37.

Pickles JO. Introduction to the Physiology of Hearing. London: Academic Press, 1988.

Ray H, Sarff LS, and Glassford FE. Sound field amplification: an innovative educational intervention for mainstreamed learning disabled students. The Directive Teacher 1984; Summer/Fall 18–20.

Salvi RJ, Henderson D, Boettcher FA, and Powers NL. Functional changes in central auditory pathways resulting from cochlear disease. In Katz J, Stecker NA, and Henderson D, Eds. Central Auditory Processing: A Transdisciplinary View. Chicago: Mosby Year Book, 1992.

Sams M, and Hari R. Magnetoencephalography in the study of human auditory information processing. In R Zappulla, LeFever FF, Jaeger J, and Bilder R, Eds. Windows on the Brain: Neuropsychology's Technical Frontiers. Ann N Y Acad Sci 1991; 620:102–117.

Sawyer DJ. The relationship between selected auditory abilities and beginning reading achievement. Lang Speech Hear Serv Schools 1981;12:95–99.

Schoeny ZG, and Hasenstab MS. Auditory processing. Short Course, Virginia Speech and Hearing Association Convention, Charlottesville, VA, 1983.

Shankweiler D, and Liberman IY. Phonology and Reading Disability: Solving the Reading Puzzle. Ann Arbor, MI: University of Michigan Press, 1989.

Sloan C. Treating Auditory Processing Difficulties in Children. San Diego, CA: College-Hill Press, 1986.

Smoski WJ, Brunt MA, and Tannahill JC. Listening characteristics of children with central auditory processing disorders. Lang Speech Hear Serv Schools 1992;23:145–152.

Sparks RL, Ganschow L, Kenneweg S, and Miller K. Use of an Orton-Gillingham approach to dyslexic/learning disabled students: explicit teaching of phonology in a second language. Ann Dyslexia 1991;41:96–118.

Spitzer JB. Central auditory evaluation protocol: a guide for training and diagnosis of lesions of the central system. Ear Hear 1983;4:221–231.

Stecker NA. Central auditory processing: implications in audiology. In Katz J, Stecker NA, and Henderson D, Eds. Central Auditory Processing: A Transdisciplinary View. Chicago: Mosby Year Book, 1992.

Stovall JV, Manning WH, and Shaw CK. Auditory assembly of children with mild and severe articulations. Folia Phoniatrica 1977;29:162–172.

Tallal P. Rapid auditory processing in normal and disordered language development. J Speech Hear Res 1976;19:561–571.

Teele D, Klein J, Chase C, Menyuk P, and Rosner B. Otitis media in infancy and intellectual ability, school achievement, speech and language at age 7 years. J Infect Dis 1990;162:685–694.

Teele D, Klein J, and Rosner B. Otitis media with effusion during the first three years of life and development of speech and language. Pediatrics 1984;74:282–287.

Totter JJ. The comprehension of time altered speech by the mentally retarded as a function of age, expressive communication competency, and rate of presentation [Ph.D. Dissertation]. State University of New York at Buffalo, 1979.

Willeford J. Assessing central auditory behavior in children: a test battery approach. In Keith R, Ed. Central Auditory Dysfunction. New York: Grune & Stratton, 1977:43–72.

Willeford J, and Burleigh JB. Handbook of Central Auditory Pro-

cessing Disorders in Children. Orlando, FL: Grune & Stratton, 1985:61–86, 138–140.

Winitz H, and Bellerose B. Phoneme generalization as a function of phoneme similarity and verbal unit of test and training stimuli. J Speech Hear Res 1963;6:380–392.

Winitz H, and Preisler L. Discrimination pretraining and sound learning. Percept Mot Skills 1965;20:905–916.

Witelson SF. Hand and sex differences in the isthmus and genu of the human corpus callosum: postmortem morphological study. Brain 1989;112:799–835.

Young ML. Neuroscience, pragmatic competence and auditory processing. In Lasky E, and Katz J, Eds. Central Auditory Processing Disorders: Problems of Speech, Language and Learning. Baltimore: University Park Press, 1983:141–162.

Yozawitz A, Bruder G, Sutton S, Sharpe L, Gurland B, Fleiss J, and Coasta L. Dichotic perception: evidence for right hemisphere dysfunction in affective psychosis. Br J Psychiat 1979;135: 224–237.

CHAPTER 33

Educational Audiology

Larry Medwetsky

What is an educational audiologist? What are the job responsibilities? In what educational settings would one be found? What student populations are served? This chapter attempts to answer the above and related questions. By reading this chapter, the reader can become better informed of the services provided by, and the challenges confronting, educational audiologists.

HISTORICAL PERSPECTIVES

Educational audiology is almost as old as audiology itself. The profession of audiology emerged during World War II as part of an overall effort to help war veterans with service-incurred hearing losses. After the war ended, rehabilitative efforts were extended to include other individuals. By the late 1940s, many schools for the deaf employed individuals whose primary responsibilities were to test hearing and fit hearing aids. Public school hearing screening programs were widespread.

Joint Committee

One of the earliest uses of the term "Educational Audiologist" is found in a 1965 report by the Joint Committee on Audiology and Education of the Deaf. This committee was composed of the American Speech and Hearing Association and the Conference of Executives of American Schools for the Deaf. A superintendent of a public residential school wrote:

> Audiology has always been, and still is, too far removed from the classroom. The audiologist generally knows too little about educational methods and yet he prescribes to parents. He has too often confused parents, caused waste of time in the education of a deaf child, and has set himself up as an educator rather than a technician. He should be an *educational audiologist* and not a clinical audiologist (Joint Committee on Audiology and Education of the Deaf, 1965:44–45).

Several important conclusions were made at the Joint Committee conference. The conclusions concerning audiologists were:

1. Audiologists generally know little about educational methods, yet often recommend various educational approaches to parents.

2. In general, audiologists have inadequate experience with, or knowledge about the deaf, particularly young deaf children. An increased emphasis needs to be placed on the education of the deaf in audiology training programs. In addition, audiologists need greater exposure to the educational and language problems imposed by deafness.

3. Because complete audiology services are not being provided to deaf children, there need to be more audiologists in educational programs for the hearing impaired.

4. Teachers want more than an audiogram. They want to know: (*a*) the child's ability to process speech auditorily and (*b*) how they can best help the student to use residual hearing.

In many ways, the above conclusions remain true today.

Rehabilitation Act

In the 1970s, legislation was passed that significantly impacted on the education of hearing-impaired children. The Rehabilitation Act of 1973 (PL 93-112, Section 504) ensured access of impaired students, elementary through college, to programs receiving federal funds. An even more important piece of legislation was "The Education for All Handicapped Children Act" (Public Law 94-142, 1975). Among its guarantees were that:

1. A free public education be available to all handicapped children between the ages of 3 and 18;

2. Handicapped children needed to be educated with nonhandicapped children to the maximal extent possible;

3. Written individualized educational programs (IEP) needed to be jointly developed by the student's teacher and parents (and the student, whenever possible). The IEPs needed to include: (*a*) an analysis of the student's present level of achievement; (*b*) short-range and annual goals; and (*c*) specific special education service requirements; and

4. The States needed to comply with these requi-

sites; failure to do so could mean a cutoff of federal special education funding.

Emergence of Mainstreaming

The above legislation coincided with emerging concerns for the education of the hard-of-hearing child. Many hard-of-hearing children were either inappropriately placed in schools for the deaf or placed in public educational facilities but receiving inadequate services. Efforts were made to ensure that the "mainstreamed" child had an adequate support system. These efforts resulted in a number of service delivery models. These models have been reviewed by the Ad Hoc Committee on Extension of Audiological Services in the Schools (ASHA, 1980) and by Berg, Blair, Viehweg, and Wilson (1986).

1. The first model is one of parent referral. The parents are, essentially, the case managers and arrange for any necessary evaluations. The parents report to the local educational authority (LEA), who then initiate intervention procedures. This model is the least costly to the school.
2. The second model is a school-based or self-contained delivery service. All necessary services are provided by the LEA. The audiologist is responsible for the assessment, intervention, coordination, follow up, and staff development. Compliance with PL 94-142 is more likely with this model, but the costs are much higher.
3. The third model is a school-community based model. Both the school and the community share in the responsibility of providing services. Clinical assessment is done outside the school setting, but the school audiologist interprets the information for the school. Costs remain high under this arrangement.
4. A fourth model is a contractual agreement model, by which the LEA contracts with community service agencies to provide audiological services. The school system is responsible for providing comprehensive services. Costs vary according to the level of services required.
5. The last model is one that has been proposed by Yater (1978) and is similar to model #3. Outside audiological assessments are used, but the school audiologist does the interpretation. The audiologist also functions as a hearing clinician, providing tutorial help in academic areas of concern. The audiologist, thus, serves as an itinerant teacher of the hearing impaired. This model is similar to an early model of educational audiology advocated by Berg (1974).

Present Status of Educational Audiology

At present, the field of educational audiology is still not well established. There seem to be four major reasons for this:

1. *Diversity of service delivery models.* There is no consensus about what educational audiology services need to be provided.
2. *Lack of specific requirements for certification.* In a survey of 43 states, Deconde Johnson (1990) reported that although most states had licensing/certification requirements for audiologists, only 13 states indicated certification was necessary to practice audiology in a school district. These results were shocking and were felt to reflect: (*a*) the absence of educational audiology services in many states, and (*b*) the inconsistency in the quality of services in others.
3. *Absence of training in educational audiology in most universities.* Typically, the most that is offered is an introductory educational audiology course or a course on education of the deaf. Hence, most audiologists lack the knowledge and training required to be competent educational audiologists. This may be one reason why Wilson-Vlotman and Blair (1986) found that educational audiologists continue to provide clinic-based services to the school population.
4. *Difficulty that educational audiologists have had in implementing change in their job situations.* Berg et al. (1986) pointed out that educational audiologists need to understand the needs of the child, teacher, parents and administrators. By learning how to best work with these four groups, the educational audiologist will obtain the necessary advocates to initiate change in the delivery of audiological services in schools.

Recognition of the above problems and the need for solutions resulted in the formation of the Educational Audiology Association in 1984. The association's goals include: (*a*) promoting the field of educational audiology; (*b*) providing support for those in the field; and (*c*) developing guidelines that will result in the delivery of services that are consistent as well as comprehensive. As part of its mandate, the Educational Audiology Association proposed a working definition of an educational audiologist:

An Educational Audiologist is a specialist who ensures that all aspects of a child's hearing and learning are maximized in order for their educational and real life capabilities to be met. The Educational Audiologist is the person responsible for the child with hearing difficulties. In many instances, this role could be one of case manager. The Educational Audiologist is qualified in the overall ramifications of sound, hearing, hearing loss, hearing aids, auditory perception (including central auditory abilities) and their impact on learning and life. The Educational Audiologist is the one responsible for identification, diagnosis, assessment, amplification programming, aural rehabilitation programming (and training when feasible) and central auditory programming. In addition, they are responsible for selection of classrooms, training of supportive personnel, parent training and support, specialist coordination, supervision of specialized testing, otologic referral, and on-going evaluations of the child's classroom and educational functioning. (cited in Blair, Wilson-Vlotman, and Von Almen, 1989:14).

SURVEYS OF AUDIOLOGISTS WORKING IN SCHOOL SETTINGS

Blair et al. (1989) surveyed full-time audiologists employed in schools. This survey was a follow up to a study conducted in 1984 (Wilson-Vlotman and Blair, 1986). A total of 203 individuals were included in the first survey and a total of 134 in the second survey. The results will be discussed under separate headings.

Demographic Characteristics

The employment settings of educational audiologists varied greatly. Most (40%) worked in public schools and in settings where self contained classrooms were available. Many audiologists, however, also worked in private day schools, residential and day schools for the hearing impaired. The ratio of educational audiologists to students was extremely variable. About half the educational audiologists worked with a total population of less than 1000 children. The lowest number of children served per audiologist were in private day schools (mean of 30 children) and in residential schools (mean of 75), whereas the greatest number of children served were in the regular public school setting (mean of 19,000).

Current Practices

Table 33.1 (from Blair et al., 1989) gives an overview of the time per month spent by educational audiologists on various tasks. The greatest decrease was in the area of audiological assessments, 35% in 1984 to 25% in 1989. Nevertheless, the percentage of time spent on amplification management increased from 14% to 23%. These results suggest that less emphasis is being given to testing and more energy to the fitting of appropriate amplification and amplification maintenance.

Blair et al. (1989) noted two other significant

Table 33.1.
Average Percentage of Time Spent by Educational Audiologists on Various Tasks (1989 Compared with 1984)[a]

Tasks	Time per Month 1989	Time per Month 1984
Diagnostic		
Screening	7.5	9.3
Audiological assessment	25.5	36.6
Central auditory assessment	1.7	2.4
Amplification Management		
Hearing aids/equipment	18.4	11.7
Earmolds	4.3	2.7
Indirect Service		
Consultation	10.3	8.8
Counseling	2.8	5.6
Direct Service		
Tutoring	4.8	7.0
Educational assessment	3.7	1.5
Leadership		
Administration	9.5	9.0
Supervision	3.5	4.2
Research	0.8	0.8
Professional growth	3.2	NR
Other	3.8	0.5

[a]From Blair et al., 1989:5.

changes over the 5-year period between the two surveys. The first is that the percentage of technicians providing screening services increased from 18% to 40%. The second is that the percentage of educational audiologists involved in central auditory testing decreased from 28% to only 16%.

Attitudes

Audiologists were also asked to evaluate their satisfaction on a number of issues. Eighty-nine percent of the participants indicated that they were moderately satisfied or very satisfied with their careers. When asked to describe the adequacy of facilities and equipment, 45% felt that they were "totally adequate" and 48% felt that they were at least moderately adequate. Only 5% felt that their facilities and the equipment available were totally inadequate. These results contrast with 1984 when 24% of the respondents felt that the accessibility to facilities/equipment was totally inadequate.

Respondents were also asked about their views on training and accreditation. At least half of the respondents felt it was important that educational audiology be accredited and that they would be willing to earn the accreditation.

Finally, the participants were asked to rank the concerns they had for the field of educational audiology. The areas of greatest concern were poor definition and misunderstanding of educational audiology, large caseloads, inadequate training, and lack of status.

Blair et al. (1989) concluded that educational audiology had too little visibility in schools and was not yet perceived as an integral part of the educational process for hearing impaired children. They felt that many administrators, and even many educational audiologists, did not understand that educational audiology services must be different from that of clinical audiology.

ROLE OF THE EDUCATIONAL AUDIOLOGIST

Clearly, educational audiologists work in a variety of educational settings, often serving different populations. These factors, in large measure, determine the audiologist's responsibilities. The primary goals, however, remain the same. These are to preserve the child's residual hearing and to maximize the child's residual hearing/auditory processing abilities. The author suggests that an educational audiologist should:

1. Identify all students with hearing loss or auditory processing disorders;
2. Develop test batteries that will be comprehensive and appropriate to the student populations served;
3. Ensure that the necessary amplification systems, when indicated, are ordered and maintained;
4. Provide inservices to staff, parents, and students;
5. Counsel both parents and students; and
6. Contribute to student placement.

Establishing an Educational Audiology Program

There are many issues that need to be addressed when establishing an educational audiology program. First, the audiologist needs to meet with all those who will impact on and be impacted by the program. Success often depends on the audiologist's ability to meet the needs/desires of students, parents, teachers, and administrators. The most important contact is another audiologist with a well-established practice. The latter will provide much information about service delivery in that region. In addition, the audiologist needs to contact a number of related-service personnel. These include: school professionals (such as the psychologist and speech/language pathologist), otolaryngologists, hearing aid dispensers, and manufacturers of equipment. Second, the audiologist needs to decide on which test procedures will be included in the test protocol and the equipment to be ordered. Third, the audiologist needs to establish a mechanism for inservicing and counseling. If the educational audiologist also wishes to be directly involved in aural habilitation, then he or she will need to meet with all those concerned for coordination of activities. Last, scheduling issues need to be resolved.

Identifying Students with Hearing Loss or Auditory Processing Disorders

Hearing-impaired students will generally be identified before the educational audiologist becomes involved. Nevertheless, many educational audiologists working in regular school systems, or in programs for physically handicapped, low-functioning or learning-disabled students, are often the first to identify a student with a hearing loss or auditory processing disorder. In these cases, identification may occur as part of a hearing/auditory processing screening program or on referral from a teacher/parent.

Audiological Assessment Procedures

Periodically, educational audiologists need to conduct comprehensive audiological assessments for all students who have been identified as having hearing losses or auditory processing disorders. A comprehensive assessment of auditory processing skills is extremely important; however, often this is underappreciated by many educational audiologists and other staff members. A comprehensive test battery allows the educational audiologist to:

1. find out the degree to which the student can process incoming information auditorily;
2. compare student performance with different amplification systems;
3. inform the teacher about what the student is able to perceive auditorily in the classroom setting; and
4. assist the teacher and speech/language pathologist in speech and auditory-training programs.

There are many speech perception tests with which to assess students. These tests vary greatly in the degree of auditory processing, memory, and cognitive skills required. For example, a score of 0% by a profoundly hearing-impaired student on an open set monosyllabic test could lead the audiologist to conclude that the student is unable to perceive speech. It is possible that had a spondee recognition task or a closed set monosyllabic word forced-choice identification task been given, the student might have actually done quite well.

Table 33.2 is a hierarchy of test procedures arranged by the degree of complexity and processing/memory skills required. These procedures can be used to test various speech stimuli (e.g., phonetic features, phonemes, words, sentences).

The educational audiologist is also responsible for monitoring middle ear status. Middle ear screenings, consisting of an otoscopic exam, tympanogram, ipsilateral reflexes, and acoustic reflectometry should be done routinely, the frequency varying as a function of

Table 33.2.
Hierarchy of Speech Perception Test Measures

I. Detection
  A. Two alternative, forced-choice detection. The speech element occurs in one interval while silence occurs in the other interval. The student must indicate in which interval the speech stimulus occurred.
  B. Open set detection. The student must indicate when the speech stimulus is heard.
II. Discrimination (Same versus Different)
  A. Presentation of two stimuli. The stimuli are the same/different in one or more specified dimensions (frequency, intensity, duration, etc.). The student states whether the two stimuli were the same/different.
  B. AXB paradigm. A and B are two different stimuli. The student must state whether X is the same as A or B. X is presented second and is one presentation away from each of the reference stimuli.
  C. ABX paradigm. The task is the same as the previous task, but while X is one presentation away from the B stimulus, it is two presentations away from the A stimulus. This increases the load on short-term memory.
  D. Oddball detection in a three-interval, forced-choice procedure. Two of the stimuli are identical and one differs. The position of the oddball varies randomly across presentations. The student needs to indicate which of the three stimuli was the oddball.
III. Identification
  A. Closed-set (forced-choice) identification. There are a minimum of two choices. The student is required to identify which of the items was spoken.
  B. Open-set recognition. The student repeats what he or she has heard.
IV. Comprehension
  A. Word associations. These include responding with a synonym or stating the category in which the word belongs.
  B. Yes/No questions
  C. WH questions (Where, What, Who, When, Why, How?)
  D. Open-ended questions
  E. Answer questions in response to a connected discourse recording

The above do not detail specialized test procedures, such as sound-symbol relations, auditory synthesis/analysis, sequencing, memory span and processing speed, that can also be assessed in hierarchial fashion.

the student population served. For example, certain student populations should be screened as often as every 3 months. These include: (a) hearing-impaired students who, because of their wearing ear molds, may have a large buildup of wax after only a few months and (b) students, such as those with Down syndrome, who are at high risk for middle ear problems. Other students, who are at less risk for middle ear problems, should be screened twice a year. However, in instances where an outer or middle ear problem is suspected, the audiologist should assess the student as soon as possible.

Amplification Programming

Amplification programming includes monitoring of classroom acoustics, as well as monitoring and maintenance of personal hearing aids and classroom systems.

Classroom acoustics have a great impact on the selection and success of amplification. The audiologist must assess the noise and reverberation levels in the classroom and decide if these might affect the student's ability to understand speech. If the answer is yes, then the audiologist needs to determine if any classroom modifications can be made and whether assistive listening devices are needed.

The audiologist might be directly involved in the fitting of personal hearing aids or only in the evaluation process. The educational audiologist needs to be aware of the advantages/disadvantages of the various prescriptive procedures. The educational audiologist should have an understanding of earmold acoustics and how different earmold modifications can influence the fitting procedure.

The educational audiologist is also responsible for advising school administrators and educators in the selection and purchase of assistive listening devices (ALDs), whether personal or classroom amplification systems, and assessing their benefits.

To ensure that personal hearing aids and ALDs are in good working order, it is necessary to establish some kind of monitoring system. To make effective use of the audiologist's time, monitoring should be carried out by a teacher or a trained staff member. Monitoring should include daily listening checks. Periodic electroacoustic evaluations are needed as well.

Inservice Training

Inservice training is provided individually or in groups. The audiologist should meet regularly with both the classroom teacher and the student's speech-language pathologist. The auditory assessment enables the audiologist to inform the teacher and speech-language pathologist about the child's auditory ability to detect, process, and comprehend the incoming speech signal (phonetic feature level up to connected discourse). In addition, the audiologist can help both of these professionals in planning the student's aural habilitation program.

Inservice workshops for all staff members are also valuable. They not only provide a chance to disseminate information but also serve to heighten staff awareness of the educational audiology services available.

Counseling

The forms of audiological counseling referred to here are discussed in a paper by Stone and Olswang (1989). These are:

1. Information sharing: providing information about a communication disorder and treatment;

2. Empathic listening: acknowledging and validating another's feelings; and

3. Problem solving: helping one examine choices and possible outcomes.

A successful educational audiology program will provide both parental and student guidance. Because students have usually been diagnosed as having a hearing loss before educational placement, parents will usually have received some form of audiological counseling. There are parents, however, who might have had difficulty absorbing all the details and still have questions. The audiologist needs to support and encourage these parents, help them in making decisions, and allow them to ask questions repeatedly.

Students should be active partners in any decision making. The more that the students understand about the auditory process, hearing aids, lipreading, and peer pressure, the more likely they are to be comfortable with their hearing impairment.

Student Placement

Of all the school professionals, the educational audiologist is the most aware of the relationship between hearing loss and its impact on auditory processing. For this reason, the educational audiologist needs to be actively involved in the admission and placement of all students who have a confirmed hearing loss or auditory processing disorder.

AUDIOLOGY PROGRAMS IN SPECIFIC EDUCATIONAL SETTINGS

The goal of this section is to detail the educational audiologist's responsibilities as a function of the particular student population served.

Day or Residential Schools for the Hearing Impaired

Assessment Procedures

Most students in a day or residential school have a bilateral severe/profound hearing loss acquired prelingually. Many audiologists are not adequately prepared for assessing and establishing auditory training programs for these students. Profoundly hearing-impaired students, especially those with a prelingual hearing loss, often do not possess the necessary auditory/speech capabilities for assessment on traditional speech perception measures (such as speech reception threshold and speech recognition in quiet/noise). The test battery usually administered consists of puretone thresholds, speech awareness thresholds, comfort and discomfort levels, and immittance audiometry. These results may be adequate for determining hearing sensitivity, dynamic range, preferred listening level, and

middle ear status but convey little information about the student's ability to process speech. It should be noted that, even with puretone testing, misleading results can be obtained. Profoundly hearing-impaired students are often assessed on audiometers having a maximal power output (MPO) of 110 dBHL. Often, the audiogram obtained indicates a corner audiogram (i.e., the thresholds derived are at frequencies below 1–2,000 Hz), when, in fact, the student has residual hearing at the higher frequencies but at intensity levels beyond the MPO of the audiometer. The results may, therefore, underestimate the degree of residual hearing and impact on successful hearing aid fitting. It is recommended that audiologists testing profoundly hearing-impaired students use audiometers having an MPO of at least 120–125 dBHL.

There are many speech perception tests that can be used to assess these students' auditory processing skills. The information obtained may be used to (a) profile a student's listening strengths and weaknesses, (b) provide baselines for auditory training, and (c) measure any gains achieved through auditory training. Table 33.3 shows a matrix, slightly modified from the one developed by Erber (1982). It summarizes the variety of speech signals a hearing-impaired child may encounter, as well as the response tasks that the child might be required to do. The response tasks are organized hierarchically according to difficulty (detection up to comprehension), while the speech stimuli are arranged by length and complexity (speech elements up to connected discourse). It is not necessary to evaluate the student's ability at each level of response difficulty (e.g., there is little benefit in establishing detection thresholds for connected discourse if a threshold for sentences has already been, or could be, obtained). Appendix 33.1 lists some of the available tests for presentation of environmental and speech stimuli. Within each level of signal complexity, the tests are ordered by response difficulty.

The clinician needs to choose tests that are appropriate for a particular student. The selection process will depend on the student's auditory abilities, as determined before and during the course of testing, and linguistic abilities.

The educational audiologist should evaluate the student's ability to perceive speech:

1. at normal speaking levels (about 45–50 dB HL) and at the student's most comfortable listening (MCL) level. Results at 45–50 dB HL tell how much the student is perceiving with his or her personal aids, in quiet, at a distance of about 5–6 feet. Testing at MCL, however, tells of the student's ability to perceive speech at a preferred listening level.

Table 33.3.
Stimulus-Response Matrix for Assessing Auditory Perception Skills in Hearing-Impaired Students[a]

Stimuli/ Response	Environmental Sounds	Speech Elements (supraseg./seg.)	Words	Sentences	Connected Discourse
Detection					
Imitation					
Discrimination					
Identification					
Comprehension					

[a] The stimuli and response tasks are arranged by order of complexity.

2. in noise (usually white noise is used but for more validity competing speech stimuli should be used).

3. in the combined auditory and visual mode. Besides greater face validity, the results obtained in the combined mode might be the only way of determining which hearing aid provides the best results. Profoundly deaf students often perform at chance levels in the auditory-only mode, which makes the comparison of different hearing aids quite difficult. Nevertheless, these students usually perform above chance in the combined mode, thus, making it easier to determine the hearing aid that provides the greatest benefit.

4. in sentence and connected discourse materials, spoken at different rates. Speech materials are often presented slowly and clearly in the clinical situation and might not reflect what actually occurs in the class. The student, therefore, might have no problems listening in the clinical setting but might have much difficulty at a typical speaking rate.

5. with the FM system, if the student uses one. Testing should be done with the FM receiver set to FM microphone only (i.e., the student picks up the teacher microphone only) and with both the FM and environmental microphones on (i.e., the FM microphone plus the microphone(s) for picking up sounds in the surrounding environment). Testing with the FM system will allow the audiologist to determine the degree to which the student's access to speech is enhanced (versus hearing aids only) in both quiet and in noise.

The audiologist also should evaluate the student's auditory and/or visual short-term memory (e.g., number of chunks recalled), as well as the student's sequencing ability. This helps to determine the student's ability to process sentences of different lengths.

A number of other nontraditional techniques can be incorporated into the assessment regimen. Psycho-acoustic testing may help determine why some severely/profoundly hearing-impaired students have good listening skills and why others have great difficulty. For example, two students might have the same audiometric thresholds, yet have very different listening abilities. These students may actually differ in their frequency or temporal resolution capabilities and/or central auditory processing skills. Psychoacoustic measurements also might be useful in (a) student placement, by serving as a predictive measure and (b) providing another way to measure gains in auditory training.

Few tests are available, at this time, that can adequately assess higher-order auditory skills in hearing impaired students. Tests, as well as programs to train in these higher-order skills, need to be developed.

It is obvious that the above assessment battery takes a long time to administer and should be given over many sessions. Many of the tests are available on tape (or can be recorded onto tape) and can be presented, via a tape recorder, in a quiet room. This allows other staff, such as teachers or speech/language pathologists, to administer parts of the test battery.

Amplification Programming

The efforts of the educational audiologist cannot be successful unless the students are fitted with the appropriate amplification systems, which, in turn, are maintained in good working order. For very young students, it may sometimes be quite difficult, if not impossible, to do hearing aid evaluations. If audiometric thresholds have been obtained, then real ear probe tube measurements should be used in fitting the hearing aids (the reader is referred to Chapter 44).

The most common assistive listening device used in the school setting is the FM-wireless system (see Chapter 42). There are a number of issues concerning FM systems of which the educational audiologist must be aware. First, many authors (Hawkins and Schum, 1985; Thibodeau, 1990; Chellappa and Ross, 1991) have shown that FM systems coupled to behind-the-ear hearing aids (directly, via a plug in audio-boot or indirectly, by magnetic induction) interact unpredictably. The hearing aid's frequency response may be altered significantly and different types of distortion may be introduced. Thus, the educational audiologist cannot simply dispense the same FM system to all students but needs to evaluate, electroacoustically, each particular combination of FM system, cords, telecoil loop, audio-boot, and hearing aid.

A second point to consider is the location of the teacher's microphone. The effect of distance and orientation between source (mouth) and receiver (teacher's microphone) is quite important. Medwetsky and Boothroyd (1991a) found that microphone placement close to the mouth (i.e., 2″ from the center of mouth and slightly off to the side) resulted in an overall intensity that was 6–8 dB higher than when the microphone was worn on the chest. Medwetsky (1991) also found that when the microphone is worn on the collar the overall intensity is also 6–8 dB lower relative to the mouth placement. Perhaps the most important finding in both studies was the observation that off-axis placement (i.e., when the microphone is not placed directly in front of the mouth) results in a decrease in intensity that is not uniform across frequencies. The drop off in the high frequencies, relative to the lows, was greater at the chest and collar than at the mouth.

Ideally, the microphone is worn on a headset, placed slightly below the lips. This placement provides the best signal/noise ratio, does not obscure the lips, and avoids unwanted popping or hissing sounds. If the teacher finds the use of a headset cumbersome, then the headset can be adapted to be worn on the neck. The reader should note, however, that when a headset is used, the orientation of microphone and mouth is the same at all times, regardless of head movement. This is not the case when the headset is worn on the neck. Those teachers who insist on wearing a lapel microphone on the chest should wear the microphone as close to the midline as possible.

A third issue, and one that has not often been addressed, is the effect that coupling (FM to the behind-the-ear hearing aid) has on the students' ability to hear their own voices. When indirect coupling is used (i.e., via magnetic induction), students must often rely on the environmental microphones of the FM-receiver to hear their own voices. Because most older students wear the FM receiver at the waist, the distance between the source (student's mouth) and the pick-up microphone is increased. Medwetsky and Boothroyd (1991a) found that the overall intensity of the speech signal at the waist was 17.5 dB less than at the mouth and that the decrease was greatest in the high frequencies. Although increasing the volume control setting on the FM receiver can partially compensate for the decrease in overall signal level, there is a similar increase in the level of background noise. A better solution to this problem is to have a microphone jack on the FM receiver and have the student wear a lapel microphone on the chest. This arrangement decreases the distance between the student's mouth and pick-up microphone, resulting in a better signal-to-noise ratio.

Maintenance of Amplification Systems

The most important component in any maintenance program is the training of staff members and parents (for home maintenance of the equipment). The teachers and parents should be trained to do (a) daily listening checks, (b) physical inspections, and (c) simple troubleshooting of amplification devices. Bess and McConnell (1981) give an excellent summary of what should be included in the listening check and physical inspection. Bess and McConnell recommend that teachers and parents have troubleshooting kits that include: a hearing aid stethoscope, battery tester, spare batteries, and pipe cleaners.

In addition to the daily checks, thorough physical inspections and electroacoustic analyses of amplification devices should be done every 2 or 3 months by the audiologist or a trained technician.

The audiologist should maintain a stock of loaner hearing aids and various accessories, such as nozzles, cords, and batteries, to allow for minor repairs to be done on the premises.

HEARING-IMPAIRED STUDENTS IN THE MAINSTREAMED SETTING

Since the passage of "The Education for All Handicapped Children Act" in 1975, increasingly greater numbers of hearing-impaired students have been mainstreamed. This, in turn, has increased the need for audiological services in the regular school systems.

In contrast to the situation in day and residential schools, mainstreamed students, seen by the audiologist, often go to different schools. This usually requires many of the students to be transported to a main site for testing. In addition, the audiologist needs to travel from site to site to see teachers, itinerant personnel, and students. This often results in the audiologist not being immediately accessible to many staff and students. The educational audiologist will, therefore, need to rely heavily on certain staff members (such as a speech/language pathologist or an itinerant teacher) to keep up to date on any audiological concerns and to follow up on audiological services (such as the maintenance of equipment).

An important audiological service in the mainstreamed setting is the inservicing of regular school teachers. Most regular school teachers do not have specific knowledge in working with the hearing impaired and, therefore, are unaware of the importance of contextual cues, facial visibility, slow speaking pace, and good lighting conditions. Initially, teachers might exhibit some anxiety in having a hearing-impaired student. The audiologist can help these teachers feel more comfortable by meeting regularly with them.

It is also a good idea to give informal workshops to the student's hearing peers. This should be done in cooperation and consultation with the hearing-impaired student, teacher, parent, and itinerant teachers. Ideally, the workshops should be given before the hearing-impaired child is enrolled in that particular class.

Another concern is in the area of classroom amplification. Because the number of students in a regular classroom is greater than that found in a day or residential school, the noise levels are usually higher. The average classroom in the regular school setting has a signal-to-noise (S/N) ratio of +4 dB and is quite reverberant (Hawkins, 1984). A favorable S/N ratio is usually not possible without some form of technological assistance. Sound field amplification is one option that has become increasingly popular with mildly hearing-impaired students, listening-disabled students, and even with normal hearing-listening students (Sarff et al., 1981; Flexer, 1989; Flexer et al., 1990). A sound field amplification system consists of a teacher-worn wireless microphone, an amplifier, a receiver, and two or more loudspeakers that are positioned to create an equal signal level throughout the room. The average S/N ratio attained with sound field amplification varies from 10–16 dB (Sarff, Ray, and Bagwell, 1981; Flexer, Millin, and Brown, 1990). The benefits of a sound field system over personal FM systems include: cost effectiveness (i.e., if several students need ALDs) and durability. In addition, the students who need this help do not "stand out" in the classroom.

Worner (1988) discussed the use of a sound field amplification system in a school for the deaf and indicated that students were able to benefit significantly from the improved S/N ratio. Results by Medwetsky and Boothroyd (1991b) indicate that a 16-dB S/N ratio, achieved by sound-field amplification, is not optimal for students with severe hearing losses (Note that because of the limited dynamic range in hearing typically found in profoundly hearing impaired individuals, achieving listening levels greater than 15 dB S/N does little to improve listening performance.). However, noise levels in classrooms in schools for the deaf typically tend to be much lower than in regular classrooms. Hence, the average S/N ratio attained with sound field amplification in schools for the deaf are likely greater than those found in regular school settings. This suggests that sound field amplification systems used in schools for the deaf might actually result in S/N ratios greater than 20 dB and, hence, support Worner's (1988) findings but further research is needed.

The reader should note that FM systems are still the system of choice for hearing-impaired students because they generally provide the best signal-to-noise ratios, but in certain cases (especially when fiscal restraint is a factor), sound field amplification might be a viable option.

In addition to the above, all services provided by the educational audiologist in the day and residential-school setting must also be provided in the mainstreamed setting.

OTHER STUDENT POPULATIONS SERVED BY EDUCATIONAL AUDIOLOGISTS

Educational audiologists often work with other student populations. These include: learning disabled, nonvocal, low-functioning students, as well as regular school children. Educational audiologists working with these student populations tend to do so on a part-time or consultant basis.

Learning Disabled Student

The term *learning disabled student* refers to a heterogeneous group of students having significant difficulties in the acquisition and use of listening, speaking, reading, writing, reasoning, or mathematical abilities (Hammill, Leigh, McNutt, and Larsen, 1981). Surveys indicate that approximately 3 percent of school-age children are learning disabled (Tucker, Stevens, and Ysseldyke, 1983). The percentage of learning-disabled children having a central auditory processing disorder is high but not precisely known. The identification and management of these problems are important because inefficient auditory processing skills may result in reading problems (DeConde, 1984) and speech and language problems (Butler, 1981). Central auditory processing (CAP) and their disorders (CAPD) refer to a variety of skills and their breakdown (see Chapter 32). The question has often been raised as to whether we are actually evaluating auditory processing skills, or assessing language comprehension and retention via the auditory modality. This may be an important theoretical issue but is irrelevant in educational audiology, since the goal of the educational audiologist is to ensure that each child adequately processes the incoming speech signal auditorily.

Willeford and Burleigh (1985) have categorized

children with CAPD into two groups. One group involves those children who have a CAPD and a language deficit. The second group includes the child with a CAPD who does not manifest a language dysfunction but does demonstrate academic and social difficulties. This child has trouble maintaining the academic pace and gaining social acceptance. A third category should be added; a number of students show evidence of a CAPD on central auditory tests, yet do not manifest academic or social difficulties. Many of these students have somehow developed compensatory strategies that allow them to do well and go "undetected." These strategies include expending a great effort to listen in class and/or relying heavily on lipreading. All students falling under these three categories can benefit from some form of auditory management program.

Many central tests are used in signifying the presence of an auditory processing disorder, however, but it is not enough to know that a student has failed one or more CAP tests. One should also determine how the student's listening disorder manifests itself. Does the student exhibit difficulties in sound-symbol relationships, decoding skills, auditory blending, auditory attention, or short-term memory? How severe are the student's listening difficulties?

In assessing learning disabled students, the audiologist must first determine whether these students, in fact, have normal hearing sensitivity. The next step requires screening for possible auditory processing problems. The "SCAN" test battery is an example of a screening procedure (Keith, 1986). The SCAN has been recorded onto audiocassette and can played on any good tape player in a quiet room. The test battery takes 20 minutes to administer. The SCAN is composed of three subtests: Filtered Words, Auditory Figure Ground, and Competing Words. The subtests have been normed on children from the ages of 3 to 11. Failure on any of these subtests suggests that the student requires more in-depth assessment. It is important to remember that the SCAN is a *screening tool* and is not meant for diagnosing an auditory processing disorder or serving as a substitute for comprehensive assessment. In addition, Keith (1986) cautions that validation research is still needed to determine the sensitivity and specificity of the SCAN. Two other popular screening tests are the Visual Aural Digit Span test by Koppitz (1975) and the Selective Auditory Attention Test by Cherry (1980). The Visual Aural Digit Span test requires the student to recall digits serially and takes less than five minutes to administer (the test is described in depth in the next section). The Selective Auditory Attention Test consists of two parts: (*1*) lists of 25 monosyllabic words prerecorded in quiet that allows the audiologist to derive a speech recognition score in percentage correct and (*2*) two equivalent lists recorded with a semantic distracter in the background, allowing for the derivation of a selective attention listening score, also in percentage correct. The lists of words are from the Word Intelligibility by Picture Identification test (Ross and Lerman, 1971). This test consists of items that are presented in a closed set format. Each test item consists of a plate of six pictures, one of which corresponds to the item presented. The test items are presented diotically, with the procedure taking approximately 8 minutes to administer. Norms are available for students from the age of 4–9 years. At present, it is not known which of the above three screening tests (or combination of tests) has the highest specificity and sensitivity for detecting students with auditory processing problems. Thus, research is needed in this area.

Once a student has been identified at risk for a listening disability by a screening test or other procedures, such as the Fisher's Auditory Problems Checklist (Fisher, 1976), a comprehensive central auditory test battery needs to be administered. Although a number of test batteries for central auditory assessment (Willeford and Burleigh, 1985; Almen, Blair, and Spriet, 1990) exist, little information is available that correlates the findings from these CAP test batteries to language/academic performance. Therefore, we must develop our own test batteries on the basis of our experience and job setting. The test battery needs to be sufficiently comprehensive so that weaknesses in any of the listening subskills will be picked up. This author has developed his own preferred test battery. The tests included and the various subskills assessed on each test are:

1. Visual Aural Digit Span

The Visual Aural Digit Span (VADS) test has been normed on students from the ages of 4–14 years (Koppitz, 1975). It is a comparative test measure in which the student is required to recall digits serially. The test stimuli are presented either visually (on cards) or auditorily, and the students are told to respond orally or by a written response. The four resultant scores are:

Input	Output	Input	Output
Visual	Oral	Visual	Written
Auditory	Oral	Auditory	Written

The results from this test allow the audiologist to determine if there are any weaknesses in serial recall, and if so, are there differences at the input and at the output stage? A difference at the output stage may indicate the effects of cross modality or the effects of increased time on short-term memory (e.g., it takes longer to write down a response than to respond verbally.). A discrepancy at the input stage indicates that the student has more difficulty processing and retaining input in one of the two modalities.

This author has noted that in auditory presentation the number of digits correctly recalled gives a good indication of the number of chunks (short-term memory span) that the student can process auditorily in everyday speech.

Another interesting way of assessing the serial recall of digits is to vary one's cadence. Usually, the digits are presented in monotone and equally spaced in time. When the numbers are grouped by cadence (e.g., 584 269), most students tend to recall one or two more digits. Learning disabled students, however, often do not show this tendency.

This author also has found that asking students to recall the auditorily presented digits in reversed order gives an indication of the student's strengths in sound-symbol relations.

2. Staggered Spondaic Word Test

The Staggered Spondaic Word (SSW) test has been normed on children as young as 5 up to the age of 60 (Katz, Yeung, and Medwetsky, 1990). Results provide information about the student's auditory decoding skills, short-term memory, sound-symbol relations and sequencing abilities. These results, in turn, can be used to predict the student's speech-in-noise ability, short-term memory for auditory content, ability to process auditory information rapidly, ability to follow directions, and related academic skills such as reading, spelling, and writing (see Chapter 17).

3. Lindamood Auditory Conceptualization Test

The Lindamood Auditory Conceptualization (LAC) has been normed on students from kindergarten to grade 7 (Lindamood and Lindamood, 1971). The Lindamood Auditory Conceptualization (LAC) assesses the student's ability to discriminate and sequence speech sounds presented in both isolation and within syllables. It is also an excellent test for assessing sound-symbol relations. The student's task is to indicate what has been heard via the manipulation of different colored blocks. Results on the LAC have been normed on students from kindergarten to grade 7. The scores achieved on the test are reliable indicators of the degree of difficulty that the student will have in reading, spelling, and writing.

4. Phonemic Synthesis Test

Norms on the Phonemic Synthesis Test (Katz and Harmon, 1982) are available down to the age of 6. This test assesses auditory decoding and the ability to blend individual phonemes in correct sequence to form a word. Results on the PST test are highly predictive of articulation, reading, spelling, and writing performance.

5. Competing Sentences Test (Willeford, 1978).

The Competing Sentences Test (CST) has been normed for students as young as age 5 years. The CST assesses auditory selective attention and divided attention for paired sentences, presented simultaneously to both ears. Paired sentences are approximately 6–8 words long and of similar content. The test can be given in two ways. In one option (selective attention), the target ear is presented with a sentence at 35 dB SL, while the other ear receives the competing sentence at 50 dB SL. The student is told, beforehand, which ear is the target and to repeat the sentence heard in that ear. In the second option (divided attention), each of these sentences is presented at 50 dB dichotically and the student is told to recall both sentences.

This author is currently working on a competing sentence test in which sentences vary from 3 to 14 words in length. This should give a better idea of the student's ability to handle sentences of various lengths.

6. Pitch Pattern Sequence Test

The Pitch Pattern Sequence Test (PPST) has been normed for students down to the age 6 (Pinheiro, 1977). Three 500-msec tones, separated by 300-msec intervals, are presented monaurally at the subject's MCL. Each test item has two high and one low pitched signals, or vice versa, that is presented in any sequence. The low-frequency tone is 800 Hz and the high-frequency tone is 1430 Hz. Subjects respond by whistling or humming, tapping on designated objects, or verbally (e.g., saying high-high-low). The results not only provide information as to pattern-perception and temporal sequencing ability but also on corpus callosum maturity.

It should be noted that none of the above tests measure sustained attention, such as required in the classroom setting. Keith (cited by Smaldino and Burk, 1990) has recently proposed a test for assessing sustained attention, the Continuous Performance Test (CPT). The CPT involves listening for and responding to target words in a string of words over approximately 10 minutes. The test holds promise, but much research is needed.

In addition to the above formal tests, the audiologist should derive information from the child's case history and meet with the student's teacher and parents.

The complete test battery listed above takes 2–3 hours to administer and, therefore, must be given over two or more sessions.

Management Techniques with Listening Disabled Students

Once testing has been completed, the audiologist needs to interpret the results and derive a profile that accurately describes the student's abilities on a number of listening subskills. In concert with the teacher and other related professionals, management techniques are then decided upon. There are a number of approaches from which to choose. One management technique is to provide parent-teacher management guidelines. These generally involve methods for controlling auditory input, such as preferential seating and visual aids. A second technique is to teach the child compensatory skills, especially those that capitalize on the visual modality. One must actually ascertain, however, that the visual modality is truly the stronger modality. It is possible that similar deficits coexist in visual perception.

A third approach involves the use of ALDs. Children with CAPD may benefit greatly from the use of FM systems or sound field amplification.

The last management technique consists of auditory perception training. There are a number of programs available (e.g., Phonemic Synthesis: Blending Sounds into Words, Precision Acoustics [Katz and Harmon, 1982]; Auditory Discrimination in Depth, DLM [Lindamood and Lindamood, 1969]). These programs usually focus on specific listening subskills. The educational audiologist must be aware of the focus of a particular training program and decide whether it suits the needs of the student.

Additional Comments

Carhart, Tillman, and Greetis (1969) found that in normal subjects a competing background consisting of one or more talkers was a more difficult listening environment than white noise. Lasky and Tobin (1973), assessing learning disabled students, found similar results. The implication from these studies is that many learning disabled children may do well on speech-in-noise tasks when the competing message consists of white noise, yet have difficulty listening in everyday situations. Hence, multitalker babble or even a single talker of similar voice pitch might be better competing signals and be more sensitive to detecting problems in background noise.

High-Functioning Nonvocal Student

High-functioning nonvocal students might include, among others, dysphasic, cerebral palsied, and brain damaged individuals. These individuals require considerable attention because they tend to exhibit a higher incidence of hearing loss, middle ear problems, and central auditory processing disorders than the general student population (Apgar and Beck, 1972). For those students possessing signing skills, assessment/management is essentially the same as for oral children. For those who do not sign, however, the test procedures will need to be modified. Before an appropriate testing strategy can be chosen, the audiologist needs certain information including the student's:

1. Communication system; that is, is the student using a communication board (with representational symbols and/or words), electronic communication aid (such as a minitypewriter), or vocal output communication aids?
2. Current level of language functioning; this information can be obtained from the teacher or the speech/language pathologist.
3. Rate of expressive language; this is important since it may introduce a memory bias into testing.

The following is a guide to various strategies that can be used to assess these students. The reader should be aware that not all strategies are applicable to a particular student (the reader is also referred to Chapter 34).

Puretone Thresholds. The audiologist can have the student respond in a variety of ways. For example, lifting one's head, shifting eye-gaze, or pointing to a yes symbol might be used as a response, depending on the child's ability.

Speech Recognition Thresholds. These can be determined by the use of a picture board.

Speech Recognition Scores. These scores can be obtained by the use of closed-set picture tests such as the Word by Picture Identification (WIPI) test (Ross and Lerman, 1970), Discrimination by Identification of Pictures (DIP) test (Siegenthaler, 1975), or the NU-CHIPS test (Elliott and Katz, 1980). Speech-in-noise testing for monosyllabic word lists simply requires the addition of noise to whatever stimulus materials are being presented. Open set testing can be done with those individuals who use minitypewriters or vocal output aids.

Sentence Recognition Scores. Although open sentence set testing is possible with those students using minitypewriters or vocal output aids, a bias may result due to the slow speed of response. The Synthetic Sentence Identification-Ipsilateral/Contralateral Competing Message tests (Jerger and Jerger, 1975) can be used as a closed-set, sentence-in-noise test as long as the student is able to read. This test requires the student to select the item heard from a randomly ordered list of ten nonsense sentences.

Central Auditory Processing Test Battery. There are a number of tests on which the non-vocal student can be assessed. These include:

1. *Visual Aural Digit Span Test.*
2. *Phonemic Synthesis Test.* The words on this test are familiar and likely to be in the student's vocabulary.
3. *Pitch Pattern Sequence Test.* The test simply requires the student to respond by indicating, in the correct sequence, the pattern of high/low tones.
4. *Lindamood Auditory Conceptualization Test.* If a student does not have the motor ability to do this test, then the student can be assessed by an eye-gaze shift from block to block.
5. *SSW Test.* The audiologist should check beforehand with the teacher to see if the words on this test are known to the child. The student's speed of response may affect the results and, therefore, needs to be considered when interpreting the scores. A bliss-symbolic approach also has been used (Glass, 1986).

If a hearing or listening disorder is identified, then management approaches appropriate to the needs of the child should be initiated. The techniques implemented are similar to those mentioned in earlier sections, although some modifications may be required.

Severe to Profound Cognitively Impaired Student

Students falling into this category include those with cognitive impairment alone and those with additional handicaps (such as deaf-blind or cognitively impaired plus motoric disability). Accurate auditory assessment of these students is difficult. Audiological reports often contain comments such as "could not test" or "the results were inconsistent." If puretone and speech thresholds have been obtained, they are likely to be su-

prathreshold. Immittance results, if the audiologist was able to place the probe tip in the student's ear, usually consist of a tympanogram; acoustic reflex thresholds are usually difficult to obtain due to the student's excessive movement (The use of acoustic reflectometry, however, provides the audiologist with a highly accurate tool for detecting the presence of middle ear effusion and requires little patient co-operation.). In summarizing the results, the audiologist might suggest Auditory Brainstem Response (ABR) audiometry (click and/or tone bursts).

There are a number of reasons why it is difficult for the clinical audiologist to obtain accurate results on the severely cognitively impaired student. First, many audiologists have had little experience testing this population. Second, the audiologist typically has a limited period of time to (*a*) review the case history, (*b*) determine an appropriate testing strategy, (*c*) do audiological conditioning, and (*d*) test the student. It is generally difficult to get these students focused and conditioned in such a short period of time. Third, the student may be fearful and become extremely agitated, making testing very difficult indeed.

Probably, the best approach is for the audiologist to take the time to initiate and supervise a conditioning program that can be carried out at the school. By working with the student and teacher on a regular basis, the audiologist will be able to find out (*a*) the child's cognitive and communicative functioning level, (*b*) the method of assessment that will be most appropriate for that child, and (*c*) the necessary modifications that will be needed.

Conditioning strategies need to be individualized. The choice of conditioning techniques needs to be decided on by both the audiologist and the teacher. Conditioning may need to be carried out every day for short periods of time, over many weeks or months. The following case illustrates the special problems that may confront the educational audiologist in carrying out a conditioning program for a particular student:

> The student is 8 years of age, cognitively functioning at the 7-month level, is totally blind but has no motor impairments. The child is suspected of having a hearing loss. Traditional conditioning by COR (conditioning by orienting response audiometry) is contraindicated because of the visual impairment. The educational audiologist observes that the student enjoys vibrotactile sensations.

This author has developed a modified VROCA (visually reinforced operant conditioning audiometry) procedure that is an extension of a technique developed by Wilson and Thompson (1984) for conditioning cognitively-impaired, hearing impaired-blind students

(Note that even though a student may be designated as being blind, the student may actually have some degree of visual acuity.). The modified procedure uses both visual and tactile reinforcers. The conditioning apparatus utilizes a touch pad that is connected to a vibrator housed underneath it. The touch pad is also wired to a brightly lit toy and an examiner on-off switch. The on-off position of the examiner switch determines whether the reinforcers can be activated. The vibrator and lit-toy can be activated by the student only when the examiner switch is in the on-position. This prevents the student from being rewarded when no sounds have actually been presented.

The student's task is to press down on the touch pad each time a sound stimulus is presented. At the beginning of conditioning, the student's hand is guided to, and pressed down on to, the touch pad each time a sound is presented. This activates the vibrator and toy. The hope is that the student will eventually make the connection between the sound presentation and depressing the touch pad for the reward. This test procedure can also be used for testing localization, by using two touch pads placed on either side of the student.

To accustom the student to the clinical setting, it is suggested that conditioning be conducted, at least occasionally, in a quiet, darkened room. Once the student has been fairly well conditioned, testing can be scheduled with the teacher and parent present, if possible. Testing should use the same techniques and equipment used to condition the student.

As with any other population, if a hearing loss is diagnosed, then the audiologist must be involved in the subsequent management. Often, such students have been diagnosed as having a hearing loss and issued hearing aids, yet the hearing aids are not being worn. The problem, usually, is that the staff members have had little or no training in the use of hearing aids. Inservices will promote greater familiarity with hearing aids, and, in turn, the hearing aids will be used more effectively.

CONCLUSION

Educational audiologists serve many student populations including: the hearing impaired, listening disabled, physically and cognitively impaired. Such students cannot be adequately served by occasional visits to a hospital or speech and hearing clinic. An effective educational audiology program requires the audiologist to conduct evaluations, provide inservice training for the staff, help develop individualized auditory and communication skill programs, ensure maintenance of hearing aids and assistive listening devices, and counsel both parents and students. The expenditure of time involved in carrying out these responsibilities precludes the audiologist from being directly involved in all of these endeavors. This limitation can be overcome by training other staff members to do hearing aid maintenance, immittance screening, and certain hearing/listening tests.

Clearly, the field of educational audiology is still developing. Universities need to develop educational audiology programs or incorporate appropriate courses into the curriculum that are relevant to the field of educational audiology. Administrative officials, both at the school board level and at the government level, need to be sensitized to the needs of hearing/listening impaired students and how many of these needs may be met by hiring more full-time educational audiologists.

The future of educational audiology appears bright. Audiologists have a greater understanding of speech processing in the hearing impaired and developmentally disabled populations and have developed useful assessment tools. Computer technology has had, and will continue to have, a great impact on educational audiology services including: hearing aid fitting, auditory assessment, and data collection. Further improvements in assistive listening devices will ensure that the effects of noise and reverberation are lessened. The full benefits of these innovations will occur, however, only when it is recognized that educational audiologists are essential to the habilitative process of hearing-impaired and listening-disabled students.

REFERENCES

Almen PV, Blair JC, and Spriet SY. Central auditory assessment. Educ Aud Assoc Newsl 1990;7(2):10–11.

American Speech-Language-Hearing Association. Ad Hoc Committee on Extension of Audiologic Services in the Schools. ASHA 1980;22:263–264.

Apgar V, and Beck J. Is My Baby All Right? A Guide to Birth Defects. New York: Trident Press, 1972.

Berg F. Educational audiology at Utah State University. J Acad Rehabil Audiol 1974;7:40–49.

Berg FS, Blair JC, Viehweg SH, and Wilson A. Educational Audiology for the Hard of Hearing Child. Orlando, Florida: Grune & Stratton, 1986.

Bess FH, and McConnell FE. Audiology, Education and the Hearing Impaired. St. Louis: CV Mosby, 1981.

Blair JC, Wilson-Vlotman A, and Von Almen P. Educational audiologist: practices, problems, directions, recommendations. Educ Aud Monograph 1989;1:1–14.

Boothroyd A. Developments in speech audiometry. Br J Aud 1968;2:3–10.

Boothroyd A. Auditory perception of speech contrasts by subjects with sensorineural hearing loss. J Speech Hear Res 1984;27(1):134–144.

Boothroyd A, Springer N, Smith L, and Schulman J. Amplitude compression and profound hearing loss. J Speech Hear Res 1988;31:362–376.

Butler K. Language processing disorders: factors in diagnosis and remediation. In Keith R, Ed. Central Auditory and Language Disorders in Children. Houston: College Hill Press, 1981.

Carhart R, Tillman TW, and Greetis ES. Perceptual masking in multiple sound backgrounds. J Acoust Soc Am 1969;45:694–703.

Chellappa M, and Ross M. Predictability of hearing aid response based on FM coupling method. Internal Report, Rehabilitation Engineering Center of Lexington Center, Inc., 1991.

Cherry RS. Selective Auditory Attention Test. St. Louis: Auditec of St. Louis, 1980.

DeConde C. Children with central processing disorders. In Hull RH, and Dilka KI, Eds. The Hearing Impaired Child in School. New York: Grune & Stratton, 1984.

Deconde Johnson C. Update on survey of state educational audiology guidelines and certification/licensure. Educ Aud Assoc Newsl 1990;7(4):4–5.

Dubno JR, Dirks DD, and Langhofer LR. Evaluation of hearing-impaired listeners using a nonsense-syllable test. II. Syllable recognition and consonant confusion patterns. J Speech Hear Res 1982;25:141–148.

Elliott LL, and Katz DR. Northwestern University Children's Perception of Speech. St. Louis: Auditec, 1980.

Erber NP, and Alencewicz CM. Audiologic evaluation of deaf children. J Speech Hear Disord 1976;41:256–267.

Erber NP. Use of the Auditory Numbers Test to evaluate speech perception abilities of hearing-impaired children. J Speech Hear Disord 1980;45:527–532.

Erber N. Auditory Training. AG Bell Association for the Deaf, Washington, 1982.

Finitzo-Hieber T, Gerlin IJ, Matkin ND, and Cherow-Skalka E. A sound effects recognition test for the pediatric evaluation. Ear Hear 1980;1:271–276.

Fisher LI. Fisher Auditory Problems Checklist. Cedar Rapids, IA: Grant Wood Area Education Agency, 1976.

Flexer C. Turn on sound: an odyssey of sound field amplification. Educ Aud Assoc Newsl 1989;5:6–7.

Flexer C, Millin JP, and Brown L. Children with developmental disabilities: the effect of sound field amplification on word identification. Lang Speech Hear Serv Schools 1990;21:177–182.

Geers AE, and Moog JS. Evaluating speech perception skills: tools for measuring benefits of cochlear implants, tactile aids, and hearing aids. In Owens E, and Kessler DK, Eds. Cochlear Implants in Young Deaf Children. Boston: Little, Brown and Company, 1989.

Glass JL. Assessing central auditory processing in children with cerebral palsy using a blissymbolic mode. Paper presented at the American Academy for Cerebral Palsy and Developmental Medicine. New Orleans, LA, 1986.

Hammill DD, Leigh J, McNutt G, and Larsen SC. A new definition of learning disabilities. Learn Disabil 1981;4:336–341.

Haskins HA. A phonetically balanced test of speech discrimination for children [Unpublished master's thesis]. Northwestern University, 1949.

Hawkins D. Comparisons of speech recognition in noise by mildly-to-moderately hearing-impaired children using hearing aids and FM systems. J Speech Hear Disord 1984;49:401–418.

Hawkins D, and Schum D. Some effects of FM-system coupling on hearing aid characteristics. J Speech Hear Disord 1985;50:132–141.

Hirsh IJ, Davis H, Silverman SR, Reynolds EG, Eldert E, and Benson RW. Development of materials for speech audiometry. J Speech Hear Disord 1952;17:321–337.

Hutchinson K. Evaluation of a basic auditory training program. Paper presented at the ASHA convention in Detroit, MI, 1980.

Jerger JF, and Jerger SW. Clinical validity of central auditory tests. Scand Audiol 1975;4:147,163.

Jerger SW, Jerger JF, and Abrams S. Speech audiometry in young children. Ear Hear 1983;4:56–66.

Joint Committee on Audiology and Education of the Deaf. Audiology and Education of the Deaf. Research Grant from the Vocational Rehabilitation Administration, Department of Health, Education and Welfare, Washington, DC, 20201, 1965.

Katz J, and Harmon C. Phonemic Synthesis: Blending Sounds Into Words. Allen, TX: Developmental Learning Materials, 1982.

Katz J, Yeung E, and Medwetsky L. SSW C*I*R: A Computer Program for Calculations, Interpretations and Recommendations of SSW Test Results. Amherst, NY: Jimm Co., 1990.

Keith RW. SCAN: A screening test for auditory processing disorders. San Antonio, TX: The Psychological Corporation, Harcourt Brace Jovanovich, Inc, 1986.

Koppitz EM. Bender Gestalt Test, Visual Aural Digit Span Test and reading achievement. J Learn Disabil 1975;8(3):32–35.

Lasky EZ, and Tobin H. Linguistic and nonlinguistic competing message effects. J Learn Disabil 1973;6(4):46–53.

Lindamood C, and Lindamood P. Auditory Discrimination in Depth. Allen, TX: Developmental Learning Materials, 1969.

Lindamood C, and Lindamood P. The Lindamood Auditory Conceptualization Test. Allen, TX: Developmental Learning Materials, 1971.

Medwetsky L. The importance of spatial and talker cues on competing sentence recall [Unpublished dissertation]. 1991.

Medwetsky L, and Boothroyd A. The effect of microphone location on the speech spectrum. Manuscript in preparation, 1991a.

Medwetsky L, and Boothroyd A. Effects of noise on speech perception by severe/profound hearing impaired as a function of different amplification techniques. Lexington Center: Internal report APD #2.6. 1991b.

Owens E, and Schubert ED. Development of the California Consonant Test. J Speech Hear Res 1977;20:463–474.

Pinheiro M. Tests of central auditory function in children with learning disabilities. In Keith R, Ed. Central Auditory Dysfunction. New York: Grune & Stratton, 1977.

Ross M, and Lerman J. A picture identification test for hearing-impaired children. J Speech Hear Res 1970;13:44–53.

Sarff L, Ray H, and Bagwell C. Why not amplification in every classroom? Hear Aid J 1981;34(October):11,52.

Siegenthaler B. Reliability of the TIP and DIP speech-hearing tests for children. J Comm Disord 1975;8:325–333.

Smaldino J, and Burk J. Evaluation of attention deficits in children. Paper presented at American Auditory Society Meeting. Seattle, WA:1990.

Stone JR, and Olswang LB. The hidden challenges in counselling. ASHA 1989;31(6/7):27–31.

Thibodeau LM. Electroacoustic performance of direct-input hearing aids with FM amplification systems. Lang Speech Hear Serv Schools 1990;21(1):49–56.

Tucker J, Stevens L, and Ysseldyke J. Learning disabilities: the expert speaks out. J Learn Disabil 1983;16(1):6–14.

Tyler RS, Gantz BJ, McCabe BF, Lowder MW, Otto SR, and Preece JP. Audiological results with two single-channel cochlear implants. Ann Oto Rhino Laryngol 1985;94:133–139.

Wepman J. Auditory discrimination test. Chicago: Language Research Associates, 1973.

Willeford JA. Sentence tests of central auditory dysfunction. In Katz, J, Ed. Handbook of Clinical Audiology, 2nd Ed. Baltimore: Williams & Wilkins, 1978.

Willeford JA, and Burleigh JM. Handbook of Central Auditory Processing Disorders in Children. New York: Grune & Stratton, 1985.

Wilson WR, and Thompson G. Behavioral audiometry. In Jerger J, Ed. Pediatric Audiology: Current Trends. San Diego: College Hill Press, 1984.

Wilson-Vlotman A, and Blair J. A survey of audiologists working full-time in school systems. ASHA 1986;28(11):33–38.

Worner WA. An inexpensive group FM amplification system for the classroom. Volta Rev 1988;90(1):29–36.

Yater VV. Educational Audiology. In Katz J, Ed. Handbook of Clinical Audiology, 2nd ed. Baltimore: Williams & Wilkins, 1978.

TEST BATTERIES

Minimal Auditory
    Capabilities Battery:

ADDRESS:

Auditec of St. Louis, 156 W. Argonne, St. Louis, MO 63122

Test of Auditory Comprehension: Foreworks, P.O. Box 9747, North Hollywood, CA 91609.

Appendix 33.1

Suggested test battery for assessing hearing impaired students. Within each level of speech stimuli, tests are arranged in order of response difficulty. Tests are selected on the basis of the student's linguistic and auditory abilities.

I. ENVIRONMENTAL SOUND TESTS

  A. Closed set, forced-choice discrimination: Minimal Auditory Capabilities (MAC) battery #4 (Auditec, 1981)

  B. Closed set, forced-choice identification:

    1. Test of Auditory Comprehension (TAC) #1. (Foreworks, 1979)

    2. TAC: #2,

    3. Iowa Cochlear Implant (ICI) test battery #7 (Tyler et al., 1985)

    4. Sound Effects Recognition Test (Finitzo-Hieber et al., 1980)

  C. Open set recognition:
ICI #3 and MAC #10. Note that the ICI subtest is an expanded version of the MAC subtest.

II. SPEECH ELEMENT TESTS

  A. Suprasegmental Features (intonation, stress, intensity, duration, # of syllables)

    1. Closed set, forced-choice identification:

      a. Pattern Perception (duration, syllables); from Low-Verbal Early Speech

      b. Perception (ESP) test battery (Geers and Moog, 1989)

      c. Auditory Numbers Test (ANT) (syllables) (Erber, 1980)

      d. Monosyllabic-Trochaic-Spondees (MTS) tests (syllables) (Erber and Alencewicz, 1976)

      e. TAC #3 (messages differ in stress, rhythm, and intonation)

      f. Speech Pattern Contrast (SPAC) test (intonation, stress) (Boothroyd, 1984)

    2. Open set recognition:

      a. ICI: #6 (syllables)

      b. ICI: #10 (male/female speaker recognition)

      c. MAC: #1 (intonation)

      d. MAC: #5 (stress)

  B. Phonetic Features

    1. Scoring is done by extrapolation of phonetic feature categories from vowel (Medwetsky, unpublished) and consonant matrices (Phoneme Identification Test: Hutchinson, 1980)

    2. Closed set, forced choice discrimination: Three Interval Forced Choice (THRIFT) test (Boothroyd et al., 1988)

    3. Closed set, forced-choice identification

      A. SPAC

      B. Nonsense Syllable Test (Dubno et al., 1982)

  C. Phonemes

    1. Vowel and Consonant Matrices. Can be evaluated by detection, discrimination, and/or identification.

    2. Closed set, forced-choice identification tests. The tests below consist of test items in which groups of words are identical except for one phoneme. Scores give an indication of the ability to identify words in a closed set; in addition, results indicate which phonemes pose difficulty for the client.

      A. MAC: #2 (medial vowels); ICI #1 (medial vowels)

      B. MAC: #7 (initial consonants); #13 (final consonants)
ICI: #2 (initial consonants); #5 (final consonants)

      C. California Consonant Test (Owens and Shubert, 1977)

Note that the items on the ICI and MAC tests listed here are the same but recorded by different speakers.

    3. Extrapolation of phoneme recognition scores from word tests: Phoneme Recognition Score from the AB Word List (Boothroyd, 1968)

III. WORDS

  A. Detection
Speech Awareness Threshold (spondees usually used)

  B. Discrimination

    1. MAC: #8 Spondee Same/Different Test

2. Wepman Auditory Discrimination Test (Wepman, 1973)

C. Identification

1. Closed set, forced-choice tests
   a. ANT
   b. Spondee Identification Test, from the ESP
   c. MTS
   d. Word Identification Subtest (from the low-verbal ESP)
   e. Body Parts (student asked to point to various body parts)
   f. Discrimination by Identification of Pictures (DIP) (Siegenthaler, 1975)
   g. Word Intelligibility by Picture Identification Test (WIPI) (Ross and Lerman, 1970)
   h. Monosyllabic Word Identification Test, from the ESP
   i. Alphabet (student asked to repeat letters from the alphabet)

2. Open set tests
   a. CID W-22 List (Hirsh et al., 1952)
   b. Pediatric Speech Intelligibility (PSI) test (Jerger et al., 1983)
   c. PBK-50 List (Haskins, 1949)
   d. AB Word List

IV. SENTENCE TESTS

1. PSI (sentence portion)
2. ICI: #8 (without context); #9 (with context)
3. CHABA Everyday Sentence test (MAC #6, Auditec)
4. The Synthetic Sentence Identification-Ipsilateral/Contralateral Competing Message test (Jerger and Jerger, 1975)

V. CONNECTED DISCOURSE

1. TAC: #7, 8, 9, 10
2. Tracking procedure

CHAPTER 34

Developmental Disabilities

Carolyn V. Young

Working with individuals who have developmental disabilities affords an opportunity to learn about many conditions that can adversely affect human development between conception and adulthood. Workers in the field of developmental disabilities continually discover new intrinsic (genetic) and extrinsic (environmental) factors which can cause mischief or even wreak havoc upon a maturing individual.

Hearing loss among persons with developmental disabilities often remains unidentified because auditory inattention is attributed to or masked by whatever is the apparent disability. Disturbing reports persist of normally intelligent, hearing-impaired persons found after many years in programs for the retarded. Typically, the persons with the losses have been assumed to "hear what they want to hear." Such misdiagnoses seem archaic in our world of advanced technology, yet they persist.

During preparation of this chapter, the editor of this text and I were reminded of epigrams we had seen on tea tags from Salada Tea Company: (1) Be careful of the theories on which you bias your opinions. (2) A little experience upsets a lot of theory. Both of us have found these maxims to be useful in our training programs and to have as much validity for Katz's work with central auditory disorders as for mine with developmental disabilities. As an introduction to this topic, some fundamental questions will be addressed. What is a developmental disability? Are many persons affected? What deficits might coexist with a hearing loss and complicate life circumstances for someone with a developmental disability? How can the audiologist help to identify neglected hearing loss in this population and provide patients and their caretakers with options for improving services?

DEVELOPMENT DISABILITY

Definition

Most people assume that "development disability" is a euphemism for "mental retardation." Actually mental retardation is only one of many conditions that may be a developmental disability. Although at least half of this diverse population is likely to be significantly impaired intellectually, the fact must be stressed that many persons with a developmental disability have normal or even greater than normal intelligence (Gollay, 1979).

In 1975 Public Law 94-103 established a categorical definition of "developmental disability" as mental retardation, cerebral palsy, epilepsy, autism or related condition impairing intelligence or adaptive behavior to such an extent as to constitute a "substantial handicap" for the affected person's normal functioning in society. Advocates for people with handicaps protested the categorization of persons with diagnostic labels rather than a description of their needs. Consequently, in 1978, the definition was revised to emphasize limitations curtailing independent living and the need for services to ameliorate the limitations. The diagnosis itself is no longer the dominating component of the definition.

The current, functional definition was passed November 6, 1978 (PL 95-602, generally known as "Rehabilitation, Comprehensive Services and Developmental Disabilities Amendments of 1978"). It was revised in October 1990 (PL 101-496, "Developmental Disabilities Assistance and Bill of Rights Act of 1990"). The term "developmental disability" means a severe, chronic disability of a person 5 years of age or older that: (1) is attributable to a mental or physical impairment or combination of mental and physical impairments; (2) is manifested before the person attains age 22; (3) is likely to continue indefinitely; (4) results in substantial functional limitations in three or more of the following areas of major life activity: self-care, receptive and expressive language, learning, mobility, self-direction, capacity for independent living and economic sulf-sufficiency; and (5) reflects the person's need for a combination and sequence of special, interdisciplinary, or generic care, treatment or other services that are of lifelong or extended duration and are individually planned and coordinated. The term "developmental disabilities" when applied to infants and young children means individuals from birth to age 5, inclusive, who have substantial developmental delay or specific congenital or acquired conditions with a high probability of resulting in developmental disabilities if services are not provided.

Number of Persons Affected

All Developmental Disabilities. The National Task Force on the Definition of Developmental Disabilities (Cerva, 1977) estimated a prevalence of 5% in the United States when all developmental disabilities were considered together. This includes approximately 8.7 million persons, of whom more than 6 million have mental retardation; 710,000 have cerebral palsy; 1 million have epilepsy; and another million have other neurologic handicaps, other than deafness and blindness (ASHA, 1971). The actual numbers of those who may have more than one condition are not well documented, but certainly many of the categories overlap.

Developmental Disability with Hearing Loss. Many persons severely handicapped by their hearing loss will not be considered multihandicapped because they lack any other evident disability. The current definition of developmental disability, however, allows eligiblility for services previously denied to persons with hearing loss if the loss imposes barriers to everyday living in at least three of the designated life activities, e.g., language, learning, and independent living.

Concomitant Conditions in Populations with Known Hearing Loss

Among students with hearing loss in special education classes in this country, approximately one-third have an additional disability (Karchmer, 1985). A little more than 30% has been a consistent prevalence figure reported over 15 years and has also been reported in Canadian schools. Nearly 10% of these children will have two or more concomitant handicapping conditions (see Figure 34.1).

Unfortunately, the audiologist's preoccupation with ears has too often obliterated awareness of the second major learning modality: vision. Thirty-eight to 58% of persons with hearing impairment have associated ocular abnormalities (Campbell et al., 1981). Approximately 65% of deaf postsecondary level students have visual problems, according to a study at National Technical Institute for the Deaf (NTID) (Johnson and Crandall, 1982). In the group found to have problems with far visual acuity ("nearsightedness"), nearly 10% had inappropriate or no corrective lenses.

Hearing Loss in Populations with Other Known Conditions

Mental Retardation. In public school programs, children in classes for the retarded have a hearing loss prevalence three times greater than normal children in the same system (Lloyd and Young, 1969).

In public schools for the mentally retarded, 15% of

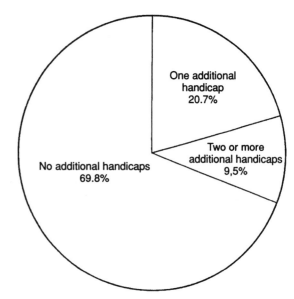

Figure 34.1. Additional handicapping conditions among 53,899 hearing impaired students. [Note: Information on additional handicapping conditions was not available for 1237 students, 2.2% of the 55,136 total reported to the 1982–1983 Annual Survey of Hearing Impaired Children and Youth.]

Table 34.1
Percentage of Hearing Impaired Children Manifesting Various Additional Handicaps, 1982–1983

Handicapping Condition	Percentage of 1982–1983 Annual Survey Population[a]
No additional handicaps	69.8
Mental retardation	8.5
Learning disability	8.1
Emotional or behavioral problem	5.6
Uncorrected visual problem	4.0
Other health impairment	3.8
Cerebral palsy	2.9
Orthopedic problem	2.6
Other	2.2
Brain damage	2.1
Heart disorder	2.0
Legal blindness	2.0
Epilepsy	1.3

[a]Column totals more than 100% because approximately 10% of the children had more than one AHC.

the children have educationally significant hearing loss (Lloyd and Moore, 1972).

In state residential institutions for the mentally retarded, 10% of both children and adults are hearing impaired (Healey and Karp-Nortman, 1975). Considering the current national trend to deinstitutionalization which leaves only the most substantially handicapped individuals in state residential programs, one can expect that this percentage would be at least doubled if it were based on statistics more recent than those on which the 1975 Healey and Karp-Nortman data were calculated.

Cerebral Palsy. Among persons with cerebral palsy, the highest incidence of hearing loss will be among those with athetosis. With improved pre- and neonatal conditions, however, the kernicterus that precipitates athetosis has declined. Specific incidences of reported hearing loss in the population with cerebral palsy have varied widely in different studies (Siegenthaler, 1987), but clearly this is a group with more loss than the normal population.

Down Syndrome. Composite studies suggest that approximately one-half to three-fourths of persons with Down syndrome are estimated to have hearing loss worse than 15dB hearing level (ANSI-1969).

Among infants with Down syndrome, approximately half will show evidence of conductive pathology (Strome, 1981).

Approximately one-fourth of adults with Down syndrome have sensory neural hearing loss (Keiser et al., 1981; Jahn and Becker, 1982).

Approximately 8% of both institutionalized (Fulton and Lloyd, 1968) as well as noninstitutionalized (Downs, 1980) persons with Down syndrome have mixed hearing loss.

Otologic management begun before the age of one is expected to reduce the prevalence of hearing loss in this population (Strome, 1981).

Other Complicating Factors

Those persons with multiple handicaps are the most likely to have disorders that would be rare in a more normal population. Audiologists who frequently evaluate hearing in these persons become accustomed to seeing unusual, yet reliable, audiometric configurations. An individual with any congenital anomaly is more likely to have a second problem, perhaps less obvious, than is someone without the first defect (Lloyd and Young, 1969). Each additional known disorder affecting a patient raises the probability that others might exist that remain to be identified. The more conspicuous a disability is, the more it tends to obscure recognition of others.

Programs with the benefit of a staff geneticist seem especially attuned to making sense out of complex symptomatology. Although familial deafness commonly represents genetic strains inherited without associated disabilities, many of the approximately 150 genetic syndromes with deafness do include other handicapping conditions (Wolff and Harkins, 1986). In the absence of genetic consultation, patients with developmental disabilities should have the advantage of a comprehensive medical examination. This can help to identify disorders that may be overlooked because the presenting problem preoccupies the diagnostician.

A hearing loss is best understood and managed only within the context of all other assets and liabilities a person might have. Because all disorders associated with hearing loss cannot possibly be covered in this chapter overview, attention will be given to those conditions most commonly seen by the audiologist serving patients with developmental disabilities.

Impaired Vision

From that ubiquitous reference, "someone's wall," I obtained the startling tidbit: "More than 50 out of every 100 Americans wear glasses—which gives you some idea of how important ears can be." The point cannot be stressed enough that information about visual status should be required for all persons with impaired hearing. Considering the frequency with which visual cues are recommended to supplement deficient auditory cues, audiologists should be more aware of visual problems that will complicate compensatory strategies for a person with both major modalities impaired. Persons with severe handicaps have a prevalence of visual impairments ranging between 75 and 95% (Cress et al., 1981), although this population has generally been dismissed as "unable to perform" on tests of visual function. Using a vision screening test developed at Parsons Research Center, Cress and her coworkers were able to obtain visual information for 90% of a population previously considered to be untestable.

> Most learning theorists concur that the vast majority—as high as 99 percent—of acquired information and knowledge is learned through the two sensory modalities of vision and audition. Impairment of both dominant modalities not only compounds the problem, but significantly changes the type of educational or rehabilitative program required, and fosters an array of learning, methodological, social psychological, and career implications (Hicks and Pfau, 1979).

For persons dependent on vision for communication, ophthalmological examination with treatment, if indicated, is critical. In addition to assessing visual acuity and identifying ocular disease, it may help in isolating the etiology of a hearing loss. Campbell et al. (1981) note that even with using an extensive battery of tests, the cause of an early onset hearing loss can remain undetermined in two-thirds of the cases. Some of these etiologies, however, can be illuminated with a thorough eye examination. Follow-up planning can then proceed more realistically, with genetic counseling provided as needed.

Cognitive and Adaptive Behavior Deficits

When both hearing loss and mental retardation afflict a person, they conspire to exert a devastating impact on language development. With intact intellectual functioning, compensatory learning schemes can be readily taught to those with sensory impairments. Nevertheless, compensatory strategies would be less likely to develop in the absence of at least high average intelligence (Sak and Ruben, 1981).

Intelligence has traditionally been ranked with IQ scores (see Appendix 34.1), but the American Association on Mental Deficiency requires that adaptive behavior must also be considered before a person is labeled as mentally retarded. Adaptive behavior includes social adjustment and judgement, self-help and communication skills, academic and vocational performance, when applicable (Grossman, 1977; ASHA Committee on Mental Retardation/Developmental Disabilities, 1982).

The lines of demarcation presumed to exist between intellectual, emotional, and affective disorders frequently become blurred outside of textbooks. Equally competent authorities, sometimes widely recognized in their respective fields, can arrive at different diagnoses for the same person. Many times individuals with severe handicaps are excluded from services at a program because what is considered to be their "primary" disability is not suitable for inclusion in the program. When more than one handicapping condition occurs in the same person, however, "multiple disabilities interact with each other in such a way that their relative effects cannot be separated" (Jones, 1982).

Neuromuscular Disorders

Since the definition of developmental disabilities was revised in 1978, many neuromuscular disorders besides cerebral palsy are considered to place one at risk to become developmentally disabled. Such disorders include, but are not limited to, early onset multiple sclerosis, hereditary progressive muscular dystrophies, childhood Huntington disease and cerebral vascular accidents incurred before age 22. Among all of the conditions involving neuromuscular problems, cerebral palsy will probably be the one seen most often by the audiologist.

The audiologist who plans to use a visual reinforcement procedure should be aware that approximately two-thirds of the population with spastic cerebral palsy may have concomitant visual defects; the population with athetoid cerebral palsy has been found to have similar visual defects but less often (Duckman, 1987). Individuals with athetoid cerebral palsy should be tested with signals presented at times that will compete

as little as possible with the 30 to 40 db of masking generated by their involuntary body movements; individuals with spastic cerebral palsy are likely to hear less well when severe spasms and abnormal reflex activity disrupt attending behavior (Mysak, 1971). The patient who is stiffened in hyperextension will probably be unable to show any reaction but frustration. The audiologist would be wise to seek consultation from a physical or occupational therapist to avoid testing techniques that might evoke abnormal reflex activity.

Unquestionably, a response task must be suited to both the cognitive and neuromuscular abilities of a patient. Generally, a parent or other caretaker can advise an audiologist what the individual with a neuromuscular disorder is able to do and not do and which position is most conducive to voluntary control. Unless the person can demonstrate some recognizable behavioral change associated with sensory stimulation, interpretation of "results" is spurious at best.

Seizure Disorders

Repeated seizures are the identifying symptom of epilepsy. Seizures are of many different types originating from erratic electrochemical impulses in various areas of the brain. They are classified as partial (focal) or generalized, depending on the pervasiveness of the neuronal misfiring in the brain. Grand mal and petit mal (absence attacks) are both generalized seizures (Epilepsy Foundation of America, 1973).

An explanation of how to differentiate generalized and partial seizures, the latter having a local origin, is beyond the scope of this chapter. The audiologist needs to be aware, however, that the bright or flickering lights often used with visual reinforcement procedures may precipitate a seizure in patients sensitive to photic stimulation (Hughes, 1981). J. Katz (personal communication, 1983) has seen some patients with seizure-like falling episodes during audiometric evaluation; these episodes appeared to be audiogenic and were associated with specific audiometric frequencies.

Occasionally, persons with developmental disabilities are so heavily medicated to quell seizure activity that they appear oblivious to their auditory environment. Though audiometric testing might be unsuccessful, tympanometry can be done readily with most such patients. The acoustic reflex, furthermore, ordinarily is not obliterated in patients receiving medications for behavior or seizure control (Evans, 1983).

Some seizure manifestations are similar to behaviors that are not seizure related. These behaviors may cause a person to seem inattentive to the auditory environment. Suspicion should be aroused by inexplicable behavior alteration, such as a sudden postural change, inappropriate pauses while talking, reduced attention span, perseverative purposeless behaviors such as picking at clothes, lip smacking or other odd facial, tongue or jaw movements (Bernstein, 1981). If such behavior is seizure related, audiologic testing will be ineffective during the seizure episodes, and the examiner must wait for the erratic brain activity to subside. Patients with such symptoms warrant referral for neurologic examination.

Stereotypy

The resourcefulness and versatility of an audiologist are rarely so taxed as when attempting to test someone with persistent, repetitious, frequently bizarre behaviors (e.g., body rocking, head swaying and finger flicking) that cannot be extinguished during an evaluation session. These behaviors are often referred to as "self-stim" (the shortened form for "self-stimulatory behaviors"), but a study of these behaviors reveals that such a term is based on a theory the veracity of which remains to be demonstrated. In an excellent overview of the topic, Baumeister (1978) has written, "Indeed, a persuasive argument may be made that stereotyped movements actually induce a state of stimulus deprivation." Psychologists generally use the term "stereotypy" to refer to this type of rhythmic, repetitive movement lacking apparent adaptive significance.

Although origins and functions of stereotypic movements remain enigmatic, their manifestations are obvious even to the casual observer and include an almost infinite variety of idiosyncratic behaviors. The problem for the audiologist is that many stereotyping individuals seem unaware of anything around them when they are preoccupied with their own peculiar, repetitious mannerisms. The problem is exacerbated when vocalizations accompany the stereotyped movements. Vocalizations will mask any test signals of lesser intensity, thereby interfering with threshold approximations, and will also create movement artifacts which obscure immittance measures.

Simply being introduced into a sound-controlled testing suite can precipitate acceleration of a patient's stereotypy. The audiologist or an assistant may need to intrude physically to subdue the stereotypy's interference with test signals. Complete restraint of movement, however, can produce increased stereotyped responding following release (Baumeister, 1978). The audiologist, therefore, can try calming the most disruptive stereotypic acts while not confining the lesser ones. Tangible reinforcement of operant conditioned audiometry (TROCA) has often been used successfully with these individuals, especially if repeat sessions can be arranged to teach the task to those who do not demonstrate proficiency within the time frame of one evaluation.

At the Institute for the Study of Developmental Disabilities, several children have been brought to the audiologist because ear problems were thought to be contributing to some self-injurious stereotypic behaviors, such as head banging, face slapping or ear poking. Often these children were very tactually defensive, especially to having someone touch their head. Immittance measures were possible only for those small enough to be restrained by clinicians. Examination by the consulting otolaryngologist was also accomplished only with the aid of strong assistants and/or sedation. Sometimes cerumen removal could not be done except under anesthesia. This procedure, which might seem extreme, resulted not only in cerumen removal, but also in the discovery of cholesteatomas in some of these children. Removal of a cholesteatoma typically did not extinguish a stereotypy, but for most of the cases the intensity of the stereotypy subsided.

Down Syndrome

Individuals with Down syndrome constitute probably the best recognized group with developmental disabilities. The incidence of Down Syndrome was formerly estimated to be 1 of 600 live births but has decreased to nearly one in 1000 live births (Buchanan, 1990). In the population of persons with mental retardation, 1 in 10 individuals can be expected to have Down syndrome (Coleman, 1980). Over 90% of persons with Down syndrome have three of chromosome no. 21, instead of the two that are normal. Hence, the syndrome's name, trisomy 21. Only part of the 21st chromosome, specifically, the distal segment of its long arm, is responsible for the phenotype (characteristic appearance) of Down syndrome (Wisniewski and Wisniewski, 1983).

Educational Potential. Many professionals, unfortunately, continue to maintain that Down syndrome foreordains one to trainable or subtrainable educational programs; however, Rynders et al. (1978) scrutinized medical and psychoeducational literature about Down syndrome from 1967 to 1976 and noted that researchers have apparently considered the condition to be uniform and often have not reported relevant or potentially relevant variables that might influence psychometric studies. These authors, additionally, reviewed findings from some early intervention programs for these children and concluded that the group spans a large range of intellectual abilities. The ultimate potential achievements are constantly expanding, and their parents may be told realistically that a baby with Down syndrome has a good chance to be psychometrically educable, that is, in the mild range of mental retardation. When proper attention is given to the auditory deficit of these children, their outlook might be even more optimistic during school years.

Precocious Aging. In later years, an accelerated aging process may lead to early neuropathological changes, including compromised immune defenses, degenerative vascular changes, recent memory loss, premature cataracts, and presbycusis (Buchanan, 1990; Wisniewski and Wisniewski, 1983). Buchanan has reported that high-frequency impairment is common in this population as early as the first decade (see Fig. 34.2).

Outer Ear Anomalies. Among newborns with Down syndrome the pinnae are more than 2 standard deviations shorter than in normal newborns (Strome, 1981); the shorter than normal longitudinal dimension is also seen in older individuals (Balkany, 1980). The outer ear is often low set (Sando et al., 1983) with the helix folded over. The external auditory meatus is typically narrow with a diameter averaging one-half to two-thirds the size of that in non-Down syndrome children of the same age (Balkany, 1980). About 40% of this population can be found to have stenotic canals, and approximately three-fourths of this group with stenosis exhibit middle ear effusion (Schwartz and Schwartz, 1978; Strome, 1981).

Middle Ear Anomalies. The middle ears of this population have been found to have ossicular malfor-

mations or erosion from chronic otitis media; deformities from both etiologies are almost indistinguishable (Balkany, 1980). Harada and Sando (1981) did histopathologic studies of temporal bones and found many abnormalities of the middle ear, the most common of which was the round window niche having a remnant of mesenchymal tissue. In this study, only one patient with mesenchymal remnants had essentially normal hearing. These investigators speculate, nevertheless, that conductive hearing loss might result from this anomaly if additional conditions are present, specifically, "complete obstruction of the round window niche by the tissue; presence of such tissue in the epitympanum and tissue surrounding the ossicles. . .; or tissue accompanied by other abnormalities, such as narrow round window niche with a small opening to the middle ear cavity."

Schwartz and Schwartz (1978) have proposed that the hypotonicity characteristic of this syndrome may involve the tensor veli palatini responsible for opening the eustachian tube. Juxtaposed to the small nasopharyngeal fossa, seen frequently in individuals with Down syndrome, the reduced tonicity of the tensor could lead to middle ear effusion unresolved by treatment. Another conjecture regarding the increased propensity for this group to develop middle ear effusion is that a vitamin A deficiency could be responsible for roughening the epithelium of the middle ear, thereby giving rise to effusion (Coleman et al., 1979).

Inner Ear Anomalies. Harada and Sando (1981) found fewer abnormalities of the inner ear than middle ear, but did find instances of endolymphatic hydrops confined to the apical turn of the cochlea. Other inner ear anomalies reported include "shortened cochlea, absence of the utriculoendolymphatic valve, hypogenesis of the posterior semicircular canal, and an enlarged bony posterior canal ampulla" (Sando et al., 1983). Wilson et al. (1983) have presented audiologic findings to support their position that "cochlear abnormality in many Down syndrome individuals seems likely." Harada and Sando (1981), furthermore, cite an article from the foreign literature which offered evidence of a good correlation between sensory-neural hearing loss and malformations of the inner ear in persons with Down syndrome.

Evoked Potentials. Studies of evoked potentials with the Down syndrome population have shown increased amplitudes of somatosensory, visual and auditory evoked potentials (Wilson et al., 1983). Wilson and his coauthors (1983) state: "Clearly our understanding of neural mechanisms which generate the ABR in Down syndrome is incomplete." These investigators found

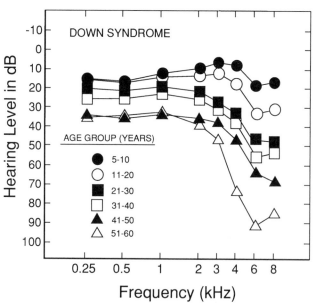

Figure 34.2. High frequency impairment. (From Buchanan LH. Early onset of presbycusis in Down syndrome. Fig. 1. Scand Audiol 1990;19(2):103–110.)

shorter latencies and steeper latency-intensity functions in Down syndrome infants than in age-matched normals. They suggest, therefore, that expected latency curves for normal infants are inappropriate for evaluating infants with Down syndrome after 6 months of age and that use of the normal curves could underestimate possible hearing loss in the Down syndrome group. Buchanan (1990) notes:

> ABR audiometry in Down syndrome should be interpreted with caution because the shortened conduction times reported in previous studies may be related to a presbycusis hearing loss with concomitant loudness recruitment.

Improved Outlook. Whereas sensory-neural impairment is more prevalent (Buchanan, 1990) than assumed before the 1990s, the widespread prevalence of conductive hearing loss reported for persons with Down syndrome (see "Hearing Loss in Populations with Other Known Conditions") may decrease as improved medical care and better living conditions are made available. A unique otolaryngologic study (Strome, 1981) directed toward otologic intervention from the first year of life for Down syndrome babies offers evidence supporting this hypothesis. Strome states that "early detection and aggressive management can significantly reduce the incidence of chronic middle ear disease" and that "less than 10% of the patients [so treated] will be left with residual conductive pathology."

One child with Down syndrome gained 2 years in her receptive language age, as measured with the Peabody Picture Vocabulary Test (PPVT) 1 year following bilateral myringotomies. That is twice the vocabulary growth an average child would have, and one must wonder whether this might be possible for more individuals with Down syndrome if their language delays were not simply attributed to their general developmental delay. A project to study pre- and postoperative PPVT scores in this population certainly has merit.

THE AUDIOLOGIST'S ROLE

Persons with developmental disabilities often get examined and re-examined, poked and prodded and programmed more than any normal person would choose. As the preceding sections of this chapter indicate, hearing loss often accompanies developmental disabilities. However, this fact does not necessarily suggest that persons with developmental disabilities should be subjected to perfunctory audiologic testing simply because some experts deem it important. A hearing screening program should be preceded by

presentations which will stress the importance of both the screening and the follow-up which must be an integral part of the program. Records or tape recording, such as those suggested in Chapter 39, designed to simulate hearing losses, can be very influential in eliciting support for a hearing screening effort. Additional rationale to support audiology services for persons with developmental disabilities may be found in the articles by Lloyd and Cox (1972) and Yaffe (1981).

Gross Hearing Screening

Individuals who either cannot be tested easily using traditional puretone screening methods or for whom audiometers are not readily accessible pose a dilemma for developmental disabilities agencies with staff interested in communication development. Audiologists often are approached by these agencies to recommend noisemakers or develop a questionnaire that can be used to help determine who might need referral for an audiologic evaluation. Occasionally, speech-language pathologists use one or both of these approaches when they work at an agency serving severely handicapped persons for whom hearing screening is mandated. Then for those individuals who show a response to the noisemaker and/or who score well on the questionnaire, the screener records a statement such as, "Gross hearing screening passed" or "Hearing appears grossly normal," signed by the professional responsible for the screening. When such a statement appears in an individual's official record, it becomes imbued with great credibility—this then has the effect of sanctioning no further testing. As a result, many who need definitive testing are deprived of the opportunity because the resident "specialist" has found nothing amiss. "Gross hearing screening" is a gross disservice to individuals with developmental disabilities and must not be tolerated.

Noisemakers. The dubious merits of noisemakers for assessing hearing status have been discussed by both Berlin (1978a) and Gerber (1982). They are not recommended for use as a test signal to determine how well a patient hears, but they may be used to see what response a patient will exhibit if he or she does hear. Another pretesting use of noisemakers is for training appropriate responses. The Waisman Center on Mental Retardation and Human Development at the University of Wisconsin-Madison has an excellent, simply written handout called, "Training Program for Play Audiometry." (This can be obtained by writing to Audiology Services, Waisman Center, 1500 Highland Avenue, Madison, WI 53706.) This is designed for use by a parent or therapist to facilitate obtaining results at the time of the audiometric evaluation.

The Questionnaire. For public relations and marketing audiology services, questionnaires and checklists can be very useful to increase the lay person's awareness of possible hearing problems. When used as a screening tool to identify persons with hearing loss, however, the validity of such questionnaires and checklists is itself a question mark. Unless a hearing loss is moderately severe, it is likely to remain undetected in persons who are institutionalized for mental illness or retardation (Rittmanic, 1971). Without adequate testing, not only are mild and moderate losses overlooked, but so too are those with normal hearing for only a limited frequency range (Ross and Matkin, 1967; Matkin, 1968; Berlin, 1978b).

Proposed Screening Guidelines

In Chicago a group of concerned professionals convened a committee to address the question of how periodic hearing screening should be implemented for persons with developmental disabilities. The screening guidelines (Young, et al., 1978) which evolved must be credited primarily to one of the participating speech-language pathologists who stressed that communication skill training be predicated on hearing level information. These guidelines for the delivery of services are included in Appendix 34.1 of this chapter as recommendations, but must be modified, of course, to fit existing resources in a community.

Regardless of modifications, premises that should be integral to the screening program include: (1) Individuals with developmental disabilities are entitled to at least what is offered to normal persons. (2) Younger children are more amenable to treatment and should receive the most frequent screening. (3) Older persons with developmental disabilities need screening less often but should be seen on some periodic basis. To depend on even knowledgeable persons to make referrals is not sufficient for meeting the needs of those with developmental disabilities. Lloyd and Cox (1972) state that in programs serving the mentally retarded, persons who need otologic care and/or who have "communicatively significant hearing impairments" are often overlooked if interdepartmental referrals are the only resource for scheduling periodic monitoring of hearing status.

A Promising Screening Technique

Speech/language pathologists should not be discouraged from doing hearing screening with persons who have developmental disabilities (ASHA, 1977), but test signals should be frequency specific. Ideally, screening should be done with an audiometer and immittance equipment, but many individuals with severe disabilities are not amenable to such screening. A preliminary investigation of an alternate procedure was done by staff at the Institute for the Study of Developmental Disabilities by using an Amplaid Reactometer, a portable instrument with narrow bands of noise at 500, 1500, and 3000 Hz, and a small speaker about the size of a softball. Results indicated that this may have promise for individuals unable to learn a conditioned response during the time available for screening at a community agency. Persons who were screened with the narrow-band noise signals and who demonstrated repeatable behavioral responses at the lowest presentation level (50 dB sound pressure level) were subsequently found to respond within normal limits during a clinical audiologic evaluation. Moreover, none of those exhibiting depressed responses with the Reactometer were within normal limits for the follow-up assessment. Since this was tried with only a limited number of patients, further investigation is warranted, but at least it was found to be much more useful than noisemakers or a checklist questionnaire for finding individuals "high risk" for hearing loss.

Borrowed Experience

Graduate training in audiology cannot possibly prepare one for the many unexpected incidents and bewildering patients seen in a clinic for developmental disabilities. Co-workers, patients and their families are likely to have "hands-on" experience which has instilled them with an expertise seldom acquired from books; this will be shared gladly if the clinician simply will ask. Certain cases are remembered for the lessons which remain, and I would like to share a few of my own so that the reader may borrow from my experience.

Exemplary Cases

The Patient with Seizures. When a patient with a seizure history comes for an audiologic evaluation, the audiologist should ask how the seizures are manifested and the extent of control provided by medication. I had imagined that seizures occurred in two forms, grand mal and petit mal, and was caught off guard when my knowledgeable assistant, Elvetta Walker, interrupted our testing session with, "Hold the warble tones. The kid is having a seizure."

I stared from the control room into the test room at our patient and my co-worker, and I saw nothing I recognized as a seizure. (I was to learn later about minor motor seizures.) Elvetta had been holding the patient's hands and waited until she felt tone return to the muscles. She then let me know I could proceed with signal presentation. After testing, Elvetta showed me that the patient's gums were hypertrophied, a side effect of a common anticonvulsant drug (Dilantin), and this had alerted her to watch for potential seizures, which she knew could be manifested in many different forms.

The Patient with Cerebral Palsy. As a neophyte working with developmental disabilities, I was bewildered by the prospect of giving a hearing test to a 3-year-old with less head control than most infants. "Mickey" had an age-appropriate receptive vocabulary, which had been assessed by cutting up the cards from the PPVT and attaching felt strips to the back of each picture so that the four items on a given page could be sufficiently separated from each other on a flannel board to permit an interpretable "eye-pointing" response. We attempted the same aproach with felt-backed spondee cards for a speech reception threshold but were unsuccessful. We had great difficulty interpreting the direction of Mickey's eye pointing because it was veiled by his uncontrollable head movements.

Never having seen anyone with such extraordinary low muscle tone, I was ready to give up; however, Mickey and his neuro-developmentally trained speech-language pathologist had a lesson to teach me. She placed him in a side-lying position, his head supported by her knee, and an earphone on his uppermost ear; he then followed her instructions to "smile and look up at me when you hear the beep." This technique enabled us to obtain reliable air- and bone-conduction thresholds at five frequencies for each ear—more than can be done with many normal 3-year-olds.

The Patient with Cognitive Deficits. Many patients with congitive limitations will require simplified instructions and even may need to be literally moved through an appropriate response. Subordinate clauses, like those beginning with "when" or "if," may not be understood. Truncated directions worked very well with one profoundly retarded youngster who enjoyed playing peek-a-boo. He was given a towel and "hidden" under it. While narrating each step of the expected task, we moved the child through it with only one- or two-word cues: "Towel on. Now listen. Wait. Beep. Towel off." The child seemed delighted with the game and complied spontaneously after only a few demonstrations. Obviously, testing must be eclectic and is probably limited more by the audiologist's ingenuity than by any lack of ability or motivation inherent in the patient.

Ground Rules

Caveats discussed in this section are irrelevant for patients only mildly incapacitated by developmental disabilities. These persons should be testable using standard adult procedures with perhaps a bit more encouragement than might be necessary with a self-referred patient. Other chapters and the accompanying reference list in this section provide a discussion of techniques and expected responses for those whose developmental levels may qualify them for pediatric procedures.

The First Might Be the Only

For patients who are severely handicapped, the clinician must first establish what response is possible for the patient, and then this response must be reinforced. Automated techniques have the distinct advantage of immediately reinforcing target behaviors. As is emphasized by Hodgson in Chapter 28, get the most important information first; an opportunity for obtaining it later can dissipate along with the patient's compliance. Specifically, what is most important can vary from patient to patient, but 2000 Hz is especially critical because it has been found to be the frequency most highly correlated with speech-recognition abilities (Boothroyd, 1978).

Time ≠ Quality

Time is no guarantee of quality. With patients who are difficult to test, the best information is usually what is obtained at the outset. Within a 1/2-hour appointment a skilled audiologist can often obtain useful results even with patients who are profoundly mentally retarded (Decker and Wilson, 1977). Several brief sessions are often more productive than a single lengthy one, but the audiologist must be able to demonstrate that future sessions will be fruitful and not simply more "could not test." Audiologists surely would be less inclined to recommend frequent re-evaluations if they were responsible for transporting patients to clinical appointments.

The Better Ear

Unquestionably, a person with unilateral hearing loss can have associated learning problems (Bess and Tharpe, 1984). Nevertheless, the person's responsiveness to the auditory environment will depend primarily upon the status of the better ear if both do not have equivalent hearing. Because sound field results will reflect the status of at least the better ear, these hearing levels can be very helpful for describing hearing status to those who must communicate with the patient. Considering the many unusual audiometric configurations found in persons with developmental disabilities, getting both high and low-frequency information in a sound field is recommended over ear-specific information for a broad-band signal such as speech. Our clinic has found Auditek's Filtered (at 500, 1000, and 2000 Hz) Echoes On Echoes tape—with its bizarre, attention-provoking, electronic signals—to be a terrific tool for eliciting responses in many otherwise auditorily oblivious patients. Of course, if the patient can maintain auditory stimulus control, earphone information should be pursued, but it is considered a lower priority than frequency-specific sound field data. When great emphasis is placed on sound field results, clinicians should recognize the advantage of warble tone signals over narrow-band noise (Wilber, 1979). Clinic staff should give special attention to monitoring levels of sound field signals. Though ANSI, as of this writing, has not published standards for warble tones or sound field narrow bands of noise, useful reference levels may be found in Chapter 6 of this text.

Interpretation of Results

Intertest Inconsistencies

When evaluating persons with developmental disabilities, the clinician often completes whatever testing is possible within the time available and finds that results do not always dovetail neatly with each other. A discussion of all possible intertest inconsistencies is not possible within space limitations here, but one of the most common is worthy of special mention.

Audiologists unfamiliar with developmental disabilities often settle for minimum levels of responses to speech signals and conclude, as has actually been reported, "Essentially normal hearing bilaterally as determined by speech audiometry. The individual should function adequately from a hearing standpoint." Adequately for whom? Certainly, the person will not function adequately if hearing levels drop precipitously for high frequencies or rise from markedly impaired low-frequency sensitivity to normal high-frequency sensitivity. Many individuals with hearing impairment retain sufficient residual auditory sensitivity within a restricted frequency range sufficient for the perception of very simple, highly predictable and often drilled commands. Consequently, appropriate responses to "stand up," "sit down," "point to. . ." and such should not be construed as evidence of normal hearing. Speech audiometry results used as the sole basis for describing hearing status can often be misleading.

Many clinicians who obtain responses for speech signals at or near normal levels but significantly poorer results for discrete frequency signals often conclude that the individual's hearing is probably consistent with the speech awareness thresholds and that the other responses are "suprathreshold." Although such an approach can placate those who bring the patient and are not worried about a hearing loss, it can have grievous consequences for the patient whose audiometric configuration is normal for some frequencies not assessed and abnormal for those that were.

How can one know a response to a particular signal is suprathreshold when the threshold has not been identified? To assume that depressed responses reflect "delayed auditory development" in an older (noninfant) individual with mental retardation is not prudent. As is well stated by Friedrich (1985), "The audiologist should be wary of operating under the assumption that a handicapped child will provide responses in a manner exactly analogous to the normal child whose chronological age corresponds to the handicapped child's developmental age." A 6-month-old normally-developing baby is quite unlike the 4-year-old child said to be at 6-month level in mental and/or motor abilities. "Delayed auditory development" has too often been used as an excuse not to pursue follow-up aggressively. The "clinical impression" one reports must be supported by the data obtained during testing. Otherwise, this impression might be contradicted subsequently when better testing is feasible.

Recommendations

The role of the audiologist with patients who have developmental disabilities should be that of a professional advisor, rather than case manager. The patient with a developmental disability will come from a family or agency program which must contend with other problems besides the patient's hearing loss. Patients do not belong to the professionals who evaluate and treat them. We should be information providers to assist patients and their caretakers in weighing options available to them. If the information offered is not explained in a manner which is consistent with what has been understood previously, the information is likely to be rejected, along with the clinician offering it.

> A parent who can build within his system a comfortable space to minister to himself and permission to skip or reject certain aspects of the habilitative process, will, in the long run, be a more effective child growth facilitator (Moses and Van Hecke-Wulatin, 1981).

AND FINALLY . . .

Developmental disabilities are as varied as snowflakes or grains of sand. Persons with developmental disabilities run the gamut from healthy to sick, agile to immobile, bright to dull, beautiful to disfigured, and lovable to alienating, but rarely either one to the exclusion of the other. They are as unique as others without developmental disabilities. Even individuals who have similar conditions will exhibit different levels of responsiveness and demonstrate different degrees of being amenable to improvement in their life circumstances. Reliance on stereotypes fosters "hardening of the categories" or "rigor categories" (Kodman, 1964). Rarely do persons fit preconceptions. This is especially true when the person is someone with developmental disabilities. For the audiologist, the patient with developmental disabilities presents challenges that are distinctive for each individual. To deal with these challenges requires an extra measure of perseverance, innovation, and sensitivity to individual assets and limitations in order to provide an accurate and, hence, useful audiologic evaluation with appropriate follow up.

REFERENCES

American Speech and Hearing Association. The developmental disabilities act. Asha 1971;13:391–393.

American Speech and Hearing Association. Issues in ethics: clinical practice by members in the area in which they are not certified. Asha 1977;19:343.

American Speech-Language-Hearing Association Committee on Mental Retardation/Developmental Disabilities. Serving the communicatively handicapped mentally retarded individual. Asha 1982;24:547–553.

Balkany JT. Otologic aspects of Down's syndrome. In Northern JL, and Downs M, Eds. Seminars in Speech, Language and Hearing, vol. 1. New York: Thieme-Stratton, 1980:39–48.

Baumeister AA. Origins and control of stereotyped movements. In Meyers CE, Ed. Quality of Life in Severely and Profoundly Mentally Retarded People: Research Foundations for Improvement. Monograph 3. Washington, DC: American Association on Mental Deficiency, 1978.

Berlin CI. Electrophysiological indices of auditory function. In Martin FN, Ed. Pediatric Audiology. Englewood Cliffs, NJ: Prentice-Hall, 1978:113–173.

Berlin CI. Superior ultra-audiometric hearing: a new type of hearing loss which correlates highly with unusually good speech in the "profoundly deaf." Otolaryngology 1978;86:111–116.

Bernstein LH. Neurological evaluation. In Frankenburg WK, Thornton SM, and Cohrs ME, Eds. Pediatric Developmental Diagnosis. New York: Thieme-Stratton, 1981.

Bess FH, and Tharpe AM. Unilateral hearing impairment in children. Pediatrics 1984;74:206–216.

Boothroyd A. Speech perception and sensorineural hearing loss. In Ross M, and Giolas TG, Eds. Auditory Management of Hearing-Impaired Children: Principles and Prerequisites for Intervention. University Park Press, 1978:117–144.

Buchanan LH. Early onset of presbyacusis in Down syndrome. Scand Audiol 1990;19:103–110.

Campbell CW, Polomeno RC, Elder JM, Murray J, and Altosaar A. Importance of an eye examination in identifying the cause of congenital hearing impairment. J Speech Hear Disord 1981; 46:258–261.

Cerva T. The demographics of developmental disabilities. Mimeographed paper prepared for the National Task Force on the Definition of Developmental Disabilities, 1977.

Coleman M. An overview of Down's syndrome. Northern JL, and Downs M, Eds. Seminars in Speech, Language and Hearing, vol. 1. New York: Thieme-Stratton, 1980:1–7.

Coleman M, Schwartz RH, and Schwartz DM. Otologic manifestations in Down's syndrome. Down's Syndrome Papers and Abstracts for Professionals 1979;2:1.

Cress PJ, Spellman CR, DeBriere TJ, Sizemore AC, Northam JK, and Johnson JL. Vision screening for persons with severe handicaps. TASH (The Association for the Severely Handicapped) J 1981;6:41–50.

Decker TN, and Wilson WR. The use of visually reinforced audiometry (VRA) with profoundly retarded residents. Ment Retard 1977;15:40–41.

Downs MP. The hearing of Down's individuals. In Northern JL, and Downs M, Eds. Seminars in Speech, Language and Hearing, vol. 1. New York: Thieme-Stratton, 1980:25–38.

Duckman RH. Visual problems. In McDonald ET, Ed. Treating Cerebral Palsy: For Clinicians by Clinicians, Austin, TX: Pro-Ed, 1987:105–131.

Epilepsy Foundation of America. Answers to the Most Frequent Questions People Ask About Epilepsy. Washington, DC, 1973.

Evans J. The effects of seizure and behavior control medications on the acoustic reflex. J Speech Hear Assoc Va 1983;24:35–43.

Friedrich BW. The state of the art in audiologic evaluation and management. In Cherow E, Matkin ND, and Trybus RJ, Eds. Hearing-Impaired Children and Youth with Developmental Disabilities: An Interdisciplinary Foundation for Services. Washington, DC: Gallaudet College Press, 1985:122–152.

Fulton RT, and Lloyd LL. Hearing impairment in a population of children with Down's syndrome. Am J Ment Defic 1968;73: 298–302.

Gerber SE. The use of noise-making toys as audiometric devices. Int J Pediatr Otorhinolaryngol 1982;4:309–315.

Gollay E. The Modified Definition of Developmental Disabilities; An Initial Exploration. Contract HEW-105-78-5003 with the Rehabilitation Services Administration, Washington, DC, 1979.

Grossman HJ, Ed. Manual on Terminology and Classification in Mental Retardation. Baltimore: American Association on Mental Deficiency, 1977.

Harada T, and Sando I. Temporal bone histopathologic findings in Down's syndrome. Arch Otolaryngol 1981;107:96–103.

Healey WC, and Karp-Nortman DC. The hearing-impaired mentally retarded: recommendations for action. Rockville, MD: American Speech-Language-Hearing Association, 1975.

Hicks W, and Pfau G. Deaf-visually impaired persons: incidence and services. Am Ann Deaf 1979;124:76–92.

Hughes JR. Epilepsy: a medical overview. In Hermann BP, Ed. Epilepsy: a Counseling Guide for Illinois. Comprehensive Program for Children with Epilepsy, Department of Neurology, U. of IL at Chicago, and the IL Dept. of Mental Health and Developmental Disabilities, 1981:53–66.

Jahn AF, and Becker A. Ear disease in adults with Down's syndrome. Paper presented at American Academy of Otolaryngology–Head and Neck Surgery Convention, New Orleans. This paper was recorded by Audio-Digest; Otolaryngology Head and Neck Surgery 1982;15:(23).

Johnson DD, and Crandall KE. The adult deaf client and rehabilitation. In Alpiner JG, Ed. Handbook of Adult Rehabilitative Audiology, ed. 2. Baltimore: Williams & Wilkins, 1982:245–249.

Jones TW. Problems in identification of multihandicapped hearing impaired students. In Holzhauer E, Hoff K, and Cherow E, Eds.

Hearing Impaired Developmentally Disabled Children and Adolescents: An Interdisciplinary Look at a Special Population. (Grant 90 DD 0005/01 from the Administration on Developmental Disabilities, Department of Health and Human Services). Rockville, MD: American Speech-Language-Hearing Association, 1982:I-23–I-29.

Karchmer MA. A demographic perspective. In Cherow E, Matkin ND, and Trybus RJ, Eds. Hearing-Impaired Children and Youth with Developmental Disabilities. Washington, DC: Gallaudet College Press, 1985:36–56.

Katz J. Personal communication, 1983.

Keiser H, Montague J, Wold D, Maune S, and Pattison D. Hearing loss of Down syndrome adults. Am J Ment Defic 1981;85:467–472.

Kodman F, Jr. The team approach to hearing problems. Maico Aud Lib 1964;2:10.

Lloyd LL, and Cox BP. Programming for the audiologic aspects of mental retardation. Ment Retard 1972;10:22–26.

Lloyd LL, and Moore EJ. Audiology. In Wortis J, Ed. Mental Retardation, vol. IV. New York: Grune & Stratton, 1972:141–163.

Lloyd LL, and Young CE. Pure-tone audiometry. In Fulton RT, and Lloyd LL, Eds. Audiometry for the Retarded with Implications for the Difficult-To-Test. Baltimore: Williams & Wilkins, 1969:1–31.

Matkin ND. The child with a marked high-frequency hearing impairment. Pediatr Clin North Am 1968;15:677–690.

Moses KL, and Van Hecke-Wulatin M. The socio-emotional impact of infant deafness; a counselling model. In Gerber SE, and Mencher GT, Eds. Early Management of Hearing Loss. New York: Grune & Stratton, 1981:243–278.

Mysak ED. Hearing disorders among the cerebral-palsied. In Travis LE, Ed. Handbook of Speech Pathology and Audiology. New York: Appleton-Century-Crofts, 1971:678–679.

Rittmanic PA. The mentally retarded and mentally ill. In Rose DE, Ed. Audiological Assessment, 1st ed. Englewood Cliffs, NJ: Prentice-Hall, 1971:369–404.

Ross M, and Matkin ND. The rising audiometric configuration. J Speech Hear Disord 1967;32:377–382.

Rynders JE, Spiker D, and Horrobin JM. Underestimating the educability of Down's syndrome children: examination of methodological problems in recent literature. Am J Ment Defic 1978;82:440–448.

Sak RJ, and Ruben RJ. Recurrent middle ear effusion in childhood: implications of temporary auditory deprivation for language and learning. Ann Otol Rhinol Laryngol 1981;90:546–551.

Sando I, Suehiro S, and Wood RP, II. Congenital anomalies of the external and middle ear. In Bluestone CD, and Stool SE, Eds. Pediatric Otolaryngology, vol. 1. Philadelphia: WB Saunders, 1983:315.

Schwartz DM, and Schwartz RH. Acoustic impedance and otoscopic findings in young children with Down's syndrome. Arch Otolaryngol 1978;104:652–656.

Siegenthaler BM. Auditory problems. In McDonald ET, Ed. Treating Cerebral Palsy: For Clinicians by Clinicians. Austin, TX: Pro-Ed, 1987:85–103.

Strome M. Down's syndrome: a modern otorhinolaryngological perspective. Laryngoscope 1981;91:1581–1594.

Wilber LA. Pure tone audiometry: air and bone conduction. In Rintelmann WF, Ed. Hearing Assessment. Baltimore: University Park Press, 1979:29–49.

Wilson WR, Folson RC, and Widen JE. Hearing impairment in Down's syndrome children. In Mencher GT, and Gerber SE, Eds. The Multiply Handicapped Hearing Impaired Child. New York: Grune & Stratton, 1983:259–299.

Wisniewski KE, and Wisniewski HM. In Reisberg B, Ed. Alzheimer's Disease. New York: Free Press (a Division of Macmillan, Inc.), 1983:319–324.

Wolff AB, and Harkins JE. Multihandicapped students. In Schildroth AN, and Karchmer MA, Eds. Deaf Children in America. San Diego: College-Hill Press, 1986:55–81.

Yaffe L. Hearing screening in a school for the severely-profoundly intellectually-impaired and multiply-handicapped students. Lang Speech Hear Serv School 1981;12:20–25.

Young CV, Colmer S, and Holloway CA. Hearing conservaton plan for individuals with developmental disabilities–proposed model. Poster session at the Illinois Speech and Hearing Association Convention, Chicago, 1978.

Appendix 34.1

Suggested Guidelines for Hearing Screening in Program Serving Developmental Disabilities

I. Anyone having developmental disabilities (DD), regardless of age, without documented hearing testing shall be considered highest priority for receiving screening services.

II. Annual hearing level and middle ear immittance screening shall be provided for:

A. Children falling in the age range during which frequent upper respiratory infections are common. Among children having DD the age range will extend to age 10.

B. Individuals older than 10 who may have DD and, as well,

    1. Persistent congestion,

    2. Frequent episodes of upper respiratory infections,

    3. Draining ears or

    4. Allergic reactions involving the ears, nose and/or throat. Annual screening shall continue until such conditions are no longer chronic and/or are being managed medically.

C. Persons considered high risk for hearing loss, specifically those with:

    1. Cleft palate,

    2. Down syndrome,

    3. Orofacial deformity or

    4. Familial history of hearing loss.

III. After the age of 10 and 2 consecutive years of having hearing status documented as within normal limits without evidence of middle ear pathology, an individual with DD shall have

A. Middle ear immittance screening annually, and

B. Hearing status screened every 3 years.

IV. Individuals being considered for a change in placement (educational or vocational) shall be scheduled for hearing screening, preferably prior to the change in placement or within 3 months of being in the new placement.

V. Individuals exhibiting regression is development and/or behavioral problems not previously characteristic for the person shall be referred for hearing screening as soon as possible.

VI. Otolaryngologic exam shall be an integral part of "hearing screening" for individuals having DD

A. Who are untestable in their community placement setting for either

    1. Hearing levels or

    2. Middle ear immittance measurements; or

B. Who yield screening data (from on-site screening in the community) indicating the need for medical examination.

Appendix 34.1
IQ Ranges for Three Frequently Used Intelligence Tests

Levels	Obtained Intelligence Quotient	
	Cattell (SD = 16)	Stanford-Binet and Wechsler Scales (SD = 15)
Mild	69–55	68–52
Moderate	51–36	54–40
Severe	35–20	39–25 (extrapolated)
Profound	19 and below (extrapolated)	24 and below

(Grossman, 1977)

CHAPTER 35

Industrial Hearing Conservation

William Melnick

The word *conservation* is defined as "a careful preservation or protection of something; the planned management of a natural resource to prevent exploitation, destruction, or neglect." *Preservation* means "to keep safe from injury, harm or destruction; to keep alive, intact, free from decay" (*Webster's,* 1989). Conservation of hearing is a major function of an audiologist. Conservation and rehabilitation (attempts to minimize the handicap of a hearing loss) form the foundation for the existence of the field of audiology. The fundamental purpose of industrial hearing conservation is not appreciably different from the aims of hearing conservation in general. There must be something unique about the industrial environment which permits us specifically to label these efforts "industrial hearing conservation." The most distinctive feature of hearing conservation in an industrial environment is that we have been able to identify a noxious agent that has a pervasive effect on the hearing of people working in this environment. The agent is intense noise.

The link between the existence of excessive noise in the environment and the production of hearing loss in people working in that environment is beyond question. Hazardous noise conditions produce destruction of auditory sensory cells, the hair cells in the cochlea (Lim and Melnick, 1971; see Figure 35.1). Sufficient destruction of these elements will produce hearing loss (Sataloff and Michael, 1973). Many of the hazardous properties of noise have been defined. Unlike many other conditions that produce sensory-neural hearing loss, a noise-related loss can be prevented. Because the physical characteristics of noise can be measured, steps can be taken to avoid hearing loss.

LEGAL BASIS

After legislation concerning protection from occupational noise exposure was written, regulations describing the minimal requirements for an acceptable industrial hearing conservation program were adopted. These government regulations stimulated the development of new conservation programs in industrial facilities which might otherwise have ignored the problem.

The courts have shown a willingness to compensate people for hearing losses that result from exposure to industrial noise. The economic realities of these legal decisions have made the problem of noise-induced hearing loss difficult to ignore.

Federal regulations of occupational noise exposure started with the Walsh-Healey Public Contracts Act in May, 1969. This Act applied to all industries having government contracts of $10,000 or more.

Under the authority of the Walsh-Healey Act, the Department of Labor (1969) issued a regulation that contained allowable levels and durations of noise exposure. Whenever these noise limits were exceeded, the regulation required "a continuing, effective hearing conservation program." In 1970, Congress passed the Occupational Safety and Health Act (OSHAct) (Williams-Steiger, 1970). One of the recommendations of Congress was that existing governmental standards be adopted to implement provisions of the Act. Consequently, the Walsh-Healey noise standard became an OSHAct standard, and was applicable not only to employers who contracted with the government but to any employer who was engaged in interstate commerce, thus covering most of the noisy industries.

In 1974, the Occupational Safety and Health Administration (OSHA) published a proposed noise regulation in the *Federal Register* (U.S. Department of Labor, 1974). This proposal set limits for noise exposure and defined, in some detail, the requirements for audiometric testing and led to an amendment to the noise standard (29 CFR Part 1910.95, U.S. Department of Labor, 1981). The amendment established the elements and procedures of an acceptable hearing conservation program, including monitoring of noise exposure, audiometric testing, record keeping, and employee education.

On March 3, 1983, a revised Hearing Conservation Amendment was published in the *Federal Register* (U.S. Department of Labor, 1983) as the "Final Rule." This amendment is the basis for the hearing-conservation component of the OSHA noise regulation in effect now.

A major reason for increased interest in industrial noise problems is the payment of compensation for occupationally caused loss of hearing. The intent of the

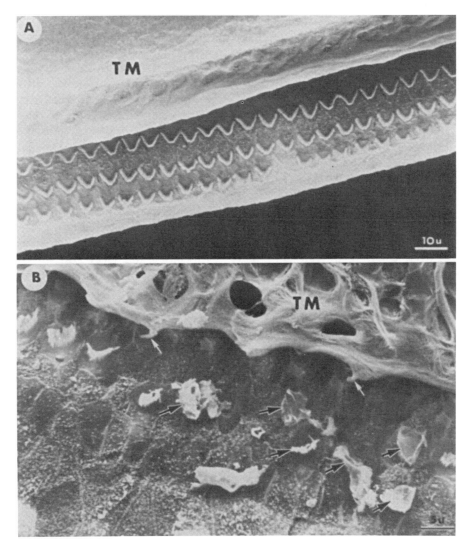

Figure 35.1. A. Scanning electron micrograph showing normal appearance of three rows of outer hair cells and tectorial membrane (*TM*). **B.** Degenerating outer hair cells (*arrows*) resulting from a 6-hour exposure to 1- to 2-kHz octave band of noise of 117-dB sound pressure level. (From Lim DJ, and Melnick W. Acoustic damage of the cochlea. Arch Otolaryngol 1971;94:294–305.)

original Workmen's Compensation Acts was to protect workers from loss of earnings and to cover medical costs arising from injuries occurring on the job. Landmark legal action has led to the inclusion of hearing loss as a compensable injury (Sataloff and Michael, 1973). In 1948, the New York Court of Appeals ruled that a person who developed a hearing loss as a result of his employment was entitled to compensation, even though there was no lost time and no loss of earnings (Slawinski v. Williams & Co., 1948). This departure from the original wage loss concept of Workmen's Compensation resulted in an increased number of claims. In 1962, a court in Georgia ruled that an employee's hearing loss resulted from a cumulative effect of a succession of injuries caused by each daily noise

insult on the ear (Shipman v. Employers Mutual Liability Insurance, 1962). This court action resulted in a decision that hearing loss was compensable under the accidental injury provisions of the Workmen's Compensation law. Wisconsin had a Workmen's Compensation Act in force since 1931 that recognized a schedule of payments for loss of hearing. The first significant number of claims under this Act was filed in 1951. After several court cases, a bill was passed in Wisconsin in 1955 to establish payment for occupational hearing loss.

A survey of workers' compensation statutes in 1985 (Fodor and Oleinick, 1986) indicated that all 50 states considered occupational hearing loss as compensable. The criteria, however, for compensable hearing loss were so restrictive in six of the states that noise-induced hearing loss essentially would not be eligible for compensation in their jurisdiction.

The activities of federal and state legislative and judicial systems have provided the motivation for development of industrial hearing conservation programs. Government activities continue, resulting in changes in laws and regulations that affect the composition of hearing conservation programs, the workers who are covered by these programs, the criteria for compensable hearing loss, and the amount of compensation to be awarded.

EFFECTS OF NOISE ON HEARING

Noise has been reported to have many effects on people working in industry, such as annoyance, decrease in working efficiency, physiologic changes in heart rate and blood pressure, and psychologic distress. More direct auditory effects include the obvious interference with speech communication produced by the masking caused by background noise, and the primary auditory effect, the capacity of noise to produce hearing loss. Industrial hearing conservation programs are, for the most part, concerned only with the loss of hearing. Thus far, no conclusive evidence has been found that physiologic effects other than hearing loss can be produced at sound levels known to be hazardous to hearing. Even if other physiologic effects are found, it is probable that these effects of noise would be eliminated incidentally by controlling the effect on hearing.

Effects of noise on hearing may be divided generally into three categories: temporary threshold shift, permanent threshold shift, and acoustic trauma (Miller, 1971; Guignard, 1973). The term *acoustic trauma* is restricted to the effects of single exposures or relatively few exposures to very high levels of sound (e.g., an explosion). In the case of acoustic trauma, the sound levels reaching the structures in the inner ear exceed the mechanical limits of those structures, frequently producing complete breakdown and disruption of the organ of Corti. People who experience these very intense noise exposures may also have ruptured eardrums and damaged ossicles. Hearing loss from acoustic trauma is to a large degree permanent. The precipitating episode is usually very dramatic and pronounced in the memory of the person experiencing the event. The person involved has no difficulty in specifying the onset of the hearing problem.

Temporary threshold shift (TTS) is a short-term effect that may follow an exposure to noise. TTS refers to an elevation in the threshold of hearing which recovers gradually after the noise exposure. Because the noise produces a transient shift in the threshold, it has

become known as TTS, or even more specifically as noise-induced temporary threshold shift (NITTS).

Permanent threshold shifts (PTS) are those hearing changes that persist throughout the life of the affected person. When a threshold shift is permanent, there is no possibility for further recovery with the passage of time after exposure. PTSs that result from acoustic trauma or a single encounter with very destructive noise exist but are relatively uncommon. More frequently, hearing loss produced by the effects of noise is a result of an accumulation of exposures repeated on a daily basis over a period of years. This kind of hearing loss is known as noise-induced. Thus, the portion of hearing loss resulting from chronic noise exposure and recovery is called noise-induced temporary threshold shift (NITTS), whereas the part that does not recover is called noise-induced permanent threshold shift (NIPTS). An excellent, thorough treatment of temporary and permanent noise-induced shifts as well as consideration of the relationship of these two auditory phenomena has been published by Kryter (1985).

Temporary Threshold Shift

Despite the large number of experiments in many laboratories throughout the world, the factors influencing TTSs and the recovery from these shifts have not been completely defined. TTS can vary hearing sensitivity from an insignificant few dB in a narrow frequency range to changes that render the ear temporarily deaf. After the termination of the noise, hearing sensitivity can return to the pre-exposure levels in a few minutes to several weeks.

Generalizations about TTS can be made from the experimental data (Miller, 1971). Low-frequency noises are not as effective in producing TTS as high-frequency noises (Ward, 1973). Noises with energy concentrated in the frequency range of 2000 to 6000 Hz produce more TTS than noises with energy elsewhere in the frequency range. Sound levels must exceed a certain intensity before the average person will experience any TTS, even for exposures as long as 8 to 16 hr. If everything else is held constant, noise levels must exceed 75dBA (75dB on the A-scale of a sound level meter) to produce TTS. Above this intensity level, TTS will increase with an increase in intensity and with an increase in the duration of the noise (Mills, 1988). There is evidence that, at least for moderate intensity levels of noise, exposure durations that exceed 8 to 16 hr may not produce any further increase in the magnitude of the threshold shift (Mills et al., 1970; Mosko et al., 1970; Melnick, 1974; Melnick and Maves, 1974). Threshold shifts become constant or asymptotic (asymptotic threshold shift, ATS). For low-level noises that produce very slight changes in threshold, most of the effect is observed in the frequency range of the noise or fatiguing sound. As the intensity of the noise increases, the frequency of maximal threshold shift occurs one-half to one octave above the frequency region of greatest concentration of noise energy (Ward, 1963). Another observation is that a noise exposure with frequent interruptions will produce less TTS than a continuous noise exposure of equivalent sound energy (Ward, 1973).

People vary considerably in their susceptibility to NITTS (Ward, 1968). For classification purposes it would be convenient if individuals were grouped into two categories—those with ears particularly susceptible and those with ears minimally susceptible—if susceptibility to TTS were to be used as a predictor of susceptibility to permanent hearing losses from noise exposure. Evidence from investigations of TTS indicates, however, that the distribution of threshold shift shows a relatively good fit to a normal distribution rather than a bimodal distribution of susceptibility (Burns, 1973).

TTS should be more than just of academic interest to those involved with industrial hearing conservation. There is usually an element of TTS which may accompany any permanent component of hearing loss after noise exposure. Hearing testing programs designed to provide evidence of the existence of permanent hearing loss must be wary of the possibility of a contaminating temporary component. This is especially true in obtaining valid pre-employment audiograms or baseline audiograms in an industrial setting. The tester must be sure that the person tested is given ample opportunity for any TTS resulting from recent noise exposure to recover.

Information from systematic investigations of the relationship of noise exposure to NIPTS is difficult to obtain. Based on the assumption that the same processes involved in the growth and recovery of NITTS are also involved in the establishment of NIPTS, TTS data have been used to predict the hazardous effects of noise (Kryter et al., 1966; Burns, 1973).

Permanent Hearing Loss

Although the precise relationship of acoustic properties of noise to the resultant hearing loss has not been described, the general relationship of noise exposure to permanent hearing loss has been fairly well established. The information regarding this relationship comes from both field studies of hearing loss in industrial environments as well as laboratory investigations of temporary threshold shift. From these investigations, four major factors have been identified that contribute to the potential hazard of noise to hearing. These factors are: (a) the overall sound level measured in dB; (b) spectral distribution (distribution of sound energy with frequency); (c) duration and distribution of noise (sound exposure during a typical work day); and (d) cumulative noise exposure in days, weeks or years (American Academy of Otolaryngology—Head and Neck Surgery, 1988). Both the physical characteristics of the noise and the temporal patterns of the noise exposure have equal importance. Noise exposure represents the integration of sound energy contained in the hazardous noise over the time that the hazardous noise is experienced.

The type of noise present in the industrial environment must also be considered. The noise might be steady-state, fluctuating, intermittent, or impulsive. Steady-state noises can be described as continuous daily exposures in which the overall levels do not vary more than ±5 dB (Guignard, 1973). Most frequently, noise encountered in industry is fluctuating, that is, the noise is continuous but levels rise and fall more than 5dB during a particular exposure period. An intermittent noise is described as being discontinuous. During the work period, the noise level may fall to low or nonhazardous noise levels between periods of hazardous noise exposure. Impulsive noise can be described as one or more short, transient, acoustical events that last less than 0.5 seconds. A single impulse is usually heard as a discrete event occurring in otherwise quiet conditions or superimposed on backgrounds of steady-state, ongoing noise.

Not surprisingly, if all the other major properties of a noise are held constant, the amount of noise-induced hearing loss will increase as the level of noise increases. This relationship is illustrated in the data published by Passchier-Vermeer (1974) and graphed in Figure 35.2. This figure shows the estimated median noise-induced hearing loss at specific audiometric frequencies as a function of the A-weighted sound level of the noise that would occur for an exposure duration of 10 years. The graph plots noise-induced hearing loss with the hearing levels being adjusted for other sources of hearing loss, such as aging, ear disease, and nonindustrial noise exposure. These data indicate greater susceptibility for the frequencies 3000, 4000 and 6000 Hz to the effects of noise. An increase in the level of noise not only increases the loss at specific test frequencies but extends the range of frequencies affected.

The extent of hearing loss and the frequency at which the loss occurs are related to the sound energy contained in the octave band just below the affected frequency. Losses at 1000 and 2000 Hz correlate best

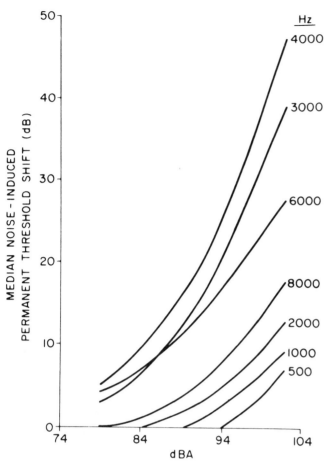

Figure 35.2. Estimated median noise-induced permanent threshold shift from 10 years of exposure to the indicated A-weighted sound levels of noise (Adapted from Passchier-Vermeer W. Hearing loss due to continuous exposure to steady-state broad-band noise. J Acoust Soc Am 1974;56:1585–1593.)

emphasizes sound in the low-frequency ranges of the audible spectrum. The A-scale attempts to approximate the sensitivity for the human ear, with the maximal weight being accorded to the frequencies in the range between 1000 and 4000 Hz. The unit of measurement with the A-weighting network is referred to as "dBA." The use of the A-scale has empirical validity because investigative evidence indicates that the ear is most susceptible to damage from frequencies in the middle of the audible range, particularly the 2000- to 3000-Hz region. Noise-induced hearing loss usually is first measurable in the 3000- to 6000-Hz range. In fact, hearing loss at 4000 Hz, or the "4000-Hz dip," has become the hallmark linking a sensory-neural hearing loss with noise as the potential etiology.

Noise-induced hearing loss will increase as the duration of exposure increases if, again, all other factors are kept constant. Investigations of industrial noise-induced hearing loss have shown that the hearing loss in the maximally affected frequency range increases exponentially as a function of duration of employment in the noisy occupation (Nixon and Glorig, 1961; Taylor et al., 1965). When the noise environment was relatively constant over a prolonged period of time, the hearing loss in the frequency range 3000 to 6000 Hz (maximally affected frequency range) increased rapidly during the first 10 years of exposure and then gradually slowed or reached a plateau. With continued exposure, there is a spread of effect to other frequencies. The development of hearing loss at these frequencies outside of the range of the maximal effect proceeds at a slower rate, and the hearing loss continues to grow over the entire period of employment.

The relationships just described in the preceding paragraphs have been based on data derived from industrial noise environments in which the exposure noise was steady or continuous for the entire exposure time. These kinds of industrial noise environments are relatively rare. More often, the noise conditions experienced by the employees are for varying periods of time, and frequently the noise is fluctuating or intermittent. Field data describing the relationship of time-varying noise to hearing loss are difficult to obtain. From the relatively few reports that have appeared, it can be generalized that the hazards of time-varying noise are significantly less than would be observed if the noise were continuous (Rudmose, 1957; Kryter, 1985).

The exact effects of the temporal pattern of exposure on hearing loss have not been described. The relationship is complicated and must consider noise levels and noise frequency as well as the infinite variety of exposure patterns. A simplifying general principle has been applied for use in the development of

with sound pressure measured in the 300 to 600 Hz octave band, whereas hearing loss at 4000 Hz is most closely related with sound pressure level in the 2000 Hz octave band (Rudmose, 1957). The shift of maximal hearing loss to the frequency range above that of the exposure frequency has been reported by investigations of both temporary and permanent noise-induced hearing losses (Ward, 1973; Kryter, 1985).

In industry, typically, the noise environments are broad band. The frequency content of broad-band noise can be analyzed by band-pass filtering, usually an octave wide. The octave band analysis has been found to be a detailed but complicated method for describing noise. A useful simplification is the application of frequency weighting networks that are incorporated in sound level meters to characterize the noise level in terms of a single number. The most frequently used filtering network is the A-weighting scale (see section on Sound Level Meters). This weighting network denoise hazard regulation. The underlying concept for guidelines that have been developed is one of equal noxiousness. Time-varying noises are described in terms of equivalent steady-state noises of relatively constant intensity for specified duration. The simplification results in a use of such quantities as equivalent sound levels or time-weighted average. The equal noxious concept involves a trading relationship of time and intensity of noise. Those who propose that noxiousness of noise be equated with sound energy contained in the noise would base the time intensity trade on the equal energy relationship. Sound energy increases by 3dB as the duration of sound exposure is doubled. The equal energy concept indicates that to maintain the same degree of noxiousness one might reduce the intensity of a specific noise by 3dB as the exposure duration is doubled. Conversely, if the overall noise level is increased by 3 dB, the duration would have to be reduced by one-half of the exposure time to maintain the same level of hazard. Because of its physical simplicity, the equal energy concept has been attractive to many people interested in noise-induced hearing loss. The major weaknesses of this approach to time-intensity trade are that the equal energy hypothesis disregards the pattern of exposure and also disregards the fact that noise is made less hazardous when that noise is interrupted.

Use of information from studies of noise-induced temporary hearing loss has led to the proposal that equal hazard be based on the ability of a noise to produce equal temporary change in hearing sensitivity (i.e., equal TTS). The proponents of this hypothesis would advise a 5-dB reduction in noise level for each doubling of the noise duration. In this case, if an acceptable noise exposure was 90 dBA for 8 hours, then a noise level of 95 dBA would be acceptable for 4 hours, 100 dBA for 2 hours, etc. This procedure for time intensity trading has become known as the "5-dB rule."

Both the 3-dB and 5-dB rules are simplifications and do not predict precisely the amount of permanent hearing loss produced in industrial environments where the noise levels fluctuate or where the noise is interrupted during the usual 8-hour work day. Both of the rules tend to be overprotective for short durations and would provide safety margins in regulations developed for hearing conservation. Thus far, the 3-dB rule has achieved greater acceptance internationally because of its basis in physical fact (equal energy), its attractiveness to instrument manufacturers, its appeal to engineers, and recent reports that the equal energy concept describes fairly well the relationship of impulse/impact noise to hearing loss (Atherley and Martin, 1971).

Damage Risk Criteria

Prevention of noise-induced hearing loss implies the ability to predict the probability of developing a hearing loss of a given magnitude when physical properties of the noise environment have been identified. Because of the many similarities in the effects of noise-produced TTS and PTS, there have been persistent attempts to demonstrate that the susceptibilities to TTS and PTS are related. If sensitivity to the temporary effects of noise could be demonstrated as an index of potential susceptibility to hearing loss, this predictor would be a major aid in industrial hearing conservation programs. Unfortunately, this relationship of TTS and PTS has not been supported by any investigations thus far. Kraak (1982) has proposed the method known as integrated TTS, which integrates the developmental and recovery period from TTS as an index for prediction; however, this technique would be rather cumbersome to apply in the field. The potential of integrated TTS as a predictor is still being evaluated. There are available predictors that have been based on a synthesis of data on noise-induced hearing loss derived from relatively well-controlled demographic field investigations. The predictive indices have become known as *damage risk criteria.*

A universal finding of all of the investigations of the effects of noise on hearing is the significant variation in the susceptibility of people to the effects of noise. In developing hazardous noise specifications, a decision must be made about the degree of hearing preservation that will be accomplished by these criteria. A criterion must be established that specifies the risk considered acceptable (Burns, 1973).

The term *damage risk criteria* has been applied both: (*a*) to the risk of acquiring a given hearing loss as a consequence of a given noise exposure and (*b*) to the particular noise limits that appear in industrial and safety standards. Strictly speaking, the term *damage risk criteria* should be used to identify a standard or rule on which a decision or judgment concerning the hazards of noise may be based. Damage risk criteria provide a method for deciding on the acceptable limits of noise exposure. Damage risk criteria should consider the amount of hearing loss that can be expected at specified audiometric frequencies in a specified percentage of people exposed to a given noise over a stated time interval (Tonndorf et al., 1979). Once the damage risk criteria have been established, then the noise exposure limits that meet the criteria can be specified. Scientists and professionals with expertise in the area of noise-induced hearing loss agree that there is sufficient information available to make reasonable approximation of the relationship of noise to hearing loss. Disagreement and debate most frequently occur when decisions must be made about how much hearing loss is acceptable, in how many people, and at what particular frequencies.

There are a number of damage risk criteria available today. Each varies according to the needs of the agency or group adopting the criterion. Proposed limits for noise exposure are at both extremes—highly restrictive and overly permissive. The EPA has proposed that no hearing loss as a result of noise exposure is acceptable and that the criterion should include measurement of hearing loss at 4000 Hz, the frequency most sensitive to the effects of noise (U. S. Environmental Protection Agency, 1974). The American Conference of Governmental Industrial Hygienists (ACGIH, 1969) considered hearing loss only in the frequencies 500, 1000, and 2000 Hz, which have been judged to have an effect on speech communication. The criterion of the ACGIH established their degree of acceptable hearing loss as less than 25 dB for the average of these three frequencies. The criterion established by the ACGIH has particular importance because these noise limits were adopted as the standard permissible exposure level in the Occupational Safety and Health Act of 1970.

The Occupational Safety and Health Administration (OSHA) of the U.S. Department of Labor, as a consequence of large scale industrial surveys that they supported, estimated the percentage of workers whose hearing loss would exceed the 25-dB average for 500, 1000, and 2000 after a working lifetime of exposure to average daily noise levels of 80, 85, and 90 dBA (U.S. Department of Labor, 1981). The risk for the 80-dBA level was estimated to be between 0 and 5%; for the 85-dBA level, this estimate increased to from 10–15%, whereas for the 90-dBA exposure level, the estimate was from 21–29%. From these surveys, it was clear that lifelong workplace exposure below 80 dBA was relatively safe to hearing, whereas the risk of substantial hearing loss begins to rise sharply at 85 dBA and higher. Adding 3000 Hz to the definition of impairment, as is now accepted by the American Medical Association and the American Academy of Otolaryngology—Head and Neck Surgery (1979), would increase the proportion of affected employees.

A more flexible approach to prediction of the effects of noise exposure on hearing is one adopted by the International Standards Organization in the development of its standard ISO 1999, Determination of Occupational Noise Exposure and Estimation of Noise Induced Hearing Impairment (ISO, 1990). The ISO standard represents the most complete summary of existing knowledge on the effects of noise on hearing sensitivity available today. This standard synthesizes

the work of Robinson and Shipton (1977) and of Passchier-Vermeer (1974). In this standard, the basic parameter for describing the effects of noise on hearing is NIPTS, which the standard defines as the difference between the distribution of hearing sensitivity in a nonnoise-exposed population and the hearing sensitivity in a noise-exposed population. The methods in the standard permit specifications in terms of NIPTS occurring for various percentages of the exposed population. Examples derived using the ISO method are indicated in Figure 35.3A, B, C and D. This figure shows the calculated NIPTS in audiogram form for the audiometric frequencies 500, 1000, 2000, 3000, 4000, and 6000 Hz for the 10th, 50th, and 90th percentiles, as a consequence of 10 years of exposure to overall noise levels of 85, 90, 95, and 100 dBA. In making these calculations, the assumption is made that the daily noise exposure is for 8 hours and the work week is comprised of 5 days. In the graphs, the 10th percentile represents the level of NIPTS which would be exceeded by 90% of the population (those showing the least affect), and the 50th percentile is the NIPTS that could be expected for half of the population. The 90th percentile, however, would be the level that would be exceeded by 10% of the exposed population (those most affected).

It must be remembered that NIPTS represents the amount of hearing loss that might be expected to be caused by noise exposure and does not represent the actual threshold hearing levels that would be measured for these segments of the population. The ISO method defines hearing threshold level as the summation of hearing level associated with age and the NIPTS estimated as a function of duration and level of the noise exposure.

To estimate the risk of sustaining hearing handicap due to noise exposure, the distribution of NIPTS would have to be converted to distributions of threshold hearing levels. To make this conversion, the hearing threshold levels of a nonnoise-exposed population of a comparable age group must be known. Calculation of threshold hearing levels of a group of people influenced by noise exposure is adjusted by the summation of the age-related threshold hearing levels for the nonnoise-exposed group and the expected NIPTS. For example, the median hearing threshold level at 4000 Hz of an unscreened group of males 40 years of age who had been working in noise levels of 95 dBA for 10 years would be calculated as follows. The median NIPTS at 4000 Hz derived using the ISO procedure for this group would be 20 dB (Figure 35.3C.). The median hearing level at this frequency for an unscreened sample of males 40 years of age estimated by the U.S. Public Health Survey for 1960–1970 was

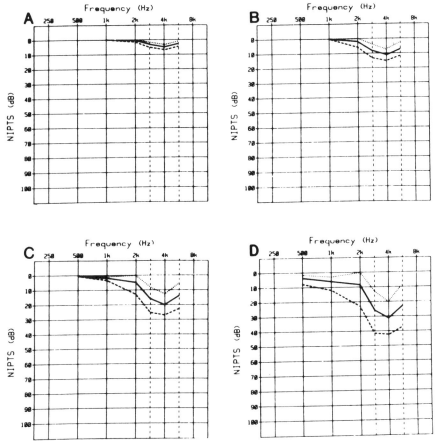

Figure 35.3. Noise-induced permanent threshold shift graphed with audiogram format. NIPTS is shown for the 10th (*dotted line*), 50th (*solid line*), and 90th (*dashed line*) percentiles. The duration of exposure is 10 years. The individual graphs A, B, C, and D represent the predicted results from exposure to 85, 90, 95 and 100dBA, respectively, as derived using ISO 1999. (From Melnick W. Auditory effects of noise exposure. In Miller MH, and Silverman CA, Eds. Occupational Hearing Conservation. Englewood Cliffs, NJ: Prentice-Hall, Inc., 1984:100–131.)

17 dB (National Center for Health Statistics, 1965). The median threshold hearing level of interest would be 20 dB plus 17 dB, or 37 dB. Similar estimates can be calculated for other percentiles, other age groups, and other exposure conditions.

The magnitude of risk calculated by this method depends on the definition of normal hearing threshold levels and the relationship of these hearing threshold levels to aging. The normal control group could be a highly screened otologically normal population or it could be drawn from a sample of people experiencing all possible factors that influence hearing sensitivity in the same way as that experienced by the noise exposed population with the exception of the occupational noise exposure. Examples of variation in risk estimates as a function of the makeup of a nonnoise-exposed population is provided by Johnson (1978). Table 35.1 represents normative groups carefully screened to eliminate all factors influencing hearing sensitivity other than the simple aging process, presbycusis. This

table shows the percentage of the population expected to exceed an average threshold hearing level of 25 dB for 500, 1000, 2000, and 3000 Hz as a consequence of being exposed to various noise levels for varying durations. A similar estimate of risk is contained in Table 35.2 where the nonnoise-exposed data were taken from threshold hearing levels for males from the 1960–1970 United States public health survey (National Center for Health Statistics, 1965). The data in these two tables clearly demonstrate that the selection of the normative population has a significant influence on the estimate of risk calculated using the standard ISO-1999.

The best known noise specifications available today are those that appear as part of the federal regulations resulting from the Occupational Safety and Health Act (Williams-Steiger, 1970) as developed by the American Conference of Governmental Industrial Hygienists (1969). These values are shown in Table 35.3 and, as can be seen, incorporate the "5-dB rule" for

Table 35.1.

Percentage of the Population Expected to Exceed 25 dB (re: ANSI 1969) for an Average of 500, 1000, 2000 and 3000 Hz as a Consequence of Exposure to Various A-weighted Sound Levels, Age and Exposure Duration, when the Age-Related Control Data Come from a Highly Screened Population[a]

Age (yr)	30	40	40	50	50	50	60	60	60	60
Exposure (yr)	10	10	20	10	20	30	10	20	30	40

Percentage Exceeding 25 dB Average

A-weighted Sound Level dBA										
Control	0	0	0	2	2	2	10	10	10	10
75	0	0	0	2	2	2	10	10	10	10
80	0	0	0	3	3	3	12	12	12	12
85	0	1	1	6	6	5	16	16	17	17
90	1	3	4	11	12	13	23	25	26	27
95	5	9	12	19	23	27	32	36	41	44
100	15	21	28	32	40	47	45	53	62	69

[a] Adapted from Johnson DL, "Derivation of Presbycusis and Noise-Induced Permanent Threshold Shift (NIPTS) to be Used for the Basis of a Standard on the Effects of Noise on Hearing," Technical Report 78-128 (Aerospace Medical Research Laboratory, Wright Patterson Air Force Base, Ohio, 1978).

Table 35.2.

Percentage of the Population Expected to Exceed 25 dB (re: ANSI 1969) for an Average of 500, 1000, 2000 and 3000 Hz as a Consequence of Exposure to Various A-weighted Sound Levels, Age and Exposure Durations, when the Age-Related Control Data are from a Nonscreened Male Group[a]

Age (yr)	30	40	40	50	50	50	60	60	60	60
Exposure (yr)	10	10	20	10	20	30	10	20	30	40

Percentage Exceeding 25 dB Average

A-weighted Sound Level dBA										
Control	0	6	6	13	13	13	27	27	27	27
75	0	6	6	13	13	13	27	27	27	27
80	0	7	7	15	15	15	28	29	29	29
85	1	10	10	19	19	19	31	32	32	33
90	3	16	17	24	26	28	36	38	39	40
95	10	24	27	32	36	40	42	46	49	53
100	23	35	42	43	50	60	52	62	71	78

[a] Adapted from Johnson DL, "Derivation of Presbycusis and Noise-Induced Permanent Threshold Shift (NIPTS) to be Used for the Basis of a Standard on the Effects of Noise on Hearing," Technical Report 78-128 (Aerospace Medical Research Laboratory, Wright Patterson Air Force Base, Ohio, 1978).

Table 35.3.

Permissible Noise Exposures[a]

Duration per Day (Hr)	Sound Level dBA Slow Response
8	90
6	92
4	95
3	97
2	100
1½	102
1	105
½	110
¼ or less	115

[a] From Part 50-204 Safety and Health Standards for Federal Supply Contracts, *Federal Register*, May 20, 1969, with correction of July 15, 1969.

time/intensity trading. The regulations specify 115 dBA to be the absolute maximal level to which anyone should be exposed, and levels beyond that should not be endured for any length of time. The percentage of the population at risk for significant hearing loss using these noise specifications has been indicated earlier in this section.

The noise specifications described in Table 35.3 pertain to continuous steady-state noise. This is cer-

tainly not the usual noise environment in industry. When the daily noise exposure is composed of periods of noise of two or more different levels, their combined effects must be considered. This kind of exposure is expressed as a noise exposure rating that is defined as the ratio of the observed duration of the dangerous noise to that duration allowable under the specifications for regulatory limits. Noise exposure is considered acceptable for all values of exposure if the combined ratios do not exceed unity, or 1. The hazard to hearing increases as the noise exposure ratio becomes progressively greater than 1. The hazardous noise rating may be calculated using the following equation:

$$C_1/T_1 + C_2/T_2 + C_n/T_n = \text{noise rating}$$

C_n indicates the total noise exposure at a specified noise level while T_n indicates the total time of an exposure permitted at that level (U.S. Department of Labor, 1983). Noise exposure can also be described in terms of a daily noise dose or the 8-hour time-weighted average sound level (TWA) (U.S. Department of Labor, 1983). The noise dose simply requires multiplying the noise rating ratio by 100. The TWA is the sound level that, if constant over an 8-hour exposure period, would result in the same measured noise dose and can be calculated in dB from the noise dose by the formula:

$$\text{TWA} = 16.61 \text{Log}_{10}(\text{dose}/100) + 90$$

For impulsive noise, the OSHA regulation states that impact noise should not exceed 140-dB peak sound pressure level.

HEARING CONSERVATION PROGRAM

Indication of the need for a hearing conservation program may be judged by simple observation of the environment. In the 1988 revision of *Guide for Conservation of Hearing in Noise,* prepared by the Subcommittee on Medical Aspects of Noise of the Committee on Hearing and Equilibrium of the American Academy of Otolaryngology—Head and Neck Surgery, the following three conditions are listed as indications of a need for such a program:

1. Difficulty in communicating by speech while in noise.
2. Head noises or ringing in the ears after working in the noise for several hours.
3. A temporary loss of hearing that has the effect of muffling speech and changing the quality of other sounds after several hours of exposure to noise.

This *Guide* further points out that pain and annoyance do not necessarily accompany hazardous noise. Pain may be felt in the ear during exposure to noise over 130 dB; however, noise-induced hearing loss may be produced at considerably lower levels.

An industrial hearing conservation program should include:

1. Noise exposure analysis;
2. Provision for control of noise exposure (including hearing protectors);
3. Measurements of hearing; and
4. Employee and employer notification and education.

Although the OSHA noise regulation retains the permissible exposure limit at 90 dBA, the 1983 amendment requires hearing conservation programs to include all workers who are exposed to 85 dBA or more.

Noise Survey

As stated earlier, whether a noise is hazardous depends on the intensity of the noise, the spectrum of the noise, the duration and distribution of exposure during a typical workday, and the overall exposure during a work life. Each of these areas must be evaluated to determine the need for instituting noise control and hearing conservation programs. Detailed analysis of the noise field is a complex, highly technical task that requires extensive training on the part of the person performing the analysis. Audiologists are typically not trained for this responsibility. The industrial audiologist, however, should be capable of conducting a noise survey. Performance of this function requires that the audiologist understand noise-measuring equipment and understand the limitations of the method of measurement he uses. Generally, a noise survey will indicate whether a hazardous noise condition does exist and whether there is a need for a more extensive, more detailed analysis of the noise, so that proper noise control procedures can be initiated. In many industrial situations, the noise survey will be conducted by an industrial hygienist or safety engineer, whereas a detailed noise analysis and noise control require the services of an acoustic engineer.

The OSHA Hearing Conservation Amendment (U.S. Department of Labor, 1983) requires employers to perform measurements of noise exposures at least once for those workers whose TWA is 85 dBA or more. The amendment further requires remeasurement when a change in equipment or a work procedure would potentially result in a significant increase in exposure. Assessment of the sound environment must include all continuous, intermittent, and impulsive noise between 80 and 130 dBA.

Most of today's rules, guidelines, and specifications for identifying hazardous noise conditions state that the A-frequency weighting network and the slow meter response on sound-level meters be used to measure noise levels. In a damage risk survey, sound-level measurements are generally required only at the position that will be occupied by the person exposed to noise. The time involved in such a survey depends on the time necessary to establish typical temporal patterns of noise exposure. If the noise is continuous and does not change from day to day, then a fairly small sample is all that is required. If, however, there are unpredictable on-off times, intermittencies and rather complex exposure patterns, then the noise survey may require many days or weeks to accomplish a meaningful description of the noise environment. If the noise is a simple continuous type then the measurements can be made simply by reading the sound level meter and recording the observation. A new sound measurement would not be necessary until there was some noticeable change in the noise source, or there was a change in the location of the worker. For the very complex noise exposure patterns that exist in many industries, however, the variation makes direct sound level measurements very difficult, and usually this kind of sound field requires the use of automatic sound recording equipment.

Surveys conducted for purposes of noise control attempt to isolate and describe a particular noise source so that appropriate and effective procedures for noise reduction can be implemented. This type of analysis requires the use of octave band or even narrower frequency band sound analyzers and are geared to pinpoint and describe individual noise source contributions. Noise control surveys also can be used to determine the amount of acoustical power output from a noise source, to enable prediction of noise levels at particular locations in a noise environment.

Sound-Level Meter. Surveying an industrial environment to determine whether the noise is hazardous requires the use of the sound-level meter. The sound-level meter consists of a microphone, amplifier, attenuator circuit, and some sort of indicating meter. Characteristics of sound-level meters are specified in ANSI Standard S1.4-1983. General purpose sound-level meters are equipped with three frequency weighting networks—A, B and C. The A-weighting network approximates the ear's response characteristics at 40 phons. The B-weighting network is intended to approximate the ear's response at 70 phons, and the C-weighting network corresponds to the ear's response at 100 phons (Earshen, 1986). The frequency characteristics of these weighting networks are shown in Figure 35.4.

Sound-level meters usually have two types of response characteristics built into the meter. These characteristics have been labeled "fast" and "slow" response. The fast response enables the meter to reach within 4 dB of its calibrated reading for 1000 Hz in 0.2 seconds. It can be used to measure levels that do not change substantially in less than 0.2 seconds. The slow response is intended to provide an averaging effect that will reduce the fluctuations of sound levels and make these noise levels easier to read. The slow setting will not provide accurate readings if the sound levels change in less than 0.5 seconds. Neither the fast nor the slow response is adequate for measuring impulse or impact types of noise. Measurement of the acoustic properties of these noises requires special equipment or special circuits in the sound-level meter.

Three basic types of microphones are used in noise measurements. These are the piezo electric, the dynamic, and the condenser microphones. Each has advantages and disadvantages, and all three may be used with sound-level meters. Those making noise measurements should be aware of the limitations of the microphone on their meter. Particularly, they should be interested in the frequency response characteristics of the microphone, the intensity range that can be covered by the microphone, the effects of temperature and humidity on the properties of the microphone and the directional characteristics.

Lack of understanding of the directional properties of microphones is a frequent source of error. A microphone calibrated for use in a random-incidence sound field should usually be held at an angle with respect to the major noise source. This angle should be specified by the manufacturer. A free field microphone is calibrated to measure sounds emanating from a source perpendicular to the microphone diaphragm. A pressure type microphone that is designed for use in a coupler for calibrating audiometers can also be used to measure noise over most of the audible spectrum. The noise, however, should be measured at a grazing incidence to the diaphragm, and the proper microphone calibration curve should be used.

Vibration of the sound-measuring equipment may cause erroneous sound-level readings. Sound-measuring equipment should, whenever possible, be mechanically isolated from any vibrating sources. Simply hand-holding the equipment or placement of it on a foam rubber pad is usually satisfactory.

Most general purpose sound-measuring instruments have built-in calibration circuits for checking electrical gain. These sound-level meters may also be used in connection with acoustical calibrators, which are either built-in or can be purchased as a separate accessory. The electrical and acoustical calibration should

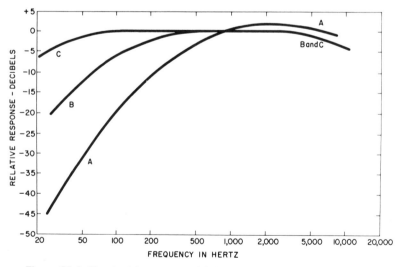

Figure 35.4. Standard frequency weighting curves for sound level meters.

be made according to the manufacturer's instructions at the beginning and end of each day's measurements. If the equipment is battery powered, a battery check should also be made at these times. These field calibration procedures are not of the highest accuracy but will serve to warn of most common instrument failures. Periodically (at least once a year), the sound-measuring equipment should be sent back to the manufacturer or to an independent acoustic laboratory for complete calibration. How often a laboratory calibration is conducted depends on the purpose of the measurements and how frequently and roughly the meter has been handled. It is a good rule of thumb that a complete calibration should be made if changes of greater than ± 2 dB are seen in the daily field calibrations (Sataloff and Michael, 1973).

The amount of noise exposure actually experienced by a given employee is difficult to measure with the usual sound-level meter. During the course of a workday, the noise environment is likely to fluctuate because of changes in the noise source, or because of changes in the employee's position in the noise field. One attempted solution to this problem is the use of personal noise dosimeters. A noise dosimeter is a type of sound-level meter that integrates the A-weighted sound pressure over a period of time and usually compares the measured exposure with a criterion sound exposure, for example with an 8-hour exposure to 90 dBA. The dosimeter is carried by the individual employee with the microphone mounted on the shoulder, on the chest, or at the ear. This device also could be used to monitor a particular area in the industrial environment. The Hearing Conservation Amendment (U.S. Department of Labor, 1983) specifies that employers must use personal monitoring when there is considerable variation in noise level over time.

Noise Control

The control of the noise environment requires highly technical skills and should be undertaken only by acoustic engineers or with the help of acoustic consultants. Noise exposure may be controlled by several methods. The most desirable method is reduction in the amount of noise produced by the source. This is not always possible or practical. Reduction of source noises can be accomplished by careful acoustic design of new equipment, modification of designs of machines in use, and by keeping the equipment in good repair.

Noise control may be achieved by reducing the amount of noise transmitted through the air or through the structure of the building. If the noise source cannot be quieted, then noise reduction can be achieved by constructing barriers between the work area and the noise source, or by sound treating work areas to reduce reverberation. A simple method to reduce the sound level at the worker's ear is to increase the distance between the worker and the noise sources. Placing noise-generating equipment on vibration mounts can reduce transmission of noise through the structural properties of the building.

Noise exposure also could be reduced through administrative or procedural changes. Work schedules could be adjusted so that noise exposures would be interrupted regularly. Personnel who are routinely exposed to high levels of noise could be rotated to other areas and/or other jobs. Work schedules might be arranged so that a minimal number of people are in a particular work area during high-noise conditions. Any procedure that reduces the noise level or reduces the total exposure time will be effective to conserve hearing.

Measurement of Hearing

The main interest of an audiologist in industrial hearing conservation, because of professional orientation, training and experience, will be in the area of hearing measurement. Audiometric examinations are the only available way to detect an individual's susceptibility to noise. By comparing the results of periodic examinations, an estimate can be made of how the employee is being affected by the noisy working environment. People who are particularly sensitive to the stresses of noise can be identified and corrective measures can be instituted before the hearing loss becomes permanent and handicapping.

An industrial hearing measurement program should involve the establishment of an individual employee's auditory sensitivity before exposure or at the initiation of the hearing conservation program. This audiometric measurement can serve as a reference for comparison with periodic follow-up tests conducted throughout the employee's participation in the program. If possible, the reference or baseline audiogram should be obtained before the employee is hired. The hearing conservation amendment (U.S. Department of Labor, 1983) requires that employers provide baseline audiograms within the first year of an employee's exposure to 85 dBA and above and then have annual audiograms for the duration of their employment in a hazardous noise environment. For employees who have been with an employer before initiation of a hearing testing program, the baseline audiogram is defined as the first audiogram taken during employment with the current employer. Periodic follow-up tests serve to monitor any subsequent changes in hearing regardless of etiology.

One of the effects of working in a noise environment is a temporary change in threshold hearing levels. Those responsible for conducting a testing program in industry should be careful to minimize the influence of temporary hearing loss on the baseline or subsequent reference audiograms. Temporary hearing loss can be minimized by allowing sufficient time for recovery of hearing sensitivity before testing the employee's hearing. Current regulations require that testing to establish a baseline audiogram be preceded by at least 14 hours without exposure to workplace noise. If it is not possible to isolate the employee from workplace noise, then this requirement can be achieved by having the employee wear effective hearing protection that would reduce the noise exposure to acceptable levels.

For use in evaluating the changes in hearing sensitivity observed as a function of annual audiometry, there must some criterion for a change to indicate that the employee is at risk for development of a noise-induced hearing loss. OSHA at first referred to this change in hearing sensitivity as a "significant threshold shift," but in the final hearing conservation amendment chose to label this change as a "standard threshold shift." OSHA defines this change in hearing sensitivity as an average shift from baseline levels of 10 dB or more at the frequencies 2000, 3000, and 4000 Hz. When such a change is observed, the employee should be retested to verify its existence. The retest will help to identify those employees who exhibited this change as a consequence of the test procedure and, thereby, reduce the number of employees requiring further action. When the repeat testing verifies the existence of a significant change, the worker involved should be notified in writing regarding this hearing loss, counseled regarding the fitting and use of hearing protection, and, when necessary, referred for further medical and audiologic evaluation in an effort to determine the etiology of the hearing loss (U.S. Department of Labor, 1983).

The hearing conservation amendment of OSHA does not specify the criteria for further medical referral. The identification of a standard (significant) threshold shift should serve to trigger "in-house" action within a given program, i.e., remedy a hazardous noise condition, poor testing technique, faulty equipment or inadequate employee education. Medical or, more specifically, otologic referral should be made for the purpose of diagnostic evaluation and treatment. The American Academy of Otolaryngology—Head and Neck Surgery (1988) defined the criteria for otologic referral as a change in the audiometric levels for either ear when compared with the baseline audiogram of: (a) more than 15 dB for the average of 500, 1000, and 2000 Hz; or (b) more than 20 dB for the average of 3000, 4000, and 6000 Hz.

Audiometers

Several types of manual puretone audiometers are manufactured (ANS S3.6-1989). For industrial testing purposes, the limited range puretone air conduction audiometer is appropriate. This type of audiometer enables measurement of threshold hearing levels from 0–70 dB HL for the frequencies 500, 1000, 2000, 3000, 4000, and 6000 Hz. For the "automatic Bekesy" audiometry, the fixed frequency type of audiometer is preferable in the industrial setting. Although once a mainstay in industrial hearing conservation programs, the Bekesy self-recording audiometer is being used less frequently and is being replaced by the microprocessor technology.

There is no simple answer to the question of whether automatic audiometers are more suitable for industrial hearing testing than manual audiometers. With the use of a manual audiometer, the tester has greater flexibility regarding the testing procedures and more control over the test situation than with the automatic variety. Some employees find that the task in manual puretone audiometry is easier to understand and perform than the automatic test. Neither of these two techniques shows an advantage over the other in terms of the time required for the test, although the use of automatic audiometers in arrays consisting of more than one test instrument will permit more efficient testing of large groups of employees. In addition, microprocessors have the advantage of reducing the time necessary for recording the testing information, for storing the test data and for making the necessary comparisons of periodic audiometric evaluations with the baseline or reference audiogram. The self-recording audiometric technique, whether it is the Bekesy type or microprocessor technology, still requires the attention of the audiometric technician. The technician can turn attention to other tasks only when certain that those being tested are responding properly. Self-recording or computerized microprocessor testing should limit the number of persons being tested at one time to that which a technician can monitor visually.

The automatic audiometers that make use of computer technology attempt to reduce procedural differences between manual measurement and automatic self-recording techniques by programming the microprocessors to carry out threshold measurements using procedures similar to that used with the manual audiometer. These devices have been available for a relatively short time and, therefore, no standards have been developed regarding their use or covering specifications for these devices. These audiometers, however, are covered by the performance specifications for audiometers contained in ANSI S3.6–1989.

Test Method

A major source of variation in manual puretone audiometry can be the test technique. People who perform these tests in industry vary widely in their audiometric background, training and experience. Because of the need to reduce this source of variance, particularly in industrial hearing conservation programs, ANSI has published a standard method for measuring puretone air-conduction threshold hearing levels, ANSI S3.21-1978 (R1986) (ANSI, 1978).

Audiometric Calibration

The test equipment is another source of possible variation in hearing test results. If threshold measurements are to be reliable and valid indications of hearing status, the audiometer must be accurately calibrated. The person doing the testing should check the audiometer daily for malfunction, listening for distortion, intermittency and extraneous noises. Federal regulations (U.S. Department of Labor, 1983) require daily testing of a person with known, stable audiometric thresholds as well as listening, by the test technician, to the audiometer's output. Changes in threshold hearing levels of greater than 10 dB, or other suspicious performance by the audiometer, require acoustic calibration.

An acoustic calibration measures the sound pressure output at 70-dB hearing level and attenuator linearity in 10-dB steps, using a 9-A coupler and a sound level meter. This type of calibration is required by OSHA at least annually. An exhaustive laboratory calibration that verifies compliance with ANSI S3.6–1969 (ANSI, 1969) is required routinely every 2 years, or if the annual electroacoustic calibration indicates an output that deviates from standard specifications by 10 dB at any test frequency. If the sound levels measured at the annual electroacoustic check exceed the specifications by ±3 dB at the test frequencies between 500 and 3000 Hz, 4 dB at 4000 Hz, or 5 dB at 6000 Hz, then an exhaustive laboratory calibration is recommended.

Test Environment

Reliable measures of hearing sensitivity require that ambient background noise levels in the test environment be sufficiently low to avoid interference with the measurement. The most recent federal regulations (U.S. Department of Labor, 1983) stipulate that the background noise levels contained in an out-of-date ANSI standard, S3.1–1960 (ANSI, 1960), are acceptable. These background noise levels will not permit the measurement of threshold hearing levels specified as ANSI-1969 (ANSI, 1989) without the potential con-

tamination of the results by masking. If a hearing testing program requires that it be possible to measure normal hearing threshold sensitivity as published by ANSI, then the background noise limits should be in agreement with those published in ANSI S3.1-1977, "Criteria for Permissible Ambient Noise during Audiometric Testing" (ANSI, 1977). These two specifications for allowable background noise levels are contained in Table 35.4. Both of these stated noise limits assume testing with earphones having attenuation properties similar to that measured for the TDH-39 earphone with MX 41/AR cushions.

Frequently, testing in an industrial situation takes place in an area of a plant or noisy factory. If an industry is sufficiently large, and there are a number of employees involved in the hearing conservation program, the situation may warrant construction of a sound-isolating test facility on the premises, or the use of a mobile test facility.

Mobile test units are particularly useful when a number of different locations are to be surveyed. At the simplest level, the mobile facility could be an enclosure in the form of an audiometric room mounted on a trailer. Nevertheless, the mobile unit may be more elaborate, containing several test rooms and including complete laboratory calibration facilities. In any case, whether the testing area is a quiet room in the industrial facility, a specially constructed sound-isolating test chamber built on the premises or a mobile testing facility, the background noise levels should be sufficiently low to test air-conduction threshold at the desired hearing level.

Test Personnel

The accuracy of the audiometric measurements generally depends on the skill of the tester. It would be desirable if an audiologist were responsible for this service, but in fact under present conditions most hearing tests are conducted by an industrial nurse or

Table 35.4.
Two Specifications of Acceptable Background Noise Levels for Audiometric Testing Tabulated as Octave Band Sound Levels (to Nearest dB)[a]

	Octave Band Center Frequency (Hz)				
	500	1000	2000	3000	4000
S3.1-1960 (Acceptable to OSHA; U.S. Department of Labor, 1983)	40	40	47	57	62
S3.1-1977 (necessary for testing ANSI-1969 normal threshold hearing levels)	22	30	35	42	42

[a]The 1977 standard is required to measure normal hearing threshold levels re: ANSI-1969.

by a technician who has minimal background in audiometry. In an effort to reduce the variation attributable to the skill and training of the technician, training programs have been devised to establish minimal educational foundations and to introduce a standard air-conduction test technique. In 1965, an Intersociety Committee (composed of the Industrial Medical Association, the American Industrial Hygiene Association, the American Association of Industrial Nurses, and the American Speech and Hearing Association) developed a 20-hour training course for the industrial audiometric technician (Maas, 1972). In 1973, the responsibility for quality control of these training programs for industrial audiometric technicians was assumed by the Council for Accreditation in Occupational Hearing Conservation (CAOHC). Clinical audiologists have been extremely active in developing and conducting these training programs. The training courses sanctioned by CAOHC provide the prospective technician with a brief background in sound, the ear, and hearing. A major part of the recommended instruction is devoted to introducing a standard procedure for measurement of puretone air-conduction thresholds, and practice in using this method. The instruction and practice include the recognition of an adequate test environment, care and maintenance of test equipment, and accurate record keeping. Successful completion of the training program qualifies the trainee for a certificate from CAOHC. Test results produced by a certified audiometric technician are legally acceptable.

OSHA requires that the audiometric tests "be performed by a licensed or ASHA certified audiologist, an otolaryngologist, or other physician, or by a technician who is certified by CAOHC or who has satisfactorily demonstrated competence in administering audiometric examinations, obtaining valid audiograms, and properly using, maintaining and checking calibration and proper functioning of the audiometers being used (U.S. Department of Labor, 1983)." Although OSHA exempts a technician who operates microprocessor audiometers from certification, that exemption does not negate the need for required testing competence.

HEARING PROTECTION

The main goal of an industrial hearing conservation program is to prevent noise-induced hearing loss. This can be accomplished by reducing the noise exposure. The best method for this reduction is to prevent the noise generation at the source. When this is not possible, the next most desirable method is to reduce the opportunity for the employee to be exposed to noise through administrative controls. There will be many

situations in which neither of these solutions to the noise problem is possible. Under these conditions, the method of choice would be to provide hearing protectors.

An effective hearing protector serves as a barrier between the noise and the inner ear, where the noise-induced damage occurs. Hearing protectors usually take one of two forms: the earmuff, which is worn over the external ear and provides an acoustic seal against the head; or earplugs, which seal the entrance to the external ear canal. The protection provided by a hearing protector depends on its design and on the physical characteristics of the person wearing the protector.

It is impossible to totally isolate the inner ear from noise by means of a hearing protector. Sound energy can reach the inner ears of persons wearing protectors by three different paths:

1. By passing directly to the cochlea through vibration of the bones and tissues of the skull (bone conduction);
2. By vibration of the hearing protector itself, which generates sound in the ear canal; or
3. By passing through leaks in the hearing protector, or around the protector because of poor fit.

The absolute limit of attenuation provided by a hearing protector depends on the sensitivity of the bone-conduction pathway.

Earplugs

There are many kinds of protectors on the market. The insert type of protector, or earplug, could be semipermanent, molded of soft rubber or soft plastic material that is sized. No single-sized molded earplug has been found that would fit the large range of ear canal sizes and shapes. Most of the accepted molded earplugs come in four or five different sizes.

Earplugs may also be malleable and made of such materials as cotton, paper, wax, glass wool, silicone putty, or slow-recovery foams. These plugs, which can be shaped by the wearer, are usually made of non-porous, easily formed materials, and they are capable of providing attenuation that compares favorably with other forms of hearing protectors. The malleable earplugs are usually designed for short-term use and are frequently disposable.

Earmuffs

Most of the muff protectors are similar in design. The protector ear cups are usually formed of a rigid, dense, imperforate material. These hard shells are fitted into soft, pliable seals, generally made of a smooth plastic envelope filled with a foam or some fluid material. The cup encloses a volume of air that is directly related to low-frequency attenuation. The inside of the ear cup is partially filled with material that absorbs high-frequency resonant noises.

Selection Factors

Most protective devices available commercially will provide sufficient attenuation to offset the hazardous noise exposures typically found in industrial environments. The chief problem has been in developing motivation for employees to wear hearing protectors. Experience has shown that no one type satisfies all employees. It is therefore a good practice to stock more than one variety of protector.

There are advantages and disadvantages to both muff and insert types of hearing protectors (Sataloff and Michael, 1973).

Advantages of Earplugs

1. Small and easily carried;
2. Can be worn conveniently;
3. More comfortable to wear in hot environments;
4. Convenient to use when the head of the wearer must be in close, cramped quarters;
5. Cost is generally significantly less than earmuffs.

Disadvantages of Insert-Type Protection

1. The semipermanent type and molded hearing protectors require more time and effort to fit;
2. The amount of protection provided by an earplug is generally less and varies considerably among wearers;
3. Can become dirty and unsanitary through use;
4. Difficult to see at a distance, making it difficult to ensure that employees are wearing them;
5. Cannot be worn by individuals with external and middle ear infections.

Advantages of Muff-type Protectors

1. A single size will fit most heads;
2. Usually more readily accepted by employee than earplugs;
3. Generally more comfortable than plugs;
4. Not as easily misplaced or lost as earplugs.

Disadvantages of Earmuffs

1. In general, more expensive than insert protectors;
2. Muff protection depends on the spring force of the head band; through usage, the force may be considerably weakened, and the protection significantly reduced.

Field Performance

Ultimately, the type of protection chosen will depend on the noise and environmental conditions in the industry. Personnel responsible for hearing protector programs should be aware of the amount of attenuation provided by the various types of protectors they intend to use. The attenuation properties listed by the manufacturer are usually the average results obtained under relatively good laboratory conditions. Information from studies of hearing protectors in use in the field indicates that actual attenuation provided by these devices is somewhat less than that specified by the manufacturer (Berger, 1986). It is a good rule of thumb to reduce these reported attenuation characteristics by 5 to 10 dB to get an estimate of actual performance in the field.

The use of single-number measurements of noise levels, such as the A-weighted sound level, has led to the development of single-number indicators of hearing protector performance. The Noise Reduction Rating (NRR) is required by the Environmental Protection Agency in its Noise Labeling Rule (U.S. Environmental Protection Agency, 1979). According to this rule, all hearing protectors must be labeled with the NRR factor. The NRR essentially reduces the attenuation attributed to a protector by subtracting 2 standard deviations from the usually specified mean performance. The NRR by virtue of this procedure is an index of protector effectiveness and could be expected by 98% of the users rather than 50% as would be the case for the mean. In actual application in hearing conservation programs, the NRR factor is simply subtracted from the A-weighted exposure level for unprotected ears yielding the protected A-weighted exposure level. For example, if the TWA for an industrial environment was measured to be 95 dBA and the NRR for a given protector was 15, the TWA for an employee using that protector would be estimated to be 80 dBA and would be judged adequate for use in that environment. The use of single-number indicators of hearing protector performance has appeal to federal regulators. OSHA lists the NRR as a convenient method for estimating the adequacy of hearing protector attenuation (U.S. Department of Labor, 1983).

The warning regarding the discrepancy between performance of protectors as listed by the manufacturers, derived under laboratory conditions, and the actual performance of the protectors under realistic industrial conditions, also applies to the NRR. Berger (1983) provided a summary of the actual protection achieved in the field. Figure 35.5 compares the NRR published by the manufacturers which uses the two standard deviation adjustment with field attenuation

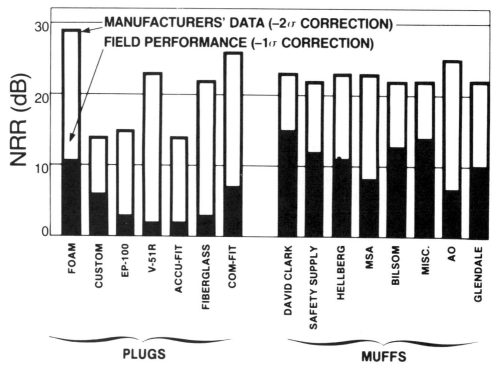

Figure 35.5. Labeled noise reduction ratings (NRR) versus real-world performance for earplugs and earmuffs. (From Berger EH. Using the NRR to estimate the real world performance of hearing protectors. Sound and Vibration 1983;17:12–18.)

data adjusted only by one standard deviation. The discrepancy is dramatic. As a consequence of his review, Berger (1986) feels a more realistic estimate of hearing protector attenuation as these devices are being used by workers would be provided by reducing the manufacturers' NRR by 10 dB.

The attenuation properties of hearing protectors as published by the manufacturers clearly overestimates the actual results and is misleading. Employers using the published NRR would be justified in believing that almost any hearing protector would reduce almost every industrial noise environment to permissible exposures. This is not necessarily the case. This erroneous belief promotes ineffective hearing conservation programs that simply distribute hearing protective devices without any attempt to educate or motivate employees regarding their use (Berger, 1986).

EDUCATIONAL COMPONENT

Education of both the employers and employees involved in a hearing conservation program is vital for the success of that program. OSHA requires that training and education sessions be given at least annually to employees exposed to 85 dBA or more. These sessions are to include information on the effects of noise on hearing, the purpose and procedures of audiometric tests and the proper selection, fitting, use and

care of hearing protectors (U.S. Department of Labor, 1983).

The educational element of hearing conservation is frequently neglected, consisting of an introductory lecture given in the orientation of new workers as well as annual, sometimes unimaginative and often unwelcome presentations. Poorly conceived and executed educational activities not only are not helpful in achieving the objectives of the program but could serve to impede its success. Nevertheless, educational contacts planned appropriately and using educational material selected judiciously can promote cooperation from all program participants.

An effective educational program involves regular activities throughout the work year. These activities should provide information about hearing conservation and the results of the local conservation program. The most successful educational events are those that are kept simple and easy to understand. Educational contacts should be kept short, with group sessions being no more than 15–25 minutes long. The objectives should be meaningful to the people involved, stressing only the information a given audience needs to know. The message should not only summarize information about the hearing conservation program but also be designed to motivate full participation. The major motivator should be avoidance of hearing loss. The educational efforts should emphasize, as clearly as possible, the handicaps imposed by hearing loss. A comprehensive educational program should include the participation of top management, medical and audiological consultants, audiometric technicians, plant nurses, front-line supervisors and foremen, union officials, as well as noise-exposed employees (Royster and Royster, 1986).

RECORD KEEPING

Keeping accurate records is important in any clinical or hearing conservation program. Records assume a particular importance in an industrial situation because of the potential for compensation and the implications for legal action. Federal and state legislation may, in fact, dictate the types of records to be maintained, the form in which these records will be kept and the length of time the records must be stored.

The employer will need to keep accurate records of noise exposure measurements. These records should include the specifications on the location, date and time the measurements were made, the noise levels obtained, and the name of the person making the measurement. The employer may also be required to keep the names of the employees and the daily noise dose experienced by each of these employees. Certainly, there is a need for records specifying the type, model, and calibration of the noise-measuring equipment.

The employer should keep accurate records of audiometric test results for all employees. At a minimum, these records should include: the name and job classification of the employee; the date of the audiogram; the name of the tester; the date of the last acoustic or exhaustive calibration of the audiometer; and an assessment of the employee's most recent noise exposure. The records of the measurements of the background noise levels in the audiometric test rooms should be maintained as well. Although not required by the most recent federal regulations, in view of the potential for legal action, it would seem wise to maintain accurate records of audiometer calibration and service.

The length of time that these records need to be retained varies from state to state and from regulation to regulation. OSHA requires that the records of noise exposure measurements shall be kept for a period of 2 years, whereas audiometric test records shall be retained for the duration of the employee's period of employment (U.S. Department of Labor, 1983).

AUDIOLOGISTS IN INDUSTRIAL HEARING CONSERVATION PROGRAMS

Initiating and maintaining an industrial hearing conservation program may involve a single professional or a group of people with relevant interests. Today, there are relatively few audiologists employed full time in industrial hearing conservation programs. More frequently, they are used in consulting roles. As a consultant, the audiologist comes in contact with industrial physicians, consulting otolaryngologists, safety engineers, industrial hygienists, industrial nurses, industrial relations and personnel managers and officials of management and unions. To function effectively in such a program, audiologists must be aware of their own skills and limitations, as well as the skills and potential services offered by each of the other members of the hearing conservation team. If an audiologist is to be a respected member of the team, he or she must understand the problems of business and industry as well as the problems of the employee who is liable to encounter hazardous noise environments. There must be a particular sensitivity to the need for maintaining test schedules that cause minimal interruption in industrial production. Audiologists can help to supply hearing testing services, can serve as educational resources for audiometric technicians and should be available as consultants to employers and employees alike. They must also be concerned with the selection and provision of hearing protection devices. The services offered by audiologists to industry will depend on the experience and training of the individual audiologist, as well as the needs of the particular industry. Audiologists should promote interest in all forms of hearing conservation, including industrial hearing conservation.

REFERENCES

American Academy of Otolaryngology—Head and Neck Surgery, Committee on Hearing and Equilibrium and the American Council of Otolaryngology, Committee on Medical Aspects of Noise. Guide for the evaluation of hearing handicap. JAMA 1979;133:396–397.

American Academy of Otolaryngology—Head and Neck Surgery Foundation, Inc. Guide for Conservation of Hearing in Noise, Rev. Ed. Washington, DC, 1988.

American Conference of Governmental Industrial Hygienists. Threshold limit values of physical agents adopted by ACGIH for 1969. Cincinnati, Ohio, 1969.

American National Standards Institute. Criteria for Background Noise in Audiometer Rooms. S3.1-1960, New York, 1960.

American National Standards Institute. Specifications for Audiometers. S3.6-1969 (R 1986), New York, 1969.

American National Standards Institute. Criteria for Permissible Ambient Noise during Audiometric Testing. S3.1-1977(R1986), New York, 1977.

American National Standards Institute. Method for Manual Puretone Threshold Audiometry. S3.21-1978(R1986), New York, 1978.

American National Standards Institute. Specification for Sound Level Meters. S1.4-1983, New York, 1983.

American National Standards Institute. Specification for Audiometers. S3.6-1989, New York, 1989.

Atherley GR, and Martin AM. Equivalent continuous noise level as a measure of injury from impact and impulse noise. Annu Occup Hyg 1971;14:11–28.

Berger EH. Using the NRR to estimate real world performance of hearing protectors. Sound and Vibration 1983;17:12–18.

Berger EH. Hearing protection devices. Chap. 10 in Berger EH, Ward WD, Morrill JC, and Royster LH, Eds. Noise & Hearing Conservation Manual, 4th ed. American Industrial Hygiene Association, Akron, OH, 1986:319–381.

Burns W. Noise and Man, 2nd ed. Philadelphia: JB Lippincott, 1973:189–251.

Earshen JJ. Sound Measurement: Instrumentation and noise descriptors. Chap. 3 in Berger EH, Ward WD, Morrill JC, and Royster LH, Eds. Noise & Hearing Conservation Manual, 4th ed. American Industrial Hygiene Association, Akron, OH, 1986:37–95.

Fodor WJ, and Oleinick A. Workers' compensation for occupational noise-induced hearing loss: a review of science and law, and proposed reforms. St Louis Univ Law J 1986;30:703–804.

Guignard JC. A Basis for Limiting Noise Exposure for Hearing Conservation. Prepared for Environmental Protection Agency, EPA-550-9-73-001-A, 4-21, 1973.

International Standard ISO-1999. Acoustics—Determination of occupational noise exposure and estimation of noise-induced impairment. International Organization for Standardization, Geneva, Switzerland, 1990.

Johnson DL. Derivation of presbycusis and noise-induced permanent threshold shift (NIPTS) to be used for the basis of a standard on the effects of noise on hearing. Technical Report 78-128, Aerospace Medical Research Laboratory, Wright-Patterson Air Force Base, Ohio, 1978.

Kraak W. Investigations on criteria for the risk of hearing loss due to noise. In Tobias JV, and Schubert ED, Eds. Hearing Research and Theory, Vol. 1. New York: Academic Press, 1982:187–303.

Kryter KD. The Effects of Noise on Man, 2nd ed. New York: Academic Press, 1985.

Kryter KD, Ward WD, Miller JD, and Eldredge DH. Hazardous exposure to intermittent and steady-state noise. J Acoust Soc Am 1966;39:451–464.

Lim DJ, and Melnick W. Acoustic damage of the cochlea. Arch Otolaryngol 1971;94:294–305.

Maas RB. Industrial noise and hearing conservation. Chap. 41 in Katz J, ed. Handbook of Clinical Audiology. Baltimore: Williams & Wilkins, 1972:772–818.

Melnick W. Human temporary threshold shift from 16-hour noise exposures. Arch Otolaryngol 1974;100:180–189.

Melnick W. Auditory effects of noise exposure. In Miller MH, and Silberman CA, Eds. Occupational Hearing Conservation. Englewood Cliffs: Prentice-Hall, 1984:100–131.

Melnick W, and Maves M. Asymptotic threshold shift (ATS) in man from 24-hour exposure to continuous noise. Ann Otol Rhinol Laryngol 1974;83:820–829.

Michael PI. Single-number performance factors for hearing protectors. In Alberti PW, Ed. Personal Hearing Protection in Industry. New York: Raven Press, 1982.

Miller JD. Effects of Noise on People. Prepared for Environmental Protection Agency, MTID 300.7, 1971:15–33.

Mills JH. Relationship of noise to hearing loss. Semin Hear 1988;9:255–266.

Mills JH, Gengel RW, Watson CS, and Miller JD. Temporary changes of the auditory system due to exposure to noise for one or two days. J Acoust Soc Am 1970;48:524–530.

Mosko JD, Fletcher JI, and Iuz GA. Growth and Recovery of Temporary Threshold Shifts Following Extended Exposure to High Level Continuous Noise. Report 911. U.S. Army Medical Research Laboratory, Ft. Knox, KY, 1970.

National Center for Health Statistics. Hearing Levels of Adults by Age and Sex, 1960–72. Vital and Health Statistics, Public Health Service Publication No. 1000-Series 11-No. 11. U.S. Government Printing Office, Washington, DC, 1965.

Nixon JE, and Glorig A. Noise-induced permanent threshold shift at 2000 cps and 4000 cps. J Acoust Soc Am 1961;33:904–908.

Passchier-Vermeer W. Hearing loss due to continuous exposure to steady-state broad-band noise. J Acoust Soc Am 1974;56:1585–1593.

Robinson DW, and Shipton MS. Tables for estimation of noise-induced hearing loss. Technical Report AC 61, National Physical Laboratory, England, 1977.

Royster LH, and Royster JD. Education and motivation. Chap. 11 in Berger EH, Ward WD, Morrill JC, and Royster LH, Eds. Noise & Hearing Conservation Manual. American Industrial Hygiene Association, Akron, OH, 1986:383–415.

Rudmose W. Hearing loss resulting from noise exposure. In Harris CM, Ed. Handbook of Noise Control. 1st ed. New York: McGraw-Hill, 1957.

Sataloff J, and Michael PI. Hearing Conservation. Springfield, IL: Charles C Thomas, 1973:70–83;161–165;315–316.

Shipman v. Employers Mutual Liability Ins. & Lockhead Corp. 1962. 125 SE (2d) 72.

Slawinski v. Williams & Co. 1948. 298 N.Y.546, 81 N.E. 2d 93, aff g 277 App. Div. 826,76 N.Y. 2d 888.

Taylor W, Pearson J, Mair A, and Burns W. Study of noise and hearing in jute weaving. J Acoust Soc Am 1965;38:113–120.

Tonndorf J, von Gierke HE, and Ward WD. Criteria for noise and vibration exposure. In Harris CM, Ed. Handbook of Noise Control. New York: McGraw-Hill, 1979:18–1 to 18–14.

United States Department of Labor. Proposed requirements and procedures, occupational noise exposure. Federal Register 39, No. 207, 1974.

United States Department of Labor. Occupational Safety and Health Administration; occupational noise exposure; hearing conservation amendment, part III. Federal Register 46, No. 11, 4078–4179, 1981.

United States Department of Labor. Occupational Safety and Health Administration; occupational noise exposure; hearing conservation amendment; final rule. Federal Register 48, No. 46, 9738–9785, 1983.

United States Environmental Protection Agency. Information on levels of environmental noise requisite to protect public health and welfare with adequate margin of safety. NTIS 550/9-74-004, Washington, DC, 1974.

United States Environmental Protection Agency. Noise labeling requirements for hearing protectors. Federal Register, Part 211, Subpart B, 4, No. 190, 56139–56147, 1979.

Walsh-Healey Public Contracts Act. Federal Register 34, No. 96, 1969.

Ward WD. Auditory fatigue and masking. In Jerger J, Ed. Modern Developments in Audiology, 1st ed. New York: Academic Press, 1963:240–286.

Ward WD. Susceptibility to auditory fatigue. In Neff WD, Ed. Contributions to Sensory Physiology, Vol. 3. New York: Academic Press, 1968:191–226.

Ward WD. Adaptation and fatigue. In Jerger J, Ed. Modern Developments in Audiology, 2nd ed. New York: Academic Press, 1973:323–328.

Webster's Ninth New Collegiate Dictionary. Springfield, MA: GC Merriam, 1989.

Williams-Steiger Occupational Safety and Health Act. PL 91-596. 1970.

CHAPTER 36

Pseudohypacusis

Frederick N. Martin

Not every patient seen in the audiology clinic is fully cooperative during the hearing evaluation. This lack of cooperation may be because the patient (*a*) does not understand the test procedure, (*b*) is poorly motivated, (*c*) is physically or emotionally incapable of appropriate responses, (*d*) wishes to conceal a handicap, (*e*) is deliberately feigning or exaggerating a hearing loss for personal gain or exemption, or (*f*) fails to respond accurately because of unconscious motivation. This chapter will describe some of the concepts underlying false or exaggerated hearing test results. It will also present some audiometric procedures that aid in the detection of inaccuracies and in the determination of a patient's true hearing thresholds.

Many terms have been used to describe a hearing loss that appears greater than can be explained on the basis of pathology in the auditory system. The most popularly used terms in the literature today are "non-organic hearing loss," "pseudohypacusis," "psychogenic hearing loss," and "malingering." Williamson (1974) cautions that such terms do not necessarily describe the same phenomenon. Inasmuch as clinicians typically do not know whether an inflated auditory threshold is the result of conscious or unconscious motivation, it seems appropriate to use generic terms. The term "pseudohypacusis," which was proposed by Carhart (1961), appears most descriptive. Both "pseudohypacusis" and "nonorganic hearing loss" will be used interchangeably in this chapter to describe responses obtained on hearing examination which are above the patient's true organic thresholds.

If one thinks of a hearing loss which is due to physical impairment in the auditory system as being "organic," then the term nonorganic is immediately clear. Many individuals with pseudohypacusis have nonorganic aspects superimposed on an organic hearing loss (Johnson et al., 1956). Audiologists must remember that their function is to determine the extent of the organic component rather than to determine the precise reason for the nonorganic results.

PSEUDOHYPACUSIS IN ADULTS

A number of factors may encourage some persons either to feign a hearing loss that does not exist or to exaggerate an existing hearing loss (Nilo and Saunders, 1976). One of these factors is financial gain. Altshuler (1982) reports that a significant amount of stress in the United States today is directly attributable to economics. The very threat of the loss of income may drive some individuals to acts of "questionable honesty" that they might not otherwise consider. Disability compensation to veterans with service-connected hearing losses constitutes a significant portion of the millions of dollars paid annually to beneficiaries of the Veterans Administration.

Other factors that may contribute to pseudohypacusis are psychosocial and include the wish to avoid undesirable situations. There may be many other "gains" that the individual may believe are afforded to hearing-handicapped persons, including excuses for ". . . lack of success, advancement in position, poor marital situation and so on" (Altshuler, 1982).

The number of persons with pseudohypacusis may be increasing since the implementation of federal laws regarding hearing safety in the workplace. Some state laws regarding noise in industry are even more stringent than federal legislation. The promise of financial reward is bound to be a factor precipitating pseudohypacusis in workers who are in danger of incurring noise-induced hearing loss. Barelli and Ruder (1970) gathered data on 162 medicolegal patients and found that 24% of the 116 workers applying for compensation proved to have a nonorganic hearing loss.

Studying social and psychologic characteristics of adult males with pseudohypacusis, Trier and Levy (1965) reported psychologic and psychiatric evaluations of patients with and without hearing complaints. The nonorganic group achieved lower scores on all measures of current socioeconomic status and scored significantly lower on measures of verbal intelligence. They showed a greater degree of clinically significant emotional disturbance. Trends of hypochondriasis were also noted, including many complaints of tinnitus. These findings are similar to other reports which state that adults with nonorganic hearing loss also manifest a reliance on denial mechanisms. Such patients appear to have a diminished sense of confidence in their ability to meet the needs of everyday life and may feel a sense of some gain by appearing to be hearing impaired.

There is disagreement over whether a nonorganic hearing loss may be psychogenic at all, or whether all exaggerated hearing thresholds are deliberately and consciously manifested with an eye toward personal gain. Beagley and Knight (1968) stated that, although psychogenic deafness is rare, it does occur and can be diagnosed if careful attention is paid to the diagnostic criteria. They summarized 21 cases of nonorganic hearing loss and specified one case as fulfilling all of the criteria for a psychiatric background. Goldstein (1966) suggests that psychogenic hearing loss does not exist as a clinical entity. He believes that all nonorganic hearing losses are consciously simulated (malingered).

Two groups of servicemen were compared by Cohen et al. (1963). One group was consistent on auditory tests and the other was not. The inconsistent group manifested deviant neurosensory signs and psychologic abnormalities, gave reports of head injuries out of proportion to the actual extent of the injury, but showed no difference from the control subjects in predisposing factors. Cohen et al. concluded that individuals who present inconsistent results on hearing tests may be influenced by psychodynamic factors.

Gleason (1958), in a study of military personnel with pseudohypacusis, found that the patient who is inconsistent on audiologic tests is likely to be deviant psychologically but not necessarily psychiatrically ill. Fifty-five percent were judged to be emotionally immature and 30% neurotic. Of 278 consecutive cases, 30% showed inconsistencies and exaggerated hearing losses and 86% of this subgroup had medically confirmed losses. The inconsistent group had many psychosomatic complaints, deviant social behavior, and in general made poor adjustments to their hearing losses. Most of these men had done poorly in school. The conclusion of this study was that in many cases of pseudohypacusis the problem is on an unconscious level to gain a favored goal, or to explain to society that the patient is blameless for inadequate social behavior. From this point of view, exaggerated hearing loss may be one symptom of a personality disturbance.

Katz (1980) cautions that certain neurologic problems can appear to be nonorganic in nature. For example, one patient who initially responded on puretone evaluation between 40 and 70 dB hearing level (HL), and eventually at levels of 20 dB, responded immediately at 15 dB to spondees. This patient was by no means a malingerer nor psychogenic. Rather he was a volunteer for a study because he was terminally ill with a tumor of the corpus callosum. He did not claim to have difficulty with hearing, nor did he exhibit any difficulty in communication.

The question arises, "Why a hearing loss?" Why does the pseudohypacusic patient select this disorder rather than back pain, headache, or some other conventional malady? Altshuler's (1982) suggestions are logical, that some incident in the lives of these patients has focused their attention on hearing. The incident may have been an ear infection, physical trauma, noise exposure, or tinnitus or hearing loss in a relative or close friend. For whatever reason, this incident is the first step toward a future nonorganic loss.

PSEUDOHYPACUSIS IN CHILDREN

A number of case reports of pseudohypacusis in children appear in the literature. Dixon and Newby (1959) reported on 40 children between the ages of 6 and 18 years with pseudohypacusis. Despite claimed hearing losses, 39 of these children were able to follow normal conversational speech with little difficulty. More recently McCanna and DeLapa (1981) reported similar findings. Most experienced audiologists can report similar experiences with marked exaggeration of hearing thresholds for puretones in the presence of normal speech reception thresholds.

There are also cases of apparent malingering with psychologic undertones. For example, Bailey and Martin (1961) reported on a boy with normal hearing sensitivity who manifested a great many nonorganic symptoms. After the audiometric examination he admitted a deliberate attempt to create the impression that he had a hearing loss. He claimed he did this so that he could be admitted to the state residential school for the deaf where his parents taught and his sister and girlfriend were students. Investigation into this boy's background revealed that he was a poor student in a high school for normal-hearing students. Hallewell et al. (1966) described a 13-year-old boy with a severe bilateral hearing loss who revealed essentially normal hearing sensitivity under hypnosis.

Cases of presumed psychogenic hearing loss have also been reported. Lumio et al. (1969) reported on three sisters whose hearing losses all appeared to develop over a period of a few months. Two of the three girls also had complaints of visual problems and were fitted with eyeglasses. All three apparently had their hearing return to normal in 1 day during a visit with their aunt. When the hearing returned the visual disorders also disappeared. These authors reported that the pseudohypacusis was due to family conflicts. They believed that it was probable that the hearing loss of the youngest child was entirely unconscious, but the other two may have been partly simulated.

Thirty-two cases diagnosed as psychogenic hearing loss are reported by Barr (1963). Although puretone audiograms showed levels in the 60- to 80-dB range, hearing for speech was considerably better than would be anticipated based on both formal and informal tests. Overall, these children were of normal intelligence but did not perform well in school. Because they were from homes where high scholastic performance was considered important, their parents willingly accepted the idea of hearing loss (based on failure of a school hearing test) as explanation of poor academic achievement. It was believed that the attention paid to the children encouraged them consciously or unconsciously to feign a hearing loss on subsequent examinations. Barr stresses that the nonorganic difficulty must be detected as early as possible before the child realizes that there are secondary gains to be enjoyed from a hearing disorder.

Sometimes children who fail school screening tests become the object of a great deal of attention. This may cause the children to continue to feign a hearing loss. A number of such school children are discussed by Campanelli (1963). These children behaved on formal tests as if they had a hearing loss but behaved normally in other situations. This study further emphasized the need for caution against preferential seating, special classes, hearing therapy, and hearing aids until the extent of the hearing problem is defined by proper audiologic diagnosis. In a study evaluating one hearing conservation program (Leshin, 1960), a number of cases of nonorganic hearing loss were discovered. A team including otologists, audiologists, medical social workers and local health department staff worked to: (a) reconcile medical, audiologic and psychosocial data to arrive at a diagnosis; (b) determine familial and environmental factors contributing to nonorganic loss, and (c) outline and implement courses of action to relieve the child's need to use pseudohypacusis as a personality mechanism.

Identification audiometry is a significant step in discovering school children with hearing disorders. There is some reason to fear that a child may fail a school test despite normal hearing due to such factors as noisy acoustic environment, improper testing technique, insufficient motivation, or poorly calibrated equipment. If attention is attracted to this incorrect failure the child may get the notion that a hearing loss provides a variety of secondary gains, such as an excuse for poor school performance. The end result may be referral to an otologic or audiologic clinic for further evaluation of hearing. Several authors (Ross, 1964; Miller et al., 1968) have stressed the need to uncover nonorganic hearing losses before referrals are made. Ross cited four cases that illustrate the problems of such referrals and the commitment to simulated hearing loss this may bring to the child.

Pseudohypacusis in children appears to occur with sufficient frequency to cause concern. Whether the notion of simulating a hearing loss comes out of a school screening failure or from some conscious or unconscious need, it must be recognized as early as possible by the audiologist to avoid a variety of unfortunate circumstances. Performance or supervision of hearing tests on young children by an audiologist may serve to avert what may later develop into serious psychologic or educational difficulties. However, the audiologist should be alert to the possibility that the problem uncovered may be one of auditory perception and not true hearing loss (Wieczorek, 1979).

INDICATIONS OF PSEUDOHYPACUSIS

The Nontest Situation

Frequently the source of referral will suggest the possibility of pseudohypacusis. When an individual is referred by an attorney after an accident that has resulted in a client's sudden loss of hearing, it is only natural to suspect that nonorganicity may play a role in test results. This is also true of veterans referred for hearing tests, the results of which decide the amount of monthly pension. It must be emphasized that the majority of patients referred for such examinations are cooperative and well meaning; however, the VA population consists of a higher risk group for pseudohypacusis than self-referred or physician-referred patients. Pseudohypacusis must be on the minds of clinical audiologists or they may miss some of the symptoms that indicate its presence.

A case history is always of value, but it is particularly valuable in compensation cases. It is obviously beneficial for examining audiologists to take the history statement themselves so that they can observe not only the responses given to questions, but also the manner in which these responses are offered. The patient may claim an overreliance on lipreading, may ask for inappropriate repetitions of words and constantly readjust a hearing aid. It is usual for hard-of-hearing patients to be relatively taciturn about their hearing problems, whereas exaggerated or contradictory statements of difficulty or discomfort, vague descriptions of hearing difficulties, and the volunteering of unasked-for supplementary information may be symptomatic of pseudohypacusis.

We sometimes see in patients with pseudohypacusis exaggerated actions and maneuvers to watch every movement of the speaker's lips, or the turning away with hand cupped over the ear, ostensibly to amplify sound. As a rule, hard-of-hearing adults face the speaker with whom they are conversing, but their watching postures are not nearly so tortuous as described above. Not all patients who intend to exaggerate their hearing thresholds create such caricatures, and even patients who do should not be condemned as having a pseudohypacusic loss on the basis of such evidence alone.

The Test Situation

During the hearing examination the pseudohypacusic patient is frequently inconsistent in test responses. A certain amount of variability is to be expected of any individual; however, when the magnitude of this variability exceeds 10 dB for any threshold measurement one must consider the possibility of nonorganicity. With the exception of some unusual conditions it can be expected that the cooperative patient will give consistent audiometric readings.

Two types of patient error are frequently seen in the clinical testing of puretone thresholds. These are false-positive and false-negative responses. When the subject does not respond at levels at or slightly above true thresholds, this constitutes a false-negative response. False-negative responses are characteristic of pseudohypacusis. Frequently, the highly responsive patient will give false-positive responses, signaling that a tone was heard when none was presented at or above threshold. False-positive responses, although sometimes annoying, are characteristic of a conscientious responder.

Feldman (1962) points out that the patient with pseudohypacusis does not offer false-positive responses during silent periods on puretone tests. Chaiklin and Ventry (1965a) found that only 22% of their group of adult subjects with nonorganic hearing loss gave a "false alarm" whereas 86% of those with organic loss gave false-positive responses. Thus one simple check for nonorganicity is to allow silent intervals of a minute or so from time to time. A false alarm is more likely to indicate that the patient is trying to cooperate and believes that a tone was introduced. Extremely slow and deliberate responses may be indicative of a nonorganic problem because most patients with organic hearing losses respond relatively quickly to the signal, particularly at levels above threshold (Wood et al., 1977).

The Audiometric Configuration

A number of authors have suggested that an audiometric pattern emerges that is consistent with pseudohypacusis. Some have described this pattern as a relatively flat audiogram showing an equal amount of hearing loss across frequencies (Semenov, 1947; Fournier, 1958). Others have suggested that the "saucer-shaped audiogram" similar to a supraliminal equal loudness contour is the typical curve illustrating non-

organicity (Doerfler, 1951; Carhart, 1958; Goetzinger and Proud, 1958). However, Chaiklin et al. (1959) observed that saucer-shaped audiograms can also occur in true organic hearing losses and that these curves are seen infrequently in nonorganic hearing loss. They concluded that there is no typical puretone configuration associated with nonorganic hearing loss. Because the patient with nonorganic hearing loss may attempt to give responses that are of equal loudness at all frequencies, ignorance of the manner in which loudness grows with respect to intensity at different frequencies does suggest that the result should be a saucer-shaped audiogram. The logic of this is apparently not borne out in fact.

In a study of 64 men with nonorganic hearing loss and 36 men with true organic loss, Ventry and Chaiklin (1965) asked a panel of three experienced audiologists to judge the configurations of the audiograms. Saucer-shaped curves appeared in only 8% of the nonorganic cases and were also seen in true organic losses. This research indicates, as many experienced audiologists have observed, that the saucer audiogram has limited use in identifying pseudohypacusis.

Test-Retest Reliability

One indication of nonorganicity is lack of consistency on repeated measures. Counseling the patient about inaccuracies may encourage more accurate responses; however, if this counseling is done in a belligerent way it can hardly be expected to increase cooperation. Sometimes a brief explanation of the test discrepancies encourages improved patient cooperation. By withholding any allegations of guilt on the part of the patient the audiologist can assume personal responsibility for not having conveyed the instructions properly. This provides a graceful way out for many patients even if they are highly committed to nonorganic loss. Berger (1965) found that some children can be coaxed into "listening harder," thereby improving results on puretone tests.

Although these suggestions are usually useful when working with civilian populations, exceptions exist when testing military personnel. When counseling and cajoling fail to eliminate symptoms of pseudohypacusis, direct confrontation may be made. Patients may be told that exaggeration of thresholds is a violation of the Universal Code of Military Justice and therefore a court martial offense. Personal communication with audiologists working in military installations reveals that such methods may be very effective indeed. Veterans with service-connected hearing losses may have their pensions interrupted until examining audiologists are satisfied with test results.

Shadow Curve

It is generally agreed that a patient with a severe hearing loss in one ear will hear a test tone in the opposite ear if the signal is raised to a sufficient level during a puretone test. The sound travels to the non-test ear by bone conduction. For an air-conduction signal the levels required for contralateralization range from 40 to 70 dB, depending on frequency (Zwislocki, 1953). The interaural attenuation, the loss of energy of the sound due to contralateralization, is much less for bone conduction than for air conduction. With the vibrator placed on the mastoid process there is almost no interaural attenuation, although it can be as much as 20 dB for the higher frequencies in some cases. If a person has no hearing for air conduction or bone conduction in one ear, the audiogram taken from the bad ear would suggest a moderate conductive loss. Unless clinical masking is applied to the better ear a "shadow curve" should be expected. A complete discussion of interaural attenuation, the shadow curve and masking is presented in Chapter 8.

It may seem advantageous to a patient feigning a hearing loss to claim that loss in only one ear. Appearing to have one normal ear is convenient because individuals need not worry about being "tripped up" in conversation by responding to a sound that is below the admitted threshold. In this way all hearing can occur in the "good ear" and the claim can be made that hearing is poor in the "bad ear." Normal activities can be carried on for the unilaterally hearing-impaired individual without any special speechreading abilities.

The naive pseudohypacusic patient may give responses indicating no hearing in one ear and very good hearing in the other ear. The lack of contralateral response, especially by bone conduction, is a very clear symptom of unilateral nonorganic hearing loss and offers a good reason why all patients should be tested initially without masking, even if it appears obvious at the outset of testing that masking will be required later in the examination.

SRT and Puretone Average Disagreement

The speech recognition threshold (SRT) is generally expected to compare favorably with the average of the best two of the three thresholds obtained at 500, 1000, and 2000 Hz (Siegenthaler and Strand, 1964). Lack of agreement between the puretone average (PTA) and the SRT, in the absence of explanations such as slope of the audiogram or poor word discrimination (Noble, 1973) is symptomatic of nonorganic hearing loss. Carhart (1952) was probably the first to report that in confirmed cases of nonorganic hearing loss the SRT is *lower* (better) than the PTA. Ventry

and Chaiklin (1965) reported that the SRT-PTA discrepancy identified 70% of their patients with confirmed pseudohypacusis; in each case the SRT proved to be at least 12 dB lower than the PTA. The lack of SRT-PTA agreement is often the first major symptom of pseudohypacusis. Persons exaggerating their thresholds undoubtedly use some kind of a loudness judgment to maintain consistency throughout testing. In attempting to remember the loudness of a suprathreshold signal previously responded to, one might easily become confused between puretone and spondaic word levels. Very little research has been carried out to explain why the discrepancy generally favors the SRT. It might be that the loudness of speech is primarily associated with its low frequency components. According to the equal loudness contours, the low frequencies grow more rapidly than tones in the speech frequencies. This speculation is supported by the work of McLennan and Martin (1976), who concluded that when puretones of different frequencies are compared in loudness against a speech signal, the difference between them is a function of the flattening of the loudness contours. Hirsh (1952, p 212) likens the phon lines to loudness recruitment in that the low frequency sounds increase in loudness more quickly per dB than the midfrequencies. Ventry (1976) explains the difference between the sensations of loudness for speech and puretones on the basis of their different sound pressure level references:

SPECIAL TESTS FOR PSEUDOHYPACUSIS

One function of audiologists is to determine the organic hearing thresholds for all of their patients, including those with pseudohypacusis. It is not simply a matter of gathering evidence against the nonorganic patient to prove a case. This is sometimes necessary but unfortunately too common, for the unmasking of nonorganic cases should not be an end in itself. Although it is easier to make a diagnosis on cooperative patients in terms of their hearing thresholds, the lack of cooperation does not justify disinterest in the patient on the part of the audiologist.

There are tests that prove the presence of pseudohypacusis, those that approximate the true threshold and those that actually quantify the patient's threshold without voluntary cooperation. Discussion of tests for pseudohypacusis will follow.

QUALITATIVE TESTS

Automatic Audiometry

Jerger (1960) described the diagnostic usefulness of automatic audiometry.

In Bekesy audiometry the locus of auditory lesion is

determined by comparison of the threshold tracings obtained with continuous and periodically interrupted tones. Patients with nonorganic hearing loss sometimes manifest a distinct Bekesy pattern (Jerger and Herer, 1961) with the tracings for interrupted tones showing poorer hearing than for continuous tones. This nonorganic type of tracing was called type V. The same kind of tracing in patients with pseudohypacusis was reported by Resnick and Burke (1962). Since these original reports type V patterns have been reported for pseudohypacusic adults (Stein, 1963) and children (Peterson, 1963).

Although the type V tracing has not been completely explained, the work of Rintelmann and Carhart (1964) suggests that it is related to the patients' own internal standard for most comfortable loudness or to their recalled loudness for a sustained tone. Hattler (1968) indicated that the type V tracing may be attributed to differential effects of memory upon the loudness of sustained and interrupted puretones. In any case, normal-hearing subjects require greater intensity for interrupted tones to match the loudness of continuous tones.

Hattler (1970) altered the normal pulsed-tone duty cycle (200 msec on, 200 msec off) to 200 msec on, 800 msec off. He called this the lengthened-off-time (LOT) test. The LOT test has the effect of increasing the tracing level of the interrupted tones for pseudohypacusic patients but has no effect on the tracings of normal listeners or organic hypacusics. LOT identified 95% of a series of nonorganic cases whereas type V tracings using the standard 50% duty cycle identified only 40%.

Chaiklin (1990) modified the traditional LOT procedure using a signal that is decreased, rather than increased in intensity. Calling the method DELOT, he found it more than 29% more sensitive than LOT in identifying pseudohypacusis.

Rintelmann and Harford (1967) stated that the type V Bekesy classification should be based on sweep frequency rather than fixed frequency tracings. They define the type V as a separation of pulsed and continuous tracings for at least two octaves with a minimum of a 10-dB separation between midpoints. Using these criteria they found type V tracings in none of their series of normal-hearing subjects, 2% of their patients with conductive hearing loss, 3% of their sensory-neural group, and 76% of their nonorganic group. These figures speak well for the procedure in identifying pseudohypacusis using strict criteria for classification. The criteria described above have been validated in other research (Ventry, 1971).

The effects of sophistication and practice on type V tracings were studied by Martin and Monro (1975). In three groups of normal-hearing subjects simulating a hearing loss the LOT procedure was consistently superior to standard-off-time in the elicitation of type V patterns. Subjects who were familiarized with the principle of the type V pattern did better than those who were not informed. A third group was allowed practice with the procedure while observing the action of the pen of the Bekesy audiometer and did consistently better in producing organic types of Bekesy tracings than either of the other two groups. A recommendation was made that in cases of suspected pseudohypacusis the continuous tones should be compared to both the standard-off-time and LOT tones, and the two pulsed-tone tracings should be compared to each other to increase the efficiency of this test. They concluded that practice and sophistication assist subjects in avoiding the type V pattern when they are trying to simulate a hearing loss.

To add greater difficulty in Bekesy tracings for pseudohypacusic patients, Hood et al. (1964) developed a technique called BADGE (Bekesy ascending-descending gap evaluation). The patient tracks threshold for a fixed frequency over a 1-min period for a continuous tone. The level is set at 0 dB HL and the tone is automatically increased in intensity until the subject presses the key, indicating that the tone has been heard. This is called the continuous ascending test. After 1 min of tracing, the pen is replaced to 0 dB HL and the audiometer is set to the automatic pulse mode. A 1-min trace is then obtained in the pulsed ascending condition. Following these tracings the tone is switched off and the pen is set in a position so that the tone is at a level 30 to 40 dB above the pulsed ascending tracing or at the maximum output of the audiometer, whichever is lower. The tone is then switched on in the pulse mode and the patient tracks threshold for 1 min. This is called the pulsed descending test. Hood et al. (1964) found that using a combination of pulsed and continuous, ascending and descending modes of tracing apparently destroys the pseudohypacusic patient's yardstick for the level selected to simulate as threshold. Using this method a number of subjects gave positive BADGE results, but did not show a type V tracing. The test obviously confuses the nonorganic patient and therefore is useful in identification of exaggerated hearing thresholds.

A high incidence of type V tracings reported among otherwise cooperative listeners unaccustomed to Bekesy audiometry suggests that this type of tracing may not be a good indicator of pseudohypacusis (Hopkinson, 1965; Stark, 1966). It has been suggested (Price et al., 1965) that a psychologic but not necessarily psychopathologic explanation may be offered for the type V tracing. Although very wide pen excursions during Bekesy audiometry may be seen in hypacusic patients, Istre and Burton (1969) reported on a patient with pseudohypacusis with swings up to 45 dB. They believed that the wide Bekesy swings may be diagnostic because the normal swing is usually 6 to 16 dB (assuming an attenuation rate of 2.5 dB/sec). It seems unwarranted to assume pseudohypacusis on the basis of swing width alone because this can be caused by factors other than nonorganicity, such as reaction time (Suzuki and Kubota, 1966) and personality (Shepherd and Goldstein, 1968).

Dean et al. (1976) used Bekesy audiometry with tonal durations of 20 and 500 msec to scrutinize the phenomenon of temporal integration in pseudohypacusic patients. Differences among tracings for the two pulsing tones and for a continuous tone did prove diagnostic for pseudohypacusis.

Arguments over the usefulness of Bekesy audiometry techniques for diagnosis of pseudohypacusis are bound to continue. It can be said at this point, however, that the LOT and BADGE tests are certainly of value, although it must be recognized that they do not indicate the true threshold. Although a type V tracing may suggest nonorganicity and the need for further tests, it is not evidence of pseudohypacusis in and of itself.

The Doerfler-Stewart (D-S) Test

Most subjects find it difficult to maintain consistent suprathreshold responses to auditory signals in the presence of several levels of noise in the same ear. This known difficulty was the principle of the test that was developed by Doerfler and Stewart in 1946. The D-S test was designed to detect bilateral pseudohypacusis by presenting successive levels of sawtooth noise and spondaic words through both channels of a speech audiometer. Although cooperative patients continue to repeat spondees even with noise levels slightly above threshold, patients who exaggerate their thresholds for both the speech and noise become confused. Perhaps because of the complexity of the D-S test, it is rarely used today (Martin and Morris, 1989).

Lombard Test

Speakers monitor their vocal intensity by means of auditory feedback. When masking is applied to their ears and threshold is raised, it is normal for people to speak more loudly in an effort to monitor their voices. This is called the Lombard voice reflex. Theoretically there should be no change in vocal intensity unless the noise is well above the speaker's threshold, masking the normal auditory feedback.

The Lombard test is performed by having the patient read a passage into a microphone while wearing earphones. Ideally, a lavalier microphone is suspended from the patient's neck because it maintains a constant distance from the speaker's lips. As the reading progresses, the level of noise is increased gradually into both ears. If the patient's microphone is fed to the volume unit (VU) meter of the audiometer, then the individual's speech levels can be monitored visually by the clinician (Simonton, 1965). If the Lombard effect is observed, it can be said that the noise was heard by the speaker. Further quantification of this test has not been possible.

Delayed Auditory Feedback (DAF)

The phenomenon of delayed speech feedback has been known for some years. When a subject speaks into the microphone of a tape recorder, has that signal amplified and played back through earphones, the result is simultaneous auditory feedback and is not unlike what most of us experience as we monitor our voices auditorily. When the feedback is mechanically or electronically delayed by approximately 200 msec, the result is a change in vocal rate and intensity (Black, 1951) and sometimes an increase in vocal loudness if the playback level is high enough to produce the Lombard effect. The ideal delay time recommended by Hanley and Tiffany (1954) for audiometric purposes is 180 msec.

When used as a test for pseudohypacusis the intensity of the recorded signal is controlled by the audiometer. One common procedure is to have the patient read a typed selection several times with no feedback followed by reading with DAF. A recommended reading time for the passage is 30 sec (Hopkinson, 1978). The initial reading time, clocked with a stopwatch, is compared to the reading time under the DAF condition. The starting level should be 0 dB HL and increased in 10-dB steps with each reading. A change in reading time of 3.5 sec may be considered a positive sign that the patient has heard her or his own speech and that the delay has caused the change (McGranahan et al., 1960).

Although some reports of reading time changes with DAF at low sensation levels have been reported, there are many people who seem to be able simply to ignore the delay in feedback of their voices. There has been little research in recent years on speech DAF, but the high variability has led to little use of this procedure. If the reading time change or change in vocal intensity can be stated with sureness, and the level at which this occurs is below the patient's admitted threshold for continuous discourse or at a low sensation level, the finding is obviously one of initially exaggerated results. Failing this, the DAF test has limited usefulness.

Swinging Story Test

For some time a procedure has been available to identify the presence of unilateral pseudohypacusis. The test requires the use of a twin channel speech audiometer. A story is read to a patient with portions directed above the threshold of the normal ear (e.g., 10 dB above the SRT) through one channel, other portions below the threshold of the "poorer ear" (e.g., 10 dB below the SRT) and portions through both channels simultaneously. One example of a good story for this purpose is seen in Figure 36.1 (Martin, 1986).

For the test to work the story must be presented rapidly, including rapid switching from channel 1 to channel 2 to both channels. Although this can be done using monitored live voice, an easier method is to use a prerecording on magnetic stereo tape. A calibration tone recorded on each channel allows for adjustment of the VU meters before the test begins.

Upon completion of the recording the patient is simply asked to repeat the story. Information directed to the "good" ear or both ears is to be expected. Any remarks from the *bad ear* column must have been heard below the patient's admitted threshold for speech and prove that the threshold for that ear has been exaggerated. All that can be determined from a positive result is that hearing is better in the poorer ear than what the patient has volunteered, providing evidence of pseudohypacusis.

One of the advantages of the swinging story shown in Figure 36.1 is that the theme changes when the *bad ear* column is included or excluded, adding to the complexity of the challenge to the pseudohypacusic patient. Because the patient must concentrate on the story and commit it to memory, it is less likely that the individual will be able to remember which material was presented to the "bad" ear. It is a good idea to make an audio tape recording of the patient's response to be certain that the interpretation is accurate.

Low Level Phonetically Balanced (PB) Word Tests

PB word tests are routinely performed at 30 to 40 dB above the SRT because most clinicians find that this usually approaches the PB max. Some clinicians routinely do performance-intensity functions for PB words (PI-PB) but this is usually reserved for special cases, such as for determination of site of lesion. Normally low word discrimination scores are expected at low sensation levels.

Hopkinson (1978), in interpreting the PI-PB functions reported by Harris (1965), suggests that normal-hearing individuals should reveal PB word scores approximately as follows:

Sensation Level	Discrimination Score
5 dB	25%
10 dB	50%
20 dB	75%
28 dB	88%
32 dB	92%
40 dB	100%

Snyder (1977) reported that unusually high PB word scores can be obtained on pseudohypacusic patients at levels slightly above their admitted thresholds. In performing low level PB word tests monitored live voice has been recommended at hearing levels of 20 and 40 dB. High scores certainly suggest normal hearing for speech.

Ascending-Descending Methods

The use of both an ascending and descending approach to puretone threshold measurements was recommended as a rapid and simple procedure (Harris, 1958). A more than 10-dB difference between these two measurements suggests a nonorganic problem because the two thresholds should be identical. Personal use of this procedure indicates that this difference is often as large as 30 dB for pseudohypacusic patients. For patients with nonorganic loss the ascending method generally reveals better thresholds than the

BAD EAR	BOTH EARS	GOOD EAR
1.	Lyons stalked dangerous prey	in the jungle
2. carrying his rifle confidently.	His animal instincts	and years of experience
3. enhanced by schooled intelligence	led him confidently	through the thicket.
4. Jim Lyons had been	long known as	the cleverest hunter in the jungle.
5. Except for those	on four feet,	Lyons never came home unsatisfied
6. or empty-handed.	Deer were his favorite prey	because of their succulent meats
7. and handsome pelts.		

Figure 36.1. Example of a swinging story test.

descending approach. The Harris test is quick and easy to perform with the simplest clinical audiometer and is the basis for the BADGE test described earlier. Kerr et al. (1975) modified Harris' original procedure and suggested that the test is improved slightly by performing the descending portion in 10-dB rather than 5-dB steps. Cherry and Ventry (1976) have further altered this procedure using a modified method of limits.

Pulse-Count Methods

Some tests may be carried out by presenting a number of puretone pulses in rapid succession and asking the patient to count and recall the numbers of pulses that were heard. The intensity of the tones may be varied above and below the admitted threshold of the tone in one ear (Ross, 1964) or above the threshold in one ear and below the threshold in the other ear (Nagel, 1964). If the originally obtained thresholds are valid the patient should have no difficulty in counting the pulses. Inconsistency should occur only if all the tone pulses are above threshold and the patient has to sort out the number of louder ones from the number of softer ones. This can be very difficult to do.

Yes-No Test

Frank (1976) described a test for pseudohypacusis that would seem too simple to work; nevertheless, it often does. The test is intended for children but has occasionally been useful with naive adults. The patient is simply told to say "yes" when a tone is heard and "no" when a tone is not heard. The tone is presented at the lowest limit of the audiometer and increased in intensity in 5-dB steps. Some patients, in an attempt to convince the examiner of poor hearing, will say "no" to tones that are heard below the level selected to be "threshold." Of course, a "no" response that is time locked with the introduction of a tone is clear evidence that the tone was heard, barring occasional false-positive responses. A similar procedure was described by Nolan and Tucker (1981). The audiologist must decide when such a procedure is best used with a given patient.

Stenger Test

One of the best ways to test for unilateral nonorganic hearing is by use of the Stenger test. The Stenger principle states that when two tones of the same frequency are introduced simultaneously into both ears, only the louder tone will be perceived.

Since its introduction as a tuning fork test more than 80 years ago the Stenger test has been modified many times. If unilateral nonorganic hearing loss is suspected, the Stenger test may be performed quickly as a screening procedure. This is most easily done by introducing a tone of a desired frequency into the better ear at a level 10 dB above the threshold and into the poorer ear at a level 10 dB below the admitted threshold. If the loss in the poor ear is genuine, the patient will be unaware of any signal in the poor ear and will respond to the tone in the good ear readily, because at 10 dB above threshold it should be easily heard. Such a response is termed a negative Stenger, indicating that the poorer ear threshold is probably correct.

If patients do not admit hearing in the bad ear and are unaware of the tone in the good ear, they simply do not respond. This is a positive Stenger which proves that the postulated threshold for the "poorer" ear is incorrect. A positive Stenger results because the tone is above the true threshold in the "bad" ear and precludes hearing the tone in the good ear.

The screening procedure described above rapidly identifies the presence or absence of unilateral nonorganic hearing loss if there is a difference in admitted threshold between the ears of at least 20 dB. The test is most likely to be positive in nonorganic cases with large interaural differences (exceeding 40 dB) or large nonorganic components in the "poorer" ear (Chaiklin and Ventry, 1965b).

A positive result on the Stenger test does not identify the true organic hearing threshold. To obtain threshold information the Stenger test can also be performed by seeking the *minimum contralateral interference levels*. The procedure is as follows: The tone is presented to the good ear at 10 dB sensation level (SL). There should be a response from the patient. A tone is presented to the bad ear at 0 dB HL, simultaneously with the tone at 10 dB SL in the good ear. If a response is obtained the level is raised 5 dB in the *bad ear*, keeping the level the same in the good ear. The level is continuously raised in 5-dB steps until the subject fails to respond. Because the tone is still above threshold in the good ear the lack of response must mean that the tone has been heard loudly enough in the bad ear so that the patient experiences the Stenger effect and is no longer aware of a tone in the good ear. Being unwilling to respond to tones in the bad ear, patients simply stop responding. The lowest hearing level of the tone in the bad ear producing this effect is the minimum contralateral interference level, and should be within 20 dB of the true threshold.

In one study (Peck and Ross, 1970) the Stenger test was performed on 35 normal-hearing subjects feigning a total hearing loss in one ear. Ascending and descending methods of tone presentation were used. No differences in the interference levels were observed between the two methods. The interference levels were found to be within 14 dB of the true thresholds, resulting in the general conclusion that the Stenger test can identify the general hearing threshold of the poor ear in a unilateral nonorganic hearing loss. This conclusion was supported by Kintsler et al. (1970), who found that the Stenger test correctly identified 25 of 31 cases of nonorganic hearing loss.

Because their results were better than suggested by the study of Chaiklin and Ventry (1965b), Kintsler et al. (1972) replicated the Chaiklin and Ventry study, which had found the Stenger not to be a good identifier of nonorganic hearing loss. They noted a close correspondence between positive Stenger test results and pseudohypacusis. In conflict with this, Hattler and Schuchman (1971) found that of 225 patients with nonorganic hearing loss the Stenger test was applicable only in 57% of the cases and had the poorest efficiency of all the tests tried even when applicable, correctly labeling only one-half of the patients with pseudohypacusis.

Monro and Martin (1977) found that the Stenger test, using the screening method, was virtually unbeatable on normal-hearing subjects feigning unilateral hearing losses. Martin and Shipp (1982), using a similar research method, found that as sophistication and practice with the Stenger test are increased, patients are less likely to be confused by low contralateral interference levels.

The studies cited above illustrate that the accuracy and efficiency of the Stenger test continue to be contested. Although the Stenger, like most tests, has certain shortcomings, most regard it as an efficient test for quick identification of unilateral nonorganic hearing loss. The only equipment required for the test is a puretone audiometer with separate hearing level dials for the right and left ears. To be sure, if the test is performed by an inexperienced clinician a series of patterns and rhythms of tone introductions may betray the intentions of the test to an alert patient.

Modified Stenger Test

More than four decades ago Taylor (1949) reported on the use of a modification of the puretone Stenger test using spondaic words. The Stenger principle holds for speech stimuli if words, like spondees, are presented via both channels of a speech audiometer simultaneously. All of the criteria for application of the puretone Stenger test apply to the modified version; that is, the SRT should be at least 20 dB different between ears and the greater the interaural difference and closer to normal one ear hears the better the test

works. A two-channel audiometer with one VU meter is easiest to use with monitored live voice presentation.

Subjects are instructed simply to repeat every spondee they hear. The words are presented 10 dB above the better ear SRT and 10 dB below the poorer ear SRT. If the patient continues to repeat the words the modified Stenger is considered to be negative, providing no evidence of pseudohypacusis. If the patient does not repeat the spondees under these conditions, then the screening test has been failed and the minimum contralateral interference level should be sought.

To determine the minimum contralateral interference level, the sensation level of 10 dB should be maintained in the better ear. The hearing level dial controlling the intensity at the poorer ear should be set to the lowest limit of the audiometer. Each time a spondee is presented and repeated by the patient, the level in the poorer ear should be raised 5 dB. The lowest hearing level dial setting in the poorer ear at which the patient stops repeating two or more spondees correctly is considered to be the minimum contralateral interference level and is above the threshold for that ear. The precise threshold cannot be known, but minimum contralateral interference levels have been noted as low as 15 dB above the SRT of the poorer ear. Certainly, if the minimum contralateral interference level is as low as 30 dB HL it may be assumed that hearing for speech is normal.

Experienced clinicians can manipulate the modified Stenger in a variety of ways. The speech itself can be less formal than spondaic words and may consist of a series of instructions or questions requiring verbal responses from the patient. The signal to the better ear may be randomly deleted on the chance that patients may be "on to" the test and may be repeating words they hear in their poorer ears (but will not admit to it) because they believe that words are also above threshold in their better ears (even though they do not hear them). To paraphrase an old saw, "experience is the mother of invention."

Martin and Shipp (1982) found that sophistication with the speech Stenger test resulted in higher minimum contralateral interference levels, which can lead the unsuspecting clinician to accept exaggerated SRT as correct. Because there is no way to control for any knowledge about the modified Stenger that a patient brings to the examination, the alert clinician is wary of contamination of test results that such knowledge may cause.

Acoustic Immittance Measurements

No procedure in recent years has had such a profound influence on diagnostic audiology as immittance measurements. Chapters 19 through 21 provide details on this subject. Among the many valuable contributions that immittance testing brings to our field is the detection of pseudohypacusis. This section is devoted to the use of tympanic membrane measurements of compliance and ways in which they may help in the detection of pseudohypacusis.

The acoustic reflex threshold is the immittance measurement that is of greatest value in the diagnosis of pseudohypacusis. The elicitation of this reflex at a low SL has been construed to suggest the presence of a cochlear lesion. If the SL (the difference between the reflex threshold and the voluntary puretone threshold) is extremely low (5 dB or less) it is difficult to accept on the basis of organic pathology. (Lamb and Peterson, 1967). Feldman (1963) cited a patient with a unilateral nonorganic hearing loss, who demonstrated acoustic reflexes in the "poor ear" below the patient's voluntary threshold. If the audiologist is certain that no artifact contaminates the readings, the suggestion that the acoustic reflex may be achieved by a tone that cannot be heard must be rejected, and a diagnosis of pseudohypacusis may be made.

More than merely identifying pseudohypacusis, acoustic reflex measurements may be useful in actual estimation of thresholds. Jerger et al. (1974) describe a procedure based on the work of Niemeyer and Sesterhenn (1974) in which the middle ear muscle reflex thresholds for puretones are compared to those for wide-band noise and low and high frequency filtered wide-band noise. The procedure, which is referred to as SPAR (sensitivity prediction from the acoustic reflex), approximates the degree of hearing loss, if any, as well as the general audiometric configuration. Details of this procedure may be found elsewhere, but it certainly appears that this method may have use in estimating thresholds of patients with pseudohypacusis.

There is no way to know how many patients with pseudohypacusis appear to have a conductive hearing loss. Of course, the middle ear muscle reflex measurement cannot be used in cases with nonorganic components overlying even the mildest of conductive problems (Alberti, 1970) since contralateral reflexes are absent in both ears when even one ear has a conductive disorder. Tympanometry can be used to suggest middle ear disorders, in such cases.

The elaborateness of middle ear measurements, including the instructions for the patient to be quiet and immobile, may have the effect of discouraging nonorganic behavior if this test is performed early in the diagnostic battery. It is often good practice to perform middle ear measurements as the first test on adults and cooperative children. They are asked to sit quietly and are told that the measurements made will reveal a great deal about their hearing. I have no hesitancy in recommending this approach in general and believe it is a useful deterrent to pseudohypacusis.

QUANTITATIVE TESTS

Despite the considerable interest that has been generated and the appeal of the previously mentioned tests, none so far has provided the most sought after information. They lack the ability to provide the true threshold of audibility in patients who will not or cannot cooperate fully. For measures of true threshold our profession has tended to turn to electrophysiologic procedures, often with considerable disappointment. Procedures that suggest or reveal threshold will now be reviewed.

Electrodermal Audiometry (EDA)

Once the most popular test for pseudohypacusis and formerly required on virtually all veterans seeking compensation for hearing loss is electrodermal audiometry (EDA). A survey by Martin and Morris (1989) shows that this procedure has fallen into disuse. The abandonment of EDA is due to the use of noxious stimuli (electric shocks) as the unconditioned stimuli that were paired with puretones or speech as the conditioned stimuli. According to the model, once conditioning was established by pairing conditioned unconditioned stimuli, the unconditioned response (drop in electrical skin resistance) to the shock would be seen in addition to a conditioned response in reaction to the tone or speech alone.

Because of the discomfort and possible liabilities involved with this procedure and the concern on the part of some audiologists regarding the validity of EDA, its popularity showed a steady decline.

Auditory Evoked Potentials (AEP)

The recent enthusiasm for AEP has resulted in the recommendation that they be used as objective tests for *all* patients complaining of noise-induced hearing loss (Heron, 1968). It has been called the "crucial test" in diagnosis of pseudohypacusis (Knight and Beagley, 1970). As an example of the enthusiasm generated for AEP, Alberti (1970) found that results obtained from this technique and from voluntary puretone testing agree within 10 dB, and recommends that AEP be used with any uncooperative patients.

The evoked response procedure just described allows the use of puretones because it looks, via an electroencephalograph and averaging computer, at the later components of the evoked response (50–300 msec). Examination of the earlier components, probably arising from the brainstem, constitutes the procedure called auditory brainstem response (ABR).

ABR has the advantage of the easy application of surface electrodes plus the fact that the response is stable and repeatable (Schulman-Galambos and Galambos, 1975). Disadvantages include the necessity of using clicks as stimuli.

Berlin (1978) indicates that ABR, in combination with electrocochleography, tympanometry, and acoustic reflexes, forms a powerful test battery for noncooperative patients (such as small children). It seems logical to extend this conclusion to pseudohypacusic patients.

ABR may have the effect of eliminating or determining the presence of nonorganic overlays on true organic hearing losses. The mere elaborateness of the procedure along with the suggestion that hearing can be measured without patient cooperation might have a deterring effect on the would-be malingerer.

Even in the hands of experienced clinicians high correlations between evoked response and voluntary thresholds are not always found (Rose et al., 1972), and so caution should be used in interpreting ABR data. Obviously, further research and clinical reports will determine the value of ABR as a diagnostic tool for pseudohypacusis.

Delayed Auditory Feedback (DAF)

General dissatisfaction has been expressed with DAF because it does not reveal the true threshold of the patient with pseudohypacusis. A procedure has been described that uses the delayed feedback notion with puretones, and which can be administered to patients who appear unwilling or unable to give accurate readings on threshold audiometry (Ruhm and Cooper, 1964).

Puretone DAF requires the use of a special apparatus, some variations of which are now commercially available. The patient is asked to tap out a continuous pattern, such as four taps, pause, two taps, pause, etc. (————□——□————). The electromagnetic key on which the patient taps is shielded from the individual's visual field. After the patient has demonstrated the ability to maintain the tapping pattern and rhythm, an audiometer circuit is added so that for each tap a tone pulse is introduced into an earphone worn by the patient. The tone has a duration of 50 msec at maximum amplitude but is delayed by 200 msec from the time the key is tapped. If the tone is audible its presence causes the subject to vary the tapping behavior in several ways, such as a loss of tapping rhythm, a change in the number of taps or an increase of finger pressure on the key.

It has been demonstrated (Ruhm and Cooper, 1962) that changes occur in tapping performance at sensation levels as low as 5 dB and are independent of test tone frequency and manual fatigue (Ruhm and Cooper, 1963). Once a subject has demonstrated key-tapping ability, any alterations seen after introduction of a delayed puretone must be interpreted as meaning that the tone was heard.

Not all researchers have found the 5-dB SL change in tapping performance using puretone DAF. Alberti (1970) found that tapping rhythms were disturbed in general at 5 to 15 dB above threshold, but has observed variations as great as 40 dB. He reported that some subjects are difficult to test with this procedure because they either cannot or will not establish a tapping rhythm, a problem that I have also observed. At times patients appear to fail to understand the instructions and at other times complain that their fingers are too stiff to tap the key.

Two studies (Monro and Martin, 1977; Martin and Shipp, 1982) show puretone DAF to be extremely resistant to effects of previous test knowledge and practice, with tones of low sensation levels. Experience apparently plays a role at suprathreshold levels with unpracticed subjects. The subjects without practice showed many more time and pattern errors than those with practice (Cooper and Stokinger, 1976). Practice notwithstanding, the puretone DAF procedure is considerably less time consuming than many of the electrophysiologic methods and has been found to be accurate, reliable and simple (Robinson and Kasden, 1973).

TEST SEQUENCE

During routine audiometrics the precise order in which tests are done probably does not have a significant effect on results. Pseudohypacusic patients attempt to set a level above threshold as a reference for consistent suprathreshold responses (Hood et al., 1964; Armbruster, 1982). For this reason threshold tests should be performed before suprathreshold tests. Structured tests (greater examiner participation) tend to lead to less hearing loss exaggeration than nonstructured tests (e.g., Bekesy audiometry) (Armbruster 1982).

The following test order has proved useful in examining patients with suspected pseudohypacusis. (a) Immittance measures; (b) SRT, including the modified Stenger test in unilateral cases; (c) Air conduction thresholds, including the Stenger test if indicated; (d) Speech discrimination tests using PB word lists at low sensation levels; (e) Bone conduction thresholds; (f) Pure tone DAF; (g) ABR.

DISCUSSION

In the vast majority of cases the detection of pseudohypacusis is not a difficult task for the alert clinician. The more challenging responsibility of the audiologist is to determine the patient's organic thresholds of hearing. The difficulty of this task increases as the cooperation of the patient decreases. Some pseudohypacusic patients are overtly hostile and unwilling to modify their test behavior even after counseling (Ventry et al., 1965).

It is not likely that a single approach to diagnosis and resolution of pseudohypacusis is forthcoming, although there are certain points on which we should all agree. For example, it is far better to discourage exaggeration of hearing thresholds at the outset of testing than to detect these exaggerations later. Once nonorganicity is observed the audiologist is faced with the responsibility of determining the true organic thresholds. Tests that may aid in deterring pseudothreshold responses include all the electrophysiologic and electroacoustic procedures. In my own opinion, acoustic immittance measurements should be accomplished initially in all routine audiologic assessments, thereby discouraging some pseudohypacusis. Puretone DAF and the Stenger test are quick and easy to perform and allow the patient to realize that the examiner has methods of determining puretone thresholds even without patient cooperation.

There are times when audiologists believe that their patients with pseudohypacusis should be referred for psychologic or psychiatric guidance. Such decisions should not be made recklessly or arbitrarily, but rather after considerable thought. Suggestions of this nature must be made carefully because of the unfortunate stigma that may be associated with psychologic referrals.

Great care must be taken in writing reports about patients with suspected pseudohypacusis. It must be borne in mind that once individuals have been diagnosed as "malingering," "uncooperative" or "functional" their reputations and prestige may be damaged. To label a patient in such ways is a grave matter because it implies deliberate falsification. Such labels are difficult to expunge and may be tragically unjust. The only way an audiologist can be absolutely certain that a nonorganic patient is truly a malingerer is for the patient to admit to the intent and most experienced audiologists would probably agree with Hopkinson (1967) that such admissions are rare indeed. Value judgments are not within the purview of the audiologist and should be avoided.

Counseling sessions should be carried out after all audiologic evaluations. Counseling the pseudohypacusic individual is naturally more difficult than counseling patients with organic hearing disorders. Children may be told only that their hearing appears to be normal (if this is believed to be the case) despite audiometric findings to the contrary. Parents should be warned not to discuss their children's difficulties in their presence or to provide any secondary rewards that may accrue to a hearing loss. Pseudohypacusic adults may simply have to be told that a diagnosis of the extent of the hearing disorder cannot be made because inconsistencies in response preclude accurate diagnosis. If a referral for psychologic evaluation or guidance is indicated, clinicians must choose their words extremely carefully lest the patient be offended. It is at this point that audiology must be practiced as more of an art than a science.

REFERENCES

Alberti P. New tools for old tricks. Ann Otol Rhinol Laryngol 1970;79:900–907.

Altshuler MW. Qualitative indicators of nonorganicity: informal observations and evaluation. In Kramer MB and Armbruster JM (eds.) Forensic Audiology. Baltimore: University Park Press. 1982;5:50–68.

Armbruster JM. Indices of exaggerated hearing loss from conventional audiological procedures. In Kramer MB and Armbruster JM (eds.) Forensic Audiology, Baltimore: University Park Press. 1982;6:69–95.

Bailey HAT Jr and Martin FN. Nomorganic hearing loss: case report. Laryngoscope 1961;71:209–210.

Barelli PA and Ruder L. Medico-legal evaluation of hearing problems. Eye Ear Nose Throat Mon 1970;49:398–405.

Barr B. Psychogenic deafness in school children. Int Audiol 1963;2:125–128.

Beagley HA and Knight JJ. The evaluation of suspected nonorganic hearing loss. J Laryngol Otol 1968;82:693–705.

Berger K. Nonorganic hearing loss in children. Laryngnoscope 1965;75:447–457.

Berlin CI. Electrophysiological indices of auditory function. In Martin FN (ed.) Pediatric Audiology. Englewood Cliffs, NJ: Prentice-Hall. 1978;113–173.

Black JW. The effect of delayed side-tone upon vocal rate and intensity. J Speech Hear Disord 1951;16:56–60.

Burgoon JD, Buller DB, and Woodall WG. Nonverbal Communication: The Unspoken Dialogue. New York: Harper and Row. 1989.

Campanelli PA. Simulated hearing losses in school children following identification audiometry. J Aud Res 1963;3:91–108.

Carhart R. Speech audiometry in clinical evaluation. Acta Otolaryngol (Stockh.) 1952;41:18–42.

Carhart R. Audiometry in diagnosis. Laryngoscope 1958;68:253–279.

Carhart R. Tests for malingering. Trans Am Acad Ophthalmol Otolaryngol 1961;65,437.

Chaiklin JB. A descending LOT-Bekesy screening test for functional hearing loss. J Speech and Hearing Disorders 1990;55:67–74.

Chaiklin JB and Ventry IM. Patient errors during spondee and pure-tone threshold measurement. J Aud Res 1965a;5:219–230.

Chaiklin JB and Ventry IM. The efficiency of audiometric measures used to identify functional hearing loss. J Aud Res 1965b;5:196–211.

Chaiklin JB, Ventry IM, Barrett LS, and Skalbeck GS. Pure-tone threshold patterns observed in functional hearing loss. Laryngoscope 1959;69:1165–1179.

Cherry R and Ventry IM. The ascending-descending gap: a tool for identifying a suprathreshold response. J Aud Res 1976;16: 281–287.

Cohen M, Cohen SM, Levine M, Maisel R, Ruhm H, and Wolfe RM. Interdisciplinary pilot study of nonorganic hearing loss. Ann Otol Rhinol Laryngol 1963;72:67–82.

Cooper WA and Stokinger TE. Pure-tone delayed auditory feedback: effect of prior experience. J Am Aud Soc 1976;1: 164–168.

Dean LA, Wright HN, and Valerio MW. Brief-tone audiometry in pseudohypacusis. Arch Otolaryngol 1976;102:621–626.

Dixon RF and Newby HA. Children with nonorganic hearing problems. Arch Otolaryngol 1959;70:619–623.

Doerfler LG. Psychogenic deafness and its detection. Ann Otol Rhinol Laryngol 1951;60:1045–1048.

Doerfler LG and Stewart K. Malingering and psychogenic deafness. J Speech Disord 1946;11:181–186.

Feldman AS. Functional hearing loss. Marco Aud Lib Ser 1962; 1:119–121.

Fournier JE. The detection of auditory malingering. Trans Beltone Inst Hear Res 1958;8.

Frank T. Yes-no test for nonorganic hearing loss. Arch Otolaryngol 1976;102:162–165.

Froeschels E. Psychic deafness in children. Arch Neurol Psychiatry 1944;51:544–549.

Gleason WJ. Psychological characteristics of the audiologically inconsistent patient. Arch Otolaryngol 1958;68:42–46.

Goetzinger CP and Proud GO. Deafness: examination techniques for evaluating malingering and psychogenic disabilities. J Kans Med Soc 1958;59:95–101.

Goldstein R. Pseudohypoacusis. J Speech Hear Disord 1966;31: 341–352.

Hallewell JD, Goetzinger CP, Allen ML, and Proud GO. The use of hypnosis in audiologic assessment. Acta Otolaryngol (Stockh.) 1966;61:205–208.

Hanley CN and Tiffany WR. An investigation into the use of electromechanically delayed side tone in auditory testing. J Speech Hear Disord 1954;19:367–374.

Harris DA. A rapid and simple technique for the detection of nonorganic hearing loss. Arch Otolaryngol 1958;68:758–760.

Harris JD. Speech audiometry. In Glorig A (ed.) Audiometry Principles and Practices. Baltimore: Williams & Wilkins 1965;7: 151–169.

Hattler KW. The Type V Bekesy pattern: the effects of loudness memory. J Speech Hear Res 1968;11:567–575.

Hattler KW. Lengthened off-time: a self-recording screening device for nonorganicity. J Speech Hear Disord 1970;35:113–122.

Hattler KW and Schuchman GI. Efficiency of the Stenger, Doerfler-Stewart and lengthened off-time Bekesy tests. Acta Otolaryngol (Stockh.) 1971;72:262–267.

Heron TG. Industrial deafness and the summed evoked potential. S Afr Med J 1968;42:1176–1177.

Hirsh I. The Measurement of Hearing. New York: McGraw-Hill. 1952;212.

Hood WH, Campbell RA, and Hutton CL. An evaluation of the Bekesy ascending descending gap. J Speech Hear Res 1964; 7:123–132.

Hopkinson NT. Type V Bekesy audiograms: specification and clinical utility. J Speech Hear Disord 1965;30:243–251.

Hopkinson NT. Comment on pseudohypoacusis. J Speech Hear Disord 1967;32:293–294.

Hopkinson NT. Speech tests for pseudohypacusis. In Katz J (ed.) Handbook of Clinical Audiology, ed 2. Baltimore: Williams & Wilkins. 1978;25:291–303.

Istre CO and Burton M. Automatic audiometry for detecting malingering. Arch Otolaryngol 1969;90:326–332.

Jerger J. Bekesy audiometry in analysis of auditory disorders. J Speech Hear Res 1960;3:275–287.

Jerger J and Herer G. An unexpected dividend in Bekesy audiometry. J Speech Hear Disord 1961;26:390–391.

Jerger J, Burney L, Mauldin L, and Crump B. Predicting hearing loss from the acoustic reflex. J Speech Hear Disord 1974;39: 11–22.

Johnson KO, Work WP, and McCoy G. Functional deafness. Ann Otol Rhinol Laryngol 1956;65:154–170.

Katz J. Type A and functional loss. SSW Newslett 1980;2:5.

Kerr AG, Gillespie WJ, and Easton JM. Deafness: a simple test for malingering. Br J Audiol 1975;9:24–26.

Kintsler DP, Phelan JG, and Lavender RB. Efficiency of the Stenger tests in identification of functional hearing loss. J Aud Res 1970;10:118–123.

Kintsler DP, Phelan JG, and Lavender RB. The Stenger and speech Stenger tests in functional hearing loss. Audiology 1972;11: 187–193.

Knight J and Beagley H. Nonorganic hearing loss in children. Int Audiol 1970;9:142–143.

Lamb LE and Peterson JL. Middle ear reflex measurements in pseudohypacusis. J Speech Hear Disord 1967;32:46–51.

Leshin GJ. Childhood nonorganic hearing loss. J Speech Hear Disord 1960;25:290–292.

Lumio JS, Jauhiainen T, and Gelhar K. Three cases of functional deafness in the same family. J Laryngol 1969;83:299–304.

Martin FN. Introduction to Audiology, ed 3. Englewood Cliffs, NJ. 1986;343–364.

Martin FN and Monro DA. The effects of sophistication on Type V Bekesy patterns in simulated hearing loss. J Speech Hear Disord 1975;40:508–513.

Martin FN and Morris LJ. Current audiological praactices in the U.S. In The Hearing Journal 1989;42:25–42.

Martin FN and Shipp DB. The effects of sophistication on three threshold tests for subjects with simulated hearing loss. Ear Hear 1982;3:34–36.

Martin NA. Psychogenic deafness. Ann Otol Rhinol Laryngol 1946;55:81–89.

McCanna DL and DeLapa G. A clinical study of twenty-seven children exhibiting functional hearing loss. Lang Speech Hear Serv Schools 1981;12:26–35.

McGranahan LM, Causey D, and Studebaker GA. Delayed side tone audiometry (abstr.) Asha 1960;2:357.

McLennan RO and Martin FN. On the discrepancy between the speech reception threshold and the pure-tone average in nonganic hearing loss. Houston: Poster Session at the American Speech and Hearing Association Convention, 1976.

Miller AL, Fox MS, and Chan G. Pure tone assessments as an aid in detecting suspected nonorganic hearing disorders in children. Laryngoscope 1968;78:2170–2176.

Monro DA and Martin FN. Effects of sophistication on four tests for nonorganic hearing loss. J Speech Hear Disord 1977;42: 528–534.

Myklebust HR. Auditory Disorders in Children. New York: Grune & Stratton, 1954.

Nagel RF. RRLJ—a new technique for the noncooperative patient. J Speech Hear Disord 1964;29:492–493.

Niemeyer W and Sesterhenn G. Calculating the hearing threshold from the stapedius reflex threshold for different sound stimuli. Audiology 1974;13:421–427.

Nilo ER and Saunders WH. Functional hearing loss. Laryngoscope 1976;86:501–505.

Noble WG. Pure-tone acuity, speech-hearing ability and deafness in acoustic trauma: a review of the literature. Audiology 1973; 12:291–315.

Nolan M and Tucker I. Functional hearing loss in children. J Br Assoc Teachers Deaf 1981;5:2–10.

Peck JE and Ross M. A comparison of the ascending and the descending modes for administration of the pure-tone Stenger test. J Aud Res 1970;10:218–220.

Peterson JL. Nonorganic hearing loss in children and Bekesy audiometry. J Speech Hear Disord 1963;28:153–158.

Price LL, Shepherd DC, and Goldstein R. Abnormal Bekesy tracings in normal ears. J Speech Hear Disord 1965;30:139–144.

Resnick DM and Burke KS. Bekesy audiometry in nonorganic auditory problems. Arch Otolaryngol 1962;76:38–41.

Rintelmann WF and Carhart R. Loudness tracking by normal hearers via Bekesy audiometer. J Speech Hear Res 1964;7:79–93.

Rintelmann W and Harford E. Type V Bekesy pattern: interpretation and clinical utility. J Speech Hear Res 1967;10:733–744.

Robinson M and Kasden SD. Clinical application of pure tone delayed auditory feedback in pseudohypacusis. Eye Ear Nose Throat Mon 1973;52:91–93.

Rose DE, Keating LW, Hedgecock LD, Miller KE, and Schneurs KK. A comparison of evoked response audiometry and routine clinical audiometry. Audiology 1972;11:238–243.

Rosenberger AI and Moore JH. The treatment of hysterical deafness at Hoff General Hospital. Am J Psychiatry 1946;102: 666–669.

Ross M. The variable intensity pulse count method (VIPCM) for the detection and measurement of the pure tone threshold of children with functional hearing losses. J Speech Hear Disord 1964;29:477–482.

Ruhm HB and Cooper WA Jr. Low sensation level effects of pure tone delayed auditory feedback. J Speech Hear Res 1962;5: 185–193.

Ruhm HB and Cooper WA Jr. Delayed feedback audiometry. J Speech Hear Disord 1964;29:448–455.

Schulman-Galkambos C and Galambos R. Brain stem auditory evoked responses in premature infants. J Speech Hear Res 1975;18:456–465.

Semenov H. Deafness of psychic origin and its response to narcosynthesis. Trans Am Acad Ophthalmol Otolaryngol 1947;51: 326–348.

Shepherd DC and Goldstein R. Intrasubject variability in amplitude of Bekesy tracings and its relation to measures of personality. J Speech Hear Res 1968;11:523–535.

Siegenthaler BM and Strand R. Audiogram–average methods and SRT scores. J Acoust Soc Am 1964;36:589–593.

Simonton KM. Audiometry and diagnosis. In Glorig A (ed.) Audiometry: Principles and Practices. Baltimore: Williams & Wilkins, 1965;9:185–206.

Snyder JM. Characteristic patterns of etiologic significance from routine audiometric tests and case history. Maico Aud Lib Ser 1977;15:Rept. 5.

Stark EW. Jerger types in fixed-frequency Bekesy audiometry with normal and hypacusic children. J Aud Res 1966;6:135–140.

Stein L. Some observations on Type V Bekesy tracings. J Speech Hear Res 1963;6:339–348.

Suzuki T and Kubota K. Normal width in tracing on Bekesy audiogram. J Aud Res 1966;6:91–96.

Taylor GJ. An experimental study of tests for the detection of auditory malingering. J Speech Hear Disord 1949;14:119–130.

Trier T and Levy R. Social and psychological characteristics of veterans with functional hearing loss. J Aud Res 1965;5:241–255.

Truex EH. Psychogenic deafness. Conn State Med J 1946;10: 907–915.

Ventry I. A case for psychogenic hearing loss. J Speech Hear Disord 1968;33:89–92.

Ventry IM. Bekesy audiometry in functional hearing loss: a case study. J Speech Hear Disord 1971;36:125,141.

Ventry IM. Pure tone-spondee threshold relationships in functional hearing loss: a hypothesis. J Speech Hear Disord 1976; 41:16–22.

Ventry IM and Chaiklin JB. Functional hearing loss: a problem in terminology. Asha 1962;4:251–254.

Ventry IM and Chaiklin JB. Evaluation of pure tone audiogram configurations used in identifying adults with functional hearing loss. J Aud Res 1965;5:212–218.

Ventry I, Trier T, and Chaiklin J. Factors related to persistence and resolution of functional hearing loss. J Aud Res 1965; 5:231–240.

Wieczorek R. School-age malingerers. SSW Newslett 1979;1:4.

Williamson D. Functional hearing loss: a review. Maico Aud Lib Ser 1974;12:33–34.

Wood TJ, Goshorn EL, and Peters RW. Auditory reaction times for functional and nonfunctional hearing loss. J Speech Hear Res 1977;20:177–191.

Zwislocki J. Acoustic attenuation between the ears. J Acoust Soc Am 1953;25:752–759.

CHAPTER 37

Presbycusis

Barbara E. Weinstein

The demographic changes in the makeup of the American population are enormous, having considerable implications for utilization of health care services (NCHS, 1987). People are living longer. Although the elderly presently comprise 12% of the population, by the year 2030 they will comprise as much as 32% of the total population—approximately two and one-half times the size of today's population of older adults (DHHS, 1990). The chief population growth among older Americans is in individuals over 85 years. In the 25-year period between 1976 and 2000, the proportion of young old persons (those below 75 years) is projected to increase by 23%. The percentage between 75–84 years will increase by 57%, and the proportion of persons over 85 years will increase by 91% (DHHS, 1990). Within each of these age groups, the rate of increase for females is remarkably greater than that for males.

The demographic shifts coupled with biomedical and technological advances have changed the health status of Americans. The prevalence of chronic conditions increases with age. In general, increasing age is associated with increased impairment in the senses and in orthopedic problems (Kane, Ouslander, and Abrass, 1989). Eighty percent of persons over 65 years suffer from at least one chronic condition, and the proportion suffering from multiple chronic conditions is high as well, increasing dramatically as a function of age (Kane et al., 1989). The ability to function in the face of multiple interacting problems is a challenge to the elderly and to health care providers charged with assessing and maintaining their health and functional status.

DEMOGRAPHICS OF HEARING LOSS

Arthritis, hypertension and hearing loss are the three most commonly reported chronic problems in the elderly (NCHS, 1987). Visual impairment is the ninth and tinnitus the tenth most common chronic condition among persons over 65 years. Hearing loss affects a substantial number of elderly persons, approximately 30% of noninstitutionalized persons over 65 years of age and 70–80% of residents of nursing facilities (Schow and Nerbonne, 1980). Hearing loss tends to increase with age, with 33% of those 65–74 years, 45% of persons between 75–84 years, and 62% of persons over 85 years of age reporting a hearing problem (NCHS, 1987). It is projected that by the year 2050, approximately 60% of elderly persons will report a hearing problem. As is evident from the studies of Moscicki, Elkins, Baum and McNamara (1985), Gates, Cooper, Kannel, and Miller (1990), among others, severity and prevalence of hearing loss in the aged varies as a function of the population characteristics, the test protocol, the instruments used to assess hearing status, and the test environment.

Moscicki et al. (1985) conducted an audiometric based epidemiologic study of hearing in 935 men and 1358 women over 57 years of age. Estimates based on the traditional definition of hearing loss, that is puretone average in the better ear greater than 25dBHL, yielded a prevalence of 31%. The mean puretone average in the better ear was 19 dBHL (SD = 16 dBHL). Individuals over 70 years of age were more likely than persons under 60 years to have a hearing loss in the speech frequencies (Moscicki et al., 1985). Gates et al. (1990) broadened the database of Moscicki et al., (1985) by re-evaluating 1662 subjects from the original Framingham Cohort. The prevalence of hearing loss in their sample was comparable, 29% using the criterion of a puretone average (PTA) >26 dB HL. The prevalence of hearing loss was significantly greater in men (33%) than in women (27%).

The age effect is apparent in studies using a nursing facility sample, as well. The rate of hearing loss among persons living in nursing facilities is on the order of 82% when hearing loss is defined as a PTA >25dBHL (Schow and Nerbonne, 1980). Seventy percent of persons 70–79 years, 92% of persons 80–89 years of age, and nearly 100% of persons over 90 years of age reportedly had a hearing impairment. Overall, the mean puretone average in the better ear of their sample was 40 dB HL (SD = 16 dB HL). The fact that Schow and Nerbonne's (1980) sample was considerably older than that of Moscicki et al. (1985) may account in part for the significant difference in mean hearing levels across the two samples.

The audiogram characterizing the sample described by Moscicki et al. (1985) is comparable to that of

Gates et al. (1990). Overall, hearing levels are within normal limits at frequencies ranging from 250–2000 Hz, sloping gradually to the level of a mild high-frequency hearing loss in women and to the level of a moderate hearing loss in men. The configuration is gradually sloping for women and abruptly falling for men (Moscicki et al., 1985). It is apparent from the cross-sectional design used by Moscicki et al. (1985) that hearing threshold levels tend to decrease dramatically with increasing age for both males and females.

The data for these two studies were comparable. Mean hearing threshold levels tended to increase with increasing frequency for males and females with mean hearing threshold levels showing remarkable similarity. Further, hearing levels tended to decline with increasing age, being most pronounced in the high frequencies. Gates et al. reported that 29% of the subjects had sharply sloping audiograms, 29% had flat audiograms, 36% had gradually sloping audiograms, whereas 6% had rising audiograms.

Harford and Dodds (1982) reported similar trends in their sample of 527 ambulatory senior citizens. The hearing levels reported by Harford and Dodds (1982) were slightly poorer across frequencies than those reported by Moscicki et al. (1985) and Gates et al. (1990). The differences may be due to procedural variables, as the testing by Harford and Dodds (1982) was conducted in a quiet environment in a residential hotel or a senior center rather than in a sound-treated room.

Brant and Fozard (1990) conducted a longitudinal study of change in puretone thresholds over a 20-year period in a homogeneous sample of 813 males participating in the Baltimore Longitudinal Study of Aging (BLSA). Examination of the audiograms conducted on the subjects revealed three interesting trends. First, the rate of change in thresholds measured in sound pressure level (SPL) was more dramatic in the speech frequencies (500–2000 Hz) than at 8000 Hz. The most significant change in thresholds began between 40 and 50 years of age, continuing into the 80s. Second, there was significant variability in the amount of change in hearing threshold levels among subjects at each age for all frequencies tested (Brant and Fozard, 1990). They concluded that age, rather than the presence of otological disease, accounted for the changes in hearing threshold levels noted in the majority of their subjects.

Finally, Schow and Nerbonne (1980) tested a sample of 202 residents of nursing facilities. Overall, mean hearing levels across frequencies were poorer than those that emerged in the studies by Moscicki et al. (1985) and Harford and Dodds (1982). Mean hearing threshold levels were consistent with a moderate hearing loss in the low to mid frequencies gradually sloping to the level of a moderately severe high-frequency hearing loss. The sample described by Schow and Nerbonne was older, accounting in large part for the more significant hearing loss across frequencies.

In conclusion, the following trends are clear from the audiometric based studies on prevalence and severity of hearing loss in the aged:

1. Age is a significant risk factor for hearing loss with mean hearing levels increasing as a function of age.
2. Hearing levels in men are slightly poorer than those of women, especially in the high frequencies.
3. The prevalence of hearing loss is somewhat higher in nursing facilities, most likely because of the mean age of residents.

ETIOLOGIES OF HEARING LOSS IN OLDER ADULTS

A number of factors have been linked to hearing loss in older adults. These include age, metabolic disorders, vascular disorders, renal disease, medications, medical treatments, and noise exposure. Moscicki et al. (1985) speculated that some of the minor risk factors for hearing loss vary according to sex. The risk factors for women include history of Meniere's disease and family history of hearing loss. In contrast, the risk factor for men is history of noise exposure.

Presbycusis

The term *presbycusis* refers to hearing loss associated with the aging process. In their recent report, the Committee on Hearing, Bioacoustics and Biomechanics (1988) defined presbycusis as the sum of hearing losses that results from several varieties of physiological degeneration including insults due to noise exposure, insults due to exposure to ototoxic agents, and insults due to medical disorders as well as medical treatments. A number of scientists have advanced the possibility of a genetically determined predisposition to age-related hearing loss (Gilad and Glorig, 1979; CHABA, 1988).

Schuknecht (1964) postulated four distinct types of presbycusis on the basis of postmortem histologic findings in cochlear and retrocochlear structures. Each of the four types of presbycusis, namely, sensory, neural, metabolic and mechanical is associated with a particular audiometric pattern; however, the relative frequency of each type of presbycusis is unknown. Similarly, although each form of presbycusis is associated with distinct pathological changes and audiometric patterns, varying combinations of the four types of presbycusis and their audiologic manifestations do emerge (Gulya, 1991). Finally, the exact mechanism of loss for each of Schuknecht's type of presbycusis is still a subject of considerable debate among researchers.

Sensory presbycusis is characterized by hair cell loss and atrophy of the auditory nerve in the basal turn of the cochlea. The degenerative changes tend to begin in middle age and progress slowly. It is manifested by a steeply sloping, high-frequency hearing loss with a proportional reduction in word recognition ability. Neural presbycusis is associated with primary degeneration of neurons and nerve fibers, with the greatest loss in the basal cochlea (Schuknecht, 1964). Neural presbycusis is typified by a loss of speech recognition ability that is out of proportion with hearing loss for puretones (White and Regan, 1987). The term *phonemic regression*, coined by Gaeth (1948), implies a disproportionate loss of speech understanding ability relative to the audiogram.

The pathology of metabolic or strial presbycusis involves atrophy of the stria vascularis (Schuknecht, 1964). The functional manifestation of metabolic presbycusis is a flat audiogram with equal hearing loss across frequencies. Speech understanding ability tends to remain intact despite the puretone loss (White and Regan, 1987). Finally, mechanical or cochlear-conductive presbycusis involves stiffening of the basilar membrane which interferes with sound transmission within the cochlea (Schuknecht, 1964). The hearing loss is slowly progressive, with a sloping configuration.

Studies of brainstem elements within the central auditory pathways and of the cerebral cortex have yielded mixed results depending in large part on the animal used to study the pathological changes (Gulya, 1991). In general, alterations in the central auditory structures including the ganglion cells in the ventral cochlear nucleus, the dorsal cochlear nucleus, the superior olivary complex, and the inferior colliculus have been reported (Gulya, 1991). Brody (1955) demonstrated a substantial decrease in the cell population most pronounced in the superior temporal gyrus. The functional correlates of the anatomical changes within the central auditory pathways have been difficult to delineate.

Although the changes in the auditory system associated with age are most pronounced in the inner ear and central auditory pathways, the structures of the outer and middle ears are susceptible to degeneration, as well. Rosenwasser (1964) noted structural changes in the tissue and skin lining the external auditory meatus which often manifest as cracking or bleeding of the skin. While these changes are of little functional significance, they are a source of annoyance to older persons wearing hearing aids. The ceruminal glands in the external auditory canal reportedly atrophy and undergo decreased activity (Regan and White, 1987). Clinically, these changes are often manifest by excessive accumulation of cerumen in the ears of older persons.

Covell (1952), Etholm and Belal (1974), and Rosenwasser (1964) reported age-related changes within structures of the middle ear. Specifically, the tympanic membrane reportedly undergoes stiffening, the incudomalleal and incudostapedial joints of the ossicles undergo progressive degeneration, and the tensor tympani and stapedius muscle atrophy with age (Etholm and Belal, 1974; Covell, 1952). Although the impedance characteristics of the middle ear may be affected by the changes in the middle ear, hearing sensitivity is not.

Noise-Induced Hearing Loss

The inner ear of older adults may also be susceptible to degeneration from exposure to excessive noise. This degeneration associated with the hair cells in the lower basal turn of the cochlea is distinct from deterioration due to "pure" presbycusis. The audiometric configuration associated with noise exposure, however, is difficult to separate from the patterns typically attributable to age (CHABA, 1988). Excessive noise exposure can present audiometrically as a loss of puretone sensitivity in the regions ranging from 3000–6000 Hz or as a steeply sloping high-frequency hearing loss. Rosen, Bergman, Plester, Mofty and Sati (1962) reported that environmental factors, such as living in a noise-free versus an industrialized society, can influence the extent of the high-frequency hearing loss that emerges in older persons. Individuals living in a noise-free environment have better hearing in the high frequencies than persons living in industrialized societies (Rosen et al., 1962). The extent to which hearing loss in older persons is attributable to noise rather than age cannot be predicted from the audiogram at this time. There is, however, support for the observation that age and exposure to noise can have a synergistic effect (Moscicki et al., 1985).

Ototoxicity

Because elderly persons often suffer from a number of chronic and acute medical conditions, they are frequently prescribed many drugs (Kane et al., 1989). Multiple drug regimens tend to predispose persons to adverse drug reactions that include hearing loss. Antimicrobials, such as aminoglycosides that include gentamycin, streptomycin, and tobramycin, are a common cause of ototoxicity. Selected diuretics (furosemides), analgesics (aspirin), antiarrhythmics (quinidine), and antihypertensives (reserpine) have been reported to produce hearing loss as well (White and Regan, 1987). Several age-related biological and physiological factors interact to determine the resultant action of ototoxic medications. The factors that influence drug pharmacology include drug absorption, drug distribution, drug metabolism and renal function (Kane et al., 1989). Unfortunately, the effects of age-related changes are often difficult to predict.

The hearing loss due to ototoxicity manifests itself as a sensory neural hearing loss most pronounced in the high frequencies. Often, the ototoxic effect exacerbates the auditory impairment associated with aging. Audiometrically, it is difficult to specify the extent to which the hearing loss is due to extrinsic factors, such as ototoxins, or to intrinsic factors, such as biologic and physiologic aging.

Selected medications commonly prescribed for the elderly also produce symptoms of tinnitus in isolation or in combination with hearing loss. Such agents as erythromycin and lidocaine have been reported to produce tinnitus. Similarly, reserpine, furosemide, and lithium reportedly produce tinnitus in selected elderly patients (Regan and White, 1987). It is helpful for the audiologist to be acquainted with medications taken by their elderly patients so they may assist in uncovering the etiology of these often disabling symptoms.

Metabolic Conditions and Vascular Disease

The prevalence of renal disease, diabetes mellitus, and hypertension are high in the elderly. Although the incidence of hearing loss in persons suffering from these medical conditions is variable, the configuration and type of loss is consistently high frequency bilateral and sensory neural. It is difficult to isolate the etiology of hearing loss in these individuals because the drugs taken to control the conditions may be ototoxic. The hearing loss characterizing persons suffering from chronic renal failure and diabetes mellitus often fluctuates in severity depending on the individual's medical condition. Accordingly, hearing status in each ear and the adequacy of a given amplification device should be closely monitored.

Senile Dementia

Senile dementia is a clinical syndrome involving a loss of intellectual function and memory, which is sufficient to interfere with social or occupational function (NIH, 1987; Kane et al., 1989). Reversible causes of dementia account for some 20–30% of all cases of de-

mentia. Eye and ear disorders have been isolated as one of eight potential causes of reversible dementia (NIH, 1987). Uhlmann, Larson, Rees, Koepsell and Duckert (1989a), Weinstein and Amsel (1986), and Uhlmann, Rees, Psaty and Duckert (1989b) reported the prevalence of hearing impairment to be higher in a sample of adults with a diagnosis of dementia than in a comparable sample free of the diagnosis. The discrepancy in prevalence is apparent among older adults living in the community and in institutions.

Weinstein and Amsel (1986), Uhlmann et al. (1989a), and Peters, Potter and Scholer (1988) also reported the severity of hearing loss to be greater in subjects with a diagnosis of dementia than in an age-matched group free of cognitive impairment. Uhlmann et al. (1989a) noted an increased risk of dementia with increased hearing loss. The pathophysiological mechanism underlying the relation between hearing loss and dementia remains elusive. The fact that unidentified or unremediated hearing loss may contribute to cognitive dysfunction, however, underlines the importance of determining auditory status in persons with a diagnosis of dementia.

PSYCHOSOCIAL RAMIFICATIONS OF HEARING LOSS

The burden of illness associated with hearing impairment in the elderly is currently being defined. Selected studies have demonstrated that hearing loss has an adverse effect on functional status, on quality of life, on cognitive function, and on emotional, behavioral, and social well-being (Uhlmann et al., 1989a; Weinstein and Ventry, 1982; Mulrow, Aguilar, Endicott et al., 1990a). Bess, Lichtenstein, Logan et al. (1989) assessed the relation between hearing loss and functional/psychosocial status in 153 elderly subjects. After a hearing screen, subjects were referred by primary care internists. Approximately 30% of subjects had normal hearing (0–16 dB HL), 35% had a slight loss, 25% had a mild loss, and 11% had hearing levels in excess of 41 dB HL. All subjects completed the Sickness Impact Profile (SIP), a 136-item standardized questionnaire that assesses physical and psychosocial function. The higher the SIP score, the greater the perceived functional impairment. Table 37.1 displays the mean score on the SIP for a representative sample of older adults with selected chronic conditions (Bess, Lichtenstein, Logan, 1990). The finding that the mean score on the SIP for older adults with significant hearing impairment is greater than the score reported for a sample of heart transplant recipients is noteworthy.

Bess, Lichtenstein, Logan, et al. (1989) found that hearing loss accounted for a significant proportion of

Table 37.1
Mean Score on the Sickness Impact Profile (SIP) for a Sample of Adults with Selected Chronic Conditions[a]

Chronic Condition	Mean Score on SIP
Unimpaired adult population	2–3
Heart-transplant recipients	9–10
Hearing-impaired elderly (PTA <41 dB HL)	13
Hearing-impaired elderly (PTA >/= 41 dB HL)	17
Chronic obstructive pulmonary disease	24–25
Terminally ill cancer and stroke patients	30–40

[a] From Bess et al. (1989).

the variation in physical, psychosocial, and overall function after controlling for selected demographic variables such as age, number of illnesses, and number of medications. Specifically, the mean SIP score increased as a function of level of hearing impairment, thus suggesting that progressive hearing impairment in the aged is associated with progressive self-reported physical and psychosocial dysfunction (Bess et al., 1989; Bess et al., 1991b). For example, the mean score on the Physical subscale of the SIP was 3 (SD = 7) for those with no hearing impairment to 19 (SD = 16) for persons with hearing levels which exceed 40 dB HL. The observation that hearing loss is associated with increased dysfunction in the elderly has considerable implication for early identification and management of the elderly hearing impaired. Therefore, the study should be replicated on samples of older adults drawn from such different populations as senior citizen centers (i.e., "well elderly") and homebound or institutionalized individuals.

Mulrow, Aguilar, Endicott et al. (1990a) conducted a cross-sectional study of 204 elderly male veterans selected from a primary care clinic. The study was designed to assess the association between hearing impairment and quality of life. Quality of life was defined according to two disease-specific and three generic measures that have been standardized on older adults (Mulrow et al., 1990a). The disease-specific measures were the Hearing Handicap Inventory for the Elderly (HHIE), which assesses the self-perceived emotional and social effects of hearing impairment, and the Quantified Denver Scale of Communication Function (QDS), which quantifies the perceived communication difficulties secondary to hearing impairment (Mulrow et al., 1990a). The generic measures included: the Short Portable Mental Status Questionnaire (SPMSQ), which yields information about cognitive function; the Geriatric Depression Scale (GDS), which assesses affect; and the Self-Evaluation of Life Function (SELF), which assesses function in several domains including physical disability, social satisfaction, aging, depression, self-esteem, and personal control.

Mulrow et al. (1990a) reported that hearing loss was associated with significant social, emotional, and communication handicaps as mean scores on the HHIE and QDS were significantly higher for the hearing-impaired group than for the nonhearing-impaired group. In contrast, mean scores on the GDS and the SELF did not differ for the groups with and without a hearing impairment. Similarly, mental status was intact for both groups of subjects. As the extent of the perceived social and emotional dysfunction was considerable for their sample (i.e., 66% had HHIE scores indicative of severe handicap; 16% had mild to moderate handicaps), the authors concluded that hearing loss has an adverse effect on quality of life; however, they also cautioned about the generalizability of their results.

Finally, self-perceived hearing handicap in the emotional and social realm also bears a significant relationship with functional status and central auditory processing ability. Bess, Lichtenstein and Logan (1991b) reported a significant relation between hearing handicap as measured using the screening version of the HHIE (HHIE-S) and the subscales of the SIP. They found that persons with severe hearing handicaps demonstrated greater dysfunction in the physical and psychosocial domains than persons with no hearing handicap. For example, the mean score on the psychosocial subscale of the SIP was 22 in persons with severe HHIE-S scores greater than 24, whereas the mean score among those with no handicap was 4. Similarly, the mean score on the physical dimension of the SIP of those with significant hearing handicaps was 18 versus a mean score of 4 among persons reporting no hearing handicap.

Jerger, Oliver, and Pirozzolo (1990) studied the impact of central auditory processing disorders as measured by performance on selected speech tests on self-perceived hearing handicap on a sample of 122 elderly subjects. The major trend that emerged from their investigation was that across all hearing-level categories, individuals whose performance on the either the Synthetic Sentence Identification Test (SSI), Speech Perception in Noise Test (SPIN), or Dichotic Sentence Identification (DSI) was indicative of a central auditory processing disorder perceived a greater hearing handicap than those without a central auditory processing disorder. Jerger et al. (1990) concluded that the finding that CAPD may influence self-perceived hearing handicap over and above that explained by peripheral hearing loss has implications for intervention strategies for the elderly.

In sum, data are accumulating to document the psychosocial handicap associated with hearing loss in the elderly. Available data suggest that the SIP and communication-specific indices, such as the Hearing Handicap Inventory for the Elderly, provide the audiologist with a composite picture of the older adult's functional capacity. In conjunction with audiometric data, this information may assist in program planning, in gauging progress in intervention, and in quantifying outcome. As the psychosocial impact of hearing loss cannot be predicted from the audiogram, the audiometric assessment should include some objective measure of functional status.

COMMUNICATION HANDICAP ASSOCIATED WITH HEARING LOSS

Speech tests are essential to the evaluation of the elderly as they offer the clinician a means of assessing receptive communication function in a quasisystematic manner, using material and procedures that vary in complexity (Olsen and Matkin, 1991). Specifically, speech tests yield objective, easily quantifiable information about (a) acoustic confusions deriving from the hearing loss, (b) recognition ability in selected listening situations, and (c) the ability to recognize selected materials including monosyllabic words and sentences. Theoretically, the latter information provides the clinician with information about client function in everyday listening situations. In addition to information about communication efficiency, speech tests provide differential diagnostic information relating to site of lesion and assist in decisions regarding hearing aid candidacy and the selection of personal hearing aids. Finally, data on speech understanding are used to determine the extent to which the aging process, changes in the auditory periphery, changes in the central auditory nervous system or cognitive factors account for deficits in speech understanding, which many older hearing impaired persons exhibit.

The treatment of speech understanding in the elderly in the following sections represents a departure from approaches adopted by other authors on the same topic. Specifically, in the sections that follow, an attempt is made to answer systematically the research questions that have dominated the research in this area over the past few decades.

First, to what extent can deficits in speech understanding be explained by age? Early studies using elderly subjects revealed that speech recognition scores in the elderly decline with increasing age and that their performance on monosyllabic word recognition tests is poorer than that which can be predicted from the audiogram (Gaeth, 1964; Blumenfeld et al., 1969; Jerger, 1973; Goetzinger et al., 1961). Subsequent investigations have revealed that the foregoing studies may have been confounded by some design problems.

For example, word recognition scores of subjects with normal hearing were compared with scores obtained by subjects whose hearing levels were depressed yet "considered to be normal for the subject's age." Further, the presentation level of some of the speech materials may have been insufficient to overcome the high frequency hearing loss characterizing selected subjects, thereby reducing performance on word-recognition tests (Gordon-Salant, 1987). Stated differently, a presentation level of 30–40 dB SL re ST may underestimate actual speech discrimination ability of individuals with the typical presbycusic hearing loss (Marshall, 1981). Subsequent investigators have compared performance of subjects matched for hearing levels, using a variety of presentation levels that yield a valid estimate of PB-max including an adaptive estimate of PB-Max, 50 dB SL re ST or 95 dB SPL (Beattie and Warren, 1983; Gang, 1976; Kamm, Morgan and Dirks, 1983). In general, performance of young adults is comparable to older persons when recognition ability is assessed in quiet and at a sufficient intensity to overcome the attenuating effects of the hearing loss across the high frequencies (Marshall, 1981). For example, when elderly hearing-impaired listeners with high-frequency hearing loss are matched with a young hearing-impaired control group with a similar configuration, speech-recognition ability in quiet is comparable for the two groups (Townsend and Bess, 1980; Kasden, 1970). The weak correlation between age and word-recognition ability, coupled with the strong correlation between hearing sensitivity and word-recognition ability, corroborates the hypothesis that peripheral hearing loss, rather than age, influences performance on speech tasks (Townsend and Bess, 1980; Weinstein and Ventry, 1983).

Gordon-Salant (1987) compared recognition scores for the NU-6 word lists in quiet at 80 dB SPL and 90 dB SPL of young and elderly listeners with normal hearing and mild-moderate high-frequency sensory neural hearing loss. In general, there were no differences in performance between the young and elderly subjects at either presentation level. Jerger and Hayes, (1977) also reported that when speech recognition ability is assessed at suprathreshold levels (i.e., PB-max), performance is equivalent across hearing-impaired subjects between 35 and 85 years of age. Finally, Bess and Townsend (1977) found that when elderly and young subjects with flat audiometric configurations and hearing levels <50 dB HL are contrasted, performance on monosyllabic word recognition tasks in quiet is comparable. However, there was a significant decline in speech intelligibility among subjects in the oldest age group, (i.e., over 70 years of age) with hearing levels in excess of 49 dB HL (Bess and Townsend, 1977). In sum, it appears from the foregoing studies that age-effects are not manifest for normal-hearing and hearing-impaired elderly subjects when monosyllabic words are presented under ideal listening conditions.

Next, to what extent does degradation in the form of noise, reverberation, or speeded speech contribute to breakdowns in word recognition ability in older adults?

In general, it appears that when the listening task is made more difficult, speech-recognition ability tends to decline in aging subjects. Dubno, Dirks, and Morgan (1984) used an adaptive procedure to assess speech-recognition performance of young and elderly listeners with normal hearing and mild sensory neural hearing loss. Specifically, Dubno et al. (1984) contrasted the signal-to-babble ratios (S-B Rs) at which young, elderly normal, or hearing-impaired listeners achieve a 50% criterion score for high/low predictability items from the Speech Perception in Noise Test (SPIN). In general, irrespective of intensity level, normal and hearing-impaired subjects over 65 years required more advantageous S-B Rs to achieve a 50% criterion score on the low predictability sentences than did their younger counterparts (Dubno et al., 1984). Gordon-Salant (1987) compared speech-recognition performance of young and elderly normal-hearing subjects and subjects with mild to moderately-severe high-frequency hearing loss, in fixed-noise conditions, and utilizing an adaptive noise paradigm. Monosyllabic word materials with an open response (i.e., NU-6) and closed set (Modified Rhyme Test, MRT) format were presented in the presence of multi-talker babble at 80 and 95 dB SPL. According to Gordon-Salant (1987), age effects are task dependent and become most pronounced in conditions utilizing the S-BR adaptive paradigm. Specifically, speech-recognition performance on the adaptive S-BR procedure was significantly poorer for normal and hearing-impaired elderly subjects for both sets of stimuli at each presentation level. In contrast, only when the MRT was presented in a fixed noise paradigm did significant differences in mean percent recognition scores emerge between the older hearing-impaired older subjects as compared with the young hearing-impaired group. Also using a sample of adults with cochlear lesions, Jerger and Hayes (1977) found the age effects to be task dependent. They examined the effect of age on monosyllabic word-recognition ability and on speech-recognition ability, using the ipsilateral competing SSI. The latter materials were presented in ipsilateral speech competition. In general, performance for the sentence materials decreased significantly with increasing age, with the decrements becoming most pronounced after

age 65 (Jerger and Hayes, 1977). Orchik and Burgess (1977) confirmed the task dependence of scores on speech-recognition tests in elderly listeners with essentially normal hearing. They found the age effect to be most pronounced when synthetic sentences (SSI) were presented in unfavorable message to competition ratios (i.e., MCR > −10).

Nabalek and Robinson (1982) examined the effects of reverberation on speech-recognition ability by using the MRT. Monaural and binaural speech perception abilities were presented in three reverberant conditions, a small room, a medium-sized auditorium, and a large listening area, such as a church. Hearing levels of subjects (10–72 years) were essentially normal at 250–2000 Hz; however, in the higher frequencies (4–8 KHz) the older subjects demonstrated a minimal sensory neural hearing loss. In general, at the longer reverberation times, older subjects exhibited significantly greater deficits in speech recognition than did the younger subjects. The data of Helfer and Wilber (1990) verify that elderly listeners with and without hearing loss experience difficulty understanding speech in reverberant conditions. Utilizing nonsense syllables as the test stimulus, they too found that older subjects showed decrements in understanding nonsense syllables distorted by noise and reverberation. The difficulty understanding the nonsense syllables was also apparent when statistically controlling for the potential effects of hearing loss on performance.

Finally, the sensitivity of time-compressed speech tasks, wherein the temporal domain is altered without producing spectral distortion to the effects of age, is a matter of controversy. Specifically, the data of Konkle, Beasley and Bess (1977), Sticht and Gray (1969), and Schon (1970) suggest that irrespective of presentation level, and percent time-compression, elderly subjects perform more poorly than younger subjects on time-compressed speech tasks utilizing monosyllabic words. However, subjects in the foregoing studies were not well matched for hearing level in the higher frequencies (Gordon-Salant, 1991), and thus the results may have been contaminated. In fact, when elderly and young subjects were matched for hearing level, Otto and McCandless (1982) found recognition of time-compressed monosyllabic words to be comparable.

In sum, research on recognition of speech materials presented in less than optimal conditions suggests that the effects of age varies as a function of the complexity of the task. In general, sentence-recognition ability in noise appears to decline with increasing age. The elderly require a more favorable S-B ratio to achieve 50% recognition of selected speech materials, and they experience decrements in performance with increasing reverberation times. The extent to which alterations in the temporal domain affect speech-recognition performance remains an area of controversy.

What is the contribution of cognitive status, peripheral factors and central auditory function to deficits in speech understanding in the elderly?

Stach, Spretnjak, and Jerger (1990) reported an increase in the prevalence of central presbycusis, defined operationally according to patterns of performance on the SSI and/or PB word lists, as a function of age, when controlling for degree of hearing loss. In fact, 17% of persons 50–54 years of age showed evidence of central presbycusis versus 90–95% of those 80 years or older (Stach et al., 1990). In light of the high prevalence of deficits on tests of central auditory processing ability, Jerger, Jerger, Oliver and Pirozzoli (1989) attempted to determine the extent to which cognitive factors or peripheral hearing loss may account for central auditory processing disorders (CAPD) in the elderly. Jerger et al. (1989) administered a battery of speech audiometric measures and a neuropsychologic test battery (e.g., tests of visual/auditory reaction time, memory scales, personality inventories) to a sample of 130 subjects ranging in age from 51–91 years. In general, subjects displayed a mild sloping to the level of a moderate, high-frequency sensory neural hearing loss (all subjects had PTAs < 50 dB HL). The prevalence of cognitive deficits in their sample was 41%, and the prevalence of CAPD was 50%. Only 27% of subjects demonstrated a cognitive deficit combined with a central auditory processing disorder, suggesting that CAPD can exist in the absence of cognitive decline and cognitive decline can exist without CAPD (Jerger et al., 1989). Jerger et al. (1989) also found that degree of hearing loss did not contribute significantly to decrements in performance on tests of central auditory processing ability. In light of their findings, Jerger et al. (1989) concluded that their results did not "support the hypothesis that decline in speech understanding in the elderly can be explained as the consequence of concomitant cognitive decline" (p. 79).

To what extent does response criterion influence performance on speech recognition tasks?

Botwinick (1969) reported that the elderly are more conservative than younger adults in perceptual tasks requiring decision making. Marshall (1981) speculated that use of a more cautious response criteria may influence performance on speech-recognition task. Gordon-Salant (1986) and Jerger, Johnson, and Jerger (1988) applied signal-detection theory to determine the influence of listening strategy on speech recognition scores. Gordon-Salant (1986) compared the response criteria of young and elderly normal and hearing-impaired listeners on closed and open-set speech-recognition tasks. The young subjects ranged in age from 18 to 40 years, and the older ones were 65 to 75 years. Young and old hearing-impaired subjects had sensory neural hearing loss in the high frequencies, which was mild to moderate in degree. The NU-6 word lists and the California Consonant Test (CCT) were used to assess speech-recognition ability at 80 and 95 dB SPL. The level of multitalker babble of the SPIN was adjusted to the S-B ratio at which 50% criterion was achieved. Subjects were compared on their ability to judge the accuracy of their responses on the speech-recognition task and on the criterion values adopted for responding under the four listening conditions (i.e., 80/90 dB SPL, NU-6/CCT). In general, irrespective of hearing status and listening condition, young and elderly subjects were comparable in their judgments of response accuracy. Judgments of accuracy were higher for all groups using an open-set response task (NU-6) than for the closed-set format (CCT). Subjects were, however, more confident in their responses to the NU-6 than the CCT materials. An age effect was noted for the normal-hearing and hearing-impaired subjects in terms of response criterion. That is, elderly subjects showed a less cautious response criterion than their younger counterparts when asked to judge the accuracy of their responses on word-recognition measures (Gordon-Salant, 1986).

In a follow-up to Gordon-Salant's (1986) work, Jerger, Johnson, and Jerger (1988) attempted to determine the extent to which listening strategy (i.e., lax or strict) impacts on speech audiometric test results. The subjects in their study ranged in age from 53 to 83 years and presented with mean PTAs that did not exceed 55 dB HL in either ear. Speech materials included phonemically balanced monosyllabic words, synthetic sentences (SSI), and the low and high probability sentences (SPIN). A test of dichotic sentence identification (DSI) was also administered (Jerger et al., 1988). Based on their listening strategies during a criterial categorization task, subjects were divided into three criterion groups; namely, lax, intermediate and strict. Performance on the speech measures was then contrasted across groups. Their findings indicated that after controlling for degree of high-frequency hearing loss, listening strategy had little impact on scores on selected speech-recognition tasks (Jerger et al., 1988). Although using different methodology, the data of Jerger and colleagues with the data of Yantz and Anderson (1984) found response criterion values to be comparable in young and elderly subjects. The bulk of work in the area would suggest that response bias differences do not influence speech recognition scores. Procedural differences and subject variables, however, render definitive conclusions about the impact of response criteria on performance on speech recognition tasks premature.

To what extent do speech-recognition measures correlate with self-perceived hearing handicap?

One purpose of speech recognition testing is to predict the impact of hearing loss on performance in everyday life situations. In an effort toward external validation of scores on speech-recognition tasks, a number of researchers have attempted to correlate scores on a variety of speech measures to scores on self-assessment scales that quantify the extent of perceived hearing handicap experienced by hearing-impaired listeners. The premise underlying these investigations is the incomplete relationship between hearing impairment data measured audiometrically and hearing handicap data measured using self-assessment techniques. Clinically, it is apparent that individuals with minimal hearing loss often experience significant handicap, whereas persons with moderate hearing loss may not perceive themselves as being handicapped. Data on the relation between word-recognition ability and perceived handicap confirm that scores on speech measures account for little of the variability in the perception of communication difficulties and in the perception of the psychosocial ramifications of hearing loss. Interestingly, correlations between puretone measures and self-assessed hearing handicap are stronger (Weinstein and Ventry, 1983; Berkowitz and Hochberg, 1971) than those between impairment data and handicap scores. The weak correlations are a consistent finding across populations, settings and self-assessment scales, suggesting that speech understanding tests are not representative of experience in everyday listening conditions (CHABA, 1988; Weinstein and Ventry, 1983; Berkowitz and Hochberg, 1971; McCartney, Maurer, and Sorenson, 1976).

Finally, Jerger, Oliver, and Pirozzolo (1990) found that scores on central auditory processing tests correlate with self-perceived hearing handicap, defined by performance on the Hearing Handicap Inventory for the Elderly. They reported that on the average, older adults with CAPD rated themselves as being more handicapped than subjects without CAPD. In sum, the large standard error associated with scores on handicap scales used with adults, coupled with the minimal relation between self-perceived handicap and word-recognition ability, underlines the role of handicap scales in helping clinicians gain insight into the effects of hearing loss on patient function.

CONCLUSIONS AND IMPLICATIONS OF STUDIES ON SPEECH RECOGNITION ABILITY IN THE ELDERLY

The following excerpts taken from selected studies on word-recognition ability in the elderly can be used to sum up the findings to date. These are as follows:

1. Listeners of differing age groups perform similarly on speech-recognition tasks in quiet when matched for equivalent hearing loss (Townsend and Bess, 1980).
2. If the role of the audiologist includes helping the patient gain insight into his communicative problem, testing should be designed to describe the communicative handicap as completely as possible. In terms of hearing and understanding everyday speech, speech discrimination testing in quiet does not provide the necessary data to do so, regardless of the test used (Orchik and Burgess, 1977).
3. Test procedures most likely to reveal deficits due to the effect of age alone are the assessment of S-B ratio yielding a particular criterion score or the assessment of percent-correct recognition performance for speech materials presented in degraded conditions (Gordon-Salant, 1987).
4. Handicap questionnaires can provide complementary information and useful clinical insights not obtained with word- or sentence-identification tests (Tyler and Smith, 1983).
5. The purpose of the speech discrimination task (e.g., reveal age effects, quantify problems in everyday listening conditions) should dictate the materials, presentation level, response format, test paradigm, and conditions under which the speech recognition performance is assessed (Carhart, 1965). "Assessment of speech recognition performance in the elderly should incorporate procedures that are sensitive to age-related processing problems" (Gordon-Salant, 1987, p. 281).

OVERVIEW OF PERFORMANCE ON IMMITTANCE AND AUDITORY BRAINSTEM RESPONSE (ABR) TESTS

Immittance

The immittance test battery administered to evaluate the status of the middle ear system in older adults generally includes tympanometry, static admittance, and acoustic stapedial reflex tests. Because of the importance placed on this diagnostic information, it is appropriate for the audiologist to consider the effects of age on the interpretation of test results. Conflicting data continue to exist on the effect of age on static admittance values, the tympanometric pressure peak (TPP), and acoustic stapedial reflex measures. Table 37.2 represents an attempt at combining data from available studies to summarize the effects of age on performance on selected acoustic immittance measures.

In general, static admittance values that yield information about the status of the middle ear system in its quiescent state do not appear to undergo a clinically significant change as a function of the aging process (Gordon-Salant, 1987). Static acoustic compliance appears to decline systematically as a function of the aging process, yet reported values are within the range considered to be normal for young adults, and thus separate norms are probably not warranted (Gordon-Salant, 1991; Jerger, Jerger, and Maudlin, 1972; Nerbonne, Bliss, and Schow, 1978). There is a dearth of data on effect of age on the tympanometric pressure peak (TPP), or the value in air pressure (daPa) that corresponds to the ear canal pressure producing the maximal peak. There is, however, some limited information that suggests that eustachian tube function, as represented by excessive negative middle ear pressure on the typanogram, is inadequate in selected aged individuals (Bess et al., 1991; Gordon-Salant, 1991).

There is some disagreement among investigators about the effect of age on acoustic reflex thresholds.

Jerger, Hayes, Anthony and Maudlin, 1978; Jerger, Jerger, and Maudlin (1972) reported a systematic decline in reflex thresholds with increasing age; Osterhammel and Osterhammel (1979) reported no change in acoustic stapedial reflex thresholds (ARTs) with age when thresholds were reported in dB HL, whereas Wilson (1981) reported an increase in thresholds with age, most notably for an activator signal of 4000 Hz. A number of investigators have reported that ARTs for broadband noise stimuli are elevated in the elderly (Silman, 1979; Silman and Gelfand, 1981; Wilson and Margolis, 1991). In their comprehensive discussion of age and the acoustic reflex, Wilson and Margolis (1991) concluded that the changes in acoustic reflex thresholds to tonal activators at or below 2000 Hz are too small to be considered statistically significant. Age-related increases in thresholds for high-frequency tonal activators and for broadband noise are, however, of statistical and clinical significance (Wilson and Margolis, 1991).

ABR

As older adults are at risk for medical problems (e.g., vascular disorders) associated with ABR abnormalities, and more often than not present with some degree of peripheral hearing loss, it behooves the audiologist to be aware of the interaction between age and absolute latency measures, waveform morphology, and the latency-intensity function. As an extensive discussion of the effect of age on each of the ABR indices is beyond the scope of this chapter, the discussion will be limited to latency measures as they are considered the most valid and reliable diagnostic of the ABR measures (Musiek, 1991).

Data on the interaction between chronologic age and the absolute latency of waves I through V are inconclusive. Beagley and Sheldrake (1978) studied a sample of 70 subjects whose hearing was within normal limits for age. Their data suggested a nonsignificant prolongation in the latency of Waves I through V, with no significant prolongation in the wave I–V interval, using click stimuli presented at 60, 70, 80 dB SL. Jerger and Hall (1980) examined the change in Wave V latency as a function of increasing age in a large sample of subjects with normal hearing and sensory neural hearing loss. They reported a modest (0.2 msec) increase in the absolute latency of Wave V in older subjects with normal hearing. Wave V latency showed little change as a function of age in those subjects with sensory neural hearing impairment. In contrast, Rowe (1978), and Harkins and Lenhardt (1980), among other investigators, reported a modest increase in the absolute latency

Table 37.2
Effect of Age on Performance on Immittance Tests

Test	Effect of Age on Performance
Static admittance values	No significant age effect, as static immittance values appear to be within the range considered to be normal for young adults.
Tympanometry	No significant effect, as 95% of ears had pressure between +/− 100 mm H$_2$O.[a]
Eustachian tube function tests	Pressure-equalization studies show ventilating inefficiency in a small proportion of older adults.
Acoustic reflex thresholds	No evidence of a systematic age effect, for tonal activators below 2000 Hz.[b,c] Small age-effect apparent (i.e., elevated reflex levels) when broadband noise is the activator signal.[c]
Acoustic-reflex decay test	No evidence of an age effect on tests of acoustic-reflex decay.[a,c]

[a] Gates et al. (1990).
[b] Gordon-Salant (1991).
[c] Wilson and Margolis (1991).

of Waves I, III and V in the older subjects as compared with the younger sample.

More recently, Jerger and Chmiel (1991) reported that for clinical purposes, the latency of the ABR waveforms, using signals presented at 80 dB nHL, are resistant to age effects. Similarly, Ottaviani, Maurizi, D'Alatri, and Almadori (1991) contend that the shift in the latency of the ABR waveforms seen in selected older subjects is due to the configuration of the hearing loss in the higher frequencies rather than age. Specifically, Ottaviani et al. (1991) reported no significant difference in the absolute latency of waves I, III and V and in the I–III and I–V interpeak intervals between presbycusic subjects and young subjects with cochlear hearing loss.

In sum, a review of selected studies to date suggest a slight (0.1–0.2 msec), if any, increase in the absolute latency of Waves I, III and V with age. Brewer (1987), Otto and McCandless (1982) and Ottaviani et al. (1991) hypothesized that high-frequency hearing sensitivity may account in part for the apparent shift in latency of selected waveforms. Finally, according to Hyde (1985), Brewer (1987) and the ASHA Working Group on Auditory Evoked Potential Measurements (1988), hearing level at 4000 Hz may influence the absolute latency of selected waves (e.g., Wave V). Specifically, when the hearing level at 4000 Hz exceeds 50 dB HL in subjects over the age of 50, "the effects of aging and hearing loss on absolute latency should be considered" (ASHA Working Group on Auditory Evoked Potential Measurements, 1988, p. 22).

IDENTIFICATION OF THE ELDERLY HEARING IMPAIRED

It is apparent from epidemiological and clinical studies that hearing loss is prevalent among older adults, that the structural changes in the aging auditory system have significant functional and psychosocial implications for the older adult, and that hearing loss and its manifestations are readily quantifiable. It is also clear that the elderly do benefit from hearing aids, and the earlier the intervention, the more likely the negative effects of hearing loss can be ameliorated. The latter considerations make hearing loss an important target for screening. According to Mausner and Kramer (1985), the major purpose of screening is to identify individuals who have a high probability of having the target disorder and start the person on the road to successful management (Cadman, Chambers, Feldman, and Sackett, 1984). As persons with chronic conditions demonstrate poor compliance with prescribed interventions, the major challenge facing the audiologist mounting a screening program is to adopt a test that not only identifies older persons presenting with

the target behavior but also incorporates strategies that will encourage compliance.

A major focus of clinical geriatrics is evaluating, restoring, or maintaining an individual's functional status, as well as diagnosing a chronic medical condition (Kane et al., 1989). Because the chronic diseases so prevalent among older adults cannot be eliminated, specialists in geriatrics are emphasizing the importance of early identification and remediation of impairments so that they do not become functional disabilities (Lachs, Feinstein, Cooney et al., 1990). The fact that ability to function despite the existence of an impairment is a central focus of geriatric care has prompted investigation into the efficacy of puretone and/or self-assessment measures as tools for identifying the hearing-impaired elderly. Additionally, the imperfect relationship between audiometric data and perceived hearing handicap has influenced some investigators to supplement a puretone screen with a handicap assessment. Before presenting data on selected screening protocols, a brief discussion of the issues surrounding the selection of an "ideal screening test" for the elderly is in order.

Ventry and Weinstein (1983) recommended supplementing a puretone screen with a self-assessment scale as a means of identifying elderly persons with a functionally handicapping hearing impairment that requires audiologic intervention. They advocated a 40 dB HL fence at 1000 and 2000 Hz as the pass-fail criterion for the population of adults over 64 years of age. The screening version of the Hearing Handicap Inventory for the Elderly (HHIE-S) is the self-assessment scale recommended to supplement the puretone screen. Several researchers have attempted to validate the protocol, using different criteria against which to judge its adequacy.

Weinstein (1986) reported on the outcome of a study wherein all older adults completing the combined 40 dB HL puretone and HHIE-S handicap screen underwent a complete audiologic evaluation to validate the recommended protocol. Using the audiologist's recommendation for medical or audiologic intervention (e.g., hearing aid, annual evaluation) as the gold standard, Weinstein (1986) reported a sensitivity of 85% and a specificity of 64% when the handicap and puretone screen were combined. The specificity of the handicap screen alone (83%) was comparable to that of the puretone screen (77%). The sensitivity of the puretone screen was 72% versus 65% for the handicap screen. Assuming a 40% prevalence of hearing loss among older adults, the predictive value of a positive outcome was highest for the HHIE-S screen (71%), and the predictive value of a negative screening outcome was highest for the combined impairment-handicap screen (87%). According to their positive predictive value, using the HHIE-S screen, 71% of persons failing the HHIE-S screen would be classified as having a hearing problem requiring audiologic attention. In contrast, a negative predictive value of 81% for the combined approach would suggest that 81% of persons who passed the combined puretone and handicap screen would not have been classified as having a problem requiring audiologic intervention. Despite problems in the design of the latter validation study, the yield from a 40 dB HL puretone screen, and/or a handicap screen, was high enough to justify its use until a more valid procedure becomes available (Weinstein, 1986).

Lichtenstein, Bess, and Logan (1988a) attempted to determine the usefulness of the Ventry and Weinstein (1983) protocol in selected primary care settings in Tennessee. The tools for the identification of hearing impaired elderly individuals included the HHIE-S and the Welch-Allyn audioscope. The audioscope is a hand-held otoscope combined with an audiometer that delivers selected tones (i.e., 20, 25, and 40 dB HL) at frequencies of 500, 1000, 2000, and 4000 Hz (Lichtenstein et al., 1988a). All subjects underwent a hearing screening in a Physician's Office and at the Bill Wilkerson Hearing and Speech Center. Fifty-eight percent of the subjects undergoing the hearing screen kept appointments at the hearing center for complete audiologic testing to determine the reliability and validity of the screening protocol administered in the physician's office (Lichtenstein et al., 1988). The gold standard against which the validity of the screening tests was judged was the presence of hearing levels in excess of 40 dB HL at 1000 or 2000 Hz in both ears, or a 40 dB loss at 1000 and 2000 Hz in one ear. The sensitivity, specificity, predictive values, and test accuracy associated with the screening tests are as follows. First, the sensitivity associated with the audioscope was quite high (i.e., 94%). Next, the specificity of the HHIE-S, when scores indicated a significant hearing handicap, was quite high (i.e., 96–98%), as well. Individuals with HHIE-S scores in excess of 24 had a posttest probability of hearing loss of 84% (Lichtenstein et al., 1988). Third, the best test accuracy (i.e., 83%) was achieved when HHIE-S and the audioscope were used in combination. In a companion study, Fino, Bess, and Lichtenstein (1989) reported that elderly individuals who obtained a score in excess of 24 on the HHIE-S were the most likely persons to purchase amplification. In contrast, individuals who passed the audioscope screen (40 dB HL at 1000 and 2000 Hz) but were considered hearing aid candidates were unlikely to seek hearing aid rehabilitation. Based on the outcomes of their studies, Lichtenstein, Bess, and Logan (1991)

concluded the following: (1) the HHIE-S is a robust test for screening elderly individuals with handicapping hearing impairments; (2) the greatest test accuracy in identifying hearing impairment was found when the two tests are combined; and (3) persons should be considered in need of referral to an audiologist when they fail the audioscope and have an HHIE score greater than 8 or they pass the audioscope and have an HHIE score greater than 24.

Schow, Smedley, and Longhurst (1990) described the outcome of a large scale study of adults designed to validate a puretone screen and the 10-item Self-Assessment of Communication (SAC) scale as a tool for screening adults for the presence of self-reported communication difficulties. Subjects were screened at selected health fairs and additional unspecified locations throughout Idaho. The puretone protocol used on all subjects, irrespective of age, was 25 dB HL at 1000 and 2000 Hz and 30 dB HL at 4000 Hz. Inability to hear a tone at any one frequency was deemed a fail (Schow et al., 1990). A score of 18/19 was considered a failure for most subjects on the SAC. The criterion standard against which the validity of their screening protocol was judged was level of puretone hearing. In contrast to the studies described by Weinstein (1986) and Lichtenstein et al. (1988a), the conclusions of Schow and his colleagues are based on puretone tests conducted on only those individuals who failed the screen. The diagnostic characteristics of their protocol (i.e., sensitivity/specificity values) were relatively comparable to those of Weinstein (1986) and Lichtenstein et al. (1988a). Unfortunately, the design of their study did not include a follow-up test on all subjects irrespective of the outcome of the screen (i.e., those who passed and failed). Thus, the generalizability and validity of their conclusions regarding sensitivity, specificity, and predictive accuracy are limited.

In sum, the foregoing investigations support the validity of the use of both self-assessment tools and puretone checks in screening programs designed to identify hearing-impaired older adults requiring audiologic services. The ideal puretone criterion for screening older adults remains a matter of controversy because of: (1) the lack of a consensus among professionals regarding the purposes of a screening test used with older adults; (2) the lack of agreement on the independent standard against which to judge the validity of a puretone screening protocol; and (3) the dearth of large-scale studies wherein the frequency and hearing levels used for screening are contrasted across groups and clinical settings. It should be noted that irrespective of the protocol, follow-up surveys of elderly individuals who fail a hearing screen suggest that the majority fail to pursue the provider's recommendation for treatment in the form of amplification (Jupiter, 1989; Koike and Johnston, 1989; Schow et al., 1990; Fino et al., 1989). Finally, the success of a screening program is determined in large part by the likelihood of compliance with recommendations for diagnostic and treatment procedures (Weinstein, 1986; Mausner and Kramer, 1985). In view of the low compliance rate among older adults, an additional research focus should be on developing programs that will promote attitudes that may increase the likelihood of compliance with the provider's treatment recommendations.

TEST BATTERY APPROACH FOR USE WITH THE ELDERLY

The foregoing sections of the chapter suggest that there is considerable variability among older adults in the etiologies of their hearing losses, in their reaction to hearing impairment, and in their performance on word-recognition tests and on physiologic measures. Accordingly, the audiologist must approach each client on an individual basis and select from an array of tests the one that best meets the needs of the client and the needs of the professional. In general, the older adult should be assessed in a comprehensive fashion, viewing both the diagnostic and rehabilitative implications of the test performance together (Kane et al., 1989).

Kane et al. (1989) emphasized the fact that physical, psychologic and socioeconomic factors interact in a complex way to influence their functional status and performance on diagnostic tests. Accordingly, they opine that although traditional measures of health status are useful in uncovering the etiology of a condition and in identifying a treatable disorder, measures of function are "often essential in determining overall health, well-being and the need for health and social services" (Kane et al., 1989, p. 49). Further, as decrements in hearing are associated with declines in physical and psychosocial function and an impoverished quality of life, it behooves audiologists to incorporate global measures of functional health status and a communication-specific self-assessment scale into the test battery (Bess, Logan, and Lichtenstein, 1990; Mulrow, Aguilar, Endicott et al., 1990).

In light of the above considerations, assessment of the older adult should begin with a comprehensive case history. The case history should be administered in a systematic fashion. The clinician should view it as an opportunity to learn about the client's attitudes toward hearing loss and hearing aids, and as a chance to gain insight into the communication specific difficulties attributable to hearing loss (Gordon-Salant, 1991). Every effort should be made to uncover auditory symptoms and the medical conditions that may underly their etiology. As elderly people are often treated with a number of medications that may affect the auditory or vestibular mechanisms, a detailed medication history is critical (Kane et al., 1989). Often, input from a caregiver or family member can be helpful at the end of the assessment, when the audiologist makes his or her management decisions. We must have a great deal of patience during our interactions with our older hearing-impaired clients. Further, audiologists should be sensitive to the concerns of elderly persons which often are not focused on their ears. For example, ongoing medical, social or psychologic problems may impact on their performance and reactions to our recommendations (Kane et al., 1989). Finally, it is imperative that we approach the older person with the conviction that improvement is possible.

As "function is the common language of geriatrics," techniques for uncovering the functional impact of hearing impairment must be a routine component of the test battery (Kane et al., p. 49). Self-assessment scales, which quantify the perceived effects of hearing loss on daily life, have emerged as instruments that can reliably uncover the functional impacts of unremediated hearing loss. Information gleaned from responses to items comprising selected self-assessment scales can assist in the assessment process and in management decisions. A variety of scales that yield estimates of the degree to which hearing loss is perceived to impact on communication and psychosocial function have evolved for use with older hearing impaired adults. Table 37.3 contains a list of handicap scales that have been standardized on the elderly. In selecting a self-assessment scale, the audiologist should consider its reliability and content validity. Further, the instrument selected by the clinician should fit the purposes and setting for which it is intended (Kane et al., 1989). Detailed descriptions of available instruments and principles involved in their selection can be found in Weinstein (1984) and Demorest and Walden (1984). Many audiologists continue to dismiss the contribution of information contained in responses to handicap scales. Their value, however, in screening, in assessing the functional impact of hearing loss, as a prognostic indicator, in monitoring patient status and as an outcome measure are quite clear (Bess, Logan, and Lichtenstein, 1991).

Puretone air and bone conduction thresholds are at the heart of the audiologic test battery providing information about hearing status and the need for medical and/or rehabilitative intervention. The clinician should be alert to the high incidence of impacted cerumen and collapsed ear canals in this population. Routine test procedures are advocated, when the client's mental, cognitive and physical health status allow. Table 37.4 contains a list of modifications that may be

Table 37.3
Overview of Selected Self-Assessment Scale Applicable to Older Hearing-Impaired Adults

Scale	Content
The Hearing Measurement Scale (HMS) (Noble and Atherly, 1970)	42-item scale yielding information about communication ability, personal opinions about the effects of hearing loss, and sensitivity for non-speech sounds. Originally designed for use with persons with noise-induced hearing loss.
The Hearing Handicap Inventory for the Elderly (HHIE) (Ventry and Weinstein, 1982)	25-item scale yielding information about the perceived social and emotional effects of hearing loss. Standardized for use with the elderly.
The Screening Version of the Handicap Inventory for Elderly (HHIE-S) (Ventry and Weinstein, (1983)	10-item scale designed to elicit information quickly and reliably about the perceived psychosocial effects of hearing loss on the elderly.
The Self-Assessment of Communication (SAC) (Schow and Nerbonne, (1982)	10-item scale to quantify perceived communication difficulties and reactions to hearing loss. Standardized on young and older adults.
Quantified Denver Scale (QDS) (Mulrow et al., (1990)	25-item questionnaire to assess perceived communication difficulties from hearing loss. Efficacy with the elderly has recently been addressed.
Sickness Impact Profile (SIP) (Bergner, Bobbitt, Carter and Gilson, (1981)	136-item questionnaire that provides information about the overall functional health status of adults.

Table 37.4
Modifications in the Standard Test Battery[a]

Behavior	Test Modification
Slow Response Time	Slow down rate of tonal presentation allowing the patient's behavior to dictate the pace of the evaluation.
Poor Memory	Repetition and simplification of test instructions. Use of gestures to facilitate understanding of instructions. Extended opportunity for practice. Frequent conditioning/reconditioning trials.
Movement Deficits	Evaluate different strategies for responding before initiating testing. Select response that requires the least amount of effort and is the most natural. Be consistent in choice of response behavior to avoid confusion and frustration.
Failing attention, distractable	Reduce length of tonal presentation allowing the patient's behavior to dictate the pace of the evaluation.

[a] Modified from Weinstein (1990).

necessary with selected clients. The author has found some of the modifications invaluable with confused patients and the frail elderly.

Speech tests should include assessment of spondee thresholds and word-recognition ability. The purpose of the speech test should dictate the procedure. Word-recognition tests provide diagnostic information, tips for counseling, and are often helpful when reaching management decisions. For diagnostic purposes, age-appropriate norms are essential for reaching diagnostic conclusions. For example, Gang (1976) suggested that the magnitude of the rollover index, which is considered a diagnostic indicator, varies somewhat with age. Further, in deciding on a presentation level for word-recognition tests, keep in mind that it is important to compensate for a high-frequency hearing loss to ensure audibility of the high-frequency speech spectrum (Gordon-Salant, Gates, Cooper, Kannel, et al. (1990).

With regard to counseling applications, comparing performance on speech tests presented with and without visual cues can often convince older adults of the contribution of speech reading to speech understanding. Similarly, comparing scores on speech-recognition tasks in quiet to scores on speech tests administered in the presence of competition can help convince the older adult of the actual communication handicap hearing loss imposes. Finally, supplementing routine monosyllabic word lists with high-frequency word lists can also help the hearing impaired to appreciate the manner in which deprivation of high frequency cues can compromise speech-recognition ability. The author considers acceptance and realistic assessment of the impact of hearing loss critical to the success of rehabilitative intervention with the hearing-impaired elderly. Speech tests have a great deal of potential in the latter regard.

Finally, the value of the immittance test for uncovering middle ear pathology, the role of vestibular function tests in the assessment of older adults at risk for falls and instability due to age-related declines in response to sudden movements, and the utility of ABR in site of lesion determinations should be self-evident (Brummel-Smith, 1990).

CONCLUDING REMARKS

The expansion of the nation's elderly population dictates that they be allowed to "function in the mainstream of American life to the extent of their full potential" (Reichel, 1983, p. 9). Remediation of the chronic conditions (e.g., hearing loss) that afflict 80% of older adults is a big step toward the goal of promoting independence and enhancing functional abilities. When one considers the enormous growth in the older population, and the increase in prevalence of hearing loss forecast for the year 2000, the role that audiologists will have to play is self-evident. In fact, audiology is central to the goal of increasing to 60% the number of persons over 65 years routinely evaluated for vision, hearing, cognition, and functional status (U.S.D.H.H.S., 1990).

The U.S. Public Health Service (1990) is committed to the view that early identification of chronic conditions (e.g., hearing loss) and corresponding intervention will reduce the magnitude of functional disability older adults will develop. The goal of this chapter was to facilitate realization of the goals of the U.S.P.H.S. and to help audiologists enhance the quality of life of older adults.

REFERENCES

American Speech Language Association. The Short Latency Auditory Evoked Potentials. ASHA Audiologic Aging Group on Auditory Evoked Potential Measurement, 1988.

Beagley H, and Sheldrake J. Differences in brainstem response latency with age and sex. Br J Audiol 1978;12:69–77.

Beattie R, and Warren V. Slope characteristics of CID W-22 word functions in elderly hearing-impaired listeners. J Speech Hear Disord 1983;48:119–127.

Bergner M, Bobbitt R, Carter W, and Gilson B. The Sickness Impact Profile: developments and final revision of a health status measure. Med Care 1981;14:57–67.

Berkowitz A, and Hochberg I. Self-assessment of hearing handicap in the aged. Arch Otolaryngol 1971;93:25–28.

Bess F, and Townsend T. Word discrimination for listeners with flat sensorineural hearing losses. J Speech Hear Disord 1977;42:232–237.

Bess F, Lichtenstein M, and Logan S. Functional impact of hearing loss on the elderly. ASHA Reports. 1990.

Bess F, Lichtenstein M, and Logan S. Audiologic assessment of the elderly. In Rintelmann W, Ed. Hearing Assessment, 2nd ed. Austin, TX: Pro-Ed, 1991a.

Bess F, Lichtenstein M, and Logan S. Making hearing impairment functionally relevant: linkages with hearing disability and handicap. Acta Otolaryngol (Stockholm) Suppl 1991b;476:226–231.

Bess F, Lichtenstein M, Logan S, Burger M, Nelson E. Hearing impairment as a determinant of function in the elderly. J Am Geriatr Soc 1989;37:123–128.

Bess F, Lichtenstein M, Logan S, Burger M. Comparing criteria of hearing impairment in the elderly: a functional approach. J Speech Hear Res 1989;32:795–802.

Blumenfeld V, Bergman M, and Milner E. Speech discrimination in an aging population. J Speech Hear Res 1969;12:210–217.

Botwinick J. Disinclination to venture response versus cautiousness in responding: age differences. J Genet Psychol 1969;115:55–62.

Brant L, and Fozard J. Age changes in pure tone hearing thresholds in a longitudinal study of normal human aging. J Acoust Soc Am 1990;88:813–820.

Brewer C. Electrophysiologic measures. In Mueller HG, and Geoffrey V, Eds. Communication Disorders in Aging: Assessment and Management. Washington, DC: Gallaudet University Press, 1987:334–381.

Brody H. Organization of the central cortex: Study of aging in human cerebral cortex. J Compar Neurol 1955;102:511–556.

Brummel-Smith K. Introduction. In Kemp B, Brummel-Smith K, Ransdell J: Geriatric Rehabilitation. Boston: College Hill Press, 1990.

Cadman D, Chambers L, Feldman W, and Sackett D. Assessing the effectiveness of community screening programs. JAMA 1984;252:1580–1585.

Carhart R. Problems in the measurement of speech discrimination. Arch Otolaryngol 1965;82:253–260.

Committee on Hearing, Bioacoustics and Biomechanics. CHABA Working Group on Speech Understanding. Speech understanding and aging. J Acoust Soc Am 1988;83:859–895.

Corso J. Age and sex differences in puretone thresholds. Arch Otolaryngol 1963;77:383–405.

Covell W. Histological changes in the aging cochlea. J Gerontol 1952;7:173–177.

Demorest M, and Walden B. Psychometric principles in the selection, interpretation and evaluation of communication self-assessment inventories. J Speech Hear Disord 1984;49:226–241.

Downs M, and Glorig A. Mild hearing loss in the aging. Hear Instruments 1988;39:28–33.

Dubno J, Dirks D, Morgan D. Effects of age and mild hearing loss on speech recognition in noise. J Acoust Soc Am 1984;76:87–96.

Etholm B, and Belal A. Senile changes in the middle ear joints. Ann Otol Rhinol Laryngol 1974;23:49–54.

Fino M, Bess F, and Lichtenstein M. Factors differentiating elderly hearing aid users and nonusers. Poster session at Annual Meeting of the American Academy of Audiology, 1989.

Frattali C, Cherow E, and Cole L. Healthy People 2000: Promoting Health for the Nation. ASHA 1991;33:30–37.

Gaeth J. A study of phonemic regression associated with hearing loss, [Unpublished doctoral dissertation]. Evanston, IL: Northwestern University, 1948.

Gang R. The effects of age on the diagnostic utility of the rollover phenomenon. J Speech Hear Disord 1976;41:63–69.

Gates G, Cooper J, Kannel W, Miller N. Hearing in the elderly: the Framingham Cohort, 1983–85. Part I. Basic audiometric test results. Ear Hear 1990;11:247–256.

Gilad O, and Glorig A. Presbycusis: The aging ear (Part I). J Am Aud Soc 1979;4:195–206.

Goetzinger C, Proud G, Dirks D, and Embrey J. A study of hearing in advanced age. Arch Otolaryngol 1961;73:662–674.

Gordon-Salant S. Effects of aging on response criteria in speech-recognition tasks. J Speech Hear Res 1986;29:155–162.

Gordon-Salant S. Basic hearing evaluation. In Mueller H, and Geoffrey V, Eds. Communication Disorders in Aging: Assessment and Management. Washington, DC: Gallaudet University Press, 1987a.

Gordon-Salant S. Age-related differences in speech recognition as a function of test format and paradigm. Ear Hear 1987b;8:277–282.

Gordon-Salant S. The Audiologic Assessment. In Ripich D, Ed. Handbook of Geriatric Communication Disorders. Austin, TX: Pro-Ed, 1991.

Gulya J. Structural and physiological changes of the auditory and vestibular mechanisms with aging. In Ripich D, Ed. Handbook of Geriatric Communication Disorders. Austin, TX: Pro-Ed, 1991.

Hall J. Effects of age and sex on static compliance. Arch Otolaryngol 1979;105:153–156.

Harford E, and Dodds E. Hearing status of ambulatory senior citizens. Ear Hear 1982;3:105–109.

Harkins S, and Lenhardt M. Brainstem auditory evoked potentials in the elderly. In: Poon LW, Ed. Aging in the 1980's: Psychological Issues. Washington, DC: American Psychological Association, 1980:101–112.

Helfer K, Wilber L. Hearing with aging and speed perception in reverberation and noise. J Speech Hearing Res 1990;33:149–155.

Herbst K, and Humphrey C. Hearing impairment and mental state in the elderly living at home. Br Med J 1980;281:903–905.

Hyde M. The effect of cochlear lesions on the auditory brainstem responses. In Jacobson J, Ed. The Auditory Brainstem Response. San Diego, CA: College Hill Press, 1985:13–146.

Jerger J, Jerger S, and Maudlin L. Studies in impedance audiometry. I. Normal and sensorineural ears. Arch Otolaryngol 1972;89:513–523.

Jerger J. Audiological findings in the aging. Adv Otorhinolaryngol 1973;20:115–124.

Jerger J, and Hayes D. Diagnostic speech audiometry. Arch Otolaryngol 1977;96:513–523.

Jerger J, Hayes D, Anthony L, and Maudlin L. Factors influencing prediction of hearing level from the acoustic reflex. Monogr Contemp Audiol 1978;1:1–20.

Jerger J, and Hall J. Effects of age and sex on auditory brainstem response. Arch Otolaryngol 1980;106:387–391.

Jerger J, Johnson K, and Jerger S. Effect of response criterion on measures of speech understanding in the elderly. Ear Hear 1988;9:49–56.

Jerger J, Jerger S, Oliver T, and Pirozzolo F. Speech understanding in the elderly. Ear Hear 1989;10:79–89.

Jerger J, Oliver T, Pirozzolo F. Impact of central auditory processing disorder and cognitive deficit on the self-assessment of hearing handicap in the elderly. J Am Acad Audiol 1990;1:75–81.

Jerger J, and Chmiel R. Effect of age on auditory evoked potentials. Paper presented at the Third Annual Convention of the American Academy of Audiology, 1991.

Jupiter T. A community hearing screening program for the elderly. Hear J 1989:14–17.

Kamm C, Morgan D, and Dirks D. Accuracy of adaptive procedure estimates of PB-max level. J Speech Hear Disord 1983;48:202–209.

Kane R, Ouslander J, and Abrass I. Essentials of Clinical Geriatrics, 2nd ed. New York: McGraw-Hill Information Services Company, 1989.

Kasden S. Speech discrimination in two age groups matched for hearing loss. J Aud Res 1970;10:210–212.

Koike K, and Johnson A. Follow-up survey of the elderly who failed a hearing screening protocol. Ear Hear 1989;10:250–253.

Konkle D, Beasley D, and Bess F. Intelligibility of time-altered speech in relation to chronological aging. J Speech Hear Res 1977;20:108–115.

Lachs M, Feinstein A, Cooney L, Drickamer M, Marottoli R, Pannill F, and Tinetti M. A simple procedure for general screening for functional disability in elderly patients. Ann Intern Med 1990;112:699–706.

Lichtenstein M, Bess F, Logan S. Validation of screening tools for identifying hearing-impaired elderly in primary care. JAMA 1988a;259:2875–2878.

Lichtenstein M, Bess F, and Logan S. Diagnostic performance of the Hearing Handicap Inventory for the Elderly (Screening version) against differing definitions of hearing loss. Ear Hear 1988b;9:209–211.

Lichtenstein M, Bess F, Logan S, and Burger M. Deriving criteria for hearing impairment in the elderly: A functional approach. J Am Acad Audiol 1990;1:11–22.

Lichtenstein M, Bess F, and Logan S. Screening the elderly for hearing impairment. In Ripich D, Ed. Handbook of Geriatric Communication Disorders. Austin, TX: Pro-Ed, 1991.

Marshall L. Auditory processing in aging listeners. J Speech Hear Disord 1981;46:226–240.

Mausner J, and Kramer S. Mausner & Bahn Epidemiology: An Introductory Text. Philadelphia: WB Saunders, 1985.

McCartney J, Maurer J, and Sorenson F. A comparison of the Hearing Handicap Scale and the Hearing Measurement Scale with standard audiometric measures on the geriatric population. J Aud Res 1976;15:51–58.

Moscicki E, Elkins E, Baum H, McNamara P. Hearing loss in the elderly: an epidemiologic study of the Framingham Heart Study Cohort. Ear Hear 1985;6:184–190.

Mulrow C, Aguilar C, Endicott J, Velez R, Tuley M, Charlip W, and Hill J. Association between hearing impairment and the quality of life of elderly individuals. J Am Geriatr Soc 1990a;38:45–50.

Mulrow C, Aguilar C, Endicott J, Tuley M, Velez R, Charlip W, Rhodes M, Hill J, and DeNino L. Quality of life changes and hearing impairment: results of a randomized trial. Ann Intern Med 1990b;113:188–194.

Musiek F. Auditory evoked responses in site of lesion assessment. In Rintelmann W, Ed. Hearing Assessment, 2nd ed. Austin, TX: Pro-Ed, 1991.

Nabalek A, and Robinson P. Monaural and binaural speech perception in reverberation for listeners of various ages. J Acoust Soc Am 1982;71:1242–1248.

National Center for Health Statistics (NCHS). Current estimates from the National Health Interview Survey: United States, 1987. Vital and Health Statistics. Series 10. Public Health Service, Washington: U.S. Government Printing Office, 1987.

National Institute on Aging. Senility reconsidered. JAMA 1980;244:259–263.

Nerbonne M, Bliss A, and Schow R. Acoustic impedance values in the elderly. J Am Aud Soc 1978;4:57–59.

Noble W, and Atherly G. The hearing measurement scale: a questionnaire for the assessment of auditory disability. J Aud Res 1987;10:229–250.

Olsen W, and Matkin N. Speech Audiometry. In Rintelmann W, Ed. Hearing Assessment, 2nd ed. Austin, TX: Pro-Ed, 1991.

Orchik D, and Burgess J. Synthetic sentence identification as a function of age of the listener. J Am Audiol Soc 1977;3:42–46.

Osterhammel D, and Osterhammel P. Age and sex variations for the normal stapedial reflex thresholds and tympanometric compliance values. Scand Audiol 1979;8:153–158.

Ottaviani F, Maurizi M, D'Alatri, and Almadori G. Auditory brainstem responses in the aged. Acta Otolaryngol Suppl (Stockh) 1991;476:110–114.

Otto W, and McCandless G. Aging and auditory site of lesion. Ear Hear 1982;3:110–117.

Peters C, Potter J, and Scholer S. Hearing impairment as a predictor of cognitive decline in dementia. J Am Geriatr Soc 1988;36:981–986.

Rosen S, Bergman M, Plester D, El-Mofty A, and Sattis MH. Presbycusis study of a relatively noise-free population in the Sudan. Trans Am Otol Soc 1962;50:135–151.

Rosenwasser H. Otitic problems in the aged. Geriatrics 1964;19:11–17.

Rowe M. Normal variability of the brainstem auditory-evoked responses in young and old subjects. Electroencephalogr Clin Neurophysiol 1978;44:459–470.

Schon T. The effects on speech intelligibility of time compression and expression on normal-hearing, hard of hearing and aged males. J Aud Res 1970;10:263–268.

Schow R, and Nerbonne M. Hearing levels among elderly nursing home residents. J Speech Hear Res 1980;45:124–132.

Schow R, Smedley T, and Longhurst T. Self-Assessment and impairment in adult/elderly hearing screening—Recent data and new perspectives. Ear Hear 1990;11:17S–28S.

Schuknecht H. Further observations on the pathology of presbycusis. Arch Otolaryngol 1964;80:369–382.

Silman S. The effects of aging on the stapedius reflex thresholds. J Acoust Soc Am 1979;66:735–738.

Silman S, and Gelfand S. Effect of sensorineural hearing loss on the stapedius reflex growth function in the elderly. J Acoust Soc Am 1981;69:1099–1106.

Stach B, Spretnjak M, and Jerger J. The prevalence of central presbycusis in a clinical population. J Am Acad Audiol 1990;1:109–115.

Stephens SDG. Evaluating the problems of the hearing impaired. Audiology 1980;19:205–220.

Sticht T, and Gray B. The intelligibility of time compressed words as a function of age and hearing loss. J Speech Hear Res 1969;12:443–448.

Townsend T, and Bess F. Effects of age and sensorineural hearing loss on word recognition. Scand Audiol 1980;9:245–248.

Tyler R, and Smith P. Sentence identification in noise and hearing handicap questionnaires. Scand Audiol 1983;12:285–292.

Uhlmann R, Larson E, Rees T, Koepsell T, and Duckert L. Relationship of hearing impairment to dementia and cognitive dysfunction in older adults. JAMA 1989a;261:1916–1919.

Uhlmann R, Rees T, Psaty B, and Duckert L. Validity and reliability of auditory screening tests in demented and nondemented older adults. J Gen Intern Med 1989b;4:90–96.

U.S. Department of Health and Human Services, Public Health Service. Healthy People 2000: National Health Promotion and Disease Prevention Objectives. Washington, DC: U.S. Government Printing Office, 1990.

Ventry I, and Weinstein B. The Hearing Handicap Inventory for the Elderly: a new tool. Ear Hear 1982;3:128–134.

Ventry I, Weinstein B. Identification of elderly people with hearing problems. Am Speech Hear Assoc J 1983;25:37–42.

Weinstein B, and Ventry I. Hearing impairment and social isolation in the elderly. J Speech Hear Res 1982;25:593–599.

Weinstein B. Identification/management of the hearing impaired elderly. Short course presented at the Annual Convention of the American Speech-Language-Hearing Association, Washington, DC, 1985.

Weinstein B, and Ventry I. Audiometric correlates of the Hearing Handicap Inventory for the Elderly. J Speech Hear Disord 1983;48:379–384.

Weinstein B. Validity of a screening protocol for identifying elderly people with hearing problems. ASHA 1986;28:41–45.

Weinstein B, and Amsel L. Hearing loss and senile dementia in the institutionalized elderly. Clin Gerontol 1986;4:3–15.

White J, and Regan M. Otologic considerations. In Mueller G, and Geoffrey V, Eds. Communication Disorders in Aging: Assessment and Management. Washington, DC: Gallaudet University Press, 1987:36–72.

Wilson R. The effects of aging on the magnitude of the acoustic reflex. J Speech Hear Res 1981;24:406–414.

Wilson R, and Margolis R. Acoustic-reflex measurements. In Rintelmann W, Ed. Hearing Assessment, 2nd ed. Austin, TX: Pro-Ed, 1991.

Yanz J, and Anderson S. Comparison of speech perception skills in young and old listeners. Ear Hear 1984;5:134–137.

MANAGEMENT OF AUDITORY PROBLEMS

CHAPTER 38

Overview of Aural Rehabilitation

Mark Ross

The practice of aural rehabilitation (AR) permits audiologists to function in the most autonomous professional capacity possible. In AR, audiologists make their own diagnosis of the communication disorder, and then prescribe and institute a course of treatment. The first part of this chapter will be devoted to an overview of aural habilitation practices, primarily as they apply to preschool and elementary age hearing-impaired children. In the second section, the focus will be on adventitiously hearing-impaired adults.

Definitions

The term *"hearing-impaired"* is used generically, to refer to any type or degree of hearing loss (Ross and Calvert, 1967; Wilson, Ross, and Calvert, 1974). The term may be modified by an adjective, such as "mild," "moderate," "severe," or "profound" for a more precise description of the hearing loss. "Hard of hearing" refers to a condition wherein a person's primary development of communication skills was through the auditory channel, and where audition serves as the primary avenue in oral communication exchanges. In distinction, the term *"deaf"* is used to describe a person whose primary development of communication skills is through a visual modality, either sign language or speechreading, and whose primary mode for interpersonal communication is visually based. (These definitions apply to audiological deafness only; some individuals who are functionally hard of hearing prefer to identify culturally and socially with the deaf community.) Of course, there are people who do not fall neatly into one category or another. They may be children with profound audiological deafness whose proficient use of residual hearing enables them to function primarily auditorily in some, but not all, circumstances (Brackett et al., 1989). Others may be profoundly hearing-impaired adults with adventitious hearing losses or late deafened adults who have received cochlear implants. Many of these people are essentially bisensory, in that they employ vision and audition in a complementary fashion with no evident preference given to either vision or audition.

Understanding the Individual

The point of this brief excursion into academic taxonomy is to emphasize that any rehabilitative effort must begin with an understanding of the person with whom we are dealing. Hard-of-hearing people, in general, require different services than do deaf people. Audiologists, as experts in the measurement and use of residual hearing, can make a greater contribution in the rehabilitation of hard of hearing people than they can with those who are deaf. We must also remember that any type of categorization system provides only general insights and general therapeutic implications; individuals, whether called "deaf," "hard of hearing," or something in between must always be dealt with on their own terms and not as members of a category.

PRESCHOOL CHILDREN

The underlying assumption of this section is that, generally, children who are recently detected as hearing impaired should initially be trained in an auditory-verbal mode. There are different points of view in this respect and legitimate concerns about the possible consequences of this recommendation. My reasoning is as follows:

1. The overwhelming majority of hearing-impaired children have residual hearing. Only a relatively few, perhaps one per thousand, have average hearing losses in excess of 90 dB in the better ear. Moreover, it has been shown (Brackett et al., 1989) that with early and appropriate training some children with profound hearing losses can function in a primarily auditory mode. Lacking precise information about degree of residual hearing, it is prudent to assume that a particular child falls within the majority category (i.e., having a significant degree of residual hearing).
2. We cannot predict, when a child is very young, how functional the residual hearing can become with proper training. There are no infallible indicators of future auditory function when we first begin to manage a hearing-impaired child.

Actual performance after training is the only valid measure we now have.

3. Hearing is the sensory avenue upon which the development of linguistic skills is normally based. The linguistic results of this development conform with the language of the general society (Fry, 1978) and of at least 90% of hearing-impaired children's parents.

4. Given early detection and management, the suitability of an auditory-verbal mode should be evident by age three or four at the latest. A recommendation for a different communication mode can be made at this time, if indicated. Such a recommendation should not imply failure; it does recognize that children have different learning styles and different communication needs. Exceptions to this time frame (or, indeed, to the initial recommendation) can, and should, be made for children who are exhibiting extreme communicative frustration and to honor parental requests (see Chapter 47).

5. There is no convincing evidence of negative psychosocial or communicative consequences for children who transfer from an auditory-verbal mode to a manual mode at a sufficiently young age. There are a great many strong feelings on this subject and some convincing anecdotal reports with respect to specific children, but these are usually associated with unfortunate delays in shifting communication emphasis.

6. Some professionals suggest that in beginning training with a strong Total Communication (TC) approach (or philosophy) that we can have it both ways: the children's residual hearing can be stimulated with the immediate benefits of an accessible communication system. (The sub-debate that recommends an initial American Sign Language approach, rather than one utilizing Manual English, is beyond the scope of this paper.) Benefits may indeed accrue if an alternating speech and sign mode were to be used, rather than simultaneous speech and sign presentations. In this manner, the usual procedure of developing bilingual skills can be replicated. As presently practiced, however, simultaneous communication appears to expose children with incomplete and ungrammatical utterances in both the sign and speech modes (see Ross and Calvert, 1984). Issues related to simultaneous communication are further discussed in Chapters 39 and 47.

7. Finally, as audiologists our professional obligation requires that we do all we can to maximize the use of residual hearing. Although we must recognize that the consequences of our therapeutic "success" with some profoundly hearing-impaired children may mean social difficulties and problems of personal identification, these are far from inevitable (Schwartz, 1990). No matter how successful we are therapeutically, a profoundly hearing-impaired child is still going to be profoundly hearing-impaired, with all that this implies in terms of psychosocial status and communicative effectiveness. By effectively practicing our profession, however, we open up a wider array of vocational and social alternatives for these children as they mature. They can then decide how they wish to relate to the hearing and deaf worlds. This is a painful process for some of the children—life is much more comfortable when such decisions need not be made—but what choice have we? In our professional ministrations, we can do no less than our best, and we must honor the rights of parents and children to make their own life-style decisions.

Given this therapeutic orientation, let us now consider the aural habilitation needs of preschool children with congenital hearing losses. Certain conceptual and practical differences distinguish management considerations relevant to this group from those of hearing-impaired adults. Basically, these factors relate to the role that audition plays in the development of oral linguistic skills. Management procedures with children must begin as early in the child's life as possible. The reasons for such urgency in detection and management is to preclude any possibility of auditory sensory deprivation and to take advantage of the normal accelerated rate of speech and language development in the early years (Ross, 1990a). The Joint Committee on Infant Screening recommended 6 months as an ideal age of detection (Joint Committee, 1982). In reality, however, the average age of detection has hovered around 12 months for the last 10 years (Elssman, Matkin, and Sabo, 1987; Stein, et al., 1990), with management procedures ordinarily delayed until about twenty months of age.

Evidence suggests that delay in detection and management serves to depress a child's ultimate linguistic and academic performance further. Or, to summarize the research in a positive fashion: the linguistic skills of hearing-impaired children who receive early amplification and who are enrolled in parent-infant and preschool programs are usually superior to those of children whose losses are detected and managed later (Watkins, 1987; White and White, 1987; Levitt et al., 1987). Nevertheless, not all the children whose losses are detected and managed early achieve higher linguistic scores than their later detected and managed peers. As Levitt et al. (1987) point out, early detection and intervention does not in itself guarantee superior performance; it is also necessary to ensure appropriate management at all later therapeutic stages as well.

MANAGEMENT ELEMENTS

There is general agreement as to the elements of an effective rehabilitation program with congenitally hearing-impaired children. For example, clinicians rarely debate whether a child should be fit with amplification, only the particular type of system which would be of most value. The importance of early management procedures is also generally accepted. Clinicians must be much more forceful advocates of immediate measures with children than they are with adults. Delays in diagnostic tests and scheduling periods are simply not acceptable. With hearing-impaired children, time is not on our side.

Parent Involvement

The early years are not only crucial for the children but for the parents as well. It is at this time that parents must recognize, accept, and adapt to the fact that their lives and their children's lives will not be what they had hoped and dreamed. The clinician's first "client" is not the child but the parents (see Chapter 40). We must allow them to mourn the loss of their dreams and to overcome the initial shock of learning about their child. We must help them work through the denials and false hopes, and to deal with the inevitable anxieties and guilt that soon emerge. Not all parents follow a predictable course of responses to the diagnosis of deafness in their child (Luterman, 1979), but all will need the sympathetic "ear" of the clinician, the time and space to ventilate their feelings, and such information as they can absorb when they are ready to deal with the situation.

The clinician should understand that he or she is a junior partner in the therapeutic process. It is the parents who have the most at stake in the future of their child. It is their interchanges with the child that will, or will not, provide the most salient linguistic experience for the learning of language. Until entering a preschool program, the only effective way of reaching a child is through the parents (Boothroyd, 1982). This is not to say that parents should be instructed to be "teachers"; rather, they should be helped to be better parents, parents who do not distort their parenting efforts because their child is hearing-impaired. They can be helped to exploit situational opportunities in a natural manner, to further the total development of their child. Whatever therapy goals are set, they are not likely to be reached without the active involvement of the parents in the therapy process.

Sometimes the parents are so overwhelmed by having a handicapped child, so focused on putting food on the table or keeping drugs and other bad influences away from their older children, that they simply cannot deal with the situation. Sometimes the parents themselves present social problems independent of their child's. In these instances, we do what we can directly for the child, with full understanding of the constraints imposed by reality conditions.

Selecting Amplification

The young hearing-impaired child should be fit with an amplification device just as soon as it is practical. This will usually take place concurrently with the parent counseling component. Ordinarily, precise audiometric information will not be available for very young children, but this is no reason to delay the hearing aid fitting. It is not difficult to fit infants with an amplification device; after all, children are completely under the control of adults and have little awareness of their differences from other children. It will be difficult, however, to ensure: that the hearing aid remains in place (behind-the-ear (BTE) aids have a way of flopping over the ear, and the earmolds of body aids tend to be easily dislodged); that the earmolds do not cause discomfort, and that the device is providing the most appropriate pattern of amplification (Boggess, 1989).

The goal of any amplification device is to amplify a speech signal and deliver it at an appropriate suprathreshold level across frequency. The difference between the impaired threshold and the amplified speech signal is the aided sensation level, i.e., aided residual hearing. Without the assurance that we have achieved the desired audibility of speech across frequency, it is clear that the child's potential auditory linguistic development will not be reached. The desired sensation level (DSL) approach to hearing aid selection makes audibility an explicit goal in the hearing aid selection process (Ross and Seewald, 1988). Although aided thresholds are useful in determining aided audibility, a better approach is to use real-ear measures, plotting all dimensions to the same SPL scale (Seewald, Ross, and Stelmachowicz, 1987; Hawkins et al., 1989). This kind of graphic portrayal demonstrates that listening is a suprathreshold affair (unlike a graph of aided thresholds) as it presents the aided speech output in relation to unaided thresholds and to desired maximal output levels. An example of such a portrayal is given in Figure 38.1.

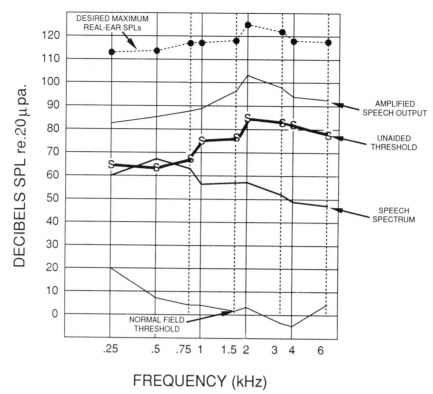

Figure 38.1. Speech spectrum, unaided thresholds, amplified speech output, and desired maximal real-ear SPLs plotted on an SPL scale. The use of the SPL scale permits viewing the direct relationship of these auditory dimensions.

The usual practice is to fit the child binaurally with BTE hearing aids, unless there are definite contraindications (e.g., a total loss of hearing in one ear, or *poorer* functioning with two aids than with just one). It is recommended that all such hearing aids include both powerful telephone coils and provision for direct audio input. Although the child may not need these auxiliary features at the time of fitting, one or both of them will be needed when an FM auditory training system is used. The evidence suggests that directional microphones would also be an advantageous feature to include (Hawkins and Yacullo, 1984).

Body aids still have an important niche to fill for some children with severe or profound hearing losses (Ross and Madell, 1988). They permit more gain before feedback occurs, and the boost in the low frequencies by the body-baffle effect can add useful acoustic information. A special instance of a body hearing aid is the FM auditory training system (see Chapter 42), wherein the FM receiver in the environmental microphone mode functions essentially as a binaural body hearing aid. In some centers, an FM system is fit as the first and primary amplification device for young children (Madell, 1988). The close proximity of the FM microphone to the talker ensures a favorable speech-to-noise ratio, perhaps the most

crucial factor underlying speech perception. Remarkable results with profoundly hearing-impaired preschool children have been reported when FM systems have been used by the children and their parents (Brackett, et al., 1989).

Preschool Programs

The advantages of early amplification and parent-infant programming can easily be dissipated unless followed up by an excellent preschool program. There are many models and not much research evidence to aid in choosing among them. However, we do know that certain elements must be included in any effective preschool program: (*a*) daily troubleshooting of hearing aid and FM systems; (*b*) FM systems used whenever the educational focus permits; (*c*) a favorable speech-to-noise ratio for as many hours per day as possible; (*d*) individual tutoring to develop communication skills; (*e*) a staff consisting of trained early childhood specialists, whose program emphasizes a cognitive and linguistic approach; (*f*) parental observation and ongoing counseling; (*g*) and integration with normal hearing children for optimal behavioral and linguistic modelling. This latter provision will also be crucial in determining the most appropriate communication mode for a particular child.

SCHOOL-AGE CHILDREN

A complete performance assessment is a necessary prerequisite to all aural habilitation activities; this includes audiological, speech and language, psychosocial, academic, and medical evaluations (Ross, Brackett, and Maxon, 1991). Understanding the auditory limitations is particularly important; no effective management program can be planned and executed unless all professionals involved understand these limitations. All hearing-impaired children, therefore, regardless of setting, should receive a comprehensive audiological assessment at least once a year. The younger elementary school children and the preschoolers may be seen more often, until their audiometric and electroacoustic (amplification adjustments) situations have been stabilized.

The great majority of hearing-impaired children are enrolled in regular school settings. This is generally an appropriate placement, and is even more so when special services are provided. Most mainstreamed children can be expected to require, and will benefit from, a full array of support services (Ross, 1990b). Even those children for whom a fully mainstreamed placement is not desirable may still benefit from the mainstream setting, provided a resource room, transitional class, or self-contained class (within the regular school) is available. For other hearing-impaired children, particularly those with the most severe hearing losses, a special school is the most appropriate (and least restrictive) educational setting. Mainstreaming is not, in itself, an educational goal for hearing-impaired children, but a process that can foster our educational goals for many of these children.

Placement decisions must be based on: (a) the results of the ongoing assessment process and (b), the child's and parent's preference. The academic and linguistic performance of fully mainstreamed children should be no more than 2 years, possibly 3 behind their peers (Brackett and Maxon, 1986). The children's oral communication skills should enable them to converse effectively with teachers and other children. A child's "oral communication attitude," the sheer desire and determination to "make it" in a regular school, has been found to be a particularly significant factor associated with successful mainstreaming (Plaster, 1981).

In addition to administering the audiological evaluation, the school-based audiologist must: (a) ensure that the proper amplification systems have been selected and are being used correctly (including troubleshooting, and making new earmold impressions); (b) sensitize the school personnel regarding the deleterious effects of poor acoustical conditions and recommend how to reduce noise and reverberation; (c)

develop, supervise or provide auditory and auditoryvisual learning experiences for the child (Berg, 1987); (d) organize and conduct in-service training programs for the school staff (Maxon, 1990); and (e) serve as the "case-coordinator" during Individual Educational Plan (IEP) processes. In other words, audiologists in school settings must serve to bridge the clinical and educational domains.

The prognosis for most hearing-impaired children is excellent, provided that they receive the appropriate auditory management and other support services. We can pinpoint the genesis of their communication problems and we know what to do about them (unlike children with other communication disorders). By ensuring that residual hearing is being employed as effectively as possible, we will have gone a long way in reducing the impact of the hearing loss.

ADVENTITIOUSLY HEARING-IMPAIRED ADULTS

An historical overview of AR should begin with the organization of the Leagues for the Hard of Hearing about 80 years ago (Green, 1990). The first chapter was organized in New York as a self-help effort by hard-of-hearing adults; its purpose was to help its members secure and retain employment by improving their communication skills (mainly lip-reading). While the Leagues for the Hard of Hearing eventually extended their outreach to include hard-of-hearing and deaf children and adults, they continued to serve adventitiously hearing-impaired adults. These agencies not only provided direct training and vocational guidance, but became important social and continuing support centers for many hard-of-hearing adults. A number of Leagues later joined together to establish the American Hearing Society.

These initial self-help aspects of AR receded with the advent of the profession of audiology after World War II (Newby, 1958). The war produced a large number of servicemen deafened by military service, a situation that resulted in a great need for hearing assessment and rehabilitative services. After the war, university training programs (mainly in Departments of Speech, Speech Correction, or Speech and Theatre) incorporated audiological training as part of the curriculum. Because the audiological roots were in rehabilitation, AR became a major focus of the curriculum. Aspiring audiologists were given academic courses in lip-reading (the term "speechreading" soon became more popular among professionals) and auditory training. These two areas were basically synonymous with what was considered AR at that time. Hearing aids were a minor part of the curriculum, mainly dealing with hearing aid evaluation (patients were to be referred to hearing aid dealers for the actual selection of the hearing aids because the sale of a product was considered unethical at that time). Students were taught how to provide information to the client, but not how to deal with the psychosocial consequences of a hearing loss.

During these years (the 1950s and the 1960s), much of the emerging professional effort focused on the development and administration of diagnostic tests. AR and associated research, while never entirely absent, became secondary professional goals. As a young profession, there was a feeling that we had to prove ourselves with "hard" research and elaborate diagnostic procedures, something very difficult to accomplish within the amorphous area of AR.

DEFINITIONS AND GOALS

In a very broad sense, any service that reduces the consequences of an adventitious hearing loss can be considered AR. Initially, however, AR was defined as speechreading, auditory training and speech conservation. While providing a hearing aid is certainly a key AR component, in the the early years of audiology this function was usually reserved for hearing aid dealers. As a matter of fact, the recognition that audiologists should dispense hearing aids was instigated by this very limitation, because of our desire to integrate hearing aid selection and follow-up into the AR process.

When audiologists are asked how they participate in AR, some will point to the selection of, and orientation to, amplification systems; others to an assessment of the handicap, along with counseling (informational and/or affective); and still others will note that they engage in direct communication therapy (the traditional areas of AR). These practices agree with the three goals of AR outlined by Montgomery and Sylvester (1984), to which most audiologists would subscribe regardless of philosophy or work environment.

1. Maximizing the reception of speech through the auditory and/or visual channels. This goal is most like the classic definition of AR, but would now also include the selection and fitting of amplification systems.
2. Reducing the impact of psychosocial factors. Such information may be derived from the one or more of the many self-assessment scales which have been developed (see Chapters 37 and 47).
3. Imparting information about hearing loss, use of hearing aids, assistive listening systems, and communication strategies.

In spite of a number of excellent textbooks on AR (Giolas, 1986; Alpiner and McCarthy, 1987; Schow and Nerbonne, 1989), we have little information on

actual AR practices, beyond the fact that most audiologists do select hearing aids. We do not know how many audiologists from different work settings engage in the various components of AR. We do not know what criteria are used to recommend any AR component; what would be the most effective AR strategies for different kinds of clients; and, finally, what constitutes "successful" AR intervention. Almost a half century after AR made its professional debut, we still clearly still have a long way to go.

THE COMPONENTS OF AN AR PROGRAM

In spite of these gaps in our knowledge, AR is not only possible, but it occurs every day. As professionals, we cannot wait until our knowledge is complete before we attend to the needs of our clients. There appears to be substantial agreement with the listing and order of the following AR components:

1. A comprehensive audiological evaluation. To develop and institute the most effective program, we must have a clear understanding of the client's hearing problems.
2. Equally important, if not more so, is the administration of a self-assessment scale. The questions in these scales permit clients to indicate the perceived impact of the hearing loss upon their everyday communication skills, as well as on the psychosocial consequences of the loss (Garstecki, 1987). These results can be used in planning an AR program that addresses the client's concerns, and as a measure of the changes brought about by any AR component (Dempsey, 1986; Ross and Weber, 1989; Malinoff and Weinstein, 1989). The increasing popularity of these scales reflect the recognition that the psychosocial and communicative impact of a hearing loss can best be rated by the clients' themselves.
3. Selection of the most appropriate electroacoustic system for a particular person, based on lifestyle, hearing loss, communication environment, and perceived difficulties. There is an overwhelming amount of literature on this topic (see Chapters 40 to 46). In this regard, the general performance superiority with binaural hearing aids is well established; a corollary concern is that if we do not provide binaural amplification, the possibility exists that the non-used ear will display further deterioration in speech perception skills (Silman, Gelfand, and Silverman, 1984; Gatehouse, 1989). Audiologists often defer to the client when it comes to accepting amplification or selecting the type of hearing aid. In an interesting article McCarthy, Mont-

gomery, and Mueller (1990) point out that, while the acceptance percentage is not quite as high when the motivating source is external pressure (e.g., a spouse or a professional), about half the client's surveyed do accept amplification when they are "pushed" a bit. The lesson for us is that we must give our clients the benefit of our knowledge in weighing the pros and cons of different kinds of systems, and then let *them* make the final decision. Too often we permit cosmetic concerns to drive the process (Ross and Madell, 1989), and do not give our clients the right to make informed decisions.

4. An adequate hearing aid orientation and follow-up program. There is some evidence that up to 30% of users discard their hearing aids in the first year of usage (Ross, 1987). This figure can be drastically reduced by an appropriate follow-up program, which includes scheduled long-term as well as short-term appointments. Possible changes in the amplification pattern and/or type of system, earmold problems, and initial adjustment experiences are all necessary aspects of a follow-up program. The particular organization and content seems less relevant than the commitment of time and resources to instruct new users in the management of their hearing aids. A particularly effective approach was described by Brooks and Johnson (1981) who trained lay counselors to manage the follow-up program, which mostly took place in the client's home.

5. Although the above four components are inherent to all AR programs, there are others that may be offered on an individual basis, depending on suitability, availability, and economic factors. Because of financial constraints—ongoing AR services are rarely funded by third party payers—some audiological service models (e.g., private practice) cannot afford to engage in AR efforts that are not directly associated with hearing aid dispensing. It is hoped that this will change in the future as more people realize that AR is as necessary as other rehabilitative services, many of which are funded by Medicare and other insurers. These additional AR components may include:
   a. Formal speechreading, auditory training, and combined mode lessons, individual or group. Although the experimental support for these classic AR components is tenuous, there is no doubt that the attitude and adjustment of people who are enrolled in these programs improve (Ross, 1987).
   b. Group sessions that provide information about hearing loss, hearing aids, assistive devices; effective communication strategies; and the psychosocial aspects of hearing loss. In addition, interchanges among the participants and spousal involvement are encouraged (Giolas, 1986).
   c. Individual counseling and informational sessions as a substitute or complement to the group meetings. Some people have hearing loss related problems that can best be addressed on an individual basis.
   d. A program devoted to hearing-related problems in the work place. An example is the Workshop to Improve Strategies for Employment (WISE) (Nadler and Pfeffer, 1989) which assists clients who are having work-related auditory problems. Topics include communication strategies, group support for reasonable assertive requests, protective laws and regulations, assistive devices in the work place, environmental manipulation, and management of individual work situations.

SELF-HELP GROUPS

In recent years, we have seen the proliferation of self-help groups for hard-of-hearing adults. Professionals should encourage and foster such groups, but as technical advisors and not as group leaders. What hard-of-hearing people can do to help themselves extends and complements what professionals can do for them. Most hard-of-hearing clients know very little about the existence of these groups when they first come to audiology centers; therefore, our assistance in making the proper connections is one of the important services that can be offered to them.

Ironically, while AR services for hard-of-hearing adults began about 80 years ago as a self-help effort (Green, 1990), its popularity declined with the advent of hearing aids (which reduced the need for the speechreading training they offered) and the involvement of the professional community in the AR process. The resurrection of self-help groups in recent years puts the primary AR responsibility where it belongs: with the involved individuals themselves.

One example of local consumer leadership is the Self Help for the Hard of Hearing (SHHH) Chapter in South Nassau, Long Island, N.Y. This group has over 170 members and the largest assistive device display that I have ever seen. In addition to monthly meetings, they publish brochures, a newsletter, and they give advice on assistive listening and alerting devices.

It should be noted that this group does not view itself as the professionals' competitors but as their adjuncts and extensions. Because they have hearing losses themselves, the SHHH members have credibility among hearing-impaired individuals, and their advice regarding professional consultation before purchasing hearing aids is generally accepted. By word of mouth and letters and articles in the local newspapers, they emphasize the fact that hearing loss is a condition to acknowledge and not to deny. Their greatest boon may be to the many adults who refuse to consider using hearing aids because they view hearing loss as an unacceptable and inadmissible condition. By their example, this consumer group helps to eliminate the stigma that the existence of a hearing loss seems to carry in our society.

GALLAUDET ELDER HOSTEL PROGRAM

Several years ago, I read an article (Bally and Kaplan, 1988) that described the Gallaudet Elder Hostel Program for hearing- impaired adults and their significant others. It reminded me of the AR program I received at Walter Reed Army Hospital almost 40 years ago. My memories of that experience have always served as the standard by which I measure other AR programs. Most have fallen far short of this standard. Recently, I spent a week at one of the Gallaudet Hostels. What I experienced was as close to an ideal AR program as is possible to find at the present time.

The activities encompassed the three goals of AR stated in the introduction to this chapter. Information was given on hearing loss and hearing aids, and included hearing evaluations and electroacoustic analysis of hearing aids, when desired. The benefits and limitations of different types of hearing aids were discussed. After this some of the participants decided to purchase new hearing aids incorporating a powerful telephone coil. A few resented the fact that their audiologists never explained advantages of a telephone coil to them, but instead immediately focused on smaller hearing aids that did not include a telephone coil.

A second activity centered on speechreading and communication strategies. What I found particularly interesting (and even personally useful) were the distinctions drawn between passive, assertive, and aggressive communication behavior. The staff continually stressed the rights of hard-of-hearing people to be reasonably assertive in order to enhance their communicative situations. Many examples were given of anticipatory strategies (how to plan ahead and make the necessary arrangements), maintenance strategies (how to stay abreast of a communication exchange), and repair strategies (what to do when communication breaks down).

The third major activity concerned the psychosocial aspects of hearing impairment. These sessions were led by a social worker skilled in working with hard-of-

hearing adults. Psychosocial problems were identified and coping strategies were analyzed. Theoretical situations were developed and discussed, and examples of the most effective coping strategies were elicited. These sessions led to many lively discussions, between the participants and the leader and among the participants themselves.

Additional activities were the rap groups for spouses, in which they expressed their frustrations and need for understanding, and social programs that reinforced the activities of the day. The fact that the group was together for a week permitted an intensity of treatment and a mutually supportive cohesiveness that is not easily replicated in other AR models. By the end of the program, it was clear that positive changes had taken place among the participants in the program.

The Gallaudet program in itself can hardly respond to the many adults who need or could benefit from AR. This demand can be addressed, in part, by combining clinical intervention and self-help groups. Possibly, it would be feasible to develop intensive 3- or 5-day AR programs on an out-patient basis. The need for AR is clear; the question is how we can best organize the most effective therapeutic models.

SUMMARY

Aural rehabilitation is an activity that derives from our professional roots and that is central to our professional mission. There is little or no dispute about the ideal content of an AR program. Hearing-impaired preschoolers, schoolchildren, and adults require different services and a somewhat different therapeutic focus. All require the best that technology has to offer and our empathetic understanding of the consequences of hearing loss. Although amplification is a key ingredient in any rehabilitative program, we must also address the psychosocial needs of both children and adults alike. It is gratifying to see that, in recent years, audiologists have begun to show a greater interest in AR. This important shift in orientation—back to our roots—is crucial; to be truly successful, AR must include the participation of audiologists.

REFERENCES

Alpiner JG, and McCarthy PA. Rehabilitative Audiology: Children and Adults. Baltimore: Williams and Wilkins, 1987.

Bally SJ, and Kaplan H. The Gallaudet University Aural Rehabilitation Elderhostels. J Acad Rehabil Audiol 1988;21:99–112.

Berg FS. Facilitating Classroom Listening: A Handbook for Teachers of Normal and Hard of Hearing Students. Boston: College-Hill/Little, Brown and Co., 1987.

Boggess J. The adequacy of hearing aid fit for severely/profoundly hearing-impaired children. J Acad Rehab Audiol 1989;22: 15–29.

Boothroyd A. Hearing Impairments in Young Children. Englewood Cliffs, N.J.: Prentice-Hall, Inc., 1982.

Brackett D, and Maxon A. Service delivery alternatives for the mainstreamed hearing impaired child. Lang Speech Hear Serv Schools 1986;17:115–125.

Brackett D, Ying E, Madell J, and Datino N. Speech perception performance of profoundly hearing-impaired children. Paper at the 1989 meeting of the New York Speech-Language-Hearing Association, Concord Hotel, Kiamesha Lake, NY, 1989.

Brooks DN, and Johnson DI. Pre-issue assessment and counselling as a component of hearing-aid provision. Br J Audiol 1981; 15:13–19.

Dempsey JJ. The hearing performance inventory as a tool in the fitting of hearing aids. J Acad Rehabil Audiol 1986;19:116–125.

Elsmann SF, Matkin ND, and Sabo MP. Early identification of congenital sensorineural hearing impairment. Hear J 1987;40: 13–17.

Fry DB. The role and primacy of the auditory channel in speech and language development. In Ross M, and Giolas TG, Eds. Auditory Management of Hearing-Impaired Children. Baltimore: University Park Press, 1978.

Garstecki DC. Self-perceived hearing difficulty in aging adults with acquired hearing loss. J Acad Rehabil Audiol 1987;20:49–60.

Gatehouse S. Apparent auditory deprivation effects of late onset: The role of presentation level. J Acoust Soc Am 1989;86(6): 2103–2106.

Giolas TG. Aural Rehabilitation. Austin, TX: Pro-Ed., 1986.

Green, R. The professional and the consumer–a partnership in hearing rehabilitation. Hear Q 1990;15(1):4–7, 14.

Hawkins DB, Morrison TM, Halligan PLW, and Cooper WA. Use of probe tube microphone measurements in hearing aid selection for children: some initial clinical experiences. Ear Hear 1989;10:281–287.

Hawkins DB, and Yacullo WS. Signal-to-noise advantage of binaural hearing aids and directional microphones under different levels of reverberation. J Speech Hear Disord 1984;49:278–286.

Joint Committee on Infant Hearing. Position Statement. Ear Hear 1982;4:3–4.

Levitt H, McGarr N, and Geffner D. Development of Language and Communication Skills in Hearing-Impaired Children. ASHA Monograph #26, Washington, DC: American Speech-Language-Hearing Association, 1987.

Luterman D. Counselling Parents of Hearing-Impaired Children. Boston: Little, Brown, and Co., 1979.

Madell J. Identification and treatment of very young children with hearing loss. Infants and Young Children, 1988;112:20–30.

Malinoff RL, and Weinstein BE. Changes in self-assessment of hearing handicap over the first year of hearing aid use by older adults. J Acad Rehabil Audiol 1989;22:54–60.

Maxon A. Implementing an in-service training program. In Hearing-Impaired Children in the Mainstream. Parkton, MD: York Press, 1990.

McCarthy PA, Montgomery AA, and Mueller HG. J Acad Am Aud Soc 1990;1:23–30.

Montgomery A, and Sylvester F. Streamlining the aural rehabilitation process. Hear Instrum 1984;35:46–50.

Nadler N, and Pfeffer E. Workshop to Improve Strategies for Employment (WISE). Paper delivered to Annual Convention of Self Help for Hard of Hearing, Washington, DC, 1989.

Newby HA. Audiology. New York: Appleton-Century-Crofts, Inc., 1958.

Plaster F. A second analysis of factors related to the academic success of hearing-impaired children in the mainstream. Volta Rev 1981;83:71–80.

Ross M. Aural rehabilitation revisited. J Acad Rehabil Audiol 1987;20:13–23.

Ross M. Implications of delay in detection and management of deafness. Volta Rev 1990a;92:69–78.

Ross M. Hearing-Impaired Children in the Mainstream. Parkton, MD: York Press, 1990b.

Ross M, and Calvert DR. The semantics of deafess. Volta Rev 1967;69:644–649.

Ross M, and Calvert DR. Semantics of deafness revisited: total communication and the use and misuse of residual hearing. Audiology 1984;9:127–148.

Ross M, and Seewald RC. Hearing aid selection and evaluation with young children. In Bess FH, Ed. Hearing Impairments in Children. Parkton, MD: York Press, 1988.

Ross M, and Madell J. The premature demise of body worn hearing aids. ASHA 1988;30:(11):29–30.

Ross M, and Weber K. Use of self-assessment scales in aural rehabilitation. Paper presented to the annual convention of Self Help for Hard of Hearing, Washington, DC, 1989.

Ross M, Brackett D, and Maxon A. Assessment and Management of Mainstreamed Hearing-Impaired Children: Principles and Practices. Austin, TX: Pro-Ed, 1989.

Schow RL, and Nerbonne MA. Introduction to Aural Rehabilitation. Austin, TX: Pro-Ed, 1989.

Schwartz S. Psychosocial management of hearing-impaired children. In Ross M, Ed. Hearing-Impaired Children in the Mainstream. Parkton, MD: York Press, 1990.

Seewald RC, Ross M, and Stelmachowicz PG. Selecting and verifying hearing aid performance characteristics for young children. J Acad Rehabil Audiol 1987;20:25–37.

Silman S, Gelfand SA, and Silverman CA. Late-onset auditory deprivation: Effects of monaural versus binaural hearing aids. J Acoust Soc Am 1984;76:1357–1362.

Stein LK, Jabaley MA, Spitz R, Stoakley D, and McGee T. The hearing-impaired infant: Patterns of identification and habilitation revisited. Ear Hear 1990;11:201–205.

Watkins S. Long term effect of home intervention with hearing-impaired children. Am Ann Deaf 1987;132:267–275.

White SJ, and White REC. The effects of hearing status of the family and age of intervention on receptive and expressive oral skills in hearing-impaired infants. In Development of Language and Communication Skills in Hearing-Impaired Children, 1987.

Wilson GW, Ross M, and Calvert DR. An experimental study of the semantics of deafness. Volta Review 1974;76:498–514.

CHAPTER 39

The Impact of Hearing Impairment

Janet R. Jamieson

The essence of a hearing loss is its effect on communication and the resulting impact on cognitive, speech, language, and psychosocial development and functioning (Vernon and Andrews, 1990). Although hearing impairment is a pervasive problem, affecting the communication of almost 21 million Americans (Hotchkiss, 1989; Schein, 1989), it is difficult to predict the impact of a hearing loss on a particular individual. This difficulty may be attributed to at least two factors. First, hearing impairments result from diverse causes, not from a single etiological agent. Second, hearing loss acts in combination with other developmentally and psychosocially significant variables to produce different outcomes in different individuals.

TERMINOLOGY

Definitions of hearing impairment vary widely in the literature and depend, to a large extent, on theoretical assumptions about the nature of hearing losses. For this reason, a brief discussion of the medical, audiological, educational, and social views of hearing impairment is in order.

The realm of medicine has traditionally viewed a hearing loss as a pathological condition, implying that a hearing-impaired individual is diseased or deviant in some way. Audiologists, however, have emphasized the effect of variables, such as the degree of hearing loss, age at onset of the hearing impairment, and age at which amplification was introduced, on the overall communication style of the individual. Audiologists have tended to refer to those who sustained profound hearing losses as "deaf," whereas persons with less severe losses have been labelled as "hard of hearing."

Educators consider the effect of the impairment on the ability to communicate when recommending educational placement. The following definitions have been adopted by the Conference of Educational Administrators Serving the Deaf (CEASD):

> A *deaf person* is one whose hearing is disabled to an extent . . . that precludes the understanding of speech through the ear alone, with or without the use of a hearing aid.
> A *hard-of-hearing person* is one whose hearing is disabled to an extent . . . that makes difficult, but does not

preclude, the understanding of speech through the ear alone, with or without a hearing aid (Frisina, 1974, p. 3).

Sociologists and linguists have another perspective. They identify the Deaf person (as opposed to hearing impaired or hard of hearing, with the capitalized term 'Deaf' denoting a cultural rather than a disability descriptor), according to parameters of cultural values and language use (Cokely and Baker, 1980; Padden, 1980). One achieves membership in the Deaf community by accepting its values, particularly the use of American Sign Language, and by associating and identifying with other Deaf people (Padden, 1980). The degree of hearing loss is not a criterion for membership in the Deaf community, and Deaf people are often unaware of the details of their Deaf friends' hearing loss. It is possible for an individual to be considered audiologically as hard of hearing, yet to be a member of the Deaf community.

In determining the impact of hearing impairment on a person's behavior, the fundamental consideration is the effect of the hearing loss on the person's ability to communicate. Thus the distinction between *deaf* and *hard of hearing* persons as suggested by CEASD will be used throughout this chapter, whereas the term *hearing impaired* will refer to individuals with any degree of hearing loss. This behavioral approach recognizes that the impact of hearing impairment can best be understood by considering the complex interaction of medical, audiological, educational, psychosocial, and linguistic variables. This chapter provides an overview of recent research regarding the impact of hearing loss on hearing-impaired children, youth, and adults. Emphasis will be placed on the effects of hearing loss on the linguistic, speech, cognitive, and psychosocial development of children, as well as on the educational, occupational, and social patterns of adults.

HEARING IMPAIRMENT AMONG CHILDREN AND YOUTH

Audition provides the primary source for the acquisition of language and speech skills in the child with normal hearing. In fact, the average child will have achieved basic competency in his or her primary language by the age of about 3 1/2 years (deVilliers &

deVilliers, 1978). The age at which a hearing loss occurs is a critical factor in determining the child's development of communicative abilities. In general, the earlier in life the hearing loss occurs, the more debilitating the effects on the child's speech and language. Therefore, it is useful to specify whether the hearing impairment is prelingual, that is, occurring before age three (Schein, 1987), or postlingual, occurring in later childhood or adulthood (Vernon and Andrews, 1990).

Precise figures on the number of hearing-impaired youth in the general population do not exist, largely because of the inconsistency in defining hearing loss (Ries, 1986). One recent study (Hotchkiss, 1989) indicated that in the mid 1980s, approximately one million American youth under 18 years of age, or slightly less than 2% of the total population, had some degree of reported hearing impairment. The overall impact that a hearing impairment will have on a child's life is greatly influenced by the age at onset, the age at which the hearing loss was diagnosed, the degree of impairment, the etiology, and, to a lesser extent, by the sex and race of the child.

Prelingually Hearing-Impaired Children and Youth

Demographics

The prevalence rates for prelingual hearing impairment vary from one country to another and often within countries (Schein, 1986). These differences have been accounted for by the summation of a variety of factors, including climate, economy, marriage patterns, and nutritional habits (Schein, 1986). Various demographic characteristics of American hearing-impaired children and youth are presented in Tables 39.1–39.4. This information was collected by the Center for Assessment and Demographic Studies (CADS) of the Gallaudet Research Institute, which annually surveys hearing-impaired children receiving special education services. Readers should be cau-

tioned, however, that because the individuals included in the survey (47,178 students in total) from which these data are drawn are primarily those whose hearing loss warrants special education intervention, the focus is on youth with a moderate-to-profound hearing loss. Thus, it is likely that students with mild and moderate losses were underrepresented.

It is often difficult to determine with accuracy the age at onset of the hearing loss. As shown in Table 39.1, this information was either not known or not reported for 34% of the students. This difficulty may be

Table 39.2
Percent Distribution of American Hearing-Impaired Students by Degree of Hearing Loss, 1988–1989

Better-Ear Average in Decibels	Percent
Total known information	100.0
Normal (<27 dB)	7.5
Mild (27–40 dB)	9.2
Moderate (41–55 dB)	11.9
Moderate severe (56–70 dB)	12.6
Severe (71–90)	18.7
Profound (>91 dB)	40.0

Center for Assessment and Demographic Studies. Annual Survey of Hearing-Impaired Children and Youth, 1988–1989. Washington, DC: Gallaudet University, 1989.

Table 39.3
Percent Distribution of Causes of Impairment for American Hearing-Impaired Students, 1988–1989.[a]

Cause	Percent
Total students	100.0
Cause unknown/unreported	49.5
At birth (out of total students)	
Heredity	26.1
Prematurity	9.4
Maternal rubella	8.1
Other complications of pregnancy	5.5
Trauma at birth	4.9
Cytomegalovirus	1.7
Rh incompatibility	1.1
Other causes before birth	8.2
After birth (out of total students)	
Meningitis	17.6
Otitis media	7.4
High fever	5.5
Infections	4.7
Trauma after birth	1.4
Measles	0.7
Mumps	0.2
Other causes after birth	4.7

[a] Because some students had more than one reported etiology, the sum of the cause specific percentages exceeds the total percentage of cases with known causes.
Center for Assessment and Demographic Studies. Annual Survey of Hearing-Impaired Children and Youth, 1988–1989. Washington, DC: Gallaudet University, 1989.

Table 39.1
Percent Distribution of American Hearing-Impaired Students by Age at Onset, 1988–1989

Age Group	Percent
Total	100.0
Information unknown/unreported	34.3
Total known information	100.0
At birth	72.0
Under 3 years	22.5
3 years or older	5.5

Center for Assessment and Demographic Studies. Annual Survey of Hearing-Impaired Children and Youth, 1988–1989. Washington, DC: Gallaudet University, 1989.

Table 39.4
Percent Distribution of American Hearing-Impaired Students by Age, Sex, and Ethnic Origin, 1988–1989

Age, Race, Sex	Percent
Age	
<3 years	2.6
3–5 years	11.4
6–9 years	25.2
10–13 years	26.0
14–17 years	24.6
>18 years	10.2
Sex	
Male	53.7
Female	46.0
Not reported	0.3
Ethnic Origin	
White	64.3
Black	17.0
Hispanic	12.9
Oriental	3.2
American Indian	0.7
Other	1.2
Multi-ethnic	0.6

Center for Assessment and Demographic Studies. Annual Survey of Hearing-Impaired Children and Youth, 1988–1989. Washington, DC: Gallaudet University, 1989.

attributed to a variety of factors, including the invisible nature of the disability and the lack of routine neonatal screening for hearing impairment. The age at onset of hearing loss is often inferred from the age at diagnosis and etiology. For example, if a child's hearing loss is diagnosed at the age of 2 years and the cause is determined to be maternal rubella, the age at onset can be inferred as prior to birth. It is clear from Table 39.1, however, that the overwhelming majority (94.5%) of students receiving special education services because of impaired hearing sustained those losses prelingually. Similar figures were reported in a recent Canadian survey, with approximately 90% of the children identified as prelingually and 10% postlingually hearing impaired (MacDougall, 1987).

Table 39.2 shows the distribution of hearing-impaired students by hearing loss. It can be seen that as degrees of hearing loss increase, so does the percentage of students. It should be noted, however, that this overall distribution of hearing loss does not hold for the general population, where prevalence tends to increase as the degree of hearing loss decreases (McDowell, Engel, Massey, and Maurer, 1981). This discrepancy is hardly surprising, as the CADS research is based on children and youth whose hearing loss is of a significance to warrant special education or rehabilitation intervention. Table 39.2 also indicates that almost 8% of the children receiving special education services because of hearing impairment actually have hearing in the normal range. It is probable that most

of these students had other communicative problems, such as central auditory processing difficulties, which led to their educational placement.

The leading causes of hearing impairment among students in the CADS survey are presented in Table 39.3. Perhaps the most striking finding concerning etiology is that the cause of hearing impairment is unknown or unreported for 50% of the students. This finding also holds true for Canadian hearing-impaired children (MacDougall, 1987). It was speculated that most of those with unknown causes probably were genetic in nature (Nance and Sweeney, 1975). Until recently, maternal rubella was reported as the leading known cause of hearing impairment among the school-age population, as a result of the rubella epidemic of 1963–1965. These students are, however, no longer school-age. Heredity and meningitis were the leading known causes of hearing loss among prelingually hearing-impaired children in the United States in 1988 (Hotchkiss, 1989). Meningitis has become the leading cause of hearing impairment after birth reported among American children. Wolff and Brown (1987) suggest that the recent development of a meningitis vaccine may sharply reduce the incidence of this disease.

The prevalence of hearing impairment also varies by age and ethnic origin of the child, as shown in Table 39.4. The small proportion of children under 3 years of age may be accounted for, at least in part, by the difficulty in obtaining an early diagnosis of hearing impairment. Similarly, the relatively small percentage of students aged 18 years and over may be explained by the fact that many in this group may have left school and, therefore, were not included in the data.

Table 39.4 also indicates that males are consistently more likely to be hearing-impaired than females, regardless of age, age at onset, and degrees of impairment (e.g., Hotchkiss, 1989; Schein, 1987). In addition the proportion of white hearing-impaired persons has been found to surpass that of the non-white population (Hotchkiss, 1989; Schein, 1987; Schein and Delk, 1974). Schein (1987) reports that explanations for this consistency have varied from genetic to economic to methodologic.

Sociocultural Implications

Although early-deafened individuals comprise only about 3% of the total hearing-impaired population (Schein, 1989), their values and culture are sufficiently different from the surrounding milieu to warrant designation as a separate and unique culture.

Hearing impairment—particularly severe to profound deafness—may be best understood by considering it as a social condition rather than a physical disability. In other words, "the medical description of deafness does not fully anticipate its social consequences" (Schein, 1987, p. 3). In general, parents provide the most important and accessible means for children to acquire social values, develop a language, and achieve a self-image separate from that of others (Clausen, 1966). That is not the case, however, for the majority of deaf children. Prelingual deafness can drastically interfere with and alter the socialization process, particularly if the parents do not themselves have a similar hearing loss.

When considered from a social perspective, deafness affects three living generations—the parents, the deaf children, and the deaf children's children (Schein, 1989). More precisely, approximately 9 out of 10 deaf children are born into families with no other deaf member (Rawlings and Jensema, 1977; Schein and Delk, 1974). Approximately 90% of marriages among prelinguistically deaf persons are to other deaf individuals (Schein and Delk, 1974). On the average, these marriages result in normally hearing offspring in about 9 out of 10 live births (Schein, 1987). Taken together, these facts have profound consequences for the sociological development of deaf persons. Frequently deaf individuals are somewhat isolated from their parents, and, in many cases, from their children as well. The Deaf community in which members share an easily accessible communication system, is, therefore, especially important to Deaf individuals in establishing and maintaining close relationships.

The Deaf Child in the Deaf Family. Deaf parents of deaf children seem to cope with the diagnosis more quickly and easily than their hearing counterparts (Meadow and Meadow, 1971). In fact, it is not unusual for deaf parents to know of their child's hearing impairment within weeks, or even days, of birth (Jamieson and Pedersen, 1993; Meadow, Greenberg, Erting, and Carmichael, 1981). The most commonly cited reasons for the easier adjustment of deaf parents include their familiarity with deafness, the accessibility of a common linguistic system for parents and child, and their membership in and support from the Deaf community. Members of the Deaf community often look inward to other members for emotional support and a shared social identity.

The primary signal of Deaf ethnicity in North America is the use of American Sign Language (ASL) (Rainer, Altshuler, and Kallman, 1963; Siple, 1978). ASL meets all the requirements of a genuine language (Stokoe, Casterline, and Croneberg, 1965); as a visual-gestural communication system, the components of each individual sign may be viewed as "sign phonemes" which correspond to sign- rather than speech-related

phenomena (Klima, Bellugi, Newkirk, and Battison, 1979; Siple, 1978). It is a common misconception to assume that there is a universal sign language: unique sign language systems have evolved wherever sufficient numbers of deaf people have been located to support a language base and language growth.

For deaf children of deaf parents, as is the case for hearing children of hearing parents, language and cognition are likely to be the natural and unconscious outcome of ordinary mother-child interaction. Recent research (Jamieson and Pedersen, 1993; Meadow et al., 1981) has underlined the similarity in interaction patterns between hearing mothers and hearing children and deaf mothers and deaf children in the degree to which communication is marked by reciprocity both in content and in turn-taking.

A comparison of the general course of ASL and oral language acquisition lends support to the notion that there may be general cognitive or linguistic universals underlying language acquisition (Siple, 1978). For example, at the phonological level, Lane, Boyes-Braem, and Bellugi (1976) and McIntire (1977) have found that deaf children acquire handshapes developmentally, in the same manner that hearing children acquire certain sounds before others.

Pettito and Marentette (1991) have found the presence of manual babbling in deaf children of deaf parents at about the same time that vocal babbling occurs among hearing children of hearing parents. It has been consistently reported that deaf children of deaf parents, who have been exposed to ASL from birth follow the same general patterns of language acquisition as do hearing children acquiring spoken language (Klima and Bellugi, 1974; Schlesinger and Meadow, 1972; Stuckless and Birch, 1966). Deaf children of deaf parents are born into the Deaf community and are surrounded by users of ASL from infancy.

The Deaf Child in the Hearing Family. Hearing parents often struggle for months before they get a medical opinion of deafness. It is not unusual for them to find that the ambiguity preceding the diagnosis is even more difficult to bear than the firm diagnosis of hearing loss (Meadow-Orlans, 1987b). Most normally hearing parents are shocked, and some traumatized, by the diagnosis of deafness in their young child. Many professionals believe that the diagnosis of a handicap in a young child evokes a response of grief that may last for years or, in some cases, never be fully resolved (Luterman, 1979; Meadow-Orlans, 1987b; Nash and Nash, 1987; Schlesinger and Meadow, 1972). This mourning reaction may be particularly difficult for parents to resolve if the cause of the hearing loss is unknown.

Meadow (1980) has suggested that deaf children of

hearing parents might become enculturated into the Deaf community and begin using ASL at one of two periods: on enrollment in a residential school for the deaf or during early adulthood. It is at critical times such as these that the deaf individual from a hearing family is most likely to encounter other people with hearing losses and develop an identity as a Deaf person. As one hearing mother remarked about her deaf son, who had become involved with the Deaf community at the age of 18: "I really feel as though they are his real family. We are his biological family, but they are his *real* family."

Language Development

The degree of hearing loss and the age at onset influence the degree to which English will be acquired. Several researchers (e.g., Curtiss, 1977; Lenneberg, 1967) have described a "critical period" for primary language acquisition, in which the neurons involved in linguistic functions lose plasticity with maturation (Seliger, 1978). It may thus be surmised that the earlier the onset of hearing loss and the more severe the degree of impairment, the greater the potential for interference in language acquisition. In addition, the process of language acquisition by hearing impaired children is also dependent, at least in part, by the form of communication used, that is, whether it is interpersonal communication or read or written English (Kretschmer & Kretschmer, 1986).

Even a slight hearing loss in infants and young children can have a significant impact on the development of language and communication skills. Although the literature on the language acquisition of hard-of-hearing children is not as extensive as that which exists on deaf children, the studies are mutually supportive. Hard-of-hearing children tend to be delayed rather than deviant in their language development, with pervasive problems noted in the areas of vocabulary deficit (Davis, 1974; Hamilton and Owrid, 1974; Ross, 1982) and syntax (Davis and Blasdell, 1975; Wilcox and Tobin, 1974). Although these children may perform adequately or even well in social contexts in which speech is directed to them, the reception and perception of incidental language poses serious problems for them. The professional literature in the education of the hearing impaired has long documented that the early onset of a severe to profound hearing loss may have devastating consequences for the development of communicative competence.

Historical Views of Language Development. In a recent review of research of the last three decades that focused on hearing-impaired subjects, Kretschmer and Kretschmer (1986) surmised that the studies could be divided into three eras: 1) that of quantitatively based

and comparative studies, 2) that dominated by linguistically based studies, and 3) that of the present focus, which represents a shift to discourse and communication studies.

The traditional studies completed during the late 1950s and 1960s usually made general, quantitative assessments of various aspects of the syntactic skills of deaf children. The results confirmed that hearing-impaired children lagged behind their hearing counterparts in measures of receptive and expressive language, but provided little insight into the language skills that these children possessed. For example, Bown and Mecham (1961) compared the performance of hearing-impaired children on the Verbal Language Development Scale with nonverbal intelligence as measured by the performance scale of the Wechsler Intelligence Scale for Children. They concluded that although verbal quotients increased with age, so did the discrepancies between these verbal scores and the performance scores, with verbal scores considerably lower than results obtained on the performance scale. Other research (e.g., Goda, 1964; Simmons, 1962) focused on frequency counts of the various parts of speech. These studies indicated that deaf children relied heavily on noun-like and verb-like words, but showed restricted understanding of words that express relationships among other words in the context of a sentence, such as prepositions, conjunctions, articles, and adjectives (Griswold and Cummings, 1974). Brannon and Murry (1966) confirmed these findings and, moreover, found that the accuracy of grammatical performance was depressed compared to that of hearing children. In retrospect, conclude Kretschmer and Kretschmer (1986), these early studies were specific about the errors and omissions in hearing-impaired children's knowledge of English but offered no insight into their knowledge of the nature of discourse.

Linguistically based research with hearing-impaired subjects, beginning in the late 1960s, emphasized the interface between syntax and semantics. In contrast to the quantitatively based research that had preceded them, these qualitative studies were important because they revealed the abilities of hearing-impaired children as effective communicators (Kretschmer and Kretschmer, 1986). For example, Skarakis and Prutting (1977) and Curtiss, Prutting, and Lowell (1979) found parallels in the basic communication-semantic categories used by both hearing and hearing-impaired children in their earliest interpersonal communications. The research also suggests that some language forms, such as questions, are acquired by hearing-impaired children in ways that do not differ significantly from the patterns of hearing children (Brown, 1984; Raffin, Davis, and Gilman, 1978;

Romanik, 1976). Thus, although it may be delayed, the early language generated by hearing-impaired children appears to approximate that of hearing children, both syntactically and semantically.

Recent interest has focused on the development of discourse-pragmatic knowledge among both hearing and hearing-impaired children. For example, Meadow et al. (1981) studied the linguistic and social interaction among hearing children and their mothers, deaf children and their deaf mothers, and deaf children and their hearing mothers. The most striking and consistent finding to emerge was the similarity in social and linguistic interaction of the deaf mother-deaf child pairs and the hearing mother-hearing child pairs. The mothers in these two groups were found to be less directive, and their children demonstrated an ability to carry on more elaborate conversations than in the hearing mother-deaf child pairs. Similar findings have been reported by Jamieson and Pedersen (1993).

By contrast, hearing mothers of deaf children have consistently been found to be more didactic, more dominant, and more intrusive, but less flexible, less permissive, and less approving in their child-directed language than hearing mothers of hearing children of comparable age (Brinich, 1980; Goss, 1970; Greenberg, 1980; Henggeler and Cooper, 1983; Meadow et al., 1981; Schlesinger and Meadow, 1972; Wedell-Monnig and Lumley, 1980). Several explanations, all arising from the communication styles of deaf and hearing parents with their deaf children, have been proposed to account for these differences. First, Schlesinger (1987) has observed a sense of powerlessness in normally hearing parents of newly diagnosed deaf children. She believes that this sense of powerlessness continues beyond infancy and becomes particularly intense when parents try to communicate with their deaf child. Unable to establish reciprocal communication, these parents may question their parenting ability and feel helpless. One measurable outcome of powerlessness in these parents, Schlesinger suggests, may be their tendency to assume control in interactions with their deaf children. A second explanation proposes that, unlike the hearing mother-hearing child and deaf mother-deaf child pairs, there is a lengthy delay in the initiation of reciprocal parent-child communication in hearing families of deaf children, resulting from delays in the diagnosis of deafness (Greenberg and Marvin, 1979). Third, Meadow-Orlans (1987a) suggests that teachers' demands to communicate orally may create pressure on hearing mothers to try to elicit responses, leading to a more dominant communication style than that which is utilized by deaf mothers. Fourth, the disruption of mother-child and teacher-child interactions often associated with deafness arise, at least in part, from the difficulty that hearing people have in shifting from an auditory to a visual orientation when interacting with deaf children (Erting, 1988; Jamieson and Pedersen, 1993; Wood, Wood, Griffiths, and Howarth, 1986). And finally, Geffner (1987) proposes that many hearing parents correct their deaf children on the basis of syntactic or articulatory errors rather than on context. The children are thus directed to focus on the form rather than on the function of language, resulting in deviant language development.

It is clear that the delay in language acquisition of deaf children of hearing parents has a pervasive effect on parent-child interactions. It also appears, however, that hearing impairment in and of itself does not preclude the development of positive mother-child interaction when both the mother and child are deaf. Taken together, results of the discourse and communication studies suggest that hearing-impaired children have the cognitive ability to develop communicative competence in a primary language.

Written Language: Reading and Writing

Reading. There is a clear relationship between the degree of hearing loss and the reading abilities of hearing-impaired children. Researchers have consistently reported that hard-of-hearing children obtain higher scores on measures of reading comprehension and vocabulary than their deaf peers (Jensema, 1975; Rogers, Leslie, Clarke, Booth, and Horvath, 1978).

Traditionally, research on the reading skills of severely to profoundly deaf children has focused on areas of perceived weakness, especially grammar, with analysis concentrated at the single sentence level (Moores, 1987; Paul and Quigley, 1990). From the early twentieth century to the present, studies have shown the limited reading performance of deaf students in relation to their hearing counterparts (Balow, Fulton, and Peploe, 1971; DiFrancesca, 1972; Goetzinger and Rousey, 1959; Pintner and Patterson, 1916; Trybus and Karchmer, 1977). However, because most of the early studies used reading tests that were designed for and normed on normally hearing students, the validity of the results may be questioned. The Center for Assessment and Demographic Studies of Gallaudet University developed testing procedures and special norms for hearing-impaired students on the Stanford Achievement Test in 1974 and again in 1983. Allen (1986), comparing performance levels on these two batteries, found that hearing-impaired students showed improved reading comprehension skills in 1983 as compared with 1974, although they continued to evidence little gain in relation to their hearing cohorts.

Research has consistently suggested that deaf students have a limited understanding of the syntax of printed English. It appears that these students have internalized the basic subject-verb-object sentence pattern of English but still demonstrate considerable difficulty with grammatical structures such as passives (Schmitt, 1966; Tervoort, 1970), complementation (Quigley, Wilbur, and Montanelli, 1976), and relative clauses (Quigley, Smith, and Wilbur, 1974). Severe to profoundly hearing-impaired students have also shown difficulty with many aspects of figurative language (Conley, 1976; Payne and Quigley, 1987).

Recently, there have been some attempts to examine hearing-impaired students' reading abilities from the perspective of discourse organization, that is, the underlying organizations of narration or expository prose. Results suggest that older students often seem to approach reading from a sentence-by-sentence approach, and might benefit from instruction in which decoding and sentence processing skills are placed within the context of understanding whole passages (Gaines, Mandler, and Bryant, 1981).

Paul and Quigley (1990) suggest that attention should be directed to the influence of a variety of reader-based variables, in addition to text-related variables, on the reading performance of hearing-impaired students. More research is needed, they suggest, on the effects of prior knowledge, metacognitive and inferencing skills, and internal coding systems used by hearing-impaired students.

Writing. Similar to the early studies on interpersonal communication and reading, quantitative studies of the writing skills of hearing-impaired students have systematically demonstrated the weaknesses of this group. Most of the research to date on deaf children's writing has focused on the product, rather than the process. Deaf children evidence limited success in written expression of English vocabulary and syntax (Geffner, 1987; Osberger, Robbins, Lybolt, Kent, and Peters, 1987). In general, the reading abilities of hearing-impaired students are superior to their writing abilities. Moores (1987) suggests that, whereas a deaf person can use compensatory strategies to understand a message when vocabulary and grammar skills are limited, the same approaches are not available when writing.

There is almost no information on how hearing-impaired children approach the process of writing. What studies do exist suggest that, like their hearing counterparts, hearing-impaired children attend to meaning rather than to form as their primary motivation for generating early compositions (e.g., Conway, 1985).

This suggests strongly that the reading and writing skills of both hearing and hearing-impaired students

can be expected to develop and grow only after an interpersonal communication system has been acquired.

Communication Systems. There has been widespread and continuing controversy concerning the primary communication system which should be used in the education of hearing-impaired children. Two basic methods of instruction may be identified in North America today, and their polarization reflects the debate. On the one hand, are the proponents of oral education, while on the other are those who advocate that deaf children should be instructed using a "total communication" approach. These two positions differ in philosophy as well as in practice: the philosophy of oral education is to enable hearing-impaired children to use residual hearing, speechreading, and speech to function later as "independent adults in a world in which people's primary mode of communication is speech" (Ling, 1984, p. 9). The total communication philosophy "endorses the right of every hearing-impaired child to communicate by whatever means are found to be beneficial" (Moores, 1987, p. 11). In practice, it allows for a combination of the oral method plus the use of signs, fingerspelling, and/or any other approach that facilitates communication for the hearing-impaired child. The total communication philosophy became dominant during the 1970s and involved the use of manually coded English sign systems, such as the Rochester Method, Seeing Essential English, Signing Exact English, Signed English, and Pidgin Sign English. In addition, Cued Speech, a manual system that provides cues for speechreading, is available although not widely used in North America.

One recent study found that preschoolers whose mothers used oral communication scored higher on measures of spoken language, whereas children whose mothers used manual communication scored higher on measures of receptive language and mother-child communication (Musselman, Lindsay, and Wilson, 1988). Strong (1988) states that because many deaf individuals have fluency in ASL, they are not linguistically impoverished, but rather lacking skills in standard English. He suggests that were deaf children to be instructed in their primary language, ASL, they might attain higher levels of academic achievement. Clearly, more investigation is needed into the long-term effects of the use of various sign systems on the development of English literacy skills. The extent of experience and opportunity that children have to communicate appears to be more critical in facilitating language growth than the actual coding system employed (Kretschmer and Kretschmer, 1986; Wood et al., 1986).

Recently, an increasing number of Deaf individuals, as well as teachers of the deaf, has come to favor a bilingual-bicultural approach to the education of deaf children. This philosophy endorses surrounding the deaf child with Deaf role models and American Sign Language, while also providing interaction with hearing adults and instructing English language use. Advocates of a bilingual-bicultural approach suggest that it emphasizes the use of language and culture in appropriate and realistic situations (Strong, 1988). Clearly, further research and evaluation than is currently available is needed on the potential of this approach for improving the language, social, and cognitive skills of deaf children.

Speech Development and Communication Mode

Wolk and Schildroth (1986) asked teachers to rate the speech intelligibility of a large sample of hearing-impaired students.

Speech intelligibility ratings were found to be systematically related to (a) the degree of hearing loss; (b) communication mode; (c) ethnic background; (d) additional handicap status; and (e) educational placement in an integrated or nonintegrated academic setting. Of these factors, the most direct correlates with speech intelligibility were degree of hearing loss and communication mode.

In general, the greater the hearing loss and the earlier it was acquired, the less intelligible the speech (Berg, 1986; Levitt, 1987). Even as early as the first few months of life, the vocalizations of hearing-impaired infants were found to differ in both quality and quantity from those of normally hearing babies (Mavilya, 1972; Menyuk, 1977). To comprehend and produce intelligible speech, it does not appear to be necessary to hear all speech sounds, although it is important to receive a substantial portion of them (Ling, 1984; Ross, 1986).

Levitt (1987) found high-frequency residual hearing to be associated with superior speech skills. The speech production and perception abilities of severe to profoundly hearing-impaired students are characterized by individual differences, but nevertheless some commonalities in their speech production errors can be described. For example, a number of studies have reported errors in respiration, rate, rhythm, stress pattern, and duration (Erber, 1982; Levitt, 1989; Ling, 1976; McGarr, 1987). Many of these problems, either singly or in combination, have an adverse effect on speech intelligibility. In addition, many deaf individuals have problems with segmental errors, including inappropriate vowel quality (Calvert and Silverman, 1983; Ling, 1976; McGarr, 1987), consonant omission (Erber, 1982; Ling, 1976), and consonant and vowel substitution (Paul and Quigley, 1990).

There are conflicting reports about the improvement of speech production skills with age among severely-to-profoundly deaf children. It appears that the speech intelligibility of older students is superior to that of younger students in auditory/oral programs (Ling and Milne, 1981; Smith, 1975), but not in total communication programs (Jensema, Karchmer, and Trybus, 1978; Osberger et al., 1987). This finding does not, however, imply a causal relationship between signing and speech skills. It is more likely that as students with high speech intelligibility used speech frequently, their reliance on signs and fingerspelling decreased. In addition, residential school placement may have contributed to increased dependence on signing and reduced use of speech.

The presence or extent of a speech problem in a hard-of-hearing child is greatly influenced by the type and degree of the hearing loss. If a child has a unilateral hearing loss, there is usually no evidence of a speech problem (Berg, 1986). Most children with a mild bilateral hearing loss will learn to speak precisely, although speech development may be delayed (Berg, 1986). It is the children with moderate-to-profound bilateral deficits, most of whom have sensory, neural, or central hearing impairments, who tend to exhibit speech problems (Berg, 1986; Ross, 1982). The speech errors of these children relate mostly to segmental features (Berg, 1986), and hence their speech is often characteristic of that of much younger normally hearing children.

Fluctuating hearing loss caused by otitis media has also been linked with speech problems, in large part because of the developmental period during which it occurs. Chronic otitis media occurs most frequently during the first three years of life and tends to be accompanied by a mild to moderate hearing loss (Klein, 1986). Children whose symptoms of chronic otitis media persist for an 8-week period have been found to be at risk for speech and language problems (Zinkus and Gottlieb, 1980). For reasons which remain unclear, the incidence rate of chonic otitis media among native Indian and Inuit populations is much higher than in other populations (Kaplan, Fleshman, Bender, Baum, and Clark, 1973; Scaldwell and Frame, 1985).

Most hearing-impaired children rely more heavily on visual cues for speech perception than do their normally hearing counterparts. The ability to speechread appears to improve with age (Geffner and Levitt, 1987) and hearing level (Erber, 1982), no doubt because each contributes to the listener's ability to exploit available language and acoustic cues. Or, as Levitt (1987) suggests, it may be that a symbiotic relationship exists between speechreading and linguistic competence: each promotes the development of the other.

Communication Preference. Wolk and Schildroth (1986) found student communication method to be very strongly related to speech intelligibility, regardless of the degree of hearing loss. The vast majority of students who are in separate programs sign, whereas the proportion of fully mainstreamed students who sign is much lower. Sixty percent of American students receiving special education services because of hearing impairment use sign and speech, 39% use an auditory/oral approach only, less than 1% use Cued Speech, with less than 1% reported as using some other means of communication (Center for Assessment and Demographic Studies, 1989). Students who relied on speaking as their primary mode were consistently rated as having intelligible speech. The opposite was true for those who relied on signing: they were rated as not intelligible. Those who used both speech and signing to communicate were equally likely to be rated as intelligible or not.

Jordan and Karchmer (1986), basing their findings on more than 46,000 hearing-impaired students, found that 66% of the prelingually hearing-impaired students used some form of sign language. Only 37% of the postlingually deafened students were reported to sign. Student signing appears most strongly associated with two factors: severity of the hearing loss and the type of classroom instruction used.

Of the students surveyed by Wolk and Schildroth (1986), white, non-Hispanic students without an additional handicap were the most likely to be rated as possessing intelligible speech. Finally, placement in an integrated setting with hearing students seems to be a consistent correlate of good speech intelligibility, regardless of degree of hearing loss (Gordon, 1987; Levitt, 1987; Wolk and Schildroth, 1986). It is not clear, however, whether intelligible speech is the result of integration or, in fact, is a central factor leading to this type of placement.

Cognitive Development and Academic Achievement

Although it is commonly accepted that the assessment of cognitive abilities is at best an inexact science, the disadvantage for hearing-impaired children when undergoing psychometric evaluation can be severe. For example, few intelligence tests have been standardized for use with a hearing-impaired population, with the result that most tests employed with these students have been standardized on hearing students. Because of communication difficulties, different administration procedures are often required when testing a hearing-impaired group, such as involving a psychometrist ex-

perienced in dealing with hearing-impaired children and avoiding the use of tests with a time limitation. In addition, caution must be made in attributing test results to the hearing loss, when indirect variables, such as complicating etiological factors or environmental deficiencies, may be the primary contributing factors.

Historical Views of Cognitive Development. Perceptions of the intellectual functioning of hearing-impaired people, particularly those who are severely to profoundly deaf, have changed over the years. The interpretation of various research findings in the twentieth century have greatly influenced educational and habilitation practices.

The work of Pintner (e.g., Pintner and Patterson, 1916) in the first part of the twentieth century led to the perception of deaf individuals as cognitively inferior. Pintner, Eisenson, and Stanton (1941) concluded that deaf children are inferior in intelligence, and set the average retardation at 10 IQ points.

In contradiction to the Pintner et al. (1941) summary of research findings, Myklebust and Brutton (1953) concluded that deaf children are not, in fact, inferior in intelligence. Their research focused on the qualitative, as opposed to strictly quantitative differences between deaf and haearing children. They reasoned that the structure of intelligence is determined, at least in part, through experience, and that deafness is a form of sensory deprivation, leading to qualitatively inferior and more concrete mental processes than those displayed by hearing individuals. Their interpretation led to the perception of deaf individuals as "concrete" in intellectual functioning, a belief that found acceptance among both researchers and practitioners, in spite of the fact that, as Moores (1987) points out, the term "concrete" was never defined. According to Myklebust and Brutton (1953):

> Deafness causes the individual to behave differently. The entire organism functions in an entirely different manner. This shift in behavior and adjustment is compensatory in nature....Deafness does not simply cause an inability in human communication. It causes the individual to see differently, to smell differently, to use tactile and kinesthetic sensation differently. And perhaps more important than all of these, but because of them, the deaf person perceives differently. As a result of all these shifts in functioning, his personality adjustment and behavior are also different. To say that the deaf person is like the hearing person except that he cannot hear is to oversimplify and to do an injustice to the deaf child. His deafness is not only in the ears, it pervades his entire being. (p. 347)

By the 1960s, leading researchers (e.g., Furth, 1964; Rosenstein 1961; Vernon, 1967) had concluded that deaf people were neither intellectually inferior nor concrete. It was obvious, however, that deaf individuals had poor English language skills. The poorer performance of deaf people on some tasks, it was reasoned, could be explained by their lack of general experience or the task emphasis on English.

Recent research (e.g., Jamieson and Pedersen, 1993; Wood et al., 1986) suggests that parents who accept their child's hearing disability are more likely to make the necessary adjustments for effective communication, such as increased reliance on the visual modality, and thereby facilitate such conversational strategies as turn-taking. Parents who are themselves hearing impaired tend to show greater acceptance of their child's deafness than do hearing parents. The performance of deaf children of deaf parents on certain problem-solving tasks has been shown to be equal to that of hearing children of hearing parents, and to far exceed that of deaf children of hearing parents (Jamieson and Pedersen, 1993). These results may be interpreted as indicating the importance of parental response to the hearing loss on the deaf child's developing cognitive abilities.

Academic Achievement. Consistent findings have been reported relating children's academic performance to severity of hearing loss (Allen, 1986; DiFrancesca, 1972; Hine, 1970; McClure, 1977; Reich, Hambleton, and Houldin, 1977; Trybus and Karchmer, 1977). Hearing-impaired children lag behind their hearing counterparts in measures of academic achievement, and hard of hearing children outperform deaf students.

On the average, academic achievement for hard-of-hearing children appears to be approximately 2 years delayed, with a slightly greater lag noted on measures of reading and somewhat less on mathematical computation (Hamp, 1972). It appears, however, that the performance of hard-of-hearing children in reading and language can approach or even match that of their hearing peers if they are provided with early amplification and auditory management.

Paradoxically, the child with a less severe hearing loss may be confronted with a conflict in the classroom not normally encountered by the deaf student. Because the hard-of-hearing child appears to hear and respond appropriately much of the time, the teacher may attribute unpredictable responses to inattentiveness and penalize accordingly.

Like hard-of-hearing children, most deaf students perform poorly on measures of reading and language, although the deficit of the latter group in both academic areas is more profound. Allen (1986), reviewing the data for the 1974 norming of the sixth edition and the 1983 norming of the seventh edition of the Stanford Achievement Test for use with hearing-impaired students, noted several other trends concerning the academic achievement of hearing-impaired students. For example, as a group, there appears to be a "leveling off" in reading achievement at about third-grade level, and there also appears to be a plateau in mathematics computation, but at about the sixth- to seventh-grade levels. Despite these low levels of achievement, however, Allen noted that as a group, hearing-impaired students have shown gain in their reading and mathematics achievement between 1974 and 1983. The cause of this improvement remains unclear, but it is possible that it may be accounted for by a variety of factors, including possible methodological differences between the two studies, as well as slight variation in student and program characteristics.

Public Law 94-142 (The Education for All Handicapped Children Act of 1975) has had a dramatic impact on special education in the United States. Under the auspices of this law, children are to be educated in the least restrictive setting. This has resulted in increasing numbers of hearing-impaired children receiving their education in local rather than residential schools. Approximately 50% of the hearing-impaired student population has some degree of academic integration in regular classrooms (Center for Assessment and Demographic Studies, 1989). Allen (1986) has found that hearing-impaired students receiving special educational services within the local schools achieve at higher levels than do students attending special schools. It is not clear, however, whether students are chosen for integration because of their superior academic performance, or whether their high levels are the result of mainstreamed placement. Schein (1989) has criticized the increased emphasis on mainstreaming on the grounds that it limits deaf children's exposure to the deaf community and deaf culture. The least restrictive academic environment does not necessarily imply a mainstream setting; for many hearing-impaired students a mainstream setting may actually be more socially and academically restrictive than residential placement. It is clear that the appropriate educational placement for a student has profound consequences, both academically and socially, and, therefore, must be determined on an individual basis.

Audiologists, speech and language pathologists, and educators increasingly stress the value of early intervention following the diagnosis of hearing impairment in a child. It appears, however, that exposure to traditional early intervention programs provides little or no lasting gains (Moores, 1985; Musselman et al., 1988). Meadow-Orlans (1987a) suggests that benefits are most likely to accrue from early intervention programs for hearing-impaired children which emphasize the following: (*a*) parent counselling; (*b*) daily hearing aid maintenance; (*c*) the development of speech and oral skills; (*d*) the inclusion of sign language; (*e*) a flexible approach in accommodating family language needs; and (*f*) the presence of deaf persons on the program staff.

Psychosocial Development

In interpreting the results of research on the psychological adjustment of hearing impaired persons, it is necessary to consider at least three critical variables: 1) the validity of the testing procedure, 2) the social context surrounding the hearing impaired individual, and 3) the etiology of the hearing loss.

As is the case with intelligence testing, when measuring aspects of personality and psychological adjustment, it is necessary that the attribute under consideration be precisely defined. Most personality tests do not possess as high a degree of validity and reliability as do measures of intelligence, and many require a relatively high level of reading ability or require considerable communication between tester and testee (Moores, 1987). It is necessary that the examiner have experience in communicating with and testing a wide variety of hearing-impaired persons before administering and interpreting the results of personality tests to them.

Second, the social-emotional adjustment of hearing-impaired persons is greatly influenced by the social context. The social reality of deafness, for example, "is primarily one in which deaf people are outsiders in a hearing world" (Higgins, 1987). Most prelingually hearing-impaired children are born to hearing parents who do not expect a disabled child. For these parents, hearing loss, and most especially deafness, is a mysterious and at times an overwhelming force with which they are, at least initially, ill-equipped to cope. As mentioned earlier, communication with the hearing-impaired child is often minimal and one-way, from parent to child. In such a situation, the child, reacting to the lack of effective communication and other negative aspects of the environment, may develop patterns of behavior that are classified as "immature" or "egocentric," for example. These behaviors should not be attributed to the hearing loss, but rather, as Moores (1987) suggests, to unsatisfactory environmental conditions that developed because a child's parents were not helped to adjust to the fact of deafness and therefore did not provide the child with sufficient environmental support to develop to his or her full potential (p. 168). Similarly, other family members, teachers, and the hearing majority will probably also engage in the same ineffective and controlling interaction patterns when interacting with the child. Thus, it can be seen that certain patterns of behavior often attributed

to hearing-impaired children and youth are only incidentally related to the hearing loss itself.

Third, some major causes of childhood hearing loss, such as rubella, meningitis, and Rh factor incompatibility, may be associated with other conditions that influence psychological adjustment (Moores, 1987). The psychological development of many hearing-impaired people is, therefore, influenced to some extent not only by the communication difficulties imposed by their hearing loss, but also by organic disorders resulting from the condition that caused their hearing loss.

Historical Views of Psychological Adjustment. Formal studies of the psychological adjustment of hearing-impaired children can be traced back to about the time psychological tests first came into use. The early, and traditionally dominant, view of the development and functioning of hearing-impaired children concentrated on the lack of hearing, identifying ways in which hearing-impaired persons, as a group, were different or "deviant" from norms or standards established for a hearing population. Given this perspective, it is not surprising that the findings of some of this early research found that the deaf and hard-of-hearing children studied were more introverted, neurotic, and submissive than their hearing peers (Pintner, 1933), immature (Myklebust, 1964), and suspicious and insecure (Levine, 1956).

The most commonly cited studies of personality characteristics of hearing-impaired individuals from the 1930s to the 1970s, however, are marred by lack of attention to some or all of the variables discussed previously. Thus, any interpretations from this body of research that suggest a loss of hearing leads to atypical behavior should be viewed with caution. Perhaps the significance of these studies lies not in the results themselves but rather in reflecting the professional outlook that dominated the practice and research with hearing-impaired children during those decades.

More recently, the trend has been more positive and holistic, with a focus on those conditions that are necessary throughout the entire life cycle for hearing-impaired persons to develop and achieve their full potential (Schlesinger and Meadow, 1972). The focus has thus shifted to assisting hearing parents in achieving a realistic acceptance of their child's hearing loss and on considering the development of the child in social context.

Personality and Behavior Disorders. Research conducted during the past two decades varies tremendously in the criteria used to define psychopathology, in the type and size of hearing-impaired samples used, and in general methodology (e.g., Gentile and McCarthy, 1973; Schlesinger and Meadow, 1972).

Nevertheless, it is generally agreed that these studies provide a more reliable and valid perspective on the psychosocial functioning of hearing-impaired children than does the earlier research. These studies are consistent in uncovering a higher prevalence of personality and behavior disorders among deaf children: 8–22% compared with rates of from 2–10% for the general population of American children (Meadow, 1980).

In general, the incidence of psychosis among hearing-impaired persons is roughly equivalent to that among the hearing population (Altshuler, 1978). There is evidence, however, that deaf people may be more suspicious (Knapp, 1948; Vernon, 1980). Vernon and Andrews (1990) suggest that much of this suspicion is reality based, having started in childhood (i.e., when hearing children use their hearing to take advantage of hearing-impaired children) and continues throughout life.

Identity problems may occur for mainstreamed hard-of-hearing children, because they neither hear as well as their classmates nor do they belong to the deaf community. Differences in interaction patterns may exist for this group as well: they appear to depend more on the teacher for mediating classroom activities than do their hearing classmates, who rely most heavily upon their peers (Kennedy, Northcott, McCauley, and Williams, 1976).

It must be emphasized that although the likelihood of psychosocial problems increases when a hearing loss is present, they are not preordained. Although most studies in this area deal with group descriptions, it is essential to consider each deaf or hard-of-hearing child individually when assessing his or her psychosocial behavior and adjustment.

Many professionals have stressed that the incidence of emotional and behavior disturbances among children and youth with a hearing loss would be much lower if two measures were taken to facilitate their optimal development. First, parents, particularly hearing parents, need early access to programs that provide the necessary emotional support and assistance in dealing effectively with their hearing-impaired child. The audiologist, usually the first professional present at the time of diagnosis, can greatly assist parents by putting them in contact with other parents of hearing-impaired children, as well as with programs that provide counselling services for parents of recently diagnosed hearing-impaired children.

Second, appropriate mental health services need to be provided for hearing-impaired children and youth with serious emotional or behavioral disturbances. Most of the mental health personnel working with deaf or hard of hearing clients have received little or no specific education in terms of the culture and communication needs of hearing-impaired persons. One obvious solution to the basic issue of communication with hearing-impaired patients is to train deaf or hard-of-hearing persons to be social workers, psychologists, and psychiatrists. Unfortunately, there is only a handful of deaf mental health professionals in North America today, and it is not unusual for deaf individuals needing mental health services to be placed on long waiting lists or not to receive the services at all.

Postlingually Hearing-Impaired Children and Youth

A child who sustains a hearing impairment after the age of three has language, communication, and educational needs that are different from those of a child whose hearing loss is prelingual. Unfortunately, the study of hard-of-hearing children, generally, and that of postlingually deafened children, represent two of the most neglected areas of research and service (Berg and Fletcher, 1970; Davis, 1986; Ross, 1982).

Demographics

A recent survey reported that only about 5% of American deaf and hard-of-hearing children had become hearing impaired after the age of three years (Center for Assessment and Demographic Studies, 1989). This figure is based on hearing-impaired students who were receiving special education services; therefore, these data may exclude those who were unidentified or those who were mainstreamed in regular education programs. Brown (1986) reported, in order of decreasing incidence, that the main causes of hearing loss after birth among both pre- and postlingually hearing-impaired children were meningitis, high fever, otitis media, infection, trauma after birth, measles, and mumps.

Postlingually hearing-impaired children comprise a small but widely disparate group, both in terms of the level of hearing and the age at onset. The challenge of meeting the educational and rehabilitative needs of this group is further complicated by the fact that many of these children are unidentified, some coping successfully and some, it is speculated, misdiagnosed as learning disabled or lazy.

For the most part, postlinguistically hearing-impaired children will have an auditorily based language developed through aural/oral interactions which occurred prior to the onset of hearing loss. For this reason, many of these children will continue to rely primarily on speaking as the preferred communication mode and the vast majority will receive instruction in an integrated academic setting. In general, the later the onset of hearing loss, the more well developed will be the overall speech perception skills and the more intelligible the speech will tend to be. Levitt (1987) found postlingually hearing-impaired children at schools for the deaf to possess far superior speech and language skills in comparison to their prelingually hearing-impaired peers. It has been found that the production of suprasegmental features tends to deteriorate over time because postlingually hearing-impaired persons do not receive adequate visual or tactile feedback and, as a consequence, their voice quality becomes monotone over time, newly learned words are often mispronounced, and there is an overall decline in quality and clarity of articulation (Vernon and Andrews, 1990). It is crucial that individuals who sustain a hearing loss after the age of three receive speech therapy to retain and build on the speech and language skills already developed.

Little is known about the academic achievement of this particular group, largely because of the sparse distribution throughout the regular school system. It seems reasonable, however, to assume that many of the patterns of cognitive functioning and psychological adjustment which are characteristic of prelingually hard-of-hearing students may also pertain to postlingually hearing-impaired children and youth.

Psychosocial Development

The acceptance of one's hearing loss is a "fundamental and highly salient facet of identity" (Rutman, 1989, p. 310). Whereas the congenitally deaf person is likely to be integrated into a supportive deaf community, the adventitiously hearing-impaired individual may not encounter similar support or role models and may therefore have difficulty with identity development. For example, Rutman (1989) suggests that when deafness occurs in adolescence or early adulthood, it may alter career choice and goals, as well as possibly lead to identity confusion and lowered self-esteem. The individual may react by denying the hearing loss, and in so doing may seriously hinder coping and adjustment processes. Vernon and Andrews (1990) suggest that although there is an initial period of shock and grief, successful adjustment can usually be attained as long as the individual and the family are provided with appropriate support and information.

Hearing-Impaired Children and Youth with Special Needs

The prevalence of additional handicapping conditions among hearing-impaired children is approximately three times as large as that in the general population, or 30% (Wolff and Harkins, 1986). Although the figures indicate fairly consistent trends over time, the

data must be treated as low estimates. In the first place, the data are based on educationally significant conditions and may exclude individuals with less severe medical conditions. In addition, the figures for the most part represent children enrolled in special education programs who have been identified as multi-handicapped, thereby excluding hearing-impaired children whose additional disabilities may not have been diagnosed. There is no way of knowing the degree to which these two criteria lead to the underrepresentation of the actual number of hearing-impaired children and youth with additional handicapping conditions.

The three most common additional disabling conditions reported among American hearing-impaired children were mental retardation (8%), specific learning disability (8%), and emotional or behavioral problems (6%). Similar figures were found among Canadian deaf and hard-of-hearing students (MacDougall, 1987). The most common physical disability for the American group was uncorrected visual problems (4%), while in the Canadian study it was legal blindness (3%). Approximately 10% of the hearing-impaired children from both groups had two or more additional handicaps, frequently derived from a single cause, as is the case with the large group of deaf youth who were victims of the rubella epidemic of 1963 to 1965.

Generally, certain causes of hearing loss, such as rubella, trauma at birth, Rh factor incompatibility, and prematurity, tend to be associated with multiple disabilities. Genetically caused hearing impairment results in the lowest prevalence of additional handicaps (Brown, 1986). The American study also suggests that males have a greater tendency to be identified as multiplihandicapped hearing impaired than do females (Brown, 1986).

The implications of these findings are profound for professionals involved in the planning and implementation of educational and habilitation programs for this population. The presence of a disability in addition to impaired hearing does not produce an additive effect; it compounds the problems exponentially (Moores, 1987). Thus, the particular needs of multiplihandicapped persons are qualitatively different from those affected by hearing impairment alone. Few professionals are specifically trained to work with these children and youth in any capacity, and the special needs of this group are often unattended (Moores, 1987). As a consequence, there is a pressing challenge to improve instruction, education, and habilitation approaches for use with these individuals, as well as to provide emotional support for their families.

Particular challenges have also been noted in the instruction and habilitation of hearing-impaired students for whom English is not the primary language used in the home environment. In the general population, a growing number of children are exposed to and acquire English as a second language (ESL) in school. For many hearing-impaired children, the primary educational goal is to develop the English language skills that hearing children bring when they first attend school. ESL hearing-impaired students, unlike other deaf children, have their first exposure to English at school. This implies that the former group of children will receive little or no reinforcement at home for the speech, vocabulary, language, and intonation that they have been taught at school. With a lack of consistent speech and language input, it is extremely challenging for these children to internalize the semantic, syntactic, phonological, and pragmatic rules of either language. For example, it has been reported that deaf children of Spanish parents are exposed to both spoken Spanish and English-based signing (Luetke-Stahlman and Weiner, 1982). These children may also be exposed to at least three different cultures: the Spanish culture of their families, the mainstream hearing culture of their teachers, and the deaf culture of their deaf role models. Little research has been conducted on improving the efficacy of intervention strategies with this group and more is urgently needed, particularly in the area of language instruction.

HEARING IMPAIRMENT AMONG ADULTS

The impact that hearing impairment has on an adult is greatly influenced by the age at which the hearing loss has been acquired. For example, a hearing loss sustained during childhood or adolescence (i.e., prevocational hearing impairment) may not be as damaging to the individual's economic future because the person had the opportunity to consider the hearing impairment when making career choices. Nevertheless, the person whose hearing loss was acquired in the midst of a career (i.e., postvocational hearing impairment) may be completely unprepared to deal with it.

Prevocationally Hearing-Impaired Adults

In 1974, Schein and Delk reported that approximately 410,000 American adults had either been born with a profound hearing loss or had acquired it before the end of adolescence. Although this number represents only a fraction of the millions of Americans with a detectable hearing impairment, the social patterns, levels of educational attainment and academic achievement, and occupational and socioeconomic status (SES) patterns differ significantly from those of postvocationally hearing-impaired adults.

Social Patterns

As mentioned earlier, approximately 90% of hearing-impaired children are born to hearing parents. Traditionally, in the case of deaf children of hearing parents, schools for the deaf have served as seedbeds for the deaf community, providing deaf children with their first exposure to others like themselves (Schein, 1989). These schools have enculturated deaf children of hearing families into Deaf culture and provided them with an easily accessible language, ASL. Residential schools are important focal points for the Deaf community, both emotionally, because many deaf individuals spent much of their childhood there, and socially, as they often provide meeting places for Deaf adult social groups. Today, with the rise in mainstreaming, many deaf children may complete their education with little or no interaction with other deaf children. Although mainstreaming decreases the opportunities for deaf children to affiliate with each other, it is unlikely that it will seriously threaten the strength of the Deaf community (Schein, 1989). Deaf persons are extremely important in the social lives of Deaf adults and remain so throughout the life span.

A minority of deaf adults do not use ASL, but instead rely primarily on speaking and speechreading when communicating (Higgins, 1980). Oral deaf adults frequently belong to an oral association of the deaf and identify and socialize primarily with other oral deaf adults or hearing persons. Still fewer oral deaf adults function in both the oral and signing deaf communities (Vernon and Andrews, 1990).

Educational Attainment and Academic Achievement

Over the last half century, the educational attainment of prevocationally hearing impaired individuals has improved considerably, although not to the extent attained by the general population (Christiansen and Barnartt, 1987). Significantly fewer deaf adults completed high school or attended college or other postsecondary institutions than did their hearing counterparts.

In a review of the socioeconomic status of deaf people, Christiansen and Barnartt (1986) found that the academic achievement of prevocationally hearing-impaired students remains quite poor. In reading comprehension, for example, the median score for deaf students aged 15–17 years was found to be equivalent to slightly above the third-grade level in the general population. Performance in mathematics was slightly better, close to a seventh-grade equivalency level. In an extensive study involving 93% of deaf American students 16 years of age and older, Mindel and Vernon (1971) found that close to 30% of this group was functionally illiterate. One positive note, however, is that although deaf students are far from catching up with the academic achievement of their hearing peers, an increasing proportion of young deaf Americans has been attending postsecondary institutions since the passage of Section 504 of the Rehabilitation Act of 1973, which requires that all institutions receiving federal support make their facilities accessible to disabled persons (Schein, 1986).

Occupational/SES Patterns

Although prevocationally deaf adults work in almost every conceivable occupation from laborers to professionals, they have tended to be concentrated in the craftsman and operative categories, far beyond the norm for the general population (Schein and Delk, 1974). Their occupational status and income tend to be lower than those of comparable groups of hearing adults. Reporting on Schein and Delk's (1978) analysis of the economic status of deaf adults between 1972 and 1977, Christiansen and Barnartt (1987) state that prevocationally deaf workers of both sexes in the United States experienced decreased labor force participation rates and increased unemployment rates relative to their hearing peers.

There have been larger and more striking differences in the principal occupations held by deaf and hearing men in comparison to those between deaf and hearing women. In 1977, approximately 30% of deaf men were employed in white collar positions, compared with 40% of hearing men. In the same year, clerical work became the predominant occupation for deaf women, although the same milestone had been reached by hearing women more than 25 years earlier. In addition, deaf workers of both sexes earned about 75% of the income of their hearing counterparts, and it appears that during the 1970s, when the most recent median income figures were reported, this relative income disadvantage increased.

Christiansen and Barnartt (1986) propose that a minority group perspective provides an appropriate explanation for the relatively low SES of deaf people. This perspective "has traditionally been applied to groups which are of lower socioeconomic status, politically powerless, culturally different, negatively stereotyped, discriminated against, and aware of this discrimination" (p. 182). This perspective focuses on the extent to which social barriers and practices handicap deaf people, rather than on deficiencies caused by the hearing loss itself.

Advocacy and Consumer Organizations

There are many organizations within the Deaf community, ranging from local clubs and sports groups to national organizations and networks. For example, the National Association of the Deaf (NAD) in the United States, the Canadian Association of the Deaf (CAD), and Deafpride, among other state, provincial, and national consumer organizations, play key roles in advancing the rights of hearing-impaired individuals and promoting their equality. Oral deaf adults also have politically and socially important organizations, such as the Oral Deaf Association of the Alexander Graham Bell Association (ODAS, AGB).

Age, education, and communication preference lead to the establishment of a large array of organizations of deaf people. Many of these groups function independently for social and practical needs, but coordinate efforts with other organizations of hearing-impaired persons for government lobbying or advocacy purposes (Schein, 1989).

POSTVOCATIONALLY HEARING-IMPAIRED ADULTS

Rutman (1989) states that persons who sustain hearing impairments after 18 years of age experience social and psychological losses. She proposes that loss of hearing in adulthood is less a problem of development, as is the case with congenitally deaf or hard-of-hearing individuals, than it is one of reorganization of an already developed personality and adjustment to altered life circumstances.

Demographics

The prevalence rate and frequency of hearing impairment vary according to the definitions and methodologies used, but two conclusions are consistently reported in any research involving demographic trends. First, the number of hearing-impaired individuals increases markedly with age. The American Speech-Language-Hearing Association reported in 1984 that significant hearing losses increased from about 4% among 35 to 54 year olds through 15% among 55 to 64 year olds to 39% among those 75 and over (Jacobs-Condit, 1984). The same report indicated that older Americans (65 years old and over) made up roughly 12% of the general population but 43% of the population with a hearing loss. Second, a rise in the frequency of hearing impairment among adults is predicted, largely because of the increase in the median age of North Americans and increased life expectancies.

Acquired Hearing Loss

Despite the high number of people who have acquired hearing losses during adulthood, relatively little research has examined the impact of the communication difficulties on the functioning and quality of life and the coping skills used by these individuals to cope with their loss (Rutman, 1989). In general, the impact that an adult-onset hearing loss will have on the life of an individual depends on the age at onset, nature, degree, and configuration of the loss, lifestyle and occupation of the person, and perceived handicap (Health and Welfare Canada, 1988). Individuals with unilateral hearing impairments have functional hearing for the acquisition of speech, language, educational, and vocational skills, and, as a consequence, their communication difficulties may be minimized by the audiologist. They may, however, experience considerable difficulty in localization or in understanding a conversation when extraneous noise is present (Giolas, 1982).

Kyle, Jones, and Wood (1985) suggest that there are three phases in the acquisition of a gradual hearing loss: first, the period before the individual acknowledges the loss and seeks medical assistance; second, the stage of acknowledging the loss and obtaining a diagnosis and referral; and finally, the subsequent accommodation, including probable hearing aid provision. Up to a quarter of this population fail to reach the second stage (Haggard, Foster, and Iredale, 1981).

In general, the problems associated with a sudden severe bilateral hearing impairment are similar to those experienced by a person with a gradual hearing impairment. The initial psychological impact of a sudden loss, however, may interfere with the adjustment process (Giolas, 1982). Sudden hearing losses cut individuals off from their normal mode of speech reception and, as a consequence, frequently lead to feelings of helplessness, depression, and confusion. Giolas (1982) recommends that, in addition to amplification and a program of speech conservation, the remediation program for this population include education about the hearing loss and emotional support for the affected individual and the family.

As mentioned previously, hearing loss is widespread among the elderly. Presbycusis, or "the handicapping effect of hearing impairment associated with the aging process" (Giolas, 1982, p. 127), may have both a conductive and a sensory neural component, with a steady decline in sensitivity to puretones, especially in the higher frequencies. For the elderly, a hearing problem may not only signify a loss of one of their senses, but may also symbolize many concerns about aging, and thus represent a very complex emotional issue. Successful use of amplification by elderly persons depends, in large part, on the nature of the hearing loss, the presence of other disabilities, and their perceptions of hearing loss and aging.

The prevalence of noise-induced, or occupational, hearing loss is rising, largely because of noise pollution in factories, as well as the increased exposure of many people to amplified music. Although occupational hearing losses may negatively affect self-esteem, family relationships, and job performance, noise-induced workers tend to be reluctant to acknowledge the hearing loss and seek professional help (Hétu, Lalande, and Getty, 1987). Rehabilitative interventions should, therefore, provide emotional support and information as well as audiological assistance.

Psychosocial Aspects

Adult-onset hearing loss "must be considered, first and foremost, a social and psychological loss which affects all communication and interpersonal interactions, and which deprives the individual of the type of social relationships, occupational goals and overall quality of life to which he or she was accustomed and which gave life meaning" (Rutman, 1989, p. 305). In the event that the hearing loss interferes with job performance, the individual may be confronted with an alteration of job requirements or even a change of career. Most of the literature on acquired hearing impairments has emphasized the social isolation reported by late-deafened adults. Successful coping is difficult, but appears to be facilitated by acknowledgement and acceptance of the hearing loss.

Advocacy and Consumer Organizations. In recent years, hard-of-hearing and deafened adults have formed advocacy and self-help groups, such as Self-Help for the Hard of Hearing, the Association of Late-Deafened Adults, and the Canadian Hard of Hearing Association. The particular goals and functions of each group are individually determined, but such organizations are similar in providing shared understanding of the experience of adventitious hearing losses, and thus provide invaluable sources of emotional support. In addition, these organizations often lobby at the local, provincial, state, and national levels on behalf of hearing-impaired adults.

SUMMARY

Hearing loss is currently the most prevalent health problem in North America and has a pervasive impact on almost every aspect of an individual's life. This impact is particularly severe for the prelingually deaf child whose emerging language, speech, social, psychological adjustment, and cognitive skills are affected. Communication, social, and academic difficulties are extensive also for children with mild to moderate losses or hearing losses sustained postlingually. Most of the research on childhood hearing impairment has focused on prelingually deaf children, with the result that there is a pressing need for further knowledge about the impact of less profound or later hearing losses on the development and adjustment of the individual. In terms of language instruction and psychological development, most recent research has stressed the importance of considering the social consequences of communication breakdown on patterns of interaction.

The presence of a disabling condition in addition to hearing impairment compounds communication difficulties exponentially. Other educational and habilitative challenges are posed by the deaf student for whom neither English nor American Sign Language is the primary language used in the home.

Adults with hearing impairments may experience communication and vocational ramifications, regardless of the age at onset of the hearing loss. Although, however, the congenitally deaf adult may be integrated into a supportive and close-knit Deaf community, the individual who acquires a hearing loss during adulthood may react with social isolation and withdrawal.

Several relatively neglected areas for basic or applied research have been identified. They include: (a) the impact of mild to moderate, as well as postlingual, hearing losses on the cognitive, linguistic, and psychological development of children; (b) the development of appropriate assessment and intervention strategies for use with multihandicapped and ESL hearing-impaired students; and (c) the social and psychological impact of adult-onset hearing loss, with a view to developing coping strategies for these individuals and their families.

In conclusion, most of the research to date suggests that the handicapping effects of hearing loss revolve around societal attitudes toward disabilities in general and communication problems in particular. Studies that focus on the strengths and abilities of hearing-impaired persons indicate that, when timely and appropriate support is provided to the individual and the family, deaf and hard-of-hearing children and adults can be as contributing and creative members of society as their hearing counterparts.

REFERENCES

Allen TE. Patterns of academic achievement among hearing impaired students: 1974 and 1983. In Schildroth AN, Karchmer MA, Eds. Deaf children in America. San Diego: College-Hill Press. 1986.

Altshuler KZ. Toward a psychology of deafness. J Communic Dis, 1978;11:159–169.

Balow B, Fulton H, Peploe E. Reading comprehension skills among hearing-impaired adolescents. Volta Rev 1971;73:113–119.

Berg FS. Characteristics of the target population. In Berg FS, Blair JC, Viehweg SH, Wilson-Vlotman A, Eds. Educational audiology for the hard of hearing child. Orlando: Grune and Stratton, 1986.

Berg F, Fletcher S. The hard of hearing child. New York: Gune & Stratton, 1970.

Bown J, Mecham M. The assessment of verbal language development in deaf children. Volta Rev 1961;63:228–230.

Brannon J, Murray T. The spoken syntax of normal, hard-of-hearing, and deaf children. J Speech Hearing Res 1966;9:604–610.

Brinich PM. Childhood deafness and maternal control. J Communic Dis 1980;13:75–81.

Brown J. Examination of grammatical morphemes in the language of hard-of-hearing children. Volta Rev 1984;86:229–239.

Brown SC. Etiological trends, characteristics, and distributions. In Schildroth AN, Karchmer MA, Eds. Deaf children in America. San Diego: College-Hill Press, 1986.

Calvert D, Silverman S. Speech and deafness, 2nd ed. Washington, D.C.: Alexander Graham Bell Association for the Deaf, 1983.

Center for Assessment and Demographic Studies. Annual survey of hearing impaired children and youth, 1988–1989. Washington, D.C.: Gallaudet University, 1989.

Christiansen JB, Barnartt SN. The silent minority: The socioeconomic status of deaf people. In Higgins PC, Nash JE, Eds. Understanding deafness socially. Springfield, IL: Charles C Thomas, 1987.

Clausen JA. Research on socialization and personality development in the U. S. and France: Remarks on the paper by Professor Chombart DeLauwe. Am Soc Rev 1966;31:248–257.

Cokely D, Baker C. American sign language: A teacher's resource text on grammar and culture. Silver Spring, MD: T.J. Publishers, 1980.

Conley J. Role of idiomatic expressions in the reading of deaf children. Ann Deaf 1976;121:381–385.

Conway D. Children (re) creating writing: A preliminary look at the functions of free-choice writing of hearing impaired kindergarteners. Volta Rev 1985;87:91–107.

Curtiss S. Genie: A psycholinguistic study of a modern-day "wild child." New York, Academic Press, 1977.

Curtiss S, Prutting C, Lowell E. Pragmatic and semantic development in young children with impaired hearing. J Speech Hearing Res 1979;22:534–552.

Davis J. Performance of young hearing-impaired children on a test of basic concepts. J Speech Hearing Res 1974;17:342–351.

Davis J. Academic placement in perspective. In Luterman D, Ed. Deafness in perspective. San Diego: College-Hill Press, 1986.

Davis J, Blasdell R. Perceptual strategies employed by normal-hearing and hearing-impaired children in the comprehension of sentences containing relative clauses. J Speech Hearing Res 1975;18:281–295.

deVilliers J, Devillers P. Language acquisition. Cambridge, MA: Harvard University Press, 1978.

DiFrancesca S. Academic achievement test results of a national testing program for hearing-impaired students (Series D, No. 9). Washington, D.C.: Gallaudet College, Office of Demographic Studies, 1972.

Erber N. Auditory training. Washington, D.C.: Alexander Graham Bell Association for the Deaf, 1982.

Erting CJ. Language policy and deaf ethnicity in the United States. Sign Lang Stud 1978;19:139–152.

Erting CJ. Cultural conflict in a school for deaf children. In Higgins PC, Nash JE, Eds. Understanding deafness socially. Springfield, IL: Charles C Thomas, 1987.

Erting CJ. Acquiring linguistic and social identity: Interactions of deaf children with a hearing teacher and a deaf adult. In Strong M, Ed. Language learning and deafness. New York: Cambridge University Press, 1988.

Frisina R. Report of the committee to redefine deaf and hard of hearing for educational purposes. Washington, D.C. (mimeo), 1974.

Furth H. Research with the deaf: Implications for language and cognition. Psychol Bull 1964;62:145–162.

Gaines R, Mandler J, Bryant P. Immediate and delayed story recall by hearing and deaf children. J Speech Hearing Res 1981;24:463–469.

Geffner D. The development of language in young hearing-impaired children. Monographs of the American Speech-Language-Hearing Association 1987;26:25–35.

Geffner D, Levitt H. Communication skills of young hearing-impaired children. Monographs of the American Speech-Language-Hearing Association 1987;26:36–46.

Gentile A, McCarthy B. Additional handicapping conditions among hearing impaired students, United States: 1971–72 (Series D, No. 14). Washington, D.C.: Gallaudet College, Office of Demographic Studies, 1973.

Giolas TG. Hearing-handicapped adults. Englewood Cliffs, NJ: Prentice-Hall, 1982.

Goda S. Spoken syntax of normal, deaf, and retarded adolescents. J Verbal Learn Verbal Behav 1964;3:401–405.

Goetzinger C, Rousey C. Educational achievement of deaf children. Am Ann Deaf 1959;104:221–231.

Gordon TG. Communication skills of mainstreamed hearing-impaired children. Monographs of the American Speech-Language-Hearing Association 1987;26:91–107.

Goss RN. Language used by mothers of deaf children and mothers of hearing children. Am Ann Deaf 1970;115:93–96.

Greenberg MT. Social interaction between deaf preschoolers and their mothers: The effects of communication method and communication competence. Dev Psychol 1980;16:465–474.

Greenberg MT, Marvin RS. Patterns of attachment in profoundly deaf preschool children. Merill-Palmer Q 1979;25:265–279.

Griswold LE, Cummings J. The expressive vocabularies of pre-school children. Am Ann Deaf 1974;119:16–28.

Haggard MP, Foster JR, Iredale FE. Use and benefit of post-aural aids in sensory hearing loss. Scand Audiol 1981;10:45–52.

Hamilton P, Owrid HL. Comparisons of hearing impairment and socio-cultural disadvantage in relation to verbal retardation. Br J Audiol 1974;8:27–32.

Hamp NW. Reading attainment and some associated factors in deaf and partially hearing children. Teach Deaf 1972;70:203–215.

Health and Welfare Canada. Acquired hearing impairment in the adult (Cat. No. H39-123/1988E). Ottawa, Ontario: Minister of Supply and Services Canada, 1988.

Henggeler SW, Cooper PF. Deaf child-hearing mother interaction: Extensiveness and reciprocity. J Pediatr Psychol 1983;8:83–95.

Hétu R, Lalande M, Getty L. Psychosocial disadvantages due to occupational hearing loss as experienced in the family. Audiology 1987;26:141–152.

Higgins PC. Outsiders in a hearing world: A sociology of deafness. Beverly Hills: Sage, 1980.

Higgins PC. The deaf community. In Higgins PC, Nash JE, Eds. Understanding deafness socially. Springfield, IL: Charles C Thomas, 1987.

Hine WD. The attainments of children with partial hearing. Teach Deaf 1970;68:129–135.

Hotchkiss D. Demographic aspects of hearing impairment: Questions and answers, 2nd ed. Washington, D.C.: Gallaudet Research Institute, 1989.

Jacobs-Condit L. Gerontology and communication disorders. Washington, D.C.: Health and Human Services, 1984.

Jamieson JR, Pedersen ED. Deafness and mother-child interaction: Scaffolded instruction and the learning of problem-solving skills. Manuscript submitted for publication, 1991.

Jensema CJ. The relationship between academic achievement and the demographic characteristics of hearing impaired children and youth (Series R, No. 2). Washington, D.C.: Gallaudet College, Office of Demographic Studies, 1975.

Jensema C, Karchmer M, Trybus R. The rated speech intelligibility of hearing-impaired children: Basic relationships and a detailed analysis (Series R, No. 6). Washington, D.C.: Gallaudet College, Office of Demographic Studies, 1978.

Jordan IK, Karchmer MA. Patterns of sign use among hearing impaired students. In Schildroth AN, Karchmer, MA, Eds. Deaf children in America. San Diego: College-Hill Press, 1986.

Kaplan GJ, Fleshman JK, Bender TR, Baum C, Clark DS. Long term effects of otitis media: A ten year cohort study of Alaskan Eskimo children. Pediatrics 1973;52:577–585.

Kennedy P, Northcott W, McCauley R, Williams SN. Longitudinal sociometric and cross-sectional data on mainstreaming hearing impaired children: Implications and preschool programming. Volta Rev 1976;78:71–82.

Klein KO. Risk factors for otitis media in children. In Kavanaugh J, Ed. Otitis media and child development. Parkton, MD: York Press, 1986.

Klima ES, Bellugi U. Language in another mode. Neurosci Res Prog Bull 1974;12:539–550.

Klima E, Bellugi U, Newkirk D, Battison R. Properties of symbols in a silent language. In Klima ES, Bellugi U, Eds. The signs of language. Cambridge, MA: Harvard University Press, 1979.

Knapp PH. Emotion aspects of hearing loss. Psychosom Med 1948;10:203–222.

Kretschmer RR, Kretschmer LW. Language in perspective. In Luterman D, Ed. Deafness in perspective. San Diego: College-Hill Press, 1986.

Kyle JG, Jones LG, Wood PL. Adjustment to acquired hearing loss: A working model. In Orlans H, Ed. Adjustment to adult hearing loss. San Diego: College-Hill Press, 1985.

Lane H, Boyes-Braem P, Bellugi U. Preliminaries to a distinctive feature analysis of handshapes in American Sign Language. Cogn Psychol 1976;8:263–289.

Lenneberg E. Biological foundations of language. New York: John Wiley and Sons, 1967.

Levine E. Youth in a soundless world. New York: New York University Press, 1956.

Levine ES. The ecology of early deafness: Guides to fashioning environments and psychological assessments. New York: Columbia University Press, 1981.

Levitt H. Interrelationships among the speech and language measures. Monographs of the American Speech-Language-Hearing Association 1987;26:123–139.

Levitt H. Speech and hearing in communication. In Wang M, Reynolds M, Walberg H, Eds. The handbook of special education: Research and practice, Vol. 3. Oxford, UK: Pergamon, 1989.

Ling D. Speech and the hearing-impaired child: Theory and practice. Washington, D.C.: Alexander Graham Bell Association for the Deaf, 1976.

Ling D. Early oral intervention: An introduction. In Ling D, Ed. Early intervention for hearing-impaired children: Oral options. San Diego: College-Hill Press, 1984.

Ling D, Milne M. The development of speech in hearing-impaired children. In Bess F, Freeman BA, Sinclair JS. Amplification in education. Washington, D.C.: Alexander Graham Bell Association for the Deaf, 1981.

Luetke-Stahlman B, Weiner F. Assessing language and/or system preferences of Spanish-deaf preschoolers. Am Ann Deaf 1982;127:789–796.

Luterman D. Counseling parents of hearing-impaired children. Boston: Little, Brown, 1979.

MacDougall JC. The McGill study of deaf children in Canada. Montreal: MacDougall, 1987.

Mavilya M. Spontaneous vocalization and babbling in hearing impaired infants. In Fant G, Ed. International symposium on speech communication ability and profound deafness. Washington, D.C.: Alexander Graham Bell Association for the Deaf, 1972.

McClure A. Academic achievement of mainstreamed hearing-impaired children with congenital rubella syndrome. Volta Rev 1977;79:379–384.

McDowell A, Engel A, Massey JT, Maurer K. Plan and operation of the second national health and nutrition examination survey, 1976–80 (Series 1, No. 15, DHSS Publication No. PHS81–1317). Washington, D.C.: National Center for Health Statistics, Vital and Health Statistics, 1981.

McGarr NS. Communication skills of hearing-impaired children in schools for the deaf. Monographs of the American Speech-Language-Hearing Association 1987;26:91–107.

McIntire ML. The acquisition of American Sign Language hand configurations. Sign Lang Stud 1977;16:247–266.

Meadow KP. Deafness and child development. Berkeley: University of California Press, 1980.

Meadow KP, Greenberg MT, Erting C, Carmichael H. Interactions of deaf mothers and deaf preschool children: Comparisons with three other groups of deaf and hearing dyads. Am Ann Deaf 1981;126:454–468.

Meadow KP, Meadow L. Changing role perceptions for parents of handicapped children. Excep Child 1971;38:21–27.

Meadow-Orlans KP. An analysis of the effectiveness of early intervention programs for hearing impaired children. In Guralnick MJ, Bennett FC, Eds. The effectiveness of early intervention for at-risk and handicapped children. New York: Academic Press, 1987a.

Meadow-Orlans KP. Understanding deafness: Socialization of children and youth. In Higgins PC, Nash JE. Understanding deafness socially. Springfield, IL: Charles C Thomas, 1987b.

Menyuk P. Effects of hearing loss on language acquisition in the babbling stage. In Jaffe B, Ed. Hearing loss in children. Baltimore: University Park Press, 1977.

Mindel E, Vernon M. They grow in silence: The deaf child and his family. Silver Spring, MD: National Association of the Deaf, 1971.

Moores D. Early intervention programs for hearing impaired children: A longitudinal assessment. In Nelson K, Ed. Children's language: Vol. V. Hillsdale, NJ: Erlbaum, 1985.

Moores DF. Educating the Deaf: Psychology: Principles and Practices, 3rd ed. Boston: Houghton Mifflin, 1987.

Musselman CR, Lindsay PH, Wilson AK. The effect of mothers' communication model on language development in preschool deaf children. Appl Psycholing 1988;9:185–204.

Myklebust H. The psychology of deafness, 2nd ed. New York: Grune & Stratton, 1964.

Mykelbust H, Brutton M. A study of the visual perception of deaf children. Acta Oto-Laryngol Suppl 1953;105:1–126.

Nance WE, Sweeney A. Genetic factors in deafness in early life. Otolaryngol Clin North Am 1975;8:19–48.

Nash A, Nash JE. Deafness and family life in modern society. In Higgins PC, Nash JE. Understanding deafness socially. Springfield, IL: Charles C Thomas, 1987.

Osberger MJ, Robbins AM, Lybolt J, Kent RD, Peters J. Speech evaluation. Monographs of the American Speech-Language-Hearing Association 1987;23:24–31.

Padden C. The deaf community and the culture of deaf people. In Baker C, Battison R. Sign language and the deaf community: Essays in honor of William C. Stokoe. Silver Spring, MD: National Association of the Deaf, 1980.

Paul PV, Quigley SP. Education and deafness. White Plains, NY: Longman, 1990.

Payne J-A, Quigley S. Hearing-impaired children's comprehension of verb-particle combinations. Volta Rev 1987;89:133–143.

Pettito LA, Marentette PF. Babbling in the manual mode: Evidence for the ontogeny of language. Science 1991;251:1493–1496.

Pintner R. Emotional stability of the hard of hearing. J Genet Psychol 1933;43:293–309.

Pintner R, Eisenson J, Stanton M. The psychology of the physically handicapped. New York: Crofts and Company, 1941.

Pintner R, Patterson D. A measure of the language ability of deaf children. Psychol Rev 1916;23:413–436.

Quigley S, Paul P. ASL and ESL? Topics Early Child Spec Educ 1984;3:17–26.

Quigley SP, Smith NL, Wilbur RB. 1974. Comprehension of relativized services by deaf students. J Speech Hearing Res 1974;17:325–341.

Quigley SP, Wilbur RM, Montanelli DS. Complement structure in the language of deaf children. J Speech Hearing Res 1976;19:448–457.

Raffin M, Davis J, Gilman L. Comprehension of inflectional morphemes by deaf children exposed to a visual English sign system. J Speech Hearing Res 1978;21:387–400.

Rainer JD, Altshuler KZ. A psychiatric program for the deaf: Experience and implications. Am J Psychiatr 1971;127:1527–1532.

Rainer JD, Altshuler KZ, Kallman FJ, Eds. Family and mental health problems in a deaf population. New York: Columbia University Press, 1963.

Rawlings BW, Jensema CJ. Two studies of the families of hearing impaired children (Series R, Number 5). Washington, D.C.: Gallaudet College, Office of Demographic Studies, 1977.

Reagan T. The deaf as a linguistic minority: Educational considerations. Harv Educ Rev 1985;55:265–277.

Reich C, Hambleton D, Houldin B. The integration of hearing-impaired children in regular classrooms. Am Ann Deaf 1977;122:534–543.

Ries P. Characteristics of hearing impaired youth in the general population and of students in special education programs for the hearing impaired. In Schildroth AN, Karchmer MA, Eds. Deaf children in America. Boston: College-Hill, 1986.

Robinson LD. Sound minds in a soundless world (DHEW Publication No. ADM 77-560). Washington, D.C.: U.S. Government Printing Office, 1978.

Rogers WT, Leslie PT, Clarke BR, Booth JA, Horvath A. Academic achievements of hearing impaired students: Comparison among selected populations. BC J Spec Educ 1978;2:183–209.

Romanik S. An investigation into deaf children's use of the interrogative form. Austral Teach Deaf 1976;17:14–28.

Rosenstein J. Perception, cognition, and language in deaf children. Excep Child 1961;27:276–284.

Ross M. Hard of hearing children in regular schools. Englewood Cliffs, NJ: Prentice-Hall, 1982.

Ross M. Aural habilitation. Austin, TX: Pro-Ed, 1986.

Rutman D. The impact and experience of adventitious deafness. Am Ann Deaf 1989;134:305–311.

Scaldwell WA, Frame JE. Prevalence of otitis media in Cree and Ojibway school children in six Ontario communities. J Am Indian Educ 1985;25:1–5.

Schein JD. Models for postsecondary education of deaf students. ACEHI 1986;12:9–53.

Schein JD. The demography of deafness. In Higgins PC, Nash JE, Eds. Understanding deafness socially. Springfield, IL: Charles C Thomas, 1987.

Schein JD. At home among strangers. Washington, D.C.: Gallaudet University Press, 1989.

Schein JD, Delk MT. The deaf population of the United States. Silver Spring, MD: National Association of the Deaf, 1974.

Schein JD, Delk MT. Economic status of deaf adults: 1972 to 1977.

In Schein JD, Ed. Progress report #12. New York: New York University, 1978.

Schlesinger HS. Effects of powerlessness on dialogue and development: Disability, poverty, and the human condition. In Heller B, Flohr L, Zegans LS. Psychosocial interventions with sensorially disabled persons. Orlando, FL: Grune & Stratton, 1987.

Schlesinger HS, Meadow KP. Sound and sign: Childhood deafness and mental health. Berkeley: University of California Press, 1972.

Schmitt P. Language instruction for the deaf. Volta Rev 1966;68:85–105.

Seliger HW. Implications of a multiple critical periods hypothesis for second language learning. In Ritchie W, Ed. Second language acquisition research: Issues and implications. New York: Academic Press, 1978.

Simmons A. A comparison of the type-token ratio of spoken and written language of deaf and hearing children. Volta Rev 1962;64:417–421.

Siple P. Linguistic and psychological properties of American Sign Language: An overview. In Siple P, Ed. Understanding language through sign language research. New York: Academic Press, 1978.

Skarakis E, Prutting C. Early communication: Semantic functions and communicative intentions in the communication of the preschool child with impaired hearing. Am Ann Deaf 1977;122: 382–391.

Smith A. Residual hearing and speech production in the deaf. J Speech Hearing Res 1975;19:795–811.

Stokoe W, Casterline D, Croneberg GG. A dictionary of American sign language on linguistic principles. Washington, D.C.: Gallaudet College Press, 1965.

Strong M. A bilingual approach to the education of young deaf children: ASL and English. In Strong M, Ed. Language learning and deafness. New York: Cambridge University Press, 1988.

Stuckless ER, Birch JW. The influence of early manual communication on the linguistic development of deaf children. Am Ann Deaf 1966;111:452–460; 499–504.

Tervoort B. The understanding of passive sentences by deaf children. In D'Arcais G, Levelt W. Advances in psycholinguistics. New York: American Elsevier, 1970.

Trybus R, Karchmer M. School achievement scores of hearing impaired children: National data on achievement status and growth patterns. Am Ann Deaf 1977;122:62–69.

Vernon M. Relationship of language to the thinking process. Arch Genet Psychiatr 1967;16:325–333.

Vernon M. Perspectives on deafness and mental health. J Rehabil Deaf 1980;13:9–14.

Vernon M, Andrews JF. The psychology of deafness: Understanding deaf and hard-of-hearing people. White Plains, NY: Longman, 1990.

Weddell-Monnig J, Lumley JM. Child deafness and mother-child interaction. Child Devel 1980;51:766–774.

Wilcox J, Tobin H. Linguistic performance of hard of hearing and normal hearing children. J Speech Hearing Res 1974;17: 286–293.

Wolff AB, Brown SC. Demographics of meningitis-induced hearing impairment: Implications for immunization of children against hemophilus influenzae type B. Am Ann Deaf 1987;131:26–30.

Wolff AB, Harkins JE. Multihandicapped students. In Schildroth AN, Karchmer MA. Deaf children in America. San Diego: College-Hill Press, 1986.

Wolk S, Schildroth AN. Deaf children and speech intelligibility: A national study. In Schildroth AN, Karchmer MA. Deaf children in America. San Diego: College-Hill Press, 1986.

Wood D, Wood H, Griffiths A, Howarth I. Teaching and talking with deaf children. Chichester, UK: John Wiley and Sons, 1986.

Zinkus PW, Gottlieb MI. Patterns of perceptual and academic deficits related to early chronic otitis media. Pediatrics 1980;66: 246–253.

CHAPTER 40

Audiologic Counseling

William R. Hodgson

A good counselor is a friendly, concerned, nonjudgmental person who listens carefully, and is sensitive to the needs of the patient. By listening to the needs and feelings of the hearing impaired person, the good counselor may help that individual to express and understand feelings and accept responsibility for making informed choices relative to rehabilitation.

The counselor explores the patient's emotions, reflecting how the patient feels about the hearing loss, the handicap of hearing impairment, and the prospect of using hearing aids. During this process, the patient is evaluating the audiologic counselor, deciding whether the audiologist has the patient's best interests at heart and is a person to be trusted.

A positive assessment enhances the probability that findings and recommendations will be accepted.

The listening skills and concerned attitude of the audiologist may be especially important when the recently fitted patient returns dissatisfied with amplification. Of course, technical adjustments to the hearing aids are important and may improve user satisfaction. Nevertheless some new users will be dissatisfied with the limitations of properly fitted and well functioning hearing aids. It is here that the support and sensitivity of the audiologist may be crucial to help the patient to work toward mastering hearing aid use, to adjust to and eventually accept amplification.

An important part of audiologic counseling consists of explaining test results and making recommendations for rehabilitation. The most common complaints of patients after visiting audiologists are "I didn't understand what they told me." Another common complaint is, "They didn't tell me." Yet, the audiologists say, "Indeed, we did tell them." Why this discrepancy? Part of the answer may lie in a suggestion from Dancer and Runnebohm (1987) that audiologists are technocratic and may focus on machines, tests, and devices rather than persons. They suggest more emphasis on training skills in effective communication. If the reader is a prospective audiologist in training, it might be wise for you to examine your communication skills and ask yourself if you feel you have or can learn effective interpersonal communication. I hope this chapter will help.

Your search for ways to communicate with the hearing impaired should include a study of what they are like—their intelligence and personality. I should warn you now, though, that the hearing impaired are not homogeneous in these respects. Studies have not shown consistent differences in intelligence or personality of particular hearing impaired groups. There is, however, one factor common to most all congenitally deaf persons: Impairment in verbal language and speech. Some of these people communicate as well as they can verbally while others use manual communication.

Most of the hearing impaired people you will encounter will have acquired hearing loss after the acquisition of language and speech and will have less than total deafness. Therefore their problem will be one of input, not output. Children in this group will have the problem of getting educated. Adults of working age who acquire hearing loss will have problems related to their occupation. The largest group you will probably see are elderly individuals who become hearing impaired. All face the need to understand, accept, and ameliorate problems associated with hearing loss. Helping them to do this is the basic job of the audiologist.

AUDIOLOGIC COUNSELING AND GUIDANCE

As used in this chapter, counseling is defined as giving information, advice and support to guide the opinions, attitudes, or behavior of hearing-impaired persons. You should remember that counseling is not an isolated activity for which a specific time is to be set aside, but an ongoing process with techniques that should be used all the time, blended in to all parts of the evaluation and followup. Audiologists should be prepared to counsel about problems relating to or stemming from hearing losses, and solutions to those problems. The audiologist must assess hearing impaired persons, listen to problems as perceived, and give appropriate information, advice, and support to reduce problems stemming from hearing loss. When audiologists encounter behavior or personality problems in the hearing impaired which do not relate directly or primarily to the hearing loss, assistance or management by a psychotherapist is needed. Such help may also be needed if problems which do primarily relate to the hearing loss seem to have generated unusual or persistent personality disorders.

Audiologic counseling and guidance apply to two major areas. One area involves logic and information; the other emotions and attitudes. Regarding the first area, the audiologist must clearly communicate information about (1) the nature and extent of the hearing disorder, (2) expected effects of the disorder on communication in various listening conditions, and (3) the remedial procedures which are feasible to reduce the magnitude of the problem. In the second area, dealing with emotions and attitudes, the audiologist seeks to facilitate acceptance and objectivity regarding the hearing loss in a way that helps the patient find solutions. Handling of these areas is not separate and must be blended in together, but factual implications in explaining test results and recommendations will be considered first.

When test results are to be explained the first decision the audiologist must make is whether to use the audiogram, tympanogram, etc., to explain the results. Student audiologists may find these props appealing and I sometimes see students trying to explain these graphs to patients who have neither the ability or interest to understand them. In making the decision whether or not to use the graphs, these factors should be considered: (1) the audiologist must ask if the patient is capable of learning to understand graphs, measurement units, etc., and how interested the patient is to learn details of the hearing loss. (2) if the audiogram is used the audiologist must take the time to explain its nature and make sure the patient understands. It should be considered whether this time could be used better in other ways. (3) the audiologist should ask how many more hearing tests the patient is likely to have as time goes by. Those who will be tested many more times (or parents of hearing impaired children) should learn to interpret audiograms.

Three key words should guide the audiologist while explaining test results and recommendations: Simplicity, redundancy, and feedback. Simplicity means straightforward explanation in lay language. The level of explanation must be consistent with the patient's ability to understand, and the audiologist must become proficient in gauging that level (some patients are very knowledgeable about sound and hearing loss). The audiologist must learn how to use simple terms and explanations without talking down to the patient. Technical terms must be avoided, or if their use is absolutely necessary, must be defined and illustrated adequately. Redundancy is an important part of teaching. When a person is learning new, complex concepts such as those associated with hearing loss, more infor-

mation will be needed than what would otherwise be minimally necessary for understanding and retention. This fact is particularly true when emotional involvement is present. Therefore, the same information must be repeated in different ways. Analogies, illustrations, and examples help. Feedback must be obtained to explore the patient's understanding, acceptance, and misconceptions. The patient's responses must be watched carefully to see when more redundancy is needed and questions must be asked to be sure the patient understands.

Emotions and feelings are the stuff dealt with in counseling. Each individual has a unique story as problems relating to hearing loss are recounted and the audiologist should listen for the emotional content. Active listening gives feedback to tell the patient the audiologist is attending to the story. The audiologist sits still, fully faces the patient and perhaps leans a little forward, maintains eye contact, nods the head - especially on emphasized points. Evaluate your listening attitude by recording a counseling session with the camera on yourself. Then watch while you fast-forward the tape. It may become clear that you were rather fidgety, played with your pencil a lot, and in general weren't very comfortable or attentive.

As described in Chapter 42, several self-assessment scales are available to probe the patient's feelings and attitudes toward the hearing loss and use of amplification. These questionnaires are useful to determine the amount of handicap the patient is experiencing, to explore how the patient feels about the hearing loss, and to reveal misconceptions. Use of these scales by both the patient and the spouse can help you to learn of problems the hearing loss is causing to each person and how realistically each looks at the problems caused by the loss and at the possibility of rehabilitation with amplification.

Psychologists tell us that people who suffer a loss often go through a sequence of emotions which may include shock, denial, projection, anger, depression, and acceptance. Whether or not you see all of these emotions in one of your patients will depend of course on what point in time you encounter the patient. This process is probably seen most clearly when parents are first told their child is hearing impaired. The initial shock and grief associated with hearing this statement is very likely to prevent parents from remembering or understanding details which follow. Therefore, subsequent counseling sessions will probably be necessary to help parents accept and understand the steps which need to be taken. On the other hand, you must realize that the adult who comes to you with a long-standing hearing loss has a chronic, not an acute problem. We already tend to be more-or-less aware of the characteristics of chronic problems before we seek professional help. The problems will have lost the emotional immediacy of an acute disorder. Most of all, we tend to "live with" chronic problems, making accomodations for the handicap they cause, rather than taking aggressive steps to treat them. Two implications: You can speak frankly (though diplomatically) about their problem with hearing impaired adults and risk little overt emotional reaction. Do not be misled by this fact to make a stark statement about a newly-detected hearing loss to the parents of a hearing impaired child. The other implication: adults with chronic hearing problems which have slowly progressed are more likely to be in the denial and projection stage of emotional reaction. Because the loss came on so slowly, giving the individual time to acclimate to it, it is very easy for the person to feel that hearing is as good as ever, but that communicants nowadays mumble and do not speak as clearly as they used to.

Information and support help people through the sequence of emotional responses. It is important for the audiologist to remember that rehabilitation requires acceptance of the presence of the hearing loss and of responsibility for doing something about it. Therefore, effective use of amplification requires that the patient accept, on an emotional level, that a hearing loss is present and it is the patient's responsibility.

Unless the patient gets help in dealing with these emotions, feelings of confusion, frustration, and anxiety are likely to predominate. The audiologist can help to reduce confusion by providing information. The more that the patient understands about hearing and hearing loss the more understandable will be the problems that are encountered and confusion will be reduced. Frustration may be reduced by instruction and demonstration regarding the things which can be done to reduce the problem. Anxiety may be associated with several sources. The patient may be reacting to the fact that the hearing aid is cosmetically unpleasant and an advertment of the hearing disorder. Introduction to others who wear hearing aids successfully (and unemotionally) and demonstration of the effectiveness of the hearing aids may help. Use of small groups during hearing aid orientation and instruction may be efficient not only in terms of audiologist hours, but also may be psychologically helpful as new hearing aid users are exposed to others with the same problem and gain experience in admitting and discussing the hearing loss.

Anxiety may be reality-based, reflecting the patient's concern about ability to afford amplification financially or ability to learn to insert and control the hearing aids. If these problems can be isolated and resolved, acceptance of the problem and improved motivation may result.

Fears and negative attitudes are not always expressed openly and explicitly. For example, the expressed fear of an elderly individual regarding doubts about the ability to learn to operate the hearing aid may be only the "tip of the iceberg," and a more general concern about inability to cope with problems may be the bigger issue. The genuine concern and listening attitude of the audiologist may lead to expression of these more general fears and steps to reduce their magnitude, resulting in the individual being able to concentrate more energy on learning effective hearing aid use.

Throughout the counseling and orientation process it is important to include "significant others" - family members and others who communicate often with the patient. They can provide physical and psychological support if they learn about the nature of sound, hearing, and hearing loss, if they understand how hearing aids work and how to work them, and if they know about the problems of hearing loss in general. Cieliczka and Moss (1989), describing an orientation program which included significant others, reported (1) reduced teaching time needed to achieve efficient hearing aid use, (2) more realistic expectations resulting in increased cooperation, and (3) more patient referrals resulting from word-of-mouth advertising. In the sections which follow, it is important to remember that inclusion of family members in the instruction and orientation process may significantly improve the prognosis for successful hearing aid use.

UNDERSTANDING THE NATURE, ADVANTAGES AND LIMITATIONS OF HEARING AIDS

Realistic expectations are crucial to successful hearing aid use. Following a survey of negative comments made by hearing aid users, Smedley and Schow (1990) concluded that unrealistic expectations were the single largest deterrent to satisfaction with hearing aids. They attributed a substantial contribution to unrealistic expectations to inflated claims in hearing aid advertising. Before hearing aid use is undertaken, it should be understood that a hearing aid is similar to a miniature public address system. That is, it functions to make sounds louder not clearer, except for the improved intelligibility associated with the increased loudness. It must be understood that hearing aids do not correct all of the problems associated with hearing loss. The prospective user must realize that a properly fitted hearing aid will make soft sounds comfortably loud and that no sounds will exceed tolerable loudness, and further, that maximum amplification will be delivered for those frequencies where the hearing loss is greatest. Beyond that, the benefits from the aid will be a function of how well the patient's ear can differentiate, or learn to differentiate, sound. The success of this depends on the patient and the ear, and not on the properly functioning hearing aid.

New hearing aid users must be advised that hearing aids function poorest in situations in which the majority of hearing-impaired individuals need them most. Persons with sensory-neural hearing losses suffer a disproportionate drop of discrimination ability in noise, relative to normal-hearing individuals (Olson and Tillman, 1968; Ross and Giolas, 1974). The hearing aid industry is trying to improve hearing aid function in noise with automatic signal processing (ASP) circuits and digital-analog hybrid programmable aids. However, a survey of elderly hearing aid users found poor function in noise the most common complaint (Smedley and Schow, 1990).

Misconceptions must be removed. Considering hearing aid use, some think aids may improve or increase hearing sensitivity. They should be informed that while auditory attentiveness and functional ability should certainly increase with hearing aid use, exercising the ear via amplification will not improve sensitivity. Conversely, there are reports of threshold shift associated with amplification (Jerger and Lewis, 1975; Darbyshire, 1976; Hawkins, 1982). While these reports are not common, they justify instructing the new hearing aid user to be alert for apparent change in hearing and to obtain regular audiologic evaluations. Routine testing probably should be done yearly for adults and semiannually for children who wear hearing aids. In short, there is no rationale for rushing into, or avoiding, initiation of amplification because of concern over change in sensitivity in either direction.

Many adults express the concern that the use of a hearing aid will make the wearer dependent on amplification to the extent that unaided hearing will subsequently be less effective. They should be assured that such is not the case. Further, it should be explained that if amplification does in fact prove useful enough for the wearer to feel dependent on the hearing aid, there is certainly no good reason to be deprived of the benefit.

Some prospective hearing aid users may have been misinformed that the nerve in their ear is dead or damaged and therefore a hearing aid will not be helpful. They should be told that, while the aid will not restore the damaged sensory mechanism, the great majority of people who wear and benefit from hearing aids have sensory-neural loss. A similar situation may exist for those with unilateral disorder, precipitous

high frequency loss or others not historically considered good hearing aid candidates. They may have been told they cannot benefit from hearing aid use. Innovations described elsewhere in this book may offer successful hearing aid use, and at least a trial should be considered.

In summary, the audiologist should listen to the patient's conceptions and misconceptions, answer questions, explain and reassure. Literature that will help patients understand hearing loss and hearing aids includes that written by Rezen and Hausman (1985) and by Combs (1987).

LEARNING EFFECTIVE HEARING AID USE

The patient should understand the need to learn proper hearing aid use. There are several facets to learning efficient use of amplification. These include such physical aspects as learning to insert and remove the aid, manipulating the controls, and putting in and removing the battery. Care and maintenance of the aid are also involved. Most importantly, learning to accept the aid and listen effectively are features in hearing aid orientation. The patient will need direction in choosing hearing aid style. In-the-ear (ITE) aids are most popular today, although sale of behind-the-ear (BTE) aids is holding steady at about 20% of the market (Mahon, 1990). The patient may want to consider BTE aids for their superior reliability and flexibility. More power and better high frequency response are also available, if needed. Cosmetic concerns are legitimate and should be considered. These may direct the patient toward ITE aids, and useful amplification can be achieved with these aids in most cases.

Physical Aspects of Hearing Aid Use

Beginning hearing aid users will have trouble putting the aid on. They should be assured that, with practice, this act will become effortless and automatic. They should be shown how to hold the hearing aid, how to insert it into the canal, and how to seat it correctly and completely. Patients should be reminded to turn the aid off before removing it, to avoid feedback. They should be told to remove the aid by grasping the earmold, not the aid itself or the tubing, or the volume control of an ITE aid.

The audiologist should explain the various controls that patients must learn to use, and show how they operate. Patients should be told where the controls should be set. Some or all of the following controls are found on hearing aids, and the patient should be taught their purpose and operation.

The Volume Control. It is essential to learn manipulation of the volume control quickly and accurately while wearing the aid in order to be able to adjust it in different acoustic environments for optimum amplification. Lack of physical dexterity, such as that caused by arthritis, may prevent patients from making these adjustments. It may be necessary to recommend an aid that is easier to manipulate.

Off-On Switch. The off-on switch is variously located. It may be incorporated in the volume control. On some aids, it is associated with the telephone switch. Some aids are turned off by partly opening the battery compartment.

Input Selector. An input selector is present on some aids. Usual settings are telecoil, microphone, and —sometimes—combined telecoil and microphone inputs. The patient must understand the purpose of these settings and their efficient use.

Tone Control. There may be a tone control which effects some change in frequency response. The preferred setting, or the acoustic circumstances in which the setting should be changed, should be taught to the patient.

Care and Maintenance

To keep earmolds of BTE aids clean and prevent accumulation of wax, they should be washed regularly in warm, soapy water. However, this activity requires that the earmold be removed from the hearing aid. Therefore, it may be difficult for some hearing aid users, those with reduced vision, neuromotor problems or advanced age. The audiologist must judge, based on observed ability, whether to recommend that the patient wash the earmold. At any rate, it should be made abundantly clear to the patient that only the mold, not the aid itself, should be washed. Futher, it should be stressed that it is important to dry the mold carefully before replacing it on the aid to remove all water from the canal. If the decision is made not to instuct the patient in washing the mold, and if another person is not available to perform this function, it may be helpful in preventing wax accumulation to recommend that the mold and aid be wiped carefully with a dry cloth or tissue after each removal. It should be stressed that ITE aids are not to be washed, and the use of a pick to remove wax should be demonstrated.

Causes of feedback should be explained to the patient. The audiologist should mention the effects of poorly fitting earmold, too much gain, or the presence of sound-reflecting surfaces close to the aid.

Patients must know the type of battery needed, how to insert the battery properly and be reminded that the aid will not function if the battery is inserted backward. Instruction should be given to buy a voltage tester, and patients should be shown how to use it to check batteries. Batteries should be checked at the end of each day and discarded if they fall below specified voltage. A new battery should be tried if speech sounds faint or unclear or if it is necessary to rotate the volume control more than usual for adequate loudness. One suggestion is to have the new hearing aid user record for a time the hours obtained from each battery after daily use of the aid has stabilized. The resultant average can serve as an alert to replacement time. Gaeth and Loundsbury (1966) demonstrated that parents are not always aware of this need. In a questionnaire asking how long children's batteries lasted, 9% of the parents indicated that the batteries lasted 12 months or more. Another 14% were apparently more honest, and admitted that they had no idea.

Elements of hearing aid care should be considered. Patients should be told not to subject the aid to excessive heat (radiators or sunlight) or humidity (hair sprays or vaporizers).

Effective Listening

Patients must first learn how to set the volume control for best listening. This setting should be made by ear, not by eye. The criterion should be comfortable loudness for existing acoustic conditions. No single volume setting can provide adequate and comfortable amplification for all daily listening conditions. Patients should learn to turn the volume up when it is quiet and down when it is noisy. They should not continuously fiddle with the volume control in an attempt to equalize loudness of each incoming signal. Rather, as they move from one general acoustic condition to another, they should adjust the gain to compensate for the overall change. The audiologist should determine a volume setting for optimum listening in quiet and assist the patient in learning to make intelligent adustments from that setting as listening conditions change. A mark should not be placed on the volume control to indicate a setting from which a patient will never vary, unless it is apparent that the patient will not be capable of learning to set the volume control accurately by listening.

Hearing aid users must acclimate themselves to the unaccustomed loudness and quiality of aided listening. During their first amplification experience, patients usually comment about the audibility of forgotten background noises and the loudness and peculiar quality of their own voice. To implement the adjustment, the patient should begin practice hearing aid use in a quiet place, listening to simple signals. The listening situation should be structured and controlled. It should progress gradually to noisy places and complex signals. That is, the final goal is performance in non-stuctured, uncontrolled situations. A possible hierarchy of listening experiences is suggested below:

1. A good beginning place for the new hearing aid user might be a quiet home living room. One person should talk about familiar, everyday things. For a child, a toy might be used which makes a sound accompanied by a visible movement. Practice listening with the sound source in different positions and at varying distances.

2. Maybe next, the listener might move to the kitchen, where the acoustics are not quite as good. Listen to one person talking or to water running at different levels, but not too loud. With children, stress the visual-auditory association.

3. Next, the patient might try listening to television in a quiet room. The first experience should be with easier situations, such as the news or programs of familiar music.

4. The aid should be worn next at a quiet dinner table.

5. Engage in conversation in a quiet room with two, then three or four other people.

6. The aid should be worn outside in a quiet place, perhaps the backyard. The goal is to acclimate to wind noise.

7. The aid may be used at church, a lecture or a play. The patient should get as close to the speakers as possible.

8. The wearer should take a quiet drive in the country, with the windows closed to reduce noise.

9. The patient should walk along the street in a quiet neighborhood.

10. The patient should take a drive with the car windows open.

11. A shopping trip should be arranged.

12. The patient should try wearing the aid at a party or in a room where a number of people are talking.

At some point along this route, patients may discover they get along as well or better without the aid. This discovery does not mean they cannot benefit from an aid, but that they may choose not to wear it under certain conditions. A careful program of experimentation will not only orient individuals to wearing a hearing aid, but will help them become efficient and intelligent hearing aid users.

While the above program is being carried out, patients should also practice listening to and identifying sounds. There are many sounds they will not have been hearing at all before using the aid. They should relearn to identify these soft sounds, or in the case of children with congenital loss, strive to learn them for the first time. There may be other sounds that could be heard without the aid. Now they will be louder and have a different quality, and patients should practice listening to them also. At the same time, they should get reacquainted with the sound of their own voice. They should strive to re-establish correct loudness control. Someone should listen to them as they practice. They should also practice adjusting the volume control quickly, unobtrusively and accurately for comfortable loudness under different listening conditions.

Along with learning effective hearing aid use, the adult hearing-impaired patient should explore other aspects of audiologic rehabilitation. Depending on the person's needs and abilities, such a program might include auditory training, speechreading instruction, assistance with effective listening strategies and assertiveness training. Additionally, many patients may benefit from information about the use of supplemental sensory aids such as telephone amplifiers, induction loops, radio-frequency amplifiers, earphones for stereo, radio or television and visual or vibratory alerting devices. The supplemental sensory aids just described may function more efficiently than conventional hearing aids in special listening situations.

Additional Requirements for Children

Additional steps in learning to use an aid are necessary for young children, especially those with severe or profound congenital loss. Such children have problems which require extensive training in listening, language and speech. These topics are covered in other chapters, and only counseling about learning hearing aid use will be covered here.

Parents of hearing-impaired youngsters should listen to the child's aid daily. To do this, they will need an individual earmold or a hearing aid stethoscope. Either can be obtained from hearing aid dispensers. Parents should be sure that speech through the aid has its usual loudness and clarity, that the aid is not generating extraneous noises and that is not intermittent in operation. Regular audiologic evaluations, including assessment of hearing aid function, are an important part of the program.

When use of amplification is first undertaken, there may be a problem keeping the aid on the child. If the child has a lot of residual hearing, the meaningfulness and utility of sound may already be obvious. Otherwise, the benefits of a hearing aid will not be immediately noticeable and the child may object to the foreign, noisy device.

Parents themselves must be convinced and committed. Sometimes parents make only a half-hearted attempt to get the child to wear the aid. For one thing, the aid is a constant reminder of the defect. Some parents are not ready to tolerate advertising to themselves and others the existence of the problem. Additionally, a good habilitation program is a lot of work, and some parents may scarcely be capable of the effort. In these cases, failure of the child to adapt readily to the aid may provide a tempting excuse to unload the burden of responsiblity and effort associated with teaching good hearing aid use. To prevent these problems audiologists must effectively explain the loss and the need for the aid. They must answer the parents' questions and support their involvement in the habilitation program. They must help parents see the long-term implications of a training program, or the consequences if no program is undertaken.

Downs (1967) recommended a step-by-step procedure for helping a child learn to accept and use an aid. With adjustments in particular cases for age, magnitude of loss and other individual problems, it should be very useful. The essence of the program is presented below. The instructions are addressed to the parents of the hearing-impaired child.

During the first week, indicate to your child that you plan for the aid to be worn for four short periods each day. Then do it; be in charge of the situation. Put in the earmold without turning the aid on. If the child does not object, play quietly for 5 minutes and remove the aid. If there is resistance, gently immobilize the child, recruiting whatever help you need. Proceed as before. As soon as the child tolerates the aid, turn it up to a low volume setting, talk quietly and play with a favorite toy for 15 minutes. Set the volume control a little higher. Play quietly for 5 minutes then take the child exploring around the house. Point out sounds. Make it clear you hear them.

During the third week, extend the periods to 30 minutes each. Turn the volume control up a little more. Place the child near you and call attention to sounds that occur.

In the fifth week, utilize four 1-hour periods of hearing aid use per day. Use the volume control recommended by the audiologist.

Thereafter, increase hearing aid use until, by the end of the second month, the child is wearing the aid during all waking hours, unless part-time use has been specified by the audiologist. Exceptions might be three 10-minute rest periods per day and during rough play outdoors. In addition to the suggestion of Downs above, other recommendations for orienting children and adults to hearing aid use may be found in

Seligman (1962), Pollack and Downs (1964), Ross and Lerman (1966), Pollack (1970), Northern and Downs (1974), Hodgson (1986), and Matkin and Hodgson (1982).

With the onset of adolescence, a time when children become more aware of appearance and concerned about being different, a long-time hearing aid wearer may reject the aid. In such instances, the following suggestions may help. The importance of the child's concern should not be belittled. An atmosphere of understanding and concern is important. Prevention, of course, is better than cure. A good training progam and a history of successful hearing aid use may reduce the tendency to reject the aid. Efforts should be made to help the child see that there is less difficulty with the aid than without it. Cosmetic appearance should be improved when possible. Parental attitudes and parent-child relationships are important. Adolescents (and other people) need a lot of support.

CONCLUSION

Different individuals approach hearing aid use with different levels and sources of motivation. The motivation of children to wear hearing aids must initially be supplied by parents. Some adults are actively interesting in improving their hearing and approach hearing aid use positively. Others have a real aversion stemming from cosmetic concern or admission of the handicap associated with hearing aid use. Still others are pushed to trial hearing aid use more by the urging of relatives than by their own concern. For all of these individuals, effective counseling and orientation are needed. Otherwise initial unsatisfactory experiences with amplification may prevent successful hearing aid use.

Perhaps it makes sense to divide potential hearing aid users into three groups. There are children born with hearing loss who face the prospect of learning language and speech with defective hearing. There are elderly people who, because of hearing loss, suffer social isolation in addition to the other problems of aging. There is another group, in between , who may be faced with the threat of failing to get an education, losing a job or changing a life style because of developing hearing loss. Amplification has potential for assisting each group with its particular problem. The audiologist has a role in helping each group to realize this potential.

REFERENCES

Cieliczka D, and Moss S. Educating significant others: key to more, and more successful, fittings. Hear J 1989;42(5):26–27.

Combs A. Hearing Loss Help. Santa Maria, CA: Alpenglow Press, 1987.

Dancer J, and Runnebohm S. Quo vadis, audiologist: Technocrat or helper. Shhh 1987;8(5), 20–23.

Darbyshire J. A study of the use of high power hearing aids by children with marked degrees of deafness and the possibility of deteriorations in auditory acuity. Br J Audiol 1976;10:74–82.

Downs M. The establishment of hearing aid use: a program for parents. Maico Aud. Lib. Ser. 1967;4.

Gaeth J, and Loundsbury E. Hearing aids and children in elementary schools. J Speech Hear Disord 1966;31:283–289.

Hawkins, D. Overamplification: a well-documented case report. J Speech Hear Disord 1982;47:382–384.

Hodgson, W. Learning hearing aid use. In Hodgson W, Ed. Hearing Aid Assesement and Use in Audiologic Habilitation, 3rd ed. Baltimore: Williams & Wilkins, 1986:217–230.

Jerger J, and Lewis, N. Bianaural hearing aids: are they dangerous for children? Arch Otolaryngol 1975;10:480–483.

Mahon, W. BTE hearing instruments. Hearing J. 1990;43(5): 11–16.

Matkin N, and Hodgson, W. Amplification and the elderly patient. Otolaryngol Clin North Am 1982;15:371–386.

Northern J, and Downs M. Hearing in Children. Baltimore: Williams & Wilkins, 1974.

Olsen W, and Tillman T. 1968. Hearing aids and sensorineural loss. Ann Otol 77, 717–727.

Pollack D. Educational Audiology for the Limited Hearing Infant. Charles C Thomas, Springfield, IL:1974.

Pollack D, and Downs, M. A parent's guide to hearing aids for young children. Volta Rev 1964;66:745–749.

Rezen S, and Hausman C. Coping with Hearing Loss. New York: Dembner Books, 1985.

Ross M, and Giolas T. Effect of three classroom listening conditions on speech intelligibility. Am Ann Deaf 1974;116:580–584.

Ross M, and Lerman J. Hearing aid selection and usage in young children. Conn Med 1966;30:793–795.

Seligman D. Hearing aid orientation for young hard of hearing children. Except Child 1962;29:268–270.

Smedley T, and Schow R. Frustrations with hearing aid use: candid observations from the elderly. Hearing J 1990;43(6):21–27.

CHAPTER 41

Room Acoustics and Speech Perception

Anna K. Nábělek and Igor V. Nábělek

SOUND FIELD IN ROOMS

Speech produced at one location in a room should be clear and intelligible everywhere in the room, but this may not always be achieved. Speech intelligibility in rooms is influenced by (a) the level of speech, (b) room reverberation and (c) background noise. The importance of each of these three factors depends on the distance of a listener from the source, because the levels of the direct and reflected sounds and the background noise vary across the room.

Level of Speech

For good intelligibility, the level of speech must be sufficiently high at any location in the room. As the human voice has limited power and the speech level decreases with distance from the source, amplification of speech often may be necessary, especially in large rooms. An amplification system should provide a reasonably uniform sound pressure level (SPL) throughout the room. Amplification systems are sometimes called public address systems. The simplest system contains a microphone, an amplifier, and a loudspeaker.

Reflections and Reverberation

Speech sound propagates from the source. Part of the sound, called the direct sound, travels directly to the listener's ears. In a room, the remaining sound strikes surrounding boundaries and objects and is reflected. Early reflections from nearby surfaces form a discrete sequence and reach the listener's ears some milliseconds, or tens of milliseconds, after the direct sound. These reflections tend to blend perceptually with the direct sound and affect the quality of the sound. The early reflections are followed by a series of multiple reflections arriving at the ears with various delays and intensities. These later reflections are spaced very closely in time and fall almost or completely on top of each other. They are perceived as a prolongation of the sound and as noise.

The succession of reflections depends on the geometry of the room, furniture and the positions of the talker and the listener. The intensity of the reflections relative to the direct sound depends on the materials with which the boundaries and objects in the room are constructed. Figure 41.1 shows an example of a sequence of a brief direct sound and its subsequent reflections.

When the sound source ceases to produce sound, the sound energy in the room does not disappear instantaneously. The energy gradually decreases whenever sound strikes surfaces and, in addition, is absorbed by the air. Eventually the sound can no longer be detected. This process of sound energy decay in a room is called reverberation. In a closed space reverberation is always present. It can be long or short depending on the rate of sound energy decay. The measure of the rate of decay, or of the reverberation, is called reverberation time (T); this is the time that is required for the SPL to decrease 60 dB after the sound from the source stops (ANSI-S1.1, 1960, R 1976). The reverberation time for a sequence of reflections is shown in Figure 41.1. It is an important but rather gross measure of reverberation, because it does not take into account the temporal distribution of the first few reflections.

For speech communication, the quality of speech is not so important as the intelligibility of speech. Speech intelligibility depends primarily on T and on the ratio between the direct and reflected energy. For describing concert hall acoustics, T is not a sufficient measure because the quality of sound of music depends greatly on the spatial and temporal distributions of the reflections as well as on the relationship between early and later reflections (e.g., Schroeder, et al. 1974).

To measure T, the test sound source is located at a place at which the sound is typically produced (e.g., the front of a classroom or a theater stage). The sound is picked up by a microphone placed at various points of interest; for example, at several different distances from the source. The test sound is switched on for a few seconds, then stopped and the sound decays. This decay is plotted by a graphic level recorder and T is determined from the rate of decay (the slope of the plot). Newer instruments, such as Bruel and Kjaer Building Acoustics Analyzer type 4417, allow for automatic reading of T.

The sounds used for T measurement are wide or narrow bands of noise, or frequency-modulated tones.

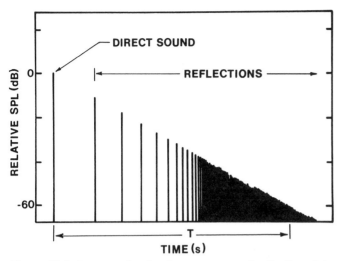

Figure 41.1. An example of a time sequence of reflections following a brief direct sound. Reverberation time (T) is shown for the 60-dB SPL decrease.

Several center frequencies of the bands are used because the absorption of room surfaces, and consequently T, are frequently dependent. The reverberation time tends to be longer below 500 Hz than above it because most materials do not absorb low frequencies well. At about 8000 Hz, T starts to decrease as acoustic energy becomes absorbed by the air. For simplicity, T is often presented as a single number. If a single number is used, its derivation should be defined. Reverberation time has been determined variously as T at 500 or 1000 Hz (Rettinger, 1973) an average of Ts over the speech frequencies (Plomp, 1976), T at 1400 Hz (Peutz, 1971), or an average of Ts at 500, 1000, and 2000 Hz (Nábělek and Pickett, 1974a). Since T in small and average-sized rooms used for speech communication is relatively uniform in range of speech frequencies, listening conditions can be fairly accurately determined by using any of the aforementioned single number Ts, room volume, and distance from the source.

Reverberation time increases with the volume of the room and decreases with the amount of sound absorption of the surfaces. That is, T is directly proportional to the volume and indirectly proportional to the absorption. The amount of absorption in rooms, and thus duration of Ts, varies greatly. In anechoic chambers, in which almost none of the acoustical energy is reflected from the walls, T approaches zero. Audiometric rooms are not completely void of reflections, especially at low frequencies; such rooms have Ts around 0.2 s. Small living rooms and offices, in which we spend most of our lives, have Ts somewhere between 0.4 s and 0.8 s. Larger classrooms, small auditoriums, and places of worship have Ts up to 1.5 s.

Longer Ts can be found in concert halls, open theaters, sports arenas, factories, and old cathedrals. Reverberant rooms which are used for special tests, such as the measurement of acoustic properties of materials and of noise emitted by machines, have hard smooth walls and Ts of 10 s or more.

The total sound energy present within any listening environment is a mixture of a direct and reflected sounds. As the direct sound declines with distance from the source while the energy of the reflections is distributed relatively evenly within the room, the ratio of the direct to reflected energy depends on the distance from the source of sound. The relationship between this ratio and speech perception will be discussed later.

In open space, without obstacles, there are no reflections and the acoustic field is "free." Close to the ground there might be reflections from the surface, however. The reflections are strong when the surface is hard, such as a concrete pavement, or very weak when the ground is covered by fresh, deep snow.

Background Noise

The sounds of speech or music which we want to hear are mixed with environmental, background noises. Noises can originate from outside or inside a room. The outside noises penetrate the room through doors, windows, walls, floors, and ceilings. They also penetrate through all openings such as ventilation ducts, leaks around doors, cracks around windows, and around partial walls. The level of noise inside a room from outside noise sources depends on the intensity of those noises, the sound insulation properties of partitions enclosing the room, and the sound absorption in the room.

In addition to the outside noises, there are noises generated inside each room. These are noises created by various human activities, music in waiting rooms, faulty fluorescent lights, ventilators, typewriters, printers, and other machines. While some human activity noises are unavoidable, others can be minimized. For example, noises made by shuffling feet can be substantially reduced by carpeting. Noisy equipment can be replaced by quieter models or contained in enclosures.

Sound Absorption

Sound absorptive materials in rooms serve two purposes: (a) they reduce reverberation time and (b) they reduce the level of the background noise. Noises spread from their sources, reaching both listeners and other objects. When the noise wave strikes the surface of material, part of the energy is reflected back into the room. The remaining energy penetrates into the material where it is either converted into heat or passes to the space at the other side of the material. For an observer in the room, the sound energy which is not reflected is eliminated from the listener's sound field because it is "absorbed" by the wall. An open window which does not reflect sound back represents perfect absorption. The greater the absorption, the larger the amount of the sound energy which is eliminated from the room.

The sound absorption coefficient is a measure of absorption of a given material. This coefficient is defined as the ratio of unreflected to incident energy. All materials absorb some energy. Materials having appreciable sound absorption coefficients (usually greater than about 0.20) are referred to as sound absorbing whereas those with very small absorption coefficients are called sound reflecting. An open window has an absorption coefficient equal to 1. Sound absorptive materials are often called "acoustic materials." This term can be misleading because it does not indicate if the material has good absorptive properties or sound insulating properties.

The absorption coefficient for most materials varies with frequency. For practical purposes, it is conventionally specified for frequencies between 125 Hz and 4000 Hz. Absorption coefficients for some commonly used materials are tabulated and can be found in various publications (e.g., Nábělek and Nábělek, 1978, p. 67). Most materials absorb more high than low frequency energy. Full, heavy draperies absorb sound better than one-layer fabrics. Carpets absorb mainly the high frequency sounds; their main application is attenuation of footsteps and shuffles. People absorb sound too, and therefore the Ts of occupied rooms are shorter than those of empty ones. A room with heavy draperies and padded furniture is less "noisy" than the same room with bare walls and hard furniture.

Absorptive materials are usually soft and porous; reflective ones are hard, dense and smooth. The insulating properties of sound absorptive materials are rather poor because the sounds easily penetrate them and pass through them to the space beyond. On the other hand, good sound insulators are poor absorbers; generally, they are made of hard materials that reflect sound back into the room.

Sound Insulation

Sound insulation pertains to the fact that only a part of the incident acoustic energy striking a partition (e.g., a door or a wall) passes through it to the other side. The rest is reflected back or dissipated in the partition as heat. The insulating properties of a material are expressed as transmission loss (TL). The TL is given by the difference between the SPL in air ("air-borne sound") at the sound source side of the partition and the SPL in air at the receiver side of the partition. The TL of the partition depends on the material, thickness, and number of layers of the partition, the frequency of the sound, and other factors. The TL of many building materials can be found in special tables (e.g., Nábělek and Nábělek, 1978, p. 64). Thick and heavy walls are good sound insulators, but thin and light partitions are not; doors and windows generally transmit more noise than do walls. Noise penetrates easily through all openings. Ceilings tend to transmit impact noises ("structure-borne noise"), for example, from footsteps. The insulation of a partition is determined by that part of it which has the smallest TL. Therefore, an expensive thick wall is useless if the door through it has poor insulating properties.

In audiometric rooms, noise insulation is provided by special materials with good sound-insulating properties. The rooms have double windows and heavy, well-sealed doors. Air is supplied through special ducts with absorptive materials and quiet ventilators.

Recommended Noise Criteria for Rooms

As a rule, people can tolerate, and may even prefer, a certain amount of background noise. The noise is considered to be acceptable if it neither disturbs room occupants nor interferes with speech communication. Acceptable noise levels for enclosures used for various types of activities were developed by Beranek, et al. (1971), and recently revised by Beranek (1989) in the form of "preferred noise criteria" (PNC) curves. The PNC curves represent the tolerance of average listeners with normal hearing to noise at frequencies between 31.5 Hz and 8000 Hz.

Excellent listening conditions, such as in concert halls, require that noise levels, expressed in terms of A-weighted averages, be no greater than 20 dB. For good listening conditions in auditoriums and drama theaters the background noise levels should not exceed 45 dB. Noise levels in shops, offices, and computer rooms, with normally operating equipment, should not exceed 60 dB. High noise levels, as they are found in many factories, are unacceptable from a communication standpoint even if safety standards are not violated. Such noise conditions are often tolerated because significant noise reduction might be too costly or even impossible (see "Industrial Hearing Conservation" Chapter).

EFFECT OF NOISE AND REVERBERATION ON SPEECH PERCEPTION—GENERAL DISCUSSION

In a room, the direct speech sound is mixed with the reverberant sound and with the background noise.

The listener's task is to decode speech from such composite sounds. The intelligibility of speech can be assessed with speech recognition (also called discrimination) tests. Test materials generally range from sentences to word and nonsense syllable lists. The results are scored as percentage of correctly identified test items. Clinically, phonetically balanced monosyllabic word tests are the most popular. The nonsense syllable tests are used primarily for studying patterns of consonant and vowel errors.

Masking by Noise

If noise is mixed with speech, then some parts of speech will be covered by the noise and become inaudible, or "masked." The masking effect of noise depends on various parameters of the noise: (a) the long term spectrum, (b) the intensity fluctuation over time, and (c) the average intensity relative to the intensity of speech. Masking is most effective by a noise which has the same long-term spectrum as the speech. The dependence of number and type of errors on the frequency range of the masking noise was demonstrated for consonants by Miller and Nicely (1955) and for vowels by Pickett (1957). Speech perception for normal-hearing listeners was affected more by steady-state noise than by fluctuating interfering signals such as competing speech (Carhart, et al., 1969; Festen and Plomp, 1990). Impulsive noises tend to be less disruptive than steady-state noises (Nábělek and Pickett, 1974a). The masking effectiveness of an impulsive noise increases with T because pauses are filled out with reverberant energy and the impulsive noise energy becomes more steady-state noise energy. The overall effects of noise on speech perception can be inferred from a speech-to-noise ratio (S/N) expressed in dB. Speech recognition scores are generally high when the S/N is high and low when the S/N is low. The term "speech to noise ratio" expresses the *ratio* of speech intensity (S) to noise intensity (N). It is a numeric that has no unit. A dimensionless unit, dB, is used for the difference between the level of the signal $Ls = 10 \log (S/l_o)$ (where l_o is a reference intensity) and the level of the noise $Ln = 10 \log (N/l_o)$. While "S/N is dB" is not quite correct, this widely used convention is employed in this chapter to avoid confusing the reader.

Pearsons et al. (1977), reported average A-weighted background noise levels at schools and at homes to be between 45 dB and 55 dB. With the average speech level of approximately 65 dB measured at 1-m distance from the mouth of the talker, the S/N in schools and homes is about +10-+20 dB (i.e., the level of speech is 10–20 dB higher than the level of the noise). Pearsons, et al. (1977), also found that teachers tended to raise their voices when the noise level was high so that they maintained the average S/N at an approximately constant +15 dB. Although these S/N ratios seem to suggest that in most schools and homes listening conditions are adequate, this may not always be the case. First, most listening takes place at distances greater than 1 m where the S/N is often much lower than at 1-m distance. Second, it is not reasonable to expect teachers to use raised voices constantly to overcome excessive noise levels. Third, since the reported results are averages, some schools and homes may have noise levels which are very low and others unacceptably high.

Often, especially for research purposes, we are interested not only in the percentage of correctly identified words in the presence of a given noise, but also which consonants and vowels are confused. Although understanding of speech does not necessarily require identification of individual phonemes (i.e., consonants and vowels), ease in phoneme identification contributes to a listener's ability to perceive speech. Most consonants are less intense and more transient than vowels, and hence more easily confused in noise than are vowels. Studies on masking by noise indicate that frequency transitions, like those which contribute to identification of consonants in syllables, are masked at lower S/N levels than constant tones (Nábělek, 1976, 1978).

Identification of various consonants is related to identification of the features of production: place (bilabial, alveolar, and velar), manner (plosive, fricative, affricative, nasal, liquid, and glide), and the presence or absence of voicing. There are seven possible types of errors: errors across one feature such as place (e.g., /p/ perceived as /t/), manner (e.g., /p/ perceived as /f/), or voicing (e.g., /p/ perceived as /b/); across two features such as place + manner (e.g., /t/ perceived as /v/), place + voicing (e.g., /p/ perceived as /d/), or manner + voicing (e.g., /p/ perceived as /v/) and across all three features (e.g., /t/ perceived as /v/). In a study by Miller and Nicely (1955), the ranking of frequency of the seven types of errors from low to high in noise was as follows: place, manner, place + manner, voicing, place + voicing, manner + voicing, and place + manner + voicing. Consonant errors in noise reported by Wang and Bilger (1973) were similarly ranked.

Vowels can be classified as monophthongs or diphthongs. All vowels are characterized by formants, i.e., spectral maxima at various frequencies. Whereas the formant frequencies in monophthongs are relatively steady during production, the formant frequencies in diphthongs change in time to cue the diphthongization. In noise, monophthongs which have similar formants are confused (Pickett, 1957; Nábělek et al.,

1992) and diphthongs are often perceived as their beginning monophthongs (Nábělek and Dagenais, 1986; Nábělek, 1988; Nábělek et al., 1992).

Masking by Reverberation

Even in quiet rooms, speech intelligibility decreases with an increase of T. This was demonstrated for normal-hearing listeners in rooms of various sizes for various speech tests (Helfer and Wilber, 1990; Peutz, 1971; Nábělek and Robinson, 1982; Neuman and Hochberg, 1983). The decline in speech recognition scores with T is gradual. For many quiet places, such as auditoriums or places of worship, a T up to 1.2 s is considered acceptable by normal-hearing listeners.

The effect of reverberation is sometimes compared to the effect of noise (Lochner and Burger, 1964; Duquesnoy and Plomp, 1980). Masking by reverberation is more complex, however, than masking by noise. Because reverberation introduces additional energy to the energy of the direct sound, the speech-corrupting "additives" exist only when speech is present, as seen in Figure 41.2. Masking by reverberation depends on the amount of reverberant energy in the room and on the rate of its decay. The stronger the reflections are, the greater the amount of reverberant energy, the slower the decay, the longer the T and, hence, the greater the masking.

Two types of sound modifications occur: speech

The term "speech to noise ratio" expresses the *ratio* of speech intensity (S) to noise intensity (N). It is a numeric that has no unit. A dimensionless unit, dB, is used for the difference between the level of the signal $L_s = 10 \log (S/I_0)$ (where I_0 is a reference intensity) and the level of the noise $L_n = 10 \log (N/I_0)$. While "S/N in dB" is not quite correct, this widely used convention is employed in this chapter to avoid confusing the reader.

sounds overlap one another (overlap masking) and the internal energy within each sound is temporarily smeared (self-masking) (Nábělek et al., 1989). The amount of overlap-masking depends on T, on the rate of speech, on the relative intensities of the preceding and following sounds and on the differences between their spectra. When speech is very rapid and/or T is long, the pauses between words become filled in with reverberant energy, and the tails of words preceding the pauses overlap with the beginning of the words following them. Intense vowels are masked relatively little by preceding low-intensity consonants, whereas consonants are substantially masked by preceding vowels or by preceding high-intensity consonants such as /s/.

Reverberation, in a manner similar to noise, affects the identification of consonants more than vowels. Nábělek and Robinson (1983) investigated errors in either noise or reverberation for consonants in syllables. In both noise and reverberation, the rank order of the seven types of errors was similar to the rank order of errors in the Miller and Nicely (1955) study. When the distributions of errors in noise and in reverberation were compared, however, it was found that the numbers of certain types of errors were not the same. In reverberation, there were relatively fewer two- or three-feature errors. Most frequently, the errors involved only one feature. This clustering of errors is not yet well understood and could be related to the particular tests used by Nábělek and Robinson.

For the vowels, as in noise, Nábělek and Dagenais (1986), Nábělek (1988) and Nábělek et al. (1992) reported that the most common errors were confusions among monophthongs with similar formants and diphthongs that were perceived as their beginning mon-

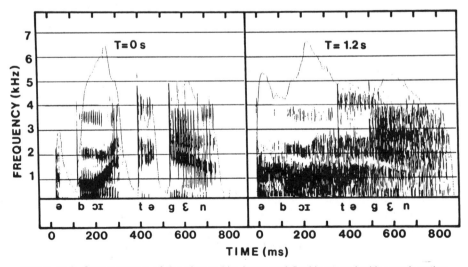

Figure 41.2. Spectrograms of the phrase "the beet again" without and with reverberation.

ophthongs (e.g., /aI/ perceived as /Ia/). Diphthongs, however, were perceived as monophthongs relatively more often in reverberation than in noise. Reverberation appears to mask the rate of formant change, which cues diphthongization, more effectively than noise.

Distance from the Source

Speech sounds received at a distance from the sound source differ from the sounds received close to the source. The following aspects of the sound depend on the distance: (a) the SPL, (b) the S/N, and (c) the ratio between direct and reflected speech energy. All three aspects can influence speech perception. At a distant location, the SPL can be too low to allow for optimal speech understanding. Also, because the SPL of speech declines with increased distance, whereas the background noise level is rather homogeneously distributed in the room, the S/N can become so unfavorable at a distant location that speech becomes unintelligible. In a well-designed room, the SPL of speech with or without amplification should be adequate in all locations so that the S/N should not decline below a value necessary for good speech understanding. In that case, the only factor which can significantly contribute to any change in speech intelligibility with a change in distance is the ratio between direct and reflected speech sounds.

The SPL of the direct sound is highest at the source and decreases 6 dB with every doubling of the distance. In Figure 41.3, the straight *line a* represents the

relative level of the direct sound as a function of the distance from the source. The level of reflected sound (*line b*) is approximately the same throughout the room but depends on the room volume and T. The total sound energy in the room is the sum of the direct and reflected sounds and its level is shown in the Figure by the *curve c*. The two lines representing direct and reflected sound levels cross at *point D*, the "critical distance" at which the levels of direct and reflected sounds are equal. The critical distance is proportional to the square root of the room volume and is inversely proportional to the square root of T. The critical distance in a medium-sized classroom, with moderate T, is about 2 m from the source. Figure 41.3 demonstrates that beyond the critical distance the SPL in a room is relatively constant due to the reflected energy. In that respect, reverberation is useful because it allows an even SPL to be maintained throughout the room except very close to the source where the SPL is the highest.

Since the ratio between the direct and reflected energy depends on the distance from the source, the question remains how speech intelligibility is affected by distance. Peutz (1971) obtained speech recognition scores at various distances from the speech source in rooms differing by volume and T. The SPL of speech was kept constant. At 1 m in front of the source, the scores were very good in all rooms. They declined gradually until a certain distance was reached beyond which the scores remained constant and independent of the distance between source and listener. Peutz found this distance to be equal to the critical distance of each room. This very important finding indicates that beyond the critical distance, the full effect of masking by reverberation takes place and remains constant. Peutz also showed that only within the critical distance, speech intelligibility may be improved by reducing the distance. These data were recently replicated by Johnson, et al. (1990), in a medium-sized classroom with normal-hearing and hearing-impaired listeners. The critical distance of the classroom was 3 m. Whereas the speech recognition score was the highest 1 m from a loudspeaker, the scores remained the same at 4 m and 8 m from the loudspeaker.

Speech Perception in Both Reverberation and Noise

We rarely converse in a very quiet place. Noisy conditions are typical for most environments. Unfortunately, when noise is combined with reverberation, speech understanding becomes difficult. For a T of 0.5 s, Peutz (1971) obtained a 95% score when S/N was +30 dB, 82% when S/N was +10 dB, and 60% when S/N was 0 dB. For a T of 1 s, the scores were 90%, 75%, and 50%, respectively. It can be concluded

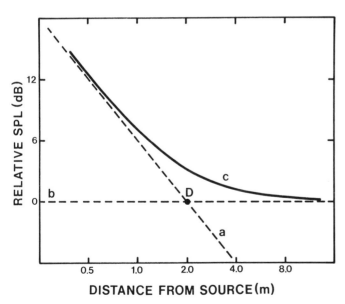

Figure 41.3. SPL in a room as a function of distance from source: (a) direct, (b) reverberant, and (c) total. Intersection of *curves a* and *b* (*point D*) defines the critical distance.

that in order to maintain high intelligibility, T in rooms with considerable noise levels should be shorter than T in quiet places and should not exceed 0.8 s for normal-hearing listeners.

Quality of Sounds in Reverberation

Reverberation also influences the quality of speech. Speech under reverberant conditions sounds muffled, or less "crisp," than without reverberation. The quality differences are small and often difficult to notice for an untrained ear. They can be noticed, however, when sounds are presented in pairs. Berkley and Allen (1993) presented pairs of speech samples with computer-simulated Ts for various positions of a microphone and loudspeaker in a small room. Listeners preferred sounds which had less reverberation and more direct energy.

For perception of music the situation is different. Music sounds better with some reverberation which is said to provide "liveliness." Optimal Ts depend on the volume of a performance hall and the type of music (Knudsen and Harris, 1980).

Localization and Reverberation

One may wonder how we can localize sources of sounds in rooms where reflections are coming to us at various angles. It has been shown by Wallach, et al. (1949), and by Haas (1951) that we localize the source according to the sound which arrives at the ears first and/or is the strongest. This is called the "precedence effect." In rooms without amplification, the first and strongest sound arriving at the ear is the direct sound which helps us to localize the source. Amplification can cause localization confusion if there is a large angle between the loudspeaker and the talker. The stronger amplified sound arrives at the listener before the direct sound and a conflict arises between visual and auditory localizations. Nevertheless, after listening for a while, we typically tend to ignore the auditory cue and rely on visual localization. In a well-designed amplification system, however, the amplified sound is delayed so that the direct sound is received by the listener first. Then the direct sound serves as the localization cue, even if it is weaker than the amplified sound.

EFFECTS OF NOISE AND REVERBERATION FOR SPECIAL LISTENERS

Many of the research studies on speech perception in noise and reverberation were conducted with groups of young, normal-hearing adults. The data which have been accumulated for other individuals, however, indicate that the norms which were developed for normal-

hearing subjects might not be appropriate for special listeners.

Special listeners are defined here as those who perform more poorly than normal-hearing young adults. Special listeners include: the hearing-impaired, children, the elderly, speech-impaired children, learning-disabled adults, and many of those for whom English is the second language. For a variety of reasons, these listeners are not able to utilize all of the information present in speech sounds. Normal-hearing listeners do not need to hear all the redundant cues for good speech understanding. Special listeners, however, may not perceive all of the cues even under ideal listening conditions. The acoustic cues which may not be available to the hearing-impaired listeners were reviewed by Pickett (1980). The elimination of redundant cues by noise and reverberation has a severe effect on speech perception for special listeners, and, therefore, for these listeners the additional loss of cues has to be prevented as much as possible. Conventional hearing aids, as well as hearing aids with amplitude compression, lack the capability to enhance selected acoustic cues (Nábělek, 1983). Hearing aids enhancing the selected cues are not yet available. The situation of normal-hearing listeners can be described as "sitting comfortably on a branch" while the situation of special listeners is like "hanging by one hand." Especially when the wind blows, hanging positions are less comfortable.

Hearing-Impaired Listeners

All of the principles of room acoustics that were discussed in the previous sections for normal-hearing listeners are applicable for hearing-impaired listeners as well, but some additional factors need to be considered. We will now examine listening conditions which are applicable for people with hearing impairment.

Hearing-impaired listeners need higher SPLs of speech than normal-hearing people in order to hear what is being said. Many hearing-impaired listeners perform very well if speech is sufficiently amplified. These individuals, however, can usually achieve high performance levels only in quiet. Conventional hearing aids and hearing aids with amplitude compression do not improve speech recognition scores either in noise or reverberation (Nábělek, 1983), and currently available hearing aids with speech processing capabilities are useful for only selected clients in selected listening conditions (Jerger, et al., 1989).

Speech perception in noise and in reverberation, by normal-hearing as well as hearing-impaired college students with moderate to profound hearing losses, was compared by Nábělek and Pickett (1974b). A similar study was carried out by Finitzo-Hieber and

Tillman (1978) with school children who had normal hearing or moderate hearing losses. The results of these studies clearly showed that hearing-impaired listeners face great perceptual difficulties in such adverse listening conditions.

Speech recognition scores decreased in noise for both the normal-hearing and hearing-impaired listeners, but there were two differences of practical importance between them. First, the impaired listeners' performance was adversely affected at S/Ns and T values which did not alter the speech perception of normal-hearing listeners. Second, since the hearing-impaired listeners performed more poorly than the normal-hearing listeners, even in the best listening conditions, their scores became unacceptably low under more adverse listening conditions. An example is given in Figure 41.4. The data points are from the Finitzo-Hieber and Tillman (1978) study with normal-hearing and moderately hearing-impaired school-age children. Monosyllabic test words were reproduced in a room with a controllable T and a babble of voices was added in some conditions to control S/N. The speech level was 25 dB above each listener's threshold for spondee words. Therefore, the speech was presented at higher levels for hearing-impaired than for normal-hearing children. In good listening conditions, without noise and reverberation, the scores for both groups were relatively high. With a S/N = +12 dB and T = 1.2 s, however, while the normal-hearing children could reasonably perform, the hearing-impaired

children's understanding of only 50% of the words was totally inadequate. With S/Ns lower than +12 dB, the scores declined even more dramatically.

Festen and Plomp (1990) investigated the effect of noise fluctuations on speech perception and found important differences between normal-hearing and hearing-impaired adults. The normal-hearing listeners' perception was most affected by steady-state noise, less by fluctuating noise such as speech babble, and least by a single interfering voice. These differences disappeared for the hearing-impaired listeners. All types of noises equally affected speech perception of the hearing-impaired listeners. Festen and Plomp suggested that this result is related to reduced temporal and frequency resolution in the impaired ears.

In both noise and reverberation, hearing-impaired listeners made consonant and vowel errors similar to those made by normal-hearing listeners (Nábělek and Robinson, 1983; Nábělek, 1988, Nábělek et al., 1992), but the hearing-impaired listeners made more errors than the normal-hearing listeners. The similarity of errors should not be surprising since both types of listeners use the same discriminatory cues (Pickett, 1980). In regard to vowel confusions, the number of errors correlated with hearing loss (Nábělek, 1988); the greater the listener's hearing loss, the greater the number of vowel errors in both noise and reverberation.

Binaural and Monaural Speech Perception.

There are individuals who have unilateral hearing losses and also individuals who have binaural hearing losses but who use only one hearing aid. Two important questions are: (a) are the speech perception abilities of one good ear different than of two good ears, and (b) is there any advantage in using binaural rather than monaural hearing aids in noisy and reverberant environments?

The speech perception abilities of people with one good ear can be inferred from speech perception data for normal-hearing listeners with one ear occluded. In reverberation alone, Nábělek and Robinson (1982) collected speech recognition scores for listeners of various ages and relatively normal hearing. A speech test, recorded in a reverberant room with various Ts ranging from 0 s–1.2 s was delivered through earphones to one or two ears. The difference between binaural and monaural scores was 5% for all Ts and all groups tested. In noise and reverberation, speech recognition scores were collected for normal-hearing by Nábělek and Pickett (1974a) and for hearing-impaired listeners by Nábělek and Pickett (1974b). In both studies a speech test was delivered to listeners sitting in a room with Ts of 0.3 s or 0.6 s, and a babble noise

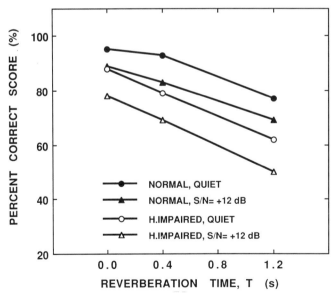

Figure 41.4. Percent words correct scores for normal-hearing and moderately hearing-impaired school-age children (adapted from Finitzo-Hieber T, Tillman TW. Room acoustics effects on monosyllabic word discrimination ability for normal and hearing-impaired children. J Speech Hear Res 1978;21:440–458).

was added to control S/N. In the binaural condition, both the normal-hearing and hearing-impaired listeners were fitted with two hearing aids. In the monaural condition, one hearing aid was replaced by an ear plug and the ear was covered by an ear muff. The mean binaural advantage for various S/Ns and Ts was about 15% for normal-hearing listeners and slightly less for hearing-impaired listeners. Similar results of the binaural advantage in noise and reverberation were reported by Plomp (1976) and Nábělek and Mason (1981) for hearing-impaired adults and by Neuman and Hochberg (1983) for normal-hearing children.

In the two-volume book, *Binaural Hearing and Amplification*, edited by Libby (1980), advantages of binaural over monaural hearing aids were extensively addressed. There are still some people, however, who have reservations about the use of binaural amplification. Such reservations are likely to be motivated by economic reasons rather than by hearing benefits. In addition, some clients do not profit from binaural amplification, but we do not yet have a quick and reliable method to identify such clients.

Individual Susceptibility.

All the results of speech perception testing in noise and reverberation have been reported in terms of mean values for groups of listeners. Such data are useful, for example, for designing schools for hearing-impaired children. Group mean data have limited value, however, when assessing an individual. Noise and reverberation affect individual speech recognition scores to different degrees. There is no clear consensus on what type of hearing-impaired listener performs poorly in such listening environments. Data indicate that individual performance is related to frequency resolution (Dubno and Dirks, 1989; Turner and Henn, 1989) and to temporal resolution (Irwin and McAuley, 1987).

Evidently speech recognition scores measured in quiet provide only limited information about the client's ability to understand speech under normal life conditions. More realistic conditions are provided when masking noise is introduced as a parameter in a battery of clinical tests. Probably an assessment of speech perception should also include susceptibility to reverberation, however, that is seldom clinically tested. This parameter has been difficult to introduce (Nábělek and Robinette, 1978). Materials for the clinical use of reverberation as a test condition are not yet commercially available, although computer-generated reverberation has been used recently to investigate the effects of reverberation on the perception of speech sounds (Berkley and Allen, 1993; Nábělek et al., 1993).

The question, indeed, is whether both noise and reverberation should be included in the test battery. According to Nábělek and Mason (1981), who measured the single and combined effects of noise and reverberation on speech perception of listeners with various configurations and degrees of binaural sensory-neural hearing losses, listeners who were greatly affected by noise also performed poorly in reverberation. The effects of noise and reverberation on an individual listener's performance were moderately correlated as both factors caused a decrease in scores. However, the combined effect of noise and reverberation could not be predicted from the performance in either noise or reverberation alone. More recently, Helfer and Wilber (1990) reported a strong relationship between puretone hearing loss and consonant recognition in quiet, noise, reverberation, and combined conditions of noise and reverberation. They also reported a significant relationship between performance in noise or quiet and in reverberation plus noise. They warned, however, that because of relatively large intersubject variability it would be unwise to assume that all individuals who perform normally on typical audiologic measures have little difficulty understanding speech distorted by room acoustics. Thus, the problem a client has in understanding dialogue in a theater, a lecture in an auditorium, or a sermon in a church may be due to the person's susceptibility to noise or reverberation or both. It follows that a test in reverberation would increase the potential value of a test battery.

Toleration of Background Noises.

Various surveys (Surr et al., 1978; Kapteyn, 1977; Franks and Beckman, 1985) indicated that background noise is one of the major reasons for dissatisfaction with hearing aids. Nábělek et al., (1991), found that full-time hearing aid users tolerated higher levels of background noise when listening to speech than listeners who used their aids only in quiet or had stopped using their hearing aids entirely. Some of these latter listeners selected very low noise levels (25 dB below the speech level) for fully satisfactory listening conditions. It is alarming that even a relatively low background noise may cause rejection or very limited use of hearing aids.

Children

It was reported in two different studies that the SPL of speech presented in quiet must be higher for young children than for young adults to achieve comparable speech recognition scores. Elliott et al. (1979), found that a 71% correct score required a 5-dB higher SPL for 5–7-year -old children than for 10-year -old children or young adults. The same 5-dB difference in the SPL for 10-year-olds and young adults was found for a 60% correct score by Nábělek and Robinson (1982). Children also performed worse than adults in noise. Elliot (1979) showed that children up to 13 years of age, with no deficits in puretone thresholds, obtained lower speech recognition scores in multi-talker noise than did older children. For example, at S/N = +5 dB, the 9-year-olds obtained about 8% lower scores than did the 17-year-olds; at S/N = 0 dB, this difference was about 27%. Under reverberant listening conditions, Nábělek and Robinson found that 10-year-old children obtained 7% lower scores than did young adults, and Neuman and Hochberg (1983) reported that the 9- and 5-year-old children had 9% and 13% lower scores, respectively, than did young adults. In both studies, binaural scores were approximately 3% higher than monaural scores, in spite of differences in speech material.

Elliott's and Neuman and Hochberg's data indicate that the younger the children are, the more they are affected by adverse listening conditions. Since their puretone thresholds are usually lower than those of young adults, their lower recognition scores are most likely related to listening skills for speech which are not yet fully developed.

ELDERLY

In several studies SPLs needed in quiet for a specific speech recognition score were compared for young and elderly listeners with relatively good hearing. Jokinen (1973) tested listeners from 20 years old to over 70 years old. He reported that a gradual increase in SPL with age was needed for a 50% recognition score. The difference between the levels for the 20–30 year olds and the elderly (over 70 years old) was 27 dB. For the same age range, Plomp and Mimpen (1979) reported a 16-dB increase in SPL for 50% score for male listeners and a 23-dB increase for female listeners with somewhat greater hearing loss than the male listeners. The data of Plomp and Mimpen are in agreement with data of Nábělek and Robinson (1982) who reported that listeners over 70 years required a 15-dB greater SPL than young adults to obtain a 60% speech recognition score. It appears that even in quiet, the SPL necessary for a given speech recognition performance depends on both age and hearing loss of the listeners. Two problems seem to be compounded in perception of speech by the elderly: hearing loss and deterioration of processing abilities.

For adverse listening conditions a reduction in speech recognition performance by the elderly was reported in many studies (Bergman et al, 1976; Duquesnoy and Plomp, 1980; Helfer and Wilber,

1990; Nábělek and Robinson, 1982). The reduction starts in the fourth decade of life. Even those older listeners who had fairly low puretone thresholds and who obtained excellent scores in good listening conditions generally performed significantly worse in noise and reverberation than did young adults.

Helfer and Wilber (1990) reported that in quiet, 70-year-old listeners with minimal hearing losses obtained a 7% lower recognition score than normal-hearing young adults. In a condition with no reverberation and S/N = +10 dB, this difference increased to 15%, and in a condition without noise and T = 1.3 s, the difference was 18%. A comparable result for listening in reverberation alone was reported by Nábělek and Robinson (1982). In the Helfer and Wilber study, in a condition with both noise and reverberation (S/N = +10 dB, T = 1.3 s), the elderly listeners' performance was 11% lower than that of the young adults. The recognition score for the elderly listeners, however, was only 44%, indicating that listening conditions became unacceptable. All Helfer and Wilber data were collected for binaural listening. Nábělek and Robinson compared scores for binaural and monaural listening in reverberation alone and found a 6% binaural advantage for the elderly listeners.

Speech-Impaired Children

Seven- and 8-year-old speech-impaired children with normal intelligence and normal puretone thresholds, obtained lower speech recognition scores in noise (S/N = +10 dB) than their normal counterparts (Elliott, 1982). All children in the Elliott study had virtually perfect scores in quiet. No data are available with this population for listening in reverberation.

Learning-Disabled Adults

In addition to speech-impaired children, Elliott (1982) compared speech perception of learning-disabled young adults and normal young adults. The performance of learning-disabled listeners was close to normal when an easy speech test was delivered in quiet or at high S/Ns. However, their performance deteriorated relative to normal listeners when the S/N was lowered to 0 dB. On a more difficult test, some handicapped persons performed normally at an S/N of +10 dB but performed very poorly at lower S/Ns. Other handicapped listeners experienced difficulty even at S/N of +10 dB. The performance of such listeners in reverberation has not yet been tested.

Non-Native Listeners

In multi-cultural societies, such as in the United States, many people communicate in non-native languages. Bergman (1980) reported differences in speech recognition scores obtained for native and non-native listeners. During his research studies in the 1960s, he observed that elderly listeners who spoke fluent but accented English obtained lower speech recognition scores than elderly listeners speaking without an accent. The difference was rather small for undistorted speech but increased to 20% for a variety of degradations, such as long reverberation (T = 2.5 s), split-band dichotic listening, and interruptions. Bergman (1980) repeated some of the studies using young Hebrew listeners (aged 20–29). The native-born Hebrew listeners' performance was compared to non-native listeners who had spoken another native language at least until age 7, but who had been speaking Hebrew for at least 13 years and were judged to be fluent in it. While undistorted sentences were perceived equally well by both groups, the scores for sentences in a babble of voices at S/N =−-3 dB were significantly lower for the non-native group. The difference was 13%. Bergman also tested elderly listeners and found that the difference in speech recognition scores in noise for native and non-native groups tended to increase with age.

Perception of speech degraded by various amounts of reverberation was tested by Nábělek and Donahue (1986) with American and non-native listeners. The native and non-native listeners were matched by gender and age. The non-native listeners were born and educated in various European and Asian countries and spoke fluent English. The criteria for the listeners were: (a) young or middle age, (b) normal hearing, and (c) at least a 94% correct speech recognition score in quiet, without reverberation. With T of 0.4 s, the non-native listeners obtained 6% lower scores; with Ts of 0.8 s and 1.2 s, they obtained 10% lower scores than the American listeners. These results indicate that non-native young and middle-age listeners who understand English very well in the absence of reverberation might have difficulty when listening in the presence of even moderate reverberation.

Takata and Nábělek (1990) compared speech perception, in either noise or reverberation, of middle-aged native Americans and Japanese listeners fluent in English using a speech test recorded by an American talker. The scores of the Japanese listeners were 8% lower than those of the American listeners in either noise (S/N =−-3 dB) or reverberation (T = 1.2 s), indicating that both noise and reverberation can be disturbing for the non-native listener.

ACOUSTIC TREATMENT OF ROOMS

We have shown in the preceding paragraphs that both noise and reverberation adversely affect speech per-

ception and that the resulting communication problem is aggravated for special listeners. Rooms which have been designed for normal-hearing listeners might have insufficient acoustics for listeners with perceptual deficiencies.

While the most intelligible speech is obtained without reverberation, complete elimination of reflections is impractical. The cost of absorptive materials and the accessibility of surfaces which can be covered by such materials limit reduction of reverberation. In addition, speech and music would sound unnatural in rooms without reverberation, since we are accustomed to listening in reverberant environments. The special anechoic rooms with no reverberation are sometimes referred to as "dead." Talking in rooms without reflections is difficult because no energy necessary for voice monitoring returns to the talker. Taking all these factors into account, Ts up to 0.5 s can be considered acceptable in rooms for special listeners.

To obtain a favorable S/N, at least +10 dB, the noise level from all outside and inside noise sources must be kept low. Schools for the deaf, speech and hearing clinics, therapy rooms, nursing homes, and other buildings used by special listeners should be built in quiet neighborhoods. If considerable outdoor noise cannot be avoided, the buildings should have double windows and double doors. Most inside noises can be substantially reduced by careful selection of quiet heating systems, ventilators, and all other equipment which must be used in the room or in adjacent spaces.

The rooms should have carpets to reduce noises made by foot traffic. Draperies, while useful, are not sufficient for controlling reverberation. Absorbing material should be mounted on suitable surfaces in the room. The best place, and usually the largest, for installing absorbing materials is the ceiling. If more absorption is needed, the materials should be placed on walls. It is usually most practical to limit the treatment of walls to areas above the reach of stretched hands to avoid damage to the absorbing material. In special cases, when absorption at low frequencies is needed, resonator-type absorbers should be used. Many new materials are being developed for application in environments where good acoustics were difficult to achieve, such as swimming pools and nursing homes.

OTHER MEANS OF REDUCING EFFECTS OF NOISE AND REVERBERATION

For many hearing-impaired persons, binaural hearing aids provide better speech perception in noise and reverberation than does a monaural aid. Some clients benefit from using hearing aids with directional microphones or with noise-reducing capabilities. Future hearing aids might have speech processors for further improving the S/N and/or dereverberation of speech.

In the present state of technology, an effective increase of S/N and reduction of the effect of T can be obtained by group amplification or assistive listening systems (Nábĕlek and Donahue, 1986; Nábĕlek et al, 1986). Speech is picked up by a microphone located close to the talker's mouth, where the direct sound has a higher level than the noise and reflected sound. Then the speech is transformed into electric signals and delivered to the listener's receiver either through wires, or electromagnetic or infrared waves. Listening systems employing the latter two principles are becoming very popular at schools for hearing-impaired children and in public places for general use (see Chapter 39 for more information).

SUMMARY

Room acoustics have a significant impact on speech communication. Speech recognition scores obtained in a quiet testing facility do not necessarily reflect the difficulties which might face the listener in everyday listening conditions. Although small rooms such as offices and classrooms have Ts which usually do not exceed 0.8 s, they might have considerable background noise levels. On the other hand, while large rooms such as auditoriums, drama theaters, and places of worship are designed to have very low background noise, their Ts (proportional to the volumes) may be 1.2 s and longer. The listening conditions in both small and large rooms can be very good for normal-hearing listeners but might not be sufficiently good for special listeners.

The SPL of speech which is sufficient for normal-hearing young adults might be too low for other listeners even in quiet listening conditions. Some special listeners, such as children, the elderly, the learning disabled, the speech-impaired, and listeners listening to non-native languages, may require speech SPLs up to 20 dB higher than do young normal adults to achieve comparable speech recognition scores. The use of amplifying systems can be a practical solution for these special listeners. Since both noise and reverberation might have adverse effects on speech perception of these listeners, the S/N in rooms should be at least +10 dB and T should not exceed 0.5 s.

The SPL for the hearing-impaired listeners can be increased by personal hearing aids. Hearing aids, however, cannot assure excellent speech perception when speech is contaminated by noise, reverberation, or both. Hearing aids amplify both speech and unwanted noise and do not remove reverberant energy from signals. Therefore, rooms for the hearing-impaired listeners should have similar specifications as rooms for the special listeners—S/N at least +10 dB and T not exceeding 0.5 s. Whereas S/N = +10 dB should secure good speech communication, many hearing aid users would require very low noise levels to fully accept hearing aids.

Individuals who have unilateral losses and hearing-impaired people who use hearing aids monaurally have greater difficulty communicating in noisy and reverberant rooms than do listeners who can use both ears. Sitting close to the source of speech is helpful. In a small classroom with moderate T, where speech is sufficiently loud in the whole space, the best conditions are found in a circle with approximately a 2-m radius from the source, within the critical distance. In a larger room, the critical distance can be somewhat greater. Nevertheless, in any case, sitting closer to the source is generally beneficial because speech becomes softer at further distances. Being close to the speaker also improves speechreading.

It has been shown that listeners with hearing losses or with other perceptual deficiencies can benefit greatly if they can receive speech signals relatively free of background noise and reverberation. Good acoustics can usually be attained if it is incorporated in building design. Modification of acoustics in existing buildings tends to be more problematic and more costly. Thought should be given to the loudness of background music in many shopping centers and waiting rooms. Such intentionally added background sounds can have negative effects on speech communication and acceptance of hearing aids. Background noises and music also could be reduced, especially for selected audiences, on radio and TV shows.

Excellent room acoustics is especially important in schools for the deaf and in therapy rooms for the variety of clients served by audiologists and speech pathologists. The client exposed to aural rehabilitation or speech therapy should receive speech samples free of background noise and reverberation.

Listening can be greatly improved even in adverse conditions by assistive listening systems, such as FM and infrared, which can deliver speech signals relatively free of background noise and room reverberation. Buildings which are built or renovated with public funds are now required to have group amplification systems available for hearing-impaired visitors. Wider use of these systems is very desirable for a variety of listeners ranging from hearing-impaired to non-native listeners. Better promotion of these systems requires development of reliable service delivery. In regard to hearing aid users, some improvements are needed in the coupling between system receivers and in-the-ear and in-the-canal hearing aids.

The hearing aids currently available on the market are not helpful for all clients and for all listening environments. Hearing aids with speech processing capabilities should be further developed. However, it is not realistic to expect that hearing aids, even with the most advanced technology, will ever be able to substitute for good listening conditions.

REFERENCES

American National Standard Acoustical Terminology. ANSI S1.1– 1960 R 1976).

Baranek LL. Balanced noise-criterion (NCB) curves. J Acoust Soc Am 1989;86:650–664.

Baranek LL., Blazier WE, and Figwer JJ. Preferred noise criterion (PNC) curves and their application to rooms. J Acoust Soc Am. 1971;50:1223–1228.

Bergman M. Aging and the Perception of Speech. Baltimore: University Park Press, 1980.

Bergman M, Blumenfeld VG, Cascardo D, Dash B, Levitt H, and Margulies MK. Age related decrement in hearing for speech. J Gerontology 1976;31:533–538.

Berkley, DA, and Allen, JB. Normal listening in typical rooms: the physical and psychophysical correlates of reverberation. Studebaker GA, Hochberg I, Eds. Acoustical Factors Affecting Hearing Aid Performance Second Edition. Boston: Allyn & Bacon, 1993:3–14.

Carhart RC, Tillman TW, Greetis ES. Perceptual masking in multiple sound backgrounds. J Acoust Soc Am 1969;45:694–703.

Dubno JR, and Dirks DD. Auditory filter characteristics and consonant recognition for hearing-impaired listeners. J Acoust Soc Am 1989;85:1666–1675.

Duquesnoy AJ, Plomp R. Effect of reverberation and noise on the intelligibility of sentences in cases of presbyacusis. J Acoust Soc Am 1980;68:537–544.

Elliott LL. Performance of children aged 9 to 17 years on a test of speech intelligibility in noise using sentence material with controlled word predictability. J Acoust Soc Am 1979;66:651–653.

Elliott LL. Effects of noise on perception of speech by children and certain handicapped individuals. J Sound Vib 1982;16:10–14.

Elliott LL, Connors S, Kille E, Levin S, Ball K, and Katz D. Children's understanding of monosyllabic nouns in quiet and in noise. J Acoust Soc Am 1976;66:12–21.

Festen JM, and Plomp R. Effects of fluctuating noise and interfering speech on the speech-reception threshold for impaired and normal hearing. J Acoust Soc Am 1990;88:1725–1736.

Finitzo-Hieber T, and Tillman TW. Room acoustics effects on monosyllabic word discrimination ability for normal and hearing-impaired children. J Speech Hear Res 1978;21:440–458.

Franks JR, Beckman N. 1985. Rejection of hearing aids: attitudes of a geriatric sample. Ear and Hearing 1985;6:161–167.

Haas H. Über den Einfluss eines Einfachechos auf die Horsamkeit von Sprache. Acustica 1951;1:49–58. Also available in English translation as: Haas H. The influence of a single echo on the audibility of speech. J Aud Eng Soc 1972;20:146–159.

Helfer KS, Wilber LA. Hearing loss, aging, and speech perception in reverberation and noise. J Speech Hear Res 1990;33:149–155.

Irwin RJ, McAuley SF. Relations among temporal acuity, hearing loss, and speech distorted by noise and reverberation. J Acoust Soc Am 1987;81:1557–1565.

Jerger J, Johnson K, Smith-Farach S. Signal processing. Hear Instr. 1989;40:12–18, 58.

Jokinen K. Presbyacusis. Acta Otolaryng. 1973;76:426–430.

Johnson CE, Nábělek AK, Asp CW. Effect of distance on normal-hearing and hearing–impaired listeners' phoneme recognition. Asha 1990;32:91(A).

Kapteyn TS. Satisfaction with fitted hearing aids. I. An analysis of technical information and II. An investigation into the influence of psycho-social factors. Scand Aud 1977;6:147–177.

Knudsen VO, Harris CM. Acoustical designing in architecture. American Institute of Physics 1980;173.

Libby ER. Binaural hearing and amplification. Chicago: Zenetron, 1980.

Lochner JPA, Burger JF. The influence of reflections on auditorium acoustics. J Sound Vib 1964;1:426–454.

Miller GA, Nicely PA. An analysis of perceptual confusions among some English consonants. J Acoust Soc Am 1955;27:338–352.

Nábělek IV. Masking of tone glides. In Hirsh SK, Eldredge DH, Hirsh IJ, Silverman SR, Eds. Hearing and Davis: essays honoring Hallowell Davis. St. Louis: Washington University Press. 1976:213-224.

Nábělek IV. Temporal summation of constant and gliding tones at masked auditory threshold. J Acoust Soc Am 1978;64:751–763.

Nábělek, IV 1983. Performance of hearing-impaired listeners under various types of amplitude compression. J Acoust Soc Am 1983;74:776–791.

Nábělek AK. Identification of vowels in quiet, noise, and reverberation: relationships with age and hearing loss. J Acoust Soc Am 1988;84:476-484.

Nabelek AK, Czyzewski Z, Crowley HJ. Vowel boundaries for steady-state and linear formant trajectories. J Acoust Soc Am 1993;94:(in press).

Nabelek AK, Czyzewski Z, Krishnan LA. The influence of talker differences on vowel identification by normal-hearing and hearing-impaired listeners. J Acoust Soc Am 1992;92:1228–1246.

Nábělek AK, Dagenais PA. Vowel errors in noise and in reverberation by hearing-impaired listeners. J Acoust Soc Am 1986;80:741–748.

Nábělek AK, Donahue AM. Comparison of amplification systems in an auditorium. J Acoust Soc Am 1986;79:2078–2082.

Nábělek AK, Donahue AM. Letowski TR. Comparison of amplification systems in a classroom. J Rehab Res Dev 1986;23:41–53.

Nábělek AK, Letowski TR, Tucker FM. Reverberant overlap and self-masking in consonant identification. J Acoust Soc Am 1989;86:1259–1265.

Nábělek AK, Mason D. Effect of noise and reverberation on binaural and monaural word identification by subjects with various audiograms. J Speech Hear Res 1981;24:375–383.

Nábělek AK, Nábělek IV. Principles of noise control. Lipscomb DM, Ed. Noise and Audiology. 1st ed. Baltimore: University Park Press, 1978:58–79.

Nábělek, AK, Pickett JM. Reception of consonants in a classroom as affected by monaural and binaural listening, noise, reverberation, and hearing aids. J Acoust Soc Am 1974a;56:628–639.

Nábělek AK, Pickett JM. Monaural and binaural speech perception through hearing aids under noise and reverberation with normal and hearing-impaired listeners. J Speech Hear Res 1974b;17: 724–739.

Nábělek AK, Robinette LR. Reverberation as a parameter in clinical testing. Audiology 1978;17:239–259.

Nábělek AK, Robinson PK. Monaural and binaural speech perception in reverberation for listeners of various ages. J Acoust Soc Am 1982;71:1242–1248.

Nábělek AK, Robinson PK. Consonant errors in noise and reverberation. J Acoust Soc Am 1983;73:S103.

Nábělek, AK, Tucker FM, Letowski TR. Toleration of background noises: relationship with patterns of hearing aid use by elderly people. J Speech Hear Res 1991;34:679–685.

Neuman AC, Hochberg I. Children's perception of speech in reverberation. J Acoust Soc Am 1983;73:2145–2149.

Pearsons KS, Bennett RL, Fidell S. Speech levels in various noise environments . Springfield, VA: National Technical Information Service PB-270 053, 1977.

Peutz VMA. Articulation loss of consonants as a criterion for speech transmission in a room. J Aud Eng Soc 1971;19:915–919.

Pickett JM. Perception of vowels heard in noises of various spectra. J Acoust Soc Am 1957;29:613–620.

Pickett JM. Current trends in basic research related to new aids for the deaf. In Levitt H, Pickett JM, Houde RA, Eds. Sensory aids for the hearing impaired . New York: IEEE Press, 1980:483–487.

Plomp R. Binaural and monaural speech intelligibility of connected discourse in reverberation as a function of azimuth of a single competing sound source. Acustica 1976;34:200–211.

Plomp R, and Mimpen AM. Speech-reception threshold for sen-

tences as a function of age and noise level. J Acoust Soc Am 1979;66:1333–1342.

Rettinger M. Acousti design and noise control . New York: Chemical Publishing Co., Inc., 1973:104.

Schroeder MR, Gottlob D, Sierbrasse KF. Comparative study of European concert halls: correlation of subjective preference with geometric and acoustic parameters. J Acoust Soc Am 1974;56:1195–1201.

Surr RK, Schuchman GI, Montgomery AA. Factors influencing use of hearing aids. Arch Otolaryngol 1978;104:723–736.

Takata Y, Nábĕlek AK. English consonant recognition in noise and in reverberation by Japanese and American listeners. J Acoust Soc Am 1990;88:663–666.

Turner CW, Henn CC. The relation between vowel recognition and measures of frequency resolution. J Speech Hear Res 1989;32: 49–58.

Wallach H, Newman EB, Rosenzweig MR. The precedence effect in sound localization. Am J Psychol 1949;62:315–336.

Wang MD, Bilger RC. Consonant confusions in noise: a study of perceptual features. J Acoust Soc Am 1973;54:1248–1266.EPGI

CHAPTER 42

Rehabilitation Technology for the Hearing Impaired

Joseph Montano

The dream of both hearing-impaired consumers and audiologists alike is for an amplification system to resolve the handicap of hearing loss. Ideally, this system would meet all hearing needs. It would reduce background noise while enhancing the quality of speech. It would be cosmetically appealing and easy to handle. It could be used in all listening environments whether they be living rooms, boardrooms, restaurants, or even, Yankee Stadium with the same level of success. Presently, however, there is no such device. Although hearing aids continue to improve in quality and versatility, they typically do not meet all of the communication needs of our patients.

Multiple factors, both acoustic and nonacoustic, influence an individual's success and failure with amplification (McCarthy, Montgomery, and Meuller, 1990). It is only through assessment and counseling that we learn about their communication needs. The information we obtain regarding the client's communication function will be pivotal when considering amplification.

The American Speech-Language and Hearing Association (ASHA) (1984) refers to aural rehabilitation as "services and procedures for facilitating adequate receptive and expressive communication in individuals with hearing impairment" (p. 37). Amplification selection is a crucial component of this aural rehabilitation process. Amplification choices are bountiful and are not limited to the hearing aid. Assistive listening devices (ALDs) can facilitate the "auditory activities of daily living" (Montano and Weinstein, 1988) by providing viable rehabilitation options.

This chapter reviews a wide varuety of ALDs that are available to supplement traditional amplification. Considerations in the selection of ALDS are discussed along with assessment and therapeutic suggestions.

ASSISTIVE LISTENING DEVICES AS REHABILITATION TECHNOLOGY

The term *assistive listening devices* has typically been used to refer to systems that (*a*) improve the signal-to-noise ratio by transmitting amplified sound directly to the hearing-impaired listener (Compton, 1990; Beaulac, Pehringer, and Shough, 1989; Vaughn, Lightfoot, and Gibbs, 1983), and (*b*) transforms sound into a vi-

sual or tactile signal (Mahon, 1985). This terminology has been addressed by both Leavitt (1989, 1987) and Compton (1990, 1993). Both authors suggested that the available technology is not limited to listening alone, many provide valuable visual and tactile representations of sound. Hence, the term *assistive listening device* appears to be restrictive. Leavitt (1987) felt that the term *rehabilitation technology for hearing impaired people* to be more appropriate. He classified systems into the following four functional categories:

Sound Enhancement Technology—specific amplification systems used to assist in the reception of sound. Included are traditional systems, such as hearing aids, as well as personal and group hardwire, infrared, induction loop and frequency modulation (FM) systems.

Television Enhancement Technology—equipment used to improve the auditory perception of a televised signal. This category includes telecaption decoding and many sound enhancement devices.

Telecommunication Technology—systems used to enhance telephone communication. Included are text telephones (TT), built-in and portable amplifiers, and induction systems.

Signal/Alerting Technology—the group of devices used to signal the presence of sound to a hearing-impaired listener. Included are visual and tactile hardwire or wireless systems, as well as hearing ear dogs.

SOUND ENHANCEMENT TECHNOLOGY

Assistive listening devices are primarily classified under sound enhancement technology. The goal of these devices is to transmit sound directly from the source to the hearing-impaired listener, in effect, decreasing the distance between the two. By negating the effects of distance, the intensity of the sound source is maintained at a constant, and hopefully, optimal listening level. This results in an improved signal-to-noise ratio. The manner in which this is accomplished distinguishes the devices.

Regardless of the manner of sound transmission, all sound enhancement technology contains the same basic components. A microphone first picks up and converts the incoming signal. An amplifier then increases the intensity of the signal. Last, the receiver converts the amplified signal back into acoustic information. The specific manner in which the signal is transmitted to the listener depends on the type of technology used.

Induction Loop Systems

The audio induction loop is one of the oldest forms of assistive listening technology in use today. These systems provide large area access to those hearing-impaired individuals who have a telecoil in their hearing aids. Audio induction loop systems are often used in schools for the hearing impaired as well as in public buildings and auditoriums.

Audio loop systems require the use of a microphone, an amplifier, a loop of wire, and a receiver. The wire surrounds an intended audience. For a large group of people, the wire may surround an entire room or a portion of a room. For individual use, an induction neckloop (a loop of shielded wire worn around the individual's neck) can be used by the hearing-impaired listener.

The input signal is picked up by a microphone, amplified and transmitted through the loop of wire. The wire generates a magnetic field, the strength of which is proportional to the input signal. The placement of another wire within the effective electromagnetic field results in the reception of the input signal. The signal is usually amplified further and, subsequently, converted into the original sound (Beaulac, Pehringer, and Shough, 1989). The electromagnetic coupling is generally accomplished through the use of the T-coil in the individual's hearing aid or through a personal-style induction amplifier.

Audio induction loop systems have a variety of applications. First, they are used successfully in situations where groups of hearing-impaired individuals gather, such as community hearing-impaired consumer group meetings. Second, induction technology can be used to couple other assistive device systems to personal hearing aids. This is accomplished through the use of the neckloop that is coupled directly to such assistive devices as hardwire, infrared and FM systems.

Induction audio loop systems are a cost-effective means of providing sound enhancement. For example, only one system is required to loop an entire room, thus providing amplification for large groups of hearing-impaired people. Installation of these systems is generally easy with little mechanical knowledge necessary. In addition, homemade induction systems can be designed from component equipment purchased at local electronic supply stores. This can result in a significant financial savings.

There can, however, be certain disadvantages associated with the use of an audio induction system. Spillover (i.e., a magnetic field generated in one room and picked by a telecoil in an adjacent room) can be a major problem. This can be particularly troublesome in settings where more than one room is looped, such as in a school for the hearing impaired.

A second possible problem is that induction systems are vulnerable to interference from a variety of sources within the designated area. These include: fluorescent lights, transformers, and electric power wires (Beck and Nance, 1989; Beaulac, Pehringer, and Shough, 1989). The resultant interference may take the form of a low-frequency hum or increased distortion.

The placement of the loop of wire within a listening environment is also extremely important. Within a given setting, there may be areas that are not reached by the electromagnetic field. This will result in "dead spots," that is, areas of no sound. When this situation occurs, one must either relocate the loop of wire or reposition the seats, if possible, in a different manner. Note that, stronger loop systems may be necessary for large-area amplification.

Telecoil capability between the various styles of hearing aids can also vary greatly, with the performance of the telecoil having a direct relationship with the successful use of induction technology. Historically, postauricular hearing aids have possessed superior induction capability. This is primarily due to the availability of space within the hearing aid. Most in-the-ear and canal-style hearing aids, because of space limitations, do not possess a telecoil, thus, eliminating their use in an induction loop environment. Even when a telecoil is present, their effectiveness is often limited. This problem can sometimes be overcome through the use of an individual induction receiver that is interfaced between the hearing aid and the electromagnetic field.

Hardwire Systems

Hardwire personal amplification systems provide a direct physical connection from the sound source to the listener. These systems couple the sound source via a microphone, amplifier, and external receiver through the use of hardwire (Fig. 42.1). The microphone is placed by the desired sound source. The signal is amplified through the body of the instrument and transmitted to the listener. The hardwire coupling can be achieved through the use of earphones, earbuds, or, if the listener wears hearing aids with a telecoil, via an induction neck loop. Note that the sound source may be coupled to an intervening amplification system, followed by coupling to the earphones.

Direct audio input (DAI) is considered a manner of hardwire coupling. The connection from the sound source to the listener is achieved by plugging an input

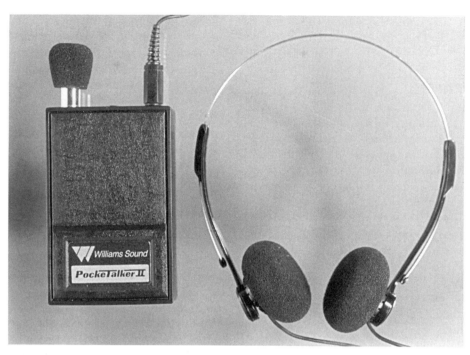

Figure 42.1. Williams Pocketalker. This example of a hardwire amplification system can be coupled with a headphone (as shown) or a neckloop for use with magnetic induction.

cord from the sound source or subsequent amplification system, directly into a hearing aid via a boot or audio shoe (Fig. 42.2) (Beck and Nance, 1989). DAI systems are currently available for many postauricular-style hearing aids, particularly moderate to high power instruments as well as certain in-the-ear-style aids. Hearing aid manufacturers provide the input cords and audio shoe for their specific models. To avoid an electrical impedance mismatch, knowledge of the coupling microphone or input sound source is necessary for the proper interfacing of the equipment.

Hardwire systems may provide an economical means of amplification. Prices for these systems can vary from as low as only a few dollars to over one hundred dollars. Certain systems can be purchased from local electronics stores, catalogue stores, mail order, and television ads. If the audiologist dispenses such hardwire systems, the reader is advised to evaluate these instruments before recommending them to patients. Because these products have not been designated as medical devices by the FDA, there are no gain, output, distortion, or frequency response specifications required. In fact, this information is not even available on many of the commercially available products.

Personal hardwire amplification systems can be used clinically in a number of ways. Table 42.1 provides examples of how these systems can be used in a variety of settings. They can be used as a source of

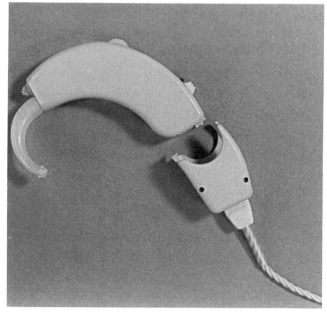

Figure 42.2. Direct audio input can allow a hearing aid to be used with an external microphone or other input sources. (Shown: Oticon E 38P hearing aid with direct audio input boot and cord).

temporary amplification in such places as schools, hospitals, nursing facilities, and physicians' offices. Their ease of operation, generally large volume controls and batteries, make them simpler to manage than many hearing aids. This can be a significant advantage when

Table 42.1
Uses of Hardwire Systems

Nursing Homes
These systems can be provided as loaners to those residents who have lost their hearing aids, or to those residents who await the receipt of their own systems.
Physicians' Offices
Devices can assist the health care provider and hearing-impaired patient both in the history intake and the provision of medical information
Automobiles
Portable systems can be used in cars to enhance communication and reduce the interference of wind and street noise.
Family
Hardwire systems can be particularly helpful for one-to-one communication, especially at social gatherings where there can be a great deal of background noise.

considering amplification options for individuals with manual dexterity problems and physically handicapping conditions. Weinstein and Amsel (1986) reported on the successful use of hardwire personal amplification systems with dementia patients in long-term care. They found that these systems provided amplification to patients who would have been unable to manage a hearing aid.

The major disadvantage to the use of hardwire systems is the limitation imposed by the direct wire connections. Although the systems are small and portable, direct wire coupling from the sound source to the listener may contraindicate their use in such large areas as auditoriums and meeting halls. In addition, when used with large groups, care needs to be taken to avoid accidental falls from wires positioned along the floor.

Infrared Systems

Infrared systems provide another means of sound enhancement. Infrared systems do not use a hardwire connection. The sound that is picked up by the microphone is converted into infrared light waves through the use of diodes, which then are dispersed throughout the listening environment. The receiver, worn by the hearing-impaired listener, transforms the infrared light waves back into an auditory signal. The receiver also serves as an amplifier and can be adjusted to a desired listening level (Fig. 42.3).

Infrared systems can be coupled in a variety of ways. First, standard headsets or insert earphones can be worn by individuals who have a mild hearing loss and do not wear hearing aids. Second, induction technology can be used by those individuals who have hearing aids equipped with telecoils. Third, direct audio input can be used by those individuals whose hearing aids have the necessary interfacing boot or shoe.

Infrared systems can be used for large area or personal amplification. Large area systems are commonly found in theaters, auditoriums and places of worship. Each infrared device is designed for the particular area of use. The number of infrared diodes used to transmit the desired signal is directly related to the size of the listening environment. A large auditorium requires significantly more diodes then required in a small conference center or living room. Personal systems are designed primarily for home use The transmitter provides a signal whose strength is sufficient for use only in a small area such as a living room or bedroom.

Infrared systems are frequently used clinically as a recommended device to enhance the sound from a television. They need not, however, be limited to only this application as can be seen in Table 42.2. One of the most beneficial aspects of this technology is its usage in theaters. This has allowed many hearing-impaired individuals to pursue an entertainment option previously unavailable to them. Since many hearing-impaired people are unaware of these various options, audiologists are encouraged to inform their clients of the benefits available to them.

The major disadvantage of infrared systems is that they can be used only in enclosed rooms. This is because infrared light waves cannot pass through or bend around obstacles. In addition, infrared systems cannot be used outdoors. The transmitted light waves

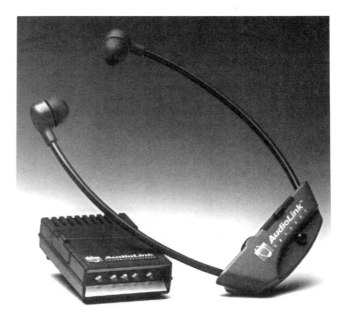

Figure 42.3. Personal infrared systems can provide enhanced listening, particularly for television enjoyment. (Shown: The Audio-Link™ Infra Red System) (Photo provided by the National Captioning Institute.)

Table 42.2
Uses of Large Area and Personal Infrared Systems

Theaters
   Infrared systems can be made available to impaired patrons at local theaters and movie houses, thus, making entertainment more accessible.
Television
   Personal infrared systems can be easily installed for use at home. Use of such a system does not affect TV volume; therefore, viewing with friends and family is possible.
Business
   Infrared systems can be installed in offices and conference rooms to allow the hearing-impaired worker to participate in meetings.
Worship
   Places of worship can have receivers available for the participants of religious services.

would intersperse among the naturally occurring light waves present outdoors, thus, destroying the transmitted signal. For sound enhancement needs that extend beyond a single room or to the outdoors, FM technology is the preferred method.

FM Systems

As mentioned earlier, FM systems provide a wireless means of transmitting the sound source to the listener. The auditory signal is picked up by a microphone and is transmitted in the form of radio frequency modulated carrier waves to a personal receiver that is worn by the hearing impaired listener

(Fig. 42.4). Each FM system consists of a transmitter with a specific radio carrier frequency, an antenna, and a compatible receiver. The Federal Communication Commission (FCC) has allocated the frequency region of 72 to 76 MHz as the Auditory Assistance Band for assisting hearing-impaired persons with communication (Beaulac, Pehringer, and Shough, 1989). This frequency region has typically been divided into 32 subregions, thus allowing for 32 different transmitting frequencies.

There are essentially two types of FM systems. The first of these is a complete system consisting of: (1) an FM microphone located on the transmitter with associated antenna; (2) an environmental microphone on the FM receiver; and (3) an amplifier sufficiently powerful to allow the receiver to function as a hearing aid.

The environmental microphones are located either in the receiver or in "dummy" hearing aids (microphones only) worn at ear level. The complete FM system is frequently the amplification system of choice for use in educational settings.

The second type of FM system, often referred to as a personal FM system, involves the coupling of the FM system to the client's personal hearing aids. The FM system in this case functions as an assistive listening device. Direct or indirect coupling can be used with personal FM systems. Direct coupling includes the use of earphones, insert earbuds, external receivers with earmolds, or direct audio input to the hearing aid. In this latter approach, the FM receiver is hardwired to an

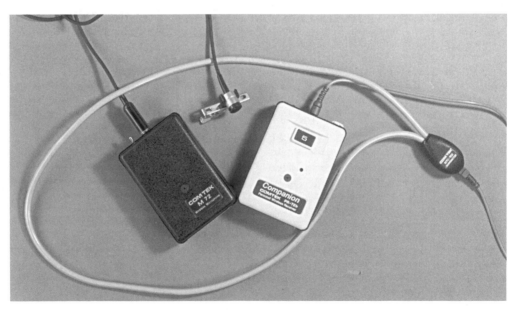

Figure 42.4. FM technology allows effective amplification in various listening situations. Signal-to-noise ratios are increased, thereby improving communication in areas of background noise.

(Shown: ComTek AT 72 transmitter, receiver, microphone, and induction neckloop)

electronic plug attached directly to the hearing aid. Indirect coupling with a client's existing hearing aid can be achieved by magnetic induction, either through the use of a neckloop or a silhouette miniloop lying flat against the hearing aid. Care needs to be taken when indirect coupling is used. Researchers have shown that indirect coupling via telecoil loop or direct coupling via direct audio boot may alter the frequency response obtained at the output (Thibideau and Saucedo, 1991; Thibideau, McCaffrey, and Abrahamson, 1988; and Hawkins and Schum, 1985). When the latter occurs, it is usually due to an impedance mismatch between the various electronic components. Hence, the electroacoustic characteristics of the personal hearing aid may not be preserved. Therefore, an electroacoustic evaluation of the effects of indirect or direct coupling should be done before FM usage.

Recently, FM systems have been developed that use FM sound field technology as a means of providing amplification (Sarff, 1981). In this situation, the speaker wears a microphone and portable transmitter. The speaker's voice is transmitted on the FM carrier signal and is picked up by a receiver-amplifier that is placed somewhere in the room. The receiver-amplifier, in turn, is connected by hardwire to a number of loudspeakers strategically placed within the room to produce an equally loud signal throughout the room. For those capable of benefiting (such as preschool and kindergarten children, minimally hearing-impaired, or CAPD children), this system provides a nonintrusive means of increasing the signal-noise ratio. (Flexer, 1993). Another advantage of this system is that it can be more cost effective than other FM systems. For further information regarding the classroom use of FM amplification, the reader is referred to Chapter 33 of this text.

FM systems have been used successfully with various hearing- and listening-impaired populations. FM systems have not only been shown to be effective with severely or profoundly hearing-impaired populations but also with children who exhibit unilateral hearing loss (Cargill and Flexer, 1991; Bess, 1986), central auditory dysfunction (Stach, Loisette, and Jerger, 1987) minimal hearing loss and children with developmental disabilities (Flexer, Millin and Brown, 1990). Increasingly, they are becoming the ALD of choice in schools for the hearing impaired, mainstream settings, early intervention programs, as well as among hearing-impaired adults. Recently, the American Speech-Language and Hearing Association (1991) recommended the use of complete FM systems with hearing-impaired infants to enhance direct language stimulation.

Because of the use of radio waves, FM systems are not subject to the limitations found with hardwire and infrared systems. They can be used outdoors as well as in classrooms, auditoriums, and living rooms. They can be used for interpersonal communication or linked with tape recorders or televisions.

There are, however, some disadvantages to the use of this system. FM systems can pick up interference from signals passed along the same FM carrier waves. For example, many paging systems (beepers) have their carrier frequency within the FCC-designated band of 72–76 MHz and, thus, may interfere with the FM transmission. Another problem may occur if duplicate FM channels are used. In this case, only the stronger signal will be picked up by the receiver. This is known as the "captive effect." Proper training is necessary for teachers to ensure appropriate usage of these systems.

Finances may be a consideration when recommending the use of FM systems. Although there is a wide range in the cost of these devices, they are significantly more expensive than hardwire amplification.

FM systems can be used in a variety of ways, from primary amplification to as assistive listening device for use in a classroom or theater. Table 42.3 describes some uses of FM technology.

TELEVISION ENHANCEMENT TECHNOLOGY

Television plays an important role in the lives of many individuals. It can be a source of information and education as well as provide an economical means of entertainment. It can provide daily activities for individuals confined to home or can be the source for

Table 42.3
Uses of FM System

Classrooms
  FM systems can be used in classes for the hearing-impaired as well as in mainstreamed classes for improving signal-to-noise ratio. They can also be used as auditory trainers for speech therapy.
Employment
  Use of these systems can help improve communication at meetings and for one-to-one situations. A conference microphone can allow greater participation.
Infants
  FM systems can help provide direct language stimulation between the parent and the hearing-impaired child.
Travel
  Any travel that requires listening to a tour guide presentation can be improved by the use of wireless FM.
Adult Education
  FM systems have been used for adult continuing education, as well as for use in college lecture hall settings.
Arenas
  Theaters, arenas, and places of worship can have FM system technology available.

creative play in a child's school yard. Nevertheless for hearing-impaired individuals and their families, it can be a source of great frustration.

Television enhancement technology consists of those devices that are used to improve a hearing-impaired individual's perception of a televised auditory signal. These devices, many within the sound enhancement technology classification described earlier, can transmit a television's audio signal directly to a listener, while maintaining a normal television volume, or produce a visual representation of the auditory signal. Systems that do not interrupt the normal television volume are especially practical for they allow family and friends to watch television at their own preferred loudness level.

Sound enhancement technology can be easily adapted for use in television viewing. The signal can be transmitted to the listener via hardwire, infrared, or FM systems and can linked to the hearing aid through the use of magnetic induction. Microphone placement for use with sound enhancement systems may be at the site of the television's external speaker or through the use of an output jack.

For many individuals with severe/profound hearing impairment or poor speech recognition ability, the use of sound enhancement technology is not sufficient. These individuals require visual information to supplement or replace the audio signal. The process by which this is accomplished is known as closed captioning. Closed captions are hidden subtitles that are provided in one band of the televised signal. To visualize these subtitles, either an external decoder or a decoder chip built into the television is required. Telecaption decoders are commercially available at major department stores as well as through the National Captioning Institute (NCI). The NCI is a nonprofit corporation that provides closed captioning services to the television and movie industry.

The amount of closed captioned programming has increased significantly over the years and is now available for many programs on the major networks and cable stations. In addition, most videotapes and even some music videos provide captioning for their hearing-impaired viewers. A list of closed captioned videotapes is available through NCI.

TELECOMMUNICATION TECHNOLOGY

Telephone communication is a major component of the auditory activities of daily living. In the past, the only amplification option available to hearing aid users was via magnetic induction. A telecoil loop was present within the handset of the telephone, the presence of which resulted in magnetic field leakage of the ongoing telephone signal. Activation of the T-switch on the hearing aid allowed the listener to pick up the magnetic field, convert it to an electric signal and amplify it through the hearing aid. An additional benefit of this system was the reduction of environmental noise since the use of the T-switch disengaged the environmental microphone. Today, however, there are a variety of amplification methods available to hearing-impaired individuals. This is especially pertinent because of the increased popularity of in-the-ear and in-the-canal aids, many of which do not have a telecoil. This fact creates a greater demand for alternative amplification products.

One event that had a great impact on the development of telecommunication technology for the hearing impaired was the Carter Phone Decision in 1968. This federal mandate permitted products not manufactured by AT&T to be used on AT&T lines. It resulted in the market being flooded with a wide array of telephones, many of which were not built to any standard (Slager, 1989). Consequently, many manufacturers eliminated the induction loop from the handset, thus, creating incompatibility with hearing aids. Hearing-impaired consumer groups worked to ensure telephone accessibility for all hearing-impaired individuals. The lobbying efforts have been quite successful with the passage of a number of recent laws. The latest, the Americans with Disabilities Act—1990 (ADA-1990) mandates telephone accessibility for all individuals with disabilities.

Today, there are a variety of amplification systems available for telephone use. Deciding which telecommunication technology is best suited for a particular hearing-impaired individual requires not only an understanding of the specific hearing loss but an awareness of the various styles and telephone systems in existence. Many of the telephone amplification devices require the use of modular phones, that is, phones that have detachable receivers and input jacks.

There are three common styles of telephone amplifiers: amplified handsets, in-line amplifiers, and portable strap-on amplifiers. Amplified handsets require the use of a modular telephone. These devices increase the loudness of the incoming telephone signal. They contain a volume control located in the body of the handset and adjustments are made by the listener. Typical amplified handsets have either a rotary or touch panel volume control. Other models may come equipped with an additional push button volume boost to increase the signal (Fig. 42.5).

In-line amplifiers are interfaced between the body of the telephone and the handset. Modular telephones

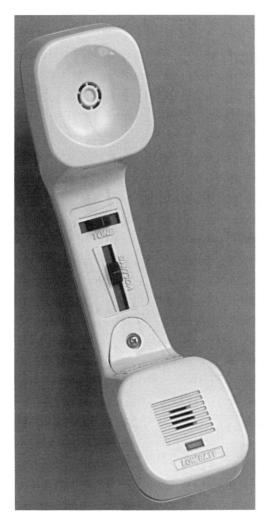

Figure 42.5. The AT&T Model K65 is an example of an amplified telephone handset. The listener has the capability to increase the loudness and change the tone of the incoming telephone call. (Shown: AT&T Model K 65) (Photo provided by AT&T.)

allow the amplification device to be connected to the base of the telephone where the handset is normally attached. A standard handset is then connected directly to the amplifier. As with the amplified handsets, a rotary volume control is used to adjust the desired loudness of the signal (Fig. 42.5).

Portable strap-on amplifiers are available for use on a variety of phones. They are small, portable systems that can be used by individuals who travel and who use several different telephones. This style of amplifier frequently requires the use of an induction system to provide amplification. Therefore, they should be used only on hearing aid compatible telephones. The AT&T strap on amplifier, however, can be used not only to provide amplification but also for converting a

nonhearing aid compatible telephone into an induction system (Fig. 42.6).

Amplification devices may not always be able to provide the necessary amplification for individuals with severe/profound hearing loss or poor speech recognition. For these individuals, visual systems are available to help make telephone communication accessible. Text Telephones (TT) also known as Telephone Devices for the Deaf (TDD) or Teletypewriters (TTY), are based on teletypewriter technology and transmit visual signals over the standard telephone line. It is necessary that both parties have TT systems to communicate. As one person types his message, the signal is transmitted along the telephone line and is decoded at the other end by the TT receiver. The message is seen on a line screen built into the TT (Fig. 42.7).

Many states have initiated TT relay systems to increase phone communication for hearing-impaired people. The use of a relay system allows hearing-impaired TT users to communicate through an outside operator with a non-TT party. That is, the individual with the TT types a message that is picked up by a telephone operator. The operator then relays

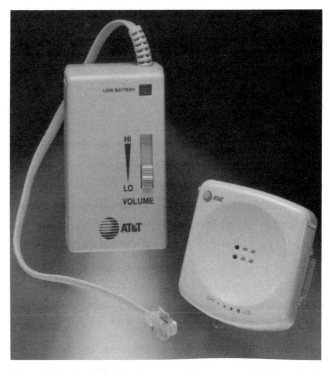

Figure 42.6. Portable telephone amplifiers are available for use in travel and business. In-line amplifiers are frequently used on home and business telephone systems. (Shown: The AT&T Portable Amplifier II and the AT&T Auxiliary Amplifier) (Photo provided by AT&T.)

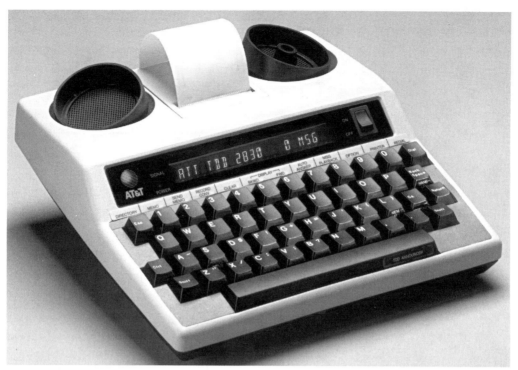

Figure 42.7. The use of a text telephone (TT) allows telephone communication for individuals who are unable to hear or understand speech over the phone. Individual state relay systems and the use of a TT make telephone communication accessible. (Shown: AT&T TDD 2830) (Photo provided by AT&T.)

the message by voice to the non TT party. The latter, in turn, speaks to the operator who then relays the message via TT to the TT party. This eliminates the need for both parties having a TT, thereby increasing accessibility of telephone communication. The ADA-1990 mandates that companies offering telephone service to the general public must offer relay services to hearing-impaired consumers who use TTs.

SIGNAL/ALERTING TECHNOLOGY

Auditory activities of daily living, such as hearing a doorbell or a telephone ring, waking to an alarm clock, or listening for a baby cry, may not be heard by many hearing-impaired individuals and may therefore be a source of great anxiety and frustration. This has led to the development of signal/alerting technology for the purpose of alerting hearing-impaired persons to the presence of environmental signals. Alerting can be done through the use of auditory (amplified), visual, or tactile signals. Alerting devices can be simple individual units for use with a single telephone or doorbell, or multi-line systems using FM transmission for signal detection throughout an entire living environment.

Larose, Evans, and Larose (1989) described three methods of sound pick-up used in alerting device tech-

nology: sound-activated systems, direct connect systems, and induction systems. Sound-activated systems detect the presence of sound through nearby microphone placement. The microphone is connected to an electronic switching mechanism. Any sound that is picked up by the microphone and exceeds a predetermined level results in the activation of the electronic switching mechanism. This, in turn, causes electric current to flow to an interfaced signal device, such as a lamp or vibrator. Sound-activated systems are frequently portable and are advantageous to hearing-impaired individuals who travel. A disadvantage of this system is that ambient noise can result in numerous false signals. Many of these devices have a sensitivity setting that is used to preset the necessary loudness of the signal before the switching mechanism can be activated. This may help to reduce the false signal responses, but it does not generally eliminate the problem.

Direct connect systems are electronically interfaced to the signal source and are activated directly by the electrical system of the equipment (such as those of a telephone and doorbell). The use of this type of pick up system eliminates the false signals that can occur with sound-activated systems. It is a more permanently installed system, however, and therefore reduces its portability.

Induction sound pick-up utilizes electromagnetic energy created by the signal source. These systems are generally interfaced with the desired signal through the use of a suction cup. The electromagnetic signal created at the source triggers the switching mechanism of the induction pick-up, then activates the signal device. Coupling the system through the use of a suction cup can result, however, in inconsistent response or nonresponse due to the possible removal or displacement of the suction device. These systems are frequently portable and suitable for travel.

In addition to the above alerting technology, programs have become available to train hearing ear dogs. These dogs are professionally trained to alert their hearing-impaired owner to a number of different sounds in a variety of listening situations (Polk, 1991). The dog and the owner must train together at a specified training setting and, for a period of time, within the owner's home environment. The hearing dog's responsibility is to attract the attention of the owner when they hear the doorbell, telephone, fire alarm, etc. and lead them to the source of the sound. Table 42.4 describes a variety of uses for signal alerting devices.

REHABILITATION TECHNOLOGY AS PART OF THE AURAL REHABILITATION PROCESS

Assessment

The puretone audiogram provides the audiologist with information that pertains to the degree and nature of a person's hearing impairment. It does not, however, provide information regarding the effects of the hearing loss on a person's behavior and daily functioning. Understanding an individual's performance in the auditory activities of daily living can help determine the need for rehabilitative devices.

Table 42.4
Uses of Signal/Alerting Technology

Alarm Clocks can be set up to activate a lamp or strobe light to awaken a hearing-impaired person. A pillow vibrator or bed shaker can also be used if needed.

Telephone systems can be designed to activate lights in various rooms in a home. They can also be used to trigger a control device that can activate a vibrotactile wristband.

Baby cry systems can be used to alert a hearing-impaired parent to the sound of a crying child. These systems can be visual or vibrotactile. Vibrotactile wristbands can be used to alert the hearing-impaired person to such signals as a baby cry, doorbell and telephone.

Travel can be enhanced by the use of a portable alerting device that can be used to indicate the presence of a hotel telephone ring or emergency alarm, such as a smoke detector. The portable feature is important because few hotel chains have these devices available for their hearing-impaired guests.

Self-assessment inventories and hearing handicap scales have been developed that enable the audiologist to explore further the behavioral effects that a hearing impairment may have on a person's functioning. These diagnostic tests can provide valuable information in planning a patient's rehabilitation program. Understanding the needs of the patient who is being assessed, why the assessment is being performed, and what information needs to be obtained is critical in deciding which scale to choose (Demorest and Walden, 1984). Weinstein (1984) summarized many of the available self-assessment scales available for use by the audiologist.

The information obtained from any of the assessment scales not only provides the audiologist with the basis for choosing rehabilitation goals, including the selection of rehabilitation technology but can also be used in counseling. It is through the counseling process that one can learn of and remediate the difficulties experienced.

In addition to self-assessment scales, needs assessment questionnaires have also been developed. These questionnaires allow the audiologist to determine the technology that would be most beneficial to the patient as well as ascertain the equipment already being used by the client. Moore and Compton (1990) developed a comprehensive needs questionnaire that can provide the audiologist with information concerning the clients's use of hearing aids, problem listening situations, signal alerting situations, devices already in use, and devices available in the community (Appendix 42.1). Needs assessment can be performed in a paper/pencil format or through patient history and interview.

Rehabilitation Considerations For Hearing-Impaired Patients

Recommendations for rehabilitation need to be made according to the specific needs of each individual patient. As mentioned previously, assessment scales, needs questionnaires and counseling are all crucial components to any successful rehabilitation program.

Part of this rehabilitation process should include the selection of rehabilitation technology. The selection of rehabilitation technology should be considered as part of the hearing aid evaluation process. That is, we not only need to decide whether the client needs hearing aids but at the same time we need to consider whether the client would benefit from any additional rehabilitation technology. Decisions regarding ALDs may, in fact, influence the hearing aid selection process. For example, assessing the need for sound enhancement technology may factor into the decision regarding the use of a T-switch on a hearing aid.

A number of factors, therefore should to be considered when determining the rehabilitation technology needs of an individual. These include:

1. Degree of hearing loss;
2. Type of hearing aids to be worn;
3. Hearing aid options (such as inclusion of a T-switch, direct audio input, or some special circuitry (CROS aid));
4. Financial concerns; and
5. Family support.

After the initial selection process, rehabilitation goals need to be developed that encompass the areas such as: hearing aid orientation, speech reading, auditory training, and coping strategies. For further information regarding aural rehabilitation, the reader is referred to Chapters 38-49 of this text.

ASSISTIVE LISTENING DEVICE CENTER

Rehabilitation technology can be found in various settings, such as: speech and hearing centers, universities, schools for the hearing impaired (Fellendorf, 1982), hospitals (Montano and Weinstein, 1988), community centers and consumer organizations. Killingsworth (1989) describes three models of assistive listening device dispensing programs commonly found in the United States: the university setting, the assistive listening device den, and the hearing aid dispensary.

Three Models

University settings tend to provide information sessions to members of the community followed by product demonstration. These sessions may be staffed by volunteers, university personnel, or graduate students.

The second model consists of an assistive listening device "den" that is staffed by volunteers who are trained and supervised by audiologists. A variety of rehabilitative technology systems are displayed with demonstrations provided to both patients and members of the community.

The third model is the hearing aid dispensary. In this model, systems are recommended as well as sold. This model generally integrates assistive listening devices into the hearing aid evaluation process. The devices are available for demonstration directly in the dispenser's office.

An example of a hospital-based rehabilitation technology program was described by Montano and Weinstein (1988). They reported on an assistive listening device program that was run within a metropolitan specialty care hospital. The program contained both a rehabilitation session as well as access to a rehabilitation technology center for the hearing impaired. The rehabilitation session consisted of: (a) review of audiometric findings; (b) hearing aid check/orientation; (c) administration of self-assessment inventories; (d) counseling; and (e) demonstration of rehabilitation technology. The assistive listening device center was set up to resemble a typical living room equipped with various devices. The room was designed to create a comfortable environment for counseling and to enable the patient to experience assistive listening devices as they would within their homes.

Rehabilitation Technology and the Audiologist

The Americans with Disabilities Act of 1990 requires that employment, transportation, public accommodations, state and local government, and telecommunications become more accessible to the hearing impaired. Rehabilitation technology will play an important role in the creation of barrier-free environments for the hearing impaired. Auditoriums and large public meeting places will need to provide amplification for those participants requiring it. Telephones will need to be hearing aid compatible. Employers will not be able to discriminate against a hearing-impaired employee and will need to provide the necessary equipment to permit job performance. To create these "barrier free" communication environments, audiologists will have to play an important role in providing the necessary assistive technology to the hearing-impaired consumer, employers, and public facilities.

Assistive listening devices have already gained considerable popularity within the hearing-impaired community. Consumer organizations such as the Self Help for Hard of Hearing People, Inc. (SHHH) have been strong advocates for their use. SHHH has established a national database that lists the approximately 8000 cultural, recreational, educational, and religious settings that provide assistive systems. Appendix 42.2 provides a resource list indicating sources and distributors of rehabilitation technology for the hearing impaired.

Information concerning rehabilitation technology continues to expand. Journal and textbook publications have included chapters and articles on assistive listening devices. Many university programs in audiology include discussions of assistive listening devices in their graduate curriculum; however, the inclusion of rehabilitation technology into everyday audiology practice has generally been limited.

Malinoff, Kisiel, Kisiel and Dygert (1989) reported on a survey of 921 hearing aid providers who were asked to rank the services they felt were most important to their practices. Assistive listening devices and aural rehabilitation were felt to be the two least important services. Respondents in this study included: private practice audiologists, otolaryngologists, hospital-based dispensing audiologists, and hearing instrument specialists. Cranmer (1991) reported that assistive listening devices accounted for approximately 1.6% of hearing aid dispensers' gross sales for 1990. Both of these reports sadly suggest that assistive listening devices to the hearing impaired still play a minimal role in the amplification process. It is hoped that reports such as these as well as empirical research will educate audiologists about the usefulness of ALDS and aural rehabilitation in general.

REFERENCES

American Speech-Language and Hearing Association. The use of FM amplification instruments for infants and preschool children with hearing impairment. ASHA 1991;32(Suppl 5):1–2.

American Speech-Language and Hearing Association. Definition of and competencies for aural rehabilitation. ASHA 1984;26:37–41.

Beaulac DA, Pehringer JL, and Shough LF. Assistive listening devices: Available options. Semin Hear 1989;10:11–29.

Beck LB, and Nance GC. Hearing aids, assistive listening devices and telephones: Issues to consider. Semin Hear 1989;10:78–89.

Bess FH. The unilaterally hearing impaired child: A final comment. Ear Hear 1986;7:52–54.

Cargill S, and Flexer C. Strategies for fitting FM units to children with unilateral hearing loss. Hear Instrum 1991;42:26–27.

Compton C. Assistive devices: An overview. ADA Feedback 1990; Winter:19–29.

Compton C. Assistive technology for deaf & hard of hearing people. In J. Alpiner, & P. McCarthy (Eds). Rehabilitative Audiology Children & Adults. Baltimore: Williams & Wilkins, 1993, pp. 441–469.

Cranmer KS. Hearing instrument dispensing—1991. Hear Instrum 1991;42:6–13.

Demorest M, and Walden B. Psychometric principles in the selection, interpretation, and evaluation of communication self assessment inventories. JSHD 1984;49:226–240.

Flexer C. Management of hearing in an educational setting. In J. Alpiner, P. McCarthy (Eds.). Rehabilitative Audiology Children & Adults. Baltimore: Williams & Wilkins, 1993; pp 176–210.

Flexer C, Millin J, and Brown L. Children with developmental disa-

bilities: The effect of sound field amplification on word identification. LSHSS 1990;21:177–182.

Fellendorf G. A model demonstration center of assistive devices for hearing impaired people. Acad Rehabil Audiol 1982;15:70–82.

Hawkins DB, and Schum DJ. Some effects of FM system coupling on hearing aid characteristics. JSHD 1985;50:132–141.

Killingsworth CA. Using assistive devices in hearing health care practice. Semin Hear 1989;10:103–120.

Larose GM, Evans MP, and Larose RW. Alerting devices: Available options. Semin Hear 1989;10:66–77.

Leavitt RJ. Considerations for use of rehabilitation technology by hearing impaired persons. Semin Hear 1989;10:1–10.

Leavitt RJ. Promoting the use of rehabilitation technology. ASHA 1987;29:28–31.

Mahon WJ. Assistive devices and systems. Hear J 1985;38:7–14.

Malinoff R, Kisiel D, Kisiel S, and Dygert P. The dispensing of hearing instruments: A study on industry structures and trends. Hear Instrum 1990;41:12–14.

McCarthy PA, Montgomery AA, and Mueller HG. Decision making in rehabilitative audiology. J Am Acad Audiol 1990;1:23–30.

Montano JJ, and Weinstein B. Assistive listening devices: The people who use them. Paper presented at ASHA Convention, Boston, MA, 1988.

Moore J, and Compton C. Communication Needs Questionnaire. Washington, DC: Gallaudet University, Department of Audiology and Speech Language Pathology, 1990.

Polk A. Hearing dogs: Concept reality. Notes of the Proceedings 6th International SHHH Convention, 1991:64–66.

Sarff L. An innovative use of free field amplification in classrooms. In Roeser R, and Downs M, Eds. Auditory Disorders in School Children. New York: Thieme Stratton, 1981:263–272.

Slager RD. Romancing the phone: The adventure continues. Semin Hear 1989;10:42–56.

Stach BA, Loisette LH, and Jerger JF. FM system use with central auditory processing disorder. Paper presented at ASHA Convention. New Orleans, LA, 1987.

Thibideau L, and Saucedo K. Consistency of electroacoustic characteristics across components of FM systems. JSHR 1991;34:628–635.

Thibideau LM, McCaffrey H, and Abrahamson J. Effects of coupling hearing aids to FM systems via neck loops. J Acad Rehabil Audiol 1988;21:49–56.

Vaughn GR, Lightfoot RK, and Gibbs SD. Assistive listening devices part III; SPACE. ASHA 1983;25:33–39.

Weinstein B. A review of hearing handicap scales. Audiology 1984;9:91–109.

Weinstein B, and Amsel L. The relationship between dementia and hearing impairment in the institutionalized elderly. Clin Gerontol 1986;4:3–15.

Appendix 42.1.

Name _____ CLIENT NO. _____

DATE _____

COMMUNICATION NEEDS QUESTIONNAIRE

Whether you use a hearing aid or not, you may hear fairly well in some situations while having to strain to hear in others. Your answers on this questionnaire will help point to ways to help you hear better in as many situations as possible.

Read the statements and questions below. Place a check mark by the statements that are true for you and answer the questions. You may have to complete some of the statements by filling in information in the middle or at the end of the statement. PLEASE FEEL FREE TO MAKE COMMENTS OR ASK QUESTIONS **ANYWHERE** ON THE QUESTIONNAIRE.

HEARING AID(S)

_____ I DO NOT OWN A HEARING AID; I AM INTERESTED IN FINDING OUT IF ONE CAN HELP ME.

_____ I DO NOT OWN A HEARING AID; I AM NOT INTERESTED IN GETTING A HEARING AID AT THIS TIME BECAUSE (Write in the reason you are not interested in getting a hearing aid at this time.):

_____ I OWN A HEARING AID NOW BUT DO NOT USE IT BECAUSE (Write in the reason you don't use your hearing aid.):

_____ I OWNED A HEARING AID AT ONE TIME; I QUIT USING THE HEARING AID BECAUSE (Write in the reason you stopped using your hearing aid.):

[IF YOU _DO NOT_ USE A HEARING AID NOW, SKIP TO THE NEXT SECTION CALLED "PROBLEM LISTENING SITUATIONS".]
I OWN A(N)

_____ BEHIND-THE-EAR HEARING AID.

_____ IN-THE-EAR HEARING AID.

_____ IN-THE-CANAL HEARING AID.

_____ BODY HEARING AID.

_____ EYEGLASS HEARING AID.

_____ OTHER (Explain)

_____ I OWN A HEARING AID AND USE IT (Mark how often you use the hearing aid.):

_____ all day long every day.

_____ off and on during the day.

_____ only a few times a week.

_____ only on special occasions.

_____ I WOULD USE MY HEARING AID MORE OFTEN IF (Write in ways you think your hearing aid could work better for you.):

_____ I USE MY HEARING AID WHEN LISTENING ON THE TELEPHONE BY:

_____ using the "T" (telecoil switch).

_____ holding the telephone receiver next to the hearing aid microphone.

IF YOU HAVE PROBLEMS USING YOUR HEARING AID ON THE TELEPHONE, EXPLAIN WHY:

_____ I DON'T USE MY HEARING AID WHEN TALKING ON THE TELEPHONE BECAUSE (Write in the reason you don't use your hearing aid on the telephone.):

PROBLEM LISTENING SITUATIONS

I WOULD LIKE TO HEAR BETTER IN THE FOLLOWING SITUATIONS: (CHECK ALL THAT APPLY.)

_____ over the telephone when I am at home

_____ over the telephone when I am at work

_____ over the telephone when I am travelling, at other people's homes, at pay phones, etc.

_____ television: regular broadcast stations only

_____ television: broadcast stations plus cable and/or VCR

_____ with one other person sitting at home (den, living room, dining room, at mealtime, watching television, etc.)

_____ while riding or driving in the car

_____ with people with whom I transact personal business (doctor, nurse, attorney, banker, insurance or real estate agent, etc.)

_____ with one or two other people in social situations (visiting, playing cards or boardgames, etc.)

_____ at work with my employer, employees, co-workers

_____ eating out (restaurant, cafeteria, etc.)

_____ in a small family group at home

_____ in a small discussion group (5 people or less)

_____ in a small recreation/leisure group (cards, boardgames, handiwork, etc.)

_____ at a small dinner party

_____ in a place of worship (church, synagogue, meeting room)

_____ at a meeting where there is one main speaker at a time.

_____ at a meeting where there is a panel discussion

_____ at a lecture where there is audience participation

_____ in a classroom

_____ at a lecture or other presentation

_____ in a movie theatre

_____ at the theatre (live play)

_____ at concerts or other live musical/dramatic programs

_____ OTHER situations in which I would like to be able to hear better (Write in your answer(s)):

THREE OF THE MOST DIFFICULT LISTENING SITUATIONS FOR ME ARE:
(Add more if you want to.)

1)

2)

3)

SIGNALING AND ALERTING SITUATIONS

I WOULD BE INTERESTED IN A DEVICE WHICH WOULD HELP ME HEAR:

_____ MY TELEPHONE RING

_____ MY DOORBELL

_____ MY ALARM CLOCK

_____ MY SMOKE OR BURGLAR ALARM

_____ A BABY OR BEDRIDDEN PERSON CALLING ME FROM ANOTHER ROOM

_____ A STOVE OR MICROWAVE OVEN TIMER

_____ MY WASHER OR DRYER OR OTHER APPLIANCE

_____ OTHER

IF YOU ALREADY USE ONE OR MORE OF THE ABOVE DEVICES, PLACE AN ASTERISK (*) BY EACH DEVICE YOU USE.

SPECIAL COMMUNICATION DEVICES I ALREADY USE

(IF YOU DO NOT USE ANY SPECIAL COMMUNICATION DEVICES NOW, SKIP AHEAD TO THE NEXT SECTION TITLED "SPECIAL LISTENING DEVICES AVAILABLE IN MY COMMUNITY".]

I ALREADY OWN AND USE THE FOLLOWING DEVICES (fill in or circle brand names):

_____ amplified handset for the telephone

_____ in-line telephone amplifier (connects between receiver and body of phone)

_____ portable telephone amplifier (Radio Shack, AT&T, etc.)

_____ portable telephone adapter for "T" switch (Rastronics, Phonear)

_____ TDD (TTY)

_____ direct earphone connection to TV, radio, tape player, dictaphone

_____ remote microphone which plugs into hearing aid

_____ personal hardwired listening device (Pocketalker, Audex, RadioShack)

_____ AM/FM/TV Band radio:

_____ next to chair and turned up

_____ next to chair with neck loop and hearing aid on "T"

_____ hearing aid plugged directly into radio earphone jack

_____ infrared listening system for TV (Sennheiser, Audex, SoundPlus, RadioShack, etc.)

_____ FM listening system (Comtek, Phonic Ear, Telex, Williams Sound, etc.)

_____ loop system for TV (using hearing aid on "T")

_____ loop system for classroom or meeting room (using hearing aid on "T" or special telecoil receiver with earphones)

_____ Closed captioned decoder

_____ OTHER (Please name or describe any other special listening devices you use.):

IF YOU USE COMMUNICATION DEVICES, USE THIS SPACE TO EXPLAIN HOW OFTEN YOU USE THEM AND HOW MUCH THEY HELP YOU. ALSO, BE SURE TO INCLUDE PROBLEMS YOU HAVE EXPERIENCED WHILE USING THESE SYSTEMS:

SPECIAL LISTENING SYSTEMS AVAILABLE IN MY COMMUNITY

A SPECIAL LISTENING DEVICE IS AVAILABLE AT THE FOLLOWING PLACES I GO TO: (FOR EACH PLACE, INCLUDE THE TYPE OF DEVICE INSTALLED, IF YOU KNOW IT: I=infrared; F=FM; L=audio loop; H=hardwired. Eg.: _F_ Church/Synagogue means that an FM system is located at your church or synagogue. If you do not know the type of system installed, just place a checkmark.)

_____ CHURCH/SYNAGOGUE
_____ THEATRE (LIVE PLAYS AND CONCERTS)
_____ MOVIE THEATRE
_____ COMMUNITY THEATRE
_____ OTHER (Write in other places that have special listening devices.):

_____ I *HAVE* TRIED TO USE ONE OR MORE OF THESE DEVICES.
_____ I *HAVE NOT* TRIED TO USE ANY OF THESE DEVICES BECAUSE:
    _____ I do not know how to find out about using the device.

_____ I hear well enough with my own hearing (+ hearing aid).
_____ I do not think it will help.
_____ I do not know if it will help.
_____ I do not know if it will help.
_____ I feel self-conscious about using the device in public.
_____ OTHER (Write in any other reason you may not have used these hearing devices.):

ADDITIONAL COMMENTS

On the back of this page, please feel free to add any information you feel would be important in helping us to understand your listening needs:

More J, and Compton C. 1988.

Appendix 42.2.

REHABILITATION TECHNOLOGY RESOURCE LIST

Resources Centers:
Alexander Graham Bell Association
1537 35 Street NW
Washington, DC 20007
Voice and TT (202) 337-5220

Gallaudet University
National Information Center on Deafness
800 Florida Avenue NE
Washington, DC 20002-3625
Voice (202) 651-5051 TT (202) 651-5052

Hearing and Speech Center of Rochester
1000 Elmwood Avenue
Rochester, NY 14620
Voice (716) 271-0680 (TT (716) 442-2988

Manhattan Eye Ear and Throat Hospital
Department of Communication Disorders
210 E. 64 Street
New York, NY 10021
Voice and TT (212) 605-3740

National Technical Institute for the Deaf
One Lomb Memorial Drive
Rochester, NY 14623
Voice (716) 475-6400 TT (716) 475-2181

New York League for the Hard of Hearing
71 W. 23 Street
New York, NY 10010
Voice (212) 741-7650 TT (212) 255-1932

Self Help for Hard of Hearing People, Inc. (SHHH)
7800 Wisconsin Avenue
Bethesda, MD 20814
Voice (301) 657-2248 TT (301) 657-2249

Manufacturers and Distributors:
SE = Sound Enhancement Technology
TE = Television Enhancement
TC = Telecommunication Technology
SA = Signal Alerting Technology

American Loop Systems   SE
43 Davis Road, Suite 2
Belmont, MA 02178
(617) 776-5667

AT&T National Special Needs Center TC, SA, SE
2001 Route 46 East
Parsippany, NJ 07054-1315
(800) 233-1222 TT (800) 833-3232

Audex   SE
713 N. 4 Street
Longview, TX 75601
(908) 753-7058

Audio Enhancement   SE
Com Tek
1746 W. 12600 S.
Riverton, UT 84065
Voice and TT (800) 383-9362

Hal Han Co.   SE, TE, TC, SA
35-53 24 Street
Long Island City, NY 11106
(718) 392-6260

Harc Mercantile, Ltd.   SE, TE, TC, SA
PO Box 3055
Kalamazoo, MI 49003-3055
Voice and TT (800) 445-9968

HEAR YOU ARE, Inc.   SE, TE, TC, SA
4 Musconetcong Avenue
Stanhope, NJ 07874
Voice and TT (201) 347-7662

HITEC   SE, TE, TC, SA
8205 Cass Avenue
Darien, IL 60559
Voice and TT (800) 288-8303
           (708) 963-5588

International Hearing Dog, Inc.   SA
5901 East 89 Avenue
Henderson, CO 80640
Voice and TT (303) 287-3277

Krown Research, Inc.   TC
129 Sheldon Street
El Segundo, CA 90245
Voice and TT (213) 322-3202

National Captioning Institute   TE, SE
5203 Leesburg Pike
Falls Church, VA 22041
Voice or TT (703) 998-2416

National Flashing Signal Systems   SA
8120 Fenton Street
Silver Spring, MD 20910
Voice and TT (301) 589-6671

Oval Window Audio   SE
33 Wildflower Court
Nederland, CO 80466
Voice and TT (303) 447-3607

Phone TTY   TC, SA
202 Lexington Avenue
Hackensack, NJ 07601
Voice (201) 489-7889
RR (201) 489-7890

Phonic Ear, Inc.   SE
3880 Cypress Drive
Petaluma, CA 949-7600
Voice and TT (800) 772-3374

Plantronics   TC
345 Encinal Street
Santa Cruz, CA 95060
(408) 426-5858

Quest Electronics   SA
510 So. Worthington Street
Oconomowoc, WI 53066
Voice (800) 245-0779
TT (800) 558-9526

Radio Shack   SE, TE, SA
1800 One Tandy Center
Fort Worth, TX 76102
(817) 390-3700

Red Acre Farm Hearing Dog Center SA
Box 278
109 Red Acre Road
Stow, MA 01775
Voice and TT (508) 897-8343

SEHAS, Inc.   SE, TE, TC, SA
533 Peachtree Street NE
Atlanta, GA 30308
(800) 241-2465

Siemens Hearing Instruments, Inc.   SE, TE
10 Constitution Avenue
Piscataway, NJ 08855 (800) 766-4500

Silent Call Corp.   SA
PO Box 868
Clarkston, MI 48347-0868
Voice (313) 391-1710
TDD (313) 391-1799

Sonic Alert   SA
1750 W. Hamlin Road
Rochester Hills, MI 48309
(313) 656-3110

Telex Communications, Inc.   SE
9600 Aldrich Avenue So.
Minneapolis, MN 55420
(800) 328-3102

Ultratec, Inc.   TC, SA
450 Science Drive
Madison, WI 53711
Voice and TDD (800) 482-2424

Wheellock, Inc.   SA
273 Branchport Avenue
Long Branch, NJ 07740
(908) 222-6880

Williams Sound Corp.   SE, TE, TC
10399 West 70 Street
Eden Prairie, MN 55344
Voice and TDD (800) 328-6190

SENSORY AIDS AND COMMUNICATION TRAINING

CHAPTER 43

Characteristics and Use of Hearing Aids

Wayne J. Staab and Samuel F. Lybarger

HISTORY AND TYPES OF HEARING AIDS

Hearing and History and Development

The function of a hearing aid is to amplify sounds to a degree and in a manner that will enable a hearing-impaired person to utilize his or her remaining hearing in an effective manner. Although there may be some exceptions, a hearing aid must also be cosmetically acceptable to be effective.

Mechanical Hearing Aids

Perhaps the first amplification system to be used was the **hand cupped behind the ear;** not too acceptable cosmetically, but providing approximately 14 dB of amplification at about 1500 Hz as measured on a manikin (de Boer, 1984). Next in order of invention came such acoustic amplifiers as horns, speaking tubes, etc. These were in use as early as the seventeenth century and were still available in the early part of this century.

Electric Hearing Aids

Mechanical hearing aids were followed, starting about the turn of the century, by **carbon hearing aids,** which were based on the principles of the telephone. **Vacuum-tube hearing aids** appeared about 1938 and offered much greater amplification possibilities, wider frequency response and lower harmonic distortion. Today's hearing aids are based on the invention of the **transistor** by Bell Telephone Laboratories and introduced into hearing aids in the 1950s. This development made possible much smaller size, far lower battery cost, and a flexibility of design never before possible. The parallel development of hearing aid components, such as microphones, receivers, capacitors and integrated circuits, contributed equally to today's hearing aid technology. The reader is referred to Watson and Tolan (1949), Berger (1984), and Mahon (1990) for in-depth historical information.

Contemporary Hearing Aids

A block diagram of a contemporary hearing aid is shown in Figure 43.9, but will be described here simply as follows: Sound is picked up by the microphone and converted to an electrical signal corresponding to the sound pressure variations. A transistor amplifier stage (field effect transistor) is usually contained within the microphone housing. The signal is then amplified by the main amplifier and delivered to a receiver (earphone) that converts the greatly amplified electrical signal back to sound. The amplifier, in addition to providing a desired maximum amount of amplification, is generally equipped with a gain control (volume control) operable by the user. It may also provide for other adjustments, such as frequency, output, and other controls that can be preset. An important function of the amplifier, in combination with the receiver and ear coupling system (consisting of any tubing or other acoustic elements used as well as the molded plastic part made to fit the ear), is to limit the maximum amount of sound pressure that the hearing aid can deliver. This is done to avoid exceeding the user's level of discomfort. A more detailed explanation of hearing aid function is provided later in this chapter under "characteristics of hearing aids."

Types of Hearing Aids: Hearing Aids by Manner of Placement

In-the-Ear Hearing Aids

The availability of very small, efficient electret microphones, correspondingly small receivers, integrated circuits (ICs), and further battery miniaturization has facilitated packaging the entire hearing aid within the concha and ear canal. The reality with these in-the-ear (ITE) or in-the-canal (ITC) hearing aids, is that the smaller the aid, the less electronic flexibility, the smaller and fewer the user controls, the fewer the acoustical modifications possible, and the smaller the battery. Nevertheless, the smaller the aid, the greater the opportunity to utilize the natural enhancements provided by the pinna, and possibly of the ear canal itself. The electronics generally are housed in a hard plastic, although soft materials are sometimes used for the canal portions. Figure 43.1 shows different styles of in-the-ear and in-the-canal hearing aids.

Custom ITE. ITE aids are mostly of the "custom" type with components built into a shell made from an impression of the user's ear. These are identified as full concha, low profile, and half concha instruments, depending on their physical location and dimensions within the concha.

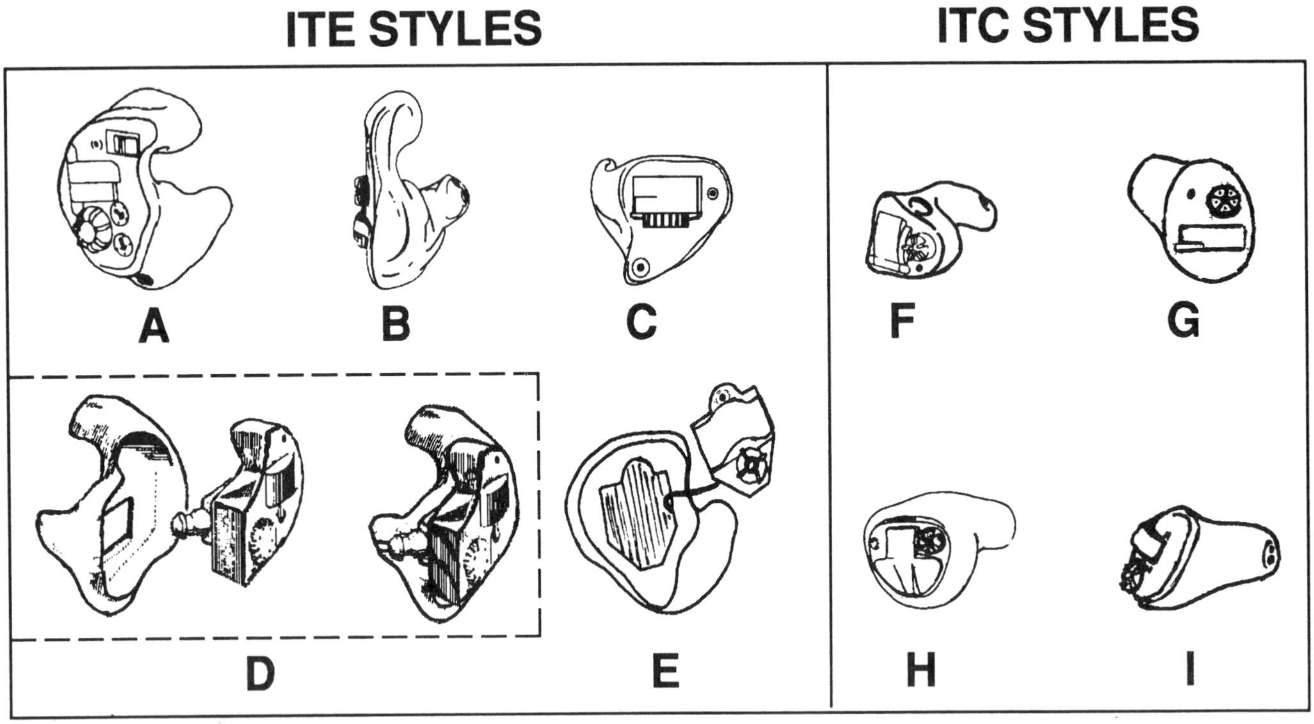

ITE STYLES   ITC STYLES

Figure 43.1. Examples of in-the-ear (ITE): (*A*) full concha, (*B*) low profile, (*C*) half concha, (*D*) custom modular, (*E*) stock modular, and in-the-canal (ITC): (*F*) mini, (*G*) regular, (*H*) custom modular, and (*I*) stock hearing aids.

The *full concha* is the most commonly used type. Using the entire concha volume provides maximal space, and therefore allows greatest flexibility to fabricate the aid, including complex circuit designs, venting, and trimmer controls. Its size and shape assist in reducing internal feedback problems and hold it securely in place. These aids use mostly the size 13 cell as the power source as of this date.

The *low profile* has the same general configuration as the full concha but is intended to provide less protrusion from the concha. As a result, it has substantially less space in which to place components, and thus is more restricted in its ability to contain complex circuitry. The battery source is usually the 312 size, although sometimes, a size 13 is used. The electronics are similar to those found in a custom ITC aid.

The *half concha* (half shell, lower concha custom) ITE occupies the concha cavum and the canal of the ear and thus is more restrictive in its electronic options. The battery is usually a 312 size and the electronics are generally those found in a custom ITE aid.

Modular ITE. These aids are built into a case of fixed shape that fits into a matching depression in a custom earmold. Built as production items, they offer the potential for better quality control but currently suffer from size and shape limitations that affect cos-

metics and functional integration of the hearing aid and earmold. The modular ITE is similar in its power supply source and electronics to the custom ITE.

Successful use of ITE aids is reduced dramatically for average losses (500, 1000, 2000 Hz) beyond 70 dB (Wernick, 1985), mainly due to feedback problems resulting from the close proximity of the microphone and receiver. Also, when the average loss is less than 35 dB, the probability of the aid being returned for credit increases significantly because of the difficulty in noticing significant benefit due to normal low-frequency hearing. This is because the desire to use as large a vent as possible (to attenuate low frequency amplification), while obtaining the amplifier gain needed at higher frequencies, is difficult without acoustic feedback. Additionally, venting may not always resolve a negative perception about one's own voice or eliminate a "stuffed up" listening sensation.

Negative patient reactions to the use of wide range receivers in ITE aids may result from their reduced sensitivity, leading to amplifier overload distortion at relatively low output levels. Physically active persons may find the ITE, especially the full concha, to be the most secure in position. The half concha may require more frequent repositioning, especially if the canal curvature is not sufficient to hold it in position.

In-the-Canal Hearing Aids

Perimeatal ITC Hearing Aids. Using miniature-sized components, the perimeatal ITC hearing aid has most of its components placed within the concha, but some in the cartilaginous portion of the ear canal. The microphone opening is located at the outer portion of the concha. Because of their size and location, the ITC aids do not allow the wide range of dispenser or user fitting adjustments found in more spacious and easily-reached BTE or even ITE hearing aids. They do, however, provide some advantage in gain at higher frequencies due to acoustic resonance in the un-blocked concha and to their depth of insertion into the ear canal. The very small receivers used may provide an extended upward frequency response compared with larger receivers.

ITC aids are mostly of the "custom" type with components built into a shell made from an impression of the user's ear. Custom-molded aids are of the "regular" and "mini" canal types—with the mini canal distinguished by being "smaller" and fitting more deeply into the cartilaginous part of the ear canal. Certain custom-molded ITCs might be considered "custom-modular" because they allow alternate electronic modules to be substituted by the dispenser without having to violate the sealed housing. Others are of the traditional "modular" type, which are built into a case of fixed shape that fits into a matching depression in a custom earmold. Still other ITC aids are of the "stock" variety, using standard shapes in an attempt to fit into an ear canal without requiring a user's ear impression (Staab, 1985a). The ITC hearing aid uses a 312 or the even smaller 10a size cell (the latter used in the "mini" canal hearing aid).

Peritympanic ITC Hearing Aids. Peritympanic ITC hearing aids have all their electronics entirely within the external auditory canal and terminate close to the tympanic membrane (Figure 43.2). Because of the depth of insertion, peritympanic ITC approaches offer a number of benefits for hearing aid users. The ITC, when fitted within the bony portion of the ear canal, and terminated within approximately 4 mm of the tympanic membrane, results in the following benefits: cosmetics, reduced gain/output requirements, greater high-frequency gain, increased hearing aid headroom, reduction or elimination of the occlusion effect, security of fit, sound bore cerumen control, improved performance in noise, feedback reduction, and normal telephone use (Staab, 1992). Some of these same benefits have been reported by other researchers as well (Zwislocki, 1953; Berger, 1988; Killion, Wilber, and Gudmundsen, 1988; Orchik, Cowgill and Parmely, 1990; Staab and Finlay, 1991). Nevertheless, the ear

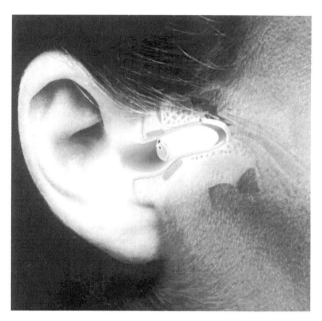

Figure 43.2. Peritympanic ITC hearing instrument (Courtesy of Philips Hearing Instruments, Mahwah, NJ)

impression-taking procedures required to fabricate an instrument for fitting this close to the tympanic membrane require greater skill and knowledge about the condition of the ear drum and of the external auditory canal.

ITC aids are more limited in gain and output than ITE aids (due to use of smaller transducers and to difficulty in isolating the components). The small receiver, however, provides an extended high-frequency range that may help some but sound "tinny" to others. Wernick and Hodgson (1984) found that canal aids produce less high-frequency amplification due to microphone location than full concha aids having comparable canal lengths. Nevertheless, because canal aids often have longer canal lengths (providing deeper insertion), these fittings often result in lower gain requirements and provide additional high-frequency response. Constraints due to size exist in circuit limitations and trimmer controls, and inability to use vents large enough to provide significant acoustical modification (including the elimination of occlusion effects with perimeatal ITC aids) are considered disadvantages. Concerns about ITC hearing aids often revolve around the difficulty in adjustment of the small volume control, and of difficulty in insertion and removal, especially by those with dexterity problems, although Murphy (1981) reports on data that question the magnitude of this as a problem. Undoubtedly, telephone use is much more effective with an ITC than with an ITE because of less feedback due to a smaller vent size, a more favorable microphone location, and the larger air volume under the telephone receiver. The significance of perceived cosmetics cannot be overstated.

The use of an ITE or ITC is based on both acoustic factors and the client's individual needs. These instruments provide for the shortest transmission distance from the hearing aid receiver to the eardrum, and thus may provide somewhat smoother responses than BTE aids and place the first peak in the response between 2 and 3 kHz (tending to replace the ear canal resonance lost when an earmold or hearing aid closes the ear canal). Additionally, the microphone location within the ear reduces wind noise interference, provides some directionality, and enhances high-frequency sounds in the 2- to 5-kHz region (Wiener and Ross, 1946; Shaw, 1966; Griffing and Preves, 1976). They, therefore, require less amplifier gain than for outside-the-ear microphone locations. Eyeglass placement and removal is often facilitated by the use of custom-molded products, while fluid discharge from the ears often precludes these type fittings. Custom-molded hearing aids for infants and/or children are viable from a fit/retention perspective and from a shell remake perspective (Curran, 1990).

Behind-The-Ear Hearing Aids

Behind-the-ear (BTE) hearing aids, also commonly referred to as over-the-ear (OTE) or postauricular hearing aids are designed to fit behind the pinna. Rugged and easily serviced, they are available in a wide selection of amplification values, for mild to profound hearing impairments. Although these aids are available in a variety of sizes, there is usually sufficient space in them for several electroacoustic adjustments such as frequency response, output, gain, AGC knee control, etc. Figure 43.3 shows a BTE aid that has several dispenser fitting adjustments in addition to the user-operated controls.

Body-Worn Hearing Aids

Body-worn (conventional, pocket) hearing aids require a separate air- or bone-conduction receiver connected to the hearing aid by a cord (Figure 43.3). Primary uses are for extreme hearing impairments in an effort to supply sufficient gain without feedback, or for persons who have difficulty manipulating smaller, ear-level units. Because of their size, these hearing aids often have a variety of user controls and dispenser adjustments. Receivers used on body-worn aids ordinarily do not have as much high-frequency range as smaller receivers, but this is seldom a problem with extremely severe hearing losses.

Eyeglass Hearing Aids

In the eyeglass hearing aid the microphone, amplifier and receiver are built into the eyeglass temples (side pieces). Introduced in 1955, the entire aid is now contained on one side. The primary disadvantage is the need to combine optics with the hearing aid (styles, hinge types, colors, etc). Although reported as an outgrowth of eyeglass aids that confined components to the portion of the eyeglass temple behind the pinna, Lybarger (1989), in rechecking dates, suggested that these two hearing aid types developed independently. The construction of an eyeglass hearing aid is shown in Figure 43.3.

Implantable Hearing Aids

Implantable hearing aids consist of cochlear, mastoid, and middle ear implants. Cochlear implants are covered in detail in Chapter 46. Mastoid and middle ear implants have not yet received extensive usage.

Hearing Aids by Mode of Operation

Single-band vs. Multi-band Hearing Aids.

Single-band hearing aids process the audio signal through a single circuit path, whose processing characteristics affect certain aspects of, or the entire, frequency range (i.e., high pass filters, AGC [automatic gain control], SSPL controls, etc.). Multiple band hearing aids have two or more circuit paths and allow for adjustments to be made separately within two or more frequency bands within the hearing aid. These are more common in programmable hearing aids.

Special Feature Hearing Aids

CROS and Its Variations. The original purpose for CROS (Contralateral Routing of Offside Signals), as reported by Harford and Barry (1965) was to pick up sound on the side of an unaidable or "dead" ear and route it to the good ear on the other side, thus, overcoming the head shadow effect. The signals are then directed from the receiver into the good ear by a tubing or nonoccluding type earmold extending into the open ear canal (Figure 43.4). The signal transmission can occur through wires behind the neck or concealed in eyeglass frames, or via a wireless transmitter and receiver combination. The benefit is especially noticeable for being able to pick up sound from the poor ear side in noisy environments. When the hearing on the good ear has a slight high-frequency loss, the CROS functions even better (Harford and Dodds, 1966).

The basic CROS concept has been utilized subsequently to overcome certain other problems relating

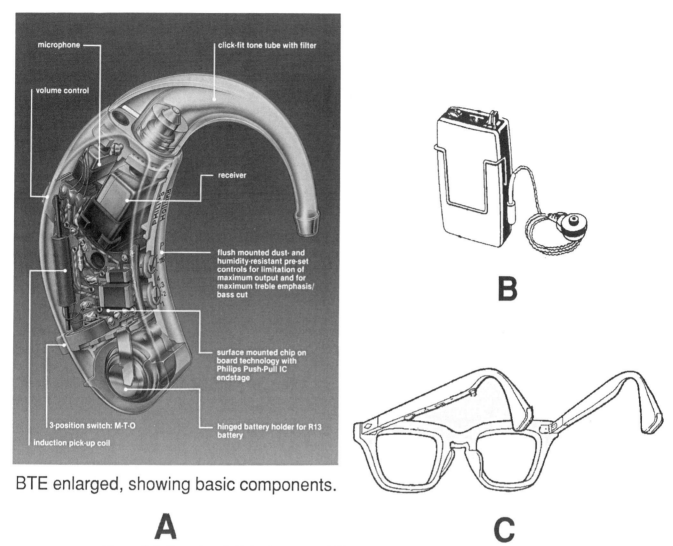

BTE enlarged, showing basic components.

microphone

volume control

receiver

click-fit tone tube with filter

flush mounted dust- and humidity-resistant pre-set controls for limitation of maximum output and for maximum treble emphasis/ bass cut

surface mounted chip on board technology with Philips Push-Pull IC endstage

3-position switch: M-T-O

induction pick-up coil

hinged battery holder for R13 battery

A

B

C

Figure 43.3. Examples of: (*A*) behind-the-ear (BTE), (*B*) body-worn (BW), and (*C*) eyeglass (EG) hearing aids (BTE drawing courtesy of Philips Hearing Instruments, Mahwah, NJ)

to hearing aid use. One of its most important advantages occurs in bilateral, high-frequency hearing losses where hearing in the low frequencies is nearly normal and drops off rapidly above some middle frequency such as 1000 Hz. Dunlavy (1968) and Wolfe (1968) were among the first to have reported tremendous success with these losses with the CROS. The success results from the almost complete elimination of gain at low frequencies when sound is delivered into an open ear canal through a plastic tube projecting a short distance into the ear canal. For example, Lybarger (1968) reported the CROS response in an actual ear to be much superior to that indicated by a coupler. The sound pressure level gain at the eardrum with the CROS aid vs. no aid, was zero or small for frequencies below 800 Hz. At higher frequencies, the gain re-

mained relatively uniform over the 1000–5000 Hz range at an average of approximately 30 dB.

An additional advantage of having the microphone and receiver separated by the head (using the head shadow), reduced the potential for feedback and permitted additional gain and output to be obtained with an ear-level unit (POWER CROS).

A subsequent finding utilizing the CROS concept of delivering the signal to the good ear by tubing only or nonoccluding earmolds was that low frequencies entered the open ear canal directly with little amplification, whereas good high-frequency amplification was provided. This led to a flurry of uses of nonoccluding ear coupling devices to provide additional high frequencies in an effort to provide more "natural" sound and high-frequency emphasis to the hearing aid user.

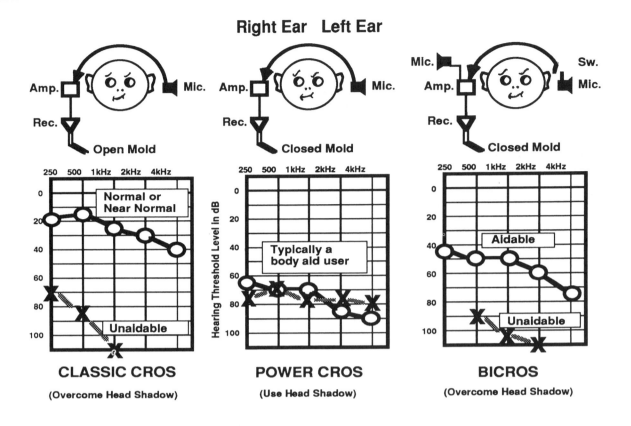

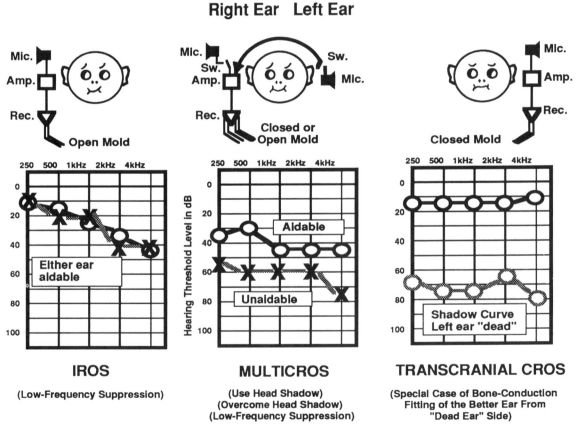

Figure 43.4. Major types of CROS type hearing aids. Sound transmission can occur via wires or by means of RF (radio frequency) transmission (no wires).

When used without the cross-over mechanics, the fitting is referred to as an IROS (Ipsilateral Routing of Signal) fitting and is in reality a standard hearing aid with a nonoccluding or "free-field" earmold on the same side—not truly a CROS variation. IROS can be very beneficial for mild to moderate, falling, sensory neural losses and adapts itself especially well for binaural use. Because of the escape of sound from the open ear canal to the microphone, however, the amount of usable gain before feedback that occurs is much less than in the CROS application and depends largely on the degree of occlusion of the earmold coupling used.

Other common uses of CROS variations include the BICROS and MULTICROS. The BICROS (Harford, 1966) arrangement is utilized when one ear is essentially unaidable and the better ear has an aidable hearing loss. Two microphones are used, one on each side of the head. The signal picked up by the unaidable ear (off-side mic) is transmitted to the better ear side, combined with the input from the microphone on that side, amplified, and delivered to the better ear, usually using a closed or smaller vented earmold to avoid feedback. The MULTICROS consists of instruments which, by means of a user-operated switch, can be used as either CROS, BICROS, or monaural hearing aids. A user-controlled switch shuts off the microphone on either side or activates both microphones when in the BICROS position. It can provide an advantage when an interfering signal is coming from one side by allowing the user to shut off the microphone on that side.

Many variations of CROS have been presented (Delk, 1975; Dunlavy, 1968; Staab, 1978; Johnson, 1982). Most of the variations concern the locations of sound pick-up to overcome or to utilize head shadow, or the methods of earmold coupling. A recent variation, however, deserves mention—that of the Transcranial CROS (Sullivan, 1988). This variation requires that the *better ear* have fairly good hearing and provides amplification to the *unaidable* ear via a standard hearing aid. The attempt is to provide sufficient air-conducted stimuli in the unaidable ear to set the skull into motion (generating a bone-conducted stimulus) to drive the better ear cochlea (Sullivan, 1988; Miller, 1989). This is feasible because of the low interaural attenuation (0 to 10 dB) provided by the head for bone-conducted stimuli (Hood, 1960). It is essentially a bone-conduction fitting to the better ear. A variation of this transcranial CROS approach is the use of a three-microphone system (CROS-PLUS); a complete hearing aid to the unaidable ear, plus a complete BICROS arrangement. Reports of better distance hearing and understanding in noise along with localization have been reported with this arrangement (Hable et al., 1990).

Nonadaptive vs. Adaptive Hearing Aids

Nonadaptive hearing aids include circuitry that does not change the basic performance of the hearing aid once its controls (functions) are set. Tone and output trimmers and fixed-function switches best identify this category (Staab, 1991).

Adaptive hearing aids include circuitry that has a processing function that alters the performance of the aid during changing input signal environments. These signal modifications are triggered mostly by frequency and/or intensity changes. Automatic Gain Control (AGC), Automatic Signal Processing (ASP), and adaptive noise filter circuits in hearing aids are the most common examples. A block diagram of a hearing aid with an adaptive noise filter circuit is illustrated in Figure 43.5.

Analog Hearing Aids

Analog hearing aids allow for the representation of a continuously changing physical variable (i.e., sound)

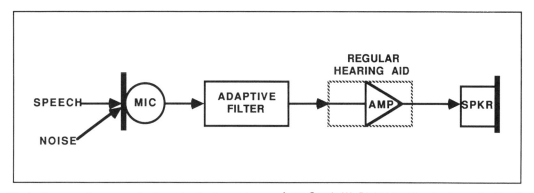

Figure 43.5. Block diagram of a computer-based adaptive noise rejection circuit added to a standard hearing aid circuit (Adapted from Staab W. Digital hearing instruments. Hearing Instruments 1987;38:18–26.)

by another physical variable (i.e., electrical current). Almost all contemporary hearing aids are analog in nature. Analog developments have not yet been exhausted and will be the dominant circuit used in hearing aids for the next few years. Figure 43.9 illustrates the function of a basic analog circuit.

Programmable Hearing Aids

Programmable hearing aids feature conventional amplifiers and filters controlled by an external digital source. Other terms used to describe this mode of operation hearing aids include: digitally programmable hearing aids, quasi-digital hearing aids, and analog hearing aids with digital control. These may be more accurately described as VLSI (very large scale integration) analog circuits controlled by digital means. The two primary components consist of a hearing aid that contains a CMOS (complimentary metal oxide semiconductor), RAM (random access memory), or EEPROM (electrically erasable programmable read only memory) memory module and an external microprocessor (computer) to access those memory locations within the chip which represent different electroacoustical performances. The memory module replaces the conventional trimmer potentiometer functions in the hearing aid and provides more varied and precise control (Staab, 1988a). Literally, from hundreds to millions of hearing aid performance characteristics can be identified, depending on the programmable system involved. The selected electroacoustical performance is maintained by either volatile (loses its memory), or nonvolatile (maintains its memory) means during periods of hearing aid malfunction or non-use. Figure 43.6 identifies features available with today's programmable hearing aids, recognizing that different companies' systems perform at least some of the functions described in slightly different ways. Some programmable systems are very simple to use and extremely portable, whereas others are quite complex and not portable. Some allow little or no control of the hearing aid characteristics by the hearing aid wearer, whereas others allow for the wearer to control performance in certain environments via a remote control they carry with them. It is expected that programmable hearing aids will become increasingly important during the next several years.

Digital Hearing Aids

True digital hearing aids are not commercially available at the time of this writing even though the first wearable digital hearing aid was demonstrated in 1983 (Nunley, Staab, Steadman, Wechsler, and Spencer, 1983) and a preliminary version sold in 1987 (Nicolet). Digital hearing aids are distinguished from programmable (quasi-digital) hearing aids in at least three ways: (1) the input signal is digitized; (2) digital signal processing circuitry (DSP chip) is used in the hearing aid; and (3) they can be designed to "make decisions" (Staab, 1991). In essence, the digital hearing aid is a wearable computer. It uses digital signal processing

Various Components/functions Available in Today's Programmable Hearing Aids

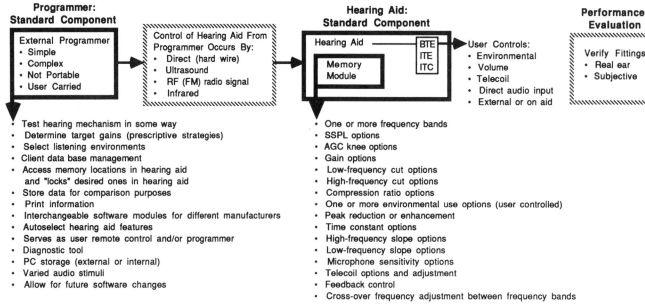

Figure 43.6. Examples of different features available with today's programmable hearing aids.

(DSP) as a sampling technique to eliminate the need for conventional analog components (i.e., transistors, precision resistors, capacitors, diodes) by implementing in software the hardware devices in which those components normally are used.

Very simply, the digital hearing aid diagram illustrated in Figure 43.7 is further explained:

1. Sound pressure impinging onto the microphone diaphragm is changed into an electrical analog voltage.
2. The electrical analog signal is low-pass filtered to avoid a condition called "aliasing," which can cause distortions.
3. The filtered electrical analog signal is "sampled and held" so that it no longer contains an infinite number of different values.
4. The sampled electrical analog amplitudes are converted to digital (binary) numbers using the A/D (analog to digital) converter. This is in the form of positive or negative electrical voltages.
5. The central processing unit (CPU) or microprocessor is a single silicon chip computer with instructions that cause the computer to mathematically manipulate the data in some predetermined way.
6. A memory maintains the program that retains the sequence of calculation operations and also maintains intermediate results.
7. The computed digital output (binary numbers) is converted back into an analog signal using a (D/A) converter.
8. A low-pass filter eliminates spurious frequency components.
9. Electrical analog impulses are converted into output sound pressure by the hearing aid receiver.

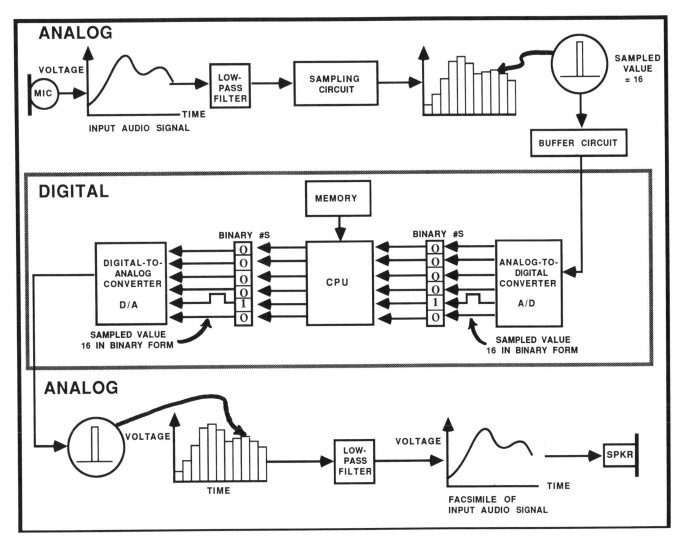

Figure 43.7. Digital hearing aid block diagram. See text for explanation of function. (Adapted from Staab W. Digital/programmable hearing aids—an eye towards the future. Br J Audiol 1991;24: 243–256.)

Basic advantages of DSP relate to the potential of developing and tailoring a device, with software only (program), to meet the needs of the hearing impaired. DSP allows for the possibility of improved methods to solve background noise and feedback problems, for greater flexibility and control of response and performance characteristics, repeatability, stability of performance, rapid prototyping capability, potentially lower implementation costs, potential to eliminate moving parts, and improved control of filters (Staab, 1985b).

Although the theoretical advantages of true digital signal processing in hearing aids are numerous, major obstacles hinder its practicality at this time. These relate primarily to the: (a) large housing requirements; (b) low battery life due to high current drain; (c) cost in down-sizing; and (d) lack of understanding of specific signal processing needs of the hearing-impaired auditory system.

Hearing Aid Systems by Mode of Presentation

Air-Conduction and Bone-Conduction Hearing Aids

Electrical hearing aids fall into two categories based on the output transduction: air-conduction or bone-conduction. Both are similar until the last transduction stage of the amplified signal where they are converted into usable stimuli for the hearing aid user.

The *air-conduction hearing aid* is designed to change electrical energy (amplified) back to acoustical energy and direct it into the ear canal. Almost all hearing aids are of this type. The *bone-conduction hearing aid* is designed to change the electrical energy (amplified) into mechanical vibration which, when applied directly to the head, stimulates the entire skull. The use of bone-conduction aids is limited to situations where a large (30–50 dB) air-bone gap exists, or where there is a chronic discharge from an ear that prevents the use of an air-conduction receiver. Additionally, even when a significant air-bone gap exists, the use of a more powerful air-conduction aid may be preferable to the use of a bone-conduction aid. When used, bone-conduction hearing aids are available in a very limited number of eyeglass, body-worn, or BTE styles. For the eyeglass version the bone vibrator is placed in the hearing aid paddle behind the ear. The necessary static force for efficient operation is supplied by adjusting the eyeglasses to fit rather tightly. Although not having as much output as the body-worn or BTE bone-conduction versions, the eyeglass arrangement is very convenient to use and quite acceptable cosmetically. For the body-worn or BTE versions, the bone-conduction vibrator is attached to a headband and placed behind the pinna in much the same manner as for bone-conduction audiometric testing.

Monaural vs. Binaural

A **monaural hearing aid** is one complete hearing aid fitted to a single ear. A **binaural hearing aid** has two separate and complete hearing aids, one for each ear. One complete hearing aid with a receiver to each ear is considered a **pseudobinaural hearing aid.** The pseudobinaural (Y-cord) arrangement is usually reserved for body-worn hearing aids.

Sales and Use Trends

Figure 43.8 provides eleven-year trend information relative to hearing aid sales by type in the United States and Canada (HIA, 1986; HIA, 1992). Of significance to this chapter are the changes in sales of hearing aid types rather than the number of total sales involved. Additionally, since 1984, CROS variation sales dropped to such low levels that they were no longer specifically identified. In the last such reporting of these instruments, they constituted 1.2% of the sales in 1983 (HIA, 1984). The increasing application of IROS and binaural amplification (even with gross asymmetry between ears), has led to a decrease in CROS use. Programmable hearing aids, introduced in 1989 and initially available in BTE versions, have contributed to the maintenance of BTE unit sales.

CHARACTERISTICS OF HEARING AIDS

Hearing Aid Components and Basic Controls

The advance of hearing aid technology and subsequent sound quality has been possible primarily because of consistent improvement in hearing aid components. Improved acoustic and electrical performance, reduced size, and greater reliability have resulted. Following is a description of the typical construction and operation of some of the major components. A block diagram of a hearing aid is presented in Figure 43.9 for reference.

Power Supply

The amplification provided by the hearing aid derives its "power" from the hearing aid battery. Generally, the greater the gain and the output requirement of the hearing aid (resulting in a higher current drain), the greater the battery's mAh (milliampere-hour) capacity must be, and the larger the physical size. Hearing aid batteries (mostly single cells) are currently of two main types; zinc-air or mercury, even though some states are in the process of outlawing mercury use in batteries.

Zinc-air cells constitute approximately 63% of all hearing aid battery sales and mercury sales 36% (Duracell, 1990). An attractive feature of zinc-air cells is their reported long shelf life, because they are not

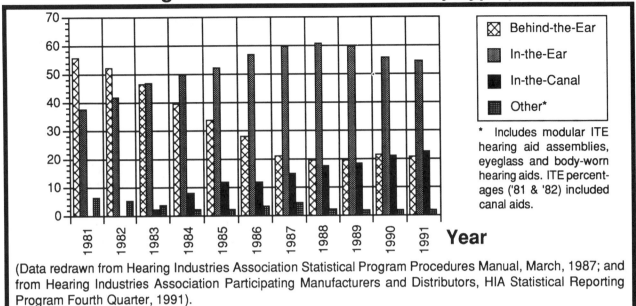

Percent Hearing Aids Sold in U.S. & Canada by Type (1981-1991)

Legend:
- ⊠ Behind-the-Ear
- ▨ In-the-Ear
- ■ In-the-Canal
- ▦ Other*

* Includes modular ITE hearing aid assemblies, eyeglass and body-worn hearing aids. ITE percentages ('81 & '82) included canal aids.

(Data redrawn from Hearing Industries Association Statistical Program Procedures Manual, March, 1987; and from Hearing Industries Association Participating Manufacturers and Distributors, HIA Statistical Reporting Program Fourth Quarter, 1991).

Figure 43.8. Eleven-year hearing aid sales trends, by type.

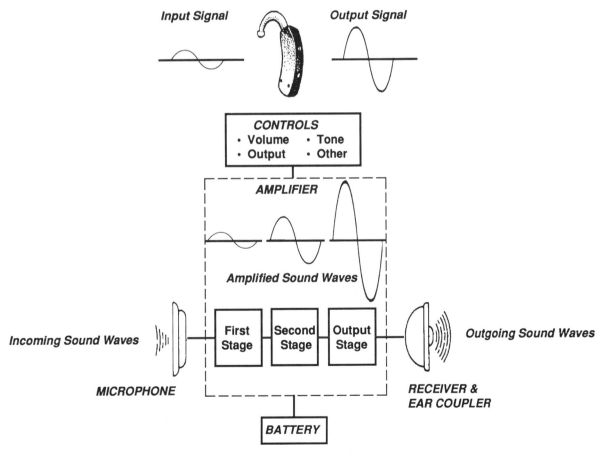

Figure 43.9. General block diagram of a hearing aid. The diagram is essentially the same for other type hearing aids as well as for the BTE shown.

activated until a tape seal is removed from small holes in the cell through which air enters to initiate activation. Also, zinc-air cells of a given size will last approximately twice as long as their mercury counterpart. However, because zinc-air cells are air activated, a potential drawback can occur when they are used with aids having high current drain (such as push-pull or AGC circuits) or with aids functioning at their maximum gain and output levels, even if they don't have high current drain. The problem is identified as an intermittency, motorboating, or pumping action. The situation can be likened to "a pump sucking air." The demand on the cell is great enough that the air activation is not sufficient to accommodate the hearing aid's required current drain, even though it's trying to. A new family of zinc-air cells is being evaluated currently to resolve this problem. It is possible that the fault may not rest completely with the cell but may sometimes result from the designer's choice of too small a battery for the current needed. Staab (1982) has also reported that under combined conditions of high temperature and high humidity, chemicals can leak through the air holes in the cell and interfere with its function, and hence, that of the hearing aid. It is for these reasons that hearing aid manufacturers often use mercury cells when evaluating suspected hearing aid problems. Another feature of zinc-air cells that can create problems is that after the seal has been removed, the cell begins to discharge slowly, even when the hearing aid is not in use.

Other type batteries, such as silver oxide or nickel cadmium, are not used to any significant extent as power supplies for hearing aids. Although silver oxide cells have the highest voltage of the cells mentioned, the high cost of silver and their relatively short operating life have rendered them unacceptable except for the highest output/gain hearing aids operating at their maximums. Although the rechargeable (nickel cadmium or Nicad) batteries have been used, they have not gained wide acceptance, partly because of the need for daily recharging in many cases and because of the user's uncertainty as to the battery's condition of charge. The number of times hearing aid-size nickel cadmium batteries can be recharged is limited, leading to the need to change them periodically. They have been used successfully, however, with auditory trainer type body-worn aids where supervision is available.

Hearing aid cells have a relatively flat discharge rate; that is, the voltage does not drop much during the cell's useful life (Figure 43.10). The cell's capacity is rated in mAh for typical load currents. If the current drain of an aid is known, an estimate of expected cell life can be calculated by dividing the cell's capacity in mAh by the current drain in milliampers (mA). This formula works well for class A amplifiers because the current drain is constant, regardless of where the volume control is set or what the input levels to the hearing aid are. Class B amplifiers, however, have a battery life that is very difficult to predict. (A discussion of amplifier classes occurs later in this chapter). Hearing aids with class B push-pull amplifiers do not have constant current drain; instead, the drain is

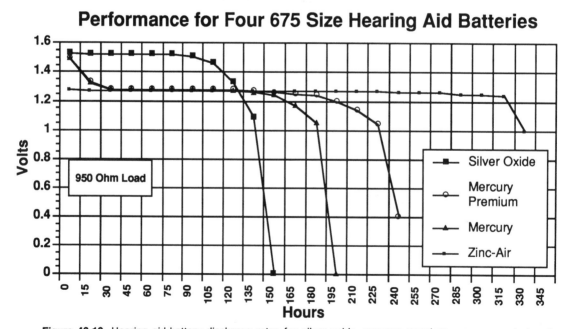

Figure 43.10. Hearing aid battery discharge rates for silver oxide, mercury premium, mercury, and zinc-air batteries, illustrating that the voltage remains fairly constant during the cell's useful life.

greater with high input levels, high gain levels, high ambient noise levels, and with extended low-frequency response range amplification. Current drain ranges of from 3 to 15 mA are not uncommon for class B push-pull, high output/gain hearing aids. Nominal voltages and capacity ranges for some commonly used hearing aid battery types are given in Table 43.1. The nominal voltage is a suitable approximate value of voltage used to identify a battery system and is printed on the package. This differs from the open circuit voltage that is measured across the terminals of a cell or battery when essentially no external current is flowing.

Table 43.1.
Approximate Battery Voltages and Capacities

Battery Type	Nominal Voltage Volts	Capacity mAh
Zinc-air 10A	1.3	50–60
Zinc-air 230	1.3	50–60
Zinc-air 536	1.3	50
Silver 312	1.5	37–40
Mercury 312	1.3	45–60
Zinc-air 312	1.3	100–120
Silver 13	1.5	75–80
Mercury 13	1.3	85–100
Zinc-air 13	1.3	170–230
Silver 76/675G	1.5	180–190
Mercury 675	1.3	180–270
Zinc-air 675	1.3	400–550
Mercury 401	1.3	800–1300

To estimate battery life:

$$\text{Hours} = \frac{\text{Milliampere hours (mAh)}}{\text{Current drain (mA)}}$$

Example: the 312 Zinc-air type battery has a capacity of 110 mAh. A hearing aid with current drain (mA) at 0.5 mA will give approximately 220 hours usage.

Transducers

The microphone and receiver in a hearing aid are transducers. They are devices that are activated by power in one form and convert, or transduce, that power into another form.

Microphones. The microphone (input transducer) converts the sound pressures that impinge upon its diaphragm into small analog electrical signals. Microphones used in wearable hearing aids have utilized a number of principles over the years, beginning with carbon microphones and crystal (piezoelectric) microphones in the late 1930s. The electromagnetic microphone with its low output impedance was introduced in a 1946 body aid and became a natural choice for transistor amplifiers in the early 1950s. Limitations of the electromagnetic microphone included poor low-frequency response and relatively high sensitivity to mechanical shock and vibration.

In today's hearing aids, the **electret microphone** (Killion and Carlson, 1974) has almost universally been used since 1971 for hearing aids because of its good sensitivity, excellent wide band frequency response and sound quality, tiny size, reliability, low internal noise and insensitivity to mechanical vibration. The word "electret" is similar in derivation to "magnet" but applies to an electric instead of a magnetic field. The electret itself is not a microphone but is a very thin fluorocarbon plastic with a metallic coating that holds or stores a permanent electric charge—it is an electrical capacitor (Figure 43.11). As the diaphragm vibrates due to the action of sound waves entering the sound inlet, a voltage is generated between the backplate electrode (conducting plate on which the

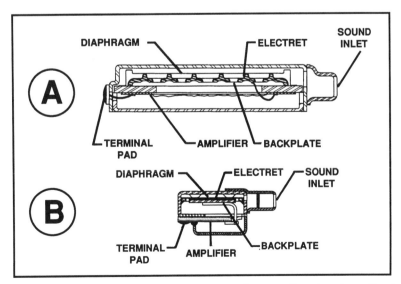

Figure 43.11. Diagram showing principle of construction of an electret microphone. **A,** diagram for a larger microphone. **B,** diagram for a smaller microphone (Courtesy of Knowles Electronics, Inc., Itasca, IL)

electret is mounted) and the diaphragm, which acts as the other electrode of the capacitor. This small voltage is then amplified by a field effect transistor (FET) located inside the microphone housing and delivered to the input terminals of the main amplifier. Electret microphones now allow for frequency response shaping by providing a variety of cut-off frequency options for selective de-emphasis of low-frequency input and are a primary means used today to alter the frequency response of hearing aids. It is interesting to note that between 1953 and 1987 microphones were reduced in volume by a factor of 172, and receiver volume was reduced by a factor of 28 (Carlson et al., 1989)—tremendous reductions in size for both.

Categories. Hearing aid microphones can be categorized as either pressure (omnidirectional) or pressure gradient (directional). **Pressure (omnidirectional)** mi-

crophones have a single port that delivers sound to the front of the microphone diaphragm. If tested in a free field, a pressure microphone picks up sound equally from all directions and thus has a circular polar sensitivity pattern. When worn in or over the ear, however, it is no longer omnidirectional except at low frequencies. The upper left view in Figure 43.12 shows a typical polar pattern for such a microphone in free field and also as tested in a hearing aid on a KEMAR (Knowles Electronics Manikin for Acoustic Research) manikin ear. The curves were made at a frequency of 2000 Hz.

Pressure gradient (directional) hearing aid microphones, subminiaturized about 1968, have *two* spaced ports. The forward port leads to the front of the diaphragm and the rear port to the back of the diaphragm. A diagram of a directional microphone is

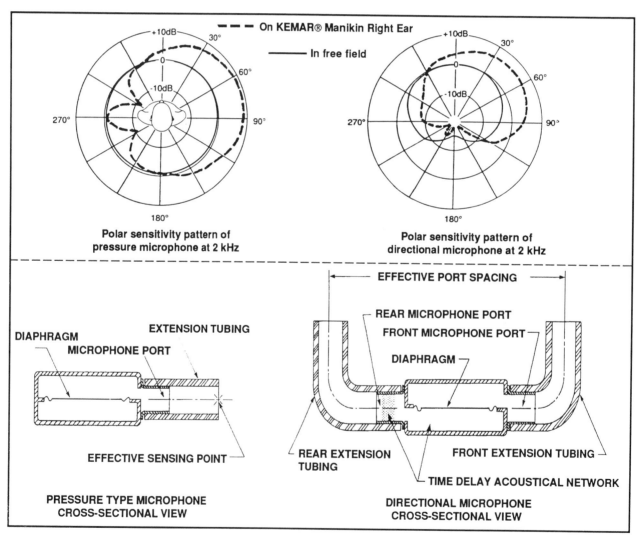

Figure 43.12. Differences in pressure (omnidirectional) and directional microphones used in hearing aids, including their polar plots. The lower portion of the figure diagrams the principles of the pres-

sure and directional microphones. (Courtesy of Knowles Electronics, Inc., Itasca, IL) shown in the lower view of Figure 43.12. As worn, sound from directly behind entering the rear port is delayed about 57 microseconds by an acoustical network before reaching the back of the microphone diaphragm. To reach the forward port, usually about 16 mm away from the rear port, time is required. The sound gets to the front of the diaphragm at about the same time as that from the rear port reaches the back of the diaphragm and vibratory forces on the diaphragm cancel. This cancellation action does not take place for sounds coming from the front. When tested in free field, a directional microphone usually has a heart-shaped polar pattern (a cardioid), as shown in the upper right free field measurement of Figure 43.12. When worn on the head, the directional sensitivity is considerably altered (dashed line on KEMAR). Sound from the rear is substantially reduced, but the greatest sensitivity lies at about 45° from the front instead of directly ahead. (Another method used to investigate the directional properties of hearing aids on a manikin is the use of the Directivity Index. This is the calculated improvement in signal to random noise ratio expected over that for an omnidirectional aid in free-field, the source being at 0° incidence, Beck, 1983). Two other useful indices are the Undirectional Index (the ratio of front-to-rear hemisphere energy) and the Distance Index (the square root of the Directivity Index, indicating relative to omnidirectional, how much further from the source the same signal-to-noise ratio can be maintained). Binaural aids of either pressure or directional types may have directional advantages.

Directional hearing aids have good directionality at low frequencies and directionality is maintained up to around 4000 Hz. They have a response curve with an upward slope of about 6 dB per octave to about 3000 Hz. The sensitivity can thus be substantially lower at low frequencies than for a pressure microphone. This may give improved results in noise that could be attributed to directionality. Nielsen (1972) has written a detailed explanation of the action of a directional microphone, information on the design and operation of small directional microphones was contributed by Carlson and Killion (1974), and design changes required to optimize directional microphone performance on the head as compared to free-field performance was published by Madaffari (1983).

The degree of attenuation of sounds from the rear is related to the environmental acoustics. Studebaker et al. (1980) demonstrated that the amount of directionality decreased as room reverberation time increased; some directional aids had essentially omnidirectional characteristics in highly reverberant environments. They stated further that typical audiometric test rooms are not good environments in which to evaluate the relative effectiveness of directional hearing aids.

Lentz (1972a) and Madison and Hawkins (1983) reported on speech discrimination performance with directional aids under different S/N ratios in a reverberant room. Madison and Hawkins reported a 3.4 dB improvement with the directional aid (as measured by the speech level required to obtain a 50% score on an NU-6 word list in the presence of a 65-dB SPL babble type noise) in an anechoic environment versus the reverberant environment. Still, all subjects showed a directional microphone advantage in the moderately reverberant room. While Lentz (1972b) looked at speech discrimination as a result of S/N ratio and found improved performance with the directional aid, he noted that in extremely reverberant environments, this advantage could possibly disappear. Because a reverberant condition is a more realistic environment, the performance of the directional microphone hearing aid may not be as advantageous under real life conditions as assumed.

In studies evaluating user preference, Mueller et al. (1983) reported significantly better results with directional microphone versus omnidirectional microphone hearing aids in noise, when used binaurally, and when used with vented earmolds. Hawkins and Yacullo (1984) showed that their hearing-impaired subjects had an 8 dB improvement in noise under binaural plus directional aided listening compared with monaural omnidirectional hearing aids. Many users, however, cannot tell the difference or may prefer omnidirectional aids (Mueller et al., 1983; Sommers, 1979; Mueller, 1981). For those who can tell the difference, the primary reason for the successful use of directional hearing aids is the result of directionality and noise suppression (Staab, 1978).

Alternate Inputs. Although not transducers, other inputs are sometimes used in hearing aids in addition to the microphone. The most frequently used is the telephone induction pick-up coil, frequently called the **telecoil.** The telecoil consists of a core of high permeability metal around which is wound a coil of a large number of turns of fine enameled wire. The alternating magnetic leakage field around most telephone receivers induces a voltage in the telecoil, which is then amplified. Better telephone reception is obtained because the microphone is usually switched off and, thus, does not pick up local ambient noise. Also, the frequency response of the system is smoother than that which occurs when acoustic coupling from the telephone receiver to the microphone is used. The telecoil mode is also used for induction loop systems. Since 1989, Federal Communications Commission

Rule 68.4 requires that all telephones sold for use in the United States have adequate magnetic field strength for telecoil operation. In May, 1992, the Federal Communications Commission ordered that telephones in all areas of the workplace, all telephones in hotel and motel rooms, all telephones in rooms in hospitals, residential health care facilities for senior citizens, convalescent homes and prisons be hearing aid compatible by May 1, 1993, where these establishments have 20 or more employees. Telephones in these same areas, for establishments that have fewer than 20 employees, need to be hearing aid compatible by May 1, 1994.

Still other hearing aids have provision for electrical inputs, using plugs or special contacts to make the connections into the amplifier. These inputs might be from FM radio receivers worn on the person or from tape recorders, televisions, etc.

Receivers. Also identified as earphones, speakers, or as output transducers, these convert the amplified electrical signal from the hearing aid to an acoustic or vibratory output. Receivers may be of the air-conduction or bone-conduction types.

Magnetic type **air-conduction receivers** are especially well suited to function with the low supply voltage amplifiers found in hearing aids because they operate efficiently directly from the output stage. Windings in magnetic receivers can be made to have the desired electrical impedance for different amplifier designs.

Receivers for ear level hearing aids (ITE, ITC, BTE and eyeglass) are generally of the balanced-armature magnetic type because of the high performance that can be achieved in an unbelievably small space. Figure 43.13 is a diagram of an *internal subminiature receiver.*

A reed (armature) of magnetically permeable metal is made an electromagnet by the alternating signal current in the coil of fine wire around it. Its free end is alternately attracted to or repelled from the small but powerful permanent magnets. Its vibration is transmitted by a tiny rod to the diaphragm and sound is developed in the adjacent cavity, from which it is transmitted through the outlet to the ear coupling system. The acoustic output from the receiver diaphragm matches the original acoustic input in waveform but has been intensified by the hearing aid's amplifier. The smaller receivers have a very wide range and can amplify up to 6000 Hz and above. Although this is considered favorable by many for better sound fidelity and for improved speech discrimination, especially when used with an extended low frequency response (Pascoe, 1975; Skinner and Karstaedt, 1979; Beck et al., 1980; Sung and Sung, 1980), these wide range receivers are less sensitive and more prone to feedback than larger receivers. Because smaller receivers fit the space requirements of ITE and ITC hearing aids, their future is assured. Circuitry is being developed to counter the sensitivity and feedback concerns.

Recently, the *integrated receiver* concept has become a reality (Carlson, 1988, 1989; Ditthardt, 1990), having been developed by Knowles Electronics for hearing aids. It is called an integrated receiver because it contains the output stage amplifier. Additional information is available in this chapter under the "amplifier" and "headroom" sections.

The *"button" receiver* used with body-worn hearing aids operates like a miniature telephone receiver and is of the magnetic type. Signal current in a coil, on a core of permeable magnetic metal, modulates the pull of a permanent magnet on a round diaphragm of mag-

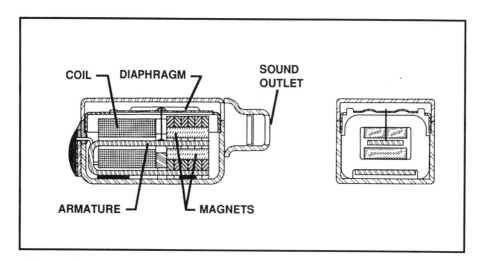

Figure 43.13. Diagram showing construction of a balanced-armature, internal, subminiature air-conduction receiver (Courtesy of Knowles Electronics, Inc., Itasca, IL)

netic metal and causes it to vibrate. Sound is developed in a small cavity adjacent to the diaphragm and is transmitted to the earmold system.

Bone-conduction receivers (vibrators, oscillators) operate on the "reaction" principle and are designed to vibrate their housings (cases) rather than setting up sound waves in the air. A mass, free to vibrate inside an enclosed case, is caused to do so by a magnetic driving system (Figure 43.14). The vibrations of the mass are transmitted through the supporting spring and armature to the case and then to the skin and bony structure of the head. The use of a bone-conduction receiver is limited mainly to situations where there is a large air-bone gap. Its response above 4 kHz may not be as good as that in small balanced-armature air-conduction receivers.

Amplifiers

The amplifier increases the amplitude of the weak electric AC voltages picked up by the microphone (Figure 43.9). It may have a number of stages of amplification. Today's hearing aids achieve amplification primarily through the use of transistors. (For a full discussion of the transistor and its function the reader is referred to any of a number of electronics books). Essentially, the transistor can be considered to be a semiconductor resistor that regulates current or acts as a conversion device. For example, in a hearing aid, it converts the current supplied by the battery into the desired output current; the total amplification being controlled by the microphone input current.

Amplifier Types. Hearing aid amplifiers are typically of the monolithic integrated circuit (IC) or of the hybrid IC; sometimes a combination of the two.

The concept of the *IC* is that of having all required circuit elements built into a single monolithic block or chip. In the IC amplifier, the components used to form the amplifier (transistors, diodes, capacitors, and resistors) are formed on a silicon chip to give the desired electronic performance. The magnitude of the complexity and number of components has led to descriptors such as medium-scale integration, large-scale integration (LSI), and very large-scale integration (VLSI). In *monolithic circuits* the entire circuit function is formed on or within a single semiconductor material (e.g., silicon). These are the fundamental form of IC. *Thin-and thick-film circuits* are formed by depositing resistive and/or conductive films on an insulating substrate and by imposing patterns on them to form electronic elements or networks. One type of IC is shown in Figure 43.15. In most cases leads are bonded to the chip to provide the necessary external connections to the microphone, battery, receiver, other controls, and for the "outboarding" of certain capacitors or other electronics components that are too large physically to be be included in the IC, or which when applied, modify the performance of the IC. Advantages of ICs are those of small size, sealing against environmental conditions, uniform manufacturing, low electronic noise, fewer solder connections, and low power requirements. The flexibility and capability of hearing aid ICs have increased greatly in recent years.

Hybrid circuits consist of very tiny discrete circuit components soldered by special techniques to a circuit pattern on a ceramic substrate with deposited networks or onto a printed circuit board (Figure 43.15). Components may include IC chips.

Amplifier Operating Classes. Hearing aid circuits usually have three or more stages of amplification. The final (output or power) stage of a hearing aid amplifier can be identified as having class A, B, or D op-

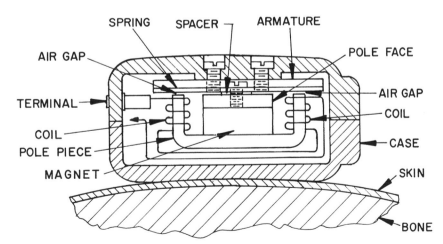

Figure 43.14. Diagram showing construction of a type of bone-conduction receiver (Courtesy of Radioear Corporation, McMurray, PA)

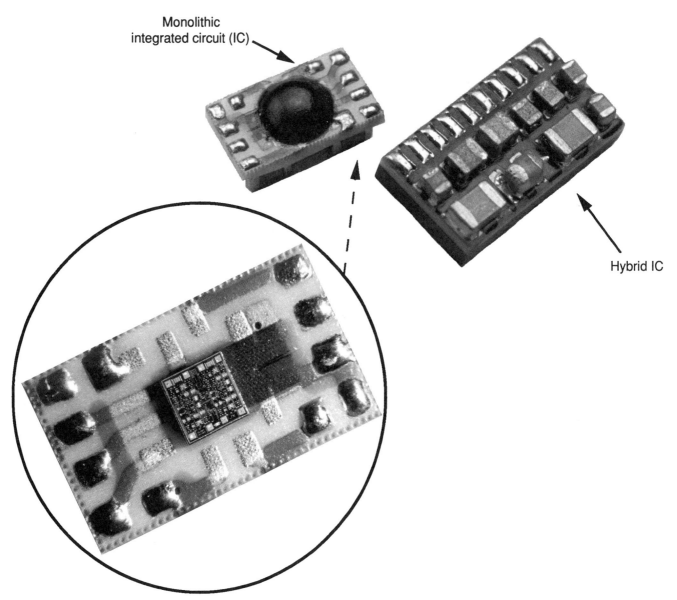

Figure 43.15. Comparison of monolithic IC (*left*) and hybrid IC (*right*) used in hearing aids. The enlargement of the IC shows its construction detail before epoxy sealing. (Courtesy of Gennum, Inc., Burlington, ON, Canada)

eration. The output amplifier interfaces with the preceding amplifier stages and provides the necessary drive to the receiver. The circuits and waveforms shown in Figure 43.16 are intended to provide a brief overview of the current drain differences among the three main types of output amplifiers used in hearing aids.

Class A (single-ended output stage amplifiers) are generally used in low gain, low power applications, where peak gain does not exceed about 50 dB. Class A amplifiers have a constant current drain, regardless of whether the input signal level is low or high (as shown by the dashed line).

When higher power requirements are desired, the amplifier is usually a push-pull type, operating in *class B*. In a push-pull configuration there are at least two active devices that alternately amplify the negative and positive cycles of the input waveform. Class B amplifiers can produce relatively high gain. They consume almost no current when no sound is entering the hearing aid and draw power only when actually amplifying. They use battery power more efficiently than does a class A amplifier. As such they do not have constant current drain. The class B output amplifying stage has a theoretical capability of providing up to four times more output signal amplitude in a hearing

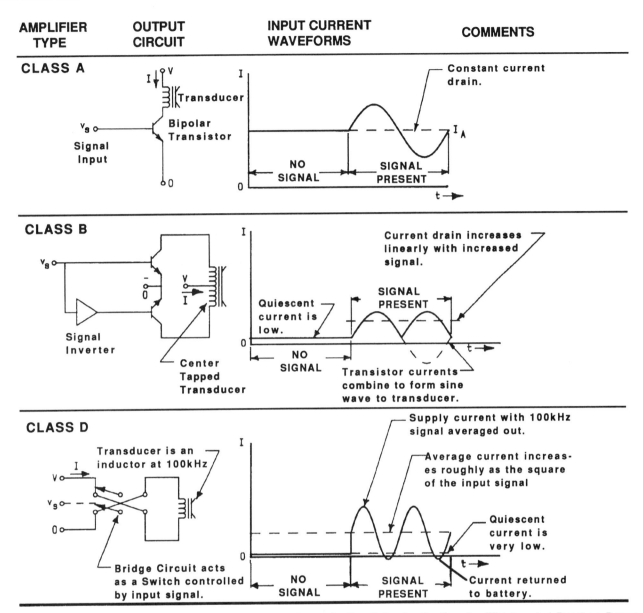

Figure 43.16. Circuits and waveforms of the three main classes of amplifiers used in hearing aids and how they can be differentiated on the basis of current drain. (Adapted from Ditthardt A. 1990. Application Notes for the Knowles EP Integrated Receiver. Report 10676-3, Knowles Electronics, Inc., Itasca, IL)

aid receiver, as compared with the single-ended output stage, before the onset of peak clipping (Preves and Newton, 1989). The class B amplifier also allows more output at high frequencies than does a class A amplifier.

Class D (pulse-width modulated) stage output amplifiers have been recently introduced into the hearing aid market (Knowles, 1988; Carlson, 1988; Ditthardt, 1990). Unlike the previous external class A or class B push-pull amplifier circuits, the class D can have its integrated output amplifier chip built *inside* the *receiver*. This IC drives the receiver from relatively low level al-

ternating current signals, which is a major departure from other receivers that are driven from external class A or class B amplifier circuits. The advantages of integrated class D receiver circuits as compared with older class B output stage designs are: (1) fewer components and required space; (2) reduced battery current; (3) higher output saturation levels and signal headroom; and (4) an increase in hearing aid reliability due to fewer external connections (Ditthardt, 1990). However, compared with state-of-the-art push-pull output amplifiers that are designed with few external components and that utilize very little current, there is little advantage to class D over class B. Thus, currently, the four advantages of class D apply more to class A. The two ways of utilizing class D versus class A include: (*a*) for the same battery current as class A, class D provides much higher SSPL90 and higher headroom; and (*b*) for the same SSPL90 as class A, class D requires much lower battery current. These are obviously the two extremes and one could operate anywhere on the continuum between the two. Thus, as always, advantages (2) and (3) are tradeoffs. The practical outcome of class D is smaller hearing aids (ITE and ITC) capable of greater gain and maximum output with less distortion due to increased headroom. Frequently, a small preamplifier chip is all that is needed to be added to the hearing aid circuitry, instead of the larger class B amplifier.

Single vs. Multiband Hearing Aid Amplifiers. Before 1987, most hearing aids utilized single band amplifiers. In these simple amplifiers, the audio signal is processed through a single circuit path, whose processing characteristics affect the entire frequency range. The only variation in frequency response provided in many of these simple amplifiers was a low-frequency tone control and a high-frequency control. Because only single pole high-pass and low-pass filters were often used for these controls, they generally affected a broad frequency range to provide a significant change in low-frequency gain and in high-frequency gain. These instruments were quite limited in capability for shaping their frequency responses to match target gain prescriptions. Frequently, with single-band hearing aid amplifiers, a dip was produced in the insertion gain response at 3000 Hz which could not be compensated for. In an effort to provide better capability with which to smooth insertion gain curves, hearing aid amplifiers were designed with an extra band of amplification in which a bandpass filter adds gain in a narrow frequency band to fill in the dip in insertion gain at 3000 Hz (Figure 43.17).

Splitting the frequency range into several bands with a multiband hearing aid circuit allows finer resolution in frequency shaping (Figure 43.17). A multiband hearing aid is somewhat like a graphic equalizer on a stereo receiver. With a graphic equalizer, the gain is individually adjustable (via sliders) in several frequency bands. A multiband hearing aid should not be confused with a multiresponse hearing aid. With a multiresponse hearing aid, the wearer can select by means of a remote control between three or four frequency responses. These different responses might be achieved with either a single-band or a multiband hearing aid amplifier. Thus, some multiband hearing aids are also multiresponse hearing aids, but not all multiresponse hearing aids are multiband hearing

aids. With a multiband hearing aid, gain is individually adjustable in several frequency bands. To accomplish this, the input signal is typically first passed through the hearing aid microphone and then through a preamplifier. Thereafter, the signal is split into several parallel bands, e.g., a low-frequency band, a mid-frequency band, and a high-frequency band. As in a graphic equalizer, the gain of each of the bands may be controlled by a potentiometer. The outputs of the three bands are summed together before the output amplifier and receiver.

The Argosy 3-channel clock™ hearing aid is unique among multiband hearing aids because of the addition of another block—the clock. The dotted lines connecting the clock to the three frequency bands and the arrows inside each frequency band box symbolize that the clock potentiometer simultaneously controls the frequency range of these bands (Figure 43.17). By varying the clock potentiometer setting, the center of the frequency range of the mid-band function of the 3-channel-clock may be shifted from about 800 Hz to about 3500 Hz.

Controls

Amplifier controls are a very important part of a hearing aid and are used to modify its basic performance. The control receiving the most wear is the **user-operated gain or volume control (VC),** which is a variable resister used to select the most effective listening level. As the volume control rotates, its resistance value varies and controls the amount of current flow between amplification stages. Volume controls on hearing aids have a *volume control taper* that can be designed to produce roughly equal increments in loudness for equal amounts of control knob rotation.

A **master adjustment of gain** is a trimmer control adjusted by the dispenser and is not the user-operated volume control. When set to a lower level, this control can be used to keep an instrument's gain below feedback, even when the user turns the volume control full-on. It can also be used to prevent overload when the SSPL90 has been reduced for tolerance reasons. Such a control usually reduces gain uniformly over the frequency range of the aid.

Electronic tone controls can alter the frequency response of the hearing aid and consist of filter networks (capacitors and resistors). Frequency response changes occur in discrete settings obtained by using a switch or by continuously variable (screwdriver) adjustment. Filter networks range from simple, passive first order filters to higher order "active" filters that allow for greater low-frequency suppression, high-frequency suppression, or suppression in any band of a multichannel hearing aid.

Hearing Instrument With Bandpass Filter Function

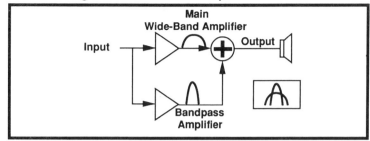

Generic 3-Band Hearing Instrument

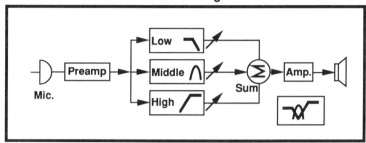

3-CHANNEL-CLOCK™ Argosy Hearing Instrument

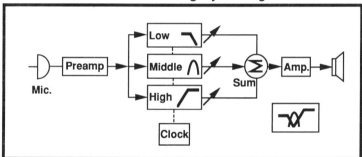

Figure 43.17. Multichannel hearing aid circuits in which gain is individually adjustable in several frequency bands. See text for explanation.

Adjustment of SSPL90 (output control) is commonly available. It is important for providing as much output capability as possible without exceeding a user's discomfort level. In some hearing aids, the range of adjustment may be on the order of 15 to 25 dB.

Other controls, such as AGC knee controls, feedback reduction circuits (mostly high-frequency gain reduction, but sometimes notch filters), etc. are also often found but will be discussed below.

Limiting Systems in Hearing Aids

Part of the function of every hearing aid is to amplify soft sounds strong enough to make them audible but not to overamplify them to produce an uncomfortable listening level. It is this upper level of amplification that limiting systems address. Every hearing aid has a maximum deliverable pressure (saturation, overload)

determined by the receiver, battery voltage, and amplifier. In practice, however, it is within the amplifier that most limiting occurs, at the saturation of the amplifier. The maximum deliverable pressure the hearing aid can produce, or its limiting level, however, can be adjusted below the level of saturation.

Concept of Linear Amplification. Linear hearing aid amplification characteristics are plotted on an input/output (IO) curve as illustrated in Figure 43.18. Linear amplification simply means that output changes always bear a direct and constant relationship to the input signal changes. As the input SPL is increased, the output SPL increases by the same number of decibels up to the point where the saturation output (SSPL) of the hearing aid is reached, after which further increases in input do not increase the output. The transfer function (or input/output characteristic) is always drawn at 45° to the horizontal if the abscissa and

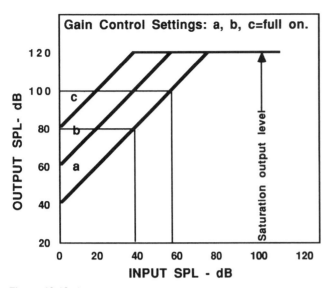

Figure 43.18. Input/output curves for a linear aid. As the gain control is advanced (from *a* to *c*), the gain in the linear portion of the curve increases, but when the saturation level is reached, no further increase occurs.

ordinate have the same scale. Linear amplification is also described as a 1:1 dB ratio over the operating range, unity slope, 45° slope, or constant gain. Any deviation from this would no longer be linear. In such a system, peak clipping of the output waveform occurs (the output is limited by means of distorting the signal and spreading the signal energy over a greater bandwidth) when the saturation output is approached and reached. (Most linear hearing aid circuits are in saturation when the input signal level reaches 90 dB SPL). At this level, considerable harmonic distortion results but in most cases presents no problem for the wearer if the aid has been selected or adjusted to have as much saturation output capability as possible without exceeding the discomfort level of the user. Recent research suggests also that linear hearing aids having a higher SSPL90, and thus high headroom, are less likely to exceed the wearer's aided uncomfortable level (UCL) than do aids having a lower SSPL90 but higher distortion (Fortune, Preves, and Woodruff, 1991). The instrument with the higher headroom and less distortion will saturate less readily, sound clearer at high levels, and will likely be worn at gain settings high enough to provide the wearer greater benefit. With respect to aided UCL, hearing aid wearers **do** equate distortion to loudness.

Limiting as a Result of Instant Output Regulation. These limiting systems include hard peak clipping and peak rounding. Both involve limiting the amplitude at a certain point but in somewhat different manners.

Hard peak clipping (PC, peak limiting) is the simplest form of output limiting and can be defined as the removal, by electronic means, of one (unsymmetrical) or both extremes (symmetrical) of alternating current amplitude peaks at a predetermined level. Class A amplifiers produce even (usually 2nd order) and odd harmonics. Push-pull amplifiers (class A or B) produce odd (usually 3rd order) harmonics. Although higher harmonics are usually more objectionable, the reason for the perceived improvement in push-pull amplifiers is that for a given output, harmonics are considerably lower than for a single-ended output amplifier (Olson, 1947). Also, as the high frequency range is increased, the more noticeable the subjective effect of harmonic distortion. Interestingly, peak clipping does not lower speech intelligibility significantly (Licklider, 1946).

Peak clipping can be accomplished by adding a resistor, connected in series, with the receiver (Figure 43.19). Two effects occur as a result of this: (1) the maximum current through the receiver is reduced so that the saturation output is reached at a lower level, and (2) only a part of the reduced output power becomes usable in the receiver—the remainder of the power is used up by the resistor. The level of limiting is determined by the value of the resistor (the higher the resistance, the lower the limiting level). Some hearing aids have a fixed level at which the output is limited (rather than to be allowed to reach its natural saturation). Others have an adjustable output level that can be controlled by manipulation of a screw or switch. Noteworthy is the fact that output reductions by peak clipping are often reflected as gain reductions by a like amount as well. (However, some amplifier designs now exist in which SSPL can be reduced via peak clipping without significantly reducing gain. This is the case, for example, with many of the Gennum class D amplifiers). Advantages of hard peak clipping are that its construction is simple and it requires very little space to accomplish very effective instantaneous output limiting. Its primary disadvantage is that harmonic and intermodulation distortion occurs above the limiting level.

Peak rounding (soft peak clipping, curvilinear compression, diode compression control, diode clipping, modified peak clipping) is a form of nonlinear amplification that is evidenced by a gradual, ever-diminishing increase in output with each successive increase in input. Limiting is achieved by adding a minimal number of components (two diodes, a capacitor and a variable resistor) to hard peak clipping circuitry to form a negative feedback loop that creates a nonlinear resistance and which most often (newer circuits now allow for appreciable reduction of SSPL90 without reducing gain) reduces both the gain and the output

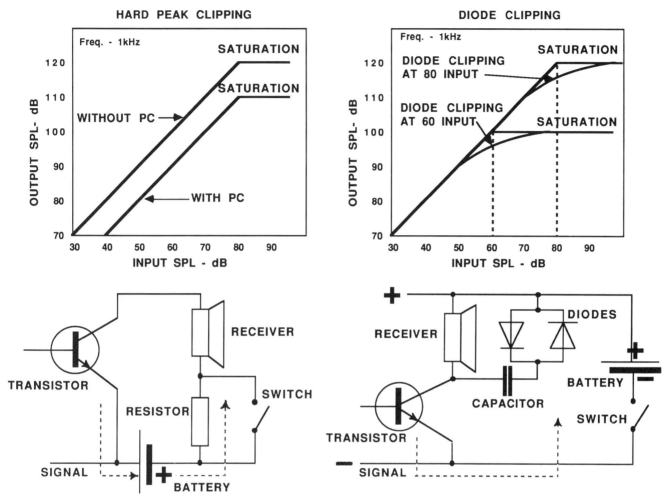

Figure 43.19. Input/output curves for peak clipping and peak rounding circuits, along with output stage circuit diagrams.

power (Figure 43.19). The variable resistor allows for the amount of negative feedback to be adjusted. The result resembles hard peak clipping in many respects, including the creation of harmonic distortion, except that the onset of clipping is gradual and the distortion arising from symmetrical peak clipping, while beginning at lower levels, is not as severe.

Limiting by Time-Dependent Gain Regulation; Feedback Circuits, Rectifier, Circuits, Adaptive Hearing Aids. *Automatic Gain Control (AGC).* These systems have a built-in monitoring circuit that automatically reduces the electronic gain of the hearing aid as a function of the magnitude of the signal being amplified. Gain is reduced by means other than peak clipping. Two major purposes of these systems are (1) to reduce the gain of an aid as the input SPL increases so that the output capability of the aid is not exceeded and distortion is thus kept low, and (2) to reduce the dynamic range of the output signal so that it is a better match to

the dynamic range of an impaired ear. Gain level is controlled automatically, thus the term **automatic gain control (AGC).** This action may be further described as the process of "compressing" a given dynamic range into a lesser dynamic range, but the descriptive circuit actions claimed by different manufacturers have led to confusion in the use of the term *compression.*

A wide variety of AGC characteristics exists in hearing aids, providing for individual differences. Figure 43.20 illustrates some of these differences. The generalized input/output curve of an AGC aid has three main components: a linear section at lower input SPLs where increments of input SPL cause equal increments in output SPL (linear); the compression section, where increments in input SPL cause smaller increments in the output SPL; and a limiting section, where increments in input SPL do not significantly increase the output SPL. Terms used to describe AGC system characteristics include:

AGC CHARACTERISTICS

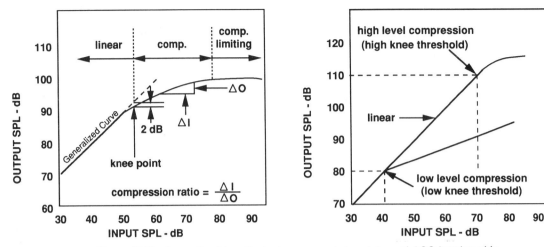

Figure 43.20. Generalized input/output curves and descriptors of AGC hearing aids.

1. **Limiting level.** The level to which the saturation output of the hearing aid is limited.
2. **AGC knee.** This is also known as the breakaway point, control threshold, compression threshold, or AGC threshold. It is the point at which the curve first departs by 2 dB on the output SPL scale from the extension of the linear portion of the curve that exists at input levels below the compression or limiting portion. The level at which the AGC knee occurs differentiates high level AGC from low level AGC systems.
3. **Compression ratio.** Identified also as the stiffness ratio or degree of compression, it is the quotient of a change in level of the input divided by the corresponding change in level at the output in the compression portion of the curve.
4. **Slewing rate.** This is the rate of gain change in msec/dB the circuit can handle.
5. **Time constants.** These are the time lags caused by the feedback circuit in stabilizing to a new gain value. The attack time refers to the length of time required for the feedback circuit to set the new gain value following a strong input signal. The release time refers to the length of time required for the reduced gain to return to normal amplification after the strong input signal is no longer present. Release times must be slower than attack times to avoid what is known as AGC flutter. If too fast, the compression action would follow the instantaneous amplitude of individual cycles, thus introducing severe waveform distortion.

Many variations of the generalized curve in Figure 43.20 exist. For example, in a compression limiting system, only the linear and the limiting section with a very high compression ratio may be present. The knee point might be at 60 to 80 dB SPL. In a wide range dynamic compression system, the knee point might be at 40 dB input SPL with a nearly constant compression ratio of 2:1 or 3:1 up to an input SPL of 80 or 90 dB.

Input-output characteristics differ with frequency. The test frequency used in the U.S. is 2000 Hz. The traditional method of showing frequency response at different input levels is to use a puretone input signal. For AGC aids, this method typically produces greater low-frequency response at high input levels than it should (blooming), because the lower gain at low frequencies is not sufficient to activate the AGC system (Ely et al., 1978). To overcome this, a high-frequency activating signal has been used while the test tone is swept across the frequency range (Studebaker, 1975; Berland, 1978). However, this method does not allow measurement in the vicinity of the activating signal frequency. A new standardized test method (anticipated to be ANSI S3.42-1992) uses a speech-shaped noise input signal to activate the AGC action appropriately over the frequency range at different input levels and produces very realistic AGC response curves. The method requires considerably more sophisticated test equipment.

The mechanism by which AGC action is achieved in the hearing aid is indicated in the diagram of Figure 43.21. A suitable sampling point in the amplifier circuit is selected. Alternating voltage from this point is fed into a level detecting device in the feedback circuit. This is usually a circuit that rectifies (changes) the AC voltage to a DC control voltage. The control voltage is fed into the variable gain type amplifier to oppose the current flow (reduce the gain) of the amplification stage(s). The amplifier gain is reduced, depending on the strength of the DC bias voltage received from the feedback detecting device. The purpose is to keep the gain of the hearing aid to a point where input plus gain does not equal saturation or exceed loudness discomfort level. When saturation is approached, the feedback circuit causes the gain to drop automatically to a level such that saturation does not occur.

The location where the monitoring circuit "samples" the output or signals to the receiver provides for classification of the AGC as either an input or as an output AGC circuit. Figure 43.22 diagrams the differences between the two. In the output-controlled AGC, excessively high input levels result in correspondingly large electrical signals arriving at the receiver. The monitor circuit will detect this at the final output of the amplifier (with the user-operated volume control at a point in the circuit preceding the sampling point) and reduce the gain of one or more of the previous stages in the amplifier to prevent the full intensity of that high level sound from being directed to the wearer. In input-controlled AGC, the sampling point is at an earlier point in the amplifier circuit, and the user-operated volume control is between it and the output stage. Because the feedback circuit occurs before the volume control, control of amplifier gain always occurs at the same input level, regardless of where the volume control is set. This forms the distinction between input and output AGC.

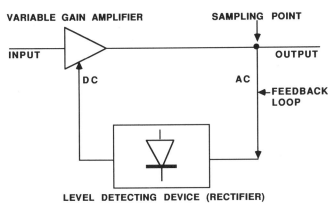

Figure 43.21. Rectification (changing an AC voltage to a DC amplification control voltage) is the mechanism by which AGC action is achieved.

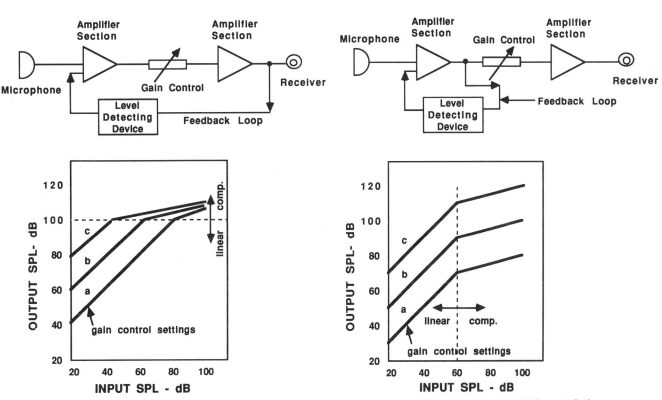

Figure 43.22. Block diagrams and input/output curves of an output- (*left*) and of an input- (*right*) controlled AGC hearing aid. Note the difference in performance as a result of gain control position.

The input-output curves of the two types are affected differently by the setting of the volume control. For output-controlled AGC, the knee point at which compression begins remains essentially constant on the output SPL scale regardless of the volume control setting (Figure 43.22). Only the gain of the aid is affected by the volume control setting; the maximal available output does not change very much, especially if the compression ratio is high. These circuits allow the dynamic range to be amplified to their maximum.

For input-controlled AGC the knee point at which compression starts remains essentially constant on the input SPL scale. Both gain and maximum available output are affected by changing the volume control position; that is, they are both increased/decreased as the volume control is increased/decreased. Input-controlled systems are more complex, involving additional circuitry, and often have a higher current drain. Fortunately, they offer less opportunity for output amplifier overload even with quite high input levels because the voltage to the output amplifier is controlled by the feedback circuit. Some hearing aids use a combination of the two types of AGC control, and still others place the volume control within the feedback loop. In other cases, multichannel compression systems have been developed with adjustable compression ratios for each channel. The difficulty in differentiating between these systems based on their *circuit electronics* has led Killion, Staab, and Preves (1990) to suggest a differentiation based on the *circuit reaction* to input levels (discussed later in this section).

Schweitzer (1979) points out that an AGC aid has an advantage over a linear aid with respect to S/N ratio at high noise levels because the gain is automatically reduced above the compression knee point for both signal and noise. For a peak clipping aid in saturation the S/N ratio would be close to zero. Still, it has generally been shown that it is important to maintain the linear portion of the hearing aid amplification over as wide a range as possible (before any limiting to satisfy the threshold of discomfort requirement) to maintain speech discrimination in noise (Sung and Sung, 1982). The implication is that the higher the threshold of discomfort (TD), and the wider the dynamic range, the higher the knee should be. Other advantages/disadvantages of the various systems is beyond the scope of this chapter, and the reader is referred to Walker and Dillon (1982), Dillon and Walker (1983), and Wernick (1985).

A major problem with AGC circuitry is that when any signal activates the monitoring circuit, the *entire* frequency spectrum is compressed. This includes the speech sounds desired to be heard as well as the loud input signal. To avoid this condition, the knee generally has to be set so that the low frequencies do not activate the AGC circuit, except at very high levels where compression is desired to limit the output to the TD.

But because the TD (and recruitment) is frequency dependent, decisions have to be reached to determine what the frequency-handling characteristics of the AGC circuit must be. Because of this consideration, a number of circuits have been introduced that attempt selective frequency or bandwidth compression through what might be called adaptive high pass filtering (Staab and Nunley, 1987; Siegelman and Preves, 1987; Kates, 1988). In these systems, AGC is achieved by using a high pass filter with a cutoff frequency that adaptively changes as a function of the input level. As the input level increases, the cutoff frequency moves upward. Another approach is through the use of multiband compressors having independent AGC circuits for each frequency band (Villchur, 1973; Waldhauer and Villchur, 1988; Hodgson and Lade, 1988, and Branderbit, 1991). Although early studies with multi-band compression systems have not been encouraging (Lippmann et al., 1981; Nábĕlek, 1983), more recent involvement seems to be holding some promising results.

Automatic gain control (AGC) action is fundamental to all circuits within the category of *limiting by time-dependent gain regulation,* even though additional functions may be incorporated. Because the circuitry is designed to act "automatically" to changes in the input stimulus and to process the incoming signals in some predetermined manner, it has more recently been termed **automatic signal processing (ASP).**

Automatic Signal Processing (ASP). A differentiation of ASP circuits can be made as follows: Those circuits that reduce gain at high levels and/or increase gain at low levels but do not change the frequency response of the hearing aid in the process, include the "traditional" automatic signal processing circuits (i.e., the AGC or compression circuits). Well-defined terms for these **fixed frequency response (FFR)** automatic signal processing circuits already exist, as indicated in Figure 43.23. More recently developed circuits that automatically change not only the gain but also the frequency response of the hearing aid as a function of the input signal are more accurately identified as **level dependent frequency response (LDFR)** circuits. Because of the variety of ways in which LDFR is performed, and because no simple, rigorous terms were used to describe their action, Killion, Staab, and Preves (1990) proposed a classification to distinguish them. This classification distinguishes among these circuits in terms of their reaction to low-level rather than high-level inputs because the former yielded easy-to-

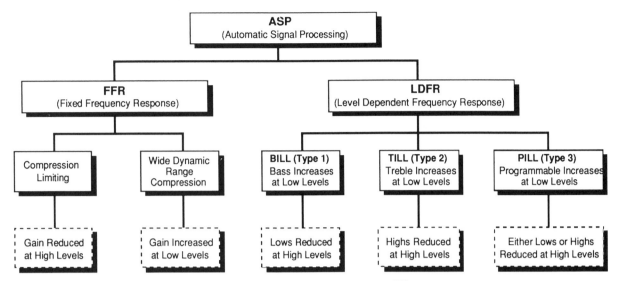

Figure 43.23. Outline of recommended classification system for ASP type hearing aids. (Adapted from Killion M, Staab W, and Preves D. Classifying automatic signal processors. Hearing Instruments, 1990;41:24–26.)

remember acronyms. (However, for those having difficulty in thinking about performance at low levels, the corresponding performance at high levels is indicated as well.).

Types of LDFR

BILL (Type 1). Bass Increases at Low Levels (bass decreases at high levels). This type of ASP describes circuits that provide relatively more bass response for low-level inputs than for high-level inputs (Figure 43.24). These circuits are intended for wearers who frequently find themselves in noisy environments, especially environments where low-frequency noise predominates. Under these circumstances there is evidence to indicate that reducing the low-frequency response may be helpful (Crain, 1988). If the overall gain of the instrument is also automatically reduced for high level inputs so as to prevent overload distortion, a further improvement is obtained (Preves and Newton, 1989).

TILL (Type 2). Treble Increases at Low Levels (treble decreases at high levels). This type of ASP describes the operation of circuits which provide relatively more treble response for low-level inputs than for high-level inputs. The K-AMP™ (Killion, 1990) is this type circuit and is intended for wearers having high-frequency hearing loss but who need more high-frequency gain for quiet sounds than they do for loud sounds. The amount of high-frequency gain that might produce a harsh or shrill sound in a linear hearing aid may become quite acceptable if the treble boost is automatically reduced for high-level inputs. If the overall gain is also automatically reduced for high input levels, it is possible to prevent audible distortion under nearly all listening conditions.

PILL (Type 3). Programmable Increases at Low Levels. This type of ASP describes the operation of circuits which provide for programmable level dependent frequency response modification in more than one amplification band and can be adjusted to provide either bass response decreases with increasing level or treble response decreases with increasing level (Waldhauer and Villchur, 1988). This form is the most versatile of the three because each of its independent processing bands can ignore strong influences in another band.

K-AMP™ Circuit. The most familiar ASP circuits for hearing aids are of the BILL type, which effectively give the most treble emphasis for loud sounds. The K-AMP type of TILL ASP works in just the opposite way, giving the most treble emphasis for quiet sounds. An automatic circuit operates an electronic volume control to make quiet sounds audible, and a tone control provides treble boost for quiet sounds. Thus, although the real-ear frequency response of a complete K-AMP hearing aid for loud sounds is essentially flat, the frequency response for quiet sounds will be high fidelity only, as perceived by the hearing-impaired listener. This type of ASP is intended for wearers with high-frequency hearing loss, when more gain is needed typically for quiet sounds, particularly at high frequencies, than for loud sounds. *(K-AMP™ is a trademark of Etymotic Research, Inc.)*

General Statement Concerning Limiting Systems

All hearing aid AGC circuits are nonlinear, and although they may vary from each other in many ways, none can be described well with a few curves or tables derived from the linear measurement techniques cur-

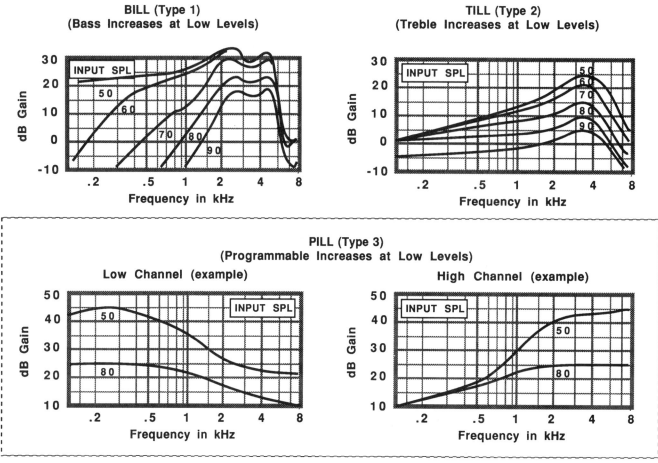

Figure 43.24. Level dependent frequency response (LDFR) circuits showing (Type 1) reduced low-frequency gain as input level increases, (Type 2) reduced high-frequency gain as input level increases, and (Type 3) either low-frequency gain reduction as input level increases, or high-frequency gain reduction as input level increases. (Adapted from Killion M, Staab W, and Preves D. Classifying automatic signal processors. Hear Instrum 1990;41:24–26.)

rently used to measure hearing aid performance. The departure from linearity of the non-AGC hearing aid is equally inscrutable and very important. The difference between a model that is well accepted and one that is not often lies in the difference in nonlinear properties that come into play during, and often after, loud inputs, which overload the amplifier of the instrument. Appropriate measurement techniques designed to measure nonlinearity must still be designed to measure AGC hearing aid systems.

Electroacoustic Distortions Affecting Hearing Aid Performance

Distortions. *Distortion* is a failure of a system to transmit or reproduce a received waveform with exactness. It refers to any signal component or characteristic present at the output of an amplifier which was not present at the input. Still, certain distortions, such as frequency distortion, are intentionally introduced

to solve specific hearing loss problems. Other distortions are not intentionally introduced and may affect hearing aid performance undesirably.

Several types of distortion of an acoustic signal are capable of being perceived by the ear; the two most common being harmonic distortion and intermodulation distortion—both forms of nonlinear distortion. Other distortions in addition to nonlinear distortion include: transient, frequency, phase, and noise. Fortunately, the influence of these types of distortion, at least as currently measured, on the successful use of today's hearing aids is probably minimal. Only the major types of distortion, and coherence as an indicator of sound quality, are therefore discussed in this section.

Harmonic distortion products (spurious signals) result when signals pass through a nonlinear amplifier. The amplifier corrupts the signal by taking a portion of the energy from the input signal and distributing it in the form of new signals, or distortion products, lying at multiples of the input signal frequency. For example, an input signal having a fundamental frequency of 500 Hz passing through a nonlinear amplifier would result in new signals formed, which are multiples of the fundamental (i.e., 1000, 1500, 2000, 2500 Hz, etc.). By separating the harmonics from the fundamental frequency in the output signal and measuring the ratio of the total value of the harmonics and the fundamental, the distortion figure can be expressed as a percentage. The greater the nonlinearity of the amplifier, the greater the amplitude of these distortion products, and the less the perceived sound quality (not necessarily intelligibility) of the hearing aid. Additionally, although the appearance of distortion in a hearing aid can indicate functional faults (e.g., defective transducers, asymmetry in the amplifier, etc.), certain intentional output limiting features against too loud a sound may result in distortion.

Intermodulation (IM) distortion (difference-frequency) is the ratio of the power of the output signal at frequencies other than those delivered to the hearing aid to the power of the signals that were applied to the hearing aid. It includes the arithmetic sums and difference tones of the input signals and their harmonics (Figure 43.25). Intermodulation distortion is illustrated by considering two input frequencies (500 and 700 Hz as examples) of equal amplitudes but not harmonically related. As a result of being passed through a nonlinear system, a complex output results with both of these frequencies present, along with their harmonics (500, 1000, 1500, and 2000; 700, 1400, and 2100 Hz). In addition, their sums and difference frequencies are generated. For example, the sum is 500 + 700 or 1200 Hz; and the difference tone is 700–500 = 200 Hz. Intermodulation distortion is explained by using two input signals, because it arises when two or more frequencies are present, such as in speech. With a complex input, such as speech

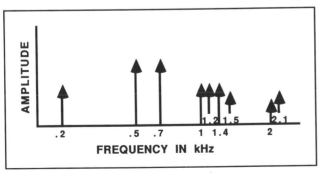

Figure 43.25. Illustration of intermodulation distortion products (sum and difference frequencies) generated by two equal amplitude signals of 0.5 and 0.7 kHz after nonlinear processing.

in high-level environmental noise, an even greater number of frequencies would be added!

Harmonic distortion components lie at frequency multiples of the fundamental, which audibly can be quite acceptable because the harmonic distortion components often coincide with the harmonic components already found in speech. Additionally, if the high-frequency response of the hearing aid is reduced, an increase of distortion can be tolerated. Nevertheless, IM distortion gives rise to sum and difference components which have no harmonic musical relationships and, therefore, can be quite annoying.

Transient distortion (response) occurs because of mechanical or electrical resonances in the hearing aid system that create oscillations of short duration when excited by a short signal burst. The distortion can result from rapid fluctuations in the amplitude or the frequency of the stimulus, or both. It is believed that the hearing aid must be highly damped, the same as the ear, to avoid ringing which masks and overshoot and which distort succeeding phonemes. Balmer (1977) states that the impaired ear can detect transient distortion and requires an average of 9 dB less gain from a good transient response aid to achieve listening comfort (and about 15% better consonant identification).

Frequency (amplitude or linear) distortion occurs when the frequency response curve of the hearing aid favors or suppresses some frequencies more than others. **Phase distortion** results when the phase angle between the fundamental frequency and any of its harmonics, or between any two frequencies of a complex wave, changes.

The effects of **hearing aid distortion and its effects on headroom** may be the single most common cause of hearing aid rejection (Preves and Newton, 1989). **Headroom** is defined as the difference in dB between the combination of the peak input level plus the gain, and the level at which peak clipping occurs. The basic concept is illustrated in Figure 43.26. The reader is referred to Preves and Woodruff (1990) for an in-depth explanation of headroom.

Agnew (1988) states that distortions created within hearing aids are thought to cause subjective judgments of poor quality and poor speech clarity. These distortions arise because of inadequate headroom that causes clipping and other types of nonlinear distortion at high input levels. The result is that hearing aids are often turned off in noisy backgrounds or are not worn at all. According to Preves and Newton, these distortions occur in all types of hearing aid saturation, whether because of linear, compression, or another type of automatic signal processing circuitry; although they are most likely to occur in linear (nonadapting)

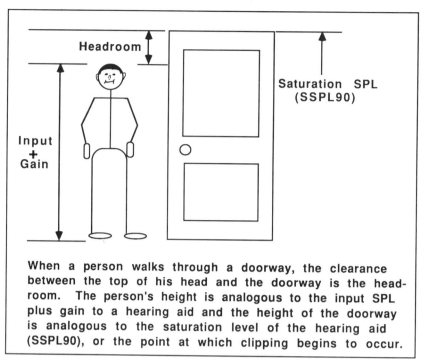

Headroom

Saturation SPL (SSPL90)

Input + Gain

When a person walks through a doorway, the clearance between the top of his head and the doorway is the headroom. The person's height is analogous to the input SPL plus gain to a hearing aid and the height of the doorway is analogous to the saturation level of the hearing aid (SSPL90), or the point at which clipping begins to occur.

Figure 43.26. Illustration of the basic concept of headroom in hearing aids. (Adapted from Preves D, and Woodruff B. Some methods of improving and assessing hearing aid headroom. Audecibel 1990;38:8–13.)

hearing aids that have a low SSPL90 and high gain. Unfortunately, because input/output functions are affected by AGC or gain reduction caused by an adaptive filter, they are not good indicators of distortion and headroom (Preves and Woodruff, 1990).

Methods used to preserve headroom include: (*a*) lowering the input SPL to the hearing aid, by use of the volume control or by the use of an AGC circuit; (*b*) raising the SSPL90 in linear aids, by using class A output stage amplifiers having lower output impedance receivers; or with class B push-pull or class D output stage amplifiers (Preves and Woodruff, 1990), or (*c*) using a combination of the above.

Because existing harmonic distortion measures (per ANSI S3.22-1987) do not necessarily correlate with sound quality, another measure has been sought that would serve as a useful quantitative indicator of subjectively observed sound quality in hearing aids. Such an indicator may be the **coherence function** (Preves and Newton, 1989; Preves and Woodruff, 1990; Dyrlund, 1989; Bareham, 1990), which describes the cumulative effect of different forms of signal corruption by a hearing aid. These authors define coherence as a direct measure of the linearity of a hearing aid and represents, in a number from 0 to 1, what part of the output signal of a hearing aid is due only to the input signal over the frequency range of interest. A coherence of 1.0 signifies "perfect" reproduction of

the input signal by the hearing aid. A coherence of 0 signifies total degradation of the input signal by the aid. At high input levels, low coherence indicates mainly the harmonic and intermodulation distortion resulting from inadequate headroom. At low input levels, low coherence indicates high levels of hearing aid amplifier noise. Figure 43.27 shows a comparison of coherence function of two different hearing aids (linear vs. ASP) to a continuous, broadband, speech-shaped random noise input signal varied from 50 to 90 dB SPL in 10 dB steps. This type stimulus is used rather than puretones because it is a more realistic stimulus. With a broad-band random noise input, all possible frequencies are presented to the hearing aid at the same time, and if the hearing aid has distortion, nonlinear combinations of some of these frequencies are created as distortion simultaneously. The top graphs show the frequency responses, and the lower graphs show the corresponding coherence. The linear aid shows that as the noise input increases, saturation is reached and the gain of the aid is reduced as a result of output clipping. Coherence drops, especially in the high frequencies (with 90 dB input at 2 kHz the coherence is 0.5, indicating that equal parts of the output signal are caused by the input signal and distortion components). In contrast, the ASP aid shows that with increasing input levels the low-frequency gain is reduced, and high frequency coherence is increased

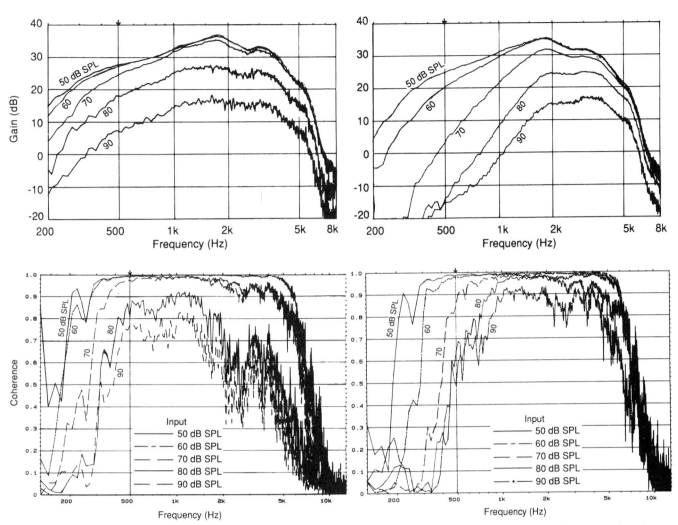

Figure 43.27. A comparison of coherence function of two different hearing aids (linear/left vs ASP/right) to a continuous, broadband, speech-shaped random noise input signal varied from 50–90 dB SPL in 10 dB steps (Courtesy of Argosy Electronics, Inc., Eden Prairie, MN)

dramatically (to almost 0.85). This indicates that 58% of the output signal has been caused by the input signal and 42% by circuit noise and distortion in the hearing aid. A "noise distortion," "true signal-to-noise ratio," or "signal-to-distortion ratio" may be computed from the coherence, and is 58%. The noise distortion formula uses a square root term: % noise & distortion = SQRT {[[1-coh]]/coh} × 100% (Preves, 1990).

Hearing Aid Noise

Amplifier noise can be added to an input signal and, thus, changes it. This noise is not a form of nonlinearity of the input signal and therefore is usually measured as a signal-to-noise (S/N) ratio. With the introduction of silicon transistors and the larger microphones then used, internal hearing aid noise has become negligible in comparison with ambient sound levels. Nevertheless, as Preves notes (1992), circuit noise complaints are still heard about state of the art circuits from hearing aid wearers having ski-slope hearing losses. Circuit noise is higher if CMOS circuitry is used, as in class D output stages, most programmable hearing aids, and many multi-channel hearing aids.

When heard, it is a buzzing or white noise in the hearing aid receiver and can be reduced by the addition of appropriate electronics. A major source of potential noise is the microphone. Because its noise is amplified by the circuitry, the inherent noise level of the microphone is one of the factors that determine the weakest signal the hearing aid can handle effectively. Also, inadequate decoupling of the battery and amplifier circuit can cause an electrical oscillation, which is described as a "motorboating" sound.

Feedback

Three types of feedback are most often identified with hearing aids. A good summary of these and other types is presented in Pollack (1980).

Acoustical feedback caused by direct sound leakage is the most common and occurs when the output signal from the hearing aid is picked up by its own microphone and reamplified. A "whistling" or "squealing" sound results. Acoustical feedback can also be due to leakage of the sound through or around an earmold or tubing, by poor acoustic isolation of either or both of the hearing aid transducers—especially under high gain usage—or by sharp resonant peaks in the hearing aid frequency response.

Mechanical feedback can occur due to mechanical vibration from the receiver to the closely spaced microphone. Rubber cushions are used to isolate the transducers from the case and from each other. To minimize mechanical feedback, the transducers within the hearing aid case are oriented so that their directions of sensitivity and maximal vibration are at right angles to each other. These positions are, however, more difficult to maintain in custom-molded hearing aid products.

Magnetic feedback can result from interaction between the telephone coil and some other magnetic field, such as that of the receiver. Careful design to avoid this is required in high gain/output hearing aids.

Acoustical Factors Affecting Hearing Aid Performance

Not only is the performance of the hearing aid altered within the hearing aid itself, but additional factors modify the signal between its source and the eardrum of the listener. Figure 43.28 adapted from Libby (1985) provides an excellent overview of these factors. He breaks these factors down into *far field effects, near field effects, hearing aid responses,* and *hearing aid plumbing.* To obtain the real ear performance at the ear of the listener, these factors must be considered because they affect the performance of the hearing aid.

Far Field Effects

Far field effects include the signal-to-noise ratio (S/N), reverberation, and direction of the sound source. The **signal-to-noise ratio** is the relationship between the

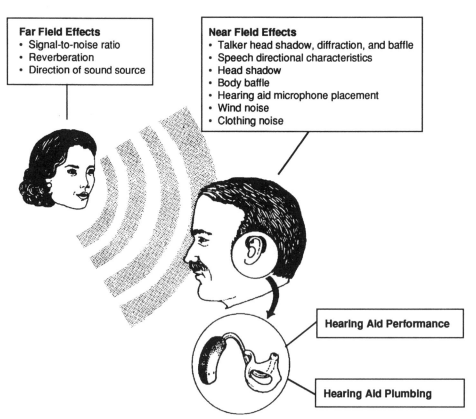

Figure 43.28. Overview of acoustical factors affecting hearing aid performance (Adapted from Libby E. Hearing instrument systems technology and performance standards. 1985:201–311. In Saudlin RE (Ed.). Hearing Instrument Science and Fitting Practices. National Institute for Hearing Instruments Studies, Livonia, MI: 1985.

intensity of the desired signal to that of the undesired signal—most frequently background or environmental noise. For example, if a signal level is 50 dB and a noise level is 45 dB, the signal to noise ratio is 50−45 or +5 dB. A S/N ratio of −5 dB means the noise is 5 dB greater than the signal. Hearing-impaired listeners require a S/N ratio from +14 to 30 dB, about 15 dB higher than required by normal hearing persons, to use their hearing as effectively as possible (Olsen and Carhart, 1967; Carhart and Tillman, 1970; Gengel, 1971; Dirks et al., 1982). The significance of the far field (distance) on the S/N ratio is well illustrated in Figure 43.29, adapted from Ross, 1986. For example, assume the ambient noise in a room to be 60 dB SPL and the talker's speech intensity at 6 inches to be 84 dB SPL. Sound pressure levels at the other distances are calculated by using the inverse square law (in which the SPL decreases by 6 dB with every doubling of distance). Because these calculations are made without the benefit of reflected sound (which would maintain a more constant SPL), they may suggest somewhat poorer results than realistically occur. Still, the example serves to illustrate well that for the more desirable S/N ratios to be approximated, the talker and hearing aid microphone must be in fairly close proximity. This can include: (*a*) moving closer to the talker; (*b*) moving the hearing aid microphone closer to the talker; (*c*) asking the talker to speak up; and (*d*) using well-designed directional microphone hearing aids (Killion, 1985).

It has also been demonstrated that a properly fitted wideband hearing aid could produce substantial assistance, giving an 18% (Pascoe, 1975) to a 22% (Skinner et al. (1982) advantage in intelligibility in noise compared with a narrower band aid. The use of binaural

aids has also been shown to provide an additional 2 to 3 dB improvement in a diffuse field (Killion, 1985). A **diffuse field** is a special sound field set up in a reverberant environment in which the amplitudes of signals in the sound field are constant over a large volume due to the addition of multitudes of standing wave patterns.

Reverberation is the persistence of sound within an enclosure after the original sound has ceased and is measured as the time in seconds for the signal to drop 60 dB, after its termination from its steady state. In an enclosure, the total sound energy present is a combination of direct sounds and their reflections. (For a full explanation of room acoustics and as it relates to intelligibility, see Chapter 41). In more reverberant enclosures the reflected sound will exceed the level of the direct sound and is more noticeable the greater the distance from the source. In general, hard, reflective surfaces and expanding room volume increase reverberation, whereas absorbent materials and smaller room volume reduce reverberation. This is due to the fact that the amount of reflective surface in an enclosure influences the amount of reflected energy and therefore reverberation time. Hodgson (1986) in reviewing several studies relating to reverberation and intelligibility, summarizes them as follows: speech intelligibility generally decreases as reverberation time increases, hearing-impaired persons perform more poorly due to reverberation than normals in adverse listening conditions, reverberation disrupts intelligibility in noise much more than in quiet environments, and that binaural performance is better than monaural in a noisy reverberant room. The implication for hearing aid use should be obvious—get close to the speaker, be situated where background noise is min-

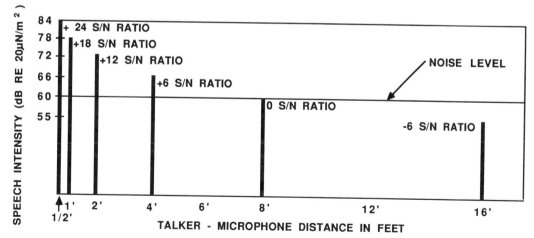

Figure 43.29. Illustration of the significance of the far field (distance) on the S/N ratio. See text for explanation. (Adapted from Ross M. Classroom amplification. In Hodgson WR, Ed. Hearing Aid Assessment and Use in Audiologic Habilitation. Baltimore: Williams & Wilkins, 1986:231–265.

imal use binaural amplification, and consider an assistive listening device.

With respect to **direction of the sound source** in a far field, localization generally occurs according to the precedence effect (localization is to sound that arrives at the ears first and/or is the strongest). Unfortunately, this concept is complicated by the fact that sounds from a far field contain reflected waves or reverberant sounds and do confuse localization. The localization of far field sounds is not easily quantified (Fletcher, 1953). However, discounting the effects of reflected waves or reverberant sounds, low frequencies spread out from the source and bend around objects in their path of travel. The amount of diffraction is dependent on the wavelength of the sound in comparison to the size of the object. High frequencies tend to travel in a straight line from the source. As a result, when a high frequency sound encounters an object in its path, an acoustic shadow is cast, and the area behind the object experiences no sound. This means that localization is more likely to occur for low frequency than for high frequency sounds because low frequency sounds have a greater likelihood of being heard. Additionally, binaural hearing and the time of arrival of a sound at each ear are strong factors in direction determination.

Near Field Effects

The effects of head shadow should be viewed from two perspectives: (1) from the effect it has on the speaker's voice and (2) the effect it has on the listener.

Speech directional characteristics show that speech sounds are very directional, with the directionality greater at high frequencies (Dunn and Farnsworth, 1939). Martin (1982) shows these reductions when recorded from the rear (180°) to be approximately as follows: (100 Hz = -5 dB; 400 Hz = -8 dB; 1000 Hz = -8 dB; 4000 Hz = -18dB; and 10,000 Hz = -18dB). The actual loss at each of the frequencies also varies with the angle of incidence. This helps explain why speech is poorly received behind a talker, especially in nonreflective environments.

Head shadow arises whenever the head is interposed between the receiving ear and the signal source, and affects mainly mid- and high-frequency sounds. The general effect is that the intensity of the signal is reduced as it passes around the head. The effect begins at about 1500 Hz with minimal attenuation and continues upward, approximating 15 dB at 5000 Hz (Staab, 1988b). As a result, high-frequency speech information is reduced when the signal is heard only from the far ear side. For speech, the overall reduction in the effective intensity caused by the head

shadow is about 6 dB (Tillman et al., 1963). The effect of this on intelligibility is a reported reduction of 23% between direct and indirect listening (Nordlund and Fritzell, (1963). The reduction would not be as great if the listener moved his or her head to eliminate the head shadow. The effect of head shadow is most noticeable in those having a nonaidable ear or for those who wear only one hearing aid. The advantage, therefore, of binaural amplification in eliminating head shadow effect can be about 25% or the equivalent of about a 6 dB improvement in S/N ratio.

Enhancement (**head baffle effect**) of the intensity of the signal can also grow when it is heard directly (without head shadow) by the near ear. Again, the magnitude is determined by the azimuth and the frequency of the signal. Sivian and White (1933) report an enhancement of approximately 5 dB when measured in a horizontal plane.

Body baffle arises from the effect of the body in a sound field and is most pronounced for body-worn hearing aids (Hanson, 1945; Romanow, 1942; and Byrne, 1983). Because of the effects of the body, a low-frequency "emphasis" of about 5 to 10 dB (smaller size body aids may account for the larger low-frequency boost) occurs near 500 Hz, with a similar reduction in hearing aid performance around 2000 Hz. Body shadow effects also occur, and when recorded from 180°, amount to an average (500, 1000, and 2000 Hz) reduction of approximately 8 dB, with the greatest reduction in the higher frequencies.

Hearing aid microphone placement has been shown to contribute significantly to hearing aid performance. A study by Lybarger and Barron (1965) found a forward-facing top-mounted microphone location to be superior to bottom-mounted microphone locations in BTE hearing aids. Of three microphone locations (in-the-ear, behind-the-ear, and over-the-ear), Berland and Nielson (1969) reported a 7 to 10 dB higher gain from 2000 Hz to 5000 Hz with the in-the-ear microphone location over the better of the two other microphone locations. This was due solely to the pinna and the microphone placement within the ear. Localization in both quiet and noise was found to be far superior for both monaural and binaural conditions with ITE microphone locations than with BTE microphone locations (Orton and Preves, 1979). Also, a seven percent superiority in speech discrimination was shown with the ITE location vs the BTE location (Randolph, Gierula, and Ross, 1977). Even on the ITE faceplate, a top-mounted microphone location was shown to have superior high-frequency response relative to other faceplate microphone locations (Staab, 1980).

When an individual wearing a hearing aid is placed

in an air stream, **wind noise** is generated by the turbulence building up around the head of the wearer, around the hearing aid, and eventually at the microphone opening. Pragmatically, the first noise source, the turbulence around the head, will never be eliminated. Wind noise is greatly dependent on wind velocity, so that a two-fold increase in wind velocity will raise the wind noise level more than 20 dB (Dalsgaard, Johansen, and Chisnall, 1967). These authors state that wind noise strongly depends on the position and shape of the microphone opening. Considerable reduction in wind noise could be obtained by altering the air stream around the microphone opening, or by positioning the microphone opening at a location where it is most protected against the wind. However, these methods influence only that part of the wind noise caused by air moving across the microphone opening and will not influence that noise generated by turbulence around the head itself.

Clothing noise relates only to body-worn hearing aids. When the hearing aid is concealed under the clothing the movement of fabric over the microphone opening creates noise. Wearing the hearing aid outside the clothing, using a top-mounted microphone location and wearing soft textured and unstarched clothing lessens the problem (Libby, 1985).

Hearing Aid Responses

Acoustical factors that modify the hearing aid electroacoustical characteristics will be dealt with later in this chapter.

Hearing Aid Plumbing

Hearing aid plumbing is more commonly referred to as earmold acoustics. In the last edition of *HOCA,* this topic took an entire chapter; however, because of the shift in hearing aid type usage, the topic, while still important, no longer commands the same length discussion.

EARMOLDS AND EARMOLD SYSTEMS

The Earmold System

The earmold system includes the complete sound path from the exit port of the hearing aid receiver to the tip of the earpiece in the ear canal. It is longer and can be more complex in BTE and EG aids than in ITE or ITC aids, where the custom-molded shell of the aid forms the outer part of the earmold. The primary function of the earmold system is to direct sound efficiently and with the desired frequency response from the receiver to the tympanic membrane. The earmold system can have a dramatic effect on the overall performance of a hearing aid and must be given careful consideration.

Real Ear Unaided Response

The ear canal, head, and pinna have a resonance, and although differing somewhat among individuals, it measures approximately 17 dB near 2700 Hz. When an earmold is inserted into the ear, this normal resonance loses its effectiveness. A goal of some earmold acoustic modification procedures is to increase the response in the 2700 Hz region to compensate for the loss of this resonance.

Earmolds

Figure 43.30 illustrates a number of basic types of earmolds. In all cases, the earmold must be comfortable, nonallergic, and cosmetically acceptable to the user or it will not be worn. Earmolds are usually made of a hard plastic, such as acrylic, or of a durable soft plastic. Soft plastic molds are helpful in eliminating acoustic feedback with high gain aids. It should be pointed out that good earmolds can be made only from good earmold impressions. A large percentage of impressions received by earmold laboratories are extremely poor. Anyone fitting hearing aids must learn how to make a truly accurate impression. Excellent information on earmold impression techniques is available from a number of earmold laboratories.

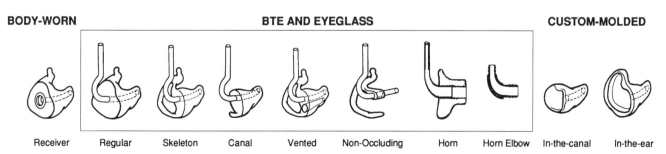

BODY-WORN   **BTE AND EYEGLASS**   **CUSTOM-MOLDED**

Receiver   Regular   Skeleton   Canal   Vented   Non-Occluding   Horn   Horn Elbow   In-the-canal   In-the-ear

Figure 43.30. Basic types of earmolds

Acoustic Elements and Analogs

Some understanding of the acoustic elements involved in an earmold system and their analog electrical counterparts can be helpful.

A property of tubes or orifices, acoustic mass or inertance, M_A, appears as **inductance** in an electrical analog circuit. For a short tube of length L and cross-section S, the inertance is $\rho L/S$, where ρ is the density of air. For a given short length, inertance decreases as the cross-section S increases. The impedance (reactance) due to inertance increases linearly with frequency. Longer tube lengths are more complex and are best treated as acoustical transmission lines, for which there are well-known electrical analogs. These require relatively complex mathematical solutions for the determination of their effects. It is easier to measure the response of actual tubing systems, and this has usually been done in this chapter.

Acoustic **compliance,** C_A, acts like a spring or electrical capacitance. It is the property of a cavity in the acoustical system. $C_A = V/\rho c^2$, where V is the volume of the cavity, ρ is the density of air, and c is the velocity of sound in air. The impedance (reactance) of an acoustic compliance decreases linearly with frequency.

Acoustic **resistance,** R_A, is similar to mechanical friction or electrical resistance. Dampers placed in the earmold system to reduce peaks in response or the friction of vibrating air against the inside walls of earmold tubing are examples of acoustic resistance. A resistive component is also present at the eardrum (Shaw, 1975, 1980).

Acoustic **impedance,** Z_A, can be thought of as opposition to the flow of acoustic energy that results from the presence of some combination of any or all of the acoustic elements described. At frequencies where positive reactance due to inertance equals negative reactance due to compliance, resonances may occur that affect impedance and cause peaks or dips in response. Units for acoustic quantities may be mks (meter-kilogram-second) or cgs (centimeter-gram-second). The latter system of units often is preferred in hearing aid systems. For more detailed information on these concepts, the reader is directed to Beranek (1954), Cox (1979), Studebaker and Hochberg (1980), and Leavitt (1986).

Earmold Systems for Body-Worn Hearing Aids

The button receiver used with body-worn aids has a nub that fits into a snap ring socket molded or pressed into the outer face of the "standard" or "receiver" type earmold. A cross-section of the system is shown in Figure 43.31A, with the acoustic elements identified. A simplified electrical analog is shown below the cross-section diagram. The magnetic transduction mecha-

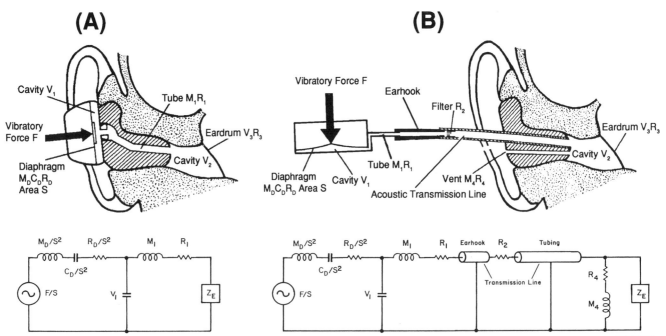

Figure 43.31. Cross-section of the earmold coupling systems for (A) body-worn hearing aids (button type systems); and for (B) BTE and EG hearing aids (tubing type systems), identifying the acoustic elements of the transmission system. Vibratory force F is proportional to the signal current through the receiver coil. In (B), the acoustic transmission line includes a flexible tube from receiver to nub and the earhook (shown straight). Analog electrical counterparts are shown below the acoustic elements. Z_E could be the impedance of an actual ear, or that of a 2-cc coupler or an ear simulator.

nism of the receiver produces an alternating force F that causes the diaphragm to vibrate when electrical signals from the hearing aid amplifier are applied. The mechanical mass, compliance, and resistance of the diaphragm strongly influence the vibratory response. Adjacent to the diaphragm is a small cavity, V_1, in which sound pressure is developed. Sound is then transmitted through the hole in the earmold. This hole, being relatively short, acts primarily as an acoustic inertance plus an acoustic resistance (M_1, R_1). The diameter and length of this hole significantly affect response.

A medium length (18 mm long by 3 mm in diameter) sound bore earmold used with a button receiver produces a response curve that is moderately flat to about 3400 Hz. A low-frequency peak at about 1000 Hz is pretty much damped out internally. An upper peak results primarily from the resonance between the compliance of cavity V_1 and the inertance M_1 of the drilled hole. When the sound bore is extended to 23.4 mm (2.4 mm in diameter), a loss of high-frequency response occurs. Too large a hole diameter would also be undesirable. The sound pressure driving the eardrum is developed in ear canal cavity V_2, having a volume of roughly 0.6 cc. The compliance of the eardrum adds an equivalent volume of about 0.8 cc and a resistance of about 350 acoustic ohms. As compared with a medium length tip, a very short tip might cause a drop in SPL of about 2 dB; a very long tip might cause an increase in SPL in cavity V_2 of about 2 dB.

Venting is not often used with high gain, high output body-worn aids, where the best possible seal is needed to prevent acoustic feedback.

Earmold Systems for BTE and Eyeglass Hearing Aids (Tubing Type Systems)

Tubing type earmold systems usually connect the earmold to a receiver located inside the hearing aid case. A sectional diagram is shown in Figure 43.31B. With tubing type systems, substantial possibilities for performance modification exist.

Sound developed in cavity V_1 is carried to the exit nub of the hearing aid through a relatively short length of small diameter flexible tubing M_1R_1. In addition to conducting sound, this tube also serves as a vibration isolator to prevent mechanical vibration of the receiver case from reaching the hearing aid case and microphone and causing feedback.

In an eyeglass aid, the visible earmold tubing (identified as the acoustic transmission line) starts at the exit nub; in BTE aids an earhook is interposed between the exit nub and the tubing. All tubing sections and earhook act as acoustic transmission lines and the effect of different tubing systems can be predicted using transmission line theory (Carlson, 1974a; White et al., 1980; Gilman, 1981). The effects can also be predicted experimentally using coupler or ear simulator measurements. At low and mid frequencies (200 to 1500 Hz), the tubing can be represented approximately as a mass that resonates with the receiver stiffness to produce a peak near 1000 Hz. At higher frequencies, the tubing produces a series of response peaks and dips (Carlson, 1974b; Cox, 1979). Acoustic resistances, or dampers, (R_2) may be placed at various locations along the tubing system. Sound passing through the tubing enters the ear canal cavity V_2. Properties of cavity V_2 explained previously for body-worn systems also apply to tubing type earmolds that occlude the ear canal. Additionally, tubing type earmold systems are often vented (M_4R_4), which affects low frequency response.

A *nonoccluding earmold* can consist of simply a piece of formed tubing projecting into the ear canal. More preferably, it consists of a "skeletalized" earmold designed to hold the tubing in place with minimal blocking of the ear canal. If no supporting structure is used, a heavier wall tubing is needed to give the necessary mechanical strength to maintain its formed shape. The nonoccluding earmold can be considered as working into cavity V_2 of a size similar to that of a closed earmold, but with a huge vent present. The small inertance of the large vent acts somewhat like a short circuit at low frequencies, and little SPL is developed in the ear canal at low frequencies. Thus, the vent performs as a low cut (high pass) filter with an upward slope of about 12 dB per octave.

The Earhook. In BTE aids, an earhook is interposed between the exit nub and the tubing. In eyeglass aids, the tubing starts at the exit nub and is typically 20 or 25 mm shorter than for BTE aids. The earhook is a semirigid acoustic connector used to provide retention of the aid over the ear and to conduct sound to the tubing portion of the earmold. Earhooks are available in a variety of sizes and materials and do influence acoustic performance. Many earhooks have a considerable taper in bore toward the tubing end and thus a very small end opening, which may not be good acoustically. However, earhooks that have minimal downward taper are available. One such earhook measured had a length of 22 mm, a starting bore of 2.25 mm and a final bore at the tubing end of 1.83 mm, averaging very nearly 2 mm. This would act acoustically very much like #13 tubing. Earhooks are available with integral dampers, although it is perhaps easier to install dampers in the tubing. A series of response modifying earhooks that provide low-pass response, a 2000 Hz notch filter, and a high pass response filter (Killion and Wilson, 1985) also exist.

Earmold Tubing. Standard sizes for earmold tubing have been established by the National Association of Earmold Laboratories (NAEL) (Blue, 1979), and are listed in Table 43.2 along with a few other available sizes. The two most commonly used sizes are #13 medium and #13 thick. Acoustically, only the inside diameter, which the tubing number identifies, has a significant effect on sound transmission. However, the thick wall tubing is often used to reduce the possibility of sound radiation that could cause acoustic feedback in high gain aids.

The effects of different tubing inside diameters (ID) are shown in Figure 43.32 as measured on a closed 2-cc coupler for a wide-band hearing aid receiver and a tubing length of 43 mm (which corre-

Table 43.2.
Standard Sizes for Earmold Tubing as Established by the National Association of Earmold Laboratories (NAEL)

Size	Normal Inside Diameter		Nominal Nominal Diameter	
	Inch	mm	Inch	mm
NAEL sizes				
No. 9	.118	3.00	.158	4.01
No. 12 standard	.085	2.16	.125	3.18
No. 13 standard	.076	1.93	.116	2.95
No. 13 medium	.076	1.93	.122	3.10
No. 13 thick	.076	1.93	.130	3.30
No. 14 standard	.066	1.68	.116	2.95
No. 15 standard	.059	1.50	.116	2.95
No. 16 standard	.053	1.35	.116	2.95
No. 16 thin	.053	1.35	.085	2.16
Other sizes				
No. 13 double wall	.076	1.93	.142	3.61
No. 15 thick wall	.059	1.50	.140	3.56
1/32 inch	.031	0.79	.094	2.39

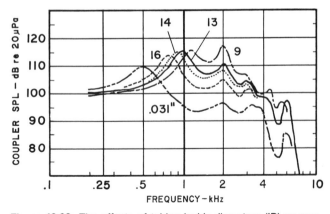

Figure 43.32. The effects of tubing inside diameters (ID) as measured on a closed 2-cc coupler for a wide-band hearing aid receiver and a tubing length of 43 mm. Tubing length is from end of earhook to reference plane of coupler. Numbers indicate NAEL tubing sizes except for 0.031-inch tubing.

sponds approximately to the typical distance from the end of an earhook to the tip of a medium length earmold). As can be seen, tubing ID could be used as a means of shifting emphasis from higher to lower frequencies or vice versa. Smaller diameter tubing can also be used as a means of reducing average saturation output and gain. Results are similar when tests are made on a closed ear simulator.

Tubing length on actual earmolds will vary over a moderate range. The effect of tubing length on receiver response is to shift the response curve peaks upward in frequency as the length decreases. In one test, the first response peak was shifted from about 850 Hz to about 1100 Hz when the tubing length was shortened from 55 to 30 mm.

Dampers. Dampers are acoustical resistances that can be placed at appropriate locations in the tubing transmission line to smooth peaks in response. Dampers made from fine plastic mesh and having resistance values of 330, 680, 1000, 1500, 2200, 3300, and 4700 acoustical ohms are available from Knowles Electronics, Inc. These fit securely at any desired location in #13 earmold tubing. In addition to the greater peak reduction resulting from greater acoustical resistance, the location of the damper in the tubing system has a strong effect, as shown in Figure 43.33. A damper placed at a distance of a quarter wavelength from the ear canal cavity will not reduce a peak at the corresponding frequency. Although the effect of a damper placed at the earmold tip can be desirable acoustically, it may become clogged with earwax in a relatively short time.

Venting. Earmolds may be vented for a number of purposes (Lybarger, 1978a):

1. *Static pressure equalization.* To provide for barometric equalization in the ear canal and possibly to relieve a "feeling of pressure." A parallel vent of about 0.025″ is recommended (0.6 mm).

2. *Low-frequency enhancement.* The mass of the vent hole and the volume in the ear canal form a resonant system. If the acoustic resistance of the vent hole is small compared with its mass, the impedance of the vented ear canal can be greater than that of the ear canal alone. When this occurs, the SPL in the ear canal can be higher at the vent resonant frequency (around 500–600 Hz) than with no vent present, with the hearing aid sounding louder. The most useful low-frequency enhancement (from 5–9 dB) occurs for a 2-mm diameter vent regardless of the earmold length (Fig. 43.34).

3. *Moderate low-frequency reduction.* As can be seen from the previous figure, considerable low-frequency reduction is obtained below 350 to 500

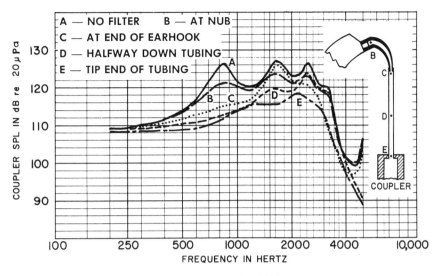

FILTER LOCATION

Figure 43.33. Effect of damper location in the tubing system. Positions *B* and *C* are those most frequently used. (From Lybarger SF. Controlling hearing aid performance by earmold design. In Larson VD, Egolf DP, Kirlin RL, and Stile SW, Eds. Auditory and Hearing Prosthetics Research. New York: Grune & Stratton, 1979:101–132.)

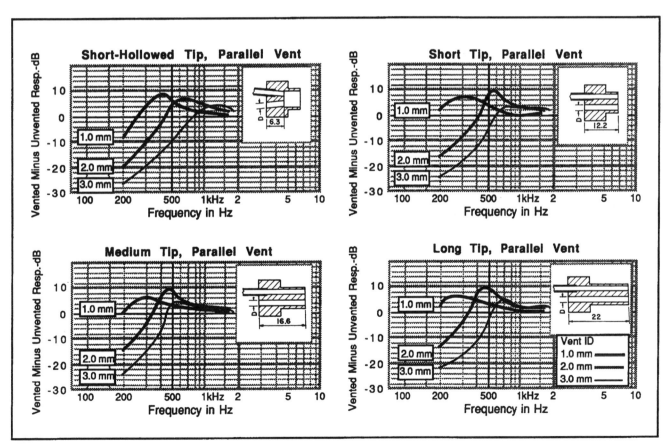

Figure 43.34. The effects of venting on BTE hearing aid performance by using various earmold lengths and three different vent sizes. Results show the vented minus unvented response in dB for a simulated earmold on a DB100 coupler. (Adapted from Lybarger SF. Controlling hearing aid performance by earmold design. In Larson VD, Egolf DP, Kirlin RL, and Stile SW, Eds. Auditory and Hearing Prosthetics Research. New York: Grune & Stratton, 1979:101–132.)

Hz, even though the enhancement occurs. The low-frequency enhancement can be eliminated while maintaining the low-frequency suppression by placing a light damping element into the vent.

4. *Strong low-frequency reduction.* A short vent, large in diameter, must be used. This effect is shown with the short-hollowed tip and 3-mm vent size.

5. *Extreme low-frequency reduction.* This is based on the use of open, or nonoccluding, earmold systems. Maximal low-frequency suppression with this type coupling is approximately 25 dB at 500 Hz (Lybarger, 1980; Staab and Nunley, 1982).

6. *Adjustability.* By varying the vent size the frequency response of the hearing aid can be adjusted to approximate specific needs. Such dispenser adjustable vents as select-a-vent (SAV) and positive-venting valve (PVV) are two commonly used systems. The range and control with these adjustable vents is questionable.

7. Venting allows the direct entrance of sound to the eardrum. A large vent, or open mold, gives nearly "normal" hearing in the lower frequencies.

An occluded earmold is unsuitable when hearing is nearly normal in the lower, but shows a significant loss in the higher, frequencies. A recommendation is made to use either a flatter response aid with a large vent, or use an aid with extended low frequency response with a closed mold.

The most common vent forms are parallel and diagonal. A parallel vent does not intersect the sound bore within the earmold, whereas a diagonal vent intersects the sound bore before the tip of the earmold. A parallel vent performs quite differently above the vent-associated resonance than does a diagonal vent. A diagonal vent produces as much as 10 dB less high-frequency response than a parallel vent (Studebaker and Cox, 1977; Cox, 1982). When a parallel vent is not possible, it is desirable to have the vent intersect the sound bore as close to the medial tip of the earmold as is possible. Additionally, Johansen (1975) reported the increased likelihood of acoustic feedback resulting with a diagonal vent.

In summary, the following can be stated: Venting provides both low-frequency enhancement and low-frequency suppression; the larger the vent the more lows are suppressed, to a maximum of about 25 dB at 500 Hz. Frequencies below about 1000 to 1500 Hz are affected, with the lower frequencies suppressed more than the mid frequencies. Venting can help reduce "fullness of ear" effect, provide static pressure equalization, allow for the direct entrance of sound, and provide some tolerance problem relief. Perceived sound quality and subjective impression of intelligibility is better than if the same response was provided with a tone control and closed earmold (Cox and Alexander, 1983).

Special BTE and EG Tubing Systems

Two-diameter Tubing Systems. In 1970, at the suggestion of H.S. Knowles, a dual tubing system to improve the high-frequency response of an eyeglass aid was introduced (Lybarger, 1972). The diameter of the tubing at the ear canal end was stepped up from the smaller diameter connected to the hearing aid exit nub to between 2.4 and 3.0 mm for a length of 16 to 25 mm. This resulted in an increase in response over the 2400 to 4000 Hz range averaging roughly 5 to 7 dB.

Two currently available two-diameter tubing arrangements, the Advanced Design Horn (ADH) by Microsonic and the Libby 3 mm "horns" give similar results. By damping out the large receiver peak around 1000 Hz and taking advantage of the additional high-frequency response mentioned in the previous paragraph, a broad peak in response near 3000 Hz is obtained that tends to compensate for the loss of canal resonance in BTE aids.

Killion (1981a) shows a series of two-diameter tubing arrangements that utilize a stepped-up tubing diameter at the ear canal end, the usual constant tubing diameter, and inserts of smaller diameter at the ear canal end when reduction of high-frequency response is desired. Figure 41.35 shows the effects of these tubing modifications.

Three-diameter Tubing Systems. Killion (1981b) developed a series of three-diameter tubing systems that included two step-ups in diameter at the ear canal end and the use of two dampers strategically placed to minimize high-frequency peaks, and that also damped the large peak near 1000 Hz. An important objective of these systems was also to extend high-frequency response and to provide suitable response curve shapes.

Figure 43.36 shows Killion's 6R12 tubing system that greatly smoothed response and maintained greater response at the high-frequency end. Tubing diameters of 1.9, 3.0, and 4.0 mm plus two 680 ohm dampers were used.

Figure 43.37 shows Killion's 8CR system that was designed to produce a broad peak around 2.7 kHz to counteract the loss of canal resonance when the ear canal was closed. Tubing diameters of 1.9 mm from the exit nub of the aid, a relatively long length of 3.0 mm and a final section of 4.0 mm were used. Dampers of 680 and 1500 ohms were added. The arrangement and a typical response are shown.

Figure 43.38 shows results recently measured using

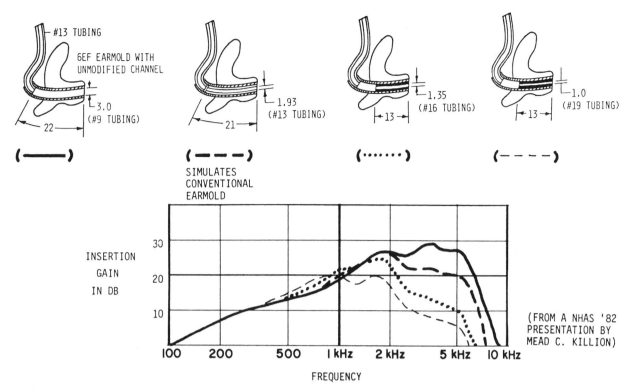

Figure 43.35. Killion 6EF earmold and hearing aid response with treble response selection inserts. The 6EF does have a 680-ohm damper at the end of the earhook to obtain these response curves. (Courtesy of Knowles Electronics, Inc., Itasca, IL)

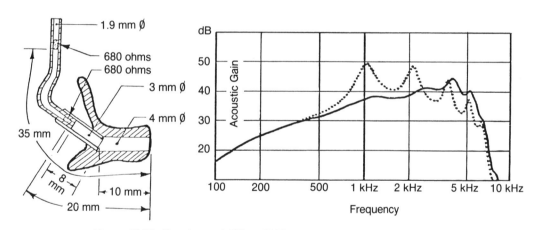

Figure 43.36. Knowles and Killion 6R12 earmold and hearing aid response (Courtesy of Knowles Electronics, Inc., Itasca, IL)

an accurately machined simulation of the 8CR system (Lybarger, 1991). The tests were made using a Knowles ED receiver with essentially constant current input and a DB100 occluded ear simulator. The undamped response shows two prominent additional peaks between 2 and 4 kHz that result from the stepped tubing design. The main peak near 1000 Hz remains, but is moved up slightly in frequency. When the two dampers are added, these peaks are smoothed and the lower frequency main peak virtually elimi-

nated to produce the broad peak desired to offset loss of canal resonance. Although the 8CR may increase gain at its broad peak compared with a single 1.9 mm tube, it is primarily a frequency response shaping system. Tests made on an occluded ear simulator show slightly less increase due to enlarged tubing sections at the canal end than observed when tests are made on a 2-cc coupler.

As originally constructed, the 8CR was difficult to assemble. Libby (1985) made available a 4-mm "horn"

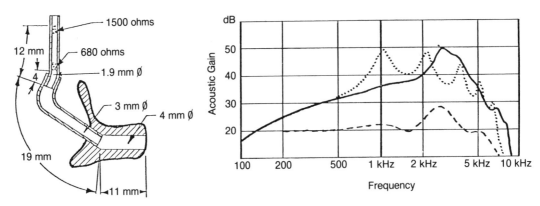

Figure 43.37. Killion 8CR earmold and hearing aid response
(Courtesy of Knowles Electronics, Inc., Itasca, IL)

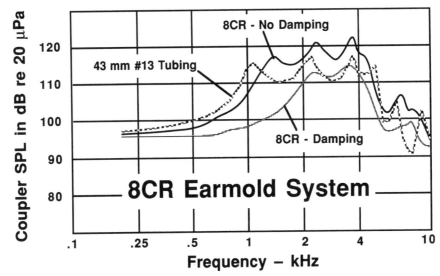

Figure 43.38. Effect of damping on a machined simulation of an 8CR system into a DB100 occluded
ear simulator and using a Knowles ED receiver (Lybarger, 1991, unpublished)

in a single molded piece that eliminated assembly problems. Undamped, this unit has almost the identical response of the undamped 8CR. With a single 1500-ohm damper at the end of the earhook, this unit gives a response quite comparable with that of the original 8CR. It should be pointed out that response to offset the loss of canal resonance can be obtained by methods other than earmold systems, for example, the use of stepped microphone response or through programmable amplifier adjustment.

To demonstrate that hearing aids really could be high fidelity devices, Killion (1981b) developed the 16KLT earmold system that extended response to about 16 kHz as shown in Figure 43.39.

Resonant and Antiresonant Earmolds. By putting a cavity in an earmold that connects with the ear canal through a tube of correct dimensions, a significant rise in high-frequency response can be obtained. Goldberg (1977) described the method of obtaining the appropriate acoustical relationship between the cavity and the tube. A high-frequency cavity arrangement described by Ely (1981) and its effect on the frequency response are shown in Figure 43.40.

If the hearing sensitivity of an ear is very much better in some limited frequency range than it is generally, an antiresonant or notch filter may be useful. A cavity in the earmold connected by a correct size and length of tube to the earmold hole forms a sidebranch that acts as a notch filter and absorbs energy at the frequency to which it is tuned. Figure 43.41 shows a construction arrangement and the type of response obtainable as described by Macrae (1982). A notch filter built into an earhook is described by Killion and Wilson (1985).

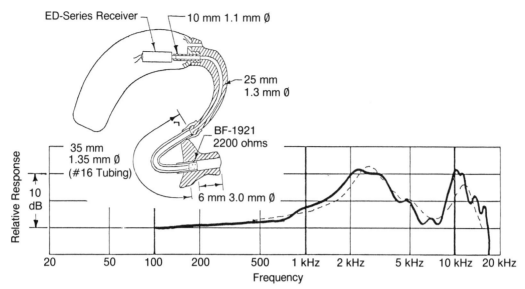

Figure 43.39. Killion 16KLT earmold and hearing aid response
(Courtesy of Knowles Electronics, Inc., Itasca, IL)

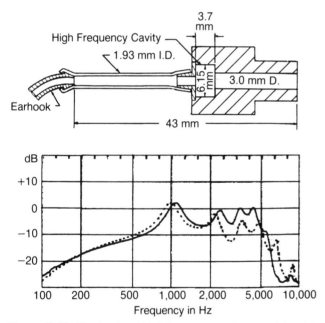

Figure 43.40. Ely simulated high-frequency cavity earmold and the effect on the insertion response of a hearing aid. The *dotted curve* is for 43 mm of no. 13 tubing; the *solid curve* shows the improved insertion response with the high-frequency cavity arrangement. (From Ely W. Electroacoustic modifications of hearing aids. In Bess FH, Freeman BA, and Sinclair JS, Eds. Amplification in Education. Washington, DC: Alexander Graham Bell Association for the Deaf, 1981:316–341.)

ITE and ITC Tubing Systems

The tubing systems in ITE or ITC aids are generally available only to the manufacturer. However, at least one system (Killion and Murphy, 1982) allows dampers to be changed by a dispenser. This is shown in Figure

43.42. Due to the rapidly decreasing size of ITE aids, this feature may not often be available. Manufacturers have a considerable range of possibilities for internal "earmold" constructions. A few comments on some of the possibilities are included here for information only.

Typically, the tubing length in an ITE aid may be on the order of 10 mm. Tubing diameters could perhaps range from 1 to 2 mm. Figure 43.43 shows the response of one Knowles ED receiver on an occluded ear simulator with 10-mm long tubing having diameters of 1.0, 1.25, and 1.85 mm. Notice that the high-frequency response increases considerably when the tubing diameter is increased. Response above 10,000 Hz is not shown.

In addition to the type of damper shown in Figure 43.42, Knowles Electronics makes three sizes of small damping screens. These have diameters of 1.78, 1.37, or 1.12 mm and are available with acoustic resistances ranging from 330 to 3300 acoustic ohms in the 1.78-mm size. The effect of 680- and 1500-ohm damper screens in a tube 10 mm long and 1.25 mm in diameter is shown in Figure 43.44. The measurements were made using a DB100 ear simulator. Note that the dampers have a considerably greater effect on the second peak than on the first.

For ITC aids, tubing length is usually shorter than for ITE hearing aids, more on the order of 4 mm in length. Maximal shortening to no tubing at all, using a Knowles Electronics ED receiver and working directly into an ear simulator, produced essentially no difference in the primary frequency peak and only a mild upward shift in the highest peak.

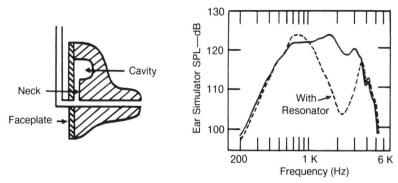

Figure 43.41. Macrae acoustic notch filter diagram and its effect on response (From Macrae J. Acoustic notch filters for hearing aids. Aust J Audiol 1982;4:71–76.)

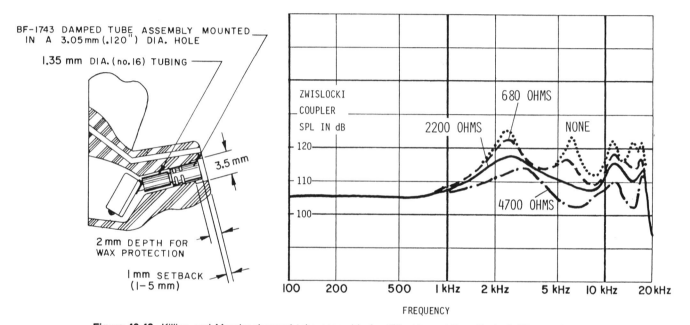

Figure 43.42. Killion and Murphy damped tube assembly for ITE aids and the effect of different damper resistances on the receiver response (Courtesy of Knowles Electronics, Inc., Itasca, IL)

It should be made clear that the previous "earmold" information on ITE and ITC aids is only to provide some general ideas. Each manufacturer has his own methods of coupling the receiver to the ear canal that provide the results that he has found successful.

TECHNICAL STANDARDS

Measurement Instrumentation and Approaches

Objectives. The ultimate objective of obtaining acoustic measurements on hearing aids is to provide data that are of maximal usefulness in selecting or adjusting a hearing aid for a particular impaired ear. Although meeting this objective is closer now than it has been in the past, much remains to be learned about the function of impaired ears, of hearing aid measurement procedures, and the interaction between the two. As Kasten and Franks (1986) point out, any attempt to cross the chasm from electroacoustic performance to suitability of the hearing aid for a listener must be done with a full understanding of the difference between real-ear and coupler measurements of hearing aid characteristics.

Other important objectives include those of assuring uniformity of quality, and to permit accurate comparison and reproducibility of hearing aid measurements by different facilities. These objectives have been realized by the development of national and international hearing aid measurement standards (Lybarger and Olsen, 1983, 1984).

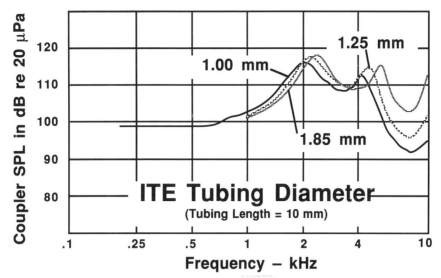

Figure 43.43. Manufacturer-controlled ITE tubing diameter effects. Response of one Knowles ED receiver on a DB100 occluded ear simulator (Lybarger, 1991, unpublished)

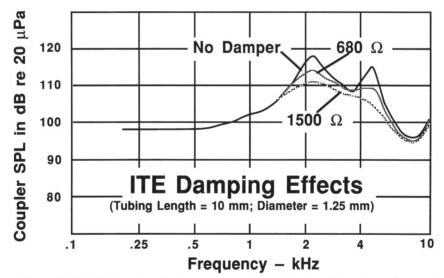

Figure 43.44. ITE damping effects as measured on a Knowles ED receiver on a DB100 occluded ear simulator (Lybarger, 1991, unpublished)

Acoustic Measurement Units Employed

The unit of sound pressure is the Pascal (Pa), equivalent to a force of 1 newton (N) per m². In all cases in this chapter, except for the determination of percentage of total harmonic distortion, sound pressure level (SPL) is used to express the root mean square (RMS) alternating sound pressure. SPL is expressed in dB, using a reference sound pressure of 20 µPa (0.00002 Pascal). This is identical with the formerly used reference pressure of 0.0002 dynes/cm². A sound pressure of 1 Pa corresponds to a SPL of 94 dB. The formula relating sound pressure (p) in Pascals and SPL in dB re 20 µN is:

$$SPL = 20 \log_{10} \frac{p}{0.00002}$$

Although dB were originally intended to express power ratios, they are rarely used in this manner for acoustics. They are conveniently used to express sound pressure, voltage and current levels and ratios, and even mechanical impedance levels relative to an appropriate reference value.

For bone-conduction measurements, the RMS alternating force level produced by a bone receiver is measured on a calibrated, standardized artificial mastoid. The reference force used is 1 µN (0.000001 newton).

Brinkmann and Richter (1977) describe a method of measuring a bone-conduction hearing aid. IEC Publication 118-9 gives standardized test procedures for such measurements.

General Measurement Arrangement for Hearing Aids

The basic principle of hearing aid measurement is simple: with the controls of the hearing aid appropriately adjusted, a suitable input signal is applied to its microphone, and the output of the hearing aid's receiver is measured and analyzed on a standardized device that is similar to a median ear acoustically; or, in the case of bone conduction, mechanically.

Figure 43.45 diagrams a hearing aid **regulation and measurement system** and illustrates the functions of important elements. A very quiet test space with sound absorbent walls is necessary. Ideally, this would be an anechoic chamber to absorb nearly all sound, but a suitable equivalent can be used. In the regulation portion of the system, the electrical test signal is developed by a sine wave (or other wave) generator. The signal passes through a compressor amplifier whose gain is determined by the output of a control microphone. The compressor circuit compensates for irregularities of the SPL in the test enclosure across the frequency range and "flattens" it so that the loudspeaker (sound source) SPL at the hearing aid microphone is constant across the frequency range. In the measurement portion of the system, the hearing aid microphone is placed at an accurately determinable test point facing the loudspeaker. Standard laboratory pressure microphones of different sizes may be used as the control microphone. The output of the hearing aid is transmitted through a specified acoustic earmold substitute to a standardized coupler or ear simulator. The SPL in the coupler or ear simulator is measured by a calibrated standard microphone. The output of this microphone is recorded versus frequency, or examined for other characteristics, such as harmonic distortion.

Acoustic Input Considerations

It is critical that a known and uniform signal be delivered to the hearing aid microphone if reproducible results are to be obtained. The methods used include one of the following:

Substitution Method. This is the oldest and perhaps the most fundamental test method. It is a method of measurement of the response of a hearing aid in which the hearing aid and the microphone, used to measure the free field sound pressure, are placed alternately at the same point (the test point) in the sound field. As used, sound waves emanate from a moderate-sized loudspeaker placed 0.5 to 2 m from the hearing aid test point. A calibrated microphone, properly oriented in terms of its free-field calibration, is placed at the test point, and the electrical input to the loudspeaker required to produce a constant SPL at that point is determined. The calibrated microphone is then removed and the hearing aid *substituted*, properly facing toward the loudspeaker. The output of the hearing aid is measured in a coupler or ear simulator and compared with the normalized sound field achieved before the hearing aid was substituted for the microphone.

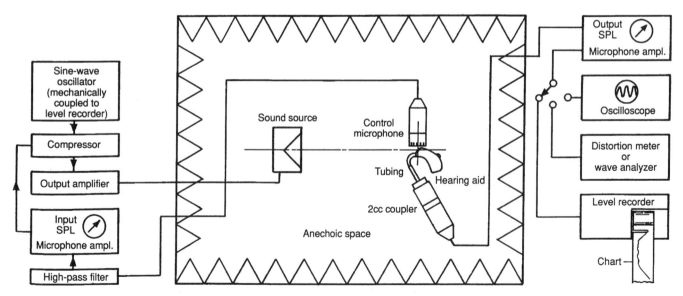

Figure 43.45. Fundamental hearing aid measurement system (Adapted from Donnelly K. Interpreting Hearing Aid Technology. Springfield, IL: Charles C Thomas, 1974).

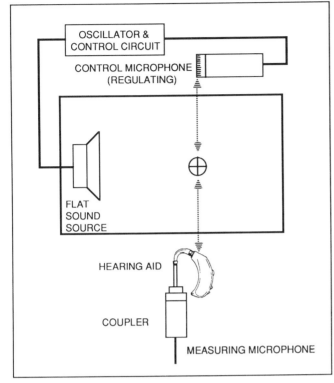

Figure 43.46. Hearing aid measurement arrangement using the *substitution* method. The control microphone measures the speaker output to produce a flat signal at the test point. The hearing aid is then *substituted* into the identical location and its output measured in a coupler or ear simulator.

A difficulty with the procedure is that because loudspeakers do not produce adequately flat responses, electrical inputs must be adjusted to the required value at each test frequency—not a simple task. Nevertheless, the availability of digital processing techniques that can store in memory and recall the information needed to supply the correct voltage to the loudspeaker at all frequencies has made the substitution method very practical. This method is especially useful for hearing aid test box and for *in situ* manikin measurements, discussed later in this chapter. Figure 43.46 diagrams the substitution method.

Comparison Method. This procedure is found in some hearing aid sound boxes but can be used also in a free field. The hearing aid is placed a short distance to one side of the test point and a standard control microphone having a flat response is placed symmetrically opposite (Figure 43.47). The assumption is that if a desired SPL is maintained at the standard control microphone, the SPL at the symmetrically situated hearing aid position will be the same. This method is referred to as a comparison method because the regulating microphone and hearing aid are in the field at the same time and the output from the hearing aid is *compared with* the SPL recorded by the regulating microphone.

Results obtained under free-field conditions using the comparison method are very nearly the same as

COMPARISON METHOD IN A SOUND BOX

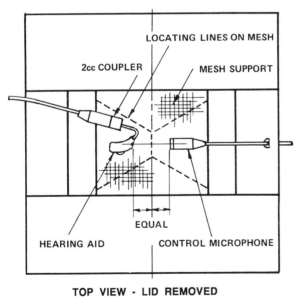

TOP VIEW - LID REMOVED

COMPARISON METHOD IN FREE-FIELD

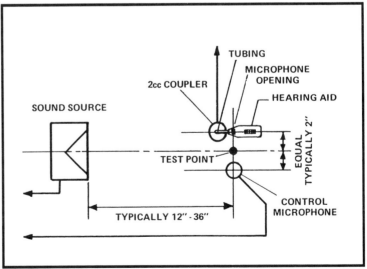

ANECHOIC SPACE

Figure 43.47. Hearing aid measurement arrangement using the *comparison* method. The *left* portion of the figure shows the arrangement used in a B&K sound box (although most other sound boxes use an equivalent substitution method), whereas the *right* side shows the arrangement used in free field. (Adapted from Donnelly K. Interpreting Hearing Aid Technology. Springfield, IL: Charles C Thomas, 1974.)

those obtained using the substitution method; however, results in a sound box using the comparison method may differ somewhat from those obtained in a free-field.

Entrance Pressure Method for Nondirectional Hearing Aids. A control microphone placed close to the hearing aid microphone sound entrance has significant advantages (Carlson, 1974b; Burkhard, 1978). The close proximity is not critical up to about 7000 Hz and the test results are practically independent of the direction of sound arrival. The method therefore offers great advantages in measuring hearing aid performance in sound boxes, where a desired progressive sound wave does not exist due to reflections from the box walls. With this procedure, the results are extremely close to those obtained under free-field conditions. The distance of the center of the sound inlet port of the hearing aid must be within the tolerances specified (Figure 43.48*A*), but the orientation can vary. If the physical structure of the aid requires a greater distance than specified, it must be as close as possible and the distance stated.

Entrance Pressure Method for Directional Hearing Aids. The configuration shown in Figure 43.48B is suitable for measuring directional aids at 0° sound incidence. To obtain reproducible results with a directional microphone aid, the distance from the sound source must be specific, the loudspeaker should not be too large, the control microphone must be small to avoid disturbing the sound flow across the microphone openings, and it must be spaced somewhat farther from the openings. Also, the frontal microphone opening must be nearer the source. To obtain really repeatable results, a highly absorbent test space, preferably anechoic, should be employed.

Tests of directional aids in sound boxes can be considered useful only for comparative tests in a particu-

lar sound box. Simpler test arrangements than shown, and which give consistently related results, are possible and may be especially useful for quality control tests.

Acoustic Output Considerations

The acoustic output of an air-conduction receiver is measured on a 2-cc coupler or on an ear simulator, depending on the nature of the measurement and on the standard test method to be followed. The purpose of the coupler or ear simulator is to simulate acoustically the average ear canal on which a hearing aid is used. The vibratory output of a bone-conduction receiver is measured on an artificial mastoid, or mechanical coupler. Common air-conduction receiver couplers and simulators are as follows:

2-cc Coupler. The 2-cc coupler (or 2 cm³) was first described by Romanow (1942) and has been used successfully since because it is simple and gives accurately reproducible results when properly used. Several forms of the 2-cc coupler are shown in Figure 43.49, each for a different measurement situation (see ANSI S3.7-1973, Method for Coupler Calibration of Earphones, and ANSI S3.7-1973 Revised, but soon to be accepted). The effective volume of the coupler cavity is 2-cc. This volume was originally intended to take into account the compliance of the ear canal/middle ear system when the canal is occluded by a hearing aid earmold. Thus, these couplers were once called "artificial ears." A leak of high acoustic impedance provides barometric equalization. Sound from the hearing aid receiver is directed into the 2-cc cavity at the center of the face of the cylindrical cavity opposite the standard microphone diaphragm. The microphone forms the other face of the coupler and simulates the tympanic membrane.

In reality, the 2-cc coupler has greater volume than

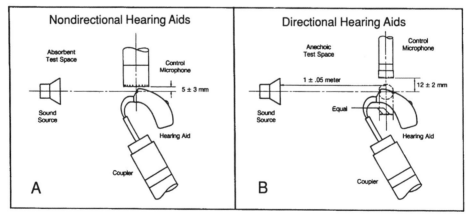

Figure 43.48. Hearing aid measurement arrangement using the *entrance pressure comparison* method for nondirectional (*A*) and for directional (*B*) hearing aids. This method is especially good for use in sound boxes where a desired sound wave does not exist due to reflections from the box walls.

2-cc COUPLER TYPES COMMONLY USED

HA-1

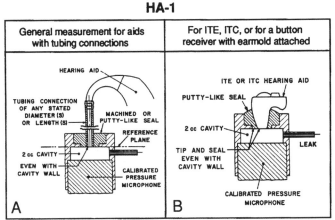

General measurement for aids with tubing connections	For ITE, ITC, or for a button receiver with earmold attached

HA-2

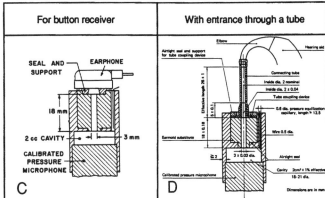

For button receiver	With entrance through a tube

HA-3

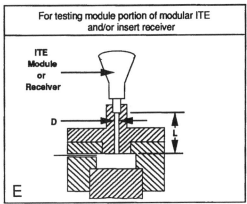

For testing module portion of modular ITE and/or insert receiver

HA-4

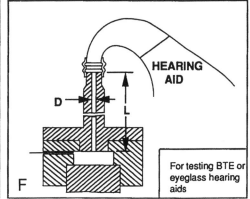

For testing BTE or eyeglass hearing aids

Figure 43.49. 2-cc couplers commonly used in hearing aid measurement. **A,** and **B,** the most generalized forms used. The relatively large opening in the sound entrance face allows almost any tubing, earmold, ITE, or ITC aid to be mounted on the coupler with a suitable formable material. **C,** for use with a button receiver. **D,** dual diameter entrance tube that has a serious disadvantage in that it does not replicate general earmold manufacturing practice. **E** and **F,** recent coupler designations for ITE modules and/or insert receivers and for BTE or eyeglass hearing aids, respectively.

median adult ears and does not incorporate any acoustic resistance. The latter fact makes it unsuitable for testing hearing aids with vented earmolds, unless the vents are closed. Many tests made on a 2-cc coupler, however, relate well to those on ear simulators or manikins. Because the 1-inch microphone usually used in the coupler falls off rapidly in response above about 8000 Hz, it is recommended that the 2-cc coupler not be used for tests above 7000 Hz unless correction is made for the microphone response.

HA-1 Earphone Coupler. This is the most generalized form of the 2-cc coupler. Because of the relatively large opening in the sound entrance face, almost any aid, including BTE, ITE and ITC aids, can be mounted on the coupler with a suitable formable seal. The end of the tubing, tip of an earmold, or hearing aid must be centered and be flush with the reference plane, or upper face of the cavity.

HA-2 Earphone Coupler. This was the original form of the 2-cc coupler and was designed to test button type receivers on body aids. The tube leading from the receiver nub has a standardized length of 18 mm (0.709 inch) and a diameter of 3 mm (0.118 inch). Results obtained with this coupler may differ from those obtained with the HA-1 coupler because of potential differences in the length and diameter of the "tube."

HA-2 Earphone Coupler with Entrance Through a Tube. This coupler arrangement has a tubing section 25 mm long by 1.93 mm in diameter (in the U.S.), followed by the 18-mm long by 3-mm diameter tube of the regular HA-2 coupler. The tube can be rigid or flexible.

At one time the HA-2 with entrance through a tube was the principal commercially available 2-cc coupler and was designed in this fashion to allow for convenient switching between body, eyeglass, and BTE aids for measurement. However, because it has a dual diameter entrance tube, it has serious disadvantages. Hearing aids measured with this coupler show considerably greater performance in the higher frequencies than would be the case with a single diameter tube. A single diameter tube coupler is much more realistic when it is considered that most earmolds are fabricated with a standard, single diameter tubing. Additionally, most special earmold systems are referenced in performance to that obtained with a constant 1.93 mm (No. 13) diameter tube all the way to the tip of the earmold. As a result, the ANSI (American National Standards Institute) S3.22-1987 method for specification of hearing aid performance allows for any of the 2-cc earphone couplers in a closed configuration and suitable for the particular hearing aid being tested, to be chosen from among those described in American National Standard S3.7-1973. The coupler and tubing used are to be stated. Lybarger (1985b) has suggested using a constant 1.93-mm diameter bore for the full 43-mm tubing length by means of an easily made adapter. It is simply inserted into the regular HA-2 coupler; a rubber socket for the button earphone nub holds and seals the adapter.

HA-3 Earphone Coupler. This is a special form of the HA-1 coupler, using a rigid or flexible sealing construction. It is intended for testing the module portion of a modular ITE hearing aid and/or nonbattery (insert) type receivers. Unless otherwise specified, the tube diameter is 1.93 mm and the length is 10 mm. The length starts at the end of the receiver tubing protruding from the module or receiver.

HA-4 Earphone Coupler (proposed). This is a variation of the HA-2 coupler and is intended for testing BTE or eyeglass hearing aids. It simulates a fitting in which the sound path bore through the earmold from the end of the earhook of the BTE aid, or from the end of the sound outlet on the eyeglass aid is assumed to have a uniform diameter of 1.93 mm and a length of 43 mm.

The 2-cc coupler has performed well for the purpose for which it was designed, the intercomparison of hearing aids. The response curves obtained with the 2-cc coupler are absolutely reproducible, making the coupler invaluable for inspection control. The coupler is also simple and robust in design—desirable features of any standard device.

The Ear Simulator. An alternate coupler that has been accepted and that more closely resembles the real ear was developed by Zwislocki (1970, 1971), and made available commercially by Knowles Electronics in 1972 as a device termed an "ear simulator." It has four acoustical networks allowing for simulation of the acoustic impedance of the human eardrum (Fig. 43.50) and

takes into account the acoustic capacitance (volume), inertance (mass), and the acoustic resistance of ears. It also more closely resembles the ear physically, with an ear canal portion of appropriate diameter and length. The reference plane, or entrance, to the ear simulator is considered to be where the tip of an average hearing aid earmold would terminate. The other end is terminated with a *type M* ½-inch condenser microphone.

The Zwislocki ear simulator allows for measurement of either vented or open canal earmolds. Also, adapters have been designed to simulate HA-1, HA-2, and HA-3 type connections so that it can be used in the same manner as a 2-cc coupler for closed earmold measurements in a hearing aid test box, although with quite different results. (The application for use with adapters is specified in International Electrotechnical Commission Publication 118-0, 1983). Data acquired in such a manner will show the hearing aid to have more high-frequency sound pressure. Although the ear simulator can be used for hearing aid measurements in a sound box, its primary use is in the KEMAR manikin (Knowles Electronics Manikin for Acoustic Research) for *in situ* measurements and for research, where its ear-like characteristics are very important.

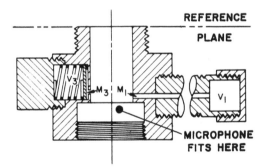

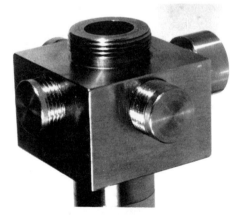

Figure 43.50. Diagram of a Zwislocki type four-branch ear simulator (*upper*). There are four resonant side branches tuned to produce a standardized acoustical input impedance similar to that of typical human ears. Photograph (*below*) shows appearance. (Courtesy of Knowles Electronics, Inc., Itasca, IL)

Ear simulator type couplers have been standardized in the U.S. (ANSI S3.25-1979) and internationally (IEC Publication 711, 1982). Slight differences exist between the two standards. However, ear simulators are not used in tests made according to FDA 1977 (Food and Drug Administration) hearing aid labeling regulations in the United States.

Comparison of the Zwislocki Ear Simulator and 2-cc Coupler Results. Sachs and Burkhard (1972) compared response curves of hearing aid receivers in real ears, on a 2-cc coupler, and on the Zwislocki ear simulator. Their tests showed the response on the ear simulator to be extremely close to the average obtained on real ears. A conversion curve showing the increase in SPL observed in the ear simulator, compared with a 2-cc coupler, is shown in Figure 43.51—a relationship that has proved quite consistent (Lybarger, 1975). Note that the sound pressure of a hearing aid developed in an ear simulator is higher at all frequencies, being about 4 dB higher in the low frequencies and increasing gradually to about 15 dB higher at 10 kHz. The relationship shown is acceptable for comparing frequency response and gain curves of hearing aids without venting or earmold changes to expected real ear performance. The Zwislocki ear simulator may be ideal for predicting the real ear saturation output of hearing aids because it presents the median middle ear impedance to the hearing aid output. With the introduction of a vent or other earmold changes, the need for measurement by an actual ear simulator arises.

The differences between the simulator and 2-cc coupler results may be related to two issues (Sachs and Burchard (1972): (1) that the smaller volume of the Zwislocki coupler produces higher sound pressures, and (2) that impedance factors above 1500 Hz, which dominate the build up of sound pressure at the eardrum, are taken into account in the Zwislocki coupler.

Descriptive Performance of the Hearing Aid

The following descriptions of air-conduction hearing aid performance, suitable for specification and toler-ance purposes, are based on procedures specified in ANSI S3.22-1987 (ASA 7-1987), Specification of Hearing Aid Characteristics. This 1987 revision of S3.22-1982 adds tolerances that are applicable for custom-made one-of-a-kind hearing aids, and becomes applicable to special purpose hearing aids having high- or low-frequency emphasis (by allowing a choice of the frequencies used in obtaining the average gain and average SSPL90.) Full details can be obtained by referring to that document. This document serves as the current Standard for meeting FDA labeling regulations for those who manufacture, repair, dispense, and distribute hearing aids in the United States. A summary of the ANSI S3.22-1987 is provided in Table 43.3, including the allowable tolerance levels.

The measurements recorded using this Standard do not include such effects as ear canal resonance and diffraction produced by the head and torso and therefore should not be expected to represent the performance of the aid under conditions of use by the wearer.

In this Standard, the **input SPL** is measured at the microphone opening for nondirectional hearing aids and for directional aids in a progressive sound field adjacent to the microphone openings. (Other measurement methods may be used if they give comparable results.) Unwanted ambient noise or stray electrical or magnetic fields, the sound source, control microphone, coupler microphone, and equipment tolerances are specified in the Standard. The **output SPL** is measured in a 2-cc coupler of a closed configuration and suitable for the particular hearing aid being tested.

Before making any measurements on a hearing aid, proper **ambient and operating conditions** should exist. Ambient conditions are met by a temperature within the range of 64 to 82° F, relative humidity not exceeding 80%, and atmospheric pressure within the range 610 to 795 mm Hg. Operating conditions involve the use of the proper supply voltage, the proper form of 2-cc coupler, the selection and statement of the acoustic connection to the coupler, etc. Although tests may be made with any basic settings of controls

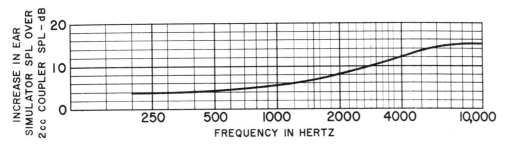

Figure 43.51. Curve showing approximate relationship of the SPL in an ear simulator to that in a 2-cc coupler.

Table 43.3.
ANSI S3.22-1987 (ASA 70-1987) Specification of hearing Aid Characteristics Summary

Characteristic	Input SPL dB re 20 μPa	Frequency (Hz)	Gain Control Setting	Presentation	Tollerance Requirements
SSPL 90 Curve	90	Frequencies between 200 and 5000	Full on	Curve State maximum value dB	No more than 3dB above mfr. stated maximum value
HFA SSPL90	90	1000, 1600, 2500	Full on	Value (dB) (3-frequency average)	Mfr. specified value ±4 dB
HFA Gull-On Gain or SPA Full-on Gain	60 or 50 (state which) 50 for AGC or where aid would overload	1000, 1600, 2500 or SPA frequencies	Full on	Value (dB) (3-frequency average)	Mfr. Specified value ±5 dB
Frequency Response	60 or 50	200–5000	Ref. Test Gain Control Pos. Set gain control back to give output SPL 17 dB less than average SSPL90, or full on for low gain and AGC aids		±4 dB in low band ±6 dB in high band
Frequency Range	60	200–5000 Line 20 dB below 3-freq. avg.	Reference Test Position	State F1 (low limit) and 12 (high limit)	For information only
Total Harmonic Distortion	70	500, 800, 1600	Reference Test Position	Number (%)	No more than 3% above mfr. specified value
Equivalent Input Noise Level, Ln	60	1000, 1600, 2500 (Avg. to get Lav)	Reference Test Position	Number (dB) Ln = L2 - (Lav - 60)	No more than 3 dB above mfr. specified value
Battery Current	65	1000	Reference Test Position	Value (mA)	No more than 20% above mfr. specified value
Telephone Pickup (Induction Coil)	10 mA/m rms magnetic field	1000	Full on	Greatest value (dB)	Within ±6 dB of mfr. specified value
Input-Output Curves (AGC only)	50 to 90 in 10 dB steps	2000	Full on	Curve Input = abscissa Curve Output = ordinate	Match specified and measured curves at 70 db input, then to be within ±5 dB of specified value
Attack and Release Times (AGC only)	Abruptly alternating between 55 and 80	2000	Full on	Values (ms)	Mfr. specified values ±5 ms or ±50%, whichever is larger.

for which test information is desired, basic settings should generally be chosen to give the widest frequency response range, the highest SSPL90, and the highest full-on gain. The user-operated gain control requires special setting procedures. It is recommended that all published curves of gain, response, or output versus frequency use a **grid plot** having a linear dB ordinate and a logarithmic abscissa scale, with the length of one decade on the abscissa scale equal to the length of 50 ± 2 dB on the ordinate scale. Curves should be developed over the frequency range from 200–5000 Hz.

Saturation SPL. It is important to know at what level a hearing aid limits its output when it receives a high-level input signal. The maximal possible level should not exceed the threshold of discomfort for a user. Conversely, too little output capability will not allow a clean signal to be delivered to an individual having a more severe hearing impairment. A practical measure of the output handling capability of a hearing aid is the SSPL90, defined as the SPL developed in a 2-cc coupler when the input SPL is 90 dB and the gain control of the hearing aid is full-on. The SSPL90 is a function of frequency, as shown by the *upper curve* of Figure 43.52. A maximum saturation level is identified on the curve and is required by the Standard.

To make it easier to categorize hearing aids on the basis of SSPL90, a three-frequency averaging method is used. The HFA-SSPL90 (high frequency average SSPL90) is defined as the average of the 1000, 1600, and 2500 Hz SSPL90 values. They are identified in Figure 43.52 as S_1, S_2, and S_3. Recognizing that some

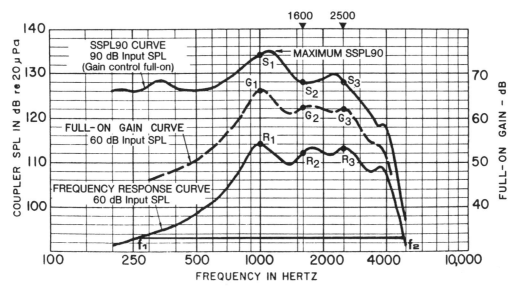

Figure 43.52. Examples of curves obtained using methods specified in ANSI S3.22-1987. The *upper curve* is the SSPL90. HFA-SSPL90 = $(S_1 + S_2 + S_3)/3$. The *dashed center curve* is a full-on gain curve, in this case made with an input SPL of 60 dB. If this curve is too close to the SSPL90 curve, or an AGC aid is tested, a lower input SPL of 50 dB is used. The HFA full-on gain = $(G_1 + G_2$ + $G_3)/3$ minus input SPL. The *lower curve* is the frequency response curve, made with the gain control at the reference test position. This is determined ordinarily by the condition that $(S_1 + S_2 + S_3)/3 - (R_1 + R_2 + R_3)/3 = 17$ dB. The frequency range is defined by locating a horizontal line 20 dB below the average value of points R_1, R_2, and R_3 or from the SPA full-on gain.

hearing aids have a frequency range that is not centered in the mid frequencies, a special purpose high-frequency average (SPA-SSPL90), using three other frequencies selected by the manufacturer, is allowed if the hearing aid meets the requirement for being called a "special purpose" hearing instrument. The Standard defines a "special purpose" hearing instrument as one whose full-on gain *at any one* of the three test frequencies (1000 or 1600 or 2500 Hz) is more than 15 dB below the maximum (peak) full-on gain *at any frequency.*

Acoustic Gain. This is defined as the difference between the output SPL in an earphone coupler and the input SPL. It is a measure of how much the input signal is amplified and is a function of frequency and the user gain control setting as well as other factors. When the gain control is set to its maximum, full-on position, and the input SPL is adjusted to a suitable value (60 dB) that will not overload the hearing aid, the full-on gain may be measured and recorded as a function of frequency (*dashed curve* in Figure 43.52). When a 60-dB input SPL possibly could overload the hearing aid (when the separation between the full-on gain curve and the SSPL90 curve is less than 4 dB at any frequency over the range from 200–5000 Hz), or when a hearing aid with automatic gain control (AGC) is being tested, a 50 dB input SPL is used. (An AGC aid is defined as one that has means other than peak clipping by which the gain is automatically controlled

as a function of the magnitude of the signal being amplified).

As in the case with SSPL90, the same three-frequencies are averaged to categorize the hearing aid on the basis of full-on gain and is referred to as the HFA full-on gain. The three values to be averaged are identified as G_1, G_2, and G_3 in Figure 43.52. As with SSPL, three different frequencies can be used to better identify the performance of the hearing aid if it meets the "special purpose" category. Their average is calculated in the same way. The newly-selected values are referred to as *SPA full-on gain.*

Frequency Response. In actual use, the gain control of a hearing aid is generally set back substantially from its full-on position. The use curve may not have the same shape as the full-on gain curve. Therefore, a standard method of establishing a gain control setting has been developed for making a response curve that is more typical of the gain control as used. The concept is to turn down the gain control so that, very roughly, the peaks of 65 dB SPL speech (which are about 12 dB higher than the long term average) do not exceed the SSPL90 capability of the aid. This new, gain control setting is referred to as the *reference test position* and is used to obtain the frequency response curve as shown in Figure 43.52. This curve is obtained with an input SPL of 60 dB, and then adjusting the gain control downward so that the HFA full-on gain or the SPA full-on gain is 17 dB below the HFA-SSPL90 or SPA-SSPL90, ±1 dB. Note that measurements of total harmonic distortion, equivalent input noise level, and battery current are also made at reference test gain control position.

Sometimes an aid may not have enough gain to permit this reduction, in which case the reference test position is the full-on position. For AGC aids, the gain control is set full-on because the compression action of the aid on the frequency response curve is minimized by using the lower input SPL of 50, instead of 60 dB.

Frequency Range. This provides a general idea of the range of frequencies over which a hearing aid might be considered to be effective and is identified in Figure 43.52. The frequency range is defined by the intersections (f_1 and f_2) of the response curve and the horizontal (*dashed line*). The location of the horizontal line is 20 dB downward from the average value of points R_1, R_2, and R_3 or from the SPA full-on gain. In the example shown, the average is 113 dB, so the horizontal line is drawn at the 93-dB level. Thus, the frequency range for the example shown is 250 to 4900 Hz.

Harmonic Distortion. The ability of a hearing aid to deliver a clean signal at the required output level is indicated by measuring its nonlinear distortion characteristics. Total harmonic distortion is a measure of nonlinearity. Numerous studies in the past have not clearly shown the expected inverse correlation between speech discrimination and harmonic distortion. Lindblad (1982) found that the average just detectable quadratic distortion (mostly second harmonic) for 21 hard-of-hearing subjects was 19%. The average just detectable cubic distortion (mostly third harmonic) was 5.7%. Moderate harmonic distortion does not degrade discrimination as much as one might expect. The experience of hearing aid engineers, however, is that low harmonic distortion at hearing aid use levels is very desirable. Fortunately, recent hearing aid advances in transducer and amplifier technology have resulted in hearing aids having such low levels of harmonic distortion (as well as other types of distortion), that it can be relegated to a position of negligible importance (Wernick, 1985).

Total harmonic distortion is measured with the hearing aid adjusted to the reference position. An input level of 70 dB at 500, 800, and 1600 Hz is used (or at frequencies corresponding to ½ the frequency of each of the three SPA frequencies) to simulate a louder than average input signal. Percentage total harmonic distortion (% THD) may be determined using either of the following methods:

In the following procedure, the amount of total harmonic distortion is measured in the output coupler by filtering out the fundamental and measuring the

RMS sum of the harmonics that remain. The percentage of total harmonic distortion (% THD) is then given by:

$$\% \text{ THD} = 100 \times \sqrt{\frac{\text{RMS sound pressure of harmonics}}{\text{RMS sound pressure of total signal}}}$$

$$= 100 \times \sqrt{\frac{p_2^2 + p_3^2 + \ldots\ldots\ldots}{p_1^2 + p_2^2 + p_3^2 \ldots\ldots}}$$

where p_1 is the sound pressure (not SPL) of the fundamental in the earphone coupler and p_2, p_3, etc. are the sound pressures of the second, third, etc. harmonics.

An alternate, and perhaps the preferred method is to measure the fundamental and each harmonic sound pressure individually. This method has the advantage of greatly reducing the effects of ambient noise. The total harmonic distortion is:

$$\% \text{ THD} = 100 \times \sqrt{\frac{p_2^2 + p_3^2 + \ldots\ldots\ldots}{p_1^2}}$$

The two methods give virtually identical results up to 20% THD. Percentage of THD values in typical hearing aids are usually in the range of 3 to 10%. For higher THD values than 20%, the latter approach should be used.

If the frequency response curve rises 12 dB or more between any distortion test frequency and its second harmonic, distortion tests at that frequency may be omitted.

Equivalent Input Noise Level, L_n. This relates to the magnitude of the internal noise generated by the hearing aid and is valid only when the ambient noise in the test space is extremely low.

With the gain control in the reference test position, coupler SPLs are measured at 1000, 1600, and 2500 Hz or at the 3 SPA frequencies (L_{av}) for an input SPL of 60 dB. The input signal is then removed and SPL is recorded (L_2) in the coupler (non frequency-specific intensity). The equivalent input noise level (L_n) is:

$$L_n = L_2 - (L_{av} - 60) \text{ dB}$$

Equivalent Input Noise Level readings can be misleading for AGC aids, especially for those with an AGC knee 50 dB or lower at the frequencies tested. This is because the gain of the aid may be much greater when no input signal is present (because the aid is not in compression) than when the input signal is present and the aid is in compression. The result is a disproportionately high L_n. Additionally, if a hearing aid has a very wide frequency band, a higher L_n may result because of the increased bandwidth and not necessarily because of internal noise.

Battery Current. Current tests are made with the

gain control in the reference test position and with a 65 dB, 1000 Hz input SPL.

Coupler SPL with Induction Coil. The sensitivity of a telecoil is made with the aid set to the "T" mode and oriented to produce the greatest coupler SPL. The aid is placed in an alternating magnetic field having a field strength of 10 mA/m rms at 1000 Hz, and the gain control full-on. A frequency response curve may be made using the same field strength and orientation. (A more realistic method for expressing the performance of telecoils is currently being developed).

Input-Output Characteristics—AGC Aids. How the output SPL varies as a function of input SPL is very important to know for AGC aids. The test procedure calls for the input SPL of a 2000 Hz tone to be varied from 50 to 90 dB in 10-dB steps and the coupler output observed. The curves are then drawn on a grid with output SPL as the ordinate and input SPL as the abscissa. This measurement is currently under revision.

Dynamic AGC Characteristics. The control of AGC function takes time. The measurement of dynamic AGC characteristics is a method to determine the attack and release times for the system to move in and out of its AGC function. With the aid's gain control set to the reference test position (full-on for AGC), a 2000 Hz input tone is abruptly alternated between 55 and 80 dB SPL. The attack time is defined as the time between the abrupt input increase and the point where the output level of the aid has stabilized to ±2dB of the steady state value for the 80 dB input SPL. The release time is defined as the time between the abrupt drop in the input signal and the point where the hearing aid's output has stabilized to ±2dB of the steady state value for the 55 dB input SPL. These times are stated in milliseconds. This measurement is currently under revision.

Other Characteristics. Standard test methods are available or under test for properties other than those listed above. Some of these include microphone probe measurements of hearing aids under actual use, reference test position setting for AGC aids, telecoil measurements, coherence testing for distortion, the use of a pseudorandom noise input for AGC aids, testing using a noise input, etc. The most important of these involves the measurement of *in situ* (hearing aid as actually worn) properties; others include the effects of battery voltage on gain, output and distortion; the measurement of intermodulation distortion; and one-third octave band analysis of internal noise.

Reasonably comparable results to the ANSI S3.22-1987 electroacoustical performance of hearing aids will be obtained using IEC Publication 118-7 (1983), *Measurement of Performance Characteristics of Hearing Aids,* which also uses a 2-cc coupler. Additionally, measurements could also be made according to the basic IEC Publication 118-0 (1983), *Hearing Aids: Measurement of Electro-Acoustical Characteristics,* but the values obtained must be interpreted quite differently because an ear simulator directly replaces the 2-cc coupler.

Automatic Hearing Aid Measurement Equipment

Digital technology is used extensively to rapidly and systematically measure hearing aid characteristics, especially as related to FDA regulations. A number of automatic test devices are available, and although they differ somewhat in their specifics, their performances can be described generally. Although an anechoic chamber or sound box can be used in which to make the measurement, the latter is the usual arrangement. (The following procedures are consistent with ANSI S3.22-1987 but do not apply to the new ANSI S3.42-1992 Standard that allows a noise input and includes the use of spectrum analysis as an alternative to swept sinusoid signal analysis.)

Anechoic Chamber. In an anechoic chamber, using a substitution method, a test point is defined within the test space at which the hearing aid microphone opening will be placed later (Fig. 43.46). First, a calibrated standard microphone is placed at the test point and properly oriented toward the loudspeaker. With a uniform voltage applied to the loudspeaker, puretones are generated and swept across the desired frequency range (These signals are a large number of closely spaced discrete frequencies to produce fairly smooth curves.). Because the loudspeaker does not have a flat response, the response is "equalized" or made flat by taking the differences from the flat response desired, and adjusting the electrical input to the loudspeaker required to maintain a flat input SPL across frequencies at the test point. (Equalization is also frequently accomplished with the entrance pressure method in real time by analyzers using two microphones as shown in Fig. 43.48*B*.) This information is stored in memory and is recalled for subsequent testing.

After equalization, the hearing aid is placed in position with its microphone opening at the test point and with the proper acoustic connection to the coupler. With the correct battery supply voltage applied to the hearing aid, the operator selects the test information desired and sets the controls of the hearing aid as required in the Standard. The automatic test device runs through the entire required program, stores, and prints the results. The only interruption in the process is for the adjustment of the hearing aid to the reference test position on certain hearing aids. To assist in this adjustment, the machine informs the operator of the average output SPL to shoot for and constantly updates this average as the gain control is adjusted by the operator to give the target value. Some devices allow for telecoil sensitivity and response to be made and printed using a calibrated magnetic field. Figure 43.53 shows the print-out for a linear hearing aid using an automatic hearing aid measurement device.

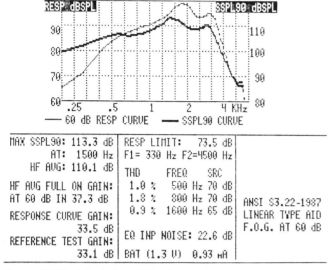

Figure 43.53. Automatic ANSI print-out for a linear hearing aid (Courtesy of Frye Electronics, Inc., Tigard, OR)

Sound Boxes. Most automatic devices for routine testing of hearing aid performance use a sound box to deliver the input signal to the aid and to reduce the entrance of ambient noise. Equalization is accomplished by using a comparison method. The use of a sound box is valid when results are equivalent or within acceptable limits to those obtained in a free-field environment (such as an anechoic chamber).

For nondirectional aids, the entrance pressure method described earlier in this chapter will be very close to those obtained under free-field conditions except at high frequencies where the shorter wave lengths of the high frequencies show some differences. However, when the sound test space is of moderate dimensions, as is usually found in most automatic test devices, a variation of the substitution method (the **equivalent substitution method**) is recommended that will give results agreeing closely with those obtained by using the pressure method, even at high frequencies. It is particularly useful for measurement systems using microprocessor or computer means to measure and control the electrical input to the loudspeaker. This procedure uses the same measurement microphone for both the input sound pressure level measurement and for the coupler. This method is diagrammed in Figure 43.54, which shows the setup for equalization of the sound source (43.54*A*), and for

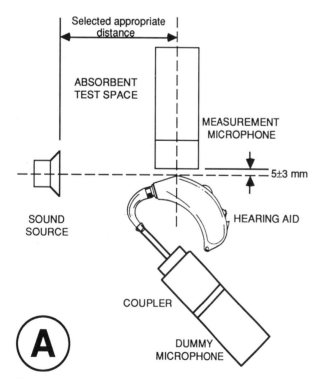

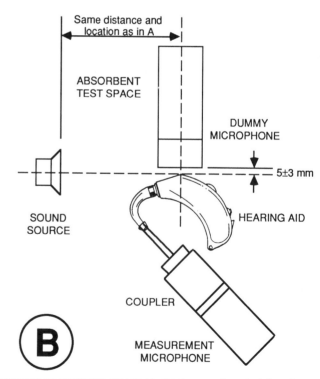

Figure 43.54. Hearing aid measuring arrangement using the *equivalent substitution method*. This is good for nondirectional aids in a small sound environment and with a system that uses micro-

processor or computer means to measure and control the electrical input to the sound source. (Adapted from ANSI S3.22-1987, Specification of Hearing Aid Characteristics.)

measurement of the hearing aid (43.54B). (This method is described in the Appendix of S3.22-1987.)

For directional aid consistency and accuracy, the entrance pressure method shown in Figure 43.48B in an anechoic test space must be used. However, for less accurate comparative tests, the sound box may be used if certain precautions are taken. Using Figure 43.48B as a reference, the front of the hearing aid, as worn, should face toward the loudspeaker in the test box (Because of the location of the loudspeaker, this is not always a simple task.). Realize also that reflections in the sound box interfere with directional aid measurement, as well as the location of the loudspeaker. When the substitution method (equalization) is used, the test point for the standard microphone and for the hearing aid microphone openings must be the same. If a control microphone is used, it should be placed as shown.

In Situ Hearing Aid Measurement.

In situ (in-place) refers to the physical testing of hearing aid performance on an actual person or on a carefully designed substitute (manikin) that has acoustic properties very close to those of a median adult. Specifically, *in situ* testing provides much better information on the gain-by-frequency and directional characteristics for the hearing aid as it is actually worn than measurements made with the S3.22-1987 standard. For example, the diffraction of the body and head of the hearing aid wearer on incident sound can significantly change the input sound pressure to a hearing aid microphone and are reflected by *in situ* measurements.

When a manikin is used, two types of measurements of a hearing aid include: (1) *direct in situ measurements,* which determine the pressure level developed in the manikin ear simulator for an equalized free field input SPL; and (2) *insertion measurements,* which determine the difference between the pressure levels developed in the manikin ear simulator with and without a hearing aid in place. Insertion measurements attempt to determine the actual acoustical assistance that a hearing aid furnishes a user.

The frequency responses obtained with a hearing aid are distinguished by whether the unaided manikin frequency response is included in (simulated *in situ* gain frequency response) or subtracted from (simulated insertion gain frequency response) the aided frequency response. When a manikin is used, the term *simulated in situ* is often applied. When comparing real ear measurements of insertion gain and *in situ* gain, insertion gain is the more preferred measurement because of ease of replication and freedom from artifacts (Preves and Sullivan, 1987).

In Situ Gain/Response. *In situ* gain (response) is the difference between the hearing aid output in SPL as measured within the ear canal as compared with the equalized free field SPL in the absence of the hearing aid wearer. It varies as a function of the position of the wearer in the free field. It does not represent the acoustical assistance provided by the hearing aid because the wearer's open ear canal resonance is included.

Insertion Gain/Response. Insertion gain (response) is the *increase* in SPL *at the eardrum* with the hearing aid in place and operating, compared with the SPL at the eardrum without the hearing aid and with the ear canal and concha unoccluded (Fig. 43.55). The unaided condition can be defined as the difference between SPL in the unoccluded wearer's ear and the reference SPL. Note that the effect of ear canal resonance and other factors is small at low frequencies but is very significant from 2 to 5 kHz. The term insertion gain, introduced by Ayers (1953), is similar in concept to the term *orthotelephonic gain* (Romanow, 1942) and *etymotic gain* (Burkhard, 1975; Killion and Monser, 1980). It has also been referred to as "real ear" or "functional" gain, and is a good indicator of how the hearing aid will amplify sound for the user. Insertion gain is influenced by the direction of incidence of the sound (Killion and Monser, 1980; Lybarger, 1985c), and by the position of the hearing aid microphone sound entrance.

The importance of insertion gain is that it agrees much more closely with subjective measures of hearing aid performance than do traditional coupler measurements. It takes into account the loss of "natural" gain due to head diffraction as well as the loss of concha and ear canal resonances when the ear canal is closed with an earmold. Insertion gain of an air-conduction hearing aid may be obtained in several ways:

a) By direct measurement on a person, using an ear probe tube microphone or a canal microphone, with and without the hearing aid;

b) By the use of an accurately designed manikin equipped with ear simulators; or

c) Approximately, by corrections applied to gain or response curves made following standardized test methods, using a 2-cc coupler or an ear simulator without a manikin.

Direct Measurements. A number of commercially available, integrated, microprocessor-based *probe microphone systems* are available to estimate functional gain electroacoustically *in situ,* and one such device is shown in Figure 43.56. These systems measure the amount by which a hearing aid changes the SPL in the external auditory meatus relative to the unaided condition. Direct measurement applications may be best

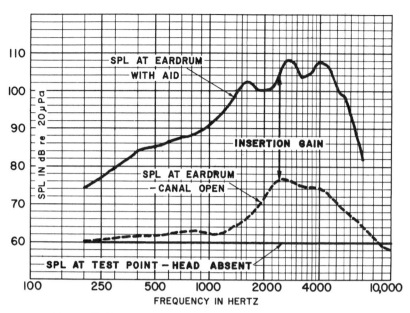

Figure 43.55. Insertion gain concept plotted (Lybarger, 1985b).

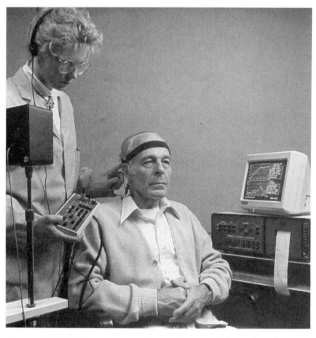

Figure 43.56. Microprocessor-based probe microphone system to measure in situ performance (Courtesy of Frye Electronics, Inc., Tigard, OR)

suited for checking *in-situ* performance and making adjustments after suitable hearing aids have been selected. A more complete discussion of the use of probe microphone systems for hearing aid selection takes place in Chapter 44.

Manufacturers of these systems have liberally adapted procedures for sound-field equalization (flattening the sound field) from ANSI and IEC standards applicable to 2-cc coupler and acoustic manikin measurements (Preves and Sullivan, 1987). A variety of real time and stored methods have been used for this equalization. In spite of this, real ear performance measured with probe microphone systems, on the average, show a high correlation between insertion gain, measured by probe microphones, and functional gain, measured behaviorally (Dillon and Murray, 1987; Harford, 1984).

Because probe microphone real ear measurements are often made in acoustically untreated rooms, a variety of nonstandardized input signals, intended to reduce standing wave artifacts, are used instead of the standard puretone signals. Creating additional measurement inconsistencies are differing signal processing approaches (filters) to improve the S/N ratio, a variety of probe microphone coupling approaches or probe tip positions, and unique resonant interactions with each ear (Harford, 1980a. 1980b; Hawkins and Mueller, 1986). Depending on the system, gain curves are displayed as real ear insertion response (REIR), real ear aided response (REAR), or both.

Manikin Measurements. Insertion gain can also be measured on an anthropometric manikin that is appropriately proportioned as an adult human and designed to provide lifelike test conditions for acoustic measurement purposes. KEMAR (Knowles Electronics Manikin for Acoustic Research, Burkhard and Sachs, 1975) is one such manikin designed for hearing aid research and engineering, and makes possible insertion gain measurements representative of those that can be expected on median adults (Fig. 43.57). It is fitted with one or two ear simulators (Zwislocki couplers) located at the ends of ear canal extensions starting at the medial end of the concha. The microphone diaphragms of the ear simulators are at positions corresponding to those of human eardrums. The pinnae are flexible, removable and of two different sizes, the larger being better for hearing aid measurements (but showing little difference in results). The response at each manikin eardrum for uniform SPL in free-field agrees quite well with Shaw's data (1974; Dirks and Gilman, 1979) for human adults at various angles of sound incidence. An extensive review of manikin measurements, and especially on KEMAR, is presented by Burkhard (1978).

An anechoic chamber is most suitable for obtaining reliable results on KEMAR. The unobstructed space from any part of the manikin to the absorbent surface should be at least 0.5 m, and a test point in the chamber should be established at a distance of 1 m from a loudspeaker that is not too large. (The smaller the sound source, the better, if adequate SPL can be

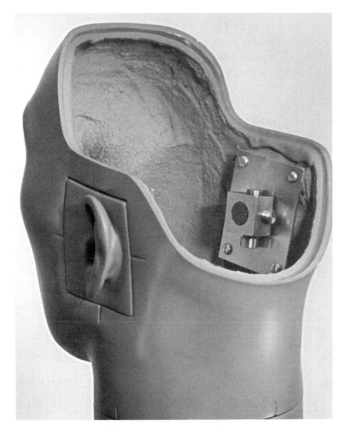

Figure 43.57. KEMAR, showing attachment of Zwislocki coupler (Courtesy, Knowles Electronics, Inc., Itasca, IL)

obtained at the manikin.) The manikin ear simulator microphone diaphragm is both measuring point and tympanic membrane substitute. For manikin measurement of insertion gain, the following procedure (of two commonly used) is recommended:

1. Produce a SPL at the selected test point that is constant with frequency (manikin absent). (A microprocessor is very effective for this purpose because the voltage required by the loudspeaker to produce the desired uniform SPL can be stored easily.) This is termed the *reference SPL*.
2. Place the manikin so that the center of the head is at the test point at an incidence of 0° to the speaker. Sound absorbing material on the sound source box, particularly on the face toward the manikin, helps to reduce reflections. The SPL at the manikin eardrum is now measured over the frequency range of interest. The difference between it and the SPL at the test point (reference SPL) is termed the *manikin unoccluded ear gain*.
3. The hearing aid is now placed on the manikin as it would be placed on a person. Turn the aid on and set its gain to the appropriate desired position.
4. By using the previously determined stored input voltages, the SPL in the manikin ear simulator is measured over the desired frequency range. The difference between the SPL produced by the hearing aid in the ear simulator and the reference input SPL is termed the *in situ gain*. The *insertion gain* is, then, the *in situ* gain minus the manikin unoccluded ear gain.

The insertion gain for most air-conduction hearing aids can be determined using the manikin. Fixtures to simulate earmolds are available for manikin testing. ITE or ITC aids cannot usually be accommodated unless the aid has been made by using an impression of the manikin ear or unless the manikin is modified.

Saturation output, full-on gain, harmonic distortion and AGC characteristics, can also be measured on a manikin. The results, of course, will not correspond to those obtained with 2-cc coupler methods required for FDA regulations, nor will they be as reliable (Teder, 1984). For research and engineering purposes, *in situ* measurement procedures by using a manikin have been standardized in IEC Publication 118-8 (1983), and in ANSI S3.35-1985. *Simulator real ear measurements (KEMAR or Zwislocki coupler) are closer to reality but represent the median, not the real ear of the individual person. As a result, they should not be applied directly to any potential hearing aid user without allowances for differences in head and torso sizes, ear canal volume, and middle ear impedance.* Insertion gain measurements made by using this procedure require expensive equipment and good expertise.

Estimation of Insertion Gain from 2-cc Coupler Measurements. Because manikin measurements are not easily performed or equipment and facilities are not available, the concept of applying corrections to 2-cc measurements has been suggested (Burkhard, 1978; Lybarger, 1978b; Killion and Monser, 1980; Longwell and Johnson, 1980; Frye, 1982; McCandless and Lyregaard, 1983). This method seems to have considerable practical value, because an approximation of the corrections needed can be visualized or derived and applied to the gain or response curves supplied with every aid measured according to ANSI S3.22-1987.

Correction values can be practical if the following precautions are observed:

1. The correction used must be for the type of aid used, taking into account the microphone sound entrance location.
2. The physical, acoustic connection from the aid to the reference plane of the coupler or ear simulator must be identical acoustically with the user's tubing and earmold.
3. Corrections are applicable to closed coupler and occluded earmold conditions on a 2-cc coupler. (Estimates of venting effects can be applied after the estimated insertion gain is determined.)
4. Corrections are average. Large individual variations may exist (Hawkins and Haskell, 1982; Hawkins and Schum, 1984).

The combination of components involved in estimating insertion gain from coupler data is as follows (modified from Lybarger, 1985a):

1. **HEAD BAFFLE.** This is the correction from free-field SPL to the SPL at the hearing aid microphone sound entrance. Madaffari (1974) gives corrections for various locations around the ear. Corrections vary depending upon the microphone locations and aid types.
2. **2-CC COUPLER RESPONSE.** This is the gain or response of the hearing aid when the input SPL is measured at the microphone sound entrance, as specified in the S3.22-1987 procedure.
3. **2-CC COUPLER-TO-EARDRUM CORRECTION.** This is the estimated correction from the 2-cc coupler to the eardrum. Data from Sachs and Burkhard (1972) may be used. If an ear simulator is used in place of a 2-cc coupler, this correction is not needed.
4. **FREE FIELD-TO-EARDRUM TRANSFORMATION.** This is the amount the SPL at the

eardrum exceeds that in free field with the ear canal open. The transformation data for 0° sound incidence given by Shaw and Vaillancourt (1985) are those used.

From the above steps, identified in Figure 43.58):
To estimate insertion gain from 2-cc coupler gain:
  Correction = (A + C − D)
  Insertion Gain = B + (A + C − D)
To estimate insertion gain from ear simulator gain (no manikin):
  Correction = (A − D)
  Insertion Gain = Ear simulator gain + (A − D)

By using the correction information above, the total estimated corrections for a BTE and an ITE aid are shown at the top of Figure 43.59. These are the corrections that must be applied to a 2-cc coupler gain or response curve to get an estimated insertion gain or response curve for these aids. An alternate way to view this is to look at the lower curves, which are the negative of the upper curves. These show the 2-cc coupler curves needed to produce a flat, zero gain insertion response. The response shown in the lower curves has been identified as CORFIG, the Coupler Response for Flat Insertion Gain. It can be seen that the correction for an ITE aid is smaller than that for a BTE aid.

Figure 43.60 shows calculated 2-cc coupler correction curves for BTE, ITE and ITC aids, using the steps described above (*solid curves*). In the case of the ITE aid, two additional correction curves, based on KEMAR measurements of actual hearing aids, are shown. The *dashed curve* was drawn from data given by Burnett and Beck (1987) and is the average for 10 different custom ITE aids. A special adapter for coupling the aids to KEMAR was used. The *dotted curve* is

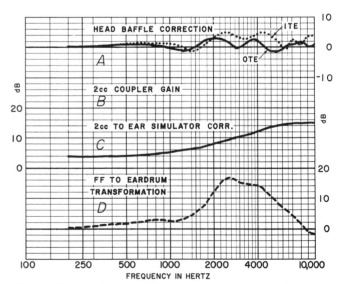

Figure 43.58. Method used to estimate insertion gain from 2-cc coupler data (Lybarger, 1985b). See text for explanation.

the average of KEMAR tests by six laboratories on one ITE aid that was made to fit the KEMAR ear canal (Lybarger and Teder, 1986). Step A for the ITC aid required the use of a free field-to-blocked ear canal transformation (Wiener and Ross, 1946). The use of this transformation was suggested by Mead Killion. Table 43.4 gives the numerical values used in plotting the curves shown. Bentler and Pavlovic (1989) have also compiled correction data. Coupler response for

flat insertion gain (CORFIG) in diffuse fields has been reported by Killion, Berger and Nuss (1987).

When applied to the 2-cc response curve of a BTE hearing aid, the corrections give the estimated insertion response, as shown in the example of Figure 43.61. The *solid curve* is the 2-cc coupler curve, and the *dashed curve* shows the estimated insertion response. The drop in response in the 3000 Hz region for the insertion gain curve suggests the desirability of a broad peak in that region as measured on a 2-cc coupler if a smooth insertion gain curve is to be obtained.

Figure 43.62 illustrates the use of CORFIG (the in-

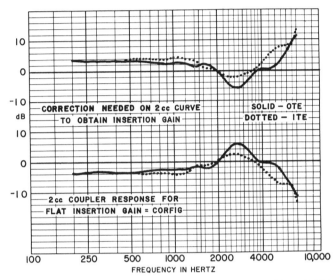

Figure 43.59. Insertion gain and CORFIG for a BTE and ITE hearing aid using the correction information from Lybarger, 1985b.

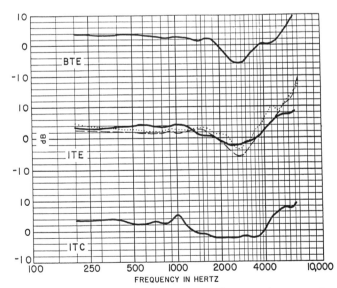

Figure 43.60. Corrections to be added to 2-cc coupler curves to get estimated insertion gain or response curves. Top (BTE); middle (ITE); bottom (ITC). For the ITE curves, the *dashed curve* was drawn from data by Burnett and Beck (1987); the *dotted curve* was drawn from data by Lybarger and Teder (1986).

Table 43.4.
Estimated 2-cc Coupler to Insertion Gain Corrections[a]

Frequency	BTE[b] (CALC)	ITE - 1[c] (CALC)	ITE - 2[d] L&T ('86)	ITE - 3[e] B&B ('87)	ITC[f] (CALC)
200	3.8	3.6	4.8	2.5	3.6
300	3.4	3.2	3.5	2.4	3.7
400	3.7	3.7	3.3	2.2	3.6
500	3.6	4.0	2.7	2.0	2.3
600	3.3	4.1	2.2	1.5	2.2
700	2.8	3.8	1.9	1.5	3.2
800	2.5	3.7	2.0	1.6	2.3
900	2.5	3.8	2.8	2.2	3.4
1000	2.7	4.2	2.8	1.6	5.1
1200	2.5	3.7	2.6	2.3	0.8
1400	1.4	1.1	3.2	2.7	-0.8
1600	2.2	0.7	3.4	2.0	-1.0
1800	1.5	0.4	1.8	0.8	-2.3
2000	-0.5	-0.6	1.5	-1.2	-2.4
2200	-2.8	-1.8	0.6	-2.7	-2.2
2400	-4.7	-2.4	-1.8	-4.6	-2.6
2600	-5.8	-2.4	-3.7	-5.7	-2.3
2800	-5.8	-2.1	-3.4	-5.6	-1.7
3000	-5.0	-1.6	-1.2	-4.3	-1.8
3200	-3.5	-1.0	-0.9	-2.6	-2.4
3400	-1.7	-0.4	2.4	-1.0	-2.2
3600	-0.5	0.5	3.5	0.5	-1.0
3800	0.3	1.3	4.5	1.8	-0.3
4000	0.5	2.5	6.7	2.8	0.6
4500	0.3	5.2	10.0	5.1	5.1
5000	1.8	6.9	8.6	6.7	6.1
5500	4.0	7.7	10.2	10.3	7.8
6000	6.5	7.6	12.6	11.6	7.3
6500	9.6	8.5	15.3	14.8	8.9
7000	11.5	13.3	18.2	19.7	11.0
7500			16.7	17.2	
8000	15.1	14.1	15.2	16.8	
9000	15.7	19.5			
10,000	17.4	20.6			

[a] Add values to 2-cc curves to obtain estimated insertion gain
[b] BTE = Calculated correction (Lybarger, 1985a; Lybarger and Teder, 1986)
[c] ITE-1 = Calculated correction (Lybarger, 1985a; Lybarger and Teder, 1986)
[d] ITE-2 = S3-48 Round Robin One aid, six labs, on KEMAR. (Lybarger and Teder, 1986)
[e] ITE-3 = Ten different ITEs on KEMAR (Burnett and Beck, 1987)
[f] ITC = Calculated correction (Lybarger, 1985a; Lybarger and Teder, 1986)

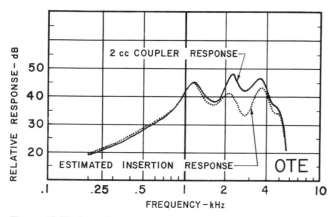

Figure 43.61. Insertion response compared with 2-cc coupler response for an OTE (BTE) aid. The 2-cc coupler curve indicates substantially better performance in the 3-kHz region than can be expected when the aid is worn. The curves above have been matched at 1kHz *after* applying the 2-cc coupler corrections of Figure 43.58.

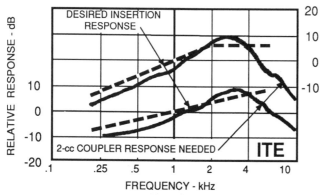

Figure 43.62. Estimated 2-cc coupler curves (*solid*) that would be required to give a 3 dB per octave rising insertion response curve (*lower dashed*) or a 6 dB per octave rising insertion response (*upper dashed*) to 2 kHz, followed by flat insertion response above that. The curves are for an ITE aid.

verse of 2-cc coupler corrections) in estimating the 2-cc coupler curve desired to meet a predetermined insertion gain response (*dashed line*) for an ITE aid. Because most hearing losses increase with frequency, a flat insertion gain response would not be desired too often. Also, although the estimating procedures described will give a better guide to the selection of an appropriate hearing aid than might be obtained by using only 2-cc coupler data, the need for final evaluation on an actual user remains important. **Of greatest importance is that even the most exact determination of insertion gain is of little value unless a definite target is established for what is needed—and that target varies based upon the fitting formulae used!**

ACKNOWLEDGMENT

Gratitude is given to all those who supplied information and data for this chapter. Special thanks to Elmer V. Carlson and Knowles Electronics, Inc. of Itasca, Illinois, for supplying data and electronic components for evaluation, and to David Preves, Ph.D. Eden Prairie, Minnesota, for comments and suggestions.

REFERENCES

Agnew J. Hearing instrument distortion: What does it mean for the listener? Hear Instrum 1988;39:10–20.

American National Standards Institute (ANSI). Methods for Coupler Calibration of Earphones. ANSI S3.7-1973, New York, 1973.

American National Standards Institute (ANSI). Methods for Coupler Calibration of Earphones. ANSI S3.7-1973 Revised, New York, 1992.

American National Standards Institute (ANSI). American National Standard for an Occluded Ear Simulator. ANSI S3.25-1979, New York, 1979.

American National Standards Institute (ANSI). Specification of Hearing Aid Characteristics. S3.22-1982, New York, 1982.

American National Standards Institute (ANSI). Methods of Measurement of Performance Characteristics of Hearing Aids Under Simulated In Situ Working Conditions. ANSI S3.35-1985, New York, 1985.

American National Standards Institute (ANSI). Specification of Hearing Aid Characteristics. ANSI S3.22-1987, New York, 1987.

American National Standards Institute (ANSI). Testing Hearing Aids With a Broad-Band Noise Signal. ANSI S3.42-1992, New York, 1992.

Ayers EW. A discussion of some problems involved in deriving objective performance criteria for a wearable hearing aid from clinical measurements with laboratory apparatus. In Proceedings of the First ICA Congress, Delft, 1953:141–143.

Balmer WF. The clarity of sound. Hear Aid J 1977;31:8, 50–52.

Bareham J. Part 2: Hearing instrument measurements using dual channel signal analysis. Hear Instrum 1990;41:32–33.

Beck LB. Assessment of directional hearing aid characteristics. Audiol Acoust 1983;22:178–191.

Beck LB, Leatherwood RW, and Punch JL. Aided low frequency responses: speech quality and speech intelligibility. Paper presented at American Speech-Language-Hearing Association Convention, Detroit, 1980.

Bentler RA, and Pavlovic CV. Transfer functions and correction factors used in hearing aid evaluation and research. Ear Hear 1989;10:58–63.

Beranek LL. Acoustic Measurements. New York: John Wiley & Sons, Inc., 1954.

Berger EH. Tips for fitting hearing protectors. Sound and Vibration, October, 22–25, 1988.

Berger KW. The Hearing Aid, Its Operation and Development, 3rd ed. Livonia, MI: National Hearing Aid Society, 1984.

Berland O. Are our testing standards misleading? Hear Instrum 1978;29:16–17.

Berland O, and Nielson TE. Sound pressure generated in the human external ear canal by a free sound field. Sound 1969;3:78–81.

Blue JV. NAEL—an important part of the team. Hear Instrum 1979;30:16.

Branderbit PL. A standardized programming system and three-channel compression hearing instrument technology. Hear Instrum 1991;42:24, 29–30.

Brinkmann K, and Richter U. Measurements on a bone-conduction hearing aid. J Audiol Tech 1977;16:66–83.

Burkhard MD. In Burkhard MD, Ed. Manikin Measurements, Conference Proceedings. Elk Grove Village, IL: Knowles Electronics, Inc. Industrial Research Products, Inc. 1975:17–18.

Burkhard MD, Ed. Manikin Measurements. Itasca, IL: Knowles Electronics, 1978.

Burkhard MD, and Sachs RM. Anthropometric manikin for acoustic research. J Acoust Soc Am 1975;58:214–222.

Burnett ED, and Beck LB. A correction for converting 2 cm^{P3} coupler responses to insertion responses for custom in-the-ear nondirectional hearing aids. Ear Hear 1987;8(5, Suppl):89S–94S.

Byrne D. Theoretical prescriptive approaches to selecting the gain and frequency response of a hearing aid. Monogr Contemp Audiol 1983;4:1–40.

Carhart R, and Tillman T. Interaction of competing speech signals with hearing losses. Arch Otolaryngol 1970;91:273–279.

Carlson EV. 1974a. Communication to ANSI Working Group S3-48.

Carlson EV. Smoothing the hearing aid response. J Aud Eng Soc 1974b;22:426–429.

Carlson EV. An output amplifier whose time has come. Hear Instrum. 1988;39:30–32.

Carlson EV. The Knowles Amplified Receiver. Report 10676-1 revision. Itasca, IL: Knowles Electronics, 1989; Inc.

Carlson EV, et al. in Heard but not seen . . . transducer technology probes the frontiers of hearing aid sound. Written by W.J. Mahon. The Hear J 1989;43:41–43, 44–48.

Carlson EV, and Killion MC. Subminiature directional microphones. J Aud Eng Soc 1974;22:92–96.

Cox RM. Acoustic aspects of hearing aid-ear canal coupling systems. Monogr Contemp Audiol 1979;1:1–44.

Cox RM. Combined effects of earmold vents and suboscillatory feedback on hearing aid frequency response. Ear Hear 1982; 3:12–17.

Cox RM, and Alexander GC. Acoustic versus electronic modifications of hearing aid low-frequency output. J Am Aud Soc 1983;4:190–196.

Crain T. Effects of an adaptive filter hearing aid on speech recognition thresholds in noise for normal-hearing and hearing-impaired listeners [Masters thesis]. University of MN Department of Communication Disorders, 1988.

Curran J. ITEs for children revisited. Hear Instrum 1990;41:40.

Dalsgaard SC, Johansen PA, and Chisnall LG. On wind noise with hearing aids. Hear Dealer 1967;Sept:10–15.

de Boer B. Performance of hearing aids from the pre-electronic era. Audiol Acoust 1984;23:34–55.

Delk JH. A Comprehensive Dictionary of Audiology, (3rd printing.) Sioux City, IA: Hearing Aid J 1975:193–195.

Dillon H, and Murray N. Accuracy of twelve methods for estimating the real gain of hearing aids. Ear Hear 1987;8:2–11.

Dillon H, and Walker G. Compression—input or output control? Hear. Instrum. 1983;34:20–21, 42.

Dirks D, and Gilman S. Exploring azimuth effects with anthropometric manikin. J Acoust Soc Am 1979;66:696–701.

Dirks DD, Morgan DE, and Dubno JR. A procedure for quantifying the effects of noise on speech recognition. J Speech Hear Disord 1982;47:114–123.

Ditthardt A. Application Notes for the Knowles EP Integrated Receiver. Report 10676-3, Itasca, IL: Knowles Electronics, Inc., 1990.

Dunlavy AR. CROS: A review of applications and fittings utilizing contralateral routing of signals. Hear Aid J 1968;21:6, 7, 30–32.

Dunn HK, and Farnsworth DW. Exploration of pressure field around the human head during speech. J Acoust Soc Am 1939;10, 184–199.

Duracell. 1990. Personal correspondence, October, Bethel, CT.

Dyrlund O. Characterization of non-linear distortion in hearing aids using coherence analysis, a pilot study. Scand Audiol 1989;18:143–148.

Ely W. Electroacoustic modifications of hearing aids. In Bess FH, Freeman BA, and Sinclair JS, Eds. Amplification in Education. Washington, DC: Alexander Graham Bell Association for the Deaf, 1981:316–341.

Ely W, Curran J, and Becker A. 1978. An investigation of blooming in AGC and peak-clipping hearing aids. Presentation at American Auditory Society Meeting, San Francisco. (Abstract in Corti's Organ, 4, 1979).

Federal Communications Commission Rule 68.4. 1989.

Federal Communications Commission Report and Order 92-217. 1992.

Fletcher H. Speech and Hearing in Communication. New York: D Van Nostrand Co. Inc., 1953.

Food and Drug Administration regulation. Federal Register 1984;49(Aug 14):32403.

Food and Drug Administration. Hearing aid devices—professional and patient labeling and conditions for sale. Federal Register 1977;42(Feb 15):9286–9296.

Fortune TW, Preves DA, and Woodruff BD. Saturation-induced distortion and its effects on aided LDL. Hear Instrum 1991; 42:37,40–41.

Frye GJ. "In situ" and "etymotic" hearing aid testing. Hear Instrum 1982;33:32–36.

Gengel R. Acceptable speech-to-noise ratios for aided speech discrimination by the hearing-impaired. J Aud Res 1971;11: 219–222.

Gilman S. An ear simulator study of resonances in occluded human ear canals. J Acoust Soc Am (Suppl 1) 1981;70:S72 (A).

Goldberg H. Earmold technology—application notes. Audiol Hear Educ 1977;3:11.

Griffing TS, and Preves DA. In-the-ear aids—part I. Hear Instrum 1976;27:22–24.

Hable LA, Brown KM, and Gudmundsen GI. CROS-plus: a physical CROS system. Hear Instrum 1990;41:27–30, 68.

Hanson WW. Baffle effect of the human body on the response of a hearing aid. J. Acoust Soc Am 1945;16:60–62.

Harford E. Bilateral CROS. Arch Otolaryngol 1966;84:426–432.

Harford E. A microphone in the ear canal to measure hearing aid performance. Hear. Instrum. 1980a;31:14–15, 32.

Harford E. Techniques and applications in hearing aids, the use of a miniature microphone in the ear canal for the verification of hearing aid performance. Ear Hear 1980b;1:329–337.

Harford E. The use of real ear measures for fitting wearable amplification. Hear J 1984;7:20–25.

Harford E, and Barry J. A rehabilitative approach to the problem of unilateral hearing impairment: the contralateral routing of signals (CROS). J Speech Hear Disord 1965;30:121–132.

Harford E, and Dodds E. The clinical application of CROS—a hearing aid for unilateral deafness. Arch Otolaryngol 1966; 83:73–82.

Hawkins DB, and Haskell GB. A comparison of functional gain and 2cm^3 coupler gain. J Speech Hear Disord 1982;47:71–76.

Hawkins DB, and Mueller HG. Some variables affecting the accuracy of probe tube microphone measurements. Hear. Instrum. 1986;37:8–12, 49.

Hawkins DB, and Schum DJ. Relationships among various measures of hearing aid gain. J Speech Hear Disord 1984;49: 94–111.

Hawkins DB, and Yacullo W. Signal-to-noise ratio advantage of binaural hearing aids and directional microphones under different levels of reverberation. J Speech Hear Disord 1984;49:278–286.

Hearing Industries Association (HIA). Special Report, 1984.

Hearing Industries Association (HIA). Statistical Report for the Quarter Ending March. New Units Sold by Type and Origin. HIA, Washington, DC, 1986.

Hearing Industries Association (HIA). Statistical Report for the Quarter Ending December. New Units Sold by Type and Origin. HIA, Washington, DC, 1992.

Hodgson WR. Speech acoustics and intelligibility. In Hodgson WR, Ed. Hearing Aid Assessment and Use in Audiologic Habilitation, 3rd ed. Baltimore: Williams & Wilkins, 1986:109–127.

Hodgson WA, and Lade KP. Digital technology in hearing instruments. Hear J 1988;41:28–34.

Hood JD. The principles and practice of bone conduction audiometry. Laryngol 1960;70:1211–1228.

International Electrotechnical Commission (IEC). Occluded Ear Simulator for the Measurement of Earphones Coupled to the Ear by Ear Inserts. Publication 711, Geneva, 1982.

International Electrotechnical Commission (IEC). Hearing Aids. Measurement of Electro-Acoustical Characteristics. Publication 118-0, Geneva, 1983.

International Electrotechnical Commission (IEC). Hearing Aids. Measurement of Performance Characteristics of Hearing Aids for Quality. Inspection for Delivery Purposes. Publication 118-7, Geneva, 1983.

International Electrotechnical Commission (IEC). Hearing Aids. Measurement of Hearing Aids Under Simulated in-Situ Working Conditions. Publication 118-8, Geneva, 1983.

International Electrotechnical Commission (IEC). Hearing Aids. Measurements of Characteristics of Hearing Aids with Bone Vibrator Outputs. Publication 118-9, 1977.

Johansen PA. An Evaluation of the Acoustic Feedback Damping for Behind the Ear Hearing Aids. Report, Research Laboratory for Technical Audiology, State Hearing Centres, Odense, Denmark, 1975.

Johnson EW. Practical experience in fitting hearing aids. Audiol Acoust 1982;21:180–204.

Kasten RN, and Franks JR. Electroacoustic characteristics of hearing aids. In Hodgson WR, Ed. Hearing Aid Assessment and Use in Audiologic Habilitation, 3rd ed. Baltimore: Williams & Wilkins, 1986;38–70.

Kates JM. Acoustic effects in in-the-ear hearing aid response: results from a computer simulation. Ear Hear 1988;9:119–132.

Killion MC. Earmold options for wideband hearing aids. J Speech Hear Res 1981a;46:10–20.

Killion MC. Smooth Insertion Gain Coupling for the EF-Series Receiver in OTE Applications. Report 10590-1. Itasca, IL: Knowles Electronics, 1981b.

Killion MC. The noise problem: there's hope. Hear Instrum 1985;36:26, 28, 30, 32.

Killion MC. A high fidelity hearing aid. Hear Instrum 1990;41: 38–39.

Killion MC, Berger E, and Nuss R. Diffuse field response of the ear. J Acoust Soc Am Suppl 1987;1:81(A).

Killion MC, and Carlson EV. A subminiature electret-condenser microphone of new design. J Aud Eng Soc 1974;22:237–243.

Killion MC, and Monser EL. CORFIG: coupler response for flat insertion gain. In Studebaker GA, and Hochberg I, Eds. Acoustical Factors Affecting Hearing Aid Response. Baltimore: University Park Press, 1980:149–168.

Killion MC, and Murphy WJ. Smoothing the ITE Response: The EF-1743 Damped Coupling Assembly. Itasca, IL: Knowles Electronics, 1982.

Killion MC, Staab WJ, and Preves DA. Classifying automatic signal processors. Hear Instrum 1990;41:24, 26.

Killion MC, Wilber LA, and Gudmundsen GJ. Zwislocki was right . . . Hear Instrum 1988;39:14–18.

Killion MC, and Wilson DL. Response-modifying earhooks for special fitting problems. Audecibel 1985;34:28–30.

Knowles Electronics, Inc. The Knowles Amplified Receiver. Knowles Report 10676-1, 1988.

Knowles HS, and Killion MC. Frequency characteristics of recent broadband receivers. J Audiol Tech 1978;17:86–89.

Leavitt R. Earmolds: acoustic and structural considerations. In Hodgson WR, Ed. Hearing Aid Assessment and Use in Audiologic Habilitation, 3rd ed. Baltimore: Williams & Wilkins, 1986:71–108.

Lentz WE. Speech discrimination in the presence of background noise using a hearing aid with a directionally-sensitive microphone. Maico Aud Aud Lib Ser 1972a;10:report 9.

Lentz WE. Assessment of performance using hearing aids with directional and nondirectional microphones in a highly re verberant room. Paper presented at American Speech-Language-Hearing Association Convention, San Francisco, 1972b.

Libby ER. Hearing instrument systems technology & performance standards. In Sandlin RE, Ed. Hearing Instrument Science and Fitting Practices. Livonia, MI: National Institute for Hearing Instruments Studies, 1985:201–311.

Licklider JCR. Effects of amplitude distortion upon the intelligibility of speech. J Acoust Soc Am 1946;18:429–434.

Lindblad AC. Detection of Nonlinear Distortion on Speech Signals by Hearing Impaired Listeners. Report TA105, Karolinska Institutet, Technical Audiology, KTH, Stockholm, 1982.

Lippmann RP, Braida LD, and Durlach NI. Study of multichannel amplitude compression and linear amplification for persons with sensori-neural hearing loss. J Acoust Soc Am 1981;69:624–634.

Longwell TF, and Johnson JH. Estimating hearing aid insertion gain from coupler gain. Hear Instrum 1980;31:20–22, 30.

Lybarger SF. Some comments on CROS. National Hearing Aid Journal 1968;21:8, 33.

Lybarger SF. 1972. Dual bore tubing arrangement. Radioear Corp. McMurray, PA.

Lybarger SF. Comparison of earmold characteristics measured on the 2-cc coupler, the Zwislocki coupler and real ears. Scand Audiol Suppl 1975;5:65–85.

Lybarger SF. Expanding the usefulness of adjustable vent inserts. Hear. Instrum. 1978a;29:18–19.

Lybarger SF. Selective amplification—a review and evaluation. J Am Aud Soc 1978b;3:258–266.

Lybarger SF. Controlling hearing aid performance by earmold design. In Larson VD, Egolf DP, Kirlin RL, and Stile SW, Eds. Auditory and Hearing Prosthetic Research. New York: Grune & Stratton, 1979:101–132.

Lybarger SF. Earmold venting as an acoustic control factor. In Studebaker GA, and Hochberg I, Eds. Acoustical Factors Affecting Hearing Aid Performance. Baltimore: University Park Press, 1980:197–217.

Lybarger SF. Earmolds. In J Katz (Ed). Handbook of Clinical Audiology, 3rd Edition. Baltimore: Williams & Wilkins, 1985a; 885–910.

Lybarger SF. 1985b. Relationship between coupler measurements of hearing aids, as required by the Food and Drug Administration (FDA) labelling regulations and the performance of an aid under actual use conditions. American Auditory Society Carhart Memorial Lecture, Atlanta. Corti's Organ. 10, No. 3.

Lybarger SF. The physical and electroacoustic characteristics of hearing aids. In J Katz (Ed). Handbook of Clinical Audiology, 3rd Edition. Baltimore: Williams & Wilkins, 1985c;849–884.

Lybarger SF. 1989. Unpublished presentation at Mayo Clinic, Rochester, MN, March 25.

Lybarger SF. 1991. Unpublished data; personal communications.

Lybarger SF, and Barron FE. Head baffle effect for different hearing aid microphone locations. Paper presented at A.S.A., St. Louis, MO, 1965.

Lybarger SF, and Olsen WO. Hearing aid measurement standards: an update and bibliography. Hear J 1983;36:19–20.

Lybarger SF, and Olsen WO. ANSI and IEC standards for hearing aid measurements. Asha 1984;26:49.

Lybarger SF, and Teder H. 2 cc coupler curves to insertion gain curves. Hear. Instrum. 1986;37:36–37, 40.

Macrae J. Acoustic notch filters for hearing aids. Austr J Audiol 1982;4:71–76.

Madaffari PL. Pressure variation about the ear. J Acoust Soc Am (Suppl.) 1974;56:S3 (A).

Madaffari PL. A comparison of directional microphone performance in free field and on a manikin. J Acous Soc Am (Suppl. 1) 1983;73:S23 (A).

Madison TK, and Hawkins DB. The signal-to-noise ratio advantage of directional microphones. Hear. Instrum. 1983;34:18.

Mahon WJ. Heard but not seen . . . transducer technology probes the frontiers of hearing aid sound. Hear J 1990;43:41–48.

Martin DW. Sound reproduction and recording systems. In Fink DG and Christiansen D, (Eds). Electronics Engineers" Handbook, 2nd Edition. New York: McGraw-Hill Book Company, 1982.

McCandless GA, and Lyregaard PE. Prescription of gain/output (POGO) for hearing aids. Hear. Instrum. 1983;34:16–21.

Miller AL. An alternative approach to CROS and Bi-CROS hearing aids: an internal CROS. Audecibel. 1989;38:29–30.

Mueller HG. Directional microphone hearing aids: a 10 year report. Hear. Instrum. 1981;32:18–20.

Mueller HG, Grimes AM, and Erdman SA. Subjective ratings of directional amplification. Hear Instrum 1983;34:14–16.

Murphy L. An investigation of the use of behind the ear and in the ear hearing aids with a geriatric population. Hear J 1981; 34:38–41.

Nábělek IG. Performance of hearing impaired listeners under various types of amplitude compression. J Acoust Soc Am 1983; 74:776–791.

Nicolet. A comprehensive instrument for clinical audiology and hearing aid fitting. Hear Instrum 1987;38:37–38, 64.

Nielsen TE. Directional microphones. Hear. Dealer 1972;23: 12–14.

Nordlund B, and Fritzell B. The influence of azimuths on speech signal. Acta Otolaryngol (Stockh) 1963;56:132–642.

Nunley J, Staab WJ, Steadman J, Wechsler P, and Spencer B. A wearable digital hearing aid. The Hear J 1983;36:29–31.

Olsen WO, and Carhart R. Development of test procedures for evaluation of binaural hearing aids. Bull Prosthet Res 1967; 10:22–49.

Olson H. Elements of Acoustical Engineering, 2nd ed. New York: D Van Nostrand, 1947.

Orchik DJ, Cowgill SP, and Parmely J. Peritympanic soft hearing instrument fitting in high frequency hearing loss. Hear Instrum 1990;41:28–30.

Orton JF, and Preves DA. Localization ability as a function of hearing aid microphone placement. Hear Instrum 1979;30:18–21, 35.

Pascoe DP. Frequency responses of hearing aids and their effects on the speech perception of hearing-impaired subjects. Ann Otol Rhinol Laryngol (Suppl 23) 1975;84:

Pollack MC. Electroacoustic characteristics. In Pollack MC, Ed. Amplification for the Hearing Impaired. New York: Grune & Stratton, 1980.

Preves DA. Expressing hearing aid noise and distortion with coherence measurements. ASHA, June/July, 56–59, 1990.

Preves DA. Personal communication, 1992.

Preves DA, and Newton JR. The headroom problem and hearing aid performance. Hear J 1989;42:21.

Preves DA, and Sullivan RF. Sound field equalization for real ear measurements with probe microphones. Hear Instrum 1987;38: 20–21, 24–26, 64.

Preves DA, and Woodruff BD. Some methods of improving and assessing hearing aid headroom. Audecibel 1990;38:8–13.

Randolph K, Gierula V, and Ross M. Hearing aid microphone location and speech discrimination: hearing impaired adults. Presented at the Annual Convention of the American Speech and Hearing Association, Chicago, IL, 1977.

Romanow FF. Methods for measuring the performance of hearing aids. J Acoust Soc Am 1942;13:294–304.

Ross M. Classroom amplification. In Hodgson WR, Ed. Hearing Aid Assessment and Use in Audiologic Habilitation. Baltimore: Williams & Wilkins, 1986:231–265.

Sachs RM, and Burkhard MD. Zwislocki Coupler Evaluation with Insert Earphones. Report 20022-1. Itasca, IL: Knowles Electronics, 1972.

Schweitzer HC. Tutorial paper: principles and characteristics of automatic gain control hearing aids. J Am Aud Soc 1979;5:84–94.

Shaw EAG. Ear canal pressure generated by a free sound field. J Acoust Soc Am 1966;39:465–470.

Shaw EAG. Transformation of sound pressure level from the free field to the eardrum in the horizontal plane. J Acoust Soc Am 1974;56:1848–1861.

Shaw EAG. The external ear: new knowledge. Scand Audiol (Suppl.) 1975;5:24–50.

Shaw EAG. The acoustics of the external ear. In Studebaker G, and Hochberg I, Eds. Acoustical Factors Affecting Hearing Aid Performance. Baltimore: University Park Press, 1980:109–125.

Shaw EAG, and Vaillancourt MM. Transformation of sound pressure level from the free field to the eardrum presented in numerical form. J Acoust Soc Am 1985;78:1120–1123.

Siegelman J, and Preves D. Field trials of a new adaptive signal processor hearing aid circuit. Hear J 1987;4:24–27.

Sivian L, and White S. On minimum audible sound fields. J Acoust Soc Am 1933;4:288–321.

Skinner MW, and Karstaedt MS. Effect of amplification bandwidth on speech intelligibility. Paper presented at American Speech-Language-Hearing Association Convention, Atlanta, 1979.

Skinner MW, Karstaedt M, and Miller J. Amplification bandwidth and speech intelligibility for two listeners with sensori-neural hearing loss. Audiology 1982;21:251–268.

Sommers M. Directional/non-directional hearing aids: one, the other, or both? Hear Aid J 1979;33:27.

Staab WJ. Hearing Aid Handbook. Phoenix, AZ: W.J. Staab, 1978:16–23.

Staab WJ. Recent advances in all-in-the-ear fitting of hearing aids. International Hearing Aid Seminar, San Diego, CA, 1980.

Staab WJ. Analysis of hearing aid repair problems. Paper presented at 1982 Jackson Hole Rendezvous, Jackson Hole, WY, 1982.

Staab WJ. Stock ITCs: a new fitting and marketing philosophy. Hear. Instrum. 1985a;36:24, 26, 28, 62.

Staab WJ. Digital hearing aids—a tutorial. Hear Instrum 1985b;36:14–24.

Staab WJ. Digital hearing instruments. Hear Instrum 1987; 38:18–26.

Staab WJ. Development of a programmable behind-the-ear hearing instrument. Hear Instrum 1988a;39:22, 24, 26, 39.

Staab WJ. Significance of mid-frequencies in hearing aid selection. The Hear J 1988b;42:23, 25–28, 30–34.

Staab WJ. Digital/programmable hearing aids—an eye towards the future. Br J Audiol 1991;24:243–256.

Staab WJ. The Peritympanic Instrument: Fitting Rationale and Test Results. The Hear J 1992;45:21–26.

Staab WJ, and Finlay B. A fitting rationale for deep canal hearing instruments. Hear Instrum 1991;42:6, 8–10, 50.

Staab WJ, and Nunley J. A guide to tube fitting of hearing aids. Hear Aid J 1982;36:25–26, 28–30, 32–34.

Staab WJ, and Nunley J. New development: multiple signal processor (MSP). Hear J 1987;41:24–26.

Studebaker GA. 1975. A broad-band noise-based method of measuring frequency response. Paper presented at the American Speech and Hearing Association Convention, Washington, DC.

Studebaker GA, and Cox RM. Side branch and parallel vent effects in real ears and in acoustical and electrical models. J Am Aud Soc 1977;3:10–17.

Studebaker GA, Cox RM, and Formby C. The effect of environment on the directional performance of head-worn hearing aids. In Studebaker GA, and Hochberg I, Eds. Acoustical Factors Affecting Hearing Aid Performance. Baltimore: University Park Press, 1980:81–105.

Studebaker GA, and Hochberg I, Eds. Acoustical Factors Affecting Hearing Aid Performance. Baltimore: University Park Press, 1980.

Sullivan RF. Transcranial ITE CROS. Hear. Instrum. 1988;39:11–12, 54.

Sung RJ, and Sung GS. Low frequency amplification and speech intelligibility in noise. Hear Instrum 1980;33:20.

Sung RJ, and Sung GS. Compression amplification: its effect on speech intelligibility in noise. Hear Aid J 1982;35:20–24.

Teder H. Repeatability of KEMAR insertion gain measurements. Hear Instrum 1984;35:16, 18, 20–22, 66.

Tillman T, Kasten R, and Horner J. Effect of head shadow on reception of speech. Paper presented at American Speech and Hearing Association, Chicago, IL, 1963.

Villchur E. Signal processing to improve speech intelligibility in perceptive deafness. J Acoust Soc Am 1973;53:1646–1657.

Waldhauer R, and Villchur E. Full dynamic range multiband compression in a hearing aid. Hear J 1988;9:19–32.

Walker G, and Dillon H. Compression in Hearing Aids: A Review and Some Recommendations. NAL Report No. 90, Australian Government Publishing Service, Canberra, 1982.

Watson LA, and Tolan T. Hearing Tests and Hearing Instruments. Baltimore: Williams & Wilkins, 1949.

Wiener F, and Ross D. The pressure distribution in the auditory canal and progressive sound field. J Acoust Soc Am 1946;18:401–408.

Wernick JS. Use of hearing aids. In Katz J, Ed. Handbook of Clinical Audiology, 3rd ed. Baltimore: Williams & Wilkins, 1985:911–935.

Wernick JS, and Hodgson WR. Canal aid vs. standard custom ITE performance. Part 1. KEMAR response analysis. Hear Instrum 1984;35:13–15.

White REC, Studebaker GA, Levitt H, and Mook D. The application of modeling techniques to the study of hearing aid acoustic systems. In Studebaker GA, and Hochberg I, Eds. Acoustical factors Affecting Hearing Aid Performance. Baltimore: University Park Press, 1980:267–296.

Wolfe A. Two audiologists' experience with CROS. National Hearing Aid Journal. 1968;21:7.

Zwislocki JJ. Acoustic attenuation between the ears. J Acoust Soc Am 1953;25:752–759.

Zwislocki JJ. An Acoustic Coupler for Earphone Calibration. Report LSC-S-7. Laboratory of Sensory Communication, Syracuse, NY, 1970.

Zwislocki JJ. An Earlike Coupler for Earphone Calibration. Report LSC-S-9. Laboratory Sensory Communication, Syracuse University, Syracuse, NY, 1971.

CHAPTER 44

Hearing Aid Fitting and Evaluation

James J. Dempsey

Selecting the proper amplification device with the appropriate characteristics has long been a challenge for the hearing health care professional. Significant advances in technology have made this selection process more difficult by increasing the variety of parameter settings under our control and placing further demand upon our ability to evaluate and determine appropriateness of these settings. It has been suggested that the audiologist working in the area of hearing aids needs to possess a unique blend of multidisciplinary skills (Hawkins, 1990a). The audiologist must be a "jack-of-all trades" to integrate information from engineers, the hearing aid industry, psychoacousticians, and other audiologists in order to provide effective amplification services for the hearing-impaired (Studebaker, 1980). The challenge is a growing one because technologic advances are occurring at a rate that exceeds our ability to fully assess or utilize these advances clinically. Our goal, therefore, should be to make the most efficient use of the available technology in order to provide the greatest benefit to the hearing-impaired population.

CANDIDACY FOR AMPLIFICATION

Adults

The characteristics that determine hearing aid candidacy for adults can be divided into audiologic factors and motivational factors. Although the audiologic information may be more readily quantifiable, the motivational information is of equal importance with regard to successful hearing aid fitting.

Audiologic Factors

The information gathered through the audiologic evaluation is necessary in order to determine candidacy for amplification. Puretone audiometric results are of importance in determining hearing aid candidacy by describing the type of hearing loss, the degree of hearing loss, and the configuration of the hearing loss. The results of speech tests, such as the speech reception threshold and uncomfortable loudness level, are also helpful in determining the dynamic range.

Dynamic range is also referred to as the range of usable hearing or the range of comfortable loudness for speech (Martin, 1986). The dynamic range is the decibel range between threshold for tones or speech and the point that the stimulus (tones or speech) becomes uncomfortably loud. The dynamic range is often significantly reduced in individuals with sensory-neural hearing losses. Elevated thresholds will necessarily shift the lower limit of the dynamic range upward. The upper limit of the dynamic range can be significantly lowered as a result of recruitment. In this manner, the dynamic range of an individual with sensory-neural hearing loss can be reduced from both directions. Individuals with sensory-neural hearing loss who have a sufficiently large dynamic range are likely to be more successful hearing aid users than those with a severely reduced dynamic range.

The dynamic range is of particular importance in hearing aid evaluations because it represents a target area for amplification. Logically, the dynamic range represents the upper and lower limits of amplification. A hearing aid that provides too much gain and has an output level that exceeds the uncomfortable listening level will be rejected by the hearing aid wearer. Wallenfels (1967) suggests that a good estimate of the most comfortable listening level is at the midpoint of the dynamic range.

Motivational Factors

Motivational factors that are part of the determination of hearing aid candidacy are often influenced by the degree of hearing handicap. As opposed to the hearing loss, which is readily quantifiable from the audiometric data, hearing handicap is more difficult to measure. It refers to the impact of the hearing loss upon an individual's communicative abilities and quality of life. To provide reliable measures of hearing handicap, self-report procedures have been developed. A more complete description of self-report procedures is provided in Chapter 48. Later in this chapter, self-report procedures will be discussed as measures of ascertaining the appropriateness of a hearing aid fitting.

The audiologist needs to be aware of the perceived need for amplification on the part of the potential hearing aid candidate. Individuals who are highly motivated and believe that they have a good deal to gain through using amplification are likely to perform well with hearing aids. It is also just as likely that those who are not motivated to use amplification and do not view themselves as having a hearing handicap will not perform well with hearing aids. Thus, degree of hearing handicap and motivation are critical factors in determining hearing aid candidacy for adults.

Children

In determining hearing aid candidacy for children, there tends to be a greater reliance on the audiologic factors and a reduced emphasis on motivational factors. In theory, any child with a significant, long-term hearing loss is a candidate for amplification. In practice, the most easily identified candidates are children with moderate, severe, or profound sensory-neural losses. Recently, there has been increased support for the use of amplification for children with mild sensory-neural losses (Maxon, 1987).

When evaluating young children, a combination of behavioral and electrophysiologic tests is recommended to determine need for amplification (Beauchaine, Barlow, and Stelmachowicz, 1990). The behavioral tests have the advantage of readily providing frequency-specific information whereas the electrophysiologic tests, such as the Auditory Brainstem Response (ABR), have the advantage of readily providing individual ear information. The profile developed from these tests provides us with an initial framework for selecting amplification characteristics. It is imperative to keep in mind, however, that a hearing aid evaluation with a young, preverbal child is an ongoing process and that all recommendations are subject to modification as further information regarding the child's hearing loss is obtained.

Although the vast majority of children whom we amplify will have sensory-neural losses, it has been suggested that amplification may also be useful with children with fluctuating hearing losses associated with conductive pathologies (Downs, 1981). This suggestion is based upon the assumption that amplification will provide a more consistent speech signal to these children and thereby reduce the impacts of the conductive component upon language acquisition and academic performance.

PRESELECTION OF AMPLIFICATION

Configuration

Binaural

Although there has been heated debate for years regarding the benefits provided by two hearing aids versus one, it is generally agreed that, unless there are significant contraindications, binaural amplification is the arrangement of choice. The source of this controversy is related to the fact that the burden of proof has been placed upon those advocating binaural amplification to provide evidence that two hearing aids are better than one (Ross, 1980). A problem exists in that advantages provided by binaural amplification are not easily demonstrated clinically (Wernick, 1985; Pollack, 1988). In addition, some hearing impaired listeners require a period of adjustment before demonstrating a binaural advantage (Nábĕlek and Pickett, 1974).

The advantages most readily apparent with binaural hearing aids are improved localization and improved speech recognition ability in noise. These binaural advantages have been repeatedly demonstrated throughout the literature when the subjects' tasks have been made sufficiently difficult (Ross, 1980; Pollack, 1988).

In spite of the above mentioned advantages, many audiologists have historically recommended monaural versus binaural amplification for a large percentage of their clients for economic reasons. The feeling of many has been that limited demonstrable improvement in aided performance in the clinic did not outweigh the additional financial burden that a second hearing aid placed upon the client. Again, the benefits of binaural amplification are difficult to measure clinically and will be more apparent in the real-world setting over time. In addition, while it is virtuous to be concerned regarding the financial burdens of our clients, it has been suggested that we can remain compassionate clinicians while allowing the cost of a second hearing aid to be primarily the responsibility of the client (Byrne, 1980; Harford, 1988).

There are also legal issues to consider in making binaural versus monaural amplification decisions. There have been recent incidences in which individuals have pursued litigation against dispensing audiologists for fitting them monaurally without informing them of the possible benefits of binaural amplification.

The advantages of binaural hearing versus monaural hearing are well documented and unequivocal. Pascoe (1985) suggests, therefore, that the question should not be are two hearing aids better than one, but, rather, can binaural advantages be achieved via amplification or not.

Monaural

When contraindications to binaural amplification exist, such as a large asymmetry in audiometric configuration, it is sometimes necessary to amplify monaurally. The obvious decision that must be made in this case is which ear to amplify. This decision, unfortunately, is more difficult than simply attempting to aid the "better ear" or the "poorer ear."

In circumstances in which a significant difference in hearing sensitivity exists between ears, the poorer ear may be selected for amplification. This decision may be made when (a) there is enough residual hearing in the poorer ear to benefit from amplification and (b) there is enough residual hearing in the better ear to function partially without amplification (Hodgson, 1981). More typically, however, when there is a significant asymmetry between ears, the better ear is chosen for amplification. For example, if someone has a profound hearing loss in the right ear and a moderate to severe loss in the left ear, the left ear will most likely be amplified.

An approach to ear selection for amplification that is more effective than "better threshold" versus "poorer threshold" is to consider the factors of dynamic range, word recognition ability, and client preference. One important consideration is to fit the ear with the wider dynamic range. That is, a client may demonstrate similar thresholds between ears but show evidence of greater recruitment in one ear versus the other. In this case, the ear with the more restricted dynamic range will be more difficult to fit successfully with a hearing aid.

We are also interested in providing the client with maximum accessibility to spoken language. Therefore, the rule of thumb to follow, based upon this premise, is to aid the ear with the best word recognition ability.

The ear preference of the client should also be considered. Many individuals will have strong preferences based upon occupational needs or handedness.

Hearing Aid Style

The following are some general considerations to be made in selecting a style of hearing aid. For a more complete description of the various types of amplification devices see Chapters 42 and 43.

Body-Worn Hearing Aids

Although body-worn hearing aids represent a very small percentage of the number of hearing aids sold annually in the United States, less than 2.3% in 1989 (Cranmer, 1990), there are still situations in which body aids continue to be useful. The advantages of body aids, compared with ear-level instruments, are the increased gain possibilities with less chance of acoustical feedback; larger controls and batteries; and greater ruggedness and durability of the instrument. For these reasons, body aids are sometimes recommended for geriatric clients with poor manual dexterity and for very young, active children.

Ear-Level Amplification

Ear-level amplification devices include behind-the-ear (BTE), in-the-ear (ITE), and custom in-the-canal (ITC) hearing aids. The acoustic and cosmetic advantages of ear-level amplification over body-worn amplification make these the devices of choice in most situations. The decision to go with an ITE or ITC hearing aid versus a BTE will be dependent upon the amount of gain necessary, the required frequency response, as well as the audiologist and client preferences. The chances of acoustical feedback are increased with an ITE or ITC hearing aid versus a BTE because of the proximity of the microphone and receiver. Therefore, a BTE will be preferable if the client needs a significant amount of gain. There are other pros and cons to each type of hearing aid, such as the availability and quality of telecoil options, which should be considered on an individual basis. In addition, many clients have a preconceived notion about the type of instrument they wish to pursue. Although this notion is almost exclusively based upon cosmetics, strong feelings on the part of the client may prove to be a decisive factor regarding successful hearing aid use.

Other Hearing Aids

Additional amplification arrangements are utilized in less typical circumstances. Instruments with bone conduction receivers have been utilized by persons with chronic conductive hearing losses caused by auditory atresias or "running ears" as a result of otitis media. Individuals with unilateral hearing loss have demonstrated significant benefits from a CROS (contralateral routing of offside signal) hearing aid arrangement in which the microphone is worn on one side of the head while the receiver is worn on the opposite side of the head. The many variations of the CROS arrangement, as well as other special applications of hearing aid amplification, are covered in more detail in Chapter 42.

FM Auditory Trainer

The hearing aid evaluation for children will often include determining the benefits of an FM auditory trainer as well as those of a personal hearing aid. The improved signal-to-noise ratio provided by FM systems has led to successful use with preverbally hearing impaired children (Madell, 1988), as well as with school-aged children. It is important to include the FM system as part of the hearing aid evaluation because there have been numerous occasions in which school systems have misinterpreted these devices as being "one-setting-fits-all" systems. Most FM auditory trainers are flexible in terms of frequency response and output characteristics and must be properly set for each individual child.

Selective Amplification

Historical Background

Once it has been determined (a) that an individual is a hearing aid candidate, (b) that a binaural or monaural arrangement is appropriate, and (c) which hearing aid style will be used, it is then necessary to determine the output and gain requirements for that individual. Selective amplification is a term that refers to the process of matching the frequency response of a hearing aid to the audiogram of an individual. The process of selectively amplifying has a long history beginning with the "mirror-fitting" technique. In the mirror-fitting approach the frequency response is set to the mirror image of the hearing loss. In this way the poorest hearing regions on the audiogram receive the greatest amplification and vice versa (Watson and Knudsen, 1940).

For several reasons, selective amplification, to the extent of "mirror-fitting," has proven to be an unsatisfactory approach to determining the frequency response and gain characteristics of a hearing aid. The primary problem is that it leads to overamplification. One basic reason for the failure of this technique is that it is based upon the concept of threshold, whereas listening is a suprathreshold phenomenon (Ross, 1978). Equal loudness contours tend to normalize at suprathreshold levels, which partially explains the overamplification provided by a mirror fit. Another problem with this technique is that the frequency response of the hearing aid, set to mirror the audiogram, is based upon measures obtained in a 2-cc coupler and does not take into account coupler/real-ear differences or insertion loss created by the presence of an earmold or an ITE.

Because the mirror fitting technique often resulted in overamplification, several procedures for selecting frequency response and gain characteristics were developed. In 1944, Lybarger proposed a procedure in which the optimal frequency response curve of a hearing aid, in dB, would be equal to "about half" of the audiogram curve (Lybarger, 1978). This was the beginning of the "one-half gain" rule which will later be shown to be the basis of many of the so-called "prescriptive techniques" currently in use.

About this same time, the classic "Harvard Report" (Davis, et al., 1946) was published. Evidence was contained in this report that refuted the notion of selective amplification. Davis, et al., found that the frequency responses that yielded the best results did not appear to be related to an individual's audiometric

configuration. They concluded that a flat frequency response or a high pass, 6 dB per octave frequency response produced optimal results for most subjects. Lybarger (1978) showed, however, that when the master hearing aid curves from the Harvard Report were converted to real-ear responses, the flat response curve dropped at about 4 dB per octave while the rising 6 dB per octave curve actually rose about 9 dB per octave below 800 Hz and was relatively flat above 800 Hz.

The principles put forth in the Harvard Report, therefore, suggested that the frequency response of a hearing aid cannot be prescribed for a particular individual. Based on the Harvard Report, Carhart (1946) concluded that the most appropriate procedure for selecting a hearing aid would be to allow the client to compare several hearing aids and to select the one that yielded the best results. This was the origin of the so-called comparative technique of hearing aid selection.

The original comparative procedure described by Carhart in 1946 was a very lengthy one involving training, counseling, and a hearing aid trial period, as well as the collecting of clinical data in the audiometric test suite. The audiometric tests suggested by Carhart included unaided measurements followed by aided measurements with three different instruments. The unaided measurements included a speech reception threshold, a measure of tolerance, and a word recognition score. The aided measurements included speech reception thresholds at full-on gain and at a most comfortable listening level (MCL); measurements of threshold of discomfort also at full-on gain and at MCL; a measurement of word recognition; and a measurement of efficiency in noise with the gain at MCL and using two types of noise. The efficiency measure was determined by presenting word recognition lists at 50 dB HL and increasing the noise levels until the words could not be repeated. The hearing aid that provided the best aided results and that most satisfied the client was the instrument of choice.

The comparative approaches that have been used for years in audiology clinics have been variations of the Carhart method. However, the original Carhart method has proven to be too time consuming. Nevertheless, many of the aided versus unaided measurements suggested by Carhart are still obtained when making comparative evaluations or as a validation criterion for the prescriptive approach.

The measurements at full-on gain suggested by Carhart are no longer obtained because they provide little information regarding the client's aided performance in real-life situations. That is, an individual should not be wearing a hearing aid at full-on gain. If it is necessary for an individual to wear an amplification device at such a high gain setting, then it is obvious that the individual requires a more powerful instrument.

The measurement of efficiency in noise has been replaced with word recognition scores obtained in a background of noise, usually at one predetermined signal-to-noise ratio. Although the reliability and validity of these procedures have been criticized in the literature (Shore, et al., 1960), open-ended monosyllabic word lists are still commonly used to obtain word recognition scores. Another modification of the Carhart technique involves the presentation level of the speech stimuli. The original method called for a presentation level of 25 dB SL re: SRT; however, today many clinicians prefer to use a fixed presentation level of 45–50 dB HL. This presentation approximates the average conversational level for speech and thus allows for generalizing to real-world situations.

Final decisions regarding hearing aid recommendation are similar to the original Carhart approach. The instrument that provides the most appropriate gain, the best word recognition score, and the most acceptable sound quality to the client is the instrument that should be selected. A problem inherent in the comparative approach, however, is that a single instrument may not meet the above criteria. That is, hearing aid "A" may provide the most appropriate gain based upon aided versus unaided SRT's, while hearing aid "B" may provide the highest word recognition score in noise, and hearing aid "C" may sound the best to the client. Without knowing how much emphasis to place on word recognition scores versus subjective preference, it is difficult to decide which hearing aid is best. Another major stumbling block to the comparative approach is the method of preselection of instruments. Traditionally, hearing aids selected for comparison have had very similar electroacoustic characteristics. This explains, at least partially, why a comparative approach often yields results with little or no discernible differences in aided performance across instruments. That is, hearing aids have often been recommended based upon very minor differences in performance or subjective preference (Harris, 1976).

PRESCRIPTIVE TECHNIQUES

There has been a recent resurgence in prescriptive hearing aid selection techniques which are based upon the notion that frequency response and gain characteristics of hearing aids should attempt to compensate for the characteristics of a given hearing loss. One factor in this renewed interest is the large number of ITE and ITC hearing aids being dispensed. These instruments most often require custom casings to be

manufactured from the earmold impressions and, because of the time and expense involved, a single instrument is generally obtained. This obviously precludes the possibility of performing a comparative hearing aid evaluation.

Lybarger

As previously mentioned, Lybarger's (1944) one-half gain rule is based on the client's audiometric thresholds. The Lybarger system allows one to select a maximum output level (referred to as maximum gain) as well as a use gain or preferred gain setting (referred to as operating gain). The maximum gain consists of operating gain plus a certain amount of reserve gain. The operating gain is based on bringing the average conversational speech level (65 dB SPL) within the most comfortable loudness (MCL) range of the listener. Lybarger's formula for operating gain in a monaural arrangement is:

$$\frac{AC\ loss}{2} + \frac{AC\ loss - BC\ loss}{4} + 5\ dB$$

AC stands for air conduction and BC stands for bone conduction. Air conduction and bone conduction loss data are puretone averages obtained for the frequencies 500 Hz, 1000 Hz, and 2000 Hz. Reserve gain consists of an additional 15 dB. The constant +5 dB is changed to −10 dB for a binaural arrangement.

Berger

Berger (1976) presented a prescriptive approach that has gained wide acceptance. The procedure is a modification of the earlier work of Lybarger. The one-half gain rule is applied to specific frequencies, as opposed to a puretone average, and operating gain is slightly greater than one-half of the hearing loss. The operating gain across the audiometric frequencies is

$$\frac{HL\ at\ 500\ Hz}{2}\ ;\ \frac{HL\ at\ 1000\ Hz}{1.6}\ ;\ \frac{HL\ at\ 2000\ Hz}{1.5};$$

$$\frac{HL\ at\ 3000\ Hz}{1.7}\ ;\ \frac{HL\ at\ 4000\ Hz}{1.9}\ ;\ \frac{HL\ at\ 6000\ Hz}{2}$$

HL stands for air conduction threshold in dB HL at a given frequency. The operating gain formula targets desired aided thresholds. The greatest gains will likely be provided for the mid-frequencies; i.e., 1000–3000 Hz. The maximum gain formula is

Maximum Gain = Operating Gain + 10 dB
Reserve Gain + Correction Factors

The correction factors vary depending upon microphone location for Body, BTE, ITE, or ITC hearing aids (Berger, 1988). Complete usage of the Berger method involves determining the sound field dynamic range for each listener. This is done by obtaining UCL's with pulsing discrete frequency signals and converting these values from dB HL to dB SPL. When the dynamic range is limited, the Berger system includes provisions for output limiting devices such as automatic gain control (AGC).

Prescription of Gain and Output (POGO)

A prescriptive system which strives for simplicity and practicality was described by McCandless and Lyregaard in 1983 and is referred to by the acronym POGO (prescription of gain and output). The POGO system is a straightforward approach to defining insertion gain and maximum power output (MPO) requirements for individuals with sensory-neural hearing losses of less than 80 dB HL. The three steps to the procedure include calculating required gain and MPO based on audiometric results; implementation of the required gain and MPO; and verification of the acoustical performance.

McCandless (1978) feels that the original one-half gain rule proposed by Lybarger provides too much low frequency amplification. This may result in poor speech intelligibility in noise due to an upward spread of masking. The POGO procedure, therefore, reduces gain at low frequencies. The insertion gain POGO formula is

.5 (HL at 250 Hz) − 10 dB; .5 (HL at 500 Hz) − 5 dB; .5 (HL at 1000 Hz); .5 (HL at 2000 Hz); .5 (HL at 3000 Hz); .5 (HL at 4000 Hz)

HL stands for air conduction threshold in dB HL at a given frequency. The formula for MPO is equal to the average UCL (in dB HL) at 500 Hz, 1000 Hz, and 2000 Hz.

$$MPO = \frac{UCL\ 500\ Hz + UCL\ 1000\ Hz + UCL\ 2000\ Hz}{3}$$

This formula provides MPO in dB HL. A 4 dB correction factor is added to this value to arrive at MPO in dB SPL as measured in a 2-cc coupler. These formulae assume a closed earmold is being used. Correction factors are used for the various types of earmold modifications (i.e., vents, horns). McCandless (1988) recommends that the aided performance of the hearing impaired individual be verified either through real-ear probe-tube microphone measurements or through frequency specific measures of functional gain (i.e., aided versus unaided thresholds).

Revised NAL

Byrne and Dillon (1986) have described a system that has come to be known as the revised NAL (National Acoustics Laboratory, Australia) procedure for selecting gain and frequency response of a hearing aid. The revised formula for calculating real-ear gain (insertion gain or functional gain) is

1. Calculate
   X = 0.05 (H500 + H1000 + H2000)
2. G 250 = X + 0.31 H 250 − 17
   G 500 = X + 0.31 H 500 − 8
   G 750 = X + 0.31 H 750 − 3
   G 1000 = X + 0.31 H 1000 + 1
   G 1500 = X + 0.31 H 1500 + 1
   G 2000 = X + 0.31 H 2000 − 1
   G 3000 = X + 0.31 H 3000 − 2
   G 4000 = X + 0.31 H 4000 − 2
   G 6000 = X + 0.31 H 6000 − 2

In this formula, G is the required insertion gain at a given frequency and H is the hearing threshold level at a given frequency. The correction factors at the end of each equation are based upon estimates of the long-term average speech spectrum. Thus, low frequencies are deemphasized and more gain is provided for the mid and high frequencies. A formula is also provided for deriving 2-cc coupler gain. As pointed out by Berger (1988), an important contribution made by the researchers at NAL is the inclusion of speech spectrum data in the gain-frequency response curve as opposed to a single estimate of average speech level such as 65 dB SPL.

Steps in using the NAL formula are similar to those described for POGO. The formula is used to calculate real-ear gain. An instrument is selected with the required frequency response and gain characteristics (as close a match as possible) and comparisons are made between the predicted real-ear gain and the real-ear measurements obtained from the hearing impaired client. Although they state that functional gain measures can be used with their system, Byrne and Dillon (1986) strongly recommend real-ear insertion gain measurements via probe-tube microphone systems to verify the aided performance.

Numerous other prescriptive hearing aid fitting techniques have been proposed (Pascoe, 1975; Cox and Bisset, 1982; Skinner, et al., 1982). A number of experimental investigations have compared the aided performance of various prescriptive techniques (Collins and Levitt, 1980; Humes, 1986). The results show that no single prescriptive procedure provides clearly superior speech intelligibility and speech quality (Sullivan, Levitt, Huang, and Hennessey, 1988). Indeed, selection of a particular prescriptive technique is often a function of what the audiologist is comfortable and familiar with.

Children

The majority of the prescriptive techniques that have been described are based upon easily obtainable measures of threshold and UCL. The use of a prescriptive technique presents a unique problem when dealing with preverbally hearing-impaired children. Seewald and Ross (1988) have developed a computer-assisted, prescriptive hearing aid fitting procedure for young hearing impaired children which they refer to as the Desired Sensation Level (DSL) method. Like the Byrne and Dillon (1986) procedure, Seewald and Ross have taken a speech spectrum-based approach to selecting amplification characteristics. A primary goal of the DSL method is to select frequency/gain characteristics that make the long-term average speech spectrum accessible across the widest possible frequency range.

The selection procedure follows the same sequential steps described earlier for POGO and the revised NAL procedures. A formula is used to specify desired electroacoustic characteristics; an instrument is selected which matches these desired responses as closely as possible; and the aided performance is verified using real-ear measurements. The specification of electroacoustic characteristics is broken down into desired sensation levels (SL's) for amplified speech and desired saturation sound pressure levels (SSPL's) of amplified speech. The desired sensation levels for amplified speech are based upon speech spectrum values proposed by Pascoe (1978), with a slight reduction in the lower frequencies to reduce possible negative effects due to an upward spread of masking. These sensation levels represent an attempt to present speech at levels sufficiently above threshold to be useful while keeping in mind the limitations imposed by the reduced residual hearing associated with sensory-neural hearing loss (Seewald, Ross, and Spiro, 1985).

As previously mentioned, a problem in hearing aid selection for preverbally hearing-impaired children is that it is difficult, if not impossible, to accurately determine UCL with these children. Seewald, et al. (1985), use predicted levels of amplified speech to select desired real-ear SSPL values. These SSPL values represent the upper limits of amplification for a particular child.

This prescriptive procedure is completely computer assisted. Once threshold data have been obtained for as many octave and interoctave frequencies as possible between 250 Hz and 6000 Hz, the data are entered

into a computer. A minimum of two thresholds is necessary to run the program. The computer, which already has stored in its memory the long-term average RMS speech spectrum, converts the threshold data from dB HL to dB SPL. The program then provides both the amount of gain required to place the speech spectrum at the desired SL's for amplified speech and the desired real-ear SSPL values.

A hearing aid and earmold combination is then selected which approximates the desired SL's and SSPL values provided by the computer program. Although functional gain measures may be used to verify appropriateness of the DSL fitting strategy, Stelmachowicz and Seewald (1991) prefer the use of probe-tube microphone measures. Since the comparison of interest with the DSL is the long-term average speech spectrum (LTSS) in the sound field versus the amplified LTSS in the ear canal, the appropriate measurement is in situ gain as opposed to insertion gain. In this case, in situ gain is defined as the sound pressure level (SPL) generated in the external auditory meatus relative to that present in the unobstructed sound field (Stelmachowicz and Seewald, 1991). Finally, some modifications of the original frequency/gain characteristics may be necessary following the comparison of the obtained in situ or functional gain measures with the predicted values.

The procedure outlined by Seewald and Ross (1988) provides a scientifically based, structured approach to selecting a first amplification device for children. Strengths of this procedure include the fact that it is speech spectrum based, it attempts to compensate for the lack of UCL information available from this population, and it is easy to implement via a personal computer.

Seewald, et al. (1985), stress that the use of a computer is not meant to replace the audiologist but merely to facilitate the process of hearing aid selection for children. Calculations that take 45 minutes to perform by hand can be carried out in less than 3 minutes with a computer.

Personal Computer Applications

The various prescriptive hearing aid selection procedures developed for adults and children are well-suited for personal computer applications. The prescriptive techniques tend to be formulae based upon thresholds and estimates of MCL and UCL, all of which are measured in dB HL, while the average speech spectrum information is measured in dB SPL. In addition, the frequency response and gain characteristics provided by the manufacturer are measured in dB SPL using either a 2-cc coupler or a Zwislocki coupler and KEMAR. Computer software programs are available that carry out conversions from dB HL to dB SPL, as well as incorporating correction factors for 2-cc coupler gain to insertion gain or functional gain (Popelka, 1983). Software programs are also available for most of the major prescriptive procedures. They provide a major savings in time and improved accuracy. A list of available software can be obtained from Computer Users in Speech and Hearing at Ohio University.

Some computer programs that are available can serve as a data base system in addition to being able to compute a particular prescription. In this case, the computer can then also be used to search for a particular model hearing aid that approximates the prescription. As Berger (1988) points out, this computerized selection procedure adds objectivity and efficiency to the hearing aid fitting process.

Target Gain

The purpose of all of the hearing aid prescriptive formulae is to provide the clinician with frequency specific target gain values. Two questions need to be answered regarding the target gain values. The first question is "What do these target gain values represent?" The second question is "With what degree of accuracy can we provide these target gain values?"

With regard to the first question, these target gain values, as presented by most of the authors of the prescriptive techniques, represent a starting point for finding the ultimate amplification that needs to be provided. From this point, finer adjustments can and should be made to the frequency response and gain characteristics of the hearing aid dependent upon the needs of a particular client.

With regard to the second question, when dealing with BTE instruments the clinician must be skillful in selecting a hearing aid that can be effectively matched to the target gain values through a combination of tone and output control adjustments as well as through earmold acoustics. When dealing with ITE instruments, the clinician must rely heavily upon the manufacturer to meet these target values. This is particularly true with ITE instruments that only have a volume control with no fitter-controlled adjustments. These instruments cannot be modified readily in the clinical setting.

The degree to which the manufacturer is able to meet the requested target values varies depending upon the individual manufacturer and the specific frequency in question. Most manufacturers will have difficulty providing adequate high frequency amplification as called for by a formula. This is particularly true

in the region of 4000 Hz and above. Mueller (1990) suggests that a very large deviation from target must be tolerated at 4000 Hz if one is to avoid returning an inordinate number of hearing aids to the manufacturer. Mueller (1990) suggests that the measured gain at 4000 Hz is typically off by 17 dB or more relative to the target value in an otherwise acceptable hearing aid. Although these large deviations from target represent present-day realities, we should not accept them as inevitable. Continual pressure placed upon manufacturers to more accurately provide the amounts of gain requested should eventually result in better agreement between target and obtained gain.

The prescriptive formulae, therefore, do not reduce the number of clinical decisions that need to be made regarding frequency response and gain characteristics. The formulae provide a structured approach to arriving at or approximating initial parameter settings.

Techniques for Fitting Digital Hearing Aids

The majority of hearing aids sold in the United States use analog signal processing. Recently, instruments have been introduced to the market that utilize either digital signal processing or, more commonly, digital control of analog processing. Compared with analog systems, digital technology allows for finer control over a broader spectrum of parameters. The flexibility provided by these digital systems offers the potential of better fitting to the individual hearing loss, but the complexity of the adjustment procedure can make these hearing aids difficult to fit (Kates, 1989).

A digitally controlled hearing aid employs an external programming unit in order to set parameters such as frequency response and gain characteristics. Once parameters are set, they are stored in digital memory. The instruments are routinely programmed at the factory, set according to the manufacturer's fitting criteria, and then shipped to the dispenser. The dispenser needs a programming unit of his own in order to adjust the instrument during fitting and to allow for comparison over various settings. Purchasing a programming unit represents a commitment on the part of the dispenser to a particular manufacturer in terms of money and product. An individualized programming package is necessary for each manufacturer's digital instrument.

A standardized programming system for digitally controlled amplification devices has recently been developed which significantly reduces the problem of committing to a single manufacturer. The Programmable Multi-Channel (PMC) system allows for the adjustment of digitally programmable hearing instruments from different manufacturers with a single programming unit (Branderbit, 1991). The programming unit utilizes interchangeable software modules developed by each manufacturer to program their hearing instruments. At the present time, nine manufacturers have developed programmable hearing instruments that can be controlled and set via the PMC system.

Several manufacturers have developed digitally controlled amplification devices with remote control units that can program different parameter settings (Pluvinage and Benson, 1988; Sandlin and Anderson, 1989). From the perspective of the hearing aid wearer, the remote control is promising in that gain can be adjusted without bringing a hand to the ear, eliminating the acoustic feedback that often accompanies manual gain adjustment. From the perspective of the hearing aid dispenser, the remote control units may allow for relatively straightforward programming of the units during the fitting process.

Verification of Aided Performance

Speech Audiometry

A number of tests employing speech stimuli have been utilized in hearing aid evaluations. For example, aided and unaided SRT's have often been compared to arrive at a single number of speech gain. Speech signals have also been used at high intensity levels in order to obtain aided and unaided UCL's. Historically, however, there has been a decided emphasis on word recognition scores (Berger, 1988).

Word recognition scores have been widely criticized in the literature for the past 30 years, beginning with the article by Shore, et al. (1960). The feeling of a significant number of researchers is that no particular speech test or speech stimulus has been demonstrated to be a valid or reliable predictor of performance with a hearing aid. Harford (1988) states that word recognition scores, as obtained traditionally in the audiology clinic, do not predict with any degree of accuracy how an individual will function with a hearing aid in everyday situations. The reason for this poor predictability is the large array of uncontrollable variables that impact on one's communicative ability. These variables include the acoustic environment, the alertness of the client, the client's ability to use visual cues, the client's command of the language, and the clarity of the speech produced by the speaker, as well as many other factors.

Despite these criticisms, some researchers continue to support the use of speech signals for limited purposes. Humes (1990), for example, acknowledges the limitations of speech stimuli for selecting from among several instruments, but supports the use of speech materials in assessing aided performance of a particular device.

Advocates of word recognition score testing would suggest that several steps be taken in order to increase the validity and reliability of these scores. These steps would include using full 50-item monosyllabic word lists, obtaining scores in noise as well as in quiet, using tape recorded stimuli, and having subjects provide written responses when possible (Ross, 1978). The speech stimuli are usually presented at levels ranging between 40–50 dB HL to approximate normal conversational level speech (Hodgson, 1981).

Functional Gain

Functional gain has been demonstrated to be an alternative to tests relying upon speech stimuli. Functional gain can be defined simply as the difference between unaided and aided sound field thresholds for warble tones or narrow bands of noise (Hawkins and Haskell, 1982). The use of warble tones or narrow bands of noise allows frequency specific values of functional gain to be obtained, most often for the frequencies 250–6000 Hz. The functional gain measures serve the important function of verifying the electroacoustic parameters derived from the various prescriptive formulae.

Several limitations of the functional gain measurement should be noted. Obviously, just as in speech audiometry, functional gain is a behavioral measurement and is subject to variables related to client participation. Also, functional gain values are obtained only at discrete frequencies with no information about what occurs between these frequencies. Finally, obtaining functional gain data can be a fairly time consuming process. This can become problematic in a busy clinical setting.

Real-Ear Measurements

Techniques are presently available that can eliminate or greatly reduce the problems just described with functional gain measurements. The development of probe-tube microphone systems during the past few years has enabled us to make measurements of aided performance in the ear (real-ear measurements). A marked interest in real-ear measurements exists because of the well-documented inadequacies of presently available coupling systems at representing the frequency response characteristics of a hearing aid in the human ear (Barlow, et al., 1988; Seewald, et al., 1985). The standard 2 cc coupler predicts better high frequency aided response, particularly in the region of 3000 Hz, than that which actually occurs when the hearing aid is worn. The Zwislocki coupler used in conjunction with the anthropometric manikin KEMAR (Knowles Electronic Manikin for Acoustic Research) represents a significant improvement over the 2-cc coupler, but still provides average data and not the real-ear response of a hearing impaired individual (Libby and Westermann, 1988).

In order to discuss real-ear measurements, one must understand the associated terminology. Schweitzer, et al. (1990), have recently proposed a consensus for real-ear measurement terms. Punch, et al. (1990), summarize several of the definitions as follows:

> **Real-ear unaided response (REUR)**—This represents the open ear canal measurement in dB minus the input signal level in dB. This measure includes the effects of ear canal resonance and the diffraction effects of the pinna and concha.
> **Real-ear aided response (REAR)**—This represents the aided ear canal measurement in dB minus the input signal level in dB. This is equivalent to in situ gain or the hearing aid gain near the eardrum.
> **Real-ear insertion response (REIR)**—This represents REAR in dB minus the REUR in dB. This is equivalent to insertion gain and is referred to as real-ear insertion gain (REIG) when measured at a specific frequency. This measure approximates the functional gain provided by an amplification device.

The REUR represents the combined effects of ear canal resonance, external ear resonance, and head diffraction effects of an individual. The REAR represents the total response of the hearing aid system, including the REUR (Pollack, 1988). REIG represents the amount of amplification provided by the hearing aid system alone and, as such, is an electroacoustic estimate of the functional gain (Preves, 1987). It is not surprising, therefore, that REIG and functional gain have been demonstrated to be highly correlated with one another (Dillon and Murray, 1987).

These real-ear measurements, REIG in particular, have proven useful in terms of verifying the electroacoustic parameters derived from the various prescriptive formulas. REIG can replace functional gain in those formulae developed prior to the availability of probe-tube microphone systems.

Several variables need to be controlled when using probe-tube measurements clinically. Loudspeaker azimuth and probe-tube placement are among the most important of these variables. Killion and Revit (1987) demonstrated a significant reduction in standard deviation of repeated measurements for a loudspeaker

placement of 45° azimuth versus the traditional 0° azimuth. With regard to probe-tube placement, the closer to the tympanic membrane the better. It is generally agreed that the probe tip should be within 5 mm of the tympanic membrane in order to measure high frequencies accurately, and also should be at least 5 mm past the tip of the earmold or the ITE. Hawkins (1990b) suggests a simple technique of inserting the tip of the probe-tube 27 mm from the tragus for adults. This is based upon average data that demonstrate a distance of approximately 35 mm from tragus to tympanic membrane in adults.

Additional uses of the real-ear measurement system have recently been proposed. Punch, et al. (1990), suggested a protocol for using real-ear measurements combined with a prescriptive formula to arrive at the desired 2-cc coupler gain for a particular individual. This is a major procedural variation from the common practice of correcting the 2-cc coupler response to arrive at a desired real-ear response. By including the REUR for a particular individual and correcting for differences in frequency responses in the coupler versus in the client's ear, individualized target coupler gain can be specified as measured in a 2-cc coupler. Because this technique provides the dispenser and the manufacturer with a common reference for specifying the responses of a hearing aid, the result should be more personalized target gain values that are more accurately obtained.

Self-Report Procedures

Another approach to verifying aided performance is through the use of self-assessment scales. As stated earlier in this chapter, many self-report procedures have been developed as reliable measures of hearing handicap. Hearing handicap refers to the impact of the hearing loss upon an individual's communicative abilities and quality of life. A number of studies have been conducted in which hearing aid benefit has been operationally defined as a reduction in hearing handicap as measured using self-report surveys pre- and post-amplification.

Tannahill (1979) demonstrated significant reduction in hearing handicap for social and situational items of the Hearing Handicap Scale (HHS) for a group of adults following a 4-week period of hearing aid use. Dempsey (1986) administered the Hearing Performance Inventory (HPI) to a group of 10 new hearing aid users prior to and 6 weeks after they obtained their instruments. Dempsey found a significant reduction in hearing handicap for those areas directly related to communication (e.g., understanding speech and intensity), but no change in the emotional domain. Dempsey suggested that further intervention, in the form of aural rehabilitation therapy, is necessary beyond providing amplification in order to demonstrate change in the emotional area.

The self-report procedure that appears to hold the greatest promise as a measure of hearing aid benefit is the Hearing Handicap Inventory for the Elderly (HHIE). Unlike the other available scales, the HHIE has been used and validated with the elderly, the population typically seen in speech and hearing clinics. The HHIE is relatively short and, therefore, is likely to maintain the attention of elderly clients while still assessing the areas of emotional, social, and situational effects of hearing loss.

Newman and Weinstein (1988) administered the HHIE prior to and following 1 year of hearing aid usage. Although they demonstrated significant reduction in hearing handicap, the authors felt that the 1-year interval may have been too long a time period for assessing benefit. A number of uncontrolled variables could have effected scores over such a long time period.

Malinoff and Weinstein (1989) administered the HHIE to a group of 45 elderly adults prior to and following 3 weeks of hearing aid use. Even over this brief time period, significant reduction in hearing handicap was demonstrated by the majority of the subjects.

The ideal time interval between administration of self-report procedures in order to measure hearing aid benefit has yet to be determined. A significant advantage of a very brief interval such as the 3-week period employed by Malinoff and Weinstein (1989) is that the information can be gathered while the hearing aid is still under a 30-day trial period. If no benefit is demonstrated, the instrument can be returned. A problem with such a brief interval, however, is that a client may not have yet adjusted to the amplification device but, in time, might show significant benefits. For this reason, as well as to determine if the improvement in hearing handicap demonstrated at 3 weeks is maintained over time, Malinoff and Weinstein are continuing to look at their subjects over a period of 3 months. As Malinoff and Weinstein suggest, the optimal time interval between administrations of self-report procedures in order to measure hearing aid benefit should remain a research priority.

SUMMARY

As alluded to throughout this chapter, the process of hearing aid fitting and evaluation is currently undergoing a metamorphosis. As ITE and ITC hearing aids rapidly replace the BTE as the most common forms of amplification being dispensed, the need to convert

from traditional comparative hearing aid evaluation procedures to prescriptive techniques increases as well. One must keep in mind, however, that the prescriptive technique provides a target gain value which is merely a structured approach for approximating initial parameter settings. The audiologist must continue to view the hearing aid evaluation as an ongoing process for determining the ideal frequency response and gain characteristics for each of their clients.

Methods of verifying aided performance have also been undergoing significant change in recent years. The advent of probe-tube microphone measurement systems has provided invaluable information regarding electroacoustic characteristics as they occur in the "real-ear." Self-report procedures have been used in an attempt to look at perceived benefit as a result of amplification on the part of the hearing aid wearer. New methods of verifying aided performance with increased face validity should remain a high priority of researchers in this area.

One technique the author is currently evaluating is the method of continuous discourse tracking. The continuous discourse tracking procedure, first described by DeFilippo and Scott (1978), involves a sender reading consecutive segments from a story and a receiver attempting to repeat each segment verbatim. When failures occur, the sender is free to employ a host of repair strategies in order to facilitate verbatim repetition. Tracking rate is most often measured in terms of words correctly repeated per minute. The reliability and validity of the tracking procedure have been criticized on the basis of uncontrolled variables such as sender, receiver, and text characteristics. In order to control some of these variables, Dempsey, et al. (1991), have developed a computer-interactive tracking procedure in which story segments are presented to the receiver via a video laser disc system and repair strategies are implemented through a computer program. In the near future this system will be used pre- and post-hearing aid fitting to look at improvements in tracking rate as a verification of hearing aid benefit.

Finally, it is the author's belief that the field of audiology is made up of equal parts science and art. The science portion of hearing aid fitting is being addressed as more and more programmable hearing aids become commercially available. These units, which employ digital technology, will likely prove efficient and accurate in terms of arriving at target gain via the various prescriptive formulae. However, the burden remains on the shoulders of the "artful" clinical audiologist to help determine the appropriateness of various parameter settings for each particular hearing aid wearer.

REFERENCES

Barlow N, Auslander M, Rines D, Stelmachowicz P. Probe-tube microphone measurements in hearing impaired children and adults. Ear and Hearing 1988;9:243–247.

Beauchaine K, Barlow N, Stelmachowicz P. Special considerations in amplification for young children. ASHA 1990;32:44–51.

Berger K. Prescription of hearing aids: a rationale. J Am Audio Soc 1976;2:71–78.

Berger K. Prescriptive hearing aid selection strategies. In Pollack M, Ed. Amplification for the hearing-impaired. 3rd ed. Orlando: Grune & Stratton, 1988:273–294.

Byrne D. Binaural hearing aid fitting: research findings and clinical application. In Libby E, Ed. Binaural hearing and amplification, Vol. II. Chicago: Zenetron, 1980:23–73.

Byrne D, Dillon H. The National Acoustics Labs (NAL) new procedure for selecting gain and frequency response of a hearing aid. Ear and Hearing 1986;7:257–265.

Carhart R. Tests for the selection of hearing aids. Laryngoscope 1946;56:78–794.

Collins M, Levitt H. Methods for predicting optimal functional gain. In Studebaker G, Hochberg I, Eds. Acoustical factors affecting hearing aid performance. Baltimore: University Park Press, 1980:341–354.

Cox R, Bisset J. Prediction of aided preferred listening levels for hearing aid gain prescription. Ear and Hearing 1982;3:66–71.

Cranmer K. Hearing instrument dispensing–1990. Hearing Instruments, 1990;41(6):4–12.

Davis H, Hudgins V, Marquis R, et al. The selection of hearing aids. Laryngoscope 1946;56:85–115, 135–163.

DeFilippo C, Scott B. A method for training and evaluating the reception of ongoing speech. J Acous Soc Am 1978;63:1186–1192.

Dempsey J. The Hearing Performance Inventory as a tool in fitting hearing aids. J Acad Rehab Audio 1986;19:116–125.

Dempsey J, Levitt H, Josephson J, Porrazzo J. A computer-interactive continuous discourse tracking procedure. J Acous Soc Am (Submitted May 1991).

Dillon H, Murray N. Accuracy of twelve methods of estimating the real ear gain of hearing aids. Ear and Hearing 1987;8:2–11.

Downs M. Contribution of mild hearing loss to auditory language and learning problems. In Roeser R, Downs M, Eds. Auditory disorders in school children. New York: Thieme-Stratton, 1981:177–189.

Harford E. Hearing aid selection for adults. In Pollack M, Ed. Amplification for the hearing-impaired. 3rd ed. Orlando: Grune & Stratton, 1988:175–212.

Harris JD. Hearing aids: current developments and concepts. In Rubin M, Ed. Hearing aids: current developments and concepts. Baltimore: University Park Press, 1976:3–6.

Hawkins D, Haskell G. A comparison of functional gain and 2 cubic centimeter coupler gain. J Speech and Hearing Disorders 1982;47:71–76.

Hawkins D. Technology and hearing aids: how does the audiologist fit in? ASHA 1990a;32:42–43.

Hawkins D. Acoustic measures of hearing aid performance. Paper presented at the Second Vanderbilt/VA Conference on Amplification for the Hearing-Impaired. 1990b.

Hodgson W. Clinical measures of hearing aid performance. In Hodgson W, Skinner P, Eds. Hearing aid assessment and use in audiologic habilitation. 2nd ed. Baltimore: Williams & Wilkins, 1981.

Humes L. An evaluation of several rationales for selecting hearing aid gain. J Speech and Hearing Disorders 1986;51:272–281.

Humes L. Prescribing gain characteristics for linear hearing aids.

Paper presented at the Second Vanderbilt/VA Conference on Amplification for the Hearing-Impaired. 1990.

Kates J. The state-of-the-art in hearing aid signal processing [Unpublished Manuscript]. New York: CUNY Graduate Center, 1989.

Killion M, Revit L. Insertion gain repeatability versus loudspeaker location: you want me to put my loudspeaker WHERE? Ear and Hearing 1987;8(suppl 5):68–73.

Libby E, Westermann S. Principles of acoustic measurement and ear canal resonance. In Sandlin R, Ed. Handbook of hearing aid amplification, Vol. I. Boston: College-Hill Press, 1988.

Lybarger S. Method of fitting hearing aids. U.S. Patent Applications S.N. 543,278. July 3, 1944.

Lybarger S. Selective amplification—a review and evaluation. J Am Audio Soc 1978;3:258–266.

Madell J. Using FM systems as the primary amplification for children with severe and profound hearing loss. Texas J Audio and Speech Path 1988;XIV(2):33.

Malinoff R, Weinstein B. Measurement of hearing aid benefit in the elderly. Ear and Hearing 1989;10:354–356.

Martin F. Introduction to audiology. 3rd ed. Englewood Cliffs: Prentice-Hall, Inc., 1986.

Maxon A. Pediatric amplification. In Martin F, Ed. Hearing disorders in children. Austin: Pro-Ed, Inc., 1987.

McCandless G. Nonlinquistic techniques of hearing aid fitting. Hearing Aid J 1978;4–48.

McCandless G, Lyregaard P. Prescription of gain/output (POGO) for hearing aids. Hearing Instruments 1983;12–16.

McCandless G. Hearing aid formulae and their application. In Sandlin R, Ed. Handbook of hearing aid amplification: Volume I. Boston: College-Hill Press, 1988.

Nábělek A, Pickett, J. Reception of consonants in a classroom as affected by monaural and binaural listening, noise, and reverberation and hearing aids. J Acous Soc Am 1974;56:628–639.

Newman C, Weinstein B. The Hearing Handicap Inventory for the Elderly as a measure of hearing aid benefit. Ear and Hearing 1988;9:81–85.

Pascoe D. Frequency responses of hearing aids and their effects on the speech perception of hearing-impaired subjects. Annals of Otology, Rhinology and Laryngology 1975;suppl 23:84.

Pascoe D. An approach to hearing aid selection. Hearing Instruments 1978;29(6):12–36.

Pascoe D. Hearing aid evaluation. In Katz J, Ed. Handbook of clinical audiology. 3rd ed. Baltimore: Williams & Wilkins, 1985:936–948.

Pluvinage V, Benson D. New dimensions in diagnostics and fitting. Hearing Instruments 1988;39(8):28–39.

Pollack M. Electroacoustic characteristics. In Pollack M, Ed. Amplification for the hearing-impaired. 3rd ed. Orlando: Grune & Stratton, 1988:21–103.

Preves D. Some issues in utilizing probe tube microphone systems. Ear and Hearing 1987;8(suppl):82–88.

Punch J, Chi C, Patterson J. A recommended protocol for prescription use of target gain rules. Hearing Instruments 1990;41:12–19.

Ross M. Hearing aid evaluation. In Katz J, Ed. Handbook of clinical audiology. 2nd ed. Baltimore: Williams & Wilkins, 1978:524–548.

Ross M. Binaural versus monaural hearing aid amplification for hearing impaired individuals. In Libby E, Ed. Binaural hearing and amplification. Chicago: Zenetron, 1980:1–23.

Ross M, Seewald R. Hearing aid selection and evaluation with young children. In Bess FH, Ed. Hearing impairment in children. Parkton, MD: York Press, Inc., 1988.

Sandlin R, Anderson H. Development of a remote-controlled, programmable hearing system. Hearing Journal 1989;42:33–36.

Schweitzer H, Sullivan R, Beck L, Cole W. Developing a consensus for "real ear" hearing instrument terms. Hearing Instruments 1990;41:28–46.

Seewald R, Ross M, Spiro M. Selecting amplification characteristics for young hearing-impaired children. Ear and Hearing 1985; 6:48–53.

Seewald R, Ross M. Amplification for young hearing-impaired children. In Pollack M, Ed. Amplification for the hearing impaired, 3rd ed. Orlando: Grune & Stratton, 1988:213–267.

Shore I, Bilger R, Hirsh I. Hearing aid evaluation: reliability of repeated measurements. J Speech and Hearing Res 1960;25: 152–170.

Skinner M, Pascoe D, Miller J, Popelka G. Measurements to determine the optimal placement of speech energy within the listener's auditory area: a basis for selecting amplification characteristics. In Studebaker G, Bess F, Eds. The Vanderbilt hearing aid report: monographs in contemporary audiology. Upper Darby, PA: Monographs in Contemporary Audiology, 1982.

Studebaker G. Fifty years of hearing aid research: an evaluation of progress. Ear and Hearing 1980;1(2):57–62.

Sullivan J, Levitt H, Huang J, Hennessey A. An experimental comparison of four hearing aid prescription methods. Ear and Hearing 1988;9:22–32.

Tannahill J. The Hearing Handicap Scale as a measure of hearing aid benefit. J Speech and Hearing Disorders 1979;44:91–99.

Wallenfels H. Hearing aids on prescription. Springfield: Charles C. Thomas, Publisher, 1967.

Watson N, Knudsen V. Selective amplification in hearing aids. J Acous Soc Am 1940;11:406–419.

Wernick J. Use of hearing aids. In Katz J, Ed. Handbook of clinical audiology, 3rd ed. Baltimore: Williams & Wilkins, 1985: 911–935.

CHAPTER 45

Hearing Aid Dispensing

Jane R. Madell

During the past 10 to 15 years, the dispensing of hearing aids has come to be recognized as a vital part of the practice of audiology. It could be argued that it now holds as important a position in this field as the diagnostic battery, which formerly had no peer. Audiologists have come to realize that dispensing hearing aids and assisting consumers to adjust to amplifications are important and rewarding parts of clinical practice.

Many of the difficulties, both for the consumer and the profession of audiology, were a result of the dispensing system in which the diagnostician and the dispenser were not the same person. The training of the audiologist and the hearing aid dealer differed greatly, and the opportunities for ongoing contact favored the individual who was minimally trained. When a hearing aid user suspected a decrease in his or her hearing, the person did not know which hearing professional to see, because in the user's eyes the distinction between the dealer and the diagnostician was generally unclear. A logical assumption on the part of the consumer might have been that something was wrong with the hearing aid, and therefore paid a visit to the dealer and not to the audiologist. In reality, a whole host of problems could have caused the client's perception of decreased communicative function. He or she may have had a change in hearing levels. Perhaps the aid was being used incorrectly, and the individual required hearing aid orientation or speechreading training. The client not knowing the options and the respective roles of the hearing-related personnel, frequently assumed that the problem was hearing aid related and would often contact the wrong person (generally the dealer). This placed the dealer in the role of case manager, a role that may be inappropriate if the dealer is not an audiologist.

The audiologist who wishes to began a hearing aid dispensing program needs to plan carefully. A detailed plan will be helpful both as a guide as well as an instrument to educate the Board of Directors of the agency, hospital or other facility and the bankers who may need to be approached if it is determined that it is necessary to borrow money (Loavenbruck and Madell, 1981).

ASSESSING THE NEED FOR HEARING AID DISPENSING

The first step in the plan is to assess the need for adding hearing aid dispensing to the audiology services currently available. Some of the questions that might be asked include: Do patients return for follow-up visits and for annual re-evaluation? Do patients get involved in aural rehabilitation? How does the existing hearing aid delivery system affect the aural rehabilitation program? Are patients satisfied with the current system? What is the relationship between the diagnostic and dispensing audiologists and hearing aid dealers? What will the public reaction be to the program? What are the likely advantages and disadvantages of initiating a hearing aid dispensing component? If students are involved in the program, how will patients be handled during student vacation? Are there state or local laws that restrict one's ability to sell a product? If it is determined that there is a need for dispensing and that it would be advantageous to the program and its patients, the following items should be considered.

Choosing the Model

A model for a hearing aid dispensing program should allow for the provision of comprehensive services including audiologic evaluation; counseling about test results; counseling about amplification and its appropriateness for the particular patient; choosing the appropriate earmold and hearing aid; making, fitting and adjusting earmolds; physical and biological checking of the aid; teaching the patient to use the aid and the mold; selling the aid; follow-up evaluations and counseling; making the necessary repairs and adjustments, as well as, demonstration and sale of assistive listening systems and aural rehabilitation.

In some settings, all of the above services will be done by the same audiologist who evaluates the patients. This model works best in private practice settings; however, this may not be the most efficient way to organize the program. In a large clinical program, it may be more economical to have one person within the program making and modifying earmolds, adjusting the aids and molds, doing minor repairs, and instructing patients in the mechanical use of the hearing aids. This person may be an audiologist or a technician. If it is a technician, then the audiologist will monitor these services, do follow-up checks, and work with patients when any problem develops. In some facilities, audiologists work both in the clinical section and in the hearing aid dispensary. Services are divided into the clinical problems, handling in the clinical section and the technical problems handled in the dispensary. Technical problems include arranging for repairs, dealing with problems of comfort with the mold and the aid, and counseling for difficulties manipulating the hearing aid. Any other difficulties are handled by the clinical section. The division of services may facilitate handling large numbers of patients quickly.

There may be some facilities where, for legal or administrative reasons, it is not possible to sell hearing aids within the program. When the audiologists at such a facility wish to dispense aids, there are two ways in which it can be handled. There are several mail order companies from which a patient can purchase a hearing aid with a trial period and warranties. The patient pays the mail order company for the aid and the audiologist for the other audiologic services. It may also be possible to find a local pharmacy or optician to sell the product and arrange for the audiologist to do the fitting and follow-up. In both cases the audiologist retains full responsibility for all professional services provided, including evaluation, fitting, and counseling.

Other models may be developed to suit the needs of an individual program. Any model chosen must provide technical assistance and cost containment to the patient.

Financial Consideration

Determining Costs. Part of the planning process involves determining the costs that will be involved in the start-up of the program. The following should be considered:

1. Purchase or rental of equipment;
2. Purchase of hearing aids (evaluation/sale);
3. Staff training costs;
4. Housing costs (especially if additional space will be needed);
5. Personnel costs;
6. Printing of forms and announcements;
7. Legal costs;
8. Accounting costs;
9. Additional insurance if necessary;
10. Funds to cover the operation of the program, including postage, phone, and other miscellaneous expenses; and

11. Start-up funds to cover expenses during the initial period before the program realizes income from the collection of fees.

Determining Fees. Part of the initial planning process includes making decisions about fee structure. It is helpful to make a list of every possible service and then determine how much will be charged for each. Some programs charge a single fee covering all services with one price for a monaural hearing aid fitting and an additional fee for a binaural fitting. Other programs charge individually for diagnostic services (audiologic evaluation, hearing aid evaluation, special diagnostic testing) and charge one fee covering the hearing aid, earmold, and fitting and counseling visits. In some settings, a certain number of postfitting visits are covered under the initial fee, with further charges for any additional visits. This procedure has the advantage of discouraging patients from coming in for services that they do not really need, but it has the disadvantage of forcing patients to consider cost whenever they are in need of assistance. Some programs charge separately for all diagnostic audiologic services and in the hearing aid dispensing program, the patients receive services at no charge during the warranty period. After the warranty expires, almost all programs charge for product-related services. There are charges for the hearing aid, earmolds, and repairs, as well as for the sale of devices to assist in daily living. Patients are not usually charged when they come in for counseling or hand holding. This system usually works well. It provides a supportive atmosphere for patients and allows the audiologist to make a realistic assessment of their rehabilitative needs. In this program, the cost of counseling is added to the cost of the hearing aid; However, if such a system is not carefully cost accounted, it can bankrupt the program. Most new hearing aid users require two to three visits in the hearing aid dispensary. One visit for fitting the aid requires about 1 hour, and two follow-up visits require about ½ hour each. Of course, there are a few patients who require significantly more visits, but they are rare.

In determining expenses, it is important to determine how much time each service requires. This expense is added to the cost of materials and to the operating expenses in determining fees. The accountant who handles other financial activities for the program should be of assistance in this procedure.

Other Planning Considerations

The initial planning should include investigation about licensing and other state laws regarding hearing aid fitting and sales. Thought should be given to methods for billing and collecting, including requirements of third-party payers. It is essential that current and potential referral sources be considered. The addition of the dispensing program to a currently existing audiology program may provide the opportunity for developing additional referral sources. It is also possible that some of the current referral sources may not wish to refer to a facility that is now dispensing hearing aids. The addition of a dispensary program may offer new opportunities for the marketing of the entire audiology program, including the hearing aid dispensing aspect (see Loavenbruck and Madell, 1981).

ORGANIZING THE DISPENSING PROGRAM

Equipment for Hearing Aid Dispensing

Most of the equipment used in hearing aid dispensing is standard audiologic equipment available in any audiology center. Some equipment, however, may not be standard in a particular center but will be essential for dispensing. Electroacoustic hearing aid test equipment must be available. Hearing aids must be checked when they first arrive at the center, before and after they are sent for repair, and when patients come into the center complaining that the hearing aid "sounds funny." Comparing electroacoustic specifications may be the only way that changes in the hearing aid performance can be identified. Fortunately, the cost of this equipment has dropped dramatically in recent years. It should be affordable in almost all settings.

Another essential piece of equipment that may need to be purchased is the hand drill and grinder. It is essential for modifying and adjusting earmolds, adjusting eyeglass hearing aids and making other adjustments. It is not possible to modify earmolds without a hand drill. Two other important pieces of equipment are a bench grinder and a hot air blower. A bench grinder is used for grinding earmolds, especially those made of hard plastic and for modifying in-the-ear (ITE) and in-the-canal (ITC) hearing aids. A hot air blower is used for bending earmold tubing and eyeglass temple tips. A match can substitute for the blower when bending tubing but not for bending temple tips.

An assortment of small tools is essential in hearing aid dispensing. Most are available in any audiology clinic that has been doing hearing aid evaluations. These include screwdrivers of different sizes, a tubing expander, long nose pliers, battery testers, and an otoscope.

Certain supplies will be needed to make minor repairs on hearing aids. These include receivers, cords and harnesses for body aids and FM systems, ear hooks of different sizes, extra battery compartments, battery testers, covers for the controls of ear-level and eyeglass aids, headbands for bone-conduction receivers, receiver washers, hearing aid cord gaskets, adapters for converting between postauricular and body aid molds and supplies for keeping behind-the-ear hearing aids from falling off the ear.

Certain items must be stocked for hearing aid maintenance. These include batteries that must be available in all sizes used in the hearing aids dispensed, air blowers for cleaning the earmolds, minilight battery testers for testing batteries of in-the-ear and behind-the-ear aids and voltage meter battery testers for testing batteries that cannot be tested on the smaller, less expensive testers. Disinfectant spray is useful for cleaning earmolds and ITE/ITC hearing aids. Dehumidifying kits should be available for patients who live in damp climates or who get a lot of moisture in their aids.

For making and modifying earmolds it is necessary to have the following: an otoscope; an earlight for inserting cotton blocks or otoblocks impression material; two impression syringe kits to make two earmolds at a time; otoblocks or cotton and thread for making blocks; and a timer to time the period the impression must stay in the ear.

Spare tubing in assorted sizes, special tubing (such as Libby horn heavy duty, and Killion acoustic tubing), dampers, and tubing cement. A linoleum knife is needed for cutting soft molds. Buffing compound is needed for smoothing down hard plastic earmolds and ITE/ITC hearing aids after grinding. Lambswool should be available for filling in vents in earmolds. To assist patients who are having difficulty inserting earmolds, it is useful to have a soothing lotion placed on the mold to make it more comfortable. A mirror to assist the patient in seeing what is happening and dummy demonstrating ears to assist in practicing getting the mold into the ear are most helpful.

It will be useful in any program seeing patients with severe to profound hearing losses to have a demonstration center in which a supply of devices that might assist them are on hand. The demonstration center is very helpful in clarifying for the patient what is available and in allowing them the opportunity to try out the devices before purchase. These devices include: a vibrating alarm clock; telephone signal lights, sound-activated alerting systems that can be used for the doorbell, phone, baby cry, smoke alarm, etc., with sound lamp or vibrator accessories and devices to amplify television; and teletypewriters (TTD). It may not be necessary for every clinic to sell all of these devices. Nevertheless it is essential that information about the devices be available, that they be available for trial, and that information be available indicating how they can be purchased (see Assistive Listening Devices, below).

Obtaining Hearing Aids for the Dispensing Clinic

Once an audiologic clinic begins to dispense hearing aids, it will be necessary to purchase all of the aids in the clinic. Consignment hearing aids are not usually available to dispensing clinics. When aids are available at no cost, on consignment, most audiologists will not hesitate to try any aids that a manufacturer might suggest. When aids are being purchased, however, the audiologist will necessarily become more selective. Decisions must be made about which manufacturers to obtain aids from, as well as the number and type of aids to carry.

There is an advantage to using only a small number of manufacturers. If you use only a few companies, they will get to know you well and will be more helpful. In addition, you will be eligible for bulk purchasing prices, especially helpful if the program is a small one that will not be ordering a large number of aids.

Not all manufacturers, however, can meet all needs. It will probably be necessary to use several manufacturers to obtain a complete line of aids. Although all manufacturers carry aids for mild and moderate losses, companies vary as to availability and quality of eyeglass aids, bone-conduction aids, power behind-the-ear aids, wired and wireless CROS (contralateral routing of signals) aids, and so forth. The audiologist will have to evaluate the patient population and determine which types of aids are needed and then investigate where they can be obtained. For special cases, aids that are not routinely stocked can be ordered for a trial, thus, enabling the audiologist to provide appropriate amplification for all clients.

Because there is usually a choice of at least two or three manufacturers for any type of hearing aid, it is important to do some investigating of the manufacturers. Determine the delivery time of aids after ordering, time for repairs, bulk purchasing discount policies, payment plans, and exchange or return policies. Some companies allow any aids purchased within one month to be included in the bulk purchase plan; others only accept aids purchased on the same purchase order. Some companies accept aids for exchange or return up to 30 days, and others allow 90 days. Some will accept the aid for exchange but will not give full credit. It might be helpful to contact other dispensing audiologists to determine what experiences they have had with the different manufacturers. Whatever decision is made can be changed in the future as experience provides new insights.

Ordering Hearing Aids. There are several options for ordering hearing aids and maintaining a stock. Aids used for evaluation purposes can be taken from this stock, dispensed when recommended and replaced. This reduces the waiting time for patients to obtain their aids, but it requires a large investment to maintain the stock. A second option is to stock only the aids used for the hearing aid evaluations and to order aids every time an aid is needed for dispensing. Very popular aids can be kept in stock, reducing time delays. A third option may be useful for small clinics that do few hearing aid evaluations. They may wish to consider not keeping any stock of aids but selecting aids for each client after the hearing evaluation and ordering them for the hearing aid evaluation. This will preclude the possibility of doing the hearing evaluation on the same day, but it will also eliminate the need for a stock of hearing aids. Any aid not recommended can be returned to the manufacturer for credit. To determine which ordering option is most appropriate, it is necessary that each clinic determine its individual needs. Is it possible to predict which hearing aids will be needed? Is it possible for patients to wait for their aids? Will patients receive their aids at the hearing aid evaluation, or will they return for a fitting? A combination of ordering options may be preferable for a particular setting.

Administrative Procedures

As in any business venture, it is essential that efficient systems be developed to deal with inventory, ordering, repairs, and accounting. It is essential to be able to keep track of what is needed and how it will be obtained. The particular system used will depend on the volume handled and the staff available. A system needs to be developed for ordering aids, including procedures to check that aids ordered have been received. A system must also be developed to keep track of aids sent out for repair. If the patient is given a loaner aid during the time his or her aid is being repaired, it is necessary to assure that the loaner aid is returned. Without such checks, loss of loaner aids can put a severe burden on any clinical program.

Although paperwork is an increased burden for all of us, it can add immeasurably to the efficiency of the operation. Exactly how much is needed in the way of paperwork will be determined by the size of the program and by the number of staff involved. The following forms are essential for any program, regardless of whether they are kept on paper or on a computer:

1. Inventory form indicating when each aid is ordered, received and sold, and the cost;
2. Medical clearance form;
3. Customer purchase agreement; and

4. Receipt forms for keeping track of hearing aids in repair and for return of loaner aids.

If the program is one in which different staff members may deal with one patient, it is necessary to have additional forms to assure that all staff members have access to information needed and to keep things from being lost. These might include any of the following:

1. Form for ordering earmolds;
2. Form for ordering hearing aids;
3. Form indicating instructions given to the patient;
4. Referral form for other services to the facility; and
5. Form recording fitting and follow-up notes.

Individual program needs will determine which forms are useful. Loavenbruck and Madell (1981, Chapter 3) discuss forms in detail. Additional information can be obtained from companies that develop business forms.

TROUBLESHOOTING PROBLEMS WITH AMPLIFICATION

Earmolds

Basic information about the different types of earmolds, how they are made, and when they are used is available in Chapter 42. it may be appropriate here, however, to offer a word of caution about molds. An earmold, an ITE or ITC hearing aid can only be as good as the impression from which it is fabricated. There are several earmold problems that can be avoided if care is taken during the impression process.

The most common earmold problem is one of insufficient volume in the ear canal. If the canal is not deep enough or full enough, the amount of usable amplification may be reduced. To avoid this problem, the canal must be packed well with cotton or an otoblock before inserting the impression material. Care should also be taken that the helix, the concha, and the tragus are sufficiently filled with impression material. If the helix and the concha are not adequately filled then there may be difficulties in retaining the mold. if the tragus portion of the mold is not sufficient full, then the tubing from a behind-the-ear aid or the receiver from a body aid might rub on the tragus and cause discomfort.

Feedback. Anyone who has worked extensively with children or adults with severe or profound hearing losses, is well aware of the difficulties that feedback can cause. Because of the necessity of using hearing aids at high power settings, an acoustic seal becomes essential for these patients. This problem is now considerably easier to solve as a result of earmold techniques such as those developed by the National Acoustic Laboratory, Sydney, Australia (Fifield et al., 1977, 1980). Space limitations do not permit a full dis-

cussion of this important topic, but the basic information can be quickly summarized. To obtain an acoustic seal, it is essential that an accurate impression be obtained and that the earmold be made to duplicate the impression without modification. Most commercial earmold material is excellent for making earmolds for patients with mild to moderately severe hearing losses because an airtight acoustic seal is not required. Silicone-based material will work well for patients with more severe losses; however, this material may not be sufficiently accurate for use with some severe or profound losses. To observe, take an earmold impression and leave it sitting on a windowsill for a day or two. The canal portion will probably begin to droop and the entire mold will settle. Therefore, by the time the earmold impression reaches the laboratory it is no longer an exact replica of the ear. The laboratory then builds the mold up to compensate for the changes in the impression. The result is an earmold that is far from an exact replica of the ear.

When it is not possible to make an earmold impression that does not cause feedback, it may be necessary to try a different type of impression material. Dental impression material is dimensionally stable and will accurately retain its shape for a long time. It is more difficult to use, but when feedback is a problem, it is worth the effort. Unfortunately, standard earmold syringes sometimes do not work well with this type of material and special syringes may be needed. Earmold impressions made with this material should eliminate almost any feedback problems. For the few patients whose feedback problems are not solved by this procedure, a three-stage earmold procedure that will solve the problem has been developed by Fifield et al. (1977). This procedure also makes use of dental impression materials and uses the pressure gauge of an impedance bridge to test the acoustic seal of the impression (Fifield et al., 1977, 1980; Loavenbruck and Madell, 1981; Madell and Gendel, 1984).

Earmold Modification. It is not uncommon for an earmold to need some adjustment when it arrives from the laboratory. It is often necessary to shorten the ear canal. For some patients, the helix portion of the canal will be uncomfortable and will need to be adjusted. If the loss is not a severe one requiring a tight acoustic seal, it is possible to remove the helix portion completely. This may make the mold easier to insert for geriatric patients. If the canal is uncomfortable and a tight fit is not required, it is also possible to reduce the size of the canal.

A very common earmold adjustment is venting. If it was not ordered when the impression was sent to the laboratory, then the mold can be vented in the office by using a hand drill. First, determine if a parallel or side vent is needed, then carefully examine the mold to determine how the vent will fit best. If the canal is a narrow one, it may be difficult to place the vent. Drilling vents requires some practice. Some people prefer to drill the vent straight from the canal portion and others prefer to drill from the exterior portion of the mold. Some find it easier to drill half the vent from the canal portion and half from the exterior portion. In any case, some time should be spent practicing drilling vents on old molds before attempting to drill vents in a patient's earmold.

Replacing tubing is another common repair. With time, tubing becomes hard and cracked and requires replacement. The old tubing needs to be removed first and can sometimes be pulled out with pliers. If the tubing has been glued in place, then placing the mold in hot water may soften the glue and facilitate removal. In some cases, it will be necessary to drill the old tubing out. After the old tubing is removed and the sound bore cleaned, new tubing can be inserted. The tubing should be set to a 90° angle at the point where it will come out of the earmold. The part of the tubing that is inserted into the canal portion of the mold can be cut at a 45° angle to facilitate insertion. To glue the tubing in place, pull it out of the canal end slightly farther than the end of the mold, add a drop of glue, and pull the tubing back into the mold. The tubing may then be cut from both ends. If the tubing is being replaced in an earmold that has been vented, be certain that the vent hole still remains. It may be necessary to redrill (Loavenbruck and Madell, 1981; Raas and Bloomgren, 1990).

Hearing Aid Repairs

Most dispensing audiologists only do minor repairs in the clinic. When the repair requires opening the case, the hearing aid is usually returned to the factory. Most hearing aid problems, however, are rather simple. A clogged earmold or tubing is a common problem and can usually be solved using warm water, a pipe cleaner and an air blower. If the debris clogging the mold is really stuck, a very small crochet hook is often useful. For ITE and ITC hearing aids, a wax loop is usually provided by the manufacturer to remove clogged wax.

Another common problem sometimes occurs when trying a hearing aid for the first time. A patient may have difficulty getting the hearing aid on the ear without twisting the tubing. If the tubing becomes twisted, then sound will be cut off. Inspection of the tubing will reveal if this is the problem, and if so, the tubing will need to be replaced and the patient reinstructed. Other common repairs include replacing the ear hook, replacing cords and receivers, and cleaning

dirt out of the controls, the microphone, and the battery contacts.

With good instruction at the time of the fitting, most patients should be able to identify and solve most hearing aid problems on their own. If the dispenser and the patient cannot solve the problem, then the aid will probably have to be returned to the factory for repair.

MODIFYING IN-THE-EAR/IN-THE-CANAL (ITE/ITC) HEARING AIDS

Modifications that are made in the office assist the dispenser in providing timely and efficient service to clients. It also permits the dispenser to determine the problem in a way that is not available when the aid is returned to the factory. For example, it is much easier to determine what is causing discomfort when the client is sitting in the office. Most manufacturers of ITE/ITC hearing aids are aware of the advantages of in-the-office repairs and are flexible if the audiologist damages the aid while attempting to make the repair.

In-the-office modifications consist of comfort changes, the use of venting and acoustic dampers to modify the acoustic signal, and minor repairs such as replacing the battery door or microphone cover. Decisions about when to vent and when to use acoustic dampers are the same for ITE/ITC hearing aids as for behind-the-ear hearing aids. Before doing any drilling or grinding of an ITE/ITC hearing aid, it is important to check the hearing aid carefully to determine where the internal parts of the hearing aid are located. This can frequently be done by holding the aid up to a strong light or by holding an otoprobe or earlight up to the canal portion of the hearing aid. Adjustments are easily made with a bench grinder that has assorted drill sizes, a buffer spindle, and a pad for polishing. Venting, shortening the canal, and removal of the helix are common adjustments that are easy to learn. An existing vent can be enlarged with a drill that is slightly larger than the vent. A new vent can be drilled if none exists. It is usually safest to drill a lateral vent because this reduces the chance of damage to the internal parts of the aid. Monomer and polymer chemicals are available to patch and repair the shells. Other glues are available for securing the receiver tubing and microphone tubing. Because the case is made of hard plastic, it will be necessary to buff it carefully after the modification is made so that it will not cause discomfort when reinserted into the client's ear. Most manufacturers provide instructions on how to modify ITE/ITC hearing aids and some will even provide old ones on which to practice. Do not hesitate to discuss this with the hearing aid manufacturers. (For further information on in-the-office modifications see Burris, 1990; Curran, 1990a, b; DeNyse, 1990; Gitles and Kaiser, 1990; Orton, 1984).

COUNSELING THE HEARING AID USER

Adjusting to Amplification

Before a patient takes a hearing aid home, it is important to ascertain that he or she can insert it, turn it on and off, and change the battery. It is not necessary to teach the patient everything in the first fitting visit. Such subjects as use of the telephone switch, tone controls, cleaning the mold, and using the battery tester can wait for a subsequent visit.

Once the audiologist is certain that the hearing aid earmold fits appropriately, the patient can try inserting it. The mold is easiest to insert when it is not attached to the hearing aid. When the patient can successfully get the mold into the ear, it can be attached to the aid. When he or she can get the aid on the ear and working, the aid may be taken home. The initial fitting appointment may take as long as an hour with some patients, whereas others will take half that time. Still others will not learn to insert the hearing aid properly in 1 hour. A recheck should be scheduled in 1 to 2 weeks to be certain that the patient can use the aid appropriately and to teach the patient anything else that is required.

Adjusting to amplification is a slow process. Some patients immediately put the hearing aid on and wear it comfortably full time, but they are certainly the exception. Even experienced hearing aid users often have difficulty with a new aid and need to learn to use it slowly, beginning with a few hours a day. A new hearing aid user will need to be begin using the aid gradually. Patients should be instructed to use the hearing aid daily, at home, in a quiet setting. They should begin using the aid between ½ and 1 hour at a time. When the aid is being used comfortably, the length of time should be increased. After it can be comfortably worn for several hours at a time, patients can begin trying to use the aid in less quiet places. It is important, however, for them to understand that listening in noisy places is going to be difficult.

To facilitate adjustment to difficult listening situations, it is important that the dispenser prepare the patient with strategies for listening at lectures, in theaters, church or temple, and groups. For instance, patients must learn to place themselves at the locations that will afford the best listening and should tell others that they have difficulty hearing and may require some assistance. This preparation of the hearing aid user is often best handled in a group situation, such as hearing aid orientation classes (Madell, 1975; Loaven-

bruck and Madell, 1981). Videotapes are available to assist in providing information that is normally covered in hearing aid orientation and speechreading classes (New York League for the Hard of Hearing, 1987, 1988; 1990a, b, c).

Checking the Aid

It is essential that the patient (or a relative) be taught to troubleshoot the hearing aid. When patients can check out the aids on their own, they are less likely to panic when something goes wrong. Most of the time they will be able to resolve the difficulty and will not need to visit the audiologist.

Patients need to know how to check controls including the on-off switch, and "M"-"T" switch and the tone control. The patient should know how to check tubing and hearing aid cords for twists, cracks or fraying, and for loose connections.

Battery-related problems must also be checked. Is the battery dead? Is it backward? Are the battery contacts dirty? The earmold or ITE/ITC hearing aid should be checked to see it if is clogged or cracked. Do the controls or switches have dirty contacts? Does moving the controls back and forth eliminate the problems?

Assistive Listening Devices (ALDs)

There are many situations that are difficult for people with hearing losses; one-to-one communication is the least of their difficulties. Hearing-impaired patients may not realize that there are solutions to their problems and, therefore, may not bring them up. (See Chapter 2 for a thorough discussion of ALDs.) It is the dispenser's responsibility to be sure that information about assistive devices is easily available.

Waking in the morning may present a problem. If a standard alarm is not loud enough, a clock radio turned to a news station may be used. If this solution is not satisfactory, a light system can be made by attaching a timer to a light. Placing a flasher disc in the socket will cause the light to flash on and off, calling more attention to the alarm. If this is not sufficient, a vibrator or a fan can be substituted for the flashing light. This same kind of light flashing system can be used to alert patients to any kind of sound needing attention, including doorbells, smoke alarms, the telephone and babies crying. Some sophisticated systems are set up to signal differently for different sound stimuli. For example, a light might flash once for the doorbell and twice for the smoke alarm.

The telephone is a serious problem for many hearing-impaired people. Telephone amplifiers are beneficial for many individuals. Some amplifiers are permanently attached to the headset, whereas others are portable. Teletypewriters are also available for those whose hearing loss is too severe to use an amplified telephone. The teletypewriter is coupled to a phone so that messages that are typed into the machine are transmitted over phone lines. Various teletypewriters, including portable ones, are now available.

Amplification systems to assist hearing-impaired people are now available in public facilities. As a result of the Americans with Disabilities Act, a growing number of theaters and lecture facilities have installed infrared listening systems, and some movie theaters have installed radio listening systems. In addition, hearing-impaired patients use assistive listening devices in classrooms and meetings. Almost all hearing-impaired people can obtain significant benefit from them (Gendel, 1978, 1980; Loavenbruck and Madell, 1981).

HEARING AID DISPENSING IN DIFFERENT WORK SETTINGS

Private Practice

Hearing aid dispensing is an integral part of almost all private practices in audiology. In this setting, patients are able to receive most of the diagnostic services available in speech and hearing centers as well as hearing aid dispensing. In most cases, the same professional provides the patient with all the services he receives. Few private practices will wish, or be able, to afford technical assistance, at least at the outset.

Community Based Clinics

Community clinics, especially those with rehabilitation programs, will find the advantages of hearing aid dispensing most inviting. Like university and hospital programs, they may experience resistance from the community in the form of pressure from hearing aid dealers. Extensive contacts will need to be made with the referral sources in the community to assure them that this added service is an advantage. Patients are not likely to be concerned about negative comments from hearing aid dealers. Those who already have relationships with hearing aid dealers, however, may be told by the dealers that there will be no after-sale service from a dispensing clinical program. Patients need to be told that follow-up will, indeed, be available and that if they choose to they may continue to receive services from their old hearing aid dealer rather than from the audiology clinic. The dispensing program should be viewed as an additional service offered by the center, which may or may not be used by the patient.

Hospital Speech and Hearing Departments

The advantages of offering a more comprehensive service often encourage hospital-based programs to add a hearing aid dispensing service. A great deal of work will probably be needed to assist the medical staff in understanding the advantages of audiologists dispensing hearing aids. The hospital pharmacy may be of assistance in developing procedures and possibly in selling hearing aids.

University Clinics

Dispensing in a university clinic offers students the opportunity to learn hearing aid dispensing as part of clinic practice (Lentz et al., 1978; Goldstein, 1979). It is now an essential aspect of training because more and more audiology facilities, in every type of employment setting, are including dispensing as part of the inservices. Dispensing in a university clinic allows students to develop essential technical, clinical, and counseling skills. A system needs to be developed, however, to keep the clinic open during vacation and holiday periods so that patients who develop hearing aid difficulties do not have to wait several weeks to receive service. Local hearing aid dealers may pressure the administration to prohibit hearing aid dispensing in the university. Extensive work will probably be needed with the university administration to assist them in understanding the importance of hearing aid dispensing in a training program.

Special attention will need to be paid to fees and billing, especially if the program has not charged fees in the past. Hearing aids cannot be given away. In addition, charging for services is a worthwhile concept for students to learn.

CONCLUSION

Hearing aid dispensing is clearly the wave of the future for audiology. Each year increasing numbers of audiologists and clinical audiology programs become involved in dispensing. Several graduate programs in audiology offer courses in hearing aid dispensing. Many others include information about hearing aid dispensing as part of the general course work on hearing aids. The very fact that a chapter on hearing aid dispensing is again included in this HOCA indicates the progress that has been made in including hearing aid dispensing as a basic service in the practice of audiology.

It is hoped that the growth of interest in hearing aid dispensing will be the first of many steps towards reinvolving audiologists in the habilitation and rehabilitation of patients with impaired hearing. In recent years, with advances in equipment and diagnostic tests, audiologists devoted more and more time to the diagnostic aspects of the profession. The involvement in dispensing forces us to more carefully assess our patients' communication needs and, hopefully, will encourage a renewed interest in aural habilitation and rehabilitation. This can have only positive effects on the profession and on the patients we serve.

REFERENCES

Brackett DB, and Madell JR. FM systems for people with impaired hearing. Hear Rehabil Q 1983;8(2):10–12.

Burris PD. Getting back to the basics: post fitting problem solving. Hear Instrum 1980;41:8–13.

Curran J. Modification of in-the-ear and in-the-canal hearing aids, Part 1. Audiology Today 1990a;2(1):27–28.

Curran J. Modification of in-the-ear and in-the-canal hearing aids, Part 2. Audiology Today 1990b;2(3):23–25.

DeNyse R. Practical modification tips for dispensers. Hear Instrum 1990;41:17–19.

Fifield D, Earnshaw R, and Smither M. A new ear impression technique. Hear Instrum 1977;28:11–12; 40–41.

Fifield D, Earnshaw R, and Smither M. A new impression technique to prevent acoustic feedback with high powered hearing aids. Volta Rev 1980;1:33–39.

Gendel JM. "Do-it-yourself" guide to devices aiding the hearing impaired. Hear Rehabil Q 1978;3:6–9.

Gender JM. Communication devices to aid the hearing impaired. Hear Rehabil Q 1980;4:4–7.

Gitles T, and Kaiser H. Tools and equipment for in-office modification. Hear Instrum 1990;41:14–16.

Goldstein DP. Audiological rehabilitation and hearing aid dispensing in a university teaching clinic. ASHA 1979;21:650–653.

Goldstein W. Assistive listening devices for individual with impaired hearing. Hear Rehabil Q 1986;11(2):4–8.

Lentz WE, Pierce BR, and Willeford JA. Dispensing hearing aids through a university training program. ASHA 1978;20: 965–969.

Loavenbruck, AM, and Madell JR. Hearing Aid Dispensing for Audiologist. New York: Grune & Stratton, 1981.

Madell JR. You and your hearing aid. Highlights Quarterly Bulletin. New York League for the Hard of Hearing. 1975;54:4–6.

Madell JR, and Gendel JM. Earmolds for patients with severe and profound hearing loss. Ear Hear 1984;5:349–351.

Marge M. The current status of service delivery systems for the hearing impaired. ASHA 1977;19:403–409.

New York League for the Hard of Hearing. Assistive Devices for the Hearing Impaired Person [Videotape]. New York: 1987.

New York League for the Hard of Hearing. Sound Advice [Videotape, Part 1, 2, and 3]. New York, 1988.

New York League for the Hard of hearing. I see what you're saying: A practical guide to speech reading: Volume 1: Fundamentals [Videotape]. New York, 1990a.

New York League for the Hard of Hearing. I see what you're saying: A practical guide to speech reading: Volume 2: Practice [Videotape]. New York, 1990b.

New York League for the Hard of Hearing. Assessment of adult speech reading ability [Videotape]. New York, 1990c.

Orton J. Perfecting your craft: The fine art of in-office ITE modification. Hear J 1984;37:7–22.

Public Citizen. Retired Professional Action Group: Paying Through the Ear. Retired Professional Action Group. Washington, DC, 1973.

Raas M, and Bloomgren M. Earmold modification techniques. Hear Instrum 1990;41:20–23.

CHAPTER 46

Cochlear Implants and Tactile Aids

Terry Hnath-Chisolm

The majority of individuals with sensory-neural hearing loss receive assistance from the use of conventional amplification. There are those, however, who appear to receive little or no benefit from hearing aids. Typically, these are individuals with puretone thresholds of 110 dB HL or greater, although some may have thresholds within the 90–109 dB HL range. Their hearing losses are characterized as "profound" and in individuals where there does not appear to be any auditory response, "total." Alternative approaches to providing these individuals with access to acoustic signals includes the use of two types of sensory aids: cochlear implants and tactile aids.

Cochlear implants are designed to provide direct stimulation to the auditory nerve. In the normal auditory system, the sound energy entering the outer ear is converted to neural signals in the cochlea. The neural signals are then transmitted along the auditory nerve and central auditory nervous system to the cortical regions of the brain for interpretation. With a severely damaged or nonfunctioning cochlea there is a breakdown at the point of conversion into neural signals. By providing stimulation to the auditory nerve, cochlear implants circumvent this problem. Currently, there are more than 3000 individuals, both children and adults, who use cochlear implants (National Institutes of Health Consensus Development Conference Statement, 1988).

Tactile aids are designed to transmit information about acoustic stimuli, especially speech, to the skin. Acoustic signals are transduced into vibratory or electrical patterns and presented in ways that are designed to make optimal use of the skin's receptive capabilities. Numerous tactile aids have been developed, either in an attempt to allow users to understand speech through touch alone or to provide supplementary cues to speechreading. Currently several devices are being marketed in the United States and are being used by over 1000 deaf individuals, including several hundred children (Levitt, 1988).

The purpose of this chapter is to provide an understanding of the development and use of cochlear implants and tactile aids in the management of hearing-impaired persons. Although there are many differences between cochlear implants and tactile aids, they share common goals. Both are intended to provide users with (a) increased access to environmental sounds; (b) increased awareness of their own voices; (c) assistance during speechreading; and, ideally, (d) the ability to recognize connected discourse through the use of the sensory aid alone. To better understand the benefits and limitations of the use of cochlear implants and tactile aids, the development and current status of each is discussed.

COCHLEAR IMPLANTS
Development

The history of electrical stimulation of the auditory system dates back to the work of Alessandro Volta in 1800. A complete description of the history of cochlear implant development is provided by Luxford and Brackman (1985). Although electrical stimulation of the auditory system had been investigated fairly regularly since the mid-19th century, it was not until 1957 that the first electrodes were implanted for the purpose of stimulating hearing. While, as Luxford and Brackman (1985) report, the recipient was not able to recognize speech by hearing alone, the implant did provide some help while speechreading and its use was preferred to silence. Positive results were reported from several experimental trials conducted in the 1960's and 1970's (e.g., Simmons, 1966; Michaelson, 1971; House and Urban, 1973). Despite widespread criticism from both the medical and research communities, extensive clinical trials with cochlear implantation began in the 1970's, primarily at the House Ear Institute in Los Angeles. By 1980, there were several research groups worldwide involved in the development and evaluation of a variety of cochlear implant systems. In the mid-to-late 1980's two devices (3M/House and Nucleus 22-channel) received approval from the Federal Drug Administration for commercial marketing, first in adults and then in children. At the present time, the number of adult cochlear implant recipients is in the thousands and several hundred children have also been implanted.

Device Characteristics

Cochlear implants are designed to restore some hearing by bypassing the defective sensory mechanism directly stimulating the auditory nerve fibers. Currently, over 25 cochlear implant systems have been developed worldwide. Although there are many differences in these systems, they all consist of several basic components as illustrated in Figure 46.1A. (To highlight similarities and differences, the basic components of tactile aids are also shown in this figure.) First, there is a microphone which picks up the acoustic signal and converts it into an electrical signal. Next is an externally worn speech coding unit. Here, the signal is manipulated into the desired electrical or digital pattern. In addition, some form of output limiting, usually compression, of the signal occurs. This is due to the narrow dynamic range of hearing for electrical stimulation. Third is a system for transmitting the signal from the processor to the internal components. Last, are surgically implanted electrodes which are capable of exciting the cochlear neurons of the auditory nerve. The electrical waveform that actually stimulates the nerve fibers is either a continuous analog current or a pulsatile coding of the original signal.

Many of the differences in the various systems are related to how the signals generated by the speech processing unit are transmitted to the nerve fibers. That is, there are differences in terms of (a) type of transmission relay system; (b) electrode configuration; (c) number of electrodes; (d) number of channels of information; and, (e) placement of electrodes. In addition, there are important differences in the ways speech is processed and coded for electrical stimulation (i.e., speech processing strategy). Table 46.1 summarizes the design characteristics of some of the cochlear implant systems currently in use in the United States.

Type of Transmission Relay System

Two methods are typically used to relay signals from the speech processing unit to the internal components of the cochlear implant system. These are percutaneous and transcutaneous. Percutaneous transmission involves a direct, hardwired connection through the skin via an external plug mounted on the skull. This type of transmission relay system was used in early

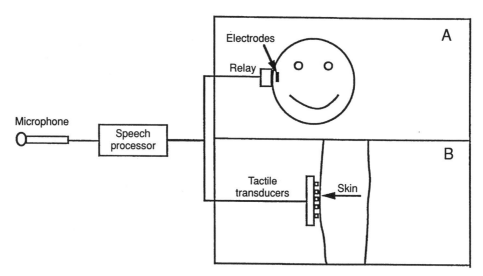

Figure 46.1. Basic components in (*a*) cochlear implants and (*b*) tactile aids.

Table 46.1.
Design Characteristics of Some Cochlear Implant Systems Used in the United States

System	Relay System	Configuration	Electrode #	Placement	Channel #	Processing Strategy
3M/House	Transcutaneous	Monopolar	1	Intracochlear	1	Filtered AM 16K Hz
3M/Vienna	Transcutaneous	Bipolar	1	Intra- or extracochlear	1	Band filtered recombined
Cochlear/Nucleus	Transcutaneous	Bipolar	22	Intracochlear	1-21	Feature
MiniMed/Clarion	Transcutaneous	Monopolar or bipolar	16 or 8	Intracochlear	1-16	Compressed analog or interleaved pulsatile
Richards Med/Ineraid	Percutaneous	Bipolar	4	Intracochlear	1-4	Band filtered

cochlear implant devices and is still in clinical use. In a transcutaneous system the signal is transmitted across the skin using either a radiofrequency link or passive magnetic induction.

The transmitter coil, which receives information from the speech coding unit, is placed outside the skin. It transmits the signal to a surgically implanted receiver coil placed under the skin on the mastoid. The receiver coil is connected to the electrode(s). The receiver coil can be either active or inactive. If inactive, it serves simply as a receiver of information. If active, then both power and information are received. The power activates circuitry within the receiver which initiates the stimulation signal to the electrode array.

Electrode Configuration

Cochlear implants rely on the fact that surviving auditory nerve fibers can be stimulated to fire by application of an externally generated electric current of sufficient strength, duration, and orientation. Thus, the stimulus in a cochlear implant system is the density of electrical current flow from an active to a ground (reference) electrode. Either of two electrode configurations is generally used in cochlear implant systems: bipolar or monopolar. A bipolar configuration consists of placing active and ground electrodes within close proximity to each other. The region of maximum current density is limited to the area near the electrode pair, resulting in a discrete number of neural fibers being stimulated. If, however, there are no stimulable neurons near the bipolar electrode pair a considerable increase in current will probably be needed to stimulate more distant ones. With monopolar stimulation the current flows from a single active electrode to a remotely placed ground electrode. The maximum current density is near the active electrode, with a relatively broad sector of neural fibers being stimulated. If there are no stimulable neurons nearby, a relatively small increase of current should allow for the activation of more distant neurons.

Number of Electrodes

Cochlear implant systems may use either a single electrode or multiple electrodes. If only one electrode is used then only monopolar stimulation is possible. When multiple electrodes are used, stimulation can be either monopolar or bipolar. If the ground electrode(s) are at a great enough distance from the active ones stimulation is monopolar. However, when the ground electrode(s) are in close proximity to the active electrodes, the stimulation is bipolar.

Number of Channels of Information

Cochlear implant systems use from one to many channels of information. The number of channels refers to the number of differentially processed signals delivered to the electrodes. It is important to note that the number of channels of information is not always synonymous with the number of electrodes. If only one electrode is used only one signal can be delivered to it. If, however, a system has multiple electrodes it can serve as either a single channel or a multichannel implant. If the same signal is delivered to each electrode or if only one electrode is selected for stimulation it is a single channel system, while if different signals are delivered to the different electrodes it is a multichannel one. In addition, transmission of information in a multichannel system can be done either serially or in parallel. In parallel transmission, information is sent to multiple electrode sites at the same time. In serial transmission, information is sent rapidly in sequence from the processor to the internal receiver, and, in turn, to the electrodes.

Placement of Electrodes

Electrode placement can be either outside or inside the cochlea. Outside, or extracochlear, placement is usually on the round window. While most devices which use extracochlear placement are single channel, multichannel extracochlear devices have also been developed. Intracochlear placement is usually through the round window into the scala tympani, with electrode depths as much as 25 mm. Usually the longer electrode depths are associated with multielectrode devices. Intracochlear placement is used more often because it allows for efficient stimulation of the auditory nerve fibers. The use of extracochlear placement, however, preserves the scala tympani for future generations of implant systems.

Speech Processing Strategies

Two basic approaches are taken to process and code speech for presentation in cochlear implant systems. In the first, an attempt is made to present all of the information in the acoustic speech signal. The task of selecting the most important elements or features is left to the auditory system. The underlying belief is that the pathologic auditory system can select the important features from the complete signal, as does the normal auditory system. The second approach involves extracting those features that are believed to be important for speech recognition from the acoustic signal and presenting them in a codified manner. This approach assumes that not only can the important speech features be identified, they also can be reliably extracted from the acoustic speech signal. Underlying this approach is the belief that the complete acoustic signal is too noisy for a pathologic cochlea. The results obtained with these approaches are discussed in the next section.

Current Status

Candidates

The majority of cochlear implant recipients are postlingually deafened adults. Typically candidates for implantation are those with puretone hearing thresholds greater than 90 dB HL, although most recipients have had hearing losses greater than 110 dB HL. More importantly, candidates should have no open set word recognition with well-fit hearing aids. In addition, candidates should not exhibit any other physical or mental contraindication. Recently, profoundly hearing-impaired individuals with hearing losses in the 90–109 dB range have also been considered as potential candidates for cochlear implantation. In addition, a few prelingually hearing-impaired adults have also received cochlear implants.

The use of cochlear implants as treatment for deafness in children appears to be increasing. The determination of cochlear implant candidacy in children is challenging, primarily due to difficulties in measuring the benefits of amplification in young children. In addition, there is lack of knowledge about the variables that contribute to successful use of cochlear implants by children. Guidelines for pediatric cochlear implants generally require a stable bilateral profound sensory-neural hearing loss with pure tone thresholds in excess of 90 dB HL. Indeed, cochlear implantation does appear to be appropriate for deaf children who do not exhibit any residual hearing, typically those with hearing thresholds well in excess of 110 dB HL (Boothroyd and Cawkwell, 1970). Many of those with thresholds in the range of 90–109 dB HL, however, can, with appropriate training, acquire phoneme recognition skills through residual hearing (Boothroyd, 1984). The rehabilitation potential of conventional amplification for this population needs to be carefully determined, on an individual basis and with appropriate training, over time.

Performance

Single Channel Systems. The first cochlear implant system to receive widespread use was the single channel intracochlear system developed at the House Ear Institute and manufactured by the 3M company. In the 3M/House system an attempt is made to provide the user with access to complete the acoustic speech signal by band-pass filtering the input signal and using it to amplitude modulate a 16 KHz sinusoidal carrier (Fretz and Fravel, 1985). Another single channel device used in the United States is the 3M/Vienna device, which has both an extra- and intracochlear version (Hochmair and Hochmair-Desoyer, 1985). In this system, the input signal to the speech processor is band-pass filtered and then split into four bands. Each band is independently balanced for loudness and then the bands are recombined to form one signal, with frequency shaping to typically provide high-frequency emphasis. Although both devices are no longer being produced in the United States (Osberger, 1990), there are many adults and children who use the 3M/House device and also a number of adult users of the 3M/Vienna implant system.

In evaluating the effectiveness of single channel cochlear implants in adults, a 1986 ASHA ad hoc committee concluded, with primary reference to the 3M/House system, that they allow for "a general awareness of sound and the recognition of few specific everyday sounds; enhancement of lipreading ability; temporal, durational, and intensity-difference (accent) cues; and pitch cues within a range below 300 Hz. Also vocal self-monitoring ability is usually improved" (Hopkinson, McFarland, Owens, et al., 1986, p. 33). The committee also found no evidence of open set speech understanding of words or sentences through use of the implant alone (without speechreading cues) by adult users of the 3M/House implant. In open set tasks, no experience is provided with test materials and there are no alternative responses from which to chose. Open set speech recognition, however, was subsequently reported for a small number of children using the 3M/House device (Berliner, Tonokowa, Dye, and House, 1989; Miyamoto, Osberger, Robbins, et al., 1989). Open set word recognition was also reported for adult users of both the intracochlear and extracochlear versions of the 3M/Vienna device (Hochmair-Desoyer, Hochmair, and Stiglbrunner, 1985; Tyler, 1988; Tyler, Moore, and Kuk, 1989).

Multichannel Systems. Several multichannel systems have been developed in which attempts are made to present all the information in the acoustic speech signal by using a "band filtering" or "vocoder" approach. In this approach, a bank of filters is used to split the incoming signal into a number of frequency bands and the output of each filter determines the electrical signal delivered to each electrode or electrode pair, placed at different points in the cochlea. Since pitch perception is related to place of stimulation along a multielectrode array rather than to rate of electrical stimulation, a given frequency will be perceived as higher in pitch if electrodes are placed toward the base of the cochlea and lower in pitch if placed toward the apex. In a sense, this strategy tries to duplicate encoding of frequency by place of stimulation as occurs in a normal cochlea.

Many multichannel cochlear implant systems developed worldwide use a band filtering approach (e.g., Banfai, Hortmann, Karczag, Kubik, and Wustrow, 1984; Chouard, Fugain, Meyer, and Chabolle, 1986; Eddington, 1983; Schindler and Kessler, 1987). Reportedly, two such systems are currently being manufactured in the United States (Osberger, 1990). One is the Ineraid, which was originally manufactured by Symbion and now is manufactured by Richards Medical Company. The system uses monopolar electrodes, percutaneous transmission, and a four channel analog signal processing strategy (Eddington, 1983).

A more recently developed system is the Clarion Multichannel system. It is the result of the collaborative work of the University of California, San Francisco, the Research Triangle Institute, and the manufacturer, MiniMed Technologies, Sylmar, California. The system is flexible in several respects including "... speech coding and processing techniques. The type of signal delivered (analog waveform or pulsatile), the temporal distribution of stimuli (simultaneous or sequential) and the stimulation mode (monopolar vs. bipolar)" (Osberger, 1990, p.38). Thus, it can be adjusted for optimal performance in each individual.

Although there are many issues, such as optimal number of channels, that need to be resolved for band filtering cochlear implant systems, overall reports on performance are encouraging. For example, recognition of environmental sounds and enhancement in speechreading performance are reported for most adult users of the Ineraid system (Parkin and Dankowski, 1986). Similar results are also reported for users of the devices that preceded the Clarion implant system (Schindler and Kessler, 1987; Wilson, Finley, Farmer, et al., 1988). More importantly, however, an estimated 50% of the users of multichannel band filtering systems demonstrate some open set speech recognition (e.g., Tyler, et al., 1989).

In contrast to the band filtering systems which present all of the speech signal, the feature extraction speech processing approach involves identifying the important features for speech recognition and reliably extracting them from the acoustic speech signal. A feature extraction strategy is used in the Nucleus 22-channel cochlear implant system developed in Australia by Tong and his colleagues (1982), and marketed in the United States by Cochlear Corporation. In its original design, the speech processor extracted an estimate of the fundamental frequency (F_o) and of the second formant (F2) center frequency. This was revised in 1985 to include an estimate of the first formant (F1) center frequency, and in the most recent version (i.e., MSP) to also include information from three high frequency bands. In addition to recognition of environmental sounds and enhancement of speechreading performance, adult users of this device have also exhibited open set speech recognition (e.g., Tyler, et al., 1989). Improvements in performance in the auditory-only condition have been reported with each new speech processing strategy used (e.g., Tye-Murray, Louder, and Tyler, 1990; Osberger, 1990). The Nucleus device is also being used in children and received marketing approval from the Federal Drug Administration in 1990. Results of initial evaluations indicate that performance is better with this device than with the 3M/House device, with an apparently larger percentage of children exhibiting open set speech recognition (Miyamoto, et al., 1989; Chute, Hellman, Parisier, and Selesnick, 1990).

Another cochlear implant system that uses a feature extraction approach is the External Pattern Input cochlear implant, developed in England (Fourcin, Douek, Moore, et al., 1983). It is a single channel extracochlear implant and the speech processor extracts voice fundamental frequency (F_o). Thus, the signal reaching the user provides voicing and timing information which can be used to effectively enhance speechreading. The investigators believe that the users of this device receive benefits similar to that obtained with other single channel implant devices. Furthermore, since it is an extracochlear device, the scala tympani is preserved for future generations of more efficient implant systems.

Comparisons. As discussed, several speech processing strategies have been incorporated in cochlear implant systems. Both the single channel presentation of the analog waveform and the multichannel band filtering, spectrum approach allow for the recognition of environmental sounds and enhancement of speechreading performance. While there are some reports of open set word recognition with the single channel systems, many users of multichannel systems demonstrate the ability to understand speech through the use of the implant alone. Similar results have also been obtained with the Nucleus feature extraction multichannel system. In addition, enhancement of speechreading performance has been found with single channel extracochlear presentation of voice F_o.

Only a few comparative studies of cochlear implant systems have been done and the results do not clearly support a conclusion of the superiority of any one speech processing strategy at this time (e.g., Dent, Simmons, White, and Roberts, 1987; Tyler, et al.,

1989; Tye-Murray and Tyler, 1989). Much of the available data, however, suggest that performance with multichannel systems, regardless of speech processing strategy, is superior to that obtained with single channel implants in both adults and children. Nonetheless, it has recently been suggested that single channel systems may be more effective than some multichannel implants in transmitting the type of acoustic speech information that may be most useful in enhancing the speechreading performance of implant users trying to understand speech in realistic situations (Rosen, Walliker, Briacombe, and Edgerton, 1989). That is, although open set speech recognition of connected discourse is the stated aim of most cochlear implant systems, in everyday situations the presence of background noise often makes speech understanding without visual cues difficult for cochlear implant users. The adverse effects of background noise are not unique to cochlear implants and the development of techniques for reducing noise is important for all sensory aids.

While it appears that most recipients benefit from the use of cochlear implants, with roughly half of the multichannel recipients estimated to have some open set word recognition, not all demonstrate the same degree of success. Indeed, there are cases where little or no benefit is demonstrated (Kishon-Rabin, Hanin, and Boothroyd, 1990). While various factors, such as number of years of deafness, age at implantation, progression of hearing loss, etc., have been associated with success, currently there are no reliable ways to predict who will do well with a cochlear implant. For example, one factor thought to be important for successful performance with a cochlear implant is the status of the residual neural population. While electrical stimulation of the promontory or round window can be used to assess nerve survival, the results are not always reliable. The development of predictive measures is an often-stated goal for future research.

One factor which can possibly influence performance is the type and amount of training given to a cochlear implant recipient. Most cochlear implant programs include some form of aural rehabilitation program. Ideally, these programs should include counseling, sensory training, and the development of appropriate communication strategies (Lansing and Davis, 1988). In addition, data indicate sensory training that occurs early after implantation is more effective than training that occurs several months after implantation (Lansing and Davis, 1988).

Sensory training typically includes both analytic (i.e., feature level) and synthetic (sentence level) level training. This training is done by "hearing" (cochlear implant) alone or by hearing in combination with speechreading. In examining the effects of analytic versus synthetic speech perception training for cochlear implant recipients, Boothroyd, Hanin, Hnath-Chisolm, and Waltzman (1987) found that subjects who received benefit, in terms of improvements in speechreading performance for open set materials, did so within 1 month of using the cochlear implant. While neither type of training resulted in any significant increases in performance in the hearing + speechreading condition, performance by hearing alone did increase as a result of intensive synthetic level training. Some of the subjects who did not initially show a great benefit from the use of the cochlear implant did demonstrate small improvements in combined hearing + speechreading performance as a result of synthetic level training, while others showed no increases in performance even with intensive training. It is possible other types of training may be more effective for those who do not demonstrate speech perception benefit from the use of a cochlear implant. Issues related to training are important to explore for users of all sensory aids.

Although most post-lingually hearing-impaired adults who receive cochlear implants have hearing losses in excess of 110 dB HL, there are some with more residual hearing. While little published data is currently available about this group's performance, there are reports of improvements in speech perception performance over that obtained with hearing aid use (Chute, 1991). It should be noted, however, that there is also data which indicates that even the "best" speech perception performance by cochlear implant users does not exceed that found in a hearing aid users with a 90 dB HL hearing losses (Hanin and Boothroyd, 1989). A definite statement about the use of cochlear implants with those with minimal residual hearing awaits the results of current experimental trials.

Another group for which there is little published data is that of pre-lingually deaf adults. These individuals, because of their lack of orientation to and memory for sound, might not be expected to do as well with cochlear implants as post-lingually deafened adults. Indeed, benefits for this group are usually limited to environmental sound recognition and visual enhancement of speech (Clark, Busby, Roberts, et al., 1987; Briacombe, et al., 1987).

Perhaps no area is more controversial than the use of cochlear implants in children. While it appears clear that cochlear implants can provide those children who have no usable residual hearing with access to the acoustic speech signal, the previously discussed issue of determining candidacy still remains. While the criteria for pediatric candidacy includes thresholds in excess of

90 dB HL, it has been reported that most children with puretone thresholds between 90 and 105 dB HL through at least 2000 Hz, using conventional amplification, exhibited better closed and open set speech recognition skills than even the highest performing multichannel implant users (Robins, Berry, Osberger, and Miyamoto, 1989). Clearly, benefits from conventional amplification need to be determined prior to implantation. Once implanted, it is important that the child receive consistent auditory, speech, and language training to maximize potential benefits.

Improvements in speech production ability have been associated with cochlear implant use by children (Kirk and Brown, 1985; Robbins, et al., 1989; Waltzman, Cohen, Spivak, et al., 1990). Although more difficult to assess, gains in linguistic development have also been observed amongst both single- and multichannel users (Kirk and Brown, 1985; Miyamoto, et al., 1989). Available data suggest greater improvements with multichannel rather than single channel devices and also with receiving the implant during early childhood. However, there is still a need for longitudinal comparative studies, with control of as many variables as possible, before drawing any conclusions about the most appropriate implant scheme for children. In addition, the difficulties in assessing the auditory capabilities of young children and the irreversible effects of surgical implantation have led researchers to question the viability of using other sensory devices, such as tactile aids, with this population (Pickett and McFarland, 1985).

TACTILE AIDS

Development

Systematic attempts to develop tactile communication aids for the deaf date back to the pioneering work of Gault in the 1920's. Several excellent reviews of this early work are available (Kirman, 1974; Levitt, 1988; Reed, Durlach, and Braida, 1982; Pickett and McFarland, 1985; Sherrick, 1984). Initially, researchers proposed to use touch as a substitute for the impaired hearing mechanism. Early devices were simple, with the speech signal transmitted directly to the skin through a single vibrator. Experimental results indicated that while these single channel devices provided only a limited amount of information about speech, they were useful in supplementing speechreading and in speech production training. In an effort to increase the amount of speech information transmitted to the skin, investigators developed a multiple vibrator system which filtered the speech signal into five frequency pass-bands and presented the output of each filter to a different vibrator. This multichannel device

can be considered the first tactile vocoder. Research with tactile vocoders revived in the 1950's due to the development of relatively compact filter banks. Results indicated that while they were capable of transmitting some speech information, they, too, served best as supplements to speechreading and in speech training.

Although the results of early tactile aid research were encouraging, their use was largely ignored, most probably due to the development and availability of wearable hearing aids. It was not until the 1980's that extensive interest in the development of tactile aids was revived. Factors which contributed to the revival of research in this area were the results of studies which indicated that many profoundly deaf individuals did not possess true hearing (e.g., Boothroyd and Cawkwell, 1970) and the growing use of cochlear implants as treatment for deafness. Many researchers believed it was natural to ask whether hearing impaired individuals could do as well with noninvasive wearable tactile aids as with surgically implanted cochlear prostheses.

The limited benefits obtained with tactile aids might lead one to question whether it is reasonable to believe that tactile communication of speech is possible. Evidence that it is comes from speech communication through unaided touch—that is, Tadoma. Tadoma is a method of communication which has been successfully used by some deaf-blind individuals. In Tadoma, the receiver monitors the movements of the speaker's articulation by placing the thumb on the speaker's lips and the other fingers on the speaker's face and neck (Reed, et al., 1982). As Reed, et al. (1982), point out, the finding that even one person can communicate successfully through the sense of touch provides "existence proof" that tactile communication of speech is possible.

Device Characteristics

All tactile aids consist of the basic components shown in Figure 46.1B. These include a microphone for picking up the acoustic signal and transducing it into an electrical signal and a unit for processing the signal and sending it to tactile transducer(s), which are capable of delivering vibratory or electrical patterns to the skin. The differences in tactile aids include: (a) type of stimulation; (b) location of stimulation; (c) number of channels of stimulation; and, (d) speech processing strategy. Device characteristics for some currently available wearable tactile aids are indicated in Table 46.2.

Type of Stimulation

Two types of stimulation are used in tactile aids: vibrotactile and electrotactile. In the more common form of

Table 46.2.
Design Characteristics of Some Wearable Tactile Aids

Device	Stimulation	Location	Channel #	Processing
Minifonator	Vibrotactile	Wrist	1	Amplitude modulation
Minivab3	Vibrotactile	Wrist	1	Amplitude modulation
Portapitch	Vibrotactile	Arm	8 or 16	Feature extraction
Tactaid I	Vibrotactile	Sternum	1	Amplitude modulation
Tactaid II+X	Vibrotactile	Wrist	2	Band filtered
Tactaid 7	Vibrotactile	Chest, abdomen, or neck	7	Band filtered
Tacticon TC-1600	Electrotactile	Abdomen	16	Band filtered
Telex KS32	Vibrotactile	Wrist(s)	2	Band filtered
Tickle Talker	Electrotactile	Fingers	5	Feature extraction

stimulation which is vibrotactile, the acoustic signal is presented to the skin using bone conduction vibrators, small solenoids, or other types of mechanical transducers. A problem associated with the use of these transducers is that the power required to drive them is high, making them relatively inefficient. In addition, when driven by strong signals these devices often emit noises which can be heard by people nearby the user. An alternative is to use electrotactile (or electrocutaneous) transducers. With these, the acoustic signal is presented to the skin as an electrical current. These transducers use less power and are relatively small. Although there is some concern about possible adverse effects of applying electric currents to the skin, electrotactile aids have been used over extended periods of time without serious side effects being reported. Results of recent studies in which electrotactile and vibrotactile devices were compared, however, have raised the possibility that vibrotactile stimulation may result in a better speech signal than electrocutaneous stimulation (Lynch, Eilers, Oller, and Cobo-Lewis, 1989; Lynch, Eilers, Oller, Urbano, and Pero, 1989). Thus, further comparative research is needed to determine the optimum transducer(s) for tactile speech aids.

Location of Stimulation

Two factors are important when considering where on the body to place a tactile aid. One is the sensitivity of different body locations to tactile stimulation and the other is the practicality of the location. The results of psychophysical studies indicate that the fingertips of the hands are the most sensitive area on a number of different measures (Weinstein, 1968). Unfortunately, the fingertips may not be a very practical location for a wearable device as manual dexterity could be limited. Possible solutions which have been suggested include the use of a "double-barreled" approach where an alerting device is attached to the fingers and connected to another display at a less conspicuous place

on the body, such as the abdomen, or to evaluate the degree of sensitivity of the pinna and outer ear canal to determine their viability as a potential site for a tactile aid (Sherrick, 1984). It may also be the case, however, that, although less sensitive than the fingertips, the response of more practical body locations is sufficient for the type of speech information being transmitted. This can only be determined by examining sensitivity and discrimination performance with wearable practical displays (e.g., Hnath-Chisolm and Medwetsky, 1988).

Number of Channels of Stimulation

Tactile aids use from one to many channels of stimulation. In single channel displays, information can be coded as changes in rate and/or amplitude of stimulation. The ability of the skin to perceive and discriminate variations in rate and amplitude, however, is relatively poor, especially when compared to the ear. For example, while the ear can respond to frequencies between 20–20,000 Hz, the skin is only responsive to frequencies between 10–1,000 Hz, with the best sensitivity at 250 Hz (Verillo, 1963). In addition, while the auditory difference limen for frequency is approximately 0.2%, vibrotactile difference limens range from 10%–25% with the best discrimination for frequencies below 100 Hz (Rothenberg, Verillo, Zahorian, Brachman, and Bolanowski, 1977). The skin also has a very narrow dynamic range (0–35 dB) when compared to the ear (0–130 dB) (Bekesy, 1959).

Multichannel tactile displays try to take advantage of the skin's sensitivity to differences in the location of stimulation. For example, if a two alternative forced-choice procedure is used, subjects can always discriminate two static pressures from one, even when the stimulators are placed side-by-side, occupying a total space of 1 mm (Johnson and Phillips, 1981). One problem with multichannel stimulation, however, is that there are marked masking effects when two or more body sites are stimulated simultaneously (Bekesy,

1959). Thus, with multichannel tactile aids, it is the ability to discriminate patterns of movement rather than location of stimulation that becomes important.

In recent studies, comparing tactile speech devices containing different numbers of multiple channels, some researchers have found better results, in terms of speech perception, as channel number is increased (Weisenberger, 1989), while others have not (Lynch, Eilers, Oller, and LaVoie, 1988). Clearly, more research is needed about the ability of the skin to resolve and process patterns of movement in order to help determine the optimum number of channels for a tactile speech display.

Speech Processing Strategies

The approaches used in developing speech processing strategies for tactile aids are the same as those discussed for cochlear implants. That is, in one approach an attempt is made to present speech information in a relatively unprocessed form, either as the time waveform in a single channel display or as a short-term time varying frequency spectrum in a multichannel display. Again, the task of distinguishing the important speech cues contained in such displays is left to the human receiver. The second approach is to extract information about specific features and present this information in a codified manner to the skin.

As Levitt (1988) points out, proponents of the first approach believe that the small improvements found with tactile aids are due to factors such as the poor design of early experimental devices, inappropriate and/or inadequate training. In this view, a person should be able to understand tactually presented speech as long as it is properly presented and sufficient training is given. Proponents of the speech feature approach argue that speech is a special code for which the auditory system serves as a unique decoder. Thus, the tactile modality should not be expected to adequately process the speech spectrum and in order for a tactile display to be successful, it needs to be simplified considerably by extracting and displaying only the most important speech cues. Supporters of this approach use the results of studies with Tadoma, in which articulatory cues allow for the understanding of continuous discourse, as evidence.

Current Status

Candidates

Typically, profound hearing-impaired individ uals who do not appear to receive adequate assistance from the use of conventional amplification are considered candidates for using tactile aids. Individuals can have post-

lingual or pre-lingual hearing losses and they can be children or adults. Since the use of a tactile aid is noninvasive and reversible, there do not appear to be any factors that would limit their use.

Performance

While numerous tactile speech displays have been developed and evaluated, to be useful clinically, the devices must be wearable. Both single and multichannel tactile aids have been developed.

Single Channel Displays. Most wearable tactile aids are single channel displays of the acoustic speech waveform. They include: Tactaid I (Audiological Engineering), Minivab3 (AB Instruments), Minifonator (Siemens), and TAM (Summitt). In evaluating and comparing the performance obtained with single channel displays, Weisenberger and Russell (1989) found them to be useful for simple auditory tasks, such as sound detection or environmental sound identification, while performance on tasks requiring access to fine-structure waveform information, such as phoneme identification, was relatively poor. In addition, the use of single channel displays was reported to result in overall improvements in connected discourse tracking, although the degree of intersubject variability was quite high (Spens and Plant, 1983). There is currently no evidence, however, that speech can be understood through the use of a single channel tactile display alone.

Multichannel Displays. Currently there are few commercially available multichannel spectrum displays. The simplest contain two channels and the input waveform is simply split into a low- and high-frequency region and delivered to separate transducers. Examples are the Tactaid II+ (Audiological Engineering) and the KS3/2 (Telex). Other devices divide the speech spectrum into a greater number of channels, such as the 7-channel Tactaid 7 (Audiological Engineering), 16-channel Tacticon Tc-1600 (Tacticon), and the 32-channel Audiotact (Sevrain-Tech, Inc.).

Comparisons. Comparisons of two channel with single channel tactile devices provide relatively equivocal results. For example, it has been shown that while for tasks in which fine-structure information would be beneficial, such as word identification, performance with Tactaid II was slightly better than with Minivab3, but for tasks which require envelope perception, such as syllable rhythm and stress, performance with Minivab3 was slightly better than with Tactaid II (Weisenberger, 1989). In addition, in terms of enhancing speechreading performance, some researchers have reported equivalent results, while others have reported better performance with two-channel, as opposed to single channel, devices (Miyamoto, Myres, Wagner, and Punch, 1987). Thus, the addition of a second channel does not appear to result in universal advantages.

When a 24-channel device was compared to a single channel one in terms of suprasegmental feature perception (i.e., syllable number and stress pattern), better results were obtained with the single channel aid (Carney and Bleacher, 1986). In addition, for the perception of segmental features performance was equivalent for the two devices (Carney, 1988). Although this may seem discouraging, in contrast to results obtained with single channel displays, some users of multichannel, spectral displays exhibit limited open set word recognition for words presented in isolation through touch alone, but only after substantial long-term training (e.g., Brooks, Frost, Mason, and Gibson, 1986a, b). In addition, there are data which suggest that multichannel devices are more effective for enhancing the perception of connected discourse (Weisenberger, 1989; Miyamoto, et al., 1987). As understanding connected discourse is the task most like real-life communication situations, these are important findings, which, in conjunction with experimental findings of limited open set word recognition (Brooks, et al., 1986a, b), suggest that further work geared toward the development of multichannel, spectral aids is warranted.

Two wearable tactile devices, which can be classified as speech feature displays, have been developed: Portapitch and the Tickle Talker. Portapitch is a vibrotactile, multichannel display of voice F_o developed by Boothroyd and his colleagues (Yeung, Boothroyd, and Redmond, 1988). Results indicate that the use of the device enhances the visual perception of phonologically significant speech contrasts (Hnath-Chisolm and Kishon-Rabin, 1988) and, with training, the visual perception of sentence length stimuli (Hanin, Boothroyd, and Hnath-Chisolm, 1988). Performance does not appear to be as good, however, as that obtained with auditory transmission of F_o, but it is not clear whether this is due to insufficient training, design limitations, or limitations in the tactile sense.

The Tickle Talker, described by Blamey and Clark (1985), is an electrotactile, multichannel display that is worn as a set of rings on the fingers of the hand. It extracts F_o, F2, and amplitude. It is similar in concept to the Nucleus 22-channel cochlear implant. F2 is coded as electrode position, F_o as pulse rate, and amplitude as electric pulse duration. Evaluation results indicate the device enhances the visual perception of phonemes, words, sentences, and connected discourse (Cowan, Alcantara, Blamey, and Clark, 1988). An analysis of the type of phonemic information transmitted indicates that users are receiving F_o information,

vowel information, and information about consonant voicing and manner (Blamey, Cowan, Alcantara, and Clark, 1988). Similar phonemic information is also conveyed through multichannel vocoder type displays (Brooks, et al., 1986a).

Regardless of type of design, it appears reasonable to conclude from the above discussion that tactile communication aids can effectively be used to enhance speechreading performance in deaf individuals. What may not be as clear is that gains in performance cannot be obtained without extensive training (e.g., Blamey, et al., 1988; Brooks, et al., 1986a, b; Hanin, et al., 1988). Recent research suggests that for adults this training should include both analytic and synthetic level tasks (Alcantara, Cowan, Blamey, and Clark, 1990; Hanin, et al., 1988).

Clearly children using tactile aids will also need systematic training. Unfortunately, clinical experience suggests this is not always the case. It is important that effective training methods be developed and implemented clinically. While children who receive cochlear implants are often provided with extra sensory and communication training, there are few programs for children using tactile aids. Yet, there is evidence that tactile aids can be effectively incorporated into speech and language training programs for deaf children (e.g., McGarr, Head, Friedman, Behrman, and Youdelman, 1986; Oller, Eilers, Vergera, and LaVoie, 1986). The integration of tactile speech aids early in a deaf child's training will potentially allow for the full benefits of tactile stimulation to be determined.

Another interesting possibility for the use of tactile aids is in combination with limited residual hearing as well as speechreading. Results of recent studies suggest that when tactile speech cues are combined with visual speech cues and those acoustic cues available to the severely-profoundly hearing-impaired individual through residual hearing, significant benefits are obtained. This has been shown for both adults (Cowan, Alcantara, Whitford, Blamey, and Clark, 1989) and children (Lynch, Eilers, Oller and Cobo-Lewis, 1989; Lynch, Eilers, Oller, Urbano, and Pero, 1989). Such "multisensory" stimulation may prove especially useful for children whose residual hearing, though limited, is too great for cochlear implantation. It may also be beneficial for those individuals who receive limited benefits from the use of cochlear implants.

COMPARISON OF COCHLEAR IMPLANTS TO TACTILE AIDS

Both cochlear implants and tactile aids are currently being used effectively in the treatment of profound hearing loss in both children and adults. Thus, it seems logical to ask how performance compares. Although few such comparative studies are currently available, more research is being conducted in this area. For example, Geers and Moog (1988) describe a 5-year longitudinal project in which the long-term use of cochlear implants, tactile aids, and conventional hearing aids by prelingually deaf children is being systematically compared. Preliminary results suggest higher performance levels for children with the Nucleus multichannel device than with single or two-channel tactile aids (Geers and Moog, 1989). Similar results are reported by Miyamoto, et al. (1989).

A comparison of performance by adults using the Nucleus multichannel implant to ones using the Tickle Talker tactile aid revealed similar performance for closed-set tasks, but an advantage for the implant in terms of a greater speechreading enhancement effect (Blamey, et al., 1988). There is great variability of performance by cochlear implant recipients, and in comparing the speechreading enhancement effect obtained with the use of a tactile display of F_o (i.e., Portapitch) to that obtained with the Nucleus device, it was found the tactile aid users did better than about one-third of the implantees (Kishon-Rabin, Hanin, and Boothroyd, 1990). However, overall performance was superior with the implant.

In a recent study, the performance of single channel adult cochlear implant users was compared to performance of artificially deafened subjects using single channel tactile aids (Carney, Kienle, and Miyamoto, 1990). The pattern of performance was similar for the perception of segmental and suprasegmental speech features, and significant quantitative differences were not found between group performance. This was somewhat surprising, since the implant users had much more experience with electroauditory stimulation than the artificially deafened subjects did with tactile stimulation.

One of the most difficult aspects of comparing tactile aid to cochlear implant performance concerns differences in "experience." Most reports of tactile aid use are "laboratory" experiments, where the subjects only use the devices for experimental purposes. Most cochlear implant subjects use their devices on a daily basis and thus have much more experience. In addition, with cochlear implants, the sensory signal is familiar as most adult implantees have had extensive auditory experience with language. Thus, when they first use their implants, these adults can draw upon auditory memory in learning to interpret the new, but "familiar" codes. In contrast, post-lingually deaf users of tactile aids do not appear to report an initial association between "hearing" and the tactile patterns they are receiving. Tactile aid users must learn to interpret

a novel, not a familiar sensory code. Thus, even more experience may be needed with tactile speech displays than with cochlear implants before optimal performance can be determined. The development of sophisticated wearable multichannel tactile displays may help provide users with this experience.

SUMMARY

Cochlear implants and tactile aids will continue to be used in the treatment of profound hearing loss. Single channel devices, of both types, can be beneficial, but multichannel devices appear to result in superior performance. Of all devices reviewed, open set recognition of continuous discourse has only been demonstrated with multichannel cochlear implants. Many questions, however, remain to be addressed. A basic understanding of how these cochlear implants and tactile aids work, their similarities and differences, and what can be expected with their use, can help the clinician in counseling clients and in making appropriate recommendations.

REFERENCES

Alcantara JL, Cowan RSC, Blamey PJ, Clark GM. A comparison of two training strategies for speech recognition with an electrotactile speech processor. J Speech and Hearing Res 1990;33:195–204.

Banfai P, Hortmann G, Karczqg S, Wustrow F. Results with eight-channel cochlear implants. Advances in Audiology 1984;2:1–18.

Berliner K, Tonokowa L, Dye L, House WF. Open-set speech recognition in children with a single channel cochlear implant. Ear and Hearing 1989;10:237–242.

Blamey PJ, Clark GM. Psychophysical studies relevant to the design of a digital electrotactile speech processor. J Acous Soc Am 1985;82:116–125.

Blamey PJ, Cowan RSC, Alcantara J, Clark GM. Phonemic information transmitted by a multichannel electrotactile speech processor. J Speech and Hearing Res 1988;31:620–629.

Boothroyd A. Auditory perception of speech contrasts by subjects with sensory-neural hearing loss. J Speech and Hearing Res 1984;27:134–144.

Boothroyd A, Cawkwell S. Vibrotactile thresholds in puretone audiometry. Acta Otolaryngologica 1970;69:381–387.

Boothroyd A, Hanin L, Hnath-Chisolm T, Waltzman S. Response of cochlear implantees to speech perception training. Paper presented at the annual convention of the American Speech-Language-Hearing Association, New Orleans, LA, 1987.

Briacombe JA, Beiter AL, Shallop JK, Martin EL, Fowler LP. Use of a multichannel cochlar implant by prelingually deafened adults. Paper presented at the annual convention of the American Speech-Language-Hearing Association, New Orleans, LA, 1987.

Brooks PJ, Frost BJ, Mason JL, Gibson DM. Continuing evaluation of the Queens tactile vocoder. II: Identification of open set words. J Rehab Res Dev 1986a;23:119–128.

Brooks PJ, Frost BJ, Mason JL, Gibson DM. Continuing evaluation of the Queens tactile vocoder. II: Identification of open set sentences and tracting narrative. J Rehab Res Dev 1986b;23:129–138.

Carney AE. Vibrotactile perception of segmental features of speech: a comparison of single channel and multichannel instruments. J Speech and Hearing Res 1988;31:438–448.

Carney AE, Bleacher C. Vibrotactile perception of suprasegmental features of speech: a comparison of single channel and multichannel instruments. J Acous Soc Am 1986;79:131–140.

Carney AE, Kienle M, Miyamoto RT. Speech perception in a single channel cochlear implant: a comparison with single channel tactile device. J Speech and Hearing Res 1990;33:229–237.

Chouard CH, Fugain C, Meyer B, Chabolle F. The Chorimac 12: a multichannel intracochlear implant for total deafness. Otolaryngologic Clinics of North America 1986;19:355–370.

Chute PM. Personal communication. 1991.

Chute PM, Hellman SA, Parisier SC, Selesnick SH. A matched comparison of single and multichannel cochlear implants in children. Laryngoscope 1990;100:25–28.

Clark GM, Busby PA, Roberts SA, et al. Preliminary results for the Cochlear Corporation multi-electrode intracochlear implant on six prelingually deaf patients. Am J Otology 1987;8:234–239.

Cowan RSC, Alcantara JL, Blamey PJ, Clark GM. Preliminary evaluation of a multichannel electrotactile speech processor. J Acous Soc Am 1988;83:2328–2338.

Cowan RSC, Alcantara JL, Whitford LA, Blamey PJ, Clark GM. Speech perception studies using a multichannel electrotactile speech processor, residual hearing, and lipreading. J AcousSoc Am 1989;85:2593–2607.

Dent LJ, Simmons FB, White RL, Roberts LA. Speech perception by four cochlear implant users. J Speech and Hearing Res 1987;30:480–493.

Eddington DK. Speech discrimination in deaf subjects with multichannel intracochlear electrodes. In Parkins CW, Anderson SW, Eds. Cochlear prostheses: an international symposium. New York: New York Academy of Sciences, 1983:244–258.

Fourcin AJ, Douek EE, Moore BCJ, et al. Speech perception with promonotory stimulation. In Parkins CW, Anderson SW, Eds., Cochlear prostheses: an international symposium. New York: New York Academy of Sciences, 1983:280–294.

Fretz RJ, Fravel RP. Design and function: a physical and electrical description of the 3M House cochlear implant system. Ear and Hearing 1985;6(suppl):14S–19S.

Geers AE, Moog J. Assistive listening devices: tactile aids/cochlear implants. Hearing Instruments 1988;39:6–9.

Geers AE, Moog J. Cochlear implants for children: how well do they work? Paper presented at the Annual Convention of the American Speech-Language-Hearing Association, St. Louis, MO, 1989.

Hanin L. Personal communication. 1990.

Hanin L, Boothroyd A. Speech pattern contrast perception with hearing aids and cochlear implants. Paper presented at the Annual Convention of the American Speech-Language-Hearing Association, St. Louis, MO, 1989.

Hanin L, Boothroyd A, Hnath-Chisolm T. Tactile presentation of voice fundamental frequency as an aid to speechreading sentences. Ear and Hearing 1988;9:335–341.

Hnath-Chisolm T, Kishon-Rabin L. Tactile presentation of voice fundamental frequency as an aid to the perception of speech pattern contrasts. Ear and Hearing 1988;9:329–334.

Hnath-Chisolm T, Medwetsky L. Perception of frequency contours via termporal and spatial tactile transforms. Ear and Hearing 1988;9:322–328.

Hochmair ES, Hochmair-Desoyer IJ. Aspects of sound signal processing using the Vienna intra- and extracochlear implant. In Schindler RA, Merzenich MM, Eds. Cochlear implants. New York: Raven Press, 1985:101–110.

Hochmair-Desoyer IJ, Hochmair ES, Stiglebrunner HK. Psychoacoustic temporal processing and speech understanding in cochlear implant patients. InSchindler RA, Merzenich MM, Eds. Cochlear implants. New York: Raven Press, 1985:291–304.

Hopkinson NT, McFarland WF, Owens E, et al. Report of the ad hoc committee on cohlear implants. ASHA 1986;28:29–52.

House W, Urban J. Long-term results of electrode implantation and electronic stimulation of the cochlea in man. American Annals of Otology, Rhinology, and Laryngology 1973;82:504–510.

Johnson K, Phillips J. Tactile spatial resolution. I: two-point discrimination, gap detection, grating resolution, and letter recognition. J Neurophysiology 1981;45:1177–1191.

Kirk K, Brown C. Speech and language results in children with a cochlear implant. Ear and Hearing 1985;6(suppl):36S–47S.

Kirman J. Tactile communication of speech: a review and analysis. Psycho Bull 1974;80:54–74.

Kishon-Rabin L, Hanin L, Boothroyd A. Lipreading enhancement by a spatial tactile display of fundamental frequency. Paper presented at the International Conference on Tactile Aids, Hearing Aids, and Cochlear Implants, at the National Acoustic Laboratories (NAL), Chatswood, New South Wales, Australia, 1990.

Lansing CR, Davis JM. Early versus delayed training for adult cochlear implant users: initial results. J Acad Rehab Audio 1988; 21:29–41.

Levitt H. Recurrent issues underlying the development of tactile sensory aids. Ear and Hearing 1988;9:301–305.

Luxford WM, Brackman DE. The history of cochlear implants. In Gray RE, Ed. Cochlear implants. San Diego: College Hill Press, Inc., 1985.

Lynch MP, Eilers R, Oller DK, Corbo-Lewis A. Multisensory speech perception by profoundly hearing-impaired children. J Speech and Hearing Disorders 1989;54:57–67.

Lynch MP, Eilers R, Oller DK, LaVoie E. Speech perception by congenitally deaf subjects using an electrocutaneous vocoder. J Rehab Res Dev 1988;25:41–50.

Lynch MP, Eilers R, Oller DK, Urbano RC, Pero PJ. Multisensory narrative tracking by a profoundly deaf subject using an electrocutaneous vocoder vibrotactile aid. J Speech and Hearing Res 1989;32:331–338.

McGarr N, Head J, Friedman M, Behrman AM, Youdelman K. The use of visual and tactile sensory aids in speech production training: a preliminary report. J Rehab Res Dev 1986;23: 101–109.

Michaelson RP. Electrical stimulation of the human cochlea. Arch Otolaryngology 1971;93:317–323.

Miyamoto RT, Myres WA, Wagner M, Punch JL. Vibrotactile devices as sensory aids for the deaf. Otolaryngology Head and Neck Surgery 1987;97:57–63.

Miyamoto RT, Osberger MJ, Robbins AJ, et al. Comparison of sensory aids in deaf children. Ann Otology, Rhinology and Laryngology 1989;98:2–7.

National Institute of Health Conference Statement: Cochlear implants (1988).

Oller DK, Eilers RE, Vegera K, LaVoie E. Tactual vocoders in a multisensory program training speech production and reception. Volta Rev 1986;88:21–36.

Osberger MJ. Audiological rehabilitaion with cochlear implants and tactile aids. ASHA 1990;32:38–43.

Parkin JL, Dankowski MK. Speech performance by patients with multichannel cochlear implants. Otolaryngology, Head, and Neck Surgery 1986;95:205–209.

Pickett J, McFarland W. Auditory implants and tactile aids for the profoundly deaf. J Speech and Hearing Res 1985;28:134–150.

Reed CM, Durlach NI, Braida LD. Research on tactile communication of speech: a review. ASHA Monographs 1982;20.

Robbins A, Berry SW, Osberger MJ, Miyamoto RT. Longitudinal evaluation of children using a tactile aid or cochlear implant. Paper presented at the annual convention of the American Speech-Hearing-Language Association, St. Louis, MO, 1989.

Rosen S, Walliker J, Briacombe JA, Edgerton BJ. Prosodic and segmental aspects of speech perception with the House/3M single channel implant. J Speech and Hearing Res 1989;32:93–111.

Rothenberg M, Verillo R, Zohorian S, Brachman M, Bolanowski S. Vibrotactile frequency for encoding a speech parameter. J Acous Soc Am 1977;62:1029–1038.

Schindler R, Kessler DK. The UCSF/Storz cochlear implant: patient performance. Am J Otology 1987;8:247–255.

Sherrick CE. Basic and applied research on tactile aids for deaf people: progress and prospects. J Acous Soc Am 1984;75:1325–1342.

Simmons FB. Electrical stimulation of the auditory nerve in man. Arch Otolaryngology 1966;84:24–76.

Spens KE, Plant GL. A "tactual" hearing aid for the deaf. Speech Transmission Quarterly Progress and Status Report 1983;1:52–56.

Tong YC, Clark GM, Blamey PJ, Busby PA, Dowell RC. Psychophysical studies for two multiple-channel cochlear implant patients. J Acous Soc Am 1982;71:153–160.

Tye-Murray N, Lowder M, Tyler R. Comparison of the F_0F2 and F_0F1F2 processing strategies for the Cochlear Corporation cochlear implant. Ear and Hearing 1990;11:195–200.

Tye-Murray N, Tyler R. Auditory consonant and word recognition among cochlear implant users. Ear and Hearing 1989;10:292–298.

Tyler RS. Open-set word recognition with the 3M/Vienna single-channel cochlear implant. Laryngoscope 1988;98:999–1002.

Tyler RS, Moore B, Kuk K. Performance of some of the better cochlear implant patients. J Speech and Hearing Res 1989;32:887–911.

Verillo R. Effect of contactor area on the vibrotactile threshold. J Acous Soc Am 1963;35:1962–1966.

von Bekesy G. Similarities between hearing and skin sensations. Psych Rev 1959;6:1–22.

Waltzman S, Cohen NL, Spivak L, et al. Improvements in speech perception and production ability in children using a multichannel cochlear implant. Laryngoscope 1990;100:240–243.

Weinstein S. Intensive and extensive aspects of tactile sensitivity as a function of body part, sex, and laterality. In Kenshalo DR, Ed. The skin senses. Springfield, Ill: Charles C. Thomas, 1968.

Weisenberger J. Tactile aids for speech perception and production by hearing-impaired people. Volta Review 1989;79–100.

Weisenberger JM, Russell AF. Comparison of two single-channel vibrotactile aids for the hearing-impaired. J Speech and Hearing Res 1989;32:83–92.

Wilson BS, Finley CC, Farmer JC, et al. Comparative studies of speech processing strategies for cochlear implants. Laryngoscope 1988;98:1069–1077.

Yeung E, Boothroyd A, Redmond C. A wearable multichannel tactile display of voice fundamental frequency. Ear and Hearing 1988;6:342–350.

CHAPTER 47

Habilitation and Education of Deaf and Hard-of-Hearing Children

Laura S. McKirdy and Michele Klimovitch

Hearing impairment leads to a broad array of symptoms that affect all aspects of speech and language to varying degrees. In general, the more severe the hearing loss, the greater the impact; but even mild hearing problems can have serious consequences for the development of language in children (Roeser and Downs, 1981; Northern and Downs, 1978; Davis, Shepard, Stelmachowicz, and Gorga, 1981).

The limitations that result from hearing loss spill over into other domains as well. Because the vast majority of hearing-impaired children are born to hearing parents (Rawlings and Jensema, 1977), there is an erosion of the fundamental channel by which children and their caregivers establish communication, i.e., the spoken word. Coupled with this inability to engage in the comfortable verbal give and take of early parent-child conversation, which in and of itself has enormous consequences for the child's emotional development, is the concommitant deep sense of grief that families experience when they learn that their child is hearing impaired. This child represents "shattered dreams" (Moses, 1985). Hearing impairment of any degree severe enough to interfere with language acquisition, or with the easy flow of conversation in any listening situation that is less than optimal, has lifelong implications. Understanding what these implications are is at the heart of designing an educational program that will enable the child to function successfully in life. To these authors who have worked with hearing-impaired individuals over the past 25 years it is also of vital importance that the hearing-impaired child develop a positive self-concept, that includes his hearing loss, and not a view of himself as an imperfect individual. This measure of self-acceptance does not imply a lessening of goals. It does, however, require acceptance of the child by the family and a willingness of all parties to make the adjustments and compensations that are necessary in light of the hearing impairment to enable the child to function to his or her fullest potential. Such a view requires that professionals assess and make recommendations for the education of each child and his or her family on the basis of what is best for that child rather than operating from a particular philosophical position. The field of education of the hearing impaired has long been torn with arguments among professionals about the best way to educate children; i.e., through an aural-oral approach alone or using a combined aural-oral plus manual communication approach (Moores, 1987).

The professionals who deal with families at the time of initial diagnosis are in a very powerful position. Families are vulnerable at this time and probably have had no prior experience with hearing loss except for perhaps an older relative who might have developed a hearing problem. Typically, the family suspects that their child has a hearing problem for about a year before having their suspicions confirmed (see Vernon and Andrews 1990 for a comprehensive discussion of the dynamics surrounding the diagnosis of hearing impairment). Once diagnosis is made, parents usually seek medical advice in the hope that the problem can be solved medically; they seek second opinions regarding the diagnosis. Eventually, they begin the process of fitting the child with hearing aids and making decisions about what will be done to educate their child. Parents must make these important decisions at the time they are the most vulnerable (Levine, 1960).

Parents initial concern about their child's hearing impairment is its effect on the development of speech. Their emphasis is on oral production without a realization of the depth of the impairment and its impact on language itself (Moores, 1987). Usually, the first people with whom they have extended conversations about hearing loss and its implications are the audiologists who made the initial diagnosis. Clinical experience has shown that their advice heavily influences families. Because hearing impairment may, directly or indirectly, affect functioning in several developmental areas as well as possibly coexisting with other handicapping conditions, the audiologist must recognize that recommendations for training and education must be made by an interdisciplinary team. The audiologist cannot and should not function autonomously.

Audiologists must have a broad understanding of the issues that are specific to hearing-impaired children. They must approach each child and family on an individual basis and must wait for the results of comprehensive interdisciplinary assessments before making any predictions or promises.

CENTRAL ISSUES IN UNDERSTANDING AND PLANNING HABILITATION

The audiologist (or any other team member) dealing with hearing-impaired children should:

1. Understand the impact of hearing loss on speech and language development (see Chapter 39 for an in-depth treatment of this issue). This includes an awareness of the impact of chronic otitis media, unilateral hearing loss, and mild to moderate degrees of hearing on learning (Roeser and Downs, 1981; Hull and Dilka, 1984; Vernon and Andrews 1990). It is of particular importance that the audiologist convey the difference between speech and language to families.

2. Be trained and experienced in the diagnosis of hearing loss in a pediatric population. This will ensure that assessment is conducted reliably and efficiently. This, in turn, will minimize the time between diagnosis of hearing loss, fitting of amplification and the initiation of intervention, a process which commonly and unnecessarily lasts 18–24 months (see Beauchaine, Barlow and Stelmachowicz, 1990).

3. Be familiar with the various amplification devices, so that the child is provided with an optimal auditory signal under a variety of listening conditions. This may mean different amplification equipment is required for different listening situations (e.g., one-to-one listening in quiet versus listening in a playgroup or classroom). Amplification systems might include personal hearing aids, FM auditory trainers, and vibrotactile devices (see Chapters 42, 43, 44, 46);

4. Be familiar with the array of educational options available to families and children, including, among others, the acoupedic approach; aural-oral approach; cued speech; total communication; American Sign Language; expectations for the child with a cochlear implant; 1:1 versus small group instruction, etc.

5. Be familiar with resources available to families within the geographic region. This is suggested because of the low incidence of profound loss, and lesser degrees of hearing loss may receive little if any special attention within local schools. Therefore, it may be necessary to look for regional resources to assist the child and the family.

6. Recognize that his or her expertise is an essential component of an interdisciplinary team approach and that the audiologist's participation is required on an ongoing basis. The role of the audiologist is a great deal more than simply the provider of an audiogram and of an amplification system. He or she needs to be an active participant in the decision making and education process and not an independent entity who functions solely from the clinic. The audiologist should help the child's teachers and therapists set expectations for listening behavior and set goals for auditory training. This includes providing information about the parts of the speech spectrum that are audible to the child, the sentence length the child can process auditorily, the rate of speech that is the most effective for that child. (See Chapter 33 for discussion of the role of the educational audiologist.)

7. Keep abreast of research regarding the effectiveness of various intervention strategies on the performance of hearing impaired children; and

8. Have knowledge and experience in how to communicate with families in a supportive and clear manner (Luterman, 1979).

INTERDISCIPLINARY TEAM ASSESSMENT

Effective planning for the hearing-impaired child can be accomplished best through the efforts of an interdisciplinary team. The team members bring expertise in their individual disciplines, combined with experience and knowledge in the special needs of hearing-impaired children. The child's parents, too, need to be included in the assessment and management process so that their strengths, needs, and priorities for their child can be addressed. The Individuals with Disabilities Education Act (IDEA) specifies components of assessment that are required to determine the child's eligibility for free appropriate public education as well as support services.

The assessment team examines functioning in several areas: (a) sensory systems; (b) fine and gross motor development; (c) cognitive abilities; (d) social/emotional status; (e) speech and language development; and (f) self-help skills.

An assessment team for a hearing-impaired child should include: (a) an audiologist; (b) a speech-language pathologist; (c) a psychologist; (d) a social worker; (e) a teacher of the hearing impaired; (f) a learning-disabilities specialist; and (g) developmental motor specialists—occupational and physical therapists; (h) family members; and (i) any medical specialists who would enhance the understanding of a child's specific needs (e.g., a pediatric neurologist, opthalmologist, otologist).

Audiologist's Role on the Team

Ideally, the audiologist should have background and training in pediatric and educational audiology, but in practice there are few such individuals. He or she is responsible for providing information about: (*a*) the type and extent of the hearing loss (e.g., conductive versus sensory neural; permanent versus intermittent; static versus progressive); (*b*) the child's amplified hearing (how much of the speech signal is within the child's range of audibility and how clear is that signal under a variety of listening conditions); (*c*) how the amplification should be set and used under a variety of listening conditions; and (*d*) how often hearing should be reevaluated, both unaided and aided, to assure that the child is receiving an optimal signal. In addition the audiologist should explain these findings to other professionals and the child's family. Figure 47.1 is a fact sheet that we have found useful when children are sent for audiological assessment. It allows us to gather information that we as habilitators and educators need. We also ask audiologists to provide information about how a child's amplification equipment should be set.

Finally, the audiologist can perform a very useful ongoing diagnostic function by working, with a child's teachers, therapists, and family. Frequently, observations outside the diagnostic setting can establish the

REQUIRED AUDIOLOGICAL INFORMATION

The following information and test results are required by our school to program effectively for your child.
1. Annual Otological Evaluation
2. Annual Audiological Evaluation
   a. Immittance testing for each ear
   b. Puretone air and bone conduction threshold testing for each ear
   c. Spondee threshold (SRT) testing for each ear
   d. Speech detection threshold testing for each ear if SRTs cannot be obtained
   e. Word discrimination scores for each ear
   f. Most comfortable and uncomfortable loudness levels for each ear
3. Semi-annual Amplification/Implant Assessment
   a. Electroacoustic analysis of each hearing aid or FM worn by child
   b. Speech processor map/tune up as necessary
   c. Warble tone sound field threshold testing (from 250–4000 Hz) for each ear and binaurally
   d. Spondee detection thresholds for each ear and binaurally
   e. Word discrimination scores for each ear and binaurally
   f. Description of earmolds
   g. Hearing aid data sheet

Figure 47.1. Information sheet given to parents before evaluation by outside specialists to ensure that the necessary information will be available for proper programming for the child.

need for adjustments of amplification equipment or bring to light a change in hearing status.

Speech/Language Pathologist

Of all team members, this group has the widest general background in the areas of speech and language acquisition and development—the areas most affected by hearing loss. It is usually the speech pathologist, in public school settings, who is called on to provide information about hearing-impaired children. Yet, a nationwide survey (Hochberg, Leavitt, and Osberger, 1983) revealed that few speech/language pathologists had special training in diagnosing and treating the hearing-impaired child. Nevertheless, they can, expand their knowledge to address the needs of the hearing-impaired child. In a subsequent section of this chapter specific diagnostic tools and strategies for the speech/language pathologist will be discussed.

In general, this professional should provide a comprehensive profile of the child's communicative functioning including the ability to understand and use language (irrespective of whether signed and/or spoken) phonologically, semantically, syntactically, and pragmatically. In addition, the assessment should address any factors that would impede the child's ability to develop communicative competence (e.g., physical factors, such as impaired oral-motor coordination, or social problems, such as extreme withdrawal). This team member should develop a plan for intervention based on the results of the assessment that includes goals for the child in three areas: (1) development of use of residual hearing (in conjunction with the audiologist); (2) development of speech (phonology, voice-pitch and melody, and rhythm); and (3) development of receptive and expressive language.

Psychologist

The psychologist's job is to define the child's current level of cognitive and social-emotional functioning as well as to give an indication of learning potential. It is of utmost importance that this assessment be conducted by someone familiar with hearing-impaired children (and their families) and with instruments that provide an unbiased assessment of competencies (see Vernon and Andrews, 1990 for a comprehensive discussion of this issue). Unless the examiner and the test selected are appropriate, a biased assessment of the child may be obtained. For example, the hearing-impaired child may have language deficits that preclude complete understanding of the directions or of the need to perform a task within time constraints. Unfortunately, there are very few psychologists with specific expertise in this area and few tests that have been normed with this population (Levine, 1974). Consequently, children are frequently diagnosed as having limiited potential when, in fact, the problem has been the administration of inappropriate tests and/or the misinterpretation of test findings by individuals who are not familiar with the working style or special communication needs of hearing-impaired children. Audiologists and speech/language pathologists should therefore, familiarize themselves with tools that are appropriate as they may well be asked for assistance in selecting tests and in determining whether an assessment accurately represents a child's level of cognitive functioning. For example, tests heavily weighted with verbal items will reflect the child's language abilities but not necessarily cognitive abilities. Zieziula (1982) Vernon and Andrews (1990), and Bradley-Johnson and Evans (1991) provide guides to the selection of tests.

Assuming that the results are valid and reliable, a comprehensive psychological test battery can offer a clear picture of a child's strengths and needs that can be extremely useful in planning the child's educational program.

Learning Disabilities Specialist

Although in some children it may be clearly shown that hearing impairment is the primary problem, data indicate that approximately one-third of hearing-impaired children have secondary disabilities that interfere with their ability to profit from instruction (Shildroth, Rawlings, and Allen, 1989). Often, these problems are not readily apparent until the child begins to have difficulty learning to read, write, or compute. In conjunction with other team members, the learning disabilities specialist can provide an analysis of the factors that may be interfering with a child's ability to master these skills and offer educational strategies for remediation.

Educator of the Hearing Impaired

Common sense dictates that this professional, by training and experience, is the team member with the most knowledge about hearing impairment and its affect on learning. Educators will be knowledgeable about the curriculum, teaching strategies, and the network of support services that can be provided to enable a hearing-impaired child to function successfully in the school environment. It is rare, however, in the authors' experience, that such individuals are called on to provide diagnostic and habilitative information, except in educational settings that specialize in hearing impairment (e.g., schools for the deaf or regional programs for the hearing impaired). The rea-

sons for this seem to be twofold. First, there is no special requirement under IDEA to include such individuals in the diagnostic process, and second, few educators of the hearing impaired are found in general educational settings. Nevertheless, with Part H of IDEA only now beginning to be implemented across the nation, the hope is that educators of the hearing impaired will be included on core teams for assessing and educating hearing impaired preschoolers.

Social Worker

Traditionally, the social worker makes the primary contact with the family and is responsible for gathering case history information. The social worker also makes observations of family dynamics as they relate to the hearing-impaired child, their attitudes about hearing loss, and the ways in which they have adapted to address the needs of the hearing-impaired child. The social worker should be familiar with hearing impairment to help develop an effective intervention plan for the child and his family. The insights provided by the social worker about the family, and its workings, will be invaluable in understanding the child in the educational setting and in setting expectations for family participation.

In addition to the above responsibilities, the social worker serves as a liaison between the school and other community/social service agencies.

Other Team Members

Occasionally, an evaluation requires the services of other professionals. A child, for example, may demonstrate problems in attention, coordination, or affect that will interfere with his or her ability to profit from instruction. Referral to appropriate professionals, such as occupational and physical therapists, pediatric neurologists, ophthalmologists, may be warranted to develop a complete understanding of the child's needs. The Conference of Educational Administrators Serving the Deaf (1989) has written a comprehensive paper, discussing the various configurations a team may take when assessing a multiply handicapped child.

Hospital, Clinic Based Assessment

The assessment team described above meets the requirements of the laws governing the education of handicapped children and is chiefly concerned with issues that are immediately relevant to the educational process. It does not, however, take into account the vital role served by the medical community in the management and correction of hearing problems. Careful medical evaluation is an integral part of the diagnostic process, while ongoing medical management is essential to ensuring that children are able to maximize their use of residual hearing. Because 50–60% of cases of congenital hearing impairment are genetically based (Vernon and Andrews, 1990), comprehensive medical evaluation is also crucial to determine if there are associated physical problems. There are certain syndromes that may have associated problems that require medical attention (e.g., hearing loss with accompanying kidney dysfunction).

A comprehensive assessment therefore, should include a medical profile as well as information specifically addressing issues that will affect the child in an educational setting. However, irrespective of the etiology, the effects of hearing impairment on speech/language acquisition and development, and on the ability to understand language day by day are educational concerns.

ASSESSMENT COMPONENTS

Audiological Evaluation

For a detailed discussion of audiological evaluation of the hearing-impaired infant and school age child refer to appropriate sections of this volume. Madell (1989) summarizes the fundamental components of an audiological assessment to be:

1. Unaided (puretone audiometry, speech recognition testing, and immittance testing);
2. Sound field testing (aided and unaided);
3. Real ear measurements;
4. Electroacoustic analysis of amplification equipment; and a
5. Comprehensive written report.

Madell (1989) discusses the importance of early and appropriate selection of an amplification system as being the single most important habilitative tool for the hearing-impaired child. She feels that even children with mild and unilateral sensory neural hearing losses should be considered candidates for amplification in early childhood because of the crucial role that hearing plays in language and speech acquisition.

Speech and Language Evaluation

The speech and language evaluation must be comprehensive as these are the areas primarily affected by hearing impairment. From the point of view of production alone, hearing impairment interferes with the subtle coordination of respiration, phonation, resonation, and articulation.

When assessing the child's speech production skills and the ability to improve speech production, four areas should be investigated: (1) auditory speech perception; (2) phonetic production; (3) phonologic produc-

tion; (4) speech intelligibility (Dunn and Newton, 1986; Osberger, 1983).

Assessment of Speech Perception

The assessment of speech perception involves two important aspects of the child's ability to receive a spoken message through hearing. First, a determination is made of the hearing level at which speech can be perceived auditorially (detection, discrimination, identification, or comprehension). Second, a determination is made of the linguistic level at which the child can comfortably perceive speech patterns and the point at which he or she has difficulty (i.e., isolated sound, syllable, word, sentence, conversation, class lecture). Tests useful for the assessment of these particular skills are the Test of Auditory Comprehension (Office of Los Angeles County Superintendent of Schools, 1976) and the Glendonald Auditory Screening Test (Erber, 1982), and the Computer Assisted Speech Perception Testing and Training Program (Boothroyd, 1987). Administration of these tests should be supplemented with observations of the student's performance in the classroom

Phonetic Assessment

A comprehensive oral-motor evaluation that might reveal any gross neurological or anatomical limitations interfering with the production of speech sounds should be conducted before completing a phonetic inventory. The phonetic inventory, traditionally, is conducted by asking the child to imitate nonsense syllables (Dunn and Newton, 1986). One inventory that is frequently used and was specifically designed for asessing hearing impaired children's speech is Ling's (1976) Phonetic Level Evaluation (PLE). The limitations of a nonsense syllable assessment are detailed by Dunn and Newton (1986 and by Abraham, Stocker, and Allen (1988).

Phonologic Assessment

Ling's (1976) phonologic assessment examines both segmental and suprasegmental skills. The segmental analysis determines whether the child is producing vowels, dipthongs, consonants, and consonant clusters correctly in a variety of word positions. The suprasegmental analysis examines the child's use of prosodic features (e.g., rhythm, stress) to express meaning. Although Ling's phonologic assessment was designed specifically for the hearing impaired, any comprehensive articulation test can give fundamental information regarding the child's phonological system. Most articulation tests, however, are not geared to examine production of suprasegmentals. This information must be gathered through observation of the child's speech in context. The reader is referred to Subtelny, Orlando, & Whitehead (1981) as well as Ling (1976) and Abraham et al. (1988) for further information regarding phonological assessment.

Speech Intelligibility

Several procedures have been used to determine whether the speech of the hearing-impaired speaker is understood by unfamiliar listeners. The simplest procedure is to have listeners write what they heard. Other techniques include use of rating scales (Subtelny, 1977) or forced choice techniques whereby the listener chooses from a set of alternatives (SPAC, Boothroyd, 1985; Speech Intelligibility Evaluation, Monsen, 1981). Carney (1986) provides a comprehensive review of this issue.

Language Assessment

There are only a few tests available that have normative data for a hearing-impaired population. Language tests normed on a hearing population to assess hearing-impaired children often necessitate adaptations, such as modification of the stimulus-response demands and the use of sign language. Such adaptations can affect test score interpretation and jeopardize the established validity and reliability of the instrument (Abraham and Stocker, 1988; Moeller, McConley, and Osberger 1982). In spite of these limitations, the assessments are useful in providing a clear picture of the child's current level of language comprehension and usage, including use of semantics, syntax, and a variety of pragmatic functions. The preferred mode of communication must be taken into account as well as the ability to alter communication depending on the needs of the audience. For example, if the child's predominant language mode is a signed system, then assessment must be conducted in that mode. Assessments that investigate the child's understanding of the printed word and his ability to express himself in writing may be included also.

Moeller (1988) states that observations before the actual evaluation permit the tester to formulate appropriate questions and to observe the unique ways in which the child uses language so that intervention priorities can be established.

Kretchmer and Kretchmer (1988) contrast product versus process assessment models in language evaluations. In product assessment models, achievement tests, tests of syntactic knowledge, vocabulary tests are used. Process assessment samples a child's performance over time and in a variety of contexts (e.g., language sampling, observations of conversation or other discourse units). Both types of assessment are necessary to plan effective intervention.

Appendix 47.1 includes language comprehension and use tests that have been developed specifically for hearing-impaired children.

Speechreading

The ability to decode speech using visual information can be assessed both formally and informally. During audiological testing of children with severely impaired hearing, the audiologist will frequently report the difference between the child's ability to discriminate phonetically balanced word lists auditorily alone and when visual cues are included. The difference score provides an indication of the contribution vision plays in clarifying the signal. Formal tools for assessing speechreading ability include tests such as How Well Do You Read Lips (Utley, 1946) and the Craig (1964) Lipreading Inventory. Yoshinaga-Itano (1988) cautions that traditional sentence speechreading tests have not been analyzed for the degree they require semantic and syntactic knowledge and may therefore be tests of linguistic ability rather than speechreading ability. She favors analysis that examines the child's ability to get the gist of a message rather than an analysis of ability to identify individual words or phonemes. DeFilippo (1990) discusses the complexity of assessment and training of speechreading and argues for its importance in helping hearing impaired individuals communicate.

Reading and Writing

Successful reading and writing skills have their foundation in knowledge and use of the language code (Laughton, 1988; Tattershall, 1988). Any limitations in language base will affect the child's ability to use that system in its printed form. The deficiencies of profoundly deaf individuals in mastering reading are widely reported (see Quigley and Kretchmer 1982 for a comprehensive review), but the more subtle influences of a less severe hearing loss are not generally recognized. There is a body of data that indicates that a hearing impairment of any degree sufficient to interfere with normal language acquisition will also seriously impede normal acquisition of reading and writing skills (Davis, Shepard, Stelmachowicz, and Gorga 1981; Berg, 1971; Trybus and Karchmer, 1977).

Assessment measures may be formal, informal, standardized, criterion-referenced, diagnostic, or teacher made. The goal of the assessment is to determine the child's knowledge and use of language and his ability to apply it to the reading and writing process so that strategies can be developed to improve reading performance.

Psychological and Psychoeducational Assessment

By law (IDEA), all materials and procedures used in evaluating a child must be in his native language. For the hearing-impaired child, the normal communication mode may be either signed or spoken language. Vernon and Andrews (1990) and Bradley-Johnson and Evans (1991) discuss, in depth, factors that must be taken into consideration when testing a hearing-impaired individual. Major factors to be considered are:

1. The majority of intelligence and personality tests rely heavily on verbal language. Administration of such tests may in actuality measure the child's knowledge of language rather than the attributes for which it was designed.
2. Hearing-impaired individuals do not respond well in timed measures because under time constraints they demonstrate a tendency to rush to complete their work (Zieziula, 1982).
3. There is poor test reliability for young hearing-impaired children (Vernon and Andrews, 1990).

Appendix 47.2 adapted from Vernon and Andrews (1990) outlines psychological and educational tests that can be used successfully with hearing-impaired children.

It sometimes happens that family members and professionals disagree about the best course of action. Some parents find it difficult to accept any recommendation that singles out their child as being different. Thus, they may refuse to have their child use a hearing aid or FM system or be unwilling to consider sign language or cued speech as educational tools. The diagnostic team and family must then decide on a course of action that represents a compromise, because without parental support any program is doomed to failure. There are occasionally instances when views are so divergent that a system of due process (a series of legal proceedings) is invoked in an attempt to reach agreement.

Team Planning

When assessment is completed, ideally all team members meet together to review the results of their testing and to develop a plan of action that meets the strengths and needs of the child and the family. When such a plan is developed by a public school, it is known as an Individualized Educational Plan (IEP) for children ages 3–21 and as an Individualized Family Service Plan (IFSP) for children ages birth through age 2

years. For the youngest children, this plan must be reviewed and updated, at least, every 6 months. For older children, the review is annual or sooner if needed. Key issues such as: (a) the educational approach that will be used and (b) the educational setting that will be most appropriate are addressed. The resources within the region are also explored.

The plan will include:

1. Long- and short-term goals;
2. A description of who will provide services;
3. How the services will be delivered (e.g., frequency, duration, individually versus group) to meet the goals;
4. An evaluation component to review whether programming has been effective; and
5. Any special support services that the child may require (e.g., FM systems, tutor-notetakers, interpreters).

MAJOR DISTINCTIONS IN EDUCATIONAL APPROACHES

After a comprehensive assessment, the team selects intervention strategies for enhancing the child's ability to understand and use language. It is generally agreed that auditory training and speech training are key elements of the education of the hearing-impaired child. The great distinction between educational approaches for hearing-impaired children is whether the approach also uses a manual form of language. Those that do not include a manual form are known as oral (or aural-oral or auditory-oral) options and may or may not include the visual support of speechreading. Information regarding each of the options will be discussed below and the reader is asked to be sensitive to issues describing philosophy versus those issues which describe methodology.

Oral Options

Within the oral options, there are subtle distinctions regarding the relative emphasis placed on the use of residual hearing and vision. The unisensory approach described below relies on residual hearing almost exclusively and speechreading occurs only in the natural context of daily living. In general, children who learn language through the oral method receive input through a combination of speechreading and amplification of sound while expressing themselves through speaking. There is no use of formal sign language or fingerspelling. Up until the early 1970s, this was the predominant method of educating hearing-impaired children in the United States, but a survey of 1,760 teachers of the hearing impaired found that only 32% were currently using an oral-only approach (Woodward, Allen, and Shildroth, 1985). The oral approach is predicated on the philosophy that language is most readily learned through audition and that "... only oral education can give children access to the auditory and/or articulatory codes on which language is based" (Ling, 1984, p. 9). The approach most nearly mirrors the normal path to speech and language acquisition. If a child is able to master language and acquire intelligible speech by using this approach, there is increased opportunity to function as normally as possible within the hearing world. The approach emphasizes integration within society in general.

Ling (1984) and Gatty (1987) report that there is much individual variability in children's ability to acquire speech by using the oral approach—some are very successful, others are not. Factors that seem to influence degree of success include the amount of residual hearing, the absence of additional handicaps, and the degree of parental involvement.

Research that has been directed at comparing students educated using an oral approach in contrast with students using other approaches has been extremely difficult to evaluate because there are self-selecting variables, i.e., children who are not successful in oral programs tend to be transferred to total communication programs (e.g., Musselman, Lindsay, and Wilson, 1988). Nevertheless, those children who do meet with success demonstrate high levels of spoken language proficiency (Jensema, Karchmer, and Trybus, 1978; Greenberg, 1980; Geers, Moog, and Schick, 1984; Luetke-Stahlman, 1988).

Unisensory Approach

The unisensory approach is a subcategory of the oral approach. It posits that oral communication skills are acquired most naturally through audition. Young children are not directly encouraged to adopt visual speechreading strategies and visual cues are withheld as much as possible. Communication training is conducted with the speaker's mouth covered so that the child relies exclusively on auditory information. The unisensory approach is also known as the acoupedic approach and its proponents include Pollack (1970, 1981, 1984), Beebe et al. (1984); and Grammatico (1975).

Cued Speech

Lying midway between oral options and options that use a manual form of language is cued speech (developed by Cornett 1967). Cued speech was developed to eliminate the ambiguities of speechreading. It uses a system of eight handshapes and four hand positions shown near the face. Two-thirds of English sounds look similar to other sounds on the lips, therefore they

are "cued" differently to enable users to decode speech phonemically. The Woodward et al. (1985) survey revealed that cued speech was used by 0.3% of the teachers.

Research concerning the use of cued speech as a tool for first language acquisition and as an educational method is gradually being generated and has shown promise for the reception of language by young children (Nicholls, 1979). It has been embraced as having a proper place within the oral education of hearing-impaired children, and it has also found a place within some total communication programs (Ling, 1984; Williams-Scott and Kipila, 1987). In our school (which is a total communication program), cued speech is used to teach phonics, to provide a visual referent for words for which there are no formal signs, for nonsense words that occur in children's rhymes and songs, and in some testing situations when the sign itself might give away the answer (e.g., the sign for "nose" is formed by pointing to the nose) (Otero, 1986). Signs that are visually descriptive of the spoken word are known as iconic signs.

Total Communication

Gustason, et al. (1972) points out that *total communication* (TC) is neither a method nor a prescribed system of instruction, but rather a philosophy. Moores (1987, p. 11) states, "A total communication philosophy endorses the right of every every hearing-impaired child to communicate by whatever means are found to be beneficial. Communication might be by speech, by signs, by gesture, by writing, or by some other means depending on the circumstances." The term, therefore, embraces all forms of communication and the selection of one form or another depends on the needs of the individual and the particular situation. In common practice, the term *total communication* has come to be synonymous with simultaneous communication, that is one in which signs and fingerspelling and speech are used together as the educational mode. Children receive input through speechreading, amplification, signs, and fingerspelling. They express themselves in speech, signs, and fingerspelling.

It is important to bear in mind that, philosophically, total communication embraces the full array of alternatives and does not endorse the use of sign language to the exclusion aural-oral communication. Ling (1984) summarizes the major tenets of a total communication philosophy as follows:

1. All visual-manual and/or auditory roles in the communication process are complementary;
2. Early identification and full acceptance of the child as a hearing-impaired individual by both

the parents and the school are necessary to ego development and self-concept;

3. Total communication should begin when the disability of deafness is first diagnosed to provide for immediate communication learning and language development; and

4. Increased learning potential is achieved with the added dimension of a multisensory approach (p. 1).

A variety of sign systems are currently in use in total communication programs. These include sign systems that have been invented to manually code English and American Sign Language.

American Sign Language

American Sign Language (ASL) is a formal visually spatially based language that meets all the linguistic requirements for definition as a language. It possesses unique semantic, syntactic, morphological, transformational, and "phonologic" (designated as cheremes) rules (Stokoe, 1958; Klima and Bellugi, 1979; Wilbur 1976). Concepts can be communicated at the same rate of transmission as spoken language (Klima and Bellugi, 1979). ASL is the third most common language in the U.S. with an estimated 500,000 users (Johnson, 1988).

There is currently heated discussion among educators of the deaf regarding the efficacy of teaching ASL as the first language for hearing-impaired children as it may be a more "natural" language for them to acquire. English would then be taught as a second language (Johnson, Liddell, and Erting, 1989). As there is incongruity between ASL and spoken language, development of oral speech and audition are not priorities. The role of the deaf community in the education and socialization of the deaf child is emphasized. Pointing to national data regarding academic deficiencies of the deaf (e.g., Trybus and Karchmer, 1977), proponents of this position argue that current methods to educate the deaf (i.e., oral methods and manually coded forms of English) have been unsuccessful for large numbers of deaf children. They hypothesize that use of ASL as the language for education and the concommitant involvement of the deaf child within the deaf community can reverse this trend.

Fingerspelling

Each of the 26 letters of the alphabet is formed with one hand. The letters are then combined to spell words. Fingerspelling has been used as an educational method both in Russia and the U.S. It is known here as the Rochester method. Speech is represented by the rapid fingerspelling of the spoken message. Quigley (1969) compared a group of 3½ to 7½ year old deaf children trained orally alone with a group that were taught by the Rochester method. The latter group was superior in speechreading, written language, and reading.

Manually Coded English

There are several systems of manually coded English (MCE) that have been developed to provide a visual word for word, morpheme for morpheme, representation of English (Wilbur, 1987). The most widely known of these systems are Signing Exact English (SEE 2) (Gustason, Pfetzing, and Zawolkow, 1972) and Signed English (Bornstein and Saulnier, 1981; Bornstein, Saulnier and Hamilton, 1980). All use ASL signs as a base but then invent signs for noncontent words (e.g., articles, affixes, suffixes, and tense markers that are omitted or coded differently in ASL). The system known as Signed English limits itself to the use of the fourteen most common English morphological markers to increase the efficiency of simultaneous speaking and signing.

Since MCE is a contrived system and not a natural language like ASL, the question has been raised as to whether it is, in fact, learnable. A study by Schick and Moeller (1992) explored this issue with a group of 13 profoundly deaf students ranging in age from 7 to 14 years. They found that MCE was indeed learnable and that the students showed expressive English skills that were comparable to a group of normal-hearing controls for many (but not all) features of English syntax and vocabulary.

Pidgin Sign English

Pidgin Sign English (PSE) exists along a continuum that has ASL at one end and English at the other. It is comprised of ASL signs used in English word order with many English grammatical markers. Studies of PSE have found that two variables control its linguistic forms. The first variable is the interpersonal context. The more formal the setting, the more English grammatical elements are incorporated. The second variable concerns the sign language competence of the normal hearing user of PSE. The more proficient the signer becomes, the more ASL is used.

Cochlear Implants

Although not specifically an educational option, the use of cochlear implants in pediatric populations presents an alternative when traditional amplification equipment has been unsuccessful. There have been very promising results reported recently regarding the auditory and speech skills of young implanted children including sound detection and discrimination of time and intensity cues (Berliner et al., 1985) and ability to understand speech without speechreading (Berliner and Eisenberg, 1987). A predictable pattern of emergence of phonemes leading to increased speech intelligibility with the multichannel implant is becoming apparent (Geers and Tobey, 1992; Osberger et al., 1993).

Children with implants are found in both oral and total communication programs, and it is incumbent on personnel to be knowledgeable about the devices and the development of auditory and speech skills for children using them (Moog and Geers, 1991; Tye-Murray, 1992). Contact with an educational specialist from a cochlear implant team can be extremely helpful (Nevins et al., 1991).

Concluding Statement

It is extremely difficult to compare research regarding the efficacy of one educational mode/philosophy with another because over the course of time those children who begin in oral-only options and are not successful find their way into total communication programs. Over a 4-year time period Musselman et al. (1988,) observed and tested 139 severe to profoundly hearing-impaired children ages 3–5 at the commencement of the study. By following the children longitudinally, they were able to record the natural movement patterns of children across educational settings as well as note their performance in various settings. They found no clearcut interactions between level of hearing, intelligence, and communication mode. Children in TC programs tended to have better receptive language skills and better mother-child communication than children in oral programs who in turn had better speech skills.

The authors, through comprehensive review of the literature and practical experience with hearing-impaired children, have come to agree with Moores (1987) with respect to selection of educational options for hearing-impaired children. Moores (1987, p. 238) stated, "If there is any chance that sole reliance on auditory-vocal communication will present a child with difficulty, oral-manual communication should be initiated immediately, since the use of oral and manual communication can facilitate development. Withholding manual communication until a child "fails" orally is a disservice to the child." Nothing that we have read or observed clinically suggests that speech and language development are in any way adversely affected by the addition of a manual component to the intervention program. We must emphasize, however, that all the components of an auditory-oral program must

be in place. That includes fastidious care of amplification equipment, emphasis on the development of residual hearing, training for the development of oral speech, and family participation and cooperation. There is no reason to wait before incorporating the use of visually supported communication. We strongly believe that language supports the development of cognition and that language is at the heart of all academic learning. Further, as language develops, the child has a base of understanding that appears to assist in deciphering the imperfect auditory code he or she receives. This in turn can help to provide a foundation for the development of residual hearing and speech. The price of waiting to see if a child will learn language through audition is too high. Waiting wastes valuable time when language could be developed. Waiting causes needless frustration and interference in parent-child interaction. Nothing is lost by adding an alternative symbolic system. Children exposed to sign language early, can develop aural-oral skills and can become effective communicators with the hearing world.

EDUCATIONAL OPTIONS FOR HEARING-IMPAIRED CHILDREN

Early Intervention

In 1986 Congress passed P.L. 99-457 The Education of the Handicapped Act Amendments that amended P.L. 94-142, The Education for All Handicapped Children Act. Final regulations were adopted in June 1989. The new law required states and territories to provide special education and related services to children aged 3 through 5 years by no later than the 1991–1992 school year, and under a separate section enabled interested states to provide early intervention services to infants and toddlers with disabilities ages birth to 2 years.

Implications of P.L. 99-457 for hearing-impaired preschoolers are twofold. First, a funding source is now available in all states that receive funds under this law to provide free and appropriate public education to hearing-impaired preschoolers ages 3 to 5 years. Second, grants are available to states to establish special programs for handicapped infants and toddler ages birth to 2 and their families and can function from a variety of bases (e.g., schools, clinics, hospitals). It is important for all professionals, who are concerned with hearing-impaired infants and toddlers, to be aware of their state's efforts in developing plans to implement 99-457 for ensuring that hearing-impaired children's needs are addressed. Diagnostic procedures and intervention need to be conducted by individuals knowledgeable about hearing impairment and the state's regulations must reflect these needs.

Early Intervention Models

Irrespective of educational philosophy, all early intervention models recognize the importance of establishing a partnership between the family and professionals. The comprehensive diagnostic process described earlier leads to the development of a "contract" between parents and professionals. This contract defines the long-term goals and the immediate objectives to be met by the early intervention program. The fundamental goal for a hearing-impaired child is the establishment of communication, including the development of audition, speech, and language. In addition, the plan addresses any secondary problems that a child may exhibit (e.g., feeding problems, or delayed fine and/or gross motor development) and outlines a course of action for their management. For hearing-impaired children born to deaf families where communication in sign language develops naturally the goals must be altered to meet the needs and priorities of the family. Often deaf families seek assistance from early intervention programs in the areas of oral speech development and auditory training.

Family education and collaboration are at the heart of an early intervention program. The role of the family in implementing the plan should be defined and consideration given to their strengths and needs. In some cases, families are so burdened by meeting the basic needs of providing food, shelter, and clothing that they have little time or energy to meet the extra needs of their hearing-impaired child. Professionals should be aware of each family's special circumstances and provide a variety of options that will ensure that each family is involved with their child as much as possible.

Early intervention programs therefore may take several forms. They may be home-based, community-based, center-based or a combination. Home-based programs involve professional(s) who travel to a family's home on a regular basis and observe and interact with the child and parent. Parent support and education are provided on an individual basis in the child's natural learning environment. This model is particularly effective for a medically fragile infant, for families with other young children at home, or for families that live a great distance from any central facility.

Community-based programs are offered in such settings as daycare facilities and Head Start programs. During the hours the child is at the facility the staff members are in fact surrogate parents and can facilitate a hearing-impaired child's learning. Even if staff is only able to ensure that a child's amplification equipment is properly used and maintained, this is a significant habilitative step.

Center-based programs can offer both an individual parent-infant program or a program providing for peer group interaction. Parental instruction and support groups are also provided by these programs. If a child requires such services as occupational or physical therapy, programming can be coordinated within the facility with the opportunity for interdisciplinary intervention.

Placement Options for Preschoolers

The transition from early intervention to preschool occurs when the child reaches chronological age 3. With the implementation of P.L. 99-457 hearing-impaired preschoolers will be guaranteed free public education; these services will probably occur within schools. Possible educational sites include: (a) general classes for preschool handicapped children which accommodate children with a variety of disabilities (experts in the area of hearing impairment may or may not be available in such settings), and (b) specialized classes that bring together hearing-impaired children and provide a program specifically designed for them implemented by professionals with expertise in the area of hearing loss.

Before making a recommendation for placement, care must be taken to determine available options. If a nonspecialized preschool for handicapped children is the option available, the composition of the class should be examined closely. The setting must be appropriately stimulating and adapted to meet the special needs of a hearing-impaired child. That is, peer communication partners may not be present in such settings and consequently there may not be consistent language modeling. This is particularly so if the child needs sign language or cues.

Some families may not avail themselves of public education and therefore may obtain habilitative therapies privately. If this is the case, then it is extremely important that all professionals working with a child coordinate efforts. Typically, the responsibility for such coordination falls upon the parent.

Irrespective of the special services provided to a child, public or private, opportunities for interaction with normally hearing children should not be overlooked. Some preschoolers may participate in a nursery school, whereas others may attend daycare in addition to the specialized program of services they receive. Proper preparation of staff will facilitate positive experiences for all concerned.

Service Continuum for School-age Hearing-Impaired Children

Transition from preschool to school-age programming generally occurs when the child is age five or six. At this transition, a comprehensive evaluation is conducted to plan for future education. The central purpose of this assessment is to determine under what conditions the child will learn best. His or her ability to understand and use language is at the heart of making this determination.

The available educational options range from placement in a specialized school setting for hearing-impaired children to placement in a mainstream classroom and include the following:

1. Self-contained classroom instruction—a special class in a residential, private, or public school designed exclusively for hearing impaired children;
2. Partial mainstreaming—hearing-impaired children spend a portion of their day in instruction with hearing children and may or may not receive support services (support services include such options as a sign language or oral interpreter, tutor, notetaker, resource room teacher, speech therapist); and
3. Full-time mainstreaming—the hearing-impaired student receives all education with hearing students and may or may not receive support services; these include any of the above options plus the possible services of an itinerant teacher.

Mainstreaming

As a result of the Individuals with Disabilities Education Act (IDEA), there has been a national thrust to prevent systematic exclusion of handicapped children from regular education programs. Increasing numbers of hearing-impaired children have been educated in regular school settings. Although the motivation for providing education in nonsegregated settings is laudable, the result for many hearing-impaired children has been disastrous. The report of the Commission on Education of the Deaf (1988) indicated that mainstreaming was inappropriately used across our nation and resulted in serious failures in education for many hearing-impaired children.

What then are the prerequisite skills a child must demonstrate to be successful in the mainstream? What support services need to be in place to make mainstreaming the option of choice? (See Ross, Brackett, and Maxon 1991 for a comprehensive discussion of mainstreaming.)

Prerequisite Factors. Earlier in this chapter the facets of a comprehensive assessment were described in detail. Such an assessment will enable the family and professionals to determine if the child is capable of handling the academic, linguistic, and social demands of a mainstream classroom.

Brackett (1978) suggests that hearing-impaired children whose language skills closely approximate the norms for normal hearing children are the ones who will fair best in mainstream classroom environments. Families and professionals need to keep in mind that the mainstream classroom is an auditory verbal environment (Flexer et al., 1989). Hearing children in mainstream classrooms have well-developed language skills even before they enter school and all instruction is conducted with the expectation of this foundation.

Although a child may be successfully mainstreamed at one point in his or her education, mainstreaming may be inappropriate at a later point. Academic and social demands increase over time. The level of classroom discourse and textbook language becomes increasingly complex in the upper primary grades. This increased complexity in language can hinder the child's ability to prosper in the mainstream. Parents need to understand that placement in the mainstream is not equivalent to the disappearance of the problems imposed by the hearing loss.

Ideally, the child's personality should be such that he or she seeks information assertively, is able to tolerate frustration, and demonstrates perseverance in learning. Preparation for mainstreaming should be thorough to ensure that the child feels secure in requesting the needed assistance in the classroom.

Support Services. Once a determination has been made that the child possesses the linguistic, academic, and personal and social skills to be mainstreamed, an array of support services are required to ensure that mainstreaming will be successful. The child cannot simply be placed in a regular classroom.

Audiological Support and Management

Hearing aids and amplification equipment need to be checked daily to ensure that they are functioning properly (Flexer, et al. 1989). Even a child with a mild hearing loss is in jeopardy when his amplification system is not working properly.

Amplification equipment should be provided that ensures the audibility and intelligibility of the speech signal in the classroom. Even the child with a mild-moderate hearing loss, who to the untrained eye may appear to hear well with his hearing aids, will miss out on the majority of unstressed consonants and noncontent words that frequently modulate the meaning of sentences (Roeser and Downs, 1981). Such children can also benefit from the use of FM equipment (see Chapter 42).

Educational Interpreters

Some children may have English language competence comparable to their hearing peers but because of the limitations of speechreading are unable to follow the teacher. Three options are available under these circumstances: oral interpreting; sign language interpreting; or manual voice interpreting (Wittier-Merithew, and Drist 1982). The interpreter extends or represents ideas, moods, thoughts, and words in the language mode that the individual uses.

The role of the educational interpreter changes considerably at different grade levels. In the earliest years, the interpreter may be involved in functions other than simply transmitting the teacher's words. For example, the interpreter may sometimes function as a teacher's helper assisting the child to complete a project, or may help facilitate interaction on the playground between the hearing-impaired child and hearing peers. The report of the National Task Force on Educational Interpreting (Stuckless et al., 1989) contains detailed information on this topic.

Tutors and Notetakers

Wilson (1982) developed a comprehensive guide to the training of tutors and notetakers and underscored the importance of their role in the education of mainstream hearing-impaired children. Their responsibilities include: (a) clarifying classroom procedures and materials; (b) reinforcing concepts gained from reading and studying; (c) keeping parents and other members of the teaching team informed about classroom activities; (d) teaching the child how to use support services effectively; (e) ensuring that the child is able to profit from such classroom materials as videotapes or movies; and (f) serving as an in-class source of information to the teacher about hearing loss and support services.

Itinerant Teacher of the Hearing Impaired

The itinerant teacher works for a limited period of time each week with individual hearing-impaired children on activities including auditory training, speech training, improving language skills, and assisting in academic subjects (Dilka, 1984). The itinerant teacher may also provide in-service training to teachers and other staff about hearing loss and its management.

Speech/Language Pathologist

In many public school settings, the speech/language pathologist may be the only individual available, on a day-by-day basis, to provide information about the hearing-impaired child to the rest of the staff; however, ideally he or she is the member of the support service team providing a comprehensive speech and language program for the child. The most beneficial speech and language program is one that uses language drawn from classroom materials and curricula as its foundation. Language training, auditory training, and speech training can all be done effectively using this approach. The child's efforts are then consistently focused on information relevant to academic success. The child can see the relationship between the work done with the speech/language pathologist and the work that must be completed in the classroom. His or her educational program is thus cohesive. (See, e.g., Blank et al., 1991; Blank et al., in press.)

Coordination of Effort

Selection and provision of support service must be followed by a coordinated effort. This is most readily accomplished if a team member is designated to serve as a case manager and is responsible for communication among professionals. Specialized staff as well as regular teaching personnel need to be aware of the efforts of their teammates. Annual inservice education also must be provided for all school personnel to familiarize them with the special needs of the mainstreamed student.

CONCLUSIONS

Several themes permeate this chapter and represent our position regarding the habilitation of hearing-impaired children. They are as follows:

1. Decision making regarding education and training of hearing-impaired children should result from interdisciplinary team assessment with collaboration of the family, the medical community, and the educational specialists.
2. All decisions regarding education and training of hearing-impaired children should take into account the impact of hearing impairment on the child's language acquisition and development. The degree of hearing loss itself is not as important as how it has affected language and speech development.
3. All decisions regarding habilitation should take into account the strengths and needs of the child and his family. Decisions should not be based on adherence to a particular philosophy.
4. When there is any doubt that a child can learn language readily through an auditory-oral mode, a sign language support system should be put in place immediately. There is no evidence to suggest that doing so will retard speech and language growth.
5. Habilitation and decisions regarding education will change as the child matures. Regular reassessment is vital to ensure the success of any program.

6. The audiologist must function as a collaborative member of the habilitative team providing key information about the child's hearing, how to optimize its use, and its potential impact on speech and language development. The audiologist should also be involved in planning goals for the development of residual hearing and ensuring that the auditory environment is favorable for establishing speech and language.

7. The speech language pathologist should be knowledgeable about speech and language acquisition in the hearing-impaired child and its impact on learning and socialization. He or she should be able to provide comprehensive speech, language, and auditory training for the hearing-impaired child, and inservice education for staff. The speech/language pathologist will probably be the central figure in providing information about hearing impairment in public school settings.

8. The provision of comprehensive support services is essential to ensure the success of any mainstream education program.

REFERENCES

Abraham S, and Stoker A. Language assessment of hearing-impaired children and youth: Patterns of test use. Lang Speech Hear Serv Schools 1988;19:160–174.

Abraham S, Stoker R, and Allen W. Speech assessment of hearing-impaired children and youth: Patterns of test use. Lang Speech Hear Serv Schools 1988;19:17–27.

Arthur G. Arthur Adaptation of the Leiter International Performance Scale. Chicago: Stoelting, 1952.

Bayley N. Bayley Scales of Infant Development. New York: Psychological Corp., 1969.

Beauchaine KL, Barlow NL, Stelmachowicz PG. Special considerations in amplification for young children. ASHA 1990;32:44–46.

Beebe H, Pearson HR, Koch ME. The Helen Beebe Speech and Hearing Center. In Ling D, Ed. Early Intervention for Hearing Impaired Children. San Diego, CA: College-Hill Press, 1984:14–63.

Berg FS. The school years. Hear Speech News 1971;39:14–20.

Berliner K, and Eisenberg L. Our experience with cochlear implants: Have we erred in our expecations? Am J Otol 1987;8:222–229.

Berliner K, Eisenberg L, and House W. The cochlear implant: An auditory prosthesis for the profoundly deaf child. Ear Hear 1985;6(Suppl 3).

Boothroyd A. Evaluation of speech production of the hearing impaired: Some benefits of forced-choice testing. J Speech Hear Res 1985;28:185–196.

Boothroyd A. CASPER: Computer Assisted Speech Perception Evaluation and Training Proceedings of the 10th Annual Conference on Rehabilitative Technology. Washington, DC, Association for Advancement of Rehabilitative Technology, 1987:734–736.

Bornstein H, and Saulnier K. Signed English: A brief follow-up. Am Ann Deaf 1981;126:69–72.

Bornstein H, Saulnier K, and Hamilton L. Signed English: A first evaluation. Am Ann Deaf 1980;125:467–481.

Brackett D. Communication modifications made to hearing impaired children in a mainstream setting [Unpublished Doctoral Dissertation]. University of Connecticut, Storrs, CN, 1978.

Carney AE. Understanding speech intelligibility in the hearing impaired. Top Lang Disord 1986;6:47–59.

Commission on Education of the Deaf. Toward equality: Education of the deaf. Washington, DC, U.S. Government Printing Office, 1988.

Conference of Educational Administrators Serving the Deaf. Assessment of multihandicapped deaf students. Am Ann Deaf 1989;134:79–83.

Connolly A, Nachtman W, and Pritchett E. Key Math Diagnostic Arithmetic Test. Circle Pines, MN: American Guidance Service, 1971.

Cornett RO. Cued Speech. Am Ann Deaf 1967;112:3–13.

Craig W. Effects of preschool training on the development of reading and lipreading skills of deaf children. Volta Rev 1964;109:280;296.

Davis J, Shepard N, Stelmachowicz P, and Gorga M. Characteristics of hearing-impaired children in public schools: Part II Psychoeducational data. J Speech Hear Disord 1981;46:130–137.

DeFilippo CL. Speechreading training: Believe it or not. ASHA 1990;32:46–48.

Dilka K. Professionals who work with the hearing impaired in school. In Hull R, and Dilka K, Eds. The Hearing Impaired Child in School. Orlando, FL: Grune & Stratton, 1984.

DuBose R, and Langley DB. Developmental Activities Screening Inventory. New York: N.Y. Times Teaching Resources Co., 1977.

Dunn C, and Newton L. A comprehensive model for speech development in hearing-impaired children. Top Lang Disord 1986;6:25–46.

Dunn L, and Markwardt F. Peabody Individual Achievement Tests. Circle Pines, MN: American Guidance Service, 1970.

Engen E, and Engen T. Rhode Island Test of Language Structure. Baltimore: University Park Press, 1983.

Erber N. Auditory Training. Washington, DC: A. G. Bell Association for the Deaf, 1982.

Flexer C, Wray D, and Ireland J. Preferential seating is not enough: Issues in classroom management of hearing-impaired students. Lang Speech Hear Serv Schools 1989;20:11–18.

Gates A, and MacGinitie ML. Gates-MacGinitie Reading Tests. New York: Teachers College Press, 1972.

Gatty J. The oral approach: A professional point of view. In Schwartz S, Ed. Choice in Deafness: A parents guide. Kensington, MD: Woodbine House, Inc., 1987.

Geers A, Moog J, and Schick B. Acquisition of spoken and signed English by profoundly deaf children. J Speech Hear Disord 1984;49:378–388.

Grammatico L. The development of listening skills. Volta Rev 1975;77:303–308.

Greenberg M. Social interaction between deaf preschoolers and their mothers: The effects of communication method and communicative competence. Dev Psychol 1980;16:465–474.

Gustason G, Pfetzing D, and Zawolkow E. Signing Exact English. Rossmoor, CA: Modern Sign Press, 1972.

Hiskey MS. Hiskey-Nebraska Test of Learning Aptitude. Lincoln, NE: Union College Press, 1966.

Hochberg I, Leavitt H, Osberger M, Eds. Speech of the Hearing Impaired: Research, Training, and Personnel Preparation. Baltimore: University Park Press, 1983.

Hull RH, and Dilka KL. The Hearing Impaired Child in School. Orlando, FL: Grune & Stratton, 1984.

Jastak J, and Jastak S. The Wide Range Achievement Test, Rev. Wilmington, DE: Jastack Associates, 1978.

Jensema CJ, Karchmer MA, and Trybus RJ. The rated speech intelligibility of hearing impaired children: Basic relationships and a detailed analysis (Series R., No. 6). Washington, DC: Gallaudet College, 1978.

Johnson HA. A sociolinguistic assessment scheme for the total communication student. J Monogr Suppl Acad Rehabil Audiol 1988;21:101–127.

Johnson RE, Liddell SK, Erting CJ. Unlocking the Curriculum. Gallaudet Research Institute Working Paper 89-3. Washington, DC: Gallaudet University, 1989.

Klima E, and Bellugi U. The Signs of Language. Cambridge, MA: Harvard University Press, 1979.

Kretchmer R, and Kretchmer L. Communication competence and assessment. J Monogr Suppl Acad Rehabil Audiol 1988;21: 5–17.

Laughton J. Perspectives on the assessment of reading. J Monogr Suppl Acad Rehabil Audiol 1988;21:101–127.

Layton T, and Holmes D. Carolina Picture Vocabulary Test. Tulsa, OK: Modern Education Corporation, 1985.

Levine E. The Psychology of Deafness. New York: Columbia University Press, 1960.

Levine ES. Psychological tests and practices with the deaf: A survey of the state of the art. Volta Rev 1974;76:298–319.

Ling D. Speech and the Hearing Impaired Child: Theory and Practice. Washington, DC: A.G. Bell Association for the Deaf, 1976.

Ling D, Ed. Early Intervention for Hearing Impaired Children: Oral Approaches. San Diego, CA: College-Hill Press, 1984.

Luetke-Stahlman B. The benefit of oral English—only as compared with signed input to hearing-impaired students. Volta Rev 1988;90:349–361.

Luterman D. Counseling Parents of Hearing-Impaired Children. Boston: Little, Brown and Co., 1979.

Madden R, Gardner E, Rudman H, Karlsen B, and Merwin J. Stanford Achievement Tests, Special Edition for Hearing-Impaired Students. Washington, DC: Gallaudet College Office of Demographic Studies, 1972.

Madell JR. Audiological assessment. The Mainstream Revisited. Paper presented New York League of the Hard of Hearing, October 26–28, 1989.

McCracken R. The Standard Reading Inventory. Klamath Falls, OR: Klamath Printing Co., 1966.

Moeller M. Combining formal and informal strategies for language assessment of hearing-impaired children. J Acad Rehabil Audiol 1988;21:73–99.

Moeller M, McConley A, and Osberger M. Evaluation of the communication skills of hearing-impaired children. Paper presented at the biannual convention of the A. G. Bell Association for the Deaf, Toronto, Canada, 1982.

Monsen R. A usable test for the speech intelligibility of deaf talkers. Am Ann Deaf 1981;126:845–852.

Moog JS, and Geers AE. Scales of Early Communication Skills for Hearing Impaired Children. St. Louis: Central Institute for the Deaf, 1975.

Moog JS, and Geers AE. Grammatical Analysis of Elicited Language—Simple Sentence Level. St. Louis: Central Institute for the Deaf, 1979.

Moog JS, and Geers AE. Grammatical Analysis of Elicited Language—Complex Level. St. Louis: Central Institute for the Deaf, 1980.

Moog JS, and Geers AE. Educational management of children with cochlear implants. Am Ann Deaf 1991;136:69–76.

Moog JS, Kuzak M, and Geers AE. Grammatical Analysis of Elicited Language—Presentence Level. St. Louis: Central Institute for the Deaf, 1983.

Moores DF. Educating the Deaf: Psychology, Principles, and Practices. Boston: Houghton Mifflin Co., 1987.

Moses K. Infant deafness and parental grief: Psychosocial early intervention. In Powell F, Finitzo-Hieber T, Friel-Patti S, and Henderson D, Eds. Education of the Hearing Impaired Child. San Diego, CA: College-Hill Press, 1985.

Musselman CR, Lindsay PH, and Wilson AK. An evaluation of recent trends in preschool programming for hearing impaired children. J Speech Hear Disord 1988;53:71–88.

Nevins ME, Kretchmer R, Chute P, Hellman S, and Parisier. Programs in action: The role of an educational consultant in a pediatric cochlear implant program. Volta Rev 1991;93:197–204.

Nicholls GH. Cued speech and the reception of spoken language. Washington, DC: Gallaudet College, 1979.

Northern JF, and Downs MP. Hearing in Children. Baltimore: Williams & Wilkins, 1978.

Office of the Los Angels County Superintendent of Schools. Test of Auditory Comprehension. North Hollywood, CA: Foreworks, 1976.

Osberger M. Development and evaluation of some speech training procedures for hearing impaired children. In Hochberg I, Leavitt J, and Osberger M, Eds. Speech and the Hearing Impaired: Research, Training, and Personnel Preparation. Baltimore: University Park Press, 1983.

Osberger MJ, Maso M, Sam L. Speech intelligibility of children with cochlear implants, tactile aids, or hearing aids. J Speech Hearing Res 1993;36:186–203.

Otero J. School successfully incorporates cued speech into total communication program. Cued Speech News 1986;19:3–5.

Pollack D. Educational Audiology for the Limited Hearing Infant. Springfield, IL: Charles C Thomas, 1970.

Pollack D. Acoupedics: An approach to early management. In Menscher G, and Gerber S, Eds. Early Management of Hearing Loss. New York: Grune & Stratton, 1981.

Pollack D. An acoupedic program. In Ling D, Ed. Early Intervention for Hearing Impaired Children. San Diego, CA: College-Hill Press, 1984:181–253.

Quigley S. The Influence of Fingerspelling on the Development of Language, Communication and Educational Achievement of the Deaf. Urbana: University of Illinois, 1969.

Quigley S, and Kretchmer RE. The Education of Deaf Children. Baltimore: University Park Press, 1982.

Quigley SP, Steinkamp MW, Power DJ, and Jones BW. Test of Syntactic Abilities. Beaverton, OR: Dormac, Inc., 1978.

Raven J. Progressive Matrices. New York: Psychological Corp., 1948.

Rawlings BW, and Jensema CJ. Two Studies of the Families of Hearing Impaired Children. Washington, DC: Gallaudet University, Office of Demographic Studies, 1977.

Reid D, Hresko W, Hammill D, Wiltshire S. Test of Early Reading Ability. Austin, TX: PRO-ED, 1991.

Roeser RJ, and Downs MP. Auditory Disorders in School Children. New York: Thieme-Stratton, Inc., 1981.

Ross M, Brackett D, Maxon A. Assessment and management of mainstream hearing impaired children: Principles and practices. Austin, TX: PRO-ED, 1991.

Schick B, and Moeller MP. What is learnable in manually coded English systems? J Appl Psycholing Res 1992;13:313–340.

Shildroth AN, Rawlings BW, and Allen TE. Hearing impaired children under age 6: A demographic analysis. Am Ann Deaf 1989;134:63–69.

Smith AJ, and Johnson RE. Smith-Johnson Non-verbal Performance Scale. Los Angeles: Western Psychological Corp., 1977.

Stokoe W. Sign language structure. Buffalo, Studies in Linguistics, occasional paper number 8, 1958.

Stuckless E, Avery JR, Hurwitz T, Eds. Educational Interpreting for Deaf Students: Report of the National Task Force on Educational Interpreting. Rochester, NY: Rochester Institute of Technology, 1989.

Stutsman R. Mental Measurement of Preschool Children. Yonkers-on-Hudson, N.Y.: World Book Co., 1931.

Subtelny J. Assessment of speech with implications for training. In Bess F, Ed. Childhood Deafness. New York: Grune & Stratton, 1977.

Subtelny J, Orlando N, and Whitehead K. Speech and Voice Characteristics of the Deaf. Washington, DC: A. G. Bell Association, 1981.

Tattershall S, Kretchmer LW, and Kretchmer RR. Assessment issues for three aspects of school communication. J Acad Rehabil Audiol Monogr Suppl 1988;21:173–197.

Trybus RJ, and Karchmer MA. School achievement status of hearing-impaired children: National data on achievement status and growth patterns. Am Ann Deaf 1977;122:62–69.

Tye-Murray N. Cochlear implants and children: A handbook for parents, teachers, and speech and hearing professionals. Washington, DC: A.G. Bell, 1992.

Utley JA. A test of lipreading ability. J Speech Hear Disord 1946;11:109–146.

Vernon M, and Andrews JF. The psychology of deafness: Understanding deaf and hard-of-hearing people. White Plains, New York: Longman, 1990.

Watkins S. SKI*HI Language development scale. Logan, UT: SKI*HI Institute, 1979.

Wechsler D. Wechsler Intelligence Scale for Children, rev. New York: Psychological Corp., 1974.

Wilbur R. The linguistics of manual language and manual systems. In Lloyd L, Ed. Communication Assessment and Intervention Strategies. Baltimore: University Park Press, 1976.

Wilbur R. American Sign Language: Linguistic and applied dimensions. San Diego: College Hill Press, 1987.

Williams-Scott B, and Kipila E. Cued Speech: A professional point of view. In Schwartz S, Ed. Choices in deafness: A parents guide. Kensington, MD: Woodbine House, 1987:23–31.

Wilson JJ. Tutoring and notetaking as classroom support services for the deaf student. In Sims D, Walter G, Whitehead R, Eds. Deafness and Communication: Assessment and Training. Baltimore: Williams & Wilkins, 1982.

Wittier-Merithew A, and Drist R. Preparation and use of educational interpreters in deafness and communication assessment. In Sims D, Walter G, and Whitehead R, Eds. Deafness and Communication: Assessment and Training. Baltimore: Williams & Wilkins, 1982.

Woodward J, Allen T, Shildroth A. Teachers and deaf Students: An ethnography of classroom communication. In Delancy S, and Tomling R, Eds. Proceedings of the First Annual Meeting of the Pacifics Linguistic Conference Eugene, Oregon, 1985:479–493.

Yoshinaga-Itano C. Speechreading instruction for children. Volta Rev 1988;90:241–260.

Zieziula FR. Assessment of Hearing Impaired People: A Guide for Selecting Psychological, Educational, and Vocational Tests. Washington, DC: Gallaudet University Press, 1982.

Appendix 47.1.

LANGUAGE TESTS DEVELOPED FOR HEARING-IMPAIRED CHILDREN

Scales of Early Communication Skills for Hearing Impaired Children (Moog and Geers, 1975)	2–8 years	Criteria referenced, observational scales of verbal and nonverbal receptive and expressive language
Test of Syntactic Abilities (Quigley, Steinkamp; Power, and Jones, 1978)	10–19 years	Test of ability to understand syntactic structures in written form
SKI-HI Language Development Scale (Watkins, 1979)	Birth to 5 years	Criteria referenced, observational scales of receptive and expressive communication and language skills
Rhode Island Test of Language Structure (Engen and Engen, 1983)	5–17+ years	Formal test of knowledge of syntactic structures
Carolina Picture Vocabulary Test (Layton and Holmes, 1985)	4–14 years	Test of child's ability to recognize signed vocabulary
Grammatical Analysis of Elicited Language-Simple Sentence Level (Moog and Geers, 1979, 1985)	3–5 years	Test of expressive language ability focusing on knowledge of syntactic structures
Grammatical Analysis of Elicited Language-Presentence Level (Moog and Geers, 1983)	3–5 years	Tests of preverbal child's ability to combine words
Grammatical Analysis of Elicited Language Complex Sentence Level (Moog and Geers, 1980)	8–12 years	Tests prompted and imitated production of 16 grammatical categories

Appendix 47.2.

PSYCHOLOGICAL AND EDUCATIONAL TESTS FOR HEARING-IMPAIRED CHILDREN
(Adapted from Vernon and Andrews, 1990)

Psychological Tests

TESTS	AGE	COMMENT
The Arthur Adaptation of the Leiter International Performance Scale (Arthur, 1952)	4–12 years	Nonverbal test best for ages 4–9
Bayley Scales of Infant Development (Bayley, 1969)	2–30 months	Well-standardized development measures for hearing children comprised of The Mental Scale, Motor Scale, and Infant Behavior Record. Meet satisfactory reliability standards and provide valuable estimates of current developmental status that may be used with hearing-impaired infants.
Developmental Activities Screening Inventory (DASI) (DuBose and Langley, 1977)	6 months–5 years	A valuable performance screening measure of cognitive development.
Hiskey-Nebraska test of Learning Aptitude (Hiskey, 1966)	3–17 years	One of the best tests available for use with hearing impaired children.
Merrill-Palmer Scale of Mental Tests (Stutsman, 1931)	2–5 years	Best as a supplemental performance measure. Requires a skilled examiner with a thorough knowledge of the psychology of hearing impairment.
Ravens Progressive Matrices (Raven, 1948)	5 years through adulthood	A supplemental measure of nonverbal intelligence.
Smith-Johnson Nonverbal Performance Scale (Smith and Johnson, 1977)	2–4 years	Excellent test for very young hearing-impaired children, norms for deaf and hearing available.
Wechsler Performance Scale for Children-Revised (Wechsler, 1974)	6–16-years	An excellent test for use with school-age hearing-impaired children. Norms exist on deaf children (Anderson and Sisco, 1977).

Educational Tests

TESTS	AGE	COMMENT
Key Math Diagnostic Arithmetic Test (Connolly, Nachtman, and Prichett, 1971)	6 years to adult	Can be individually administered in total communication. Appropriate for all ages and categories of hearing-impaired children. May need to simplify language.
Test of Early Reading Ability: Deaf or Hard of Hearing (Reid, Hresko, Hammill, and Wiltshire, 1991)	3–13	Assesses skills associated with reading in the areas of construction of meaning, the alphabet and its functions, and conventions of written language.

CHAPTER 48

Aural Rehabilitation of Adults with Hearing Impairment

Thomas G. Giolas

The last two decades have seen increased emphasis on rehabilitation programs to assist adults to cope with their hearing difficulty. Today's programs take a broad perspective and focus on the overall *handicapping effect* of hearing difficulty. Most importantly, these programs center on *communication* and the manner in which the *communication process* has been disrupted. Good verbal communication skills facilitate emotional, educational and social growth. Effective communication is the greatest problem two human beings face in interacting with each other (Shostrom, 1967). People spend a great deal of their adult lives trying to make others understand what they are saying or trying to understand what is being said to them (Fleming, 1972).

It follows, therefore, that if any *aural rehabilitative program* is to be effective it must be designed to meet the wide range of needs of the target population. The program should primarily focus on *verbal communication*. However, it should also center on ways in which a breakdown in the communication process impacts on *other everyday activities*, such as performance in the work setting, interpersonal relationships with friends and family, and personal business transactions. These areas should be dealt with directly or indirectly through referral for personal counseling. The purpose of this chapter is to present the ingredients of a program consistent with this point-of-view.

DEFINITIONS

A number of terms are currently used to describe or refer to persons who are experiencing hearing difficultly. Tables 48.1 and 48.2, from Schow and Weinstein (1990), illustrate the inconsistent use of audiologic terms by various organizations. In order to minimize the confusion, a brief discussion regarding the definition of some of these terms is in order.

The use of functional terms follows only when there is agreement on the concepts under discussion. With regard to the rehabilitation of a person with a hearing impairment, there are aspects of the problem that must be established. One deals with the organic status of the auditory mechanism, while the second addresses the effect of the *organic status* on the person's *everyday life situation*. Once these concepts are established, the diagnostic and management approaches can be planned. It should be noted that the terms used are of secondary importance. What is paramount is that the concept being discussed is readily recognizable.

With these two aspects of the problem in mind, the suggested terms offered by either The American Association of Otolaryngology (1979) or the American Speech-Language-Hearing Association (1980) appear to be the most appropriate (see Table 48.1). The terms clearly differentiate between the organic status of the auditory mechanism (Hearing Impairment) and the effect of that impairment on the communicative social and emotional status of the individual (Hearing Handicap).

More specifically, *hearing impairment* emerges as the term to be used when reference is being made to the condition of abnormal hearing and no additional information regarding the impairment is indicated; *hearing handicap* will refer to the effect of the hearing impairment on the person's everyday situation (Davis and Silverman, 1978). *Aural rehabilitation*, therefore, becomes the process by which the communication disorder specialist assists in reducing the *hearing handicap* resulting from the *hearing impairment*.

Two other terms, *hearing loss* and *deaf*, will be used and require definition. *Hearing loss* is used whenever specific reference is being made to a hearing impairment which is of particular intensity magnitude, such as a 40 dB hearing loss. The term *deaf* will refer to persons in whom the sense of hearing is nonfunctional *when used alone*, with or without amplification, for the ordinary purposes of life. Such an individual may (*a*) have been born either totally deaf or sufficiently deaf to prevent the establishment of speech and natural language; (*b*) have become deaf in childhood before language and speech were completely established (prelingual); or (*c*) have become deaf after having acquired speech and language skills (post-lingual), thus significantly impairing communication skills (Nicolosi, Harryman, and Kresheck, 1978). For further informa-

Table 48.1

Different definitions for auditory domains of disorder, impairment, handicap, and disability as specified by American Academy of Otolaryngology (AAO, 1979), American Speech-Language-Hearing Association (ASHA, 1981), and the World Health Organization (WHO, 1980),[a]

AAO, 1979	ASHA, 1981
Permanent Impairment. A change for the worse in either structure or function, outside the range of normal, is permanent impairment. The term is used here in a medical rather than a legal sense. Permanent impairment is due to any anatomic or functional abnormality that produces hearing loss. This loss should be evaluated after maximum rehabilitation has been achieved and when the impairment is nonprogressive at the time of evaluation. The determination of impairment is basic to the evaluation of permanent handicap and disability.	*Hearing impairment* is used to mean a deviation or change for the worse in either auditory structure or auditory function, usually outside the range of normal.
	Hearing handicap means the disadvantage imposed by a hearing impairment on a person's communicative performance in the activities of daily living.
	Hearing disability means the determination of a financial award for the loss of function caused by any hearing impairment that results in significant hearing handicap.
Permanent Handicap. The disadvantage imposed by an impairment sufficient to affect a person's efficiency in the activities of daily living is permanent handicap. Handicap implies a material impairment.	WHO, 1980
	Disorder occurs as a result of some type of disease process or malformation of the auditory system.
Permanent Disability. An actual or presumed inability to remain employed at full wages is a permanent disability. A person is permanently disabled or under permanent disability when the actual or presumed ability to engage in gainful activity is reduced because of handicap and when no appreciable improvement can be expected.	*Impairment* is any loss or abnormality of psychological, physiological, or anatomical structure or function.
	Disability is any restriction or lack (resulting from an impairment) of ability to perform an activity in the manner or within the range considered normal for a human being.
	Handicap is a disadvantage for a given individual, resulting from an impairment or a disability, that limits or prevents the fulfillment of a role that is normal (depending on age, sex, and social and cultural factors) for that individual.

[a] Schow (1990 p.7s) Reprinted by permission.

Table 48.2
Domains of Auditory

	Disorder	Impairment	Disability	Handicap
Definition	Pathology of the hearing organ	Abnormal function of the auditory system	Reduced abilities of the individual	Need for extra effort
				Reduced independence
Area affected	Middle ear	Auditory sensitivity recognition	Speech perception	Grade of employment
	Inner ear	Localization	Environmental awareness	Scope of employment
	Hair cells	Temporal processing	Orientation	Remuneration
	Auditory nerve	Binaural integration		Personal relations
	Brainstem			Social integration
	Auditory cortex			

[a] Schow (1990 p.7s) Reprinted by permission.

tion on this topic, the reader is referred to Chapter 39.

TARGET POPULATION

The focus of this chapter will be on individuals who acquired their hearing impairment as adults. It is believed that this group comprises the majority of hearing impaired adults and which, at the present time, is grossly underserved. The reader is referred to Chapter 38, for a historical review of aural rehabilitation programs.

THE REHABILITATION PROCESS

The purpose of rehabilitative intervention with a hearing impaired adult is to reduce the handicapping effects of hearing impairment, with special emphasis on communication performance. Accordingly, the role of the audiologist becomes that of (a) assessing the handicapping effects of hearing impairment in terms of communicative efficiency and (b) gauging the success of aural rehabilitative procedures (medical or nonmedical) in reducing these handicapping effects. This obviously involves a thorough evaluation of both hearing impairment and hearing handicap.

This orientation to the rehabilitation process requires a commitment on the part of the audiologist that goes beyond determining the extent of hearing loss and site of lesion. It means that there must be also a strong commitment to the communication and other needs of the hearing impaired person; that is, these needs cannot be met by only defining the parameters of the hearing impairment and by determining the amplification needs. The components of an aural rehabilitation program presented in this chapter are presented within the context of this orientation.

Assessment for Rehabilitation

The first step in the rehabilitation process involves assessing the handicapping effect of the hearing impairment. Basic information regarding this effect can be obtained through the administration of one or a combination of several evaluation procedures. These procedures can be categorized into three groups: (*a*) threshold measures; (*b*) suprathreshold measures; and (*c*) self-report instruments.

Threshold Measures

In terms of assessing hearing handicap, two questions can be asked on the basis of threshold measures: (*a*) to what degree has conversational speech been rendered less audible and (*b*) to what degree is it less intelligible? When puretones, rather than speech, have been used to obtain a *puretone threshold*, the answers to these questions are actually *predictions* of the handicap based on the configuration and extent of the hearing loss. Giolas (1982) found moderate correlation coefficients (averaging .57) suggesting that while there is a relationship between puretone thresholds and self-assessment of hearing handicap, this information alone is insufficient to account for the perceived hearing handicap.

However, in the hands of an audiologist with a solid background in speech production, speech perception, and hearing impairment, information obtained from puretone thresholds can provide useful data regarding speech understanding. For example, the extent to which the hearing loss involves critical frequencies necessary to receive the spoken message will influence how much difficulty an individual will have (*a*) knowing if someone is speaking to him or her, (*b*) in understanding what is said, or (*c*) in a combination of both conditions. This is illustrated in Figures 48.1 and 48.2.

Figure 48.1 represents a person with normal hearing in the lower audiometric test frequencies and reduced hearing in the higher frequencies beyond 2000 Hz. It is predicted that in a quiet setting this person will have little difficulty hearing and understanding what is being said. On the other hand, it is predicted that the person whose hearing is represented by the audiogram plotted in Figure 48.2, indicating that all audiometric frequencies are affected, will experience difficulty in both hearing and understanding speech. The vowels, with low-frequency energy concentration, and the consonants, with high-frequency energy concentration, will both be affected, resulting in an intensity and speech intelligibility problem. Ling and Ling (1978) and Van Tassell (1981) state that various phonetic features can be discrimi-

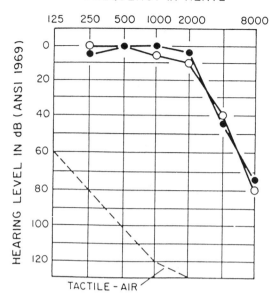

Figure 48.1. Audiogram Illustrating Normal Hearing through 2000 Hz.

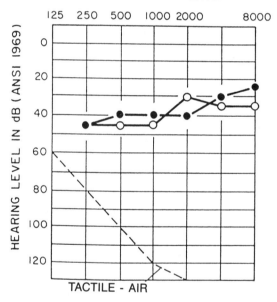

Figure 48.2. Audiogram Illustrating Reduced Hearing for All Frequencies.

nated only if hearing is present for the frequency range corresponding to the acoustic properties of the features and if the speech is sufficiently intense to reach the client's threshold in that frequency range. However, there is considerable data (Levitt, 1982) indicating that speech acoustic events as perceived by hearing impaired persons with the same hearing loss, may differ to quite a degree at suprathreshold levels, with many individuals responding unpredictably. Thus, while puretone thresholds offer the trained audiologist considerable information and insight, they have their limitations in describing hearing handicap and must never be used alone to make this judgment.

In instances when puretone threshold and suprathresholds for speech (e.g., 40 dB HL) are difficult to obtain, the *speech reception threshold (SRT)* or some modification of the procedure may well enhance the information available regarding the extent of hearing loss, and how speech is being processed. Some of these modifications include obtaining a *speech detection threshold (SDT)*, restricting the word list, pretraining with the word list to enhance familiarization.

Because response to the SRT procedure, and some of its modified forms, is sometimes more successful than response to suprathreshold speech measures, the degree to which the SRT or SDT approximates the puretone air conduction audiometric configuration can offer some insight into how well the reduced hearing is being used. For example, Sims (1982) showed that the SDT is closely related to the puretone threshold of 250 Hz. (r = .81). While the SDT does not correlate as well with other audiometric frequencies, it is a useful corroborator of low frequency.

Suprathreshold Measures

Information about the listener's response to auditory stimuli at suprathreshold levels is useful in that it provides us with an opportunity to assess the difficulty experienced by the client in understanding under various listening conditions. Preselected speech messages are presented through earphones to each ear separately or presented in a sound field. The messages are generally presented in quiet conditions at normal conversational intensity levels, as well as at levels which represent soft speech or loud speech. Sound field testing might include speech recognition accuracy with competing noise (Carhart, 1969; Olsen and Carhart, 1967; Olsen and Tillman, 1968; Tillman, Carhart, and Olsen, 1970). This noisy environment test situation should include the assessment of the listener's performance when the primary signal is directly in front of the listener and the noise on either or both sides, as well as assessment of performance when the primary signal is on one side and the competing noise is on the other side. The assessments done will depend upon the hearing loss in each ear and the ear being considered for a hearing aid. In either case, the concern is how well the listener follows everyday conversational speech in both a quiet and a noisy environment.

In addition to assessing the listener's performance with auditory cues alone, one should also assess the listener's performance with the addition of visual cues. The degree to which the listener benefits from visual cues contributes much to identifying specific problems as well as assisting in the selection of rehabilitative activities (Erber 1971; Erber 1974a, b). For example, knowing that a listener yields an extremely poor score when a speech message is presented in the absence of visual cues, but a considerably higher score when visual cues are added, offers information on how well the listener is able to integrate the incoming auditory and visual information. A visual message (e.g., words or connected speech) presented by itself will also offer additional information (Hutton, Curry, and Armstrong, 1959). It helps the clinician determine through which sensory modality the client is better able to process the incoming speech signal (auditory or visual). This information in turn helps the clinician plan an appropriate training program. It is interesting to note that Ross, et al. (1972), found that a combined visual auditory (look-listen) measure produced a higher score than adding the auditory alone (listen) measure and visual (look) alone score together to obtain information regarding the use of the contribution of each modality to the overall information process.

Appropriate amplification (Hearing Aids) plays an important role in minimizing the handicapping effects of hearing impairment. While a variety of hearing aid evaluation approaches are described in the literature (see Chapter 44), most agree on the importance of using speech materials in determining the appropriate amplification.

It is suggested that pretraining with test words occur prior to the testing session. There is no question that results obtained in this manner will be more indicative of true auditory performance; that is, the contribution of learning to do the task, to overall performance, will be minimized. This approach is actually included in some test procedures with normal hearing children (Goldman, Fristoe, and Woodcock, 1970). The rationale for such an approach with children is to minimize vocabulary deficiency as an influencing factor and to more closely test speech discrimination. An excellent discussion of the use of such an approach with severely hearing-impaired persons is found in Lloyd (1972).

Self-Report Procedures

In addition to audiometric procedures, a number of self-report test instruments have been developed to assess another dimension of hearing handicap, i.e., a person's perceptions of the handicapping effect of the hearing impairment. The impetus for the use of these instruments is a result of general dissatisfaction with the degree to which standard audiometric procedures provide concrete information about how a given hearing impairment has influenced a specific person's life situation in general, and verbal communication in particular (Noble, 1978; Giolas, 1970). Noble (1978) suggests that audiometric procedures at worst are misleading and at best inadequate when used as predictors of hearing handicap. For example, most clinicians have had the experience of dealing with two hearing-impaired persons with quite *similar* audiograms and yet quite *dissimilar* communication problems or of dealing with a person who has a low speech discrimination score obtained in the traditional manner, but who reports minimal communication difficulty.

One explanation for these discrepancies lies in the target behaviors measured by audiologic procedures (Noble, 1978). These procedures measure the ear's response to specific auditory stimuli (puretones, selected speech messages, etc.) in a laboratory setting (quiet and simulated noisy conditions).

While these procedures are appropriate when assessing hearing impairment, they are less effective when assessing communication efficiency. In the latter case, the clinician is required to infer from these results the client's performance in typical listening-speaking situations. The accuracy of these inferences depends upon how representative these laboratory conditions are of the everyday communication setting. The communication process is not only dependent upon the ear's physical status (organic impairment), but is also dependent upon a number of factors such as (*a*) with whom the person is speaking (relationship to the speaker); (*b*) under what conditions the communication act is occurring (number of speakers, environmental noise conditions); and (*c*) the purpose of the verbal intercourse (social, work, business). Consequently, it has become apparent that audiometric procedures, as they are typically administered, are not representative of most listening-speaking situations and, as a result, generate only general, predictive statements regarding how well a person will function in most real-world communication situations. For example, audiometric procedures might suggest client difficulty with the loudness of the signal or probable client difficulty with understanding speech even when it is made comfortably loud, but they fall short of describing when, where, and with whom these communication problems typically occur for the person being tested. Furthermore, they offer no information as to how the person feels about having a hearing impairment. The clinician must obtain this information if the total rehabilitative process is to be optimally effective. What is needed is an approach to assessing hearing

performance that yields data which is more than just predictive; what is needed are instruments to assess behaviors that would be expected to improve after rehabilitative intervention, e.g., the behaviors comprising the communication process and the coping strategies used by the hearing-impaired person. The new self-report instruments show promise in achieving this goal.

The basic format of these instruments consists of presenting the hearing-impaired person with a series of questions centering around a potentially handicapping condition and asking the person to judge his or her overall performance in this situation. The following sample question is taken from the hearing handicap scale developed by High, Fairbanks, and Glorig (1964).

Can you hear adequately when you are conversing with more than one person?
_____ Practically always.
_____ Frequently.
_____ As often as not.
_____ Occasionally.
_____ Almost never.

The major differences between most of these instruments lie in the purpose; scope and number of items comprising the questionnaire; and, in some cases, test administration and scoring. Table 48.3 summarizes some salient characteristics of those procedures developed since 1964. The reader is also encouraged to read Part III of Dr. W. Noble's book, *Assessment of Impaired Hearing* (1978), for an in-depth, critical analysis of various self-report procedures, including some earlier attempts at nonscaled inventories. Finally, two additional publications (Giolas, 1983; Schow and Smedley, 1990) are recommended. They expand on the complexity of the self-assessment approach, including instruments designed for the screening of hearing handicap.

COMPONENTS OF AN AURAL REHABILITATION PROGRAM

The first step of the aural rehabilitation process consists of a thorough evaluation of hearing impairment and its handicapping effect. This evaluation process will have identified the organic status of the auditory mechanism and number of potential communication difficulties experienced by a hearing-impaired person. These communication difficulties are generally associated with (*a*) the audibility of the message; (*b*) speech discrimination; (*c*) the environment, including background noise and the communication situation; and (*d*) response to auditory failure. The first step in planning a rehabilitative program is to begin by discussing

Table 48.3
Self-Report Instruments for Assessing Hearing Handicap

Instrument	Author(s)	Target Population	Assessment Focus	Items	Time (mins)
Hearing Handicap Scale (HHS), 1964	High et al.	Adult	Speech communication Environmental sounds Warning signals	20 (2 forms)	5
Hearing Measurement Scale (HMS), 1970	Noble and Atherly	Adult	Speech hearing Nonspeech acuity Localization Reaction to handicap Speech distortion Tinnitus Social effects Personal reaction to loss	53	10–40
Social Hearing Handicap Scale (SHI), 1973	Ewertson and Birk-Nelsen	Adult	Specific listening Situations	21	5
Denver Scale of Communication Function, 1974	Alpiner et al.	Adult	Family Social Vocational General Communication	25	15
Profile Questionnaire for Rating Communication Performance, 1982.	Sanders	Adult	Home Business Social environments	22	15
Denver Scale of Communication Function of Senior Citizens (DSSC), 1976	Zarnoch and Alpiner	Seniors	Attitude toward peers Socialization Communication Specific situations	35	15
Nursing Home Hearing Handicap Index, 1977	Schow and Nerbonne	Seniors in a nursing care facility	General Communication Handicap	10	—
Denver Scale of Communication Function, Modified, 1978	Kaplan et al.	Seniors	Same as DSSC	35	—
Hearing Performance Inventory (HPI), 1979	Giolas et al.	Adults	Understanding speech Intensity Social Personal Occupational Response to auditory Failure	158	30–55
Self-Assessment of Hearing, 1980	Manzella and Taigman	Elderly	To determine if audiological hearing aid needed	16	—
Hearing Problem Inventory, 1980	Hutton	Adults	Perception of hearing problems benefit from and use of aids	51	—
Communication Assessment Procedure for Seniors, 1981	Alpiner and Baker	Seniors in extended care facilities	General communication Group situations Other persons' self-concept Family	35	20–40
Self-Assessment of Communication/Significant other Assessment of Communication, 1982	Schow and Nerbonne	Elderly and spouse	Communication situations Feelings Perception of others' attitude toward handicap	20	—
HPI, Revised Form, 1983	Lamb et al.	Adults	Same as HPI	90	20
Hearing Handicap Inventory for the Elderly, 1982	Ventry and Weinstein	Elderly	Emotional Social	25 (screening form 10)	—
Hearing Aid Performance Inventory (HAPI), 1984	Walden et al.	Adult	Hearing aid benefit in daily life	64	—
Communication Profile for the Hearing Impaired (CHPI), 1986	Demorest and Erdman	Adult	Communication performance Communication importance Environment strategies Personal adjustment	145	20–40
Performance Inventory for Profound and Severe Loss, 1980	Owens and Fujikawa	Adults with severe/profound loss	Understanding speech with and without visual cues Intensity Response to auditory failure Environmental sounds Personal	74	50

— = information not reported or unavailable

with the hearing-impaired person the results of the audiometric and self-report procedures in terms of communication breakdowns. This allows the hearing-impaired person to begin gaining some insight into his or her situation, and provides the clinician with the opportunity to introduce the proposed management program in terms of the person's specific hearing problems. It also provides the client with the opportunity to indicate which problems are of sufficient importance to be included early in the rehabilitation program. In addition, a discussion regarding the handicapping effect of the hearing impairment will serve to identify problem areas and their solutions.

At this point a specific management program is outlined. For many, this program will consist of pursuing amplification through the use of a personal hearing aid(s). It will include a *hearing aid evaluation* (see Chapter 44) and *hearing aid orientation* (see Chapter 40). This phase of the aural rehabilitation program is designed to help the person make *optimal use of auditory cues.*

Optimal Use Of Auditory Cues

For persons with normal hearing, the auditory modality has played the primary role in most of their mental development. Through the spoken message, complicated information has been transmitted to facilitate the acquisition of language, speech, and academic and vocational skills. The ease with which this takes place is due in large part to the multiple redundant cues provided by verbal and nonverbal communication processes. It is because of these redundant cues (Miller, 1951) that the message becomes *predictable,* and it is this predictability which makes the transmission of information so powerful. Most cues contributing to the predictability of verbal messages are physiologic, acoustic, and linguistic parameters.

The hearing impaired person should be advised that speech predictability assists persons who have acquired a hearing impairment to compensate effectively, even though many auditory cues are diminished as a result of the disorder. With the help of amplification, many of the physiologic and acoustic cues are restored. Given an established internal language structure, special attention to situational cues, and a good preparatory set, the hearing-impaired adult is often able to function satisfactorily in most listening situations.

Because the major parameter of hearing impairment is reduced sensitivity as a function of frequency, the basic foundation of the remediation process is *amplification.* That is, the more intense the speech signal, the more content cues that become available to the listener. Consequently, the *hearing aid* emerges as the single most important component of an aural rehabilitation program for this population.

Hearing Aid Orientation

Too many hearing-impaired persons are not wearing their hearing aids at all or are using them improperly. This is primarily a function of poor management. A carefully designed program of hearing aid orientation must be an integral part of the aural rehabilitation program. The goal of such a program should be to help hearing-impaired persons receive optimal benefit from their personal hearing aid. A sample Hearing Aid Orientation program is outlined in Table 48.4. This program assumes a carefully conducted *hearing aid evaluation and fitting* procedure by a clinical audiologist.

A carefully orchestrated hearing aid orientation program is usually sufficient to start the post-lingually hearing-impaired person on the road to making optimal use of residual hearing through the use of amplification. However, some authors suggest that extensive *auditory training* can be helpful in improving speech perception (McCarthy and Alpiner, 1982). McCarthy and Alpiner define auditory training in terms of three parameters:

1. Learning to recognize auditorily those sounds which have been incorrectly discriminated.
2. Pre- and post-hearing aid orientation including adjustment to amplification.
3. Improvement of tolerance levels.

Table 48.4
Sample Hearing-Aid Orientation Program[a]

Prerequisites
  Hearing aid candidacy considerations
  Hearing aid evaluation, including selection and fitting
Introduction to the hearing aid
  How the hearing aid operates (volume switch, batteries, etc.)
  Amplification through a hearing aid (advantages and limitations)
Assessing the effectiveness of the hearing aid (during trial period)
  Observations of performance with and without the hearing aid
  Evaluation of the family member or close friend
  Pre-and postamplification measurements with self-report
    procedures
  Follow-up phone calls and clinic visits
  Joint meeting to make final decision
Handling special problems in hearing aid adjustment
  Frequent follow-up clinic visits during trial period
  Participation in aural rehabilitation groups
Long-term follow-up
  Telephone call in 3 months
  Clinic visit in 6 months

[a]Giolas (The hearing handicapped adults. Englewood Cliffs, NJ: Prentice Hall, 1982:95.) Reprinted by permission.

McCarthy and Alpiner discuss a number of auditory training activities which can be used in a group or individual setting. They stress, however, that a thorough evaluation of the person's auditory training needs must precede any management program.

Communication Strategies

Optimizing residual hearing through the successful use of a hearing aid will not completely eliminate auditory failure. Auditory failure occurs as a result of a noncorrectable distortion of the spoken message due to the hearing impairment as well as adverse environmental conditions. It becomes the responsibility of the hearing-impaired person to develop strategies to compensate for such difficulties. These strategies can be grouped into three categories: (*a*) use of visual and situational cues; (*b*) manipulation of the physical environment; and (*c*) constructive response to auditory failure.

These communication strategies are best introduced and developed in a *group setting*, where discussion and role playing can be used to demonstrate the principles involved. These *aural rehabilitation groups* provide a dynamic setting in which the interaction between peers (hearing-impaired persons), family members, and the group leader (the audiologist) generate productive discussions and, most importantly, solutions to communication problems. The emphasis placed on each category of communication strategies will vary and depends upon the group members' needs. Table 48.5 outlines the purpose and format of these groups. Activities centering on the optimal use of auditory cues are often included as part of the group activities.

Use of Visual Cues

One of the more productive compensatory communication strategies used in difficult listening situations is increased reliance on the nonverbal cues inherent in all communication settings. This strategy is based on the assumption that lip movements, facial expressions, gestures, and situational cues offer meaningful supplementary information. The visual cues accompanying oral communication, coupled with the amplified auditory cues provided by the hearing aid, can certainly enhance the process of decoding the auditory message. Consequently, the goal of many group activities is to develop a greater awareness of the value of using nonauditory cues. This heightened awareness is not difficult to develop and becomes more or less automatic with practice.

Several activities are conducted to illustrate the general advantages of using nonverbal cues. Initially, activities are designed to highlight the value of visual

Table 48.5
Aural Rehabilitation Groups

Purpose:	To provide supportive and substantive help to persons having communication problems associated with hearing impairment
Goal:	The goal is to analyze auditory failures and to develop concrete behaviors which result in improved communication
Process:	The group is used with the audiologist serving as the group leader
Rationale:	The group process provides a setting in which there is considerable exchange of information, mutual support and validation of communication problems and solutions
Format:	Role of the Group Leader 　Facilitator of discussion 　A good listener 　Expert on hearing and its disorders Session Structure 　Presentation of contest (through films, lectures, etc.) 　Supervised group discussion 　Communication strategies activities 　Home assignments Group Members 　Hearing impaired persons and a close friend or family member with whom communication is important and frequent Group Activities 　Optimal use of auditory clues 　Optimal use of visual cues 　Manipulation of environment 　Response to auditory failure

cues in general, i.e., facial expressions, gestures and situational cues. Later, activities centering around *lipreading per se* are conducted to illustrate the *supplementary* role of this type of visual cue. Some prefer the term *speechreading* to *lipreading*. Speechreading is thought to be a more comprehensive term, suggesting the use of a broader scope of visual cues (facial expressions, gestures, bodily stance, etc.) in addition to lip movements. Speechreading and the concept it conveys (the use of all visual cues for communication purposes) has merit and has general acceptance by professionals; however, lipreading is still the term generally used by the lay person. It is important that aural rehabilitation programs include emphasis on both the use of general visual cues, as well as specific cues from lip movements.

Use and Misuse of Lipreading

Care is taken to discuss the limitations of lipreading as an information channel for verbal messages. The advantages and limitations of lipreading are pointed out, with examples cited or activities conducted to illustrate each of them. Clues may be obtained from watching the lips which resolve many potential acoustic confusions. The possible confusion between the acoustically similar verbal requests "pass the cheese" and "pass the peas" could be avoided because of the obvious visible differences between *cheese* and *peas* that is seen on the lips. Contextual cues would not help to differentiate between *cheese* and *peas*, but visual cues would. Helping people become aware of the probability of this type of confusion will go a long way towards motivating them to watch the speaker. On the other hand, the limitations of depending upon lipreading alone are best illustrated by turning down the sound of the television set and suddenly noticing how little can be gleaned from the silent lip movements on the screen.

Finally, it must be emphasized that very few people with a post-lingual hearing impairment are sufficiently impaired to require total dependence on visual cues alone; they typically have sufficient residual hearing and linguistic skills to benefit most from combined visual and auditory cues. Furthermore, it is extremely difficult (if not impossible) to carry on an extensive discussion with just lipreading alone and no situational cues. The primary reasons for this are that (*a*) only approximately 70% of the speech sounds are interpretable visually and a talker can produce 13–15 speech gestures per second, but the listener's eye can only resolve 8–9 gestures per second (McCarthy and Culpepper, 1987), and (*b*) many of the sounds look alike on the lips. The reader is referred to Spitzer, Leder, and Giolas (1992) for extensive therapy plans for speechreading, including goals, objectives, success criteria, and extensive materials which include lists of visually and auditorily similar and dissimilar words and sentences.

In order to educate both the hearing-impaired persons and their families alike, they are all are invited to participate in the lipreading activities. The value lies not only in the gained awareness of the factors and skills involved in lipreading, but also in the discussions that follow. Participants are encouraged to analyze their failure and/or success with the lipreading activities along the lines of several questions. These questions include: How did they approach the task of lipreading? Did they give up when they did not understood the first few words, or did they keep trying to find contextual cues? Did they state what they thought was said and ask for confirmation? Did they ask for the whole sentence to be repeated? Did they take a guess? Opportunities are provided to practice using all of these strategies and others in a lipreading activity. The lipreading activity provides a simulation of real-life speaking-listening situations in which to practice using all (and others which may arise) of these communication strategies. Appendix 48.1 contains Guidelines for Lipreading Activities (Giolas, 1982), as well as Erick-

son's (1974) excellent suggestions for improving speechreading effectiveness.

In conclusion, lipreading activities provide a fine opportunity to present communication strategies that may be used by the hearing-impaired adult. Little or no attention should be paid to whether there is improvement in lipreading per se in that no formal lipreading tests are administered. What should be attended to is whether there is improvement in the client's approach to deciphering the auditory-visual code. Lipreading tests generally place too much emphasis on lipreading skill and not enough on the role it plays in the broader context of the communication process.

Manipulation of the Environment

The setting in which the communication act takes place plays an important role in how well a person will hear and understand what is being said. This is especially true for the hearing-impaired person whose *redundancy-factor* has been reduced by the hearing impairment. Consequently, environmental conditions, such as background noise, lighting, number of people talking, and distance from the speaker, can all contribute to auditory failure. Whenever possible, these conditions should be optimized to improve communication efficiency. Giolas (1982) outlined the following guidelines that a hearing-impaired person can follow to improve the communication environment.

1. Effect a relatively noise-free environment. This includes requesting that background music be turned down or off, closing a door to minimize corridor noise, and requesting meeting rooms with good acoustics (see Chapter 41).
2. Secure the most advantageous position relative to the speaker(s). It is always wise to arrive early so that you can have the option of sitting close to the chairperson at meetings, sitting up front at lectures, public hearings, church, etc., and be in a position to see all speakers.
3. At informal gatherings limit the number of speakers you engage in conversation at any one time. One-to-one conversations are easier than group conversations.
4. Correct poor lighting conditions in order to facilitate the use of all nonverbal cues. Dimly lit restaurants are prime examples of poor lighting conditions. Often there are better lighted tables that can be used.
5. Encourage the use of public address systems when they are available or use an assistive listening device to overcome poor listening conditions (see Chapter 42).

Response to Auditory Failure

A person's failure to understand what was said may be rectified by an attempt to repair the communication breakdown. For example, when a person misses a point being made, a simple request for it to be repeated may provide the needed information. In this example, no sustaining communication breakdown occurred because it was corrected immediately. A significant problem occurs only when an auditory failure goes unchecked and subsequent misunderstandings of what was said develops. Therefore, hearing-impaired persons must develop a repertoire of responses to auditory failure. Giolas (1982) suggested the following fairly successful responses.

1. When you are aware that you have missed something that was said, ask for it to be repeated. Repeat the portions you heard to facilitate the flow of the conversation.
2. If someone is talking unusually softly, adjust your hearing aid to hear that person better or ask the person to talk a little louder.
3. Whenever possible, inform the speaker that you have a hearing impairment and suggest what he or she can do to help you understand.
4. Avoid pretending you understood what was said. It is likely to lead to greater confusion later on.
5. If you cannot interrupt the speaker, ask someone near you to fill you in on what you did not hear.
6. Even though you feel you are missing a lot, keep trying to follow the discussion. Some nonverbal or situational cues will often emerge to get you back on the track.
7. It is helpful to ask someone near you to alert you to changes in the topic of conversation.

Table 48.6 summarizes the group activities typically included in a standard aural rehabilitation group.

Table 48.6
Examples of Group Activities Included in Aural Rehabilitation Groups

Optimal Use of Auditory Cues
    Amplification Considerations
    Hearing-Aid Orientation
Communication Strategies
    Optimal Use of Visual Cues
        Role of Redundancy
        Role of Visual Cues in General
        Role of Lipreading
            Contribute to understanding conversational speech
            Limitations
            Use of lipreading activities to develop a general approach
                to communication breakdowns
Manipulation of Environment
Response to Auditory Failure

THE REHABILITATION PROGRAM FORMAT

It is not always possible or appropriate to conduct aural rehabilitation in a group setting. Sometimes schedules do not permit a person to attend group sessions. Individuals with severe hearing losses may make participation in group discussion difficult. Still others might prefer to meet individually with the audiologist until they become more comfortable with their hearing impairment. Whether the rehabilitative process is conducted individually or within a group, the goal and principles are identical. In both situations, the clinician is interested in helping persons with a hearing impairment develop effective compensatory communication strategies. Although in the *individual* format the discussion takes place between two people (or three if the spouse can be included), the group discussion process is still used.

Individual sessions also are often conducted when personal issues associated with the hearing impairment need to be discussed. These sessions also provide an opportunity to explore communication strategies specific to individual needs.

SPECIAL CONSIDERATIONS

The Deaf Adult

As established at the outset of this chapter, the focus of this chapter is on adults who have acquired their hearing impairment as adults. The rehabilitation process that has been described assumes that the client has had numerous years of sufficient hearing to acquire normal speech and language development and that the person's mode of communication is oral. In addition, it is also assumed that the individual hears sufficiently to converse orally and understand what is being said by the clinician and the group.

While many of the principles inherent in this orientation apply to the severely-to-profoundly congenitally deafened adult, they require a much different assessment and rehabilitation format. The procedures developed at the National Technical Institute for the Deaf (NTID), and discussed by Sims (1985) in the third edition of this handbook, provide an excellent review of this topic. NTID has developed a useful *profile test battery,* that includes instruments for assessing auditory speech recognition, speechreading with and without sound, manual reception (signed English without voice or lip movement), simultaneous (signed English and speech) reception, English writing and reading and speech intelligibility. Furthermore, the NTID has designed an extensive rehabilitation program that includes a 20-hour orientation to hearing aids, a two-level auditory training program, and a speechreading program which includes word and sentence level videotaped exercises.

The same principles and procedures discussed above for the congenitally deafened adult hold true for the person with a cochlear implant. This individual requires similar, but much more intense, work on auditory training, speech production, and counseling, all of which are beyond the scope of this chapter. The reader is referred to Chapter 46 on cochlear implants and vibrotactile aids.

The reader is also referred to Spitzer, Leder, and Giolas (1992), which focuses on a modular approach to aural rehabilitation for the late-deafened adult with special emphasis on the newly cochlear implanted person. Spitzer, et al., includes comprehensive chapters on the impact of a hearing impairment on everyday life, auditory and vibrotactile training, speechreading lessons, and voice and resonance therapy. Each chapter contains a series of complete and graduated goals, objectives, and materials to address persons with low, medium, and high levels of communication difficulty.

Adult with a Sudden Hearing Loss

Generally, the problems associated with a sudden severe bilateral hearing impairment are similar to the problems exhibited by a person with a gradual hearing impairment. However, they are complicated by sudden onset and by the severity of the loss. The initial psychologic impact of such a loss is so great that resistance to aural rehabilitation is often marked. The impact of a sudden bilateral severe hearing impairment is best understood in terms of Ramsdell's (1978) three psychologic levels of hearing, i.e., primitive, signal/warning, and symbolic.

The *primitive* level of hearing provides a very important and basic contribution to a person's general feeling of security. It is the basic ingredient which creates a background of feeling, which Ramsdell (1978) calls *affective tone*. It connects people with their immediate auditory environment, helping them to feel a part of a living active world. As they become aware of the auditory background of their daily living, they are attuned to changes occurring in it, and are in a state of readiness to react appropriately. Ramsdell indicates that the primitive level relates us to the world below the level of conscious perception. It is the loss of the primitive level that causes the feeling of "deafness," and the depression that those who are suddenly deafened experience. This same reaction although to a lesser extent is experienced by those in whom severe hearing loss develops more gradually. One person who had acquired a sudden severe bilateral hearing loss reported that the sudden silence gave her the feeling

that something ominous had happened in the world and that everyone was mourning a death. As the rehabilitative process progressed, she began to understand that some of her feelings of depression were related to the "death" of her primitive level of hearing.

The *signal or warning level* of hearing is an extension of the primitive level, but operates on a more conscious level of listening. It provides valuable information about what is going on in the immediate environment and facilitates appropriate reactions. For example, normally hearing persons are constantly aware of environmental sounds within their hearing range and use them in a preparatory set manner. The security afforded by auditorily monitoring the environment and identifying the direction of sounds has a major influence on our feeling of well-being.

Finally, Ramsdell describes the level of hearing which allows people to organize auditory events into meaningful language units or symbols and then to use these symbols to communicate verbally with others. The *symbolic level* requires the best hearing ability of the three levels described and interference at this level causes a host of communication problems.

The rehabilitative process for the person with a sudden hearing impairment varies. It is determined by a number of factors, including (a) the extent and type of the hearing impairment; (b) the degree to which the person is visually oriented; (c) the person's work situation; (d) the person's general lifestyle and basic approach to personal problems; and (e) the family's understanding of the problem and overall support.

Initially, considerable time is spent talking with the hearing-impaired person and his or her family. All persons involved are provided with the opportunity to ask any and all questions regarding the status of the individual's hearing, the cause of the impairment, the management plan, and the prognosis for improvement. Throughout this discussion the audiologist strives to play a supportive role. Remedial activities are initiated as soon as possible to provide the person the family with a sense of success and progress. As the program continues, time may need to be set aside to allow for questions the individuals may have about why they feel as they do, what the future holds for them, and other concerns they may have regarding their hearing. Throughout this management program, the audiologist should be on the lookout for signs pointing to a psychologic referral.

Whenever possible, at least one family member or close friend should be included in most management sessions. This will provide both parties with an opportunity to work on new communication patterns under the supervision of the audiologist. It will also help the nonhearing-impaired person develop a better understanding of the hearing-impaired person's communication problems.

The evaluation procedures described earlier may be used with this population. In that the sudden nature of this hearing is associated with extreme anxiety, the evaluation procedure is usually spread out over a number of sessions to allow remediation to begin as soon as possible.

Amplification is tried at the earliest time. Its success depends on a variety of factors, including (a) the severity of the loss, (b) its etiology, and (c) the person's willingness to give the hearing aid a fair trial. The trial period is accompanied by intensive hearing aid orientation activities similar to those described earlier. The hearing-impaired person is helped to understand that even though the hearing aid does not restore speech to its preimpairment clarity, coupled with visual and situational cues it can help improve communication efficiency. For some people, it will contribute more to reestablishing the primitive and signal warning levels of hearing than the symbolic level.

The activities designed to foster increased use of visual cues are most important and productive with this population. Vision symbolizes a significant safety factor and represents a major approach to compensating for the hearing impairment. Most importantly, it provides a vehicle through which to present communication strategies applicable to all hearing-impaired persons. Consequently, intensive work on the use of visual cues, including speechreading, comprises a major part of the management program. Individual, as well as small group (one or two family members), sessions become the standard management format for these activities.

Adult with a Unilateral Hearing Loss

Persons with monaural hearing often exhibit communication problems and negative feelings about their impairment and the situations in which they experience communication difficulty. This is because *one good ear does not afford normal hearing for all practical purposes.*

While persons with monaural hearing do not require the extensive aural rehabilitation suggested for the bilaterally hearing-impaired adult, it should be pointed out that they will most likely have difficulty (a) localizing the direction from which sound is coming and (b) understanding speech both when the talker is located on the side of the poor ear and when there is background noise present in the listening environment. Assuming the hearing impairment is medically irreversible, the goals of the discussions are two-fold: (a) the reduction of negative emotions related to the

hearing impairment and (b) the development of effective actions in response to adverse listening situations.

The use of amplification with persons having unilateral hearing impairment has been discussed by Dempsey (Chapter 44) and Montano (Chapter 42). In instances where amplification is appropriate, hearing aid orientation will also be needed and, of course, geared to the special problems associated with monaural hearing.

Standard self-report *evaluation* procedures have not been developed to systematically assess the communication problems experienced by those with unilateral hearing impairment. Consequently, the clinician must improvise. Communication problems areas to explore with this population include whether the person has difficulty hearing or understanding speech under the following conditions:

1. When speech is presented to the impaired ear while the normal ear is partially or fully masked by extraneous noise.
2. When speech is presented to the impaired ear while no appreciable extraneous noise masks the normal ear.
3. When subject is situated in a setting which contains a great deal of extraneous noise, regardless of whether the stimulus is directed toward the good or the bad ear.
4. When subject is situated in a relatively quiet setting, regardless of whether stimulus is directed toward the good or the bad ear.
5. Difficulty distinguishing from which direction a given auditory stimulus came in the presence of considerable extraneous noise.
6. Difficulty distinguishing from which direction a given auditory stimulus came in a relatively quiet setting.

Elderly Adult

The aural rehabilitation groups described in this chapter are quite appropriate for the elderly person. In many ways, the groups' similarity in terms of age, general interests, adjustment patterns, and stage of life often makes the rehabilitation approach more effective. Because the aging process often creates a general reduction in responsiveness to verbal messages, it is sometimes advisable to reduce the group size. This in turn will reduce the potential number of verbal exchanges and make it easier for the group members to follow the group activities. If the meetings can be held in familiar settings, with members who regularly interact, and at a convenient time, aural rehabilitation groups can be the most rewarding approach to helping the older person with a hearing problem. As with all groups, care is taken to select activities commensurate with the maturity and experiences of the members. If a group of people have lived in the geographic area for many years, discussions of how things used to be and the history of old landmarks, provide an abundance of materials to implement the communication strategy activities. In that many elderly people are extremely dependent on family members and/or close friends for social outlets and transportation, it is especially important to include family and friends in the group activities. This will facilitate improvement in other aspects of their personal relationships. For more in depth discussion on this topic, the reader is referred to Chapter 49, Assisting the Older Client.

Educational Setting

More and more colleges and universities are opening their doors to the hearing-impaired student. The era of *mainstreaming* the hearing handicapped person is here and the role of the university audiology clinic is clear. It should become the home base for hearing impaired students in the college or university setting. It should work closely with the student and school personnel to determine the nature of supportive services *that* the hearing impaired student will need. This will involve a careful evaluation of the student's *hearing handicap,* with special consideration given to *educational listening situations,* as well as to the appropriate *personal* and *classroom amplification* needs. The clinic should be in a position to evaluate the student's hearing aids and explore the feasibility of using an assistive listening device in classes.

Most universities have an Office of Services for the Handicapped. The hearing-impaired person should be put in touch with such an office. These offices are often able to provide services such as tutoring, oral or manual interpreting, a note taker, special arrangements for test taking, and other services. They often work closely with State Offices of Vocational Rehabilitation and can put the hearing-impaired student in touch with this agency.

SUMMARY

The aural rehabilitative process for adults with hearing impairment has been discussed. Table 48.7 summarizes the steps of the remediation process that have been outlined in this chapter. The basic goal of this process is to reduce the handicapping effects of hearing impairment, with special emphasis on communication performance. Accordingly, the process begins with a thorough assessment of both hearing impairment and hearing handicap. Components comprising

Table 48.7
Remediation Process

PURPOSE
  To reduce the handicapping effects of hearing impairment, with special emphasis on communication performance (i.e., component of the communication process)
CONSIDERATIONS
  Nature of Hearing Impairment
  Nature of Hearing Handicap
  Appropriate Referral(s)
  Amplification Needs
  Compensatory Communication Strategy Needs
DEVELOPING AN INDIVIDUAL MANAGEMENT PROGRAM
  Discussion of test results and observations with hearing impaired person and family
  Work individually with hearing impaired person on amplification and compensatory communication strategy needs
  If needed, include an Aural Rehabilitation Group

the treatment program are described from the perspective of adults with a hearing impairment regardless of extent and onset of the hearing loss. For the most part, the rehabilitative process consists of demonstrating the need for active and aggressive listening, as well as providing opportunities to accomplish this goal.

REFERENCES

Alpiner J, Chevrette W, Glascoe G, Metz M, Olsen B. The denver scale of communication function. 1974.

Alpiner J, Baker J. Communication assessment procedure for seniors. 1980 (unpublished).

American Academy of Otolaryngology committee on hearing and equilibrium and the American Council of Otolaryngology committee on the medical aspects of noise. Guide for the evaluation of hearing handicap. JAMA 1979;241:2055–2059.

American Speech and Hearing Association (ASHA) Executive Board. On the definition of hearing handicap. ASHA 1981; 23:293–297.

Carhart R. Problems of the hearing impaired in noisy social gatherings. In Oto-Rhino-Laryngology: Proceedings of the Ninth International Congress (Mexico). Amsterdam: Excerpts Medica, 1969:564–568.

Davis AC. Hearing disorders in population: first phase finding of the MRC national study of hearing. In Lutman ME, Haggar MP, Eds. Hearing science and hearing disorders. London: Academic Press, 1983.

Davis H, Silverman SR. Hearing and deafness. 4th ed. New York: Holt, Reinhard, and Winston, 1978.

Demorest ME, Erdman SA. Scale composition and item analysis of the communication profile for the hearing impaired. J Acad Rehab Audiol 1986;29:515–535.

Erber NP. Evaluation of special hearing aids for deaf children. J Speech Hear Disord 1971;36:527–537.

Erber NP. Auditory, visual and auditory-visual recognition of consonants by children with normal and impaired hearing. J Speech Hear Res 1972;39:413–422.

Erber NP. Visual perception of speech and deaf children: recent developments and continuing needs. J Speech Hear Disord 1974a;39:179–185.

Erber NP. Effects of angle, distance and illumination on visual reception of speech by profoundly deaf children. J Speech Hear Res 1974b;17:99–112.

Erickson JG. Speech reading: an aid to communication. Danville, IL: The Interstate Printers & Publishers, Inc., 1978.

Ewertson H, Birk-Neilsen H. Social hearing handicap index: social handicap in relation to hearing impairment. Audiology 1973; 12:180–187.

Fleming M. A total approach to communication therapy. J Acad Rehab Audiol 1972;6:35–36.

Giolas TG. The measurement of hearing handicap: a point of view. Maico Audiol Libr Ser 1970;Vlll:6.

Giolas TG, Owens E, Lamb SH, Schubert ED. Hearing performance inventory. J Speech Hear Disord 1979;44:169–195.

Giolas TG. Hearing handicapped adults. Englewood Cliffs, NJ: Prentice Hall, 1982.

Giolas TG. The self-assessment approach in audiology: state of the art. Audiology 1983;8:157–171.

Goldman R, Fristoe M, Woodcock RW. Test of auditory discrimination. , MN: American Guidance Service, Inc., 1970.

High WS, Fairbanks G,Glorig A. Scale for self-assessment of hearing handicap. J Speech Hear Disord 1964;29:215–230.

Hutton CET, Curray, Armstrong MB, Semi-diagnostic test materials for aural rehabilitation. J Speech Hear Disord 1959;24: 318–329.

Hutton CL. Responses to a hearing problem inventory. J Acad Rehab Audiol 1980;13:133–154.

Kaplan H, Feeley J, Brown J. A modified Denver scale: test-retest reliability. J Acad Rehab Audiol 1978;11:15–32.

Lamb SH, Owens E, Schubert ED. The revised form of the hearing performance inventory. Ear and Hearing 1983;4:152–159.

Levitt H. Speech discrimination ability in the hearing impaired: spectrum considerations. In Studebaker GA, Bess FH, Eds. The Vanderbilt hearing report. Monographs in contemporary audiology. Upper Darby, PA, 1982.

Ling D, Ling AH. Aural habilitation. Washington, DC: Alexander Graham Bell Association for the Deaf, 1978.

Lloyd LL. The audiologic assessment of deaf students. In The Proceedings of the 45th Meeting of the Convention of the American Instructors of the Deaf. Washington, DC: U.S. Government Printing Office, 1972:585–594.

Manzella D, Taigman M. A hearing screen test. J Acad Rehab Audiol 1980;13:21–28.

McCarthy PA, Alpiner JG. The remediation process. In Alpiner JG, Ed. Handbook of adult rehabilitative audiology. 2nd ed. Baltimore: Williams & Wilkins, 1982.

Miller GA, Heise CA, Lichten D. Intelligibility of speech as a function of the context of the test material. J Exp Psychol 1951; 41:329–335.

Nicolosi L, Harryman E, Kresheck J. Terminology of communication disorder. Baltimore: Williams & Wilkins, 1978.

Noble WG. Assessment of the hearing-impaired: a critique and a new method. New York: Academic Press, 1978.

Noble WG, Atherly G. The hearing measurement scale: a questionnaire for the assessment of auditory disability. J Speech Hear Res 1970;23:470–479.

Olsen WO, Carhart R. Development of test procedures for evaluation of binaural hearing aids. Bull Prosthet Res 1967;10(7): 22–49.

Olsen WO, Tillman TW. Hearing aids and sensorineural hearing loss. Ann Otol Rhinol Laryngol 1968;77:717–726.

Owens E, Fujikawa A, The hearing performance inventory and hearing aid use in profound hearing loss. J Speech Hear Res 1980;23:470–479.

Ramsdell OA. The psychology of the hard-of-hearing and the deafened adult. In Davis H, Silverman SR, Eds. Handbook of clinical audiology. Baltimore: Williams & Wilkins, 1978.

Ross, M, Kessler M, Phillips M, Lerman J. Visual, auditory and combined mode presentations of the WIPI test to hearing-impaired children. Volta Rev 1972;74:90–96.

Sanders DA. Aural rehabilitation: a management model. Englewood Cliffs, NJ: Prentice Hall, Inc., 1982:410–416.

Schow RL, Gatehouse S. Fundamental issues in self-assessment of hearing. Ear and Hearing 1990;11(suppl 5).

Schow RL, Nerbonne MA. Communication screening profile: use with elderly clients. Ear and Hearing 1982;3:135–147.

Schow RL, Nerbonne MA. Assessment of hearing handicap by nursing home residents and staff. J Acad Rehab Audiol 1977;10:2–12.

Shostrom EL. Man the manipulator. Nashville, TN: Abington Press, 1967.

Sims DG. Hearing and speechreading evaluation of the deaf adult. In Sims DG, Walter GG, Whitehead RL, Eds. Deafness and communication: assessment and training. Baltimore: Williams & Wilkins, 1982.

Sims DG. Visual and auditory training for adults. In Katz J, Ed. Handbook of clinical audiology. 3rd ed. Baltimore: Williams & Wilkins, 1982.

Spitzer JB, Leder SB, Giolas TG. Rehabilitation of late onset deafness. Chicago: Mosby Yearbook, in press

Tillman TW, Carhart R, Olsen WO. Hearing aid efficiency in a competing speech situation. J Speech Hear Res 1970;13: 789–811.

Tillman TW, Jerger JF. Some factors affecting the spondee threshold in normal-hearing subjects. J Speech Hear Res 1959; 2:141–146.

Van Tassell DJ. Auditory perception of speech. In Davis JM, Hardick EJ, Eds. Rehabilitative audiology for children and adults. New York: John Wiley & Sons, 1981.

Ventry IM, Weinstein BE. The hearing handicap inventory for the elderly: a new tool. Ear and Hearing 1982;83:128–234.

Walden BE, Demorest ME, Hepler EH. Self-report approach to assessing benefit derived from amplification. J Speech Hear Res 1984;27:49–56.

WHO. International classification of impairments, disabilities and handicaps: a manual of classifications relating to consequences of disease. World Health Organization, 1980:25–43.

Zarnock JM, Alpiner JG. The Denver scale of communication function for senior citizens living in retirement centers. Unpublished manuscript, University of Denver. The handbook of adult audiology. Baltimore: Williams & Wilkins, 1978.

Appendix 48.1

I. *Rational.* Lipreading activities are conducted with persons who have acquired a hearing impairment in adulthood for the reasons listed below.

    A. Lipreading activities stimulate awareness of visual and situational cues in the communication setting.

    B. They provide practice using visual and situational cues as a supplementary communication strategy.

    C. They provide an activity in which the hearing-impaired person's approach to speaking situations can be observed.

II. *A basic activity.* A group of sentences, phrases, or key words are written on the chalkboard and used as a basis for working on one or all of the above goals. The message is centered around a common theme and the difficulty of the task is varied as a function of the group's proficiency or the specific goals of the activity. Some suggestions for varying the difficulty of the task are listed below.

    A. Begin with single topics (e.g., baseball).

    B. To increase difficulty add more topics (e.g., sports in general).

    C. Start with short, easily recognizable sentences, and increase length gradually.

    D. Begin by giving many cues (reduced response set), and decrease them gradually (increased response set).

    E. Go from sentences to whole stories, varying the number of cues offered.

    F. Provide for early and continued success. It is important that a positive attitude toward the effective use of visual cues be developed. The overall goal is not so much to teach lipreading per se but rather to have the group experience the value of visual cues in general.

III. *Specific goals.*

    A. Develop activities which illustrates the contributions of situational and contextual cues, gestures, facial expressions, etc.

    B. Provide experiences in observing various speakers from different views and distances.

    C. Discuss the importance of good lighting, proper distance, and looking at the speaker.

Appendix 48.2

1. Watch the speaker—not just his lips, but everything he does, expressions, gestures, and so forth.

2. Check the seating arrangement. This is particularly true in groups situations. Don't sit where the speaker will have bright lights behind him. The resulting eyestrain will make speechreading hard, and it will also put the speaker's face in a shadow. It is always best to have your back to the light. In small, informal groups, this is also important. If the room is arranged with a sofa faced by two or three chairs, it is better to sit in one of the chairs in order to have a better view of all the other speakers. If you choose the sofa, the persons on both sides of you will be difficult to speechread. In an auditorium or similar situation, sit close enough to see as well as hear as much as possible.

3. Learn the topic being discussed. When we know what a person is talking about, it is easier to follow the conversation. By following the trend of main ideas, one can contribute to the conversation and avoid making guesses that are far from the topic. When entering a group plate, always ask, "What's being discussed?"

4. Learn to look for ideas rather than isolated words. This is the hardest thing a speechreader has to do. With hearing, following ideas is natural. We don't pay attention to any specific words, we just seem to hear and synthesize. The speaker stresses the key words to make them stand out to the listener with normal hearing, an aid to following ideas. While the speechreader may not be able to take advantage of every word a speaker says, with many speakers he can become especially aware of changes in rhythm, stress, timing, and gestures that indicate the words being emphasized and the changes in meaning. By keeping alert for key words in the sentence, the speechreader can follow ideas, even if he misses some of the "verbal filling" from adverbs, prepositions, and other descriptive parts of speech. Nouns and verbs are the most important parts of speech. The other parts of speech embellish or add details that are not vitally essential. To prevent confusion, we are not suggesting that people omit various parts of speech when talking to the hard of hearing, but rather that speechreaders will do better if they do not try to identify every word. As skill advances, more details will become apparent.

5. Use the clues from the situation to help get meanings. The idea is often spelled out by the actual situation. One may also anticipate what vocabulary or phrases will probably be used. The speechreader must recognize and make use of all details in the situation.

6. Stay aware of current events. When we know something about a topic we can more readily recognize the key words, names, and so forth. Because people talk about what is on television and in the news, it will be helpful to read the daily newspaper and to be aware of the programs many people may watch, even if you don't watch television.

7. Keep informed of your friends' interests. Most of our friends have favorite topics. Much as we might desire a change, it is actually a blessing because limited content makes speechreading easier.

8. Try to relax. Don't strain to get every word or syllable. It's not important to understand every word as long as you get the idea. In fact, when you try too hard and get too tense, this will interfere with your ability to speechread.

9. Don't be afraid to guess. Some instructors call it "intelligent guessing." If we know the topic and pick out key words, we can automatically guess the rest of the speech. Some persons won't permit themselves to guess. They have to be sure; consequently, they are constantly getting lost. While they are trying to figure out a word or a phrase, the speaker has continued to talk. Meanwhile, the speech reader who is afraid to guess is concentrating on only one word at a time. By the time he has figured out the introductory remarks, the speaker has completed the story.

10. Be flexible and ready to change your mind when necessary. Because some words may look the same, you will need to get the word clues in the rest of the sentence.

11. Remember you will usually be using your remaining hearing in combination with your speechreading ability. You can get clues from both channels and use them together to understand the speaker. This will vary with each hard-of-hearing person, depending on his hearing loss or how much a hearing aid helps. Also, situations will

(continued)

---

*J. G. Erickson, *Speech Reading: An Aid to Communication* (Danville, Ill.: The Interstate Printers & Publishers, Inc., 1978), pp. xi-xiv. Reprinted by permission.

vary; you may have to rely on speechreading in some situations more than others.

12. Inform your friends that you are studying speechreading. Tell them it will help you if they don't shout or exaggerate their lip movements when they speak. They also might make a special effort not to cover their mouths and to make sure you can see their faces when they are talking.

13. Keep your sense of humor. There are times when you may confuse a word or subject and feel a little foolish. You many have to say "I sure was off on that word!" and then resume the conversation. As speechreading skills increase, this will happen less often.

14. Watch your own speech. It you talk softly, shout at others, or slur your words together, you are not presenting the model of good speech you would like others to use when talking to you.

15. Don't be afraid of speechreading. Let it become a friend. Like all good friendships, let it develop slowly. It is a skill that requires much practice, not just during lessons, but in everyday living.

CHAPTER 49

Assisting the Older Client

Raymond H. Hull

The minimum age associated with the term "aged" is ever changing due to the advances of medicine and related health maintenance. It is now becoming commonplace for individuals to live to ages that were thought impossible even 30–40 years ago. Although the boundary of life expectancy continues to expand, the effects of the aging process on one's sensory capabilities have not changed appreciably. As persons live to greater ages, we must look toward the maintenance and enhancement of these capabilities for which science has not yet provided.

One of the most frustrating sensory deficits accompanying the aging process is the deterioration of auditory function, or presbycusis. A decline in hearing and the concomitant reduction in the ability to communicate is one of the greatest problems some older persons face in attempting to cope in their everyday world. However, most older clients with presbycusis can be rehabilitated with varying degrees of success.

WHAT IS PRESBYCUSIS?

Presbycusis is a multidimensional auditory disorder that affects an estimated 60% of all persons over age 65 years (Hull, 1991). It includes (a) a gradual downward shift in threshold sensitivity across all frequencies, accompanied by a decrement in speech discrimination; and (b) a compounding decline in central auditory function that is manifested by increased difficulty in such factors as auditory fusion, auditory attention, auditory judgment, sorting behaviors, and a decline in speed of auditory closure and synthesis.

As stated, it is presently estimated by this author that as many as 60% of persons over age 65 years possess symptoms of presbycusis. However, the incidence figures vary from author to author and study to study. For example, the 1981 Health Interview Study (National Center for Health Statistics, U.S. Department of Health and Human Services, 1981) determined that the incidence of hearing loss among a sample of adults between ages 65–74 years was only 24%, and for those over 75 years, 39%. The differences in the incidence figures appear to lie not only in the definition of presbycusis, but also in the process of data gathering (Hull, 1991). Among those who reside in health care facilities, the incidence is found to be higher than the well elderly in the community. In a study by Schow and Nerbonne (1980), for example, the incidence of hearing loss among nursing home residents was found to be over 80%. An earlier study by Chafee (1967) found the incidence of hearing loss among nursing home residents to be nearly 90%%. This author has found the incidence of hearing loss among health care facility residents overall to be 87%, with variations from one health care facility to another.

No matter what the cause, or who possesses it, presbycusis is a frustrating disorder that affects many adults. Its principal effects center on breakdowns in communication which are often exacerbated because the affected individual and family may not be aware of the cause. However, the problems can often be ameliorated by an audiologist. Once the decline in auditory function is discovered, the client can be advised of the components of an aural rehabilitation program that should be of assistance in enhancing that person's communicative skills.

AURAL REHABILITATION

The aural rehabilitation process is multifaceted, ranging from the fitting of a hearing aid or other assistive listening device, to counseling techniques such as developing coping mechanisms in difficult listening situations. A comprehensive auditory rehabilitation program will not only deal with issues such as the use of compensatory visual cues in communication, but also with the enhancement of central auditory function as it relates to the speed and accuracy of auditory synthesis, tracking, and comprehension.

We have recognized for some time that any rehabilitative effort on behalf of hearing impaired older adults must be as unique and comprehensive as the hearing impairment itself (Alpiner, 1968; Pang and Fujikawa, 1969; Parker, 1969; Barr, 1970; Willeford, 1971; Fleming, Birkle, Kolman, Miltonberger, and Israel, 1973; Binnie, 1976; Colton, 1977; Tannahill and Smoski, 1978; Alpiner, 1978; Hull, 1982; Vaughn and Gibbs, 1982; Alpiner and McCarthy, 1987; Hull, 1991). The audiologist working with the geriatric client must oftenbe highly innovative. Each older person is different, with differing physiologic and psychologic problems accompanying the auditory deficit.

The information presented here should be read with this in mind, with modifications being made, if necessary, on an individual basis.

BEGINNINGS OF REHABILITATION

Hearing Aid Evaluation

Many older adults are wary at the thought of wearing a hearing aid. They may have consented to the visit in your clinic because their children have requested that they at least try a hearing aid. In some cases, spouses may have reached the limits of their tolerance for the communication breakdowns, and have demanded an evaluation to determine if a hearing aid will help. Many individuals who come for evaluation have a positive outlook, anticipating that a hearing aid will provide them with more efficient communication. Others consent to a hearing evaluation because they are hopeful that a medical problem will be discovered and cured.

Before arriving at the audiology clinic, the only knowledge that many persons have about hearing aids has come from a hearing aid dealer or hearing aid literature received in the mail. Thus, the clients must be given to understand that they are now dealing with a competent professional who is trained in the assessment of hearing and the rehabilitation of those with hearing impairment. Nevertheless, it is occasionally difficult to convince the aged person that your sole purpose is not to sell hearing aids. Additionally, in the health care facility environment, when hearing aid procedures are part of a total rehabilitation program, this minimizes the likelihood that they will be subject to high pressure sales and inappropriate fittings.

Audiologists must remember that they are probably dealing with an individual who has heard normally in the past, led a normal social life, was a major contributor to the family, may have been the primary supporter, and had many friends. Now the person may be retired and living on a fixed, smaller income. The individual may have few friends who are still living, have considerable difficulty communicating with the family because of decreased auditory function, and may be frustrated and angry at the whole process of becoming older.

The clients' frustrations in communication, along with any physical discomforts, may cause them to appear irritated or intolerant of the evaluative session. The clients may deny both the apparent auditory difficulties and the need for amplification by placing the blame on others who do not speak clearly. "People seem to mumble nowadays" is a common complaint.

Hearing aid evaluation procedures will vary with the individual client. It is important to consider the person's tolerance for the evaluation process. The procedures may need modification to compensate for a patient's physical limitations, potential fatigue or emotional response to the testing situation (Chapter 37 discusses presbycusis and the basic evaluation procedures). However, the following procedures have been found to be generally beneficial:

1. Initial test battery.
   a. Puretone air- and bone-conduction thresholds.
   b. Speech reception thresholds under phones.
   c. Assessment of auditory recognition under phones for phonetically balanced words and sentences (for example, CID Everyday Sentences).
   d. Most comfortable loudness and uncomfortable loudness levels; the latter, for tolerance and dynamic range.
2. Explaining results. The preliminary test results should be explained with regard to the degree and possible handicap of the hearing impairment.
3. Indications for a hearing aid. If the possibility of benefit from a hearing aid is evident, a discussion of that possibility should take place along with the purposes of a hearing aid evaluation.
4. Medical referral. Referral to an appropriate physician is made if there is a need for clearance for a hearing aid. He/she will send the client back for possible hearing aid fitting/aural rehabilitation services.
5. Hearing aid fitting procedures. Earmold impression(s) should be taken and an appointment made for the hearing aid fitting. Counseling regarding the use of hearing aids should continue. Appropriate test procedures at this time include:
   a. A free field speech reception threshold (SRT) unaided; and
   b. Free field speech recognition with phonetically balanced words—unaided.
   c. If the preliminary results indicate that a specific aid may benefit the person (e.g., a behind-the-ear (BTE) or in-the-ear (ITE) aid), the audiologist should instruct the client regarding the use of that aid, including how to change batteries and other such intricacies. A family member should be present in case of communication or memory problems.
6. The aid is dispensed to the client on a 30–60 day trial basis. Prefitting electroacoustic analysis of the aid(s) should be conducted, followed by a postfitting Real-Ear assessment, a free-field SRT, and speech recognition testing.

7. Hearing aid orientation and consultation. Specific instructions regarding adjustments that may be required for use of the hearing aid and variations for specific environments for trial should be shown. A few suggested environments for trial and orientation may include: (*a*) while watching television, (*b*) at church, (*c*) at any social gathering where the person would feel comfortable wearing an aid, and (*d*) while taking a walk.

The client should be instructed to wear the hearing aid only when the person desires to wear it. Emphasize that it is not necessary to wear it in all the environments suggested, but stress the desirability of trying it in as many situations as possible. Set an appointment for the client to return, or advise the person to contact the audiologist in 1 week to 1 month, depending upon the client. During the return visit, the client may be ready for further discussion regarding the benefits of amplification as it applies to specific situations, and not the generalities that were discussed during the initial evaluation the week prior.

BASIC CONSIDERATIONS IN SELECTING A HEARING AID

In discussing the utilization of hearing aids with the older client, and in selecting aids for consideration or purchase, the following should be considered.

Auditory Capabilities of the Client

Even though the puretone configuration may indicate a good prognosis for the use of amplification, auditory discrimination problems along with any central auditory processing dysfunction may reduce its effectiveness. Some elderly persons may have purchased several hearing aids from various dealers in the hope that one of them would successfully allow for more efficient communication. After spending large sums of money, the client may find that none of the aids provide sufficient benefit and, therefore, none is worn. "The dresser drawer syndrome" (Alpiner, 1974) is testimony to the caution that should be exercised in the hearing aid evaluation of the older adult.

The audiologist must look carefully at the auditory capabilities of the aged client—not so much at the fact that hearing loss is present, but at whether a hearing aid will allow for more efficient communicative function. For some younger clients, a hearing aid may be viewed as providing benefits that are at least better than nothing at all. For some elderly clients, however, the frustration resulting from an inappropriate hearing aid can be interpreted as worse than nothing at all.

Physical Capabilities of the Client

The client's manual dexterity is an important consideration in selecting the type and size of a hearing aid. The older individual fitted with a small canal hearing aid, whose less than nimble fingers cannot manipulate the gain control, will experience great frustration in attempting to wear the aid. Many elderly persons have difficulty placing the small battery in the battery compartment. If the individual is unlucky enough to drop the battery, visual and other difficulties might interfere with its retrieval. Behind-the-ear (BTE) hearing aids generally allow for easier manipulation of the controls and require a larger battery size. Convincing an older adult client to accept a hearing aid that is larger than a small ITE aid is, however, another matter. It is often difficult for the elderly client to accept the need for amplification and the wearing of a hearing aid. The thought of using a larger hearing aid may be even more difficult to accept. However, once the client determines that the ease of manipulation of the controls of the BTE aid outweigh its disadvantages of size and wearability, counseling toward its use is facilitated.

This is not to say that all elderly persons should be counseled toward the use of BTE hearing aids. This author has had a number of years of success in fitting his older clients with standard in-the-ear (ITE) hearing aids. Many active older persons can utilize smaller aids. More recent developments in refining the circuitry of all-in-the-ear aids, including programmable hearing aids, are making them more appealing for use with older adult clients. In the end, however, there is no single type of hearing aid that is most beneficial for all hearing-impaired older adults. The client and the audiologist must work together to discover the most satisfactory form.

Assistive Listening Devices

Assistive listening devices (ALDs) are of benefit to many older hearing-impaired clients. For example, infrared amplification systems are being installed in large numbers of popular theaters in the United States, in addition to churches, community centers, and other buildings. They can greatly benefit hearing-impaired older adults, including those who possess severe discrimination problems. Other devices that are commonly used include (*a*) inexpensive personal amplifiers, (*b*) hard-wired receivers for use with television or radio, (*c*) small "pocket" amplifiers for use at home or at meetings, (*d*) personal FM units coupled to the telecoil of the user's hearing aid via a magnetic loop adapter. These and other alternative listening systems have been shown to be of great assistance to the older hearing-impaired adult (Hull, 1988) (see also Chapter 42).

Hearing Aid Follow-up

It is this authors' belief that the hearing-impaired older person needs to become involved in a vital aural rehabilitation program as soon as his or her hearing loss has been diagnosed. If a hearing aid has, indeed, been recommended, then the client should be encouraged to wear it during aural rehabilitation sessions. Counseling about its use, discussions regarding the benefits and limitations of hearing aids, and suggestions for communicating in the everyday world should continue. This type of follow-up will greatly enhance the client's success in adapting to the use of amplification.

If it has been found that the client cannot effectively utilize a hearing aid, then speechreading/auditory training alternatives should be employed without the use of amplification.

REHABILITATION PROCESS

Counseling the Elderly Client

Whether or not clients can benefit from amplification, their emotional acceptance of the auditory impairment and their desire for more efficient communicative function must be of primary concern to the audiologist. If the client is unable to cope emotionally with an auditory impairment, or does not desire exploration of rehabilitation options, then it is appropriate for the audiologist to intervene as a counselor (see Chapter 40 for additional information on this topic).

The empathy shown by the audiologist in understanding the problems faced by the individual is an important first step. Most elderly clients do not want sympathy from the counseling audiologist. The young audiologist who says, "I know just how you feel" when the elderly client describes his frustrations, should expect to hear the client justifiably reply, "You do not know how I feel. You are not my age and are not experiencing my difficulties in communication." However, the audiologist must be able to relate to what the elderly person is saying through a knowledge of presbycusis and experiences in working with other older persons. The aged client may be envious of the younger audiologist and might wonder how an individual so much his or her junior could possess such knowledge and understanding. The skilled rehabilitative audiologist should be able to overcome the barriers of age and deal with the specific auditory and related problems of the aged client through the rapport that has been established. The client must be as-

sisted to realize that the audiologist is there to listen and to discuss the auditory difficulties he or she faces, and that the audiologist's purpose is to help the client learn to function more efficiently in spite of the auditory difficulties.

Motivation for some clients is difficult to develop and maintain. Motivation toward participation in aural rehabilitation programs will occur only when the client knows that the audiologist understands his or her auditory problems, concerns and frustrations. Most importantly, the aged clients must know that the audiologist feels that they can be helped to communicate more efficiently. Since aural rehabilitation can be difficult and sometimes only slightly rewarding from session to session, counseling is perhaps the most important aspect of the total aural rehabilitation process.

Group Involvement

Group counseling can be most effective. The empathy and camaraderie that often develops within groups of hearing-impaired older adult clients can be very rewarding. Many realize for the first time that others have experienced similar frustrations and problems in communication. It can be highly motivating to a person to see others with hearing impairment who are socially active individuals, who have not retreated as a result of their hearing loss. Such group involvement can work well in the community for independent older persons, and in health care facility environments for the more confined.

Peer Involvement

Peer pressure can be an effective technique for motivating the older client to attempt aural rehabilitation. Other clients who have experienced success through aural rehabilitation programs can provide great encouragement to hearing-impaired clients who may be reluctant to participate. For those who express a seeming lack of desire to participate in aural rehabilitation because of age or infirmity, encouragement from peer members of the group who would like to communicate with the potential client can work very effectively.

Family Involvement

It is desirable that the older client's family, or significant others, be involved in the counseling process regarding his or her auditory difficulties, but this is frequently not possible. For example, the older person who may be placed in a health care facility because his daughter does not have the time to provide a meaningful home environment, may also find that the family does not "have the time" to visit him frequently, or to participate in counseling activities. It is interesting, however, that difficulty communicating is occasionally given as one reason for a lack of visits. Yet, the families will not take opportunities offered them to better understand and ease this communication problem. They report that "Dad is getting confused." The term "confused" all too often takes on the connotation of "senile." It is important, however, that the family or significant others come to realize that aural rehabilitation not only involves the hearing-impaired client but themselves as well.

The following are suggested topics for discussion during the rehabilitative audiologist's meetings with family members or significant others, and the client.

1. What is presbycusis?
   a. How does it affect a person's ability to communicate?
   b. The resulting frustrations on the part of the older adults and those with whom they attempt to communicate.
2. Hearing aids.
   a. Why some older adults cannot utilize amplification on a day-to-day basis even though they appear to be hearing impaired.
   b. The benefits of amplification as part of a total aural rehabilitation program.
   c. How a hearing aid works.
3. How to communicate more efficiently with their hearing-impaired family member.
   a. Speak at a slightly greater than normal intensity.
   b. Speak at a normal rate but not too rapidly.
   c. Do not speak to the elderly client at a greater distance than 6 feet or less than 3 feet.
   d. Concentrate light on the speaker's face for greater visibility of lip movements, facial expression and gestures.
   e. Do not speak to the elderly person unless you are visible to him or her, i.e., not from another room while the person is reading the newspaper or watching television.
   f. Do not force the older person to listen to you when there is a great deal of environmental noise. That type of environment can be difficult for a younger normally hearing person, let alone an elderly individual who may also exhibit symptoms of central auditory involvement in presbycusis.

If an elderly person's ability to communicate with his family or significant others can be enhanced, then a giant step toward other successes in aural rehabilitation efforts can be made.

AURAL REHABILITATION TREATMENT SESSIONS

Speechreading/Auditory Training

No matter how motivated the older client is toward learning to communicate more efficiently, the motivation will quickly fade if traditional analytic approaches of speechreading and auditory training are utilized. Analytic instruction regarding phoneme recognition in isolation and in the context of syllables and words is also difficult, and has questionable effectiveness. Assuming that the clients involved in the aural rehabilitation program possess normal or near normal language function, more meaningful approaches for enhancing their ability to receive and interpret verbal messages can be utilized.

The use of residual hearing should be stressed. If the older client can make use of a hearing aid, then it should be worn during aural rehabilitation sessions that include speechreading instruction. If a hearing aid is not used routinely by individual clients because they have not been able to make good use of amplification, then a hearing aid is not advised during speechreading instruction. Voice, however, should still be used by the clinician. Therefore, all clients are forced to use their residual hearing. If a client appears to have the auditory capacity to wear a hearing aid, but for some reason is having difficulty adjusting to its use, then aural rehabilitation sessions provide a good atmosphere for controlled trial of various amplification devices.

Effective speechreading lessons include (a) instruction regarding visually confusing phonemes, (b) the predictability of the English language in conversational speech, (c) enhancing the ability to select important visual-auditory word clues from conversations that facilitate correct interpretation of meaning and (d) instruction in manipulating one's environment to facilitate their ability to function communicatively (Hull, 1982). Individuals with visual problems who are also hearing-impaired are not excluded from the speechreading sessions. For these persons, the sessions become useful as auditory training therapy.

Extension of the more formalized speechreading/auditory training classes may include assignments that involve, at a beginning level: (a) Speaking to at least one other person at some time during each day (e.g., for 2 minutes) before the next aural rehabilitation session. They are instructed to record any difficulties in carrying on the conversations so that the problems can be discussed at the next aural rehabilitation session. (b) Clients are given assignments to practice during special activities, e.g., at church, or the theater, at social events, or other such environments.

Nontraditional/Innovative Approaches to Aural Rehabilitation Treatment

Other components of effective aural rehabilitation sessions, as utilized by this author (Hull, 1982; 1991) involve:

Problem-Solving Sessions

Clients (or significant others) are asked to record and discuss specific situations in which they have had difficulty communicating. These situations are brought to the aural rehabilitation sessions and presented by the client (or client and spouse or significant other) who experienced them. They are then discussed by the group and audiologist (or by the client and audiologist in individual sessions). Approaches are discussed regarding possible strategies for coping with or adjusting to the situation. These can be powerful and tangible sessions for all who are involved.

Use of Time Compressed Speech

One common symptom of advancing age is the slowing of the speed of central nervous system processing of auditory-linguistic information (Marshall, 1981; Schmitt and McCroskey, 1981; Madden, 1985; and others). The use of time compression of speech has been found by this author to be an effective method through which clients can maintain or even enhance speed and precision of speech comprehension. Clients practice by listening to progressively time-compressed sentences and paragraphs, attempting over a 8-to-10 week sequence of sessions to increase their speed of comprehension of recorded speech (with corresponding accuracy). For example, clients who can increase their speech comprehension accuracy for sentences and paragraphs to 80%–90% at time-compression levels of 35% (i.e., 65% of the message received over time), have been found to similarly increase their accuracy of auditory speech recognition by as much as 24% age points (Hull, 1986). This method has been found to be a very exciting and tangible method for enhancing the speed andaccuracy of speech comprehension among individual clients who can tolerate the demands of the process.

Interactive Laser-Video Training For Increasing Speed and Accuracy of Visual Synthesis and Closure

Interactive laser-video technology has recently evolved for use in training for increased speed and accuracy of visual closure, tracking, and synthesis for olympic athletes, air force fighter pilots, and radar observers. This technology has also been found by Hull (1989a) to be an effective and motivating way of training hearing impaired adults to increase their visual compensatory skills, particularly as it relates to speed, accuracy, and visual vigilance. Clients are trained to make visual closure with greater speed and accuracy, to make rapid decisions about what is seen, and to gain skill in visual tracking.

Environment Design

Hull (1989b) describes different avenues for training hearing impaired older clients in techniques and strategies of environmental design. The clients are taught how to modify the acoustic/environment design of their homes, offices, and other communicative environments to their listening advantage. These can be important aural rehabilitation sessions in that they empower clients to modify their most difficult communication situations.

All of the above mentioned methods are bringing the aural rehabilitation process into the era of modern technology. They are not only effective, but they are also tangible and motivating forms of training for those clients who can perform these tasks. Except for the severely hearing-impaired client who might find the time-compressed speech tasks too difficult, this author has found most older clients to benefit from these techniques at least to some degree.

SPECIFIC SUGGESTIONS FOR INITIATION OF AURAL REHABILITATION PROGRAMS FOR THE OLDER CLIENT IN A HEALTH CARE FACILITY

Aural rehabilitation programs in the health care facility should be coordinated by the audiologist, but should also involve (a) the head of nursing, (b) the activity director, (c) the social worker, and (d) the nurses' aides.

Coordination is maintained by periodic meetings of the audiologist and the staff members of the center. These meetings, held at least twice per year, should have as their purpose a discussion of the maintenance and improvement of the program. The audiologist should, however, be in continual contact with the center personnel regarding the program and the progress of individual clients.

Funding

Funding of the aural rehabilitation program should come from the health care facility. Financial commitment on the center's part will encourage a more vital interest in its success. With appropriate medical referral for audiologic diagnostic services, federal health insurance programs, such as Medicare, will provide payment for audiologic evaluations whenconducted by an audiologist who is certified by the American

Speech-Language-Hearing Association, or holds the appropriate state license, and who has received a provider number for administration of such services.

Payment for services delivered at a health care facility can either be made on a per-client basis or on a fee-for-services contract (a fee for each service provided). The fee-for-services contract is generally more satisfactory. The amount is negotiated between the audiologist and the administration of the center.

Evaluation of Auditory Function

Once the administration of the facility has given its approval for the initiation of the aural rehabilitation program, the first step is to achieve an audiometric evaluation for all residents whose health and mental state allow. This first evaluation will determine the need for further evaluation, including hearing aid assessment and possible fitting.

The procedures for the initial evaluation consist of (a) puretone air-conduction thresholds under phones, (b) immittance measurements (tympanometry and acoustic reflex) for the determination of site of lesion, and (c) screening for auditory discrimination difficulties by the use of monosyllabic words (25-word list) and 10 sentences (CID Everyday Sentences). Residents who, for reasons of health and/or mobility, cannot participate in puretone threshold evaluations, a bed-side evaluation for speech understanding (at a conversational level) can be administered. For example, 25 spondaic words (NU-6), or lists of CID Everyday Sentences can be administered, once with the patient's eyes closed, and once while they are open, to obtain information regarding his or her ability to repeat monosyllabic word or sentence items with and without visual cues.

Any new residents should be evaluated within 2 weeks after admittance to the health care facility. If hearing impairment is discovered, participation in the aural rehabilitation program can be initiated early. Early intervention not only encourages greater participation in the aural rehabilitation program, but also may reduce the degree of depression affecting many elderly persons when they are placed in the health care facility. It also alerts the staff to make necessary modifications in communication for that client.

Records of Progress

Complete records must be kept on each client. Results of audiometric evaluations should be kept not only in the client's master file but also in individual files by the audiologist. Communicative and social progress should be recorded for each client who participates in the aural rehabilitation program. One method that has

been found to be successful is the use of individual clients' social progress reports which are written jointly by the head nurse, the activity director, the social worker, and the audiologist.

Increased ability to communicate will generally reflect positively upon other aspects of the elderly person's life. As elderly persons realize that communication can occur with greater efficiency, they will often become more ambulatory, show a greater desire for improved personal appearance, and be more willing to venture into the world outside of the health care facility.

In-Service Training

An aware administrative and nursing staff is necessary to maintain an effective and workable aural rehabilitation program for the older adult in the health care facility. The staff should have knowledge of (a) the nature of presbycusis; (b) the frustration of hearing impairment on the aged person; (c) approaches for support of the client; and (d) the components of the aural rehabilitation program.

One effective way of assuring that the health care facility staff is aware of these problems, and that a good working relationship is established, is through periodic in-service training. It has been found that in-service training is beneficial not only for the retirement center staff, but also for the residents themselves as continuing education seminars.

Staff

Because health care facilities traditionally have a rapid turnover in personnel, in-service training sessions should be conducted at least once every other month. The length of in-service training sessions will vary with the topic of discussion, but at least 1 hour should be allotted. To be maximally effective, the in-service training should involve nurses, nurses' aides (since they are more directly involved with the residents on a day-to-day basis), the activity director, the social worker, and the director of the retirement center. It is not necessary for the retirement center director to be involved in all in-service sessions except when individual clients are being discussed. However, to be aware of the ongoing nature of the services, the director should attend when possible.

Topics that are considered important for in-service training are:

1. How the ear functions;
2. What is presbycusis;
3. The impact of presbycusis;
4. Hearing aids, their structure, care, advantages, and limitations with this population;

5. How to troubleshoot for simple hearing aid malfunction;

6. What is aural rehabilitation;

7. How best to communicate with the hearing-impaired elderly person;

8. Staff discussions of individual hearing-impaired residents and their progress in the aural rehabilitation program; and

9. Environmental design for hearing-impaired older persons.

In essence, the in-service training provides the staff with insight into presbycusis, its complications, and information about the progress of residents participating in the aural rehabilitation program. Certainly, all new staff members and those who have questions regarding specific residents should attend the in-service training.

Residents

"In-service," or a continuing education program for health care facility residents, has been found to be an extremely valuable and effective component of the overall aural rehabilitation program. Most residents are personally interested in the process of aging and its effects on them physiologically, psychologically, and socially. Even though older persons often will not tolerate a long movie, lecture, or meeting, they will attend meetings on the process of aging. The content of this type of meeting is much the same as the in-service provided to the center personnel, with modifications that allow for personal involvement and interaction among participants. Even though the older adults in attendance may relate personal experiences regarding their own auditory difficulties, the purpose of such a program should not take on the image of group counseling.

The residents are presented information that will result in a better understanding of how the aging process may affect hearing and how it may affect them personally. The premise for these meetings is that one cannot limit the presentation of information about presbycusis strictly to those who work with older adults. It must also be taken to the older adults so that they, too, will have a better understanding of what is happening to them.

If all health care facilities within a given community work together to maintain an effective aural rehabilitation program for their residents, then its viability increases manyfold. "A Community-Wide Program in Geriatric Aural Rehabilitation" (Hull and Traynor, 1975) has been established by the University of Northern Colorado to encourage and coordinate the aural rehabilitation programs in the community. A Fellowship in Geriatric Aural Rehabilitation has also

been established by the participating health care facilities to support the education of graduate students in audiology within the UNC Audiology Program who are interested and committed to serving hearing-impaired older adults upon graduation. However, this program, as currently managed, does not cease with the health care facility, but also extends into the rest of the community. This communitywide effort is necessary if a complete aural rehabilitation program for the older adult is to exist.

PROGRAMS FOR THE WELL ELDERLY CLIENT IN THE COMMUNITY

A most efficient method for contacting older hearing-impaired persons in the community is through (a) public interest talks by audiologists, (b) newspaper articles, and (c) public service television/radio spots or interviews. Presentations can also be given at local community senior centers and the Public Health Service Well Elderly Clinics (diagnostic health clinics). If enough interest is generated, then audiology services in the form of screenings can be provided to determine which persons might require complete diagnostic evaluations, hearing aid evaluations, and entrance into an aural rehabilitation program. These screening clinics can be held, for example, at such familiar places as the local senior citizens' center or, if a mobile unit with sound-treated facilities is available, at several familiar sites for greater convenience for the older person.

The management principles which guide the aural rehabilitation program for the well older client in the community are similar to those discussed earlier in this chapter and include (a) counseling techniques, (b) considerations regarding hearing aids, (c) in-service programs, and (d) communication techniques. Modifications may be required when considering the social vitality and mobility of the well older client in the community.

Payment for diagnostic services may come from the client, or from the client's federal health insurance. Payment for aural rehabilitation services may also be covered by privateinsurances. Until it is designated as a covered benefit, however, Medicare does not presently cover auditory rehabilitation services and so payment must be made by the client or agency sponsoring the client.

AFTER REHABILITATION

The aim of aural rehabilitation efforts is to improve the communicative capabilities of hearing-impaired older adults so that they will be able to function at a higher level, both socially and personally. Some may reach a level of skill that will allow for greater ease of auditory-verbal communication between the client and family or friends, while others may make strides toward greater independence. Increased communicative function may reactivate in some an interest toward opening avenues of participation into their own social, financial, and personal worlds.

On the negative side, the audiologist must also be able to face the death of older clients. However, the audiologist should not concentrate upon the inevitability of death, but look upon rehabilitation as adding quality of life to the later years of the older client.

It is important to look beyond the fact that a longer life has been given to older adults. We have for too long looked at the gift of extended life as our ultimate goal for the aged person. If we are, indeed, adding re life to those additional years, we must also pay g₁ 'ter attention to making this additional time as productive as possible. Audiologists can assist elderly clients by their teaching and rehabilitative efforts. There are approximately 19 million individuals in the U.S. over age 65 who possess some degree of hearing impairment. With ourassistance, many can function again as more productive citizens.

REFERENCES

Alpiner J. Audiologic problems of the aged. Geriatrics 1968;18:19–26.

Alpiner J. The feasibility of rehabilitating the hearing-impaired elderly client. Paper presented at Workshop on hearing and related communication disorders among the aged, Division of Long-Term Care, Public Health Service, Department of Health and Human Services, Denver, CO, 1974.

Alpiner JG. Evaluation of Communication Function. In Alpiner J, Ed. Handbook of adult rehabilitative audiology. Baltimore: Williams & Wilkins, 1978.

Alpiner J, McCarthy P. Rehabilitative audiology: children and adults. Baltimore: Williams & Wilkins, 1987.

Barr D. Aural rehabilitation and the geriatric patient. Geriatrics 1970;25:111–113.

Binnie CA. Relevant aural rehabilitation. In Northern JL, Ed. Hearing disorders. Boston: Little, Brown, 1976:213–229.

Chafee C. Rehabilitation needs of nursing home patients: a report of a survey. Rehab Lit 1967;18:377–389.

Colton J. Student participation in aural rehabilitation programs. Acad Rehab Audiol 1977;10:31–35.

Colton J, O'Neill J. A cooperative outreach program for the elderly. Acad Rehab Audiol 1976;9:38–41.

Fleming M, Birkle L, Kolman I, Miltenberger G, Isreal R. Development of workable aural rehabilitation programs. Acad Rehab Audiol 1973;6:35–36.

Hull R. Techniques of aural rehabilitation treatment for elderly clients. In Hull R, Ed. Rehabilitative audiology. New York: Grune & Stratton, 1982;383–406.

Hull R. The use of time compression in aural rehabilitation treatment for older adults. Presentation before the Convention of the American Speech-Language-Hearing Association, Washington, DC, 1986.

Hull R. Central auditory processing and aging. Presentation before the Research Symposium on Communication Sciences and Disorders and Aging. Washington, DC, September 8–10, 1988.

Hull R. Evaluation of assistive listening devices by elderly listeners. Hearing Instruments 1988;38(7):14–18.

Hull R. Training in visual tracking and synthesis through interactive laser-video technology. Presentation before the Convention of the American Speech-Language-Hearing Association. St. Louis, 1989a.

Hull R. Environmental factors in communication with older persons. In Hull R, Ed. Communication disorders in aging. Beverly, CA: Sage Publications, 1989b:153–162.

Hull R. Techniques of aural rehabilitation treatment. In Hull R, Ed. Aural rehabilitation. San Diego, CA: Singular Publishing Goup, 1992.

Hull R, Traynor R. A community-wide program in geriatric aural rehabilitation. Asha 1975;17:33–34, 47–48.

Madden D. Age-related slowing in the retrieval of information from long-term memory. Gerontology 1985;40:208–210.

Marshall L. Auditory processing in aging listeners. J Speech-Language-Hearing Disord 1981;46:226–240.

Pang L, Fujikawa S. Hearing impairment in the aged: incidence and management. Hawaii Med J 1969;29:190–213.

Parker W. Hearing and age. Geriatrics 1969;24:151–157.

Schmitt J, McCroskey R. Sentence comprehension in elderly listeners: the factor of rate. Gerontology 1981;36:441–445.

Schow R, Nerbonne M. Hearing levels among elderly nursing home residents. J Speech and Hearing Disord 1980;45:124–132.

Tannahill JC, Smoski WJ. Introduction to aural rehabilitation. In Katz J, Ed. Handbook of clinical audiology. Baltimore: Williams & Wilkins, 1978.

Vaughn G, Gibbs S. Alternative and companion listening devices for the hearing impaired. In Hull R, Ed. Rehabilitative audiology. New York: Grune & Stratton, 1982:117–128.

Willeford J. The geriatric patient. In Rose D, Ed. Audiological assessment. Englewood Cliffs, NJ: Prentice-Hall, 1971.

AUTHOR INDEX

SUBJECT INDEX

Page numbers in italics denote figures; those followed by "t" denote tables.